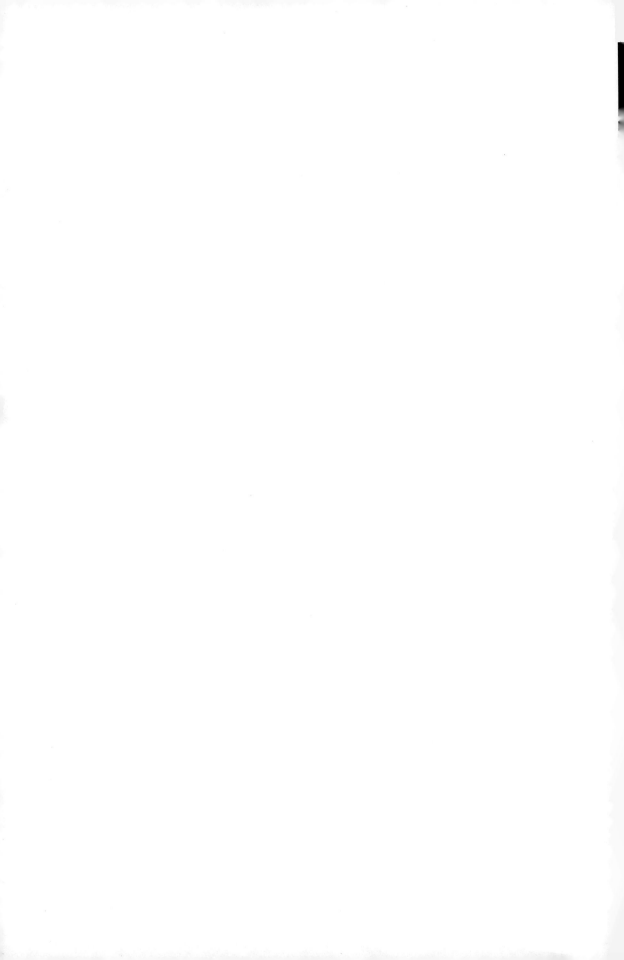

GARDNER AND SUTHERLAND'S
CHROMOSOME ABNORMALITIES
AND GENETIC COUNSELING

OXFORD MONOGRAPHS ON MEDICAL GENETICS

General Editors:

JUDITH G. HALL   PETER S. HARPER   LOUANNE HUDGKINS   EVAN EICHLER   CHARLES J. EPSTEIN (DECEASED 2011)

ARNO G. MOTULSKY (RESIGNED 2011)

GARDNER AND SUTHERLAND'S

Chromosome Abnormalities and Genetic Counseling

FIFTH EDITION

R. J. McKinlay GARDNER

ADJUNCT PROFESSOR

CLINICAL GENETICS GROUP

UNIVERSITY OF OTAGO, DUNEDIN, NEW ZEALAND

David J. AMOR

LORENZO AND PAMELA GALLI CHAIR

UNIVERSITY OF MELBOURNE

VICTORIAN CLINICAL GENETICS SERVICES

MURDOCH CHILDREN'S RESEARCH INSTITUTE

ROYAL CHILDREN'S HOSPITAL, MELBOURNE, AUSTRALIA

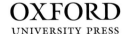

OXFORD

UNIVERSITY PRESS

OXFORD
UNIVERSITY PRESS

Oxford University Press is a department of the University of Oxford. It furthers the University's objective of excellence in research, scholarship, and education by publishing worldwide. Oxford is a registered trade mark of Oxford University Press in the UK and certain other countries.

Published in the United States of America by Oxford University Press
198 Madison Avenue, New York, NY 10016, United States of America.

Library of Congress Cataloging-in-Publication Data
Names: Gardner, R. J. M., author. | Amor, David J., author.
Title: Gardner and Sutherland's chromosome abnormalities and genetic counseling / R. J. McKinlay Gardner, David J. Amor.
Other titles: Chromosome abnormalities and genetic counseling | Oxford monographs on medical genetics ; no. 70.
Description: Fifth edition. | Oxford ; New York : Oxford University Press, [2018] |
Series: Oxford monographs on medical genetics ; no. 70 | Preceded by Chromosome abnormalities and genetic counseling / R.J. McKinlay Gardner, Grant R. Sutherland, Lisa G. Shaffer. c2012. | Includes bibliographical references and index.
Identifiers: LCCN 2017034126 | ISBN 9780199329007 (hardcover : alk. paper)
Subjects: | MESH: Chromosome Aberrations | Genetic Counseling
Classification: LCC RB155.7 | NLM QS 677 | DDC 616/.042—dc23
LC record available at https://lccn.loc.gov/2017034126

This material is not intended to be, and should not be considered, a substitute for medical or other professional advice. Treatment for the conditions described in this material is highly dependent on the individual circumstances. And, while this material is designed to offer accurate information with respect to the subject matter covered and to be current as of the time it was written, research and knowledge about medical and health issues is constantly evolving and dose schedules for medications are being revised continually, with new side effects recognized and accounted for regularly. Readers must therefore always check the product information and clinical procedures with the most up-to-date published product information and data sheets provided by the manufacturers and the most recent codes of conduct and safety regulation. The publisher and the authors make no representations or warranties to readers, express or implied, as to the accuracy or completeness of this material. Without limiting the foregoing, the publisher and the authors make no representations or warranties as to the accuracy or efficacy of the drug dosages mentioned in the material. The authors and the publisher do not accept, and expressly disclaim, any responsibility for any liability, loss or risk that may be claimed or incurred as a consequence of the use and/or application of any of the contents of this material.

9 8 7 6 5 4 3 2 1

Printed by Sheridan Books, Inc., United States of America

This book is dedicated to Jocelyn, Geoffrey, and Craig, their parents, and all other families who seek our "chromosomal advice."

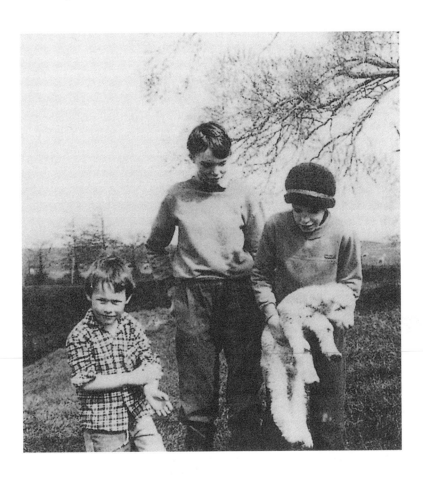

Jocelyn and Geoffrey (with lamb) have a partial trisomy for chromosome 4 long arm, and Craig, the youngest, had a 46,XY result on amniocentesis. Their father is a translocation carrier (see Fig. 5–1, lower). Craig, since married, came to the genetic clinic for confirmatory advice about his low genetic risk.

Heredity

Inescapably, this is me—the diagnosis
is cause for anger at those
who brightly say we choose our destinies.
There is no store
of courage, wit or will
can save me from myself and I must face
my children, feeling like
that wicked fairy, uninvited
at the christening, bestowing on my own,
amidst murmurs of apprehension, a most
unwanted gift—that
of a blighted mind. No one
could tell me of this curse when I
was young and dreamt of children
and the graces they would bear. Later,
it seemed that a chill morning
revealed deeper layers
of truth. For my romancing
there is a price to pay—
perhaps my children's children
will pass this tollgate after me.
My grandmothers gaze down from their frames
on my wall, sadly wondering.

—Meg Campbell

Dear DNA

In real life you're just
a tangle of white filaments
captured in a test-tube,
and your first photo is not flattering:
grey smudges like tractor tracks,
or a rusty screw. Yet
many say you are beautiful.
Online for a night

with a hundred fantastic portraits
and I'm head over heels
In love with you, DNA,
bewitched by your billions
coiled in my cells, transcribing,
replicating, mutating.
I see your never-ending dance.
A length of twisted ladder
briefly unwinds,
both strands duplicate,
each copy drifts away
on its secret mission
to make a thought, feel sunshine,
or digest this morning's porridge.
Two winding parallel threads,
a tiny tangle of gossamer
designing my life.
DNA, you are astonishing
and I am yours truly.

—Winifred Kavalieris

Genes pass on our kind
But our selves are transmitted
In words left behind.

—J. Patrick Gookin

Curiosity is a virtue, perhaps an unsung and
undervalued virtue, which should be the energizing fuel
to the thinking geneticist.

—Willie Reardon

Where is the wisdom we have lost in knowledge?
Where is the knowledge we have lost in information?

—T. S. Eliot

PREFACE TO THE FIFTH EDITION

Chromosomal disorders have been, and will always be, with us; that is a given. What is changing is our ability to recognize and detect them: detection both in terms of the subtlety of abnormalities and of the means we can use to find them. Classical cytogenetics has now well and truly given way to "molecular karyotyping," and this has been the extraordinary development of the early twenty-first century. Readers will now be as accustomed to molecular nomenclature in defining a segment, such as chr5:1-18,500,000, as they had been to the classical description, 5p14.1→pter.

The very small deletions and duplications which molecular karyotyping can now reveal have become familiar to the clinicians and counselors who see patients and families in the clinic. A large number of these are now on record, many attracting the nomenclature "copy number variant": Some are very well understood, others becoming so, and yet quite a few—variants of uncertain significance, the acronym "VOUS" in daily parlance—whose roles in human pathology are imperfectly appreciated.

Many are not in the same mold as the deletions and duplications of classical cytogenetics, in which the single defect sufficed to cause a particular phenotype, and always did so: We now need to take account of the concept of incomplete penetrance, with some microdeletions or duplications not, of themselves, always leading to an abnormal phenotype. Apparently clinically normal parents may carry the same alteration as their child with an abnormal phenotype. Digenic, or "two-hit," mechanisms may now require consideration. These were not formerly notions much entering into the assessment of chromosomal disorders; discussion apropos in the clinic presents a new challenge.

The number of "new" del/dup syndromes increases almost with each issue of the clinical genetic journals. We include a mention of a considerable number of these here (Chapter 14), not intending to create an encyclopedic resource per se but believing that such a record may provide a useful first point of contact when these cases are encountered in the clinic. Copy number variants of uncertain significance, on the other hand, we mostly take only a broad rather than a detailed view (Chapter 17); the reader will need to consult other repositories for fuller information, as their interpretations evolve.

The new (or now, established) laboratory methodologies blur the boundaries between what might have been regarded as the classic chromosomal abnormalities and Mendelian conditions. Some disorders recorded as being due not only to segmental deletion/duplication affecting a single locus but also to point mutation at that locus we continue to treat as "chromosomal"; and for most, their place in this book is secure. But one major category, the fragile X syndromes, are now seen as essentially Mendelian disorders, their historic cytogenetic-based nomenclature notwithstanding, and they no longer claim their chapter.

Peripheral blood and skin have been the tissues in common usage for chromosome analysis, with an increasing role for cells got from the convenient and painless "spit sample." Prenatal diagnosis has been based on amniocentesis and chorionic villus sampling, but latterly blastomeres from early embryos, and fetal DNA in the maternal circulation, have become targets for testing. Now we can anticipate the potential for whole genome analysis to be applied to the prenatal diagnosis of the classic aneuploidies, from a simple maternal blood sample, and this would widen such testing very considerably. Questions such as these raise ethical issues, and a literature on "chromosomal ethics" is accumulating.

As we have previously written, however marvelous may be these new ways to test for chromosomes, the concerns of families remain essentially the same. We may reproduce here the final paragraph of the Preface of the first edition of this book, from 1989, as valid now as then:

> Families pursue genetic counseling in an effort to demystify the mysterious. If they did not want to "hear it all," they would not bother with genetic counseling. Families want an honest evaluation of what is known and what is unknown, a clear explanation of all possibilities, both good and bad, and a sensitive exploration of all available information with which they can make knowledgeable decisions about future family planning. Thus, Bloch et al. (1979) succinctly convey the essence of why people go to the genetic counselor. We hope this book will assist counselors in their task.

Dunedin   R.J.M.G.
Melbourne   D.J.A.
February 2018

ACKNOWLEDGMENTS

We thank John Barber, Rachel Beddow, Amber Boys, Cyril Chapman, Jane Halliday, Jan Hodgson, Caroline Lintott, Nicole Martin, Belinda McLaren, Fiona Norris, Mamoru Ozaki, Mark Pertile, Jenny Rhodes, Sharyn Stock-Myer, and Jane Watt for their critical advice. We acknowledge Lisa Shaffer, who was a co-author of the previous edition, and much of whose work has flowed over into this edition. We have made much use of the ideograms created by Nicole Chia. The length of the Reference list, and the frequency with which we acknowledge, in legends to figures, the courtesy of colleagues whose work we use, speaks for the debt we owe to our colleagues in clinical cytogenetics worldwide.

Belatedly, R.J.M.G. thanks Ngaire Adams and Dianne Grimaldi, whose need for chromosomal teaching at Dunedin Hospital in the 1980s provided the germination for writing this book. We have appreciated the wise guidance, and the patience and forbearance of Oxford University Press, from Jeff House when this book made its first appearance, through to Chad Zimmerman and Chloe Layman in this fifth edition. R.J.M.G. thanks his wife Kelley for her patient help, once again, in document management; and the front cover art, and most of the new illustrations in this edition, have been drawn, or redrawn, by her.

CONTENTS

PART ONE

BASIC CONCEPTS

1

ELEMENTS OF MEDICAL CYTOGENETICS

CHROMOSOMES WERE first seen and named in the late nineteenth century. *Chromosome* is a combination of Greek words meaning colored (*chrom*) body (*soma*); the word was coined by the illustrious German anatomist Heinrich Wilhelm Gottfried von Waldeyer-Hartz. It was early appreciated that these brightly staining objects appearing in the cell nucleus must be the "stuff of heredity," the very vessels of our genetic inheritance. Most observers had concluded, in the earlier part of the twentieth century, that the human chromosome count was 48. It was not until the 1950s, due to technical advances, and in particular the use of a hypotonic solution to swell the cells, giving an uncluttered view of the chromosomes, that Joe Hin Tjio and Albert Levan could recognize that 46 was the correct number. This discovery spurred research into conditions in which a chromosomal cause had

hitherto been suspected, and in 1959 ("the wonderful year of human cytogenetics") came the first demonstrations of a medical application of the new knowledge, with practically simultaneous discoveries of the chromosomal basis of Down syndrome, Klinefelter syndrome, and Turner syndrome (Lejeune et al.[1] 1959; Jacobs and Strong 1959; Ford et al. 1959); these were followed soon thereafter by the recognition of the other major aneuploidy syndromes. Harper (2006) records the history, and the personalities behind the history, in his book *First Years of Human Chromosomes*—a book that should be read by every student of medical cytogenetics with an interest in how their discipline came to be. Harper points out that the practice of genetic counseling came into its own essentially upon the basis of these chromosomal discoveries: So to speak, geneticists now had "their organ."

---

1 Among the 'al.' was Marthe Gautier, who recounted, half a century following this report, her own less than fully acknowledged role in the endeavor; and Sir Peter Harper, in a commentary, and in his role as historian to the genetics community, takes an interpretative perspective upon this pioneering discovery (Gautier and Harper 2009).

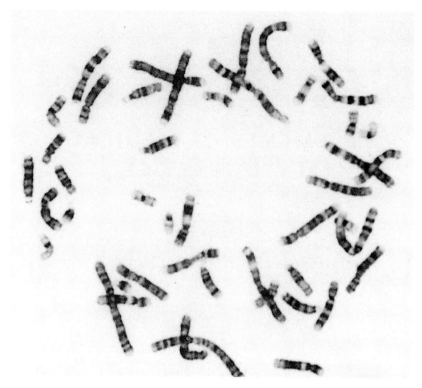

FIGURE 1–1   The appearance of banded chromosomes, from a classical cytogenetic study.

"Colored bodies" became an especially apt derivation with the development of various different staining techniques in the 1980s and 1990s, showing different parts of chromosomes in many different colors, whether true or computer-generated false colors. The images produced by this kaleidoscopic karyotyping could be rather beautiful. Black-and-white photographs were less splendid but often sufficed (Figure 1–1). Albeit that molecular methodologies have substantially taken over from classical cytogenetics, and providing a different view of the genetic material, the word *chromosome* will surely last forever.

Chromosomal Morphology

Chromosomes have a linear appearance: two arms that are continuous at the *centromere*. Reflecting the French influence in the establishment of the cytogenetic nomenclature, the shorter arm is designated *p* (for petit), and the longer is *q* (variously explained

as being the next letter in the alphabet, a mistyping of *g* (for grand), for queue, or as the other letter in the formula $p + q = 1$). In the early part of the cell cycle, each chromosome is present as a single structure, a chromatid, a single DNA molecule. During the cell cycle, the chromosomes replicate, and two *sister chromatids* form. Now the chromosome exists as a double-chromatid entity. Each chromatid contains exactly the same genetic material. This replication is in preparation for cell division so that, after the chromosome has separated into its two component chromatids, each daughter cell receives the full amount of genetic material. It is during mitosis that the chromosomes contract and become readily distinguishable on light microscopy.

Blood and buccal mucosal cells are the tissues from which DNA is extracted in routine chromosome analysis. From blood, the nucleated white cell is the tested component for microarray analysis, and in classical cytogenetic analysis, it is the lymphocyte. Buccal mucosal cells and white blood cells[2] are obtained from

---

2 In studying the saliva of patients who had received a bone marrow transplant, Thiede et al. (2000) made the observation that 74% of the DNA in saliva was actually derived from donor white blood cells rather than from recipient buccal epithelial cells. When samples were collected by cheek brush, only 21% of the DNA was donor-derived. The fact that the origin of saliva DNA is predominantly white

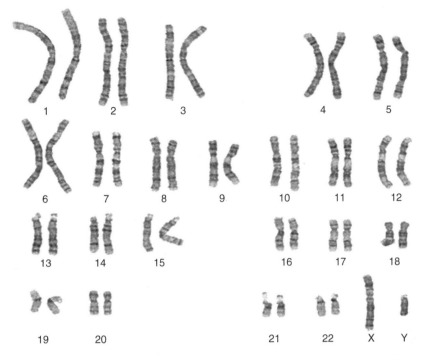

FIGURE 1–2   Chromosomes arranged as a formal karyotype, from a classical cytogenetic study.

a saliva sample. The chromosomal status of each small sample is taken as representative of the constitution of (essentially) every other cell of the body. In the case of invasive prenatal diagnosis, the cells from amniotic fluid or chorionic villi are the source material; these tissues are assumed (with certain caveats) to represent the fetal chromosomal constitution. Noninvasive prenatal diagnosis exploits the presence of fetal blood cells and DNA in the maternal circulation.

The 46 chromosomes come in 23 matching pairs and constitute the *genome*. One of each pair came from the mother, and one from the father. For 22 of the chromosome pairs, each member (each *homolog*) has the same morphology in each sex: These are the *autosomes*. The *sex chromosome* (or *gonosome*) constitution differs: The female has a pair of X chromosomes, and the male has an X and a Y chromosome. The single set of homologs—one of each autosome plus one sex chromosome—is the haploid set. The *haploid* number (n) is 23. The haploid complement exists, as such, only in the gametocytes (ovum and sperm). All other cells in the body—the *soma*—have a double set: the diploid complement

($2n$) of 46. If there is a difference between a pair of homologs, in the sense of one being structurally rearranged, the person is described as a *heterozygote*.

The chromosomes are classically distinguishable on the basis of their size, centromere position, and banding pattern. The centromere may be in the middle, off-center, or close to one end—metacentric, submetacentric, and acrocentric, respectively. The chromosomes are numbered 1 through 22, and X and Y, and are also assigned to groups A through G, according to their general size and the position of the centromere. The diagrammatic representation of the banding pattern is the *ideogram* (Appendix A). The numbering is based on size, largest to smallest (to split hairs, this order is not exact; for example, chromosomes 10 and 11 are shorter than chromosome 12, and chromosome 21 is smaller than 22).

The classical format of a chromosome display, the "*karyotype*," has the chromosomes lined up with p arms upward, in their matching pairs (Figure 1–2). Those coming from a DNA-based view may see the chromosome lying on its side, and microarray reports usually show a horizontal depiction of the chromosome arms,

---

blood cells should be kept in mind in the rare circumstance of performing a constitutional chromosome analysis on someone who has had a bone marrow transplant, and also when there is a need to test a "second tissue" (other than blood) when searching for evidence of chromosome mosaicism.

with the graph indicating duplications and deletions by a rise or a fall compared to baseline, respectively (although no one is proposing that short and long arms be renamed as left and right!). Karyotypes are described according to a shorthand notation, the International System of Human Cytogenetic Nomenclature (ISCN 2016); an outline is given in Appendix B.

Chromosomal Structure

Chromatin exists in differently condensed forms: the less condensed *euchromatin* and the more condensed *heterochromatin*. Euchromatin contains the coding DNA—the genes—while heterochromatin comprises noncoding DNA. Chromosomes are capped at the terminal extremities of their long and short arms by *telomeres*, specialized DNA sequences comprising many repeats of the sequence TTAGGG, that can be thought of as sealing the chromatin and preventing its fusion with the chromatin of other chromosomes. The *centromere*[3] is a specialized region of DNA that, at mitosis, provides the site at which the spindle apparatus can be anchored and draw each separated chromatid to opposite poles of the dividing cell. Centromeric heterochromatin contains "satellite DNA," so-called because these DNA species have different buoyant densities and produce distinct humps on a density gradient distribution. (These are not to be confused with the satellites on acrocentric chromosomes.) A separate issue, of considerable academic interest (but which we shall take no further here), is the "packaging question": how the centimeters of DNA are compacted into micron-length chromosomes, and which parts of the nucleus each chromosome occupies (Annunziato 2008; Lieberman-Aiden et al. 2009).

CHROMOSOME ABNORMALITY

Chromosomes are distributed to each daughter cell during cell division in a very precise process—precise, but prone to error. From our perspective, the two cell divisions of *meiosis*, during which the gametes are formed, are of central importance. Most of the discipline of medical cytogenetics focuses on the consequences of disordered meiosis having produced a chromosomally abnormal gamete, causing a chromosomal abnormality in the *conceptus*. A chromosome abnormality that is present from conception and involves the entire body is a *constitutional* abnormality. If an additional cell line with a different chromosomal complement arises before the basis of the body structure is formed (that is, in embryonic or pre-embryonic life) and becomes an integral part of the organism, *constitutional mosaicism* results. In this book, we concern ourselves practically solely with constitutional abnormalities. Acquired chromosomal abnormality of course exists, and indeed it is a major initiating and sustaining cause in most cancers, a fact first proposed by Boveri in 1914 and voluminously attested in the work of Mitelman et al. (2016); but this is more the field of study of the molecular pathologist than the genetic counselor.

An incorrect amount of genetic material carried by the conceptus disturbs and distorts its normal growth pattern (from zygote → blastocyst → embryo → fetus). In *trisomy*, there is three of a particular chromosome, instead of the normal two. In *monosomy*, only one member of the pair is present. Two of each is the only combination that works properly! It is scarcely surprising that a process as exquisitely complex as the development of the human form should be vulnerable to a confused outflow of genetic instruction from a nucleus with a redundant or incomplete database.

Trisomy and monosomy for a whole chromosome were the first cytogenetic mechanisms leading to an abnormal phenotype to be identified. More fully, we can list the following pathogenetic mechanisms that arise from chromosomal abnormalities:

1. A dosage effect, with a lack (deletion) or excess (duplication) of chromosomal material, whether for a whole chromosome or a part of a chromosome. This is by far the predominant category.

2. A direct damaging effect, with disruption of a gene at the breakpoint of a rearrangement

3. An effect due to the incongruent parental origin of a chromosome or chromosomal segment (genomic imprinting)

4. A position effect, whereby a gene in a new chromosomal environment functions inappropriately

5. Combinations of the above

We discuss these mechanisms in more detail in following chapters.

---

3 When considering the physical structure of rearranged chromosomes, it is useful to keep in mind the absolute requirement for a centromere to be present on every chromosome. There is also the need for each chromosome to have two telomeres, the single exception being when the rearranged chromosome forms a ring.

Autosomal Imbalance

STRUCTURAL IMBALANCE

As noted earlier, imbalance may involve the gain or loss of a whole chromosome—*full aneuploidy*—or of part of a chromosome—*partial aneuploidy*. The abnormality may occur in the nonmosaic or mosaic state. Loss (that is, monosomy) of chromosomal material generally has a more devastating effect on growth of the conceptus than does an excess of material (that is, trisomy). Certain imbalances lead to certain abnormal phenotypes. The spectrum is listed in outline in Box 1–1. Most full autosomal trisomies and virtually all full autosomal monosomies set development of the conceptus so awry that, sooner or later, abortion occurs—the embryo "self-destructs" and is expelled from the uterus. This issue is further explored in Chapter 19. A few full trisomies are not necessarily lethal in utero, and many partial chromosomal aneuploidies are associated with survival through to the birth of an infant.

Characteristically, "survivable imbalances" produce a phenotype of widespread dysmorphogenesis, and there may be malformation of internal organs and limbs. It is often in the facial appearance (*facies*) that the most recognizable physical abnormality is seen, with Down syndrome the classic example, although the physical phenotype in some cases of subtler deletion or duplication may be rather "bland." The most complex organ of all, the brain, is the most vulnerable to a less than optimal genetic constitution, and some compromise of mental and intellectual functioning, usually to the extent of an obvious deficit, is nearly invariable, at least in imbalances of classical size. With several of the (much smaller) imbalances due to copy number variants, developmental delay or mental retardation[4] with an outwardly normal physical phenotype is well recognized as a chromosomal presentation. Thus, the central concern of most people seeking genetic counseling for a chromosomal condition is that of having a child who might have a physical, intellectual, or severe social handicap.

Historically, the chromosomal basis of many syndromes was identified following analysis of groups of patients with similar phenotypes. This "phenotype-first" approach led to the identification of many of the well-known microdeletion syndromes (and of course such classic conditions as Down syndrome). With the advent of microarray analysis, new syndromes came to be identified based on their DNA aberration, a "genotype-first"

---

4 Words can be powerful, and choice of language can help, or hinder, a counseling consultation: Facts are to be conveyed clearly but also sensitively. The reader will have noticed our use of the expression "mentally retarded" in a number of places in this chapter. Some may have flinched; others may simply have accepted this as an accurate description. "Developmental delay" is a widely used term, and it can be perfectly appropriate in a pediatric setting, although less so in dealing with an adult. In the introduction to their paper on array analysis and karyotyping, Hochstenbach et al. (2009) refer to "idiopathic developmental delay (in infants <3 years of age) and mental retardation (in older children)"; this distinction acknowledges that prediction of intellectual capacity is more precise in older children. And yet "mental retardation" has acquired a pejorative and somewhat harsh sense over the years, and some will prefer to use such expressions as "intellectual disability" or "cognitive compromise." As we write elsewhere, counselors will need to know to whom they speak and what language is best to use.

approach. Representative examples of these newer syndromes are reviewed in Chapter 14.

SEX CHROMOSOMAL ABNORMALITY

Sex chromosome (gonosome) imbalance has a much less deleterious effect on the phenotype than does autosomal aneuploidy. The X chromosome is one of the larger and is gene-dense; the Y is small, comprising mostly heterochromatin, and carries very few genes. In both male and female, one, and only one, completely functioning X chromosome is needed. X chromosomes in excess of one are inactivated, as the normal 46,XX female exemplifies; her second X does, however, maintain some segments genetically active. With X chromosome excess or deficiency, a partially successful buffering mechanism exists whereby the imbalance is counteracted, in an attempt to achieve the same effect as having a single active X. In such states as, for example, XXX, XXY, XXXX, XXYY, and XXXXX, excess X chromosomes are inactivated. In the 45,X state, the single X remaining is not subject to inactivation. If an abnormal X chromosome (e.g., an isochromosome, or a deleted X) is present, then, as a rule, cells containing this abnormal chromosome as the active X are selected against, perhaps due to preferential growth of those cells in which it is the normal X that is the active one. In X imbalance, the reproductive tract and brain are the organs predominantly affected. The effect may be minimal. As for Y chromosome excess, such as XYY, there is a rather limited phenotypic consequence, but again the brain may be a vulnerable organ.

FUNCTIONAL IMBALANCE

A correct amount of chromatin does not necessarily mean the phenotype will be normal. Inappropriate inactivation, or activation, of a segment of the genome can compromise the genetic message. Some segments of the genome require only monosomic expression, and the homologous segment on the other chromosome is inactivated. If this control fails, both segments can become activated, or both inactivated, and the over- or under-expression of the contained loci can cause phenotypic abnormality. The classic example of this is genomic imprinting according to parent of origin, and we discuss this concept in Chapter 18. A rather specialized example arises with the X-autosome translocation. A segment of X chromosome can fail to be inactivated; or conversely, X-inactivation can spread into an autosomal segment (Chapter 6).

The Frequency and Impact of Cytogenetic Pathology

According to the window of observation, chromosomal disorders make a greater or lesser contribution to human mortality and morbidity. Looking at prenatal existence, the earliest window has been provided by the in vitro fertilization (IVF) clinic, from the procedure of preimplantation genetic diagnosis (Chapter 22), at which cells taken from 3- to 5-day-old embryos are subjected to genetic analysis; and an extraordinary fraction are chromosomally abnormal. After implantation (about day 6), and through the first trimester of pregnancy (to week 13), chromosomal mortality is very high, and aneuploidy is the major single cause of spontaneous abortion (Chapter 19). Perinatal and early infant death has a significant chromosomal component, of which trisomies 18 and 21 (although the latter less so in more recent times) are major elements.

As for morbidity, the brain, as mentioned above, is the most vulnerable organ, and chromosomal defects are the basis of a substantial fraction of all intellectual deficit, and many of these retarded individuals will also have structural malformations that cause functional physical disability. Among a mentally retarded population, Down syndrome is the predominant contributor in the fraction who have a classic chromosome abnormality (Phelan et al. 1996). Development of the heart is particularly susceptible to chromosomal imbalance, and in a population study from the US National Center on Birth Defects, 1 in 8 infants with a congenital heart defect had a chromosomal abnormality, with again trisomy 21 the most common of these (53%), followed by trisomy 18 (13%), 22q11.2 deletion (12%), and trisomy 13 (6%) (Hartman et al. 2011).

Adolescence is a period during which many sex chromosome defects come to light, when pubertal change fails to occur; and in young adulthood, chromosomal causes of infertility are recognized. Few new classic cytogenetic defects come to attention later in adult life, but many retarded children survive well into adulthood and some into old age, and some require lifelong care from their families or from the state. This latter group imposes a considerable emotional and financial burden. While some parents and caregivers declare the emotional return they have from looking after these individuals, for others this responsibility is a source of continuing, unresolved, if attenuated, grief.

In Table 1–1 we set out the birth incidences of the various categories of (classical) chromosomal

Table 1–1. Classical Chromosomal Rearrangements and Imbalances, Recorded in 34,910 Live Newborns in Århus, Denmark, over a Total 13-Year Period, 1969–1974 and 1980–1988

	NO. OF CASES	PER 1,000[a]	BIRTH FREQUENCY PER GROUP
Sex Chromosomes			
Klinefelter Syndrome and Variants			
47,XXY	20	1.12[b]	
47,XXY/46,XY	7	0.39	
46,XX	2	0.11	
			1 in 616 ♂
XYY			
47,XYY	18	1.01	
47,XYY/46,XY	2	0.11	
			1 in 894 ♂
XXX			
47,XXX	17	1.00	
			1 in 1,002 ♀
Turner Syndrome and Variants			
45,X	1	0.06	
45,X/46,XX and 45,X/47,XXX	3	0.18	
45,X/46,X,r(X)	1	0.06	
45,X/46,X,i(Xq)/47,X,i(Xq),i(Xq)	1	0.06	
Other Turner variant	2	0.12	
			1 in 2,130 ♀
Other			
45,X/46,XY	1	0.06	
46,XX/47,XX,del(Yq)	1	0.06	
46,XX/46,XY	1	0.06	
Total	77	2.21	1 in 453
Autosomes			
Unbalanced Forms			
Trisomy 13	2	0.06	
Trisomy 18	7	0.20	
Trisomy 21	51	1.46	
Trisomy 8	1	0.03	
Supernumerary marker, ring	25	0.72	
Deletions, duplications	6	0.17	
			1 in 379
Balanced Forms			
Robertsonian 13/14 translocation	34	0.97	
Other Robertsonian	9	0.26	
Reciprocal translocations	50	1.43	
Inversions (other than of chromosome 2)	4	0.11	
			1 in 360
Combined sex plus autosomal totals	266	7.62	1 in 131
Combined totals, excluding balanced autosomal forms	169	4.84	1 in 207

Notes: Not included in the 34,910 live newborns listing are four cases of induced abortion due to sex chromosome prenatal diagnosis, involving the karyotypes 47,XXY, 47,XYY, 47,XXX, and 45,X/46,X,del(Xq), and 15 cases of autosomal-diagnosis induced abortions, involving the karyotypes +21, +13, +18, and three different derivative chromosomes. Had these pregnancies proceeded to term, the frequencies in the relevant group category would have been marginally increased.

These figures might continue to be broadly valid into this century, except that the category of deletions and duplications will substantially increase due to the more powerful detection now offered by molecular technology.

[a]Per 1,000 male, per 1,000 female, or per 1,000 both, as appropriate. The gender-specific denominators in this study were 17,872 males and 17,038 females.

[b]An increasing incidence of XXY in recent years has been suggested, and an Australian study, including data up to 2006, arrived at a figure of 1.91 per 1,000 (Herlihy and Halliday 2008; Morris et al. 2008; Herlihy et al. 2010).

Source: From Nielsen and Wohlert (1991)

abnormality; these data are from a Danish study, one of a number that have examined this question in the later decades of the twentieth century, with largely similar findings in each. Overall, around 1 in 135 liveborn babies have a classical chromosomal abnormality, and about 40% of these are phenotypically abnormal due to the chromosome defect. If we were to look at day-5 blastocysts, the fraction with abnormality might be close to a half. Fertile adults (ascertained by virtue of having presented for noninvasive prenatal testing) have much lower frequencies of sex chromosome aneuploidy (Samango-Sprouse et al. 2016). If we studied a population of 70-year-olds, we could expect to see very few individuals with an unbalanced autosomal karyotype.

The finer the cytogenetic focus, the greater the incidence, and it is now a task for the cytogenetic epidemiologist of this century, in the microarray/molecular era, to derive new estimates of cytogenetic abnormalities in the different populations (Rosenfeld et al. 2013). The brain again declares its susceptibility, with many examples of a brain-only phenotype (intellectual disability, epilepsy, autism, psychiatric disease) due to microduplications and microdeletions detectable only on molecular karyotyping, and chromosomes 15 and 16, in particular, represented.

THE RESEARCH APPLICATION OF CYTOGENETIC PATHOLOGY

The phenotypes that result from chromosome abnormalities can point the way to discovery of the causative genes. An early example of deletion mapping is the recognition that the gene for retinoblastoma was on chromosome 13, given the association of this cancer with the 13q– syndrome. Another cancer gene to be similarly mapped was *APC* (adenomatous polyposis coli), following the observation of polyposis of the colon in an individual with mental retardation and del(5)(q22q23) (Hockey et al. 1989). The triple dose of chromosome 21 in Down syndrome was a signpost on the way to finding the β-amyloid precursor protein (*APP*) gene as one of the Alzheimer disease loci. A translocation with one breakpoint at 7q11.23 was found to disrupt the elastin gene in a family segregating supravalvular aortic stenosis. Further investigation of this locus in Williams syndrome proved this to be the site of

deletion in this condition (Nickerson et al. 1995). The gene for CHARGE[5] syndrome, *CHD7*, was discovered due to two patients with an 8q12 microdeletion (Vissers et al. 2004). We have conducted reviews of chromosomal conditions in which epilepsy and kidney disease are features, with the aim of providing leads to epilepsy genes and renal genes (Singh et al. 2002a; Amor et al. 2003).

The precision of microarray analysis, coupled with access to genome databases, now allows a much finer focus in the pursuit of causative genes. Ou et al. (2008) propose, and Ballesta-Martínez et al. (2013) support, that one of the genes *SIX1, SIX6,* or *OTX2* may be the basis of one form of branchio-oto-renal syndrome, from their study of a child with a duplication of 14q22.3q23.3. We have shown *WDR35* to be the gene for a short rib–polydactyly syndrome, having found a microdeletion on chromosome 2p24 by single nucleotide polymorphism (SNP) and copy number variant (CNV) analysis (Mill et al. 2011); and *RAB39B* to be the basis of a syndrome of early onset Parkinson disease and intellectual disability, a 45 kb deletion at Xq28 leading us to this discovery (Wilson et al. 2014).

It is a general principle that many important scientific discoveries are made serendipitously; or, as Louis Pasteur put it, "chance favors the prepared mind" (*le hasard ne favorise que les esprits préparés*). Voullaire et al. (1993) identified a small supernumerary marker chromosome (sSMC) in a child with a nonspecific picture of physical abnormality and intellectual deficit, which had no C-band positive centromere (only a constriction). Conventional wisdom has it (and indeed as we have written above) that a chromosome cannot be stably transmitted at cell division if it has no centromere. These workers studied this sSMC and discovered that it did have a simple, but nevertheless functional centromere. This observation led the way to the delineation of the "neocentromere" (p. 226).

ETHICAL AND COUNSELING ISSUES

Our focus in this book is largely on the biology of chromosomal defects, and the reproductive implications that they may entail. Certain bioethical issues, coming to be more formally defined in the late twentieth century, do, however, demand

---

5 CHARGE = coloboma, heart, choanal atresia, retardation, genital, ear.

attention. Counselors must hold fast to these requirements: (1) that they act beneficently toward their patients[6] and (2) that they strive to make their services accessible to those who may need them.

NONDIRECTIVE COUNSELING

In a Western ethos, the counselor is required to respect the autonomy of the client, and this largely translates into the principle that counseling be non-directive. Counseling may in fact never be truly non-directive, and we need to have an awareness of our own biases in order that our advice will be, as seen by those to whom we give it, valid. Rentmeester (2001) comments that since it is "impossible for human language to convey facts purely, without any spoor of values" and since "risk cannot be appreciated without consideration of values," it is neither helpful nor indeed possible to try to be value-neutral. There is a fine line between directive and detached counseling, a point well illustrated in Karp's (1983) deft essay, "The Terrible Question." Ingelfinger (1980) comments, admittedly in a somewhat different context: "A physician who merely spreads an array of vendibles in front of the patient and then says, 'Go ahead and choose, it's your life,' is guilty of shirking his duty, if not of malpractice." Rentmeester offers the refreshing advice that it is not necessarily unprofessional to answer a patient's question: "What would you do?" It is the skill of the counselor that helps clients reach the decision that is, for them, the right one, and for the clients to feel satisfied that they have done so. The subtleties and complexities of attempting to be nondirective in the setting of a prenatal diagnosis clinic are discussed by Anderson (1999), who analyzes responses of couples who did or who did not choose to have testing. She emphasizes the wide range of beliefs and values that people can have, as well as the likelihood for failed communication if these differences are not appreciated.

In some other societies, the perceived good of the group may carry more weight than the professed wishes of the individual. The degree to which one society can seek to influence practice in another is a matter of some controversy, well illustrated by the response in the West last century to the "eugenic" Chinese Maternal and Infant Health Care Law of 1994 (*Lancet* editorial 1995). The subtleties of the issue led to keenly pointed argument (correspondence in the *American Journal of Human Genetics*, 1999: Guo 1999; Chen et al. 1999; Mao 1999). Knoppers (1998) comments on the subtle boundary between the need to respect cultural, religious, and social diversity, and the imperative to adhere to tenets of generally accepted rights and ethics. More provocatively, she points to a "political and moral one-upmanship" that has colored the argument and that may confuse deciding between what is "immoral state policy or just plain common sense."

TESTING CHILDREN

To state the obvious, familial rearrangements are familial. It is very natural that parents would be concerned whether children they already have might be carriers, once an abnormality has been identified in one of them. Children, certainly, need to know their carrier status, sooner or later. It is very unfortunate (and possibly creates an exposure to legal redress) if a failure to transmit information leads to another affected child unknowingly being born elsewhere in the family. Burn et al. (1983) reported a family with a translocation having been the cause of cri du chat syndrome in two generations, the genetic information not having flowed through to the people who really needed to know it. We have had a similar experience: a family with a t(4;12) concerning which we had gone to the lengths of deriving and publishing a recurrence risk figure (Mortimer et al. 1980), and yet this information not traveling with a young man who had moved, as a child, from one country to another, and whose life was since blighted by having had a daughter with partial 4p trisomy, and whose wife had terminations due to unbalanced forms identified at prenatal diagnosis.

On the other hand, genetic counselors are attuned to the principle of not taking away a child's right to make, in the fullness of time, his or her own informed decision to learn about genetic risks he or she may face; thus, the principle is that the child's future autonomy is to be respected. The American Society of Human Genetics and the American College of Medical Genetics (1995) have determined that "timely medical benefit to the child should be the primary justification for genetic testing in children and adolescents," and it is true that

---

6 There seems no completely satisfactory word to use here, and we variably write of patients, clients, counselees, men and women, people, and "those whom we see."

a balanced chromosomal rearrangement will have no influence upon a person's physical health, other than, in due course, his or her reproductive health (and the issue is thus to be seen in a different light than testing for adult-onset disease). Questions are raised that testing could damage a child's self-esteem, distort the family's perceptions of the child, and have adverse effects upon the child's capacity to form future relationships (Clarke 1994). In France, testing a healthy child for the possibility of inheritance of a parental chromosome rearrangement may be unlawful (Hervé et al. 2015).

Parents' views are not without validity. Clayton (1995) commented that there is the possibility of conflict with parents, as physicians come increasingly to act as advocates for the child's interests, but notes further that "children are generally ill-served if their parents feel they have not been listened to"; she also draws the conclusion that this is a medico-ethical rather than a medico-legal issue. Vears et al. (2016) offer a similarly nuanced view. McConkie-Rosell et al. (1999) sought opinions from a group of 65 parents of fragile X children attending a national conference in Portland, Oregon, in 1996. They noted a "strong belief in a parental right to make the decision regarding carrier status in their children," with about half considering that they should have the right to decide when their child should be tested and informed of the result. The Genetic Interest Group in the United Kingdom gently chided the profession in commenting that "the vast majority of people are better able to understand the implications than they are often given credit for" and has enunciated the following principle: "After suitable counseling, parents have the right to make an informed choice about whether or not to have their children tested for carrier status. Ideally, children should only be tested when of an age to be involved in the decision" (Dalby 1995).

It may be that earlier concerns overstated the potential for harm: At least with respect to the Mendelian cancer-predisposing syndrome familial adenomatous polyposis, children having undergone predictive testing and receiving a positive gene test result experienced no increase in anxiety, depression, or loss of self-esteem (Michie et al. 2001). Indeed, Robertson and Savulescu (2001) see potential benefit to the child, and they support the view that, as a general rule, the parents' views should prevail, and a request for predictive testing be respected. There is also the practical point that many parents will have had a prenatal karyotype from amniocentesis or chorionic villus sampling for one of their children-to-be; and it may not seem entirely logical to decline to test their other, postnatal children. In an analogous Mendelian case, X-linked Duchenne muscular dystrophy, Helderman-van den Enden et al. (2013) go so far as to state "it is cruel to subject the parents to an ordeal, lasting years, with this dilemma [of their unborn or infant daughter possibly being a carrier]."

From the foregoing, we conclude that a conservative stance, but not an immovable one, is appropriate. Debating the issue with them, many parents will see the wisdom of the declared position of the profession and be well satisfied (and possibly relieved) with the advice to leave testing until the child can decide. Equally, there will be occasions when acquiescence to a parental request may be reasonable. Either the parent's mind is set at rest or they know of the need to raise the issue with the child at a "suitable age," which should be with the assistance of the genetic counseling clinic. The task for the counselor is to assist parents in deciding what age would be suitable for their child and to convey the information in such a way that concern for the future is kept in perspective, and the child's self-confidence is kept intact. And the pragmatic imperative: the wish to avoid family distress due to avoidable births of abnormal children in the next generation, as outlined above. Bache et al. (2007) found that 9% of carriers in Denmark, identified in childhood (or prenatally), had not been told as young adults; this observation led to a change in practice in that country, with a reminder letter being sent to the parents when their child reached the age of 18 years.

FAMILY STUDIES

More widely, the parents' siblings and cousins could be carriers. Grandparental karyotypes may be useful in knowing which branch of a family to follow. The rights of individuals could, potentially, clash with the obligation that flows from belonging to a family: "No man is an island, entire unto himself" and some may see altruism as a duty. Austad (1996) proposes that the family's right to know about "sensitive genetic information" should take precedence over the individual's right not to know. He considers it "alarming to use the principle of autonomy to renounce the co-responsibility for others, in this case, relatives"; he goes on to state that "we cannot exclude ourselves from the genetic fellowship of fate into which we are born." If counselors take pains to provide clear information and to do so sensitively, such studies should usually proceed without unfortunate consequence. A suitable approach, in most families, will be to ask the person coming to the clinic to take the responsibility of bringing the matter to the attention of relatives, with appropriate support from the counselor. A letter couched in terms that it could be shown to other family members, and providing contact points for further information, is often useful. Forrest et al. (2007) reviewed many international sources and identified these criteria seen as common obligations falling to the families, and to the counselors who see them: (1) Individuals have a moral obligation to communicate genetic information to their family members, (2) genetic health professionals should encourage individuals to communicate this information to their family members, and (3) genetic health professionals should support individuals throughout the communication process. We would add a caveat, now that microarray analysis has become the norm: The uncertainties of interpretation of many CNVs seen in routine clinical practice can complicate "cascade testing" to a degree that the exercise may become counterproductive and unhelpful.

PREDICTIVE GENE TESTING: DELIBERATE AND INADVERTENT

Counselors are very familiar with the concept of predictive genetic testing—that is, offering genetic testing to people who are presently well but who are at risk for having inherited a particular genotype that may, at some stage in adult life, be the basis of the onset of disease. Its widest application is in the fields of cancer genetics and neurogenetics. With respect to rare translocations in the balanced state that may confer a predisposition to cancer, mention is made on p. 111, and over and above the reproductive implications of individuals being tested in such families, a cancer-associated risk will need to be assessed. As for inadvertent testing, we may mention a 30-year-old woman we have seen, presenting with premature ovarian failure and having a karyotype to check for an X chromosome mosaicism, but in whom trisomy 8 and a 14q;18q translocation were seen in 3/100 cells. She was otherwise in good health. This may well have been an "accidental"

very early diagnosis of a lymphoma, and referral to a hematologist–oncologist—which was more than she had bargained for by having the test—was duly arranged. Nevertheless, although advice about a cancer risk may come as an "unwanted surprise," discovery of a chromosomal predisposition may in fact be life-saving (Heald et al. 2007).

With the increasing application of microarray technology, the likelihood of discovering an incidental abnormality may now need more frequently to be taken into account, when a chromosome test is ordered. We mention on p. 329 the 17q21.31 duplication which may be the basis of a familial dementia. Schwarzbraun et al. (2009) report their experience in testing a severely mentally retarded and mildly dysmorphic 7-year-old girl, in whom microarray revealed a de novo microdeletion (774 kb; contained 47 genes) at 17p13.1, and this deletion presumed to be the explanation for the clinical picture. One of the deleted 47 genes, however, happened to be *TP53*, and thus this deletion was considered to represent, effectively, a germline Li-Fraumeni[7] mutation. This was quite unanticipated information for the parents to deal with, and the issue was further complicated by the child's mental incapacity. Schluth-Bolard et al. (2010) consider this question, and they write

> the local Ethical Committee at the University Hospital of Lyon, France, suggested implementation of a plan to inform patients and their parents on the possibility of discovering pathology unrelated to mental retardation, and give them a month to carefully ponder on the possible consequences before signing the consent for study.

More pragmatically, they continue:

> If this period of reflection would be difficult to apply in clinical practice, the possibility of incidental findings should be discussed during pre-test counseling and information should be given during post-test counseling by a trained clinician, aware of the potential psychological impact of such findings.

Noninvasive prenatal testing (NIPT) may lead into unanticipated ethical minefields. An occasional

---

7 Li-Fraumeni syndrome is a dominantly inherited cancer-predisposition syndrome, due to *TP53* germline mutation, with severe implications. The cancers include, in early childhood, soft-tissue sarcoma; in later childhood, osteosarcoma; and in young adulthood, breast, brain, and hematological malignancy. It is controversial whether medical surveillance should be offered in childhood.

inadvertent cancer diagnosis may be made (Osborne et al. 2013). In a case reported in Sun et al. (2015), massive copy number gains of chromosome 21, and some other chromosomes, were observed, completely different from what would be seen in fetal trisomy; and in fact the diagnosis was recurrence of a follicular lymphoma. Meschino et al. (2016) report the case of a woman who had had NIPT for trisomy 21, due to the ultrasound detection of two "soft markers" for Down syndrome, and who also, as it happened, had a family history of early onset Alzheimer disease. A dup(21) was identified, which included the Alzheimer-associated *APP* locus at 21q21.3 (but not the Down syndrome critical region). Thus, she, and her unborn child, had had an unwitting predictive genetic test for a dominantly inherited dementia. Further to complicate the story, she had an identical twin sister. Meschino et al. debate the complicated issues that arose from this case, and they rehearse lessons to be taken for those in the field.

UNCERTAIN DISCOVERIES AT PRENATAL MICROARRAY

Conveying uncertainty is more difficult than giving definite information. Much experience has been accumulated in the decade or so during which microarray has become the main means of chromosome diagnosis, but not every microdeletion or microduplication is well understood. There is the complicating factor that some of these abnormalities may be pathogenic only in certain circumstances—that is, they can be nonpenetrant. This becomes a particular issue in prenatal diagnosis: If a microdeletion/duplication is a "new" finding, and not listed in any database, what does one say to the mother? Brady et al. (2014) consider this question and come down in favor of not mentioning such discoveries, and they argue that, rather than undermining parental reproductive rights, in fact this policy prevents giving a false sense of autonomy. Stark et al. (2013) and de Jong et al. (2014) reach similar conclusions. An alternative viewpoint is proposed by McGillivray et al. (2012), who suggest nondisclosure may smack of paternalism, notwithstanding the distress that an uncertain interpretation may bring to bear. Counselors are well aware of these challenges and controversies, and in a survey of US and Canadian genetic counselors, just over half had reservations about giving "ambiguous results" and saw this as an ethical issue (Mikhaelian et al. 2013).

THE STATUS OF EMBRYOS AT IN VITRO FERTILIZATION

Lejeune has commented, indeed provided extensive testimony, on the ethical distinction between abortion and discarding an unwanted embryo. At a famous court case dealing with a dispute about IVF embryos in Blount County, Tennessee, in 1989, he insisted on the point that human life commences at conception, and therefore that disposing of a zygote is, in essence, no different from the induced abortion of an established pregnancy. This argument is not necessarily seen as convincing to those pragmatic couples who choose to have preimplantation diagnosis in order to avoid the predicament of having to decide upon a course of action following prenatal diagnosis of a chromosomal abnormality at chorionic villus sampling or amniocentesis. One Catholic thinker is of the opinion that "human personhood" of the embryo does not inhere until the stage at which embryonic cells have differentiated and the primitive streak has appeared (at about the end of the second week post-conception) (Ford 1988). Prior to that time, when the "pro-embryo," as he prefers to call it, is only a *personne en devenir*, "we should resist the conceptual and linguistic temptation to attribute an unwarranted ontological unity to an actual multiplicity of developing human blastomeres." More liberally, Isaacs (2002) discusses the concept of a continuum, in which the "moral status" of the fetus increases in value through pregnancy (and indeed after birth); and some couples seem intuitively to follow this line.

Molecular methodologies, as we have already had cause to comment, bring with them ethical challenges. In a paper memorably titled "Embryos Without Secrets," Hens et al. (2013b) consider the new dimensions implied by the new methodologies. They conclude that microarray and, potentially, whole genome analysis may be a double-edged sword in the hands of those providing preimplantation genetic diagnosis (PGD), and they call for more discussion about "who should have the final say on which embryo to select." An embryo can be seen as a future person, and that being so, Hens et al. (2013a) point to an onerous responsibility upon the PGD clinician. These authors, while acknowledging the "principle of procreative beneficence" put forward by Savulescu and Kahane (2009), who consider that couples have a moral obligation (if reasonably feasible) to select the embryo whose life can be expected to be best, point out that the situation may not necessarily be straightforward. The counselor working in an IVF clinic will need to keep abreast of these complex questions and to be aware of the vulnerabilities of the couples presenting.

"GUILT" IN A CARRIER

Sometimes a chromosomal diagnosis may be made in an older child or even an adult, where the parents will have held for years to the notion that obstetric misadventure, or a virus, or some other blameable event was the cause of the child's condition. Some people find it upsetting to have to readjust or to know that they may have been the source of the abnormality. They are likely to use words such as guilt, blame, and fault. Helping these people to adjust to the new knowledge is a challenge for the counselor. They may eventually come to find the chromosomal explanation valuable and a source of some relief (as indeed some do at the outset).

INTELLECTUAL DEFICIENCY AND GENETIC ABORTION

Intellectual deficiency is a condition for which many parents are unwilling to accept a significant recurrence risk—hardly remarkable, since intellectual function is such an obvious attribute of humanness. The great majority of those who chose to have prenatal diagnosis opt for pregnancy termination[8] if a chromosomal condition implying major mental defect is identified. Some for whom abortion is not acceptable may nevertheless choose prenatal diagnosis for reassurance or for the preparedness that certain knowledge can allow. Community views on mental handicap are changing, and the late twentieth century saw something of an exodus from institutions and from special schools, as the mentally and psychologically disabled joined the "mainstream," some more successfully than others. Many syndromes, in this Internet age, have their own support groups, and these are often a source of advocacy. Counselors need to handle the tension inherent in these views and the views of parents who want to avoid having a handicapped child; and the separate conflict that parents experience when a decision is taken to terminate an otherwise wanted pregnancy. As we discussed earlier, the doctrine of nondirective counseling is a central tenet of modern practice, and it is a test of counselors' professionalism that their own views not unduly influence the advice and counsel that they give. De Crespigny et al. (1998) document the experiences and comments of a number of couples in their book *Prenatal Testing: Making Choices in Pregnancy*, intended for the lay public. Walters (1995) and Tillisch (2001) offer personal perspectives. First, Walters:

> Defending the right of women who are carrying babies with Down's syndrome to have abortions is not pleasant. Anyone who does so is likely to sound heartless, especially if they have no first-hand experience. It is even harder for me. I am the father of a Down's syndrome baby. . . . It is the most painful thing I will ever say but my wife, Karen and I wish she had had a test. If she had, we would have terminated the pregnancy. I must be a callous swine, mustn't I? . . . Her birth was a tragedy, but not so different to any tragedy that can strike out of the blue, such as a crippling accident. Just as we work to avoid other tragedies, I see nothing wrong in using Down's tests to avoid the tragedy of human handicap. . . . I know that I would rather not have existed at all than to be, like her, sentenced to a life of confusion, frustration, pain and possibly loneliness when Karen and I are gone. If I feel guilt, it is that I was responsible for her birth. To me that guilt is far worse than anything I would have felt had I prevented it.

Tillisch is the mother of a child with the del(1)(p36) syndrome (p. 269). Anomalies had been detected on ultrasonography during the pregnancy, but an amniocentesis returned a normal cytogenetic result. The child had a stormy neonatal course, and in due course the chromosomal defect was identified. Tillisch writes:

> I'm so thankful that the amniocentesis results were inaccurate. Since we didn't learn of Kasey's diagnosis until she was 9 months old, we were able to get to know, love, and admire Kasey as an individual, as our daughter. We didn't allow doctors to define her for

---

8 A sensitivity in discussing the choice of abortion may be discerned in the following conversation with her genetic counselor that Urquhart (2016) had: She writes, "'What about cases where people want to change the management of their pregnancy?' I asked, using the euphemism for abortion I had learned during our counseling sessions, 'We would have to investigate other options,' she said."

us. . . . From a mother's perspective, Kasey's future is bright. She receives treatment and will soon go to a public school. We will allow Kasey to show us her potential, rather than labeling her "severely mentally retarded" and casting her off to be locked away from society. . . . My father once asked, if I could ever make Kasey "whole," would I? Without any hesitation, I answered: absolutely not. Adding the missing genes would make Kasey a different person, a stranger.

These differing, one could say polar views of parents find some parallels in the positions of those whom we could consider as the philosophers of our profession. Lejeune, in a provocative address to the American Society of Human Genetics in 1970, deplored the application of his original cytogenetic discovery to the prenatal diagnosis of Down syndrome. Epstein (2002) reflected, some three decades later, upon Lejeune's influence, and while not stepping back from the standpoint that prenatal diagnosis is a proper and valid medical procedure, he does acknowledge (as must we) that a plurality of views exists, and that the genetics community must be sensitive to, and must respect, the range of views in the community.

Brock (1995) discusses the philosophy of "wrongful handicap," addressing the question of whether not producing a child who would suffer has harmed that potential child, and he enunciates a principle that

> individuals are morally required not to let any possible child for whose welfare they are responsible experience serious suffering or limited opportunity if they can act so that, without imposing substantial burdens or costs on themselves or others, any alternative possible child for whose welfare they would be responsible will not experience serious suffering or limited opportunity.

This position (somewhat reflecting that of Savulescu and Kahane, 2009, above) could be seen as providing an ethically based framework for making a decision to terminate an abnormal pregnancy and to conceive again.

There are some subtleties in the choice of language when fetal anomalies are uncovered by ultrasound, as de Crespigny et al. (1996, 1999) discuss. We speak of the pregnant woman as a mother, yet she is not; neither is her husband/partner as yet a father. Equally, the fetus is not a baby, not acquiring that status until ex utero existence is achieved. But of course many parents-to-be, not to mention professionals, use these words. Counselors should be sensitive to these subtleties. De Crespigny observes that if an ultrasonologist should discover a fetal defect, using the terms "baby" and "mother" may exert indirect pressure on the couple to continue the pregnancy:

> Although many women regard a fetus as a baby from the very beginning, others will be affronted if their doctor does not seem to recognize this difference between a fetus and a baby, which they may interpret as interfering with the pregnant woman's reproductive freedom.

As always, counselors will need to know their patients, and to judge the right words to use and the way to say them (Benkendorf et al. 2001).

PREGNANCY AND THE INTELLECTUALLY HANDICAPPED

One issue to test the caliber of the bioethicist (not to mention the counselor) is that of the rights of the intellectually handicapped to have children (Elkins et al. 1986a). What of the person with Down syndrome, or some partial trisomy compatible with fertility, in whom a question of procreation arises? Zühlke et al. (1994) give an example in describing a man with Down syndrome who developed a relationship with a mentally retarded girl living in the same house. She requested removal of an intrauterine contraceptive device, became pregnant, and the normal baby was brought up by the maternal grandmother. A case in Queensland, Australia, of a couple both with Down syndrome, wishing to marry and to have children, came to public attention in 2016 through a popular television program. On the one hand, the right of the handicapped person to experience parenthood is debated, and the American Academy of Pediatrics Committee on Bioethics (1990) expressed reservation about the sterilization of intellectually handicapped women on the basis of anticipated hardship to others. On the other hand, Gillon (1987) notes that normal people have the option of being sterilized, and the mentally handicapped should have the same right. The Law Lords in Great Britain concur that sterilization may be in the best interest of the handicapped person herself (Brahams 1987).

Many parents or guardians, not wishing to become "parental grandparents," favor sterilization. Some regard hysterectomy as having the double benefit of ensuring sterility and facilitating personal hygiene; others consider only reversible contraception to be acceptable. The High Court of Australia decided in 1992 that the parents of a handicapped child cannot themselves lawfully allow sterilization, but that a court authorization is required, and noted that this requirement "ensures a hearing from those experienced in different ways in the care of those with intellectual disability and from those with experience of the long term social and psychological effects of sterilization" (Monahan 1992). Ten years later, it appeared that very few unlawful sterilizations of minors were being performed in the state of Victoria (Grover et al. 2002).

When a retarded woman with a chromosomal defect is pregnant, or is pregnant by a retarded man, one or other of the couple having an unbalanced karyotype, and the pregnancy is recognized in time, the grounds for termination may be seen as substantial. The ethical issue arises over the difficulty (or impossibility) of securing the woman's informed consent versus the expressed wishes of her guardians. Martínez et al. (1993) report from Alabama a mother with cri du chat syndrome, who was severely retarded and had no speech, pregnant by an unknown male, and "although pregnancy termination had been desired by the patient's grandmother, social and legal limitations prevented access to this procedure." Some less severely affected persons (if they are able to grasp the issue) may not regard it as undesirable to have a child like themselves; on the other hand, they may have the insight to recognize their own deficiency and not wish to pass it on. We may perhaps read this into the brief report of Bobrow et al. (1992) of a man with Down syndrome fathering a child, the mother having had first-trimester prenatal diagnosis (the baby was normal). There is the concept of imagining what a retarded person would want, were he or she intellectually competent to make a decision—a concept some would regard as paternalistic (and infringing personal autonomy) and that others might see as valid and common sense. The sociology rather than the biology will exercise the counselor's mettle in this uncommonly encountered situation.

Two approaches to a modification of genetic counseling for those with intellectual disabilities have been described, and with respect to the particular example of Williams syndrome (Farwig et al. 2010). Watkins et al. (1989) teach basic facts to the counselee, using simplified language and repetition as needed. In discussion, they use yes/no rather than open-ended questions. In contrast, Finucane (1998) takes a psychosocial approach, in which a more conversational style, focusing on feelings and attitudes, takes precedence over the provision of facts. She argues that most individuals with intellectual disability reason concretely (in Piagetian terms, are in the preoperational or concrete operational periods of development, rather than in the formal operational period), do not understand numbers or quantity reliably, and tend to act egocentrically. She advises that it is important for the goals set by the genetic counselor to be limited, specific, concrete, and related to the reason for referral.

The other party is the child. Is having good parenting a right? What of a normal child born, for example, to a man carrying a dup(10)(p13p14) chromosome and a mother with idiopathic mental defect? How can the interests of the child and of the parents be resolved? This is an actual case that we have seen (Voullaire et al. 2000a): It was quite poignant as this mildly retarded man, who had some insight into his own handicap, struggled to understand how best he might be a father to his 46,XX baby, and expressed sadness at the abnormal behavior displayed by his older 46,XY,dup(10) child. The capable and willing grandmother stepped into the breach; but when the daughter is older, and assuming she is of normal intelligence, how will the realization of her parents' abnormality affect her? Whether a normal child in this sort of setting has a legal claim for "dissatisfied life" is an intriguing and as yet (to our knowledge) untested notion (Pelias and Shaw 1986).

ACCESS TO PRENATAL DIAGNOSTIC SERVICES

It would not, at present, be economically feasible or sensible to make definitive prenatal diagnosis (chorionic villus sampling or amniocentesis) available to every pregnant woman. Even among those for whom testing is, in principle, freely available, a proportion will not present, either because they are opposed to abortion, or because they have not been informed about, or have not understood, the issues involved (Halliday et al. 2001). Those who can afford it and who do not meet criteria (essentially maternal age or other particular indicators of risk) for acceptance in the public system may have the privilege of access to private testing. Mass screening methodologies (Chapter 20) are to some extent bypassing the inequity inherent in the public/private dichotomy. As NIPT, using the analysis of fetal DNA from a maternal blood sample, becomes more readily available, potentially all pregnancies could be subject to chromosomal analysis; but this ready availability will, of itself, raise a question about the need for satisfactory counseling prior to undergoing such an "easy" and seemingly routine procedure as a venepuncture (Schmitz et al. 2009; de Jong et al. 2010).

Legal barriers may arise in some jurisdictions. Abortion is (in 2017) the subject of legal review in Chile, with draft legislation proposing decriminalization on the grounds of, inter alia, "an embryo or foetus suffering from a congenital structural anomaly or a genetic disorder incompatible with life outside the womb"; the Genetic Branch of the Chilean Society of Paediatrics has suggested changing the wording to "a congenital anomaly of poor prognosis," among which they would include trisomies 13 and 18 (Pardo Vargas et al. 2016). In the United States, as Miller et al. (2000) comment, "there is perhaps no more divisive subject than abortion." Bills proposed in 2017 in the legislatures of Oklahoma and Texas, specifically naming a prenatal diagnosis of Down syndrome as not being lawful grounds for abortion, are titled the Oklahoma Prenatal Discrimination Act and the Texas Disabled Preborn Justice Act, respectively; other such bills have been proposed in other states. Donley (2013) contends that such bans would in fact be unconstitutional, and the interested reader possessed of a legal-oriented mindset is referred to her detailed and finely argued essay.

If prenatal testing is not made available, or if an abnormal result is reported but has not been passed on to the parents, the option of pregnancy termination is denied. Here, the legal concept of the "right not to be born" may be invoked (Weber 2001). The issue is controversial.[9] French courts made landmark decisions in 2000 and 2001 in which substantial financial compensation was granted to parents of children with Down syndrome. Whatever the legalities, the lesson for the counselor is that testing should be offered to those for whom it may be appropriate, and that they should be diligent and careful in ensuring that prenatal testing results are safely conveyed to the right person.

PARTICIPATION IN RESEARCH

There is much yet to learn about clinical cytogenetics, and much of this cannot be done without patient participation (a rather obvious statement, and one that applies to medicine generally). It is, of course, well enshrined that patients who are potential recruitees should be fully informed upon the implications for themselves of a study in which they might be invited to participate, and that they have the opportunity to decline, without compromise of their own health care. Having made that point, one can see a reciprocity in providing a health care service: The patient who benefits (often at the expense of the state) could be seen as having a moral duty at least to consider an invitation to be involved in a bona fide research study. And having made that point, the reality is that, rather often, patients are very willing to come forward, and they gain some satisfaction in feeling that they may be making a contribution toward the greater good: The altruism gene shines brightly in many people.

It was thus disappointing to have read in Giardino et al. (2009) (and see p. 498) that a large study on de novo rearrangements detected at prenatal diagnosis could not be properly completed, in which data on a little over a quarter-million pregnancies were accumulated, from several Italian cities, and a good number (246) of de novo rearrangements identified. Here was an opportunity to build on the remarkable work of Warburton (1991). But, as these authors write, "Unfortunately, our limited information regarding the frequency and type of clinical features associated with the prenatal detection of apparently balanced rearrangements did not allow us to improve prenatal genetic counseling by updating the risk provided so far by Warburton." One perfectly valid reason may have been the logistics: "The diagnostic laboratories, the services providing genetic counseling and follow-up and the hospitals where the births take place are not integrated, but often topographically [geographically] distant." Organizing multicenter research, and undertaking fieldwork to gather data, is certainly challenging. However, it

---

9 A claim for "wrongful life" concerning cri du chat syndrome was brought on behalf of the child in a legal case in Australia, whose birth followed a failed vasectomy (Watson 2002). The claim failed, the judge finding it impossible to compare, and to place values on, impaired existence versus non-existence.

appeared that privacy concerns trumped any other issue: "Furthermore, request of further information in the absence of a specific consensus is forbidden by the actual [present] privacy law."

And it did not escape notice that, in the same issue of *Prenatal Diagnosis* in which this paper appeared, another paper (Ramsay et al. 2009) examined the attitudes toward research participation of parents whose child had had an abnormality shown at prenatal ultrasound. To quote these authors:

> The balance falls between the possibility of causing upset to parents, particularly those with handicapped or ill children, and the possibility of gaining new knowledge that may prove important to parents deciding whether or not to continue their pregnancy after diagnosis of a fetal abnormality.

Their study in fact demonstrated that

> the great majority of respondents indicated they would be happy to be contacted to provide information on their children's health and development. . . . Research ethics committees can be reassured that the risk of causing inappropriate and unnecessary parental distress by inviting them to take part in such studies is low.

2

CHROMOSOME ANALYSIS

FOR THE FIRST HALF-CENTURY of clinical cytogenetics, analysis of chromosomes was an exercise in microscopy. This century, molecular methodologies are holding sway. But it behoves the counselor to have a good understanding of how things used to be, not least because one often needs to make reference to the historical literature. And it is, of course, an obligation to keep abreast of new developments. Modern cytogenomic (this word now entering the lexicon) reports are sophisticated documents, and those who read them, and who interpret them to patients and families, need to be well informed.

CLASSICAL CYTOGENETIC ANALYSIS

On classical methodology, chromosomes are analyzed under the light microscope, at a magnification of about 1000×. The chromosomes are stained to be visible, and a great many staining techniques were used to demonstrate different features of the chromosome. We list some of these, in particular those

with a more immediate practical application to the clinical issues we discuss in this book, or which are of historical value when referring to the older literature.

1. *Plain staining* ("solid staining"). Many histologic dyes, including Giemsa, orcein, and Leishman, stained chromosomes uniformly. Until the early 1970s, these were the only stains available.

2. *Giemsa or G-banding.* This procedure required a trypsin (protein digestion) step, and is the main staining method in use in routine classical cytogenetics. It allows for precise identification of every chromosome and for the detection and delineation of structural abnormalities. At the 400–550 band level, rearrangements down to about 5 megabases in length can be discerned, at least in regions where the banding pattern is distinctive. Its precision is increased by manipulations designed to arrest the chromosome in its more elongated state at early metaphase or prometaphase—high-resolution banding. Alternative methods to demonstrate

essentially the same morphology are quinacrine or Q-banding, and reverse or R-banding. In R-banded chromosomes, the pale staining regions seen in G-banding stain darkly, and vice versa.

3. *Constitutive or C-banding.* This technique stains constitutive heterochromatin—mainly the centromeric heterochromatin, some of the material on the short arms of the acrocentric chromosomes, and the distal part of the long arm of the Y chromosome. Constitutive heterochromatin, by definition, has no direct phenotypic effect and, in general, is devoid of active genes.

4. *Replication banding.* This technique is used primarily to identify inactive X chromatin. A nucleotide analog (BrdU) is added either as a pulse at the beginning, or toward the end of the cell cycle, to allow the cytogenetic distinction of chromatin that replicates early, from that which replicates late. It produces a banding pattern similar to that of R-banding.

5. *NOR (silver) staining.* This stain, of largely historic interest now, identified nucleolar organizing regions (NOR), which contain multiple copies of genes coding for rRNA, and which are sited on the satellite stalks of the acrocentric chromosomes.

6. *Distamycin A/DAPI staining.* This fluorescent stain identifies the heterochromatin of chromosomes 1, 9, 15, 16, and Y. A particular use was to distinguish the inverted duplication 15 chromosome from other small marker chromosomes.

7. *Fluorescence in situ hybridization* (FISH) and variations thereupon. The major cytogenetic advance of the 1990s was the ability to identify specific chromosomes, and parts of chromosomes, by in situ hybridization with labeled probes. FISH has been widely used to detect submicroscopic deletions and to characterize more obvious chromosome anomalies. The hybridization method may be direct or indirect. Direct attachment of a detectable molecule (e.g., a fluorophore) to the probe DNA enables its microscopic visualization immediately after its hybridization to the target DNA in the chromosome. The more sensitive indirect procedure requires special modification of the probe with a hapten detectable by affinity cytochemistry. The most popular systems are the biotin–avidin and digoxigenin systems. By using combinations of biotin-, digoxigenin-, and fluorophore-labeled probes, multiple simultaneous hybridizations can be done to locate different chromosomal regions in one preparation (multicolor FISH).

A more focused use of FISH is in the assessment of the structural nature of imbalances revealed by microarray analysis (see below), with the probe from the genomic region targeted to the specific region identified by the array.

8. *Comparative genomic hybridization* (CGH). In CGH, differentially labeled, fluorophore-tagged DNA from the patient and a normal control (reference sample) is applied to a metaphase slide prepared from a "standard" normal person. Relative excesses and deficiencies of patient DNA bind competitively, with respect to the control, onto the reference chromosomes, and yield different color intensities on exciting the fluorophores. This procedure has been applied to archival pathology material. "High-resolution" CGH refers not to a more stretched chromosome preparation, but to a further level of sophistication of the computer software that is used to analyze the images, by adjusting for the idiosyncratic patterns that each homolog may have. Small imbalances may be identifiable by this approach, ~10 Mb or greater, and the nature of uncertain rearrangements clarified (Knight and Flint 2000; Kirchhoff et al. 2001; Ness et al. 2002).

Chromosomes examined by various techniques are illustrated in Figure 2–1. Full detail is to be found in Gersen and Keagle (2013), Mark (2000), and Miller and Therman (2001), while Trask (2002) provides an historical span of the cytogeneticist's skill.

MICROARRAY ANALYSIS

Since the 2010s, microarray has become the first-tier clinical diagnostic test for individuals with developmental disabilities or congenital anomalies (Manning and Hudgins 2010; Miller et al. 2010). There are basically two microarray techniques in use: The first uses a CGH approach, much like that described above for chromosomal CGH; and the second uses single nucleotide polymorphisms (SNP) to assess the number of alleles in a sample. Although microarrays can differ in their genomic composition and substrates used for the analysis, most microarrays comprise thousands of spots of reference DNA sequences, applied in a precisely gridded manner upon a slide (or "chip") in which the locations can be known by computer analysis. Some commercial microarrays combine CGH and SNP detection on the same array.

Not that classical cytogenetics is likely to fade altogether from view: There are two

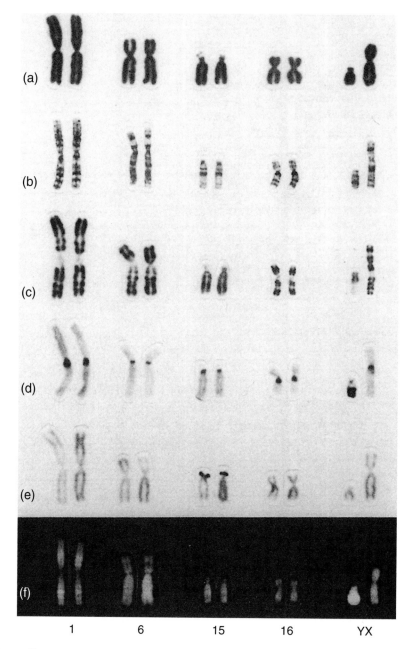

FIGURE 2–1   Chromosome pairs 1, 6, 15, 16, and Y and X stained by various techniques: plain stain (*a*), G-banding (*b*), replication banding (*c*), C-banding (*d*), Ag-NOR stain (*e*), and Q-banding (*f*).

crucial reasons for its continuing use in the laboratory. First, not all array results can give a definitive construction, and FISH is sometimes necessary to elucidate the cytogenetics. Second, the array cannot detect balanced rearrangements,[1] and recognition of the carrier state will continue to need an old-fashioned chromosome test. And third, a rather subjective "reason" is that, by continuing to work with chromosomes, the

1 Albeit that whole genome sequencing is being used to address this shortcoming (Ordulu et al. 2016; Redin et al. 2017).

molecular cytogeneticist/cytogenomicist will not lose the intuitive understanding of what chromosomes are really like, and not see them merely as theoretical constructs or computer-screen displays. As mentioned above, the reporting of microarray results is a sophisticated exercise, and counselors need to be sophisticated readers of these reports. Many laboratories now use depictions from one of the genome browsers—with a classic chromosome ideogram on its side at the top—to illustrate the precise extent of the imbalance, and noting the genes contained within this segment.

Comparative Genomic Hybridization

The fundamental principle is essentially the same as in chromosomal CGH, noted above, but using the array, rather than the metaphase spread, as substrate. Patient and control DNA are labeled in two different fluors, usually one that appears red and one that appears green. These labeled DNAs are applied to the microarray, and hybridization takes place. Typically, if the number of copies between the control and the patient are the same, the spot looks yellow (produced from an overlapping of equal amounts of red and green).[2] The fluorescent intensities of each dye are measured. If the patient has an excess at a locus (due to duplication or aneuploidy), the hybridization will more reflect the dye of the patient's DNA. If the patient has a deficiency at a locus (loss due to deletion or unbalanced translocation), the hybridization will more reflect the dye of the control DNA. These fluorescent intensities are presented as a log ratio of each of the dyes, and plotted as shown in Figure 2–2. Microarrays for CGH are typically constructed from bacterial artificial chromosomes (BACs) or oligonucleotides. Each spot represents a unique BAC or oligonucleotide. An array with 3,000 BAC spots could detect unbalanced rearrangements at a 1 Mb resolution across the entire genome (Snijders et al. 2001). The power of array-CGH over classical cytogenetics is illustrated in a study from Finland, in which approximately 20% of 150 patients with mental retardation, and whose G-banded karyotypes had previously been assessed as normal, showed a presumed pathogenic imbalance on microarray (Siggberg et al. 2010).

Single Nucleotide Polymorphism (SNP)

As with the microarrays described above, SNP arrays can be used to detect the number of alleles in a specimen. SNP arrays provide two types of information. First, the intensity of the signal arising from each SNP can be measured to produce a log ratio, similar to that produced from CGH analysis: A relative increase in signal intensity corresponds to copy number gain, and a decrease in signal intensity corresponds to deletion. Second, SNP arrays produce genotyping information: Heterozygosity, with two distinct alleles, can be distinguished from homozygosity, and from the presence of three alleles. Apparent homozygosity may indicate a loss of DNA, such as a deletion, while three alleles may indicate a gain of DNA copy number, such as a duplication or trisomy. SNP-based microarrays have the added advantage of detecting uniparental disomy when the child's results are compared to the parental genotypes. Isodisomy may be revealed, in the absence of parental samples, when the entire chromosome shows homozygosity, and chromosomal monosomy is an incompatible interpretation. The fuller information forthcoming from the SNP-array is reflected in its alternative name, 'karyomapping'.

Balanced rearranged chromosomes, as noted above, cannot be detected using any of the current routine microarray-based technologies. A (non-routine) exception is the technique of array painting. This technology combines the use of flow-sorted chromosomes to separate the two derivatives of a balanced translocation, amplifies the DNA, and applies each amplified derivative to a microarray, in order to determine the breakpoint locations and size of the segments involved (Gribble et al. 2004).

POLYMERASE CHAIN REACTION-BASED APPLICATIONS

A number of technologies are available to assess DNA copy number. These are targeted approaches to answer a specific question: How many copies of the target are present in the patient? These techniques include quantitative fluorescent polymerase

---

2 The cover art pays due homage.

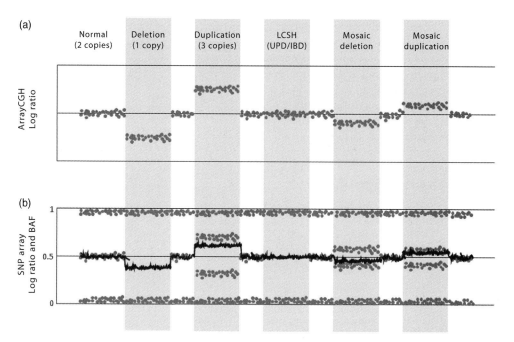

FIGURE 2–2   Interpretation of array comparative genomic hybridization (ArrayCGH) compared with SNP array. (*a*) In ArrayCGH, the signal between the test and reference sample is converted to a log ratio (gray dots) which acts as a proxy for copy number. An increase in log ratio represents a gain in copy number. (*b*) SNP arrays generate log ratio (black line) by comparing the signal intensities between different SNPs analyzed and offer an additional metric, the *B allele frequency* (BAF) (gray dots). The BAF is the component of the total allele signal (A + B) explained by a single allele (A): A BAF of 0 represents the genotype A/A or A/–, a BAF of 0.5 represents the genotype A/B, and a BAF of 1 represents the genotype B/B or B/–. Deletions result in the loss of heterozygous (A/B) genotypes, whereas duplications result in a separation of heterozygous genotypes into AA/B and A/BB. The BAF also allows for the detection of copy number neutral abnormalities such as uniparental disomy and identity by descent (IBD) which appear as absence of heterozygous (A/B) genotypes without change to the log ratio.

Source: From Alkan et al., Genome structural variation discovery and genotyping, *Nat Rev Genet* 12: 363–376, 2011. Courtesy E. E. Eichler, and with the permission of Nature Publishing Group.

chain reaction (QF-PCR) and multiplex ligation-dependent probe amplification (MLPA). QF-PCR and MLPA use specific primers to amplify segments of DNA to determine copy number and identify deletions or aneuploidy.

NEXT-GENERATION SEQUENCING

DNA methodologies based on massively parallel genomic sequencing ("next-generation sequencing," NGS) have enabled remarkable advances in mutation analysis, with the entire expressed genetic complement, the "exome," and even the whole genome, tractable to interrogation. In the cytogenetic field, NGS is now routinely applied as a highly accurate molecular counting tool, sequencing cell-free DNA circulating in the maternal plasma, and mapping each sequence read back to

its chromosome of origin. At the time of writing, chromosome microarray remains the gold standard methodology for molecular karyotyping, but NGS is a very promising up-and-coming alternative. Low-coverage genome sequencing can detect, with 100% sensitivity, copy number variants diagnosed by microarray, and the technology offers the additional benefit of detecting balanced chromosome rearrangements (Dong et al. 2014, 2016). Given that genome sequencing at higher levels of coverage offers considerable diagnostic yield for the diagnosis of sequence-level mutations, it is expected that, in time, a single NGS-based test will generate both copy-number and sequence data, and will become the first-line test for the investigation of children with developmental disabilities. NGS is also showing promise in the diagnosis of aneuploidy in preimplantation embryos (Wells et al. 2014).

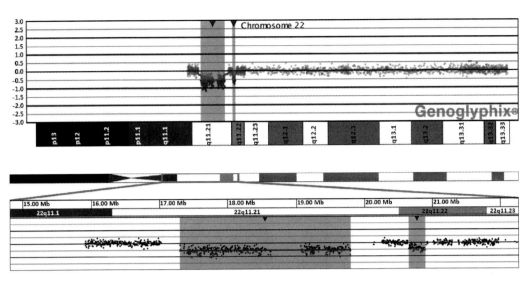

FIGURE 2–3   Plot of chromosome 22 in a patient with a 22q11 deletion performed using an oligonucleotide-based array with comparative genomic hybridization. The deletion is indicated by the shaded area, which reflects a deviation from the $\log_2$ ratio of 1 (equal to zero). Distal to the classic DiGeorge deletion is a common copy number variant (CNV).

CYTOGENETIC (OR CYTOGENOMIC) REPORTS

Chromosomal findings from molecular analyses are often presented in an intuitive pictorial form, such as, for example, the display in Figure 2–3. Although cytogenetics will continue to evolve, whatever techniques come to be used, the fundamental purpose of the cytogenetic report will of course remain the same. Descriptions about the technologies used will be important addenda to reports, because they may inform the clinician about the interpretation of the chromosome analysis and the need for further possible analysis. Reports may also include a listing of presumed significant genes in the region, a comment upon imprinting, and the likelihood of benign versus causative genomic changes. A pedantic but important point is that the genome "build" be noted.

GENETIC COUNSELING CONSIDERATIONS

In the majority of cases, the abnormalities found by molecular technologies have clear clinical relevance for the patient and the family. However, higher resolution strategies may uncover DNA changes of unclear clinical significance (as we discuss at length in Chapter 17). Such findings may lead to testing of additional family members, parents, grandparents, and sometimes siblings, to understand the relationship, if any, between the DNA alteration and the clinical phenotype or medical condition of the patient. The possibility of findings of unclear clinical significance should be discussed when ordering the test, especially in the prenatal setting. Because these molecular-based tests have the ability to interrogate the entire genome, the pretest genetic counseling should include information about uncovering unwanted information, such as loci that could predispose to cancer or to adult-onset disorders. The use of SNP arrays may uncover substantial stretches of homozygosity due to consanguineous or even incestuous relationships (Schaaf et al. 2011). These counseling caveats notwithstanding, the higher resolution potential of these new technologies will increase the detection rate of chromosome abnormalities, and will much improve our ability to make diagnoses and to provide the answers that families seek.

3

THE ORIGINS AND CONSEQUENCES OF CHROMOSOME PATHOLOGY

"WHAT WENT WRONG? And will it happen again?" These are the common questions from "chromosomal families" that bring people to the genetic clinic. We can recast these questions: "Did I, or one of us, produce an abnormal gamete? If so, why? What gamete might be produced next time? Or, if the chromosomes were normal at conception, what went wrong thereafter?" To deal intelligently with these questions, the counselor needs a broad knowledge of how gametes form, how chromosomes behave, and how the early conceptus grows.

The *classic chromosome disorders* are the full aneuploidies and the partial aneuploidies. These partial aneuploidies were of sufficient size (albeit some have been called "microdeletions"[1]) that they were detectable on microscope cytogenetics;

the phenotypes were practically always abnormal. On molecular karyotyping, the challenge arises of dealing with very small imbalances (*microdeletions, microduplications, copy number variants*), which may not always lead to clinical abnormality. The concepts of incomplete penetrance and polygenic (or at least oligogenic) inheritance have become of practical relevance in this context. Finally, *errors of imprinting* contribute a small fraction to the whole.

The broadening scope of medical cytogenetics—some now say medical cytogenomics—following upon advances in molecular methodologies has led to the distinction between chromosomal and other genetic causes of disease, formerly so clear-cut,

---

1 For the most part, we confine our use of the expressions "microdeletion" and "microduplication" to those pathogenic imbalances detectable only on molecular karyotyping, and to which the expression pathogenic copy number variant is also often applied. The word "microdeletion" had been applied to some conditions of the classical cytogenetic era, such as Prader-Willi syndrome and Smith-Magenis syndrome; these certainly were, by the standards of the day (the 1980s), very small deletions, and only just visible to very experienced microscopists. However, by molecular criteria, they would now be seen as rather large, of megabases size; whereas several of the pathogenic microdeletions and microduplications of molecular karyotyping are measured in kilobases.

now somewhat blurring at the margins. One practical definition of a chromosomal disorder might have been based on the methodology used for diagnosis—that is, any condition typically diagnosed by classical cytogenetics or by microarray. But with next-generation sequencing (NGS), that distinction would fail: NGS can be widely applied, diagnostically, to the generality of genetic disease. "Genomic imbalance" may be a more suitable, and more fundamental, definition: too much, or too little, chromosome material. Even so, the line cannot be drawn with absolute clarity between chromosomal and Mendelian disease: A Mendelian condition may be due to a complete duplication (e.g., Charcot-Marie-Tooth neuropathy, p. 327) or to a partial deletion (e.g., Pitt-Hopkins syndrome, p. 304), and thus diagnosable on cytogenomic technology. The analysis of copy number variants (CNVs)—short segments of genomic material in excess or deficiency—is generally regarded as a chromosomal exercise; Lupski (2009) and Carvalho et al. (2010) see these conditions in the category "genomic disorders." We will largely confine ourselves (Chapter 17) to those which are known to be pathogenic; but there is also blurring, here, in terms of CNVs whose harmlessness, or not, is uncertain.

We focus first upon the classic chromosomal disorders. Most of these arise at meiosis. A gamete from a 46,N person may acquire an extra (but normal) chromosome, and this would lead to a full aneuploidy in the conceptus: a trisomy or a monosomy. Or, partial aneuploidy may be due to meiotic malsegregation having taken place in gametogenesis of a 46,rea parent carrying a balanced rearrangement. De novo (that is, with normal parental karyotypes) partial aneuploidies may have been generated at a meiotic division, or at a premeiotic germ cell mitosis; where there is mosaicism, a postmeiotic event in the embryo may be implicated. Many of the microdeletions and microduplications detectable at molecular karyotyping are quite often carried

by a parent, although a number are de novo. While it may not be possible to presume with reasonable confidence where the original error lay, a theoretical consideration of the point at which a chromosomal defect arose—before, during, or after meiosis—can underpin a useful understanding. It thus behooves us to appreciate the broad processes of meiotic and mitotic cell divisions.

MEIOSIS

Meiosis in Chromosomally Normal Persons

The purpose of meiosis is to achieve the reduction from the diploid state of the primary gametocyte ($2n = 46$) to the haploid complement of the normal gamete ($n = 23$), and to ensure genetic variation in the gametes. The latter requirement is met by enabling the independent assortment of homologs (the physical basis of Mendel's second law),[2] and by providing a setting for recombination between homologs. While we do not dwell on recombination per se, this is, to the classical geneticist, a raison d'être of the chromosome: "From the long perspective of evolution, a chromosome is a bird of passage, a temporary association of particular alleles" (Lewin 1994).

The mature gamete is produced after the two meiotic cell divisions: meiosis I and meiosis II. In meiosis I, the primary gametocyte (oöcyte[3] or spermatocyte, also referred to as primordial germ cells) gives rise to two secondary gametocytes, each with 23 chromosomes.

As per the *classical description* (Figure 3–1), these chromosomes have not divided at the centromere, and they remain in the double-chromatid state. In meiosis II, the chromosomes of the secondary gametocyte separate into their component chromatids. In the male, the daughter cells produced are the four spermatids, which mature into spermatozoa. In the female, the daughter cells are the mature ovum and its polar bodies. (In fact, it is not until sperm penetration that meiosis II in the ovum is completed.) Each gamete contains a haploid set of chromosomes. The diploid complement is restored at conception with the union of two

---

2 The law of independent assortment: During gamete formation, the segregation of the alleles of one allelic pair is independent of the segregation of the alleles of another allelic pair. The exception: If two loci are close together—"linked"—on the same chromosome.

3 The reader will note the use of the umlaut, ö, in this spelling, here and throughout the book. This will serve as a reminder of the correct pronunciation, oh-oh-cyte (not oo-cyte).

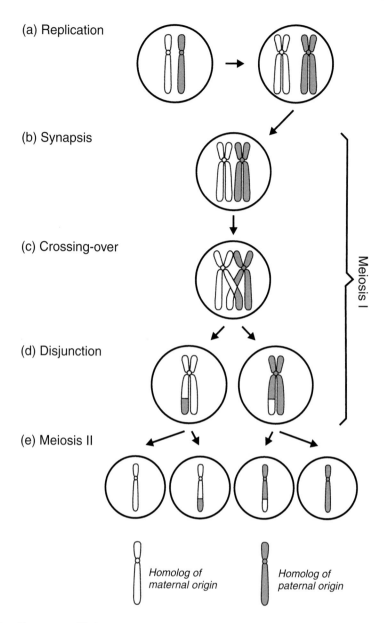

(a) Replication

(b) Synapsis

(c) Crossing-over

Meiosis I

(d) Disjunction

(e) Meiosis II

*Homolog of
maternal origin*

*Homolog of
paternal origin*

FIGURE 3–1   Chromosomal behavior during meiosis I, according to the classical model. Circles represent germ cells: at (*a*) oögonia and spermatogonia (gonocytes); at (*b–d*) primary oöcytes and spermatocytes (gametocytes); and at (*e*) secondary oöcytes and spermatocytes. One crossover has occurred between the long arms of one chromatid of each homolog. Following meiosis I, the chromosome number has halved (reduction division). In oögenesis, one of the two cells at (*d*) would be the first polar body, and would not enter meiosis II.

haploid gametes. The moment of conception, as the embryologist sees it, is not at sperm penetration, but only when the two pronuclei have fused to form a single nucleus ("syngamy").

Note that spermatogenesis divides the cytoplasm evenly, so that after meiosis II there are four gametes of equal size. The sperm head that penetrates the ovum comprises almost entirely nuclear material; the tail is cast off. In oöcytes, cytoplasmic division is markedly uneven, producing a secondary oöcyte and first polar body after meiosis I, and the mature ovum and second polar body at meiosis II. The ovum and its second polar body each has a haploid chromosome set, but the ovum retains almost all of

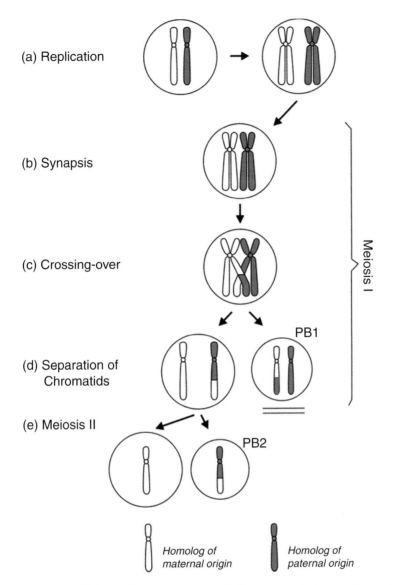

(a) Replication

(b) Synapsis

(c) Crossing-over

(d) Separation of Chromatids

PB1

(e) Meiosis II

PB2

Meiosis I

Homolog of maternal origin

Homolog of paternal origin

FIGURE 3–2   Chromosomal behavior during meiosis, specifically ovarian meiosis, according to the model of "reverse segregation." Circles represent germ cells: at (*a*) oögonia; at (*b–d*) primary oöcyte; at (*d*) first polar body (PB1); and at (*e*) secondary oöcyte and the second polar body (PB2). One crossover has occurred between the long arms of one chromatid of each homolog. The single-chromatid chromosomes separate at (*d*); this is the step that defines "reverse segregation." Meiosis II follows at (*e*). Note that the pairs of cells after meiosis II (ovum + second polar body) have homologs of *opposite* parental origin (*non*-sister chromatids). In the classical model (Fig. 3–1), the homologs in these pairs would always be of the same parental origin (sister chromatids). It was this distinction which, along with other evidence, pointed Ottolini et al. (2015) toward proposing this new model.

the cytoplasm.[4] (The chromosomes of the first polar body typically do not undergo a second meiotic division.) Another major sex difference concerns the timing of gamete maturation. In the female, meiosis is partway through, in the late prophase of meiosis I, by the eighth month of intrauterine life

---

4 Cytoplasm contains the mitochondria, and transmission of mitochondrial DNA is maternal. The mitochondrial genome has been described, somewhat whimsically, as chromosome 25, or the M chromosome. In not otherwise referring to this "chromosome," we are not seeking to deny its importance or interest!

(the actual process of recombination taking place during weeks 16–19 of fetal life). At birth, on average there are somewhat over half a million oöcytes (Bukovsky et al. 2004). Most of this pool gradually disappears, but those eggs destined to mature stay in a "frame-freeze" until they enter ovulation, some one to five decades thereafter,[5] and meiosis recommences. Testicular stem cells, on the other hand, do not begin to enter meiosis until the onset of puberty. Thereafter, millions of mature sperm are continuously produced.

We now examine more closely the details of meiosis, according to the classical model. During the final mitotic division in the primary gametocyte, the homologous pairs of chromosomes have (as with any mitosis) replicated their DNA to change from the single-chromatid to the double-chromatid stage. They now enter into the meiotic cell cycle (Figure 3–1a). As meiosis I proceeds to prophase, chromosomes conduct a "homology search" and come together and pair, with matching loci alongside each other (Figure 3–1b). This process—synapsis—continues with a more intimate pairing of the homologs, starting at the tips of the chromosomes and proceeding centrally (Barlow and Hultén 1996), and the synaptonemal complex is formed. The paired chromosomes themselves are called bivalents.[6] Synapsis sets the stage for an exchange of matching chromosome segments; this is the process of recombination, or crossing-over (Figure 3–1c). Next, desynapsis occurs (the diplotene stage), with dissociation of the synaptonemal complex and the formation of chiasmata. Now, the two homologous chromosomes disjoin and go to opposite poles of the cell. This is the anaphase stage; the orderly movement of chromosomes during this sequence is facilitated if synapsis, recombination, and chiasmata formation have proceeded normally. Finally, the cell divides into the two daughter cells (Figure 3–1d). How the chromosomes are distributed—which chromosome goes to which pole—is called segregation. Normally, each daughter cell gets one of each of the pair of chromosomes, and this is referred to as one-to-one (1:1) segregation. Uniquely in the meiosis I cell division (as classically described), daughter cells are produced with double-chromatid chromosomes.

These cells then enter meiosis II (with the exception of the first polar body, as noted above). In this cycle, the chromosomes do not replicate because they are already in the double-chromatid state. The chromosomes separate at the centromere, and the resulting single-chromatid chromosomes disjoin, one going to each pole, resembling a mitotic division (Figure 3–1e).

The foregoing, classical construction has held sway since practically the beginning of cytogenetics. The *alternative description* puts the events of meiosis I and II in the reverse order: That is, the chromosomes separate into chromatids at meiosis I and then segregate into daughter cells at meiosis II (Figure 3–2). This has been called "reverse segregation" (Ottolini et al. 2015; Webster and Schuh 2017). Certain chromosomes are more prone to take this course: chromosomes 4, 9, 11, 13, 14, 15, 16, 19, 21, and 22.

Chromosomal pathology arises when these processes of disjunction and segregation go wrong—*mal*segregation and *non*disjunction.

Malsegregation and Nondisjunction in Meiosis

Malsegregation (or missegregation) is remarkably frequent at meiosis, and in consequence many human conceptions are trisomic or monosomic. Malsegregation is a "catch-all" term; in principle, nondisjunction specifically refers to the failure of homologous chromosomes to segregate symmetrically at cell division, although in practice it is often considered (and we sometimes do) as "the inclusion of both daughter chromosomes in the same nucleus, by whatever mechanism" (Miller and Therman 2001). The process of malsegregation is described according to two models: the classical description of nondisjunction, and a modern description. Albeit that the classical model has long been seen as the typical process, in fact, as Gabriel et al. (2011) write, "it appears to be a relatively minor player" and "the received wisdom that non-disjunction [sensu stricto] is the primary mechanism leading to human aneuploidy should be reconsidered." Nevertheless, and taking a conservative

---

5 As Eichenlaub-Ritter (2012) points out, oöcytes are one of the longest-lived cells in the body.

6 Since, at the level of the chromatid, the bivalent pair contains four elements, the word tetrad can also be used in this setting; in this sense, the cell at this stage of the cycle has $23 \times 4 = 92$ chromatids. At the molecular level, the number of single DNA strands is eight.

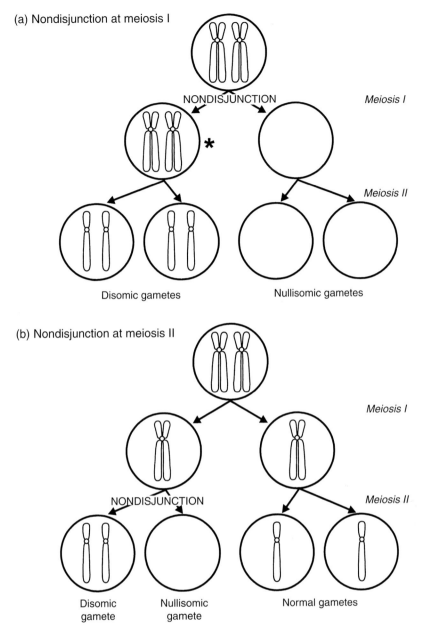

(a) Nondisjunction at meiosis I

NONDISJUNCTION

Meiosis I

Meiosis II

Disomic gametes   Nullisomic gametes

(b) Nondisjunction at meiosis II

Meiosis I

NONDISJUNCTION   *Meiosis II*

Disomic   Nullisomic   Normal gametes
gamete   gamete

FIGURE 3–3   The classical view of the mechanics of nondisjunction. The asterisked gamete reflects the complement of the oöcyte in Fig. 3–4 (*upper*). In öogenesis, one of the two cells following meiosis I would be the first polar body, which might or might not proceed to meiosis II.

viewpoint,[7] we first set out in detail the model that has appeared in textbooks for generations; but then pay due attention to the new knowledge.

The *classical description* of the mechanism of meiotic nondisjunction is as follows. In a chromosomally normal person, if the pair of homologs comprising a bivalent at meiosis I fail to separate (fail to disjoin[8]), one daughter cell will have two of the chromosomes and the other will have none. This is 2:0 segregation (Figures 3–3a and 3–4, upper). In other words, one

7   "Be not the first by whom the new are tried, Nor yet the last to lay the old aside." Alexander Pope, *An Essay on Criticism*, 1711.

8   Note that disjunction is a normal process, and nondisjunction is not; there is no such word as dysjunction.

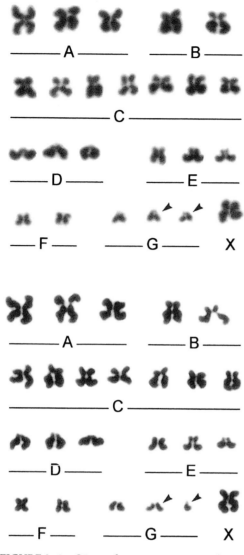

FIGURE 3–4　Oöcyte chromosomes at metaphase of meiosis II, showing nondisjunction of a G-group chromosome having occurred at the preceding first meiotic division. *Upper*, oöcyte with classical nondisjunctional disomy, showing an additional G-group double-chromatid chromosome. Possibly the arrowed pair are chromosome 21s, and the karyotype 24,X,+21. *Lower*, oöcyte with "predivisional" disomy, showing an additional G-group single chromatid. The arrowed pair may be chromosome 21s, and the karyotype 24,X,+21cht.

Source: From Kamiguchi et al. 1993, courtesy Y. Kamiguchi.

gametocyte is disomic for that homolog, and the other is nullisomic. Nondisjunction may occur in meiosis II, meiosis I having proceeded normally. In meiosis II, it is the chromatids that fail to separate (Figure 3–3b). Following these nondisjunctional errors, the conceptus, at fertilization, ends up trisomic or monosomic, assuming the other gamete to be normal (Figure 3–5a, b). Trisomy or monosomy in the offspring of normal parents is called primary trisomy or primary monosomy.

While the classical description is a useful model, in fact "*predivision*" of sister chromatids is the predominant mechanism in the female and is important in the male (Gabriel et al. 2011; Uroz and Templado 2012; Fragouli et al. 2013; Ottolini et al. 2015). Predivision refers to the "precocious" separation of chromatids during meiosis I, as initially proposed by Angell (1997), and involves three sequential events (Figure 3–6). First, the (double-chromatid) homologs fail to pair during meiosis I; or, if they do pair, they separate again before meiosis I is complete. In other words, instead of the two (double-chromatid) chromosomes existing as a conjoined bivalent, they exist as two separate univalents. Second, these univalents are prone to "predivide"—that is, the separation of the two chromatids that should (on the classical plan) happen at meiosis II, instead takes place while they are still in the first meiotic cycle. This could happen to both univalents or just the one, and these would then exist as single-chromatid chromosomes. Third, at anaphase of meiosis I, these double- or single-chromatid chromosomes segregate independently, to the oöcyte and polar body, or mature spermatocytes. The oöcyte in Figure 3–4 (lower) may be an example of asymmetric segregation due to this process, having received a double-chromatid and a single-chromatid chromosome.[9]

A process somewhat intermediate between these two mechanisms is "*achiasmate nondisjunction*," in which the homologs had never joined, and then segregate together to the same daughter cell. The end result is the same as if classical nondisjunction had occurred, but without any recombination (Uroz and Templado 2012).

The majority of human malsegregation takes place in *oögenesis*. Meiosis is overwhelmingly the site in older women (Rabinowitz et al. 2012),

---

9　Certain terminologies and nomenclature may be mentioned here. A gamete with an extra chromosome is *hyperhaploid*, with a karyotype written as, for example, 24,X,+21. A gamete missing a chromosome is *hypohaploid*. (e.g., 22,Y,–21). If, at meiosis I, the extra chromosome is present only as a single chromatid (e.g., the asterisked oöcyte in Figure 3–6), the abbreviation cht is used: thus, 24,X,+21cht. The ISCN (2016) provides nomenclature for meiotic cells, and an extra 21 at meiosis I, present as a univalent, would be denoted as MI,24,+I(21).

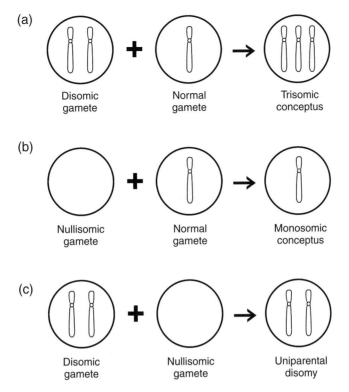

FIGURE 3–5 Aneuploid gametes producing an aneuploid conceptus (*a* and *b*), and aneuploid gametes producing uniparental disomy (*c*).

although overall, premeiotic mitotic errors contribute a fraction, with about 16% of immature oöcytes aneuploid (Daina et al. 2014). In women in their twenties, the first meiotic division is the site at which most abnormality typically arises; in women in their forties, meiosis II becomes predominant (Allen et al. 2009). Remarkably high fractions of mature oöcytes are aneuploid, at least as measured in a population of women presenting to an in vitro fertilization (IVF) clinic: In women aged 28–37 years, near a half (47%) of eggs are disomic or nullisomic, whereas in 38- to 47-year-olds, the figure rises to 78% (Fragouli et al. 2013). Certain aneuploidies show predilections for one or other meiotic stage: For example, essentially all trisomy 16 may be due to a maternal meiosis I error, whereas most trisomy 18 reflects meiotic II malsegregation.

In *spermatogenesis*, predivision and achiasmate nondisjunction are equally important malsegregant mechanisms; spermatocyte aneuploidy may be more frequent than previously considered, but the existence of a postmeiotic checkpoint may exclude most aneuploid spermatozoa from full maturation (Uroz and Templado 2012). Chromosome 21 and the X and Y are the most prone to nondisjunction in the male, whether at meiosis I or II. Only in trisomy 2 among the autosomes is there a substantial paternal contribution, with close to half reflecting a meiotic error in spermatogenesis (Hassold 1998; Robinson et al. 1999).

Given the frequency with which nondisjunction happens, it is not at all surprising that instances of *multiple aneuploidy* are known, the observed numbers during pregnancy reducing as nonviability takes its toll. In spontaneous abortions toward the end of the first trimester, double autosomal combinations, from simultaneous nondisjunctions, may be seen in the analysis of products of conception (Micale et al. 2010). As for livebirth, the reader with a sense of history will want to review the 48,XXY,+21 case described in Ford et al. (1959); a very few other cases have followed, the most common combination being trisomy 21 along with an additional sex chromosome (Li et al. 2004; Tennakoon et al. 2008). *Sequential nondisjunctions* at both meiotic divisions could lead to tetrasomy, and this is the basis of some X chromosomal polysomy (Hassold et al. 1990b; Deng et al. 1991). Complete nondisjunction is an

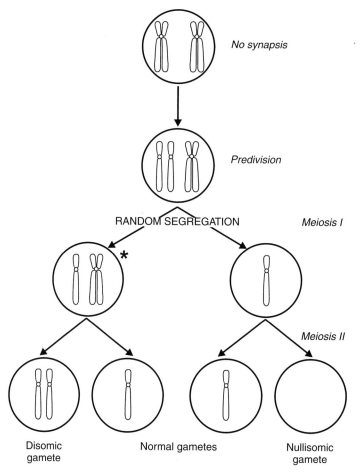

No synapsis

Predivision

RANDOM SEGREGATION

Meiosis I

Meiosis II

Disomic gamete

Normal gametes

Nullisomic gamete

FIGURE 3–6   Nondisjunction following "predivision" of one homolog into its component chromatids in meiosis I (Angell's hypothesis). The asterisked gamete reflects the complement of the oöcyte in Figure 3–3 (*lower*). In oögenesis, one of the two cells following meiosis I would be the first polar body, which might or might not proceed to meiosis II.

expression that could be applied in the case of triploidy, when this is due to the retention of the polar body within the ovum (Martin et al. 1991).

Simultaneous parental nondisjunctions, both gametes being disomic, is rare, but not unknown, and is another route to double aneuploidy, and for example Robinson et al. (2001) describe 48,+14[pat],+21[mat] in a spontaneous abortion. If one gamete is disomic and the other nullisomic, for the same chromosome, this means that one parent has contributed both members of the homologous pair, and the other none (Figure 3–5c). This is uniparental disomy due to "*gametic complementation*," an event of extreme rarity. Simultaneous errors of nondisjunction and other rearrangement would typically be quite coincidental, such as a child having

both XXY Klinefelter syndrome (maternal nondisjunction) and del(15)(q11.2q13) Prader-Willi syndrome (paternal deletion) (Nowaczyk et al. 2004).

CAUSES OF MEIOTIC NONDISJUNCTION

As discussed above, most aneuploidy due to nondisjunction arises in oögenesis. "Quality checking," which is stringently applied in the male, is poorly effective in the female, and so the maturing of an aneuploid oöcyte is not prevented; and as Hunt and Hassold (2002) comment, Nature seems to have erred in putting less protective investment into the more scarce gamete. A particular vulnerability of maternal meiosis likely lies in the degradation, over time, of factors that underpin the adhesion of the homologous chromatids of the bivalent. This failure of snug apposition leads the chromosomes to adopt unstable positions when meiosis resumes; or, homologs may become separate from each other, and this then sets the scene for predivision, or for achiasmate nondisjunction (Duncan et al. 2012; Eichenlaub-Ritter 2012). This cohesion, or its lack, is the explanation most often raised (Toth and Jessberger 2016). Other possibilities include a role for the spindle apparatus, a component of the cellular machinery which draws chromosomes to their positions in dividing cells, and its compromised function could cause aneuploidy (Howe and FitzHarris 2013). One proposed rare Mendelian basis is the *SYCP3* gene, coding for one of the synaptonemal complex proteins, mutation in which affects meiosis both in the female, to produce aneuploid oöcytes, and in the male, to cause spermatogenic arrest (Bolor et al. 2009).

While these meiosis-control factors may be the proximate cause of failed disjunction, what background attributes might lead to a loss in its integrity? Of course, older childbearing age is an obvious answer (Harton et al. 2013). A very telling insight comes from the work of Battaglia et al. (1996). These investigators sampled oöcytes at meiosis II metaphase from younger (20–25 years) and older (40–45 years) volunteers who were having normal menstrual cycles. They did not look at individual chromosomes but, rather, at the disposition of the spindle and the metaphase chromosomes as a whole. They made the most striking findings according to the ages of the women: A symmetrical and neatly arrayed complex was seen in the younger women, while in the older women the spindle was askew and the chromosomes a-jumble, as shown in Figure 3–7 (and see separate color insert). It is not difficult to accept that this structural disorganization would undermine the capacity of the chromosomes of the oöcyte then to undergo regular segregation.

Not that the young are immune. Fragouli et al. (2006a), in a paper dedicated to the memory of the 18-year-old patient whom they had studied, analyzed oöcytes harvested ahead of her chemotherapy for a marrow malignancy which, had she lived, might have enabled fertility. Of 11 oöcytes and 7 first polar bodies able to be analyzed, one egg had a single chromatid X and could have gone on to a monosomy X conception, while another egg was inferred (via its polar body) to have an additional X and 21 chromatid, and the conception could have been 48,XXX,+21. The introductory sentence of this paper is worth quoting: "Humans as a species are not as fertile as other mammals"; and, as already noted, it is in meiosis of the oöcyte that much of this (relative) weakness resides.

A search for factors that might explain the maternal age effect has been somewhat unforthcoming. An age-related accumulation of mitochondrial DNA mutations is plausibly suggested, but well short of being confirmed (Nikolaou and Templeton 2004). Variation in dietary folate input and in its metabolism has been proposed as linked to meiosis II nondisjunction, but the evidence is scant (Hollis et al. 2013). Meiosis II nondisjunction has also been put forward as associated with low socioeconomic status; but if so, the link, such as potentially poor diet or an unfavorable environment, would remain to be clarified (Hunter et al. 2013). Nevertheless, it is to be noted that meiosis II is the most age-susceptible cell division, and so these possibilities can be seen as not implausible. The several proposed factors, and the sites and times at which they may be operative, are reviewed in Eichenlaub-Ritter (2012).

An alternative to the foregoing meiosis-focused scenarios is to suppose that, at least in some cases, the error in the gamete had arisen at a premeiotic stage, and that the parent is actually a gonadal mosaic for the aneuploidy. Given the theoretical biology of gonadal embryology, and supposing that mitotic errors as gametocytes multiply might be not infrequent, this is a quite plausible supposition (see also below, Gonadal Mosaicism). This intriguing concept, with respect to oögenesis, and specifically concerning the likelihood that some Down syndrome may be due to maternal trisomy 21 gonadal mosaicism, is addressed in Kovaleva (2010), Delhanty (2011), and Hultén et al. (2013).

Meiosis in Chromosomally Abnormal Persons

The classic major category is the phenotypically normal person heterozygous for a balanced structural rearrangement (translocation, inversion, and insertion being the main forms), and meiosis can present considerable complication. A class of increasing importance is the individual who may carry a molecular-defined microdeletion or microduplication, and whose own phenotype may be normal or only mildly or subtly abnormal. Meiosis here is straightforward (albeit that the interpretation of risk is often not, as we discuss below). Rarely, we see persons who are themselves chromosomally

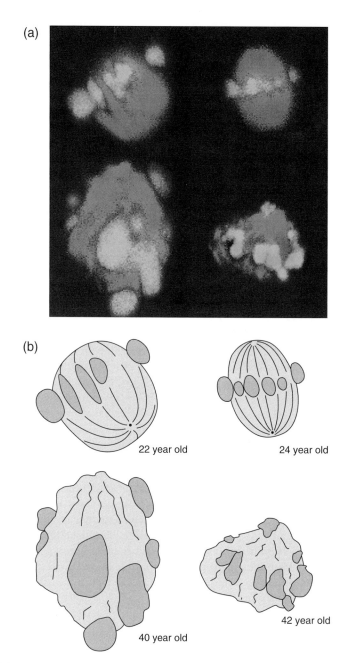

FIGURE 3–7   (*a*) Meiosis II oöcytes from younger and older women, illustrating what may be the physical basis of the maternal age effect. The microtubules of the spindle stain green, and the chromosomes stain orange. (*b*) The tracing identifies these components, and the smooth or wavy lines suggest, respectively, an intact or a degenerating spindle apparatus (the ages of the women indicated). The chromosomes are well organized at the metaphase plate at the equator of the cells in the younger women (the 22-year-old's oöcyte, on the upper left, is viewed on a tilt). In contrast, the 40-year-old's oöcyte shows the chromosomes in disarray. The 42-year-old woman's oöcyte has one chromosome, at the top, dislocated from the metaphase plate, and the disposition of the other chromosomes at the equator is not as regular as in the younger women. (*See color insert.*)

Source: From Battaglia et al., Influence of maternal age on meiotic spindle assembly in oöcytes from naturally cycling women, *Hum Reprod* 11: 2217–2222, 1996. Courtesy D. E. Battaglia, and with the permission of Oxford University Press and *Human Reproduction*.

unbalanced with either a full or a partial aneuploidy, and who are clearly phenotypically abnormal, presenting with questions of their reproductive potential. We will deal in detail with each situation in separate chapters, but we consider the broad principles here.

BALANCED CARRIERS OF CLASSIC STRUCTURAL REARRANGEMENTS

In heterozygotes for some balanced rearrangements involving only small segments, the chromosomes may "ignore" the nonhomologous material they contain, and pair (this is "heterosynapsis") and segregate much as would happen at a normal meiosis. In other balanced rearrangements, the inherent tendency to pairing dictates that homologous segments of rearranged chromosomes will align, as well as they are able, in order to achieve this ("homosynapsis"). This may require the chromosome to be something of a contortionist, forming complex configurations such as multivalents and reversed loops. According to either scenario, the stage is set for the possibility of unbalanced segregation. The gametes produced—and therefore the conceptuses that arise—are frequently imbalanced. In this context, a segmental aneuploidy is usually involved—that is, a part of a chromosome is present in the trisomic or monosomic state; or, rather frequently, a combination of trisomy for one segment and monosomy for another. Partial trisomy and partial monosomy are also referred to as *duplication* and *deletion*, respectively.

In some rearrangements, recombination presents a further hazard. Inversions and insertions may produce a new recombinant (rec) chromosome that has a different genetic composition from that of the original rearrangement. A conceptus forming from a gamete containing it would inevitably be genetically unbalanced.

CARRIERS OF MICRODELETIONS OR MICRODUPLICATIONS

These imbalances, detectable only on molecular karyotyping, are (relative to chromosome length) very small, mostly of kilobase size. They are not known to interfere with normal cell division; thus, meiosis is symmetric, 1:1—an even probability of transmitting the abnormal chromosome. These microdeletions and microduplications, sometimes called Copy Number Variants (CNVs) when pathogenicity

is in question, are to be distinguished, in practice, from the partial aneuploidies (deletions and duplications) of classical cytogenetics noted above.

FULL AND PARTIALLY ANEUPLOID INDIVIDUALS

In the individual who him- or herself has a full aneuploidy, and in whom gametogenesis is able to proceed, in theory a trivalent may form, or a bivalent and an "independent" univalent. Either could lead, effectively, to a 2:1 segregation. This appears actually to be the case in trisomy 21, whereas in sex chromosomal states (XXX, XXY, and XYY) the "third" chromosome is, as it were, disposed of, and the great majority of gametes are normal. In the person with a classic partial aneuploidy due to an unbalanced rearranged chromosome, whether 46,(abn) or 47,+(abn), the abnormal chromosome may have an even (or near-even) chance to be transmitted in the gamete.

NONDISJUNCTION IN MITOSIS AND THE GENERATION OF MOSAICISM

The purpose of a mitotic cell division is faithfully to pass on an intact and complete copy of the parental cellular genome to the progeny cells. The mitotic cycle consists of the following sequence: gap-1 period (G1) → synthesis period (S) → gap-2 period (G2) → mitosis (cell division). The G1 → S → G2 components together comprise the interphase period of the cell cycle. During the S period, the chromosomes replicate their DNA, thus converting from the single-chromatid to the double-chromatid state. Genetically active segments of chromosomes replicate earlier during the S period, while inactive segments, which include almost the entire inactivated X chromosome in the female, are late-replicating. The cell division period is further subdivided into prometaphase → metaphase → anaphase → telophase. The chromosomes condense to enter prometaphase, and condensation continues into metaphase. Metaphase chromosomes align on the equatorial plate, and the spindle apparatus becomes attached to the centromere of each chromosome, consisting of its two kinetochores. Pulled at the kinetochores (centromeres), the chromatids of each chromosome then separate (disjoin) and are drawn in opposite directions (anaphase) and arrive at the opposite poles of the cell (telophase). Then the chromosomes decondense, the nuclear membrane reconstitutes, the cytoplasm constricts and divides, and two daughter cells now exist.

A mitotic error can cause phenotypic abnormality by generating, in an initially normal conceptus, an abnormal cell line at some point during embryogenesis. If we focus on the end result, the feature distinguishing mitotic from meiotic errors is that the former typically produce a mosaic conceptus, whereas meiotic errors lead to a nonmosaic abnormality. We define constitutional chromosomal mosaicism as the coexistence, within the one conceptus, of two (or, rarely, more) distinct cell lines which are genetically identical except for the chromosomal difference between them, these cell lines having been established by the time that embryonic development is complete (the point at which the embryo becomes a fetus). Thus, the different cell lines are fixed in the individual and are a part of his or her chromosomal constitution.[10] The earlier in embryogenesis that a mitotic error occurs, the greater the likelihood for a substantial fraction of the soma to be aneuploid, leading to increasing departure from normality of the phenotype. But it is probable that many mitotically arising abnormalities lead to cell death, leaving no trace.

Considering the enormous numbers of mitoses that proceed successfully, it is clear that the ordering of chromosomal disjunction during cell division must be a marvelously robust mechanism. A complex system of interacting components underlies the mechanism; study of the "cohesinopathies," some of which present as chromosome instability syndromes (Chapter 16), has identified a number of factors that are required for well-conducted cell division. Rare instances of multiple mosaicism, which is sometimes familial, point to susceptibilities in the system. For example, Miller et al. (1990) karyotyped a child because of major physical and neurodevelopmental defects, and he had cells trisomic and monosomic for almost every chromosome, and only about a quarter were 46,XY; similar such cases are on record. The quite common finding of loss of an X or a Y chromosome in an occasional cell in an older female or male population (and more notably in centenarians) may reflect "normal" age-related anaphase lag (Russell et al. 2007) (p. 342).

Normal Zygote

Nondisjunction can occur in an initially normal (46,N) zygote, with the generation of mosaicism for a trisomic and a concomitant monosomic line, as well as the normal line (Figure 3–8a). In autosomal nondisjunction, growth of the monosomic cell line is severely compromised, and it will likely die out in early embryogenesis, leaving just the normal and the trisomic cell lines comprising the individual.[11] Mosaic Down syndrome, with the karyotype 47,+21/46,N, is the classic example. In one particular autosomal aneuploidy, trisomy 8 mosaicism, somatic nondisjunction accounts for practically all cases (Karadima et al. 1998).

Actually, about 5% of standard apparently nonmosaic 47,+21 is also due to a mitotic defect from a 46,N zygote (Antonarakis et al. 1993), with the "third" chromosome 21 equally likely to be maternal or paternal. In 3% of apparently nonmosaic 47,XXY and 9% of 47,XXX, the error was postzygotic, presumably prior to the formation of the inner cell mass (MacDonald et al. 1994). As noted above, the nature of the mosaicism can indicate the likely time of its generation. An aberrant mitosis involving the X chromosome, in an initially 46,XX zygote, may generate X and XXX cell lines, both of which would be survivable. If this happens at the first mitosis, X/XXX mosaicism would result. If at any later mitosis, a normal cell line would exist, and the mosaic state would be X/XX/XXX (Figure 3–8b). The same can happen in a 46,XY zygote, with an X/XYY or an X/XY/XYY mosaicism resulting (the gender in the embryo being determined according to the

---

10   We overlook here the question of somatic aneuploidy arising in adult life as a cause of disease, and the long-accepted concept of chromosome abnormality in a somatic cell as a step in carcinogenesis is the classic example (Oromendia and Amon 2014). The suggestion that Alzheimer disease might have a basis in mosaic trisomy 21 or X aneuploidy of some brain tissue is intriguing, but leaving open the question of the time in life at which the putative aneuploid cell line may have become incorporated (Iourov et al. 2012; Yurov et al. 2014). The bowel, an organ constantly replenishing its epithelium, accumulates microdeletions and microduplications with age (Hsieh et al. 2013).

11   A very rare example of autosomal monosomy/disomy/trisomy mosaicism was identified in the abnormal baby reported in Stefanou et al. (2006), mentioned below. Only 1 cell in 200 on blood showed 47,XY,+20, and disomy was demonstrated on buccal mucosal fluorescence in situ hybridization (FISH) and skin fibroblast analysis, but 39/50 cells from urinary sediment were monosomic.

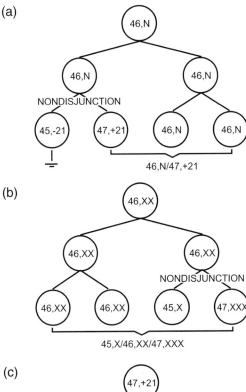

(a)

(b)

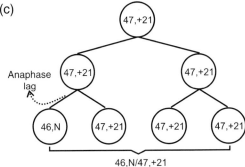

(c)

FIGURE 3–8   Generation of mosaicism.
(*a*) Postzygotic nondisjunction in an initially normal conceptus. In this example, one cell line (monosomic 21) is subsequently lost, with the final karyotype 46,N/47,+21. (*b*) Postzygotic nondisjunction in an initially normal 46,XX conceptus, resulting in 45,X/46,XX/47,XXX mosaicism. (*c*) Postzygotic anaphase lag in an initially abnormal 47,+21 conceptus; this leads to a "corrected," or "rescued," normal cell line.

sex chromosome composition of gonadal tissue). More than one mitotic error can happen, separate in time and place; for example, DeBrasi et al. (1995) identified concomitant

45,X and 47,XX,+8 (and 46,X,+8) in a woman with clinical features of both trisomy 8 and Turner syndrome, in whom the molecular study supported the hypothesis of an originally 46,XX conception.

Aneuploid Zygote

Nondisjunction can occur in a postzygotic mitosis in a conceptus that is initially trisomic for an autosome (for example, 47,+21). Thus, one copy of the homolog in question is lost. The same result may be due to the mechanism of anaphase lag.[12] This converts the trisomy in this cell to 46,N and is sometimes referred to as "correction" or "rescue." Its descendant cells are 46,N, and the karyotype of the conceptus is, for example, 47,+21/46,N (Figure 3–8c). Most mosaic trisomy/disomy 13, 18, 21, and X arises in this way—for example, 47,XXY → 46,XY/47,XXY (Robinson et al. 1995).

A conceptus with what might be called 'interchange tertiary trisomy'—that is, a 47-chromosome count, with the two translocation chromosomes and an additional copy of one of the derivative chromosomes—might generate a cell line with the balanced state, if one of the derivatives is lost postzygotically. Thus, a zygote with, for example, a 47,t(1;2),+der(1) karyotype might acquire a cell line with 46,t(1;2). If this cell line included blood-forming tissue, but if much of the soma otherwise consisted of cells with the unbalanced state, a phenotypically abnormal child could have, on blood sampling, a balanced translocation karyotype. Such a case is presented in Dufke et al. (2001); speculatively, this scenario might be a rare contributor to the apparent slight excess of abnormal children among the balanced carrier offspring of translocation carrier parents (p. 110).

Postzygotic "Correction" of Aneuploidy and Uniparental Disomy. If the conversion of trisomy to disomy occurs prior to the formation of the pre-embryo, and if the 46,N line then gives rise to the pre-embryo, the embryo will be nonmosaic 46,N. According to which one of the three

---

12 In this latter case, the chromosome fails to connect to the spindle apparatus, or is tardily drawn to its pole, and fails to be included in the reforming nuclear membrane. On its own in the cytoplasm, it will form a micronucleus and soon be lost.

chromosomes was lost, normal biparental disomy in the embryo could be restored, or uniparental disomy (UPD) could result (Figure 3–9). This is far and away the usual mechanism of UPD. It is at prenatal diagnosis, typically, that the fact of this rescue mechanism comes to be discovered, with trisomy seen at chorionic villus sampling (CVS), and disomy at a subsequent amniocentesis (Sirchia et al. 1998). Chromosome 15 is of particular concern, and Purvis-Smith et al. (1992) and Cassidy et al. (1992) provide historic illustrations in pregnancies

showing 47,+15 at CVS, with conversion to 46,N at amniocentesis; but the infants had upd(15)mat, and so they were born with Prader-Willi syndrome. Walczak et al. (2000) showed the same thing retrospectively, in demonstrating trisomy 15 by FISH on archived placental tissue.

An inference of "rescue" may be made in the case of UPD discovered because of isozygosity for a recessive gene, and an example of this is deafness due to the connexin-26 gene. Yan et al. (2007) report a child presenting with deafness due to

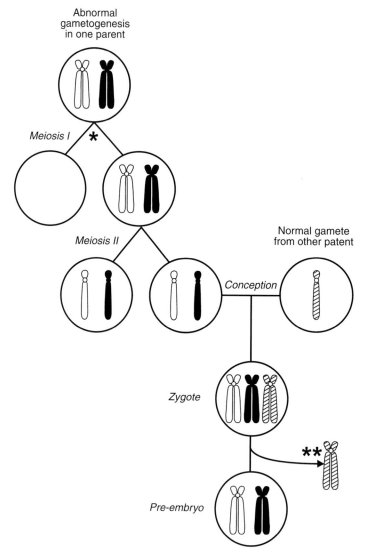

FIGURE 3–9   Uniparental disomy from "correction" of a trisomic conceptus by loss of a homolog. Nondisjunction* at meiosis I, followed by postzygotic loss** of one homolog, causes uniparental heterodisomy. (If, for example, this were chromosome 15, and the meiotic nondisjunction occurred in the mother, the child would have Prader-Willi syndrome.) Nondisjunction at meiosis II would cause uniparental isodisomy.

homozygosity for the common 35delG mutation, for which his father, but not his mother, was a carrier. As it transpired, the child had upd13(pat), with isodisomic and heterodisomic segments of chromosome 13, the segment in 13q12.1, which contains the connexin-26 locus, being one of the regions of isodisomy. Quite possibly, this had been a trisomic 13 conception but rescued due to discarding one of the chromosomes, which happened to be the maternal chromosome 13. Had it not been for the coincidence of the father's heterozygosity for the 35delG mutation, the rescue would have been entirely successful.

Postzygotic correction can also happen in the other direction, as it were: to convert a monosomic zygote into a disomic one. It is very rarely recognized (Schinzel et al. 1993). Quan et al. (1997) report a girl, 46,XX, with Duchenne muscular dystrophy due to a homozygous deletion of exon 50 of the dystrophin gene. She had homozygosity of the X chromosome for all of the tested marker loci: apparently, a complete maternal uniparental isodisomy X. Even a meiosis II nondisjunction would likely have had some heterozygosity, due to recombination at meiosis I; and so Quan et al. propose a mitotic mechanism. A 45,X0 conception, from a 22,0 sperm + 23,X egg at syngamy, underwent duplication, or possibly nondisjunction, of the single X chromosome. Unfortunately, this X chromosome carried a de novo Duchenne mutation.

Vulnerability of the First Few Mitoses

The first few mitotic divisions from the one-cell zygote are particularly vulnerable to error, and this brief period of development needs to be considered separately. Insight into this vulnerability has come from experience in the IVF laboratory. Surprisingly large fractions, about 25%–30%, of cleavage embryos subjected to preimplantation genetic diagnosis (PGD) are chromosomally mosaic, typically with complete aneuploidies (at least in a population of older women presenting to an IVF clinic). The majority of these show "chaotic mosaicism," with aneuploidies for different chromosomes in different cells, and up to 100% of cells aneuploid. Day 4 (the morula) is seen as a watershed, and mosaicisms, meiotic and mitotic, are very frequently observed (Mertzanidou et al. 2013). Coming into day 5, at

the blastocyst stage, the rate falls very considerably, presumably due either to loss of individual aneuploid cells in an embryo and ongoing survival of the normal lineages or to cessation altogether of cell division, with demise of the embryo (Fragouli et al. 2013).

Insight into the timing of the abnormality can also be gained from inference in the study of mosaic individuals. Jacobs et al. (1997), in a study of Turner syndrome, observed that patients with Xq isochromosome mosaicism hardly ever have a 46,XX cell line: Most are 45,X/46,X,i(Xq). This is what would be expected if the error happened at the very first mitosis of the initially 46,XX zygote. If it happened at the next two or three divisions, a 46,XX cell line would also have been present, 45,X/46,XX/46,X,i(Xq). If three cell lines are detected, an origin in a later mitosis can be assumed. For example, Stefanou et al. (2006) describe an abnormal infant with trisomy 20 mosaicism on blood but with a monosomic 20 cell line identified in urinary epithelial cells. The very first division of the zygote may be especially prone to error.

A separate question concerning a different type of early vulnerability relates to the generation of several independent de novo copy number variants around the time of late gametogenesis, fertilization, and the first few mitoses—the "multiple de novo CNV (MdnCNV) phenotype" (p. 382).

SOMATIC RECOMBINATION IN HOMOLOGS

Genetic exchange can take place, as a normal event, during a mitotic cycle, involving either the pair of homologous chromosomes or the sister chromatids of one chromosome. The cytogenetic demonstration of sister chromatid exchange (SCE) is rather dramatic (Figure 16–1). Should the SCE be unequal, tandem duplication and deletion lines may be generated. If the deletion line is lost, a normal/duplication mosaicism results (Rauen et al. 2001). According to the somatic extent of the abnormal cell line, the phenotype may or may not be affected.

GONADAL MOSAICISM

Cells destined to give rise to gametocytes originate from the yolk sac in early embryogenesis and migrate to the gonadal ridge on the dorsal wall of the abdominal cavity, where, along with the supporting cells, they come to comprise the tissue of the gonad (De Felici 2013). In doing so, gametocytes must replicate many times, going through about 30 cycles of division in the male. Thirty cycles produces 2^{30} (about 1,000,000,000) progeny cells, and the potential for error exists at each cell division contributing to this population. These errors could be nondisjunctions or the production of structural rearrangements. Consider this startling statistic: The total length of the seminiferous tubule in a man is about half a kilometer, a third of a mile (Johnson et al. 1998). If a mutation were to occur in a spermatogonium in, for example, the twentieth cycle of division, its progeny would then go through 10 more cycles and comprise 2^{10} (about 1,000) cells. This would be only a millionth (1,000/1,000,000,000) of the ½ km of tubule—a mere ½ mm. So a man mosaic in such a way would have a risk of only 1 in a million to father a conception with this particular abnormality, given the a priori improbability of the fertilizing sperm coming from this imperfect ½ mm. From similar reasoning, a defect arising at the tenth cycle could affect half a meter of tubule and carry a risk of 1 in 1,000. Oögonia need go through a lesser number of mitotic cycles (about 22), but the same principles broadly apply. Hultén et al. (2013) controversially suggest mitotic errors during ovariogenesis are inevitable and that "most women may be trisomy 21 ovarian mosaics."[13]

DETECTING MOSAICISM

A classic chromosome test on any normal person— a routine analysis from a sample of peripheral blood—would probably get a normal result (46,N). We would conclude from an analysis of a dozen or so cells from one specialized tissue that the rest of the soma is also 46,N. In most of the person's tissue, this will be truly the case. But the body comprises a vast number of cells—ten trillion (10^{13}) or so— which required a vast number of mitoses for their generation. The dozen cells checked in the laboratory are only a ten-billionth of a percent of all the person's cells, and we routinely (and, for practical purposes, not unreasonably) regard this minute fraction as a valid representative of the remaining

99.9999999999%. Notwithstanding, we can surely suppose that one or more errors will have happened, during one or some of the many mitoses, and these will have produced a chromosomally abnormal cell line, and the person is really a chromosomal mosaic. It seems plausible to imagine that unrecognized islands of mosaicism, involving a tiny number of cells—only a few thousand, perhaps—could well be a frequent state. Almost certainly, somewhere in their soma, everyone may be such a mosaic (and see footnote 10); but this fascinating academic matter is not a question much raised in the genetic counseling clinic.

For more clinically relevant degrees of mosaicism, and if blood may not necessarily reflect the karyotype elsewhere in the body, what other tissues are available for analysis? Skin fibroblasts are a more "basic" tissue, and skin biopsy has long been performed in the pursuit of a diagnosis of mosaicism. A particular case is that of the Pallister-Killian syndrome, due to 12p isochromosome (p. 505), which usually cannot be diagnosed on blood, and thus skin biopsy, or other non-blood tissue, is a necessary procedure (Cobben et al. 2013). Chorionic villi and amniocytes are the tissues assessed at prenatal diagnosis, and "confined placental mosaicism" is a well-recognized category. Other somatic tissues amenable to study, and thus allowing recognition of mosaicism, are the buccal mucosal cell and the urinary epithelial cell (Reddy and Mak 2001; Stefanou et al. 2006). In saliva samples, leukocytes are the predominant cell type (Thiede et al. 2000). Classical cytogenetics can (if the tested tissue is representative) show mosaicism unequivocally, with the recognition of two different karyotypes, but this is dependent on there being enough cells in the less frequent line for the observation to be made. In molecular karyotyping, detection is a subtler exercise, and it is based on an appreciation of a quantitative shift in the $\log_2$ graph, or, if single nucleotide polymorphism array is the methodology, the genotyping pattern may be revealing; but in principle, mosaicism that might have passed muster on classical analysis can be picked up (Repnikova et al. 2012). A rather different question is mosaicism in the preimplantation embryo (as discussed above).

---

13 Hultén and colleagues had made this extraordinary suggestion, and one which would overturn much of the received wisdom about the generation of trisomy, in studying ovarian tissue from apparently normal female fetuses and observing a very low-level trisomy 21 mosaicism. They hypothesized that the maternal age effect might be due to a different maturity of the trisomic oöcyte. While a similar study due to Rowsey et al. (2013) failed to confirm this observation, the argument continues (Hultén et al. 2014).

CHIMERISM

Chimerism, which is to be distinguished from mosaicism, is the coexistence of more than one cell line in an individual, due to the union of two originally separate ("sibling") conceptions (Chen et al. 2013f).[14] It could be imagined that twin blastocysts happen to make contact and then fuse, and this may be the more typical scenario. Since four gametes will have contributed to the person, we may hear the expression "tetragametic" chimerism. Alternatively, but likely very rarely, there might have been two sperm fertilizing an ovum and a polar body. A 46,XX//46,XX or 46,XY//46,XY chimera would most probably present as a normal female or male, whereas 46,XX//46,XY could manifest an abnormality of sexual differentiation (p. 539). An extraordinary example of chimerism is recorded in Wiley et al. (2002) of a malformed stillborn with 47,XY,+21//47,XX,+12.

The discovery of chimerism can cast a most remarkable light in certain cases in which parenthood is being tested. A mother apparently "could not have been" the mother of two of her three sons, when she and the family underwent HLA (immune histocompatibility) testing ahead of a planned kidney transplant. But it transpired that she was a tetragametic 46,XX//46,XX chimera. Her ovaries presumably comprised tissue from both fused conceptuses, but blood-forming tissue came from only one: Thus, she could have children who had neither of her blood-test HLA haplotypes (Yu et al. 2002). Similarly, a father who "failed" a paternity test from a son conceived at IVF—Could this have been a laboratory mix-up?—turned out himself to be a tetragametic 46,XY//46,XY chimera. The child came from sperm due to tissue deriving from the father's absorbed fraternal co-twin, and his genetic profile was that of a nephew of his father (Baird et al. 2015).

The more usual form is "confined" chimerism, in which only one tissue—that is, blood—possesses the two cell lines. This is due to twin-to-twin (or feto-fetal) transfusion, when dizygous twins have intimately opposed placentae, allowing vascular connections ("anastomoses") to form between them, with marrow colonization by the other twin's hematogenous cells. Sudik et al. (2001), for example, describe a woman typing XY in almost all (99%) of peripheral lymphocytes, but she was 46,XX on three other tissues, including ovarian; she had had a twin brother, who had died as a neonate. Somewhat stretching the analogy, Bianchi (2000) makes the intriguing suggestion that, due to the retention and persistence of fetal blood cells following delivery, every mother is, in a sense, a hematologic (micro) chimera.

TWINNING

Dizygous twinning is more frequent in mothers in their late thirties, and so it is not remarkable that occasionally twins are born, one with normal chromosomes and the other with a maternal-age-related aneuploidy. Monozygous twinning could happen in an abnormal conception just as in a normal one, and the occasional instance of twins concordant for an abnormal karyotype is to be expected (Schlessel et al. 1990). Rather more remarkable is the case of monozygous twins discordant for karyotype—clearly, the adjective "identical" is inappropriate here! Rogers et al. (1982) studied monochorionic twin brothers, one 46,XY and the other 47,XY,+21 with Down syndrome, in whom genetic analysis supported a diagnosis of monozygosity. In this type of twinning, the assumption is that either an initially 47,XY,+21 conceptus underwent splitting, with loss of a chromosome 21 then occurring in one of the newly created embryos, or, vice versa, a mitotic nondisjunction occurred in one monozygous embryo from an initially normal conception. A number of similar cases are on record, including monozygous twins of opposite gender (Lewi et al. 2006; Stemkens et al. 2007; Zech et al. 2008).

Perhaps the most extraordinary circumstance of discordance in monozygous twins concerns the acardiac (that is, lacking a heart) fetus. Trisomy 2 is one of the aneuploidies observed (Mihci et al. 2009). An initially normal conceptus might generate a trisomy 2 cell line that then separates and produces the co-twin, or an initially trisomic conceptus gives rise to a "corrected" lineage. It is only the presence of the normal twin that allows the acardiac co-twin to survive, with placental vascular connections providing

---

14 For the record, the chimera of classical mythology was "in the forepart a lion, in the hinder a serpent, and in the midst a goat." Note the // descriptive format.

blood circulation from normal to abnormal twin.[15] We have seen such a case due to trisomy 3, with the affected acephalic, acardiac fetus of barely recognizable human form (McGillivray et al. 2004).

STRUCTURAL REARRANGEMENT

The following classical structural rearrangements may be listed: translocations, insertions, inversions, isochromosomes, duplications, deletions, and complex rearrangements. These may be very obvious on classical karyotyping or, for smaller deletions or duplications (3–5 Mb), may have required high-resolution banding for identification. With molecular karyotyping, imbalances of submicroscopic size, typically measured in kilobases, are detectable (Gu et al. 2008). As noted above, "microdeletion" and "microduplication" are used here to describe these kilobase- or low Mb-size imbalances when clearly pathogenic, while "copy number variant" is the expression when pathogenicity is uncertain or practically excluded.[16] All arose de novo at one point—whether with the index case in whom the abnormality was discovered, or in a parent or more distant ancestor, with a balanced or unbalanced form transmitted thereafter in the family. Jacobs (1981) derived the following mutation rates for the generation of de novo classical rearrangements: 1.6×10^{-4} per gamete for the balanced reciprocal translocation, and 2.9×10^{-4} per gamete for unbalanced rearrangements. Concerning CNVs, the mutation rate for larger (>500 kb) microdeletions/duplications is 6.5×10^{-3} per gamete (Itsara et al. 2010). In other words, out of 100,000 gametes, 16 will have a balanced and 29 an unbalanced de novo classical rearrangement, while 650 will have a de novo larger CNV.

The illegitimate breakage and reunion that produces these rearrangements is typically due to the apposition of nonmatching (nonhomologous) chromosomal segments, but which do happen to contain DNA sequences with a high degree of homology ("low copy repeats"). These are called "paralogous sequences," and they are also known as "duplicons" and "segmental duplications." The process is called non-allelic homologous recombination (NAHR), and it applies to both classical and molecular-defined rearrangements (Itsara et al. 2012). Specific palindromic AT-rich sequences comprise the basis of "hot spots" at 11q23, 17q11, and 22q11, leading to the recurrent translocations t(11;22) and t(17;22) due to breakpoints at these sites (Kurahashi et al. 2010). Most breakpoints are in nontranscribed DNA, and thus, for the most part, contribute no untoward effect per se upon the phenotype. We discuss possible mechanisms of formation in more detail in the appropriate chapters.

Setting in Which De Novo Rearrangement Occurs

While mutations causing chromosomal rearrangement could, in principle, occur during either meiosis or mitosis, and in the gonad of either sex, in fact, different chromosomal forms differ in this respect. Most Robertsonian translocations arise in oögenesis, at a maternal meiosis (Bandyopadhyay et al. 2002). Microdeletions/duplications can occur in both gonadal types, and mostly at a meiosis, at least inasmuch as the common cases of 7q11, 15q11q13, and 22q11 may be considered to be representative (Thomas et al. 2010). On the other hand, spermatogenesis is the setting for almost all de novo non-Robertsonian reciprocal rearrangements, and both meiosis and premeiotic mitoses may be the site (Höckner et al. 2012).

Balanced, Apparently Balanced, and Unbalanced Rearrangements

Structural rearrangements can be balanced, with the correct amount of genetic material in a cell, or unbalanced, with a deletion and/or duplication of genetic material. Arguing somewhat circularly, in the phenotypically normal person it is inferred that although such an individual's genetic material is in a different chromosomal arrangement, it is present in the correct (balanced) amount and functioning properly. It is irrelevant to the person's health, other than his or her reproductive health. It may be helpful in explaining this to think of the person's genome as a recipe book—a series of instructions for everything that is genetically determined. If an error occurs in the pagination (a translocation) and, for example, pages 17–24 are inserted between pages 36 and 37, the recipes are all still there; they are still perfectly capable of being read. If a sequence of

---

15 This is called twin reverse arterial perfusion (TRAP).
16 But note that many writers will refer to known pathogenic small imbalances as CNVs.

pages is inserted upside down (an inversion), one need only turn the book around to read them.

If a phenotypically abnormal person has a rearrangement that is balanced on classical laboratory study, one can only speak, at the cytogenetic level, of the rearrangement being "apparently balanced." In the case of an associated intellectual deficit, one can suggest (and specifically in a de novo case), but not state with certainty, that the observed phenotype may be due to the identified karyotype. In some, the clinical picture, in light of knowledge of the chromosomal breakpoints, may inform interpretation. Consider the well-known *PMP22* gene at 17p11.2, the basis of Charcot-Marie-Tooth and pressure-sensitive neuropathy (p. 327). Nadal et al. (2000) studied a mother and son, both of whom presented with pressure-sensitive neuropathy. The classical cytogenetic study showed them to be heterozygotes for the apparently balanced translocation t(16;17)(q12;p11.2). Applying the technology of the day, the chromosome 17 breakpoint was shown to have been sited actually within the *PMP22* gene. This disruption would have led to a functional haploinsufficiency, which is known to be the basis of pressure-sensitive neuropathy. Point proven.

Molecular karyotyping may cast light on previously ill-understood pictures and, for example, reveal a submicroscopic microdeletion/duplication (Feenstra et al. 2011). The more abnormal the phenotype, the greater the likelihood of detecting imbalance. The extraordinary sophistication of whole genome sequencing may offer yet further precision of interpretation (Ordulu et al. 2016). A rearrangement that is balanced at the genomic level may yet lead to a phenotypic consequence due to gene disruption or due to "position effect." As examples of the former, as well as the *PMP22* case just mentioned, Dupont et al. (2013) identified a *COL2A* disruption in a family with Stickler syndrome, the affected persons having inherited a rcp(12;15)(q13;q22.2); and Luukkonen et al. (2012) showed that a translocation breakpoint within an intron of the *neurotrimin* gene was the basis of aortic disease in a family segregating a t(10;11)(q23.2;q24.2). Utami et al. (2014) analyzed breakpoints in translocation or inversion patients from four families, with respectively t(9;17)

(q12;q24), t(6;8)(q16.2;p11.2), inv(X)(p21q25), and inv(5)(q22q35.1). They identified disruptions in five genes located at one or both breakpoints, of very plausible role in the clinical phenotypes. The determinations were at the nucleotide level of precision; for example, in the apparently balanced t(9;17) (q12;q24), seen in a father and his two children with poor speech development, the rearrangement had actually generated deletions at chr9:77,767,265-77,767,269 and chr17:79,257,250-79,260,287. These deletions occurred within the sequences of the *GNAQ* and *RBFOX3* loci on chromosomes 9 and 17, respectively, with the rearrangement causing disruption of these genes, both of which have a high brain expression.

Concerning position effect, one of the earliest examples is of the *SOX9* gene at 17q25.1: Chromosomal rearrangement in the vicinity can result in loss of long-range regulation and hence nonexpression of the (intact) gene, with sex reversal, campomelic dysplasia, and Pierre Robin syndrome possible phenotypic consequences (Gordon et al. 2014) (Figure 14–2). A similar example is a t(2;7) (p25.1;q22) in which two loci contributing to limb formation, *DLX5* and *DLX6*, on one side of the 7q22 breakpoint, were separated from their controlling element, *DYNC1I1*, on the other side, with a split hand and foot malformation resulting (Lango Allen et al. 2014). The opposite effect is overexpression of a gene, and David et al. (2013) discuss a t(8;13) (q23.3;q21.31) in a family with trichorhinophalangeal syndrome, proposing that an enhancer element at 13q21.31 came to lie upstream of the *TRP1* gene at 8q23.3, influencing its activity such that it overexpressed, and this led to the development of the syndrome in heterozygous family members. (This may be considered as a form of "epigenetic" effect, and we discuss this concept below.)

MICRODELETIONS AND MICRODUPLICATIONS OF INCOMPLETE PENETRANCE AND VARIABLE EXPRESSIVITY

While the classic chromosome disorders are characterized by complete penetrance,[17] the picture with

---

17 *Penetrance* is a quantitative descriptor and refers to the percentage fraction of a particular genetic cohort who show phenotypic abnormality. In such a population, in which the fraction is less than 100%, we may speak of *incomplete* penetrance; in a single individual showing no abnormality, this is *nonpenetrance*. *Expressivity* is qualitative, and reflects the range of clinical manifestation, in those in whom a condition has been penetrant. It may sometimes become a matter of semantics whether a subtly abnormal person is considered to represent nonpenetrance or penetrance with very mild expressivity.

the molecular-defined microdeletions/duplications is different. Some carriers may display no clinical abnormality, and yet a child of theirs may have presented with obvious symptomatology. If the "normal" parent is studied more closely, microsigns of the phenotype associated with that imbalance may be discerned; but they remain within the range of what is considered normal in the general population, and they can function as independent, productive adults. These normal parents are considered to be nonpenetrant with respect to the imbalance in question. It is more particularly with autism and nondysmorphic intellectual disability that these matters apply.

The basis of this variation may lie in the coexistence of another microdeletion/duplication or CNV, most likely on another chromosome, and inherited quite coincidentally. Each imbalance might not suffice to cause a phenotype on its own, but the two together may add up to abnormality. This is the "two-hit" hypothesis (Girirajan et al. 2010; Coe et al. 2012; Gau et al. 2012). Most often, one hit (the first hit) will be the more important, and the second hit could be due to any one of a number of different "lesser" imbalances, which typically would warrant being called no more than a CNV, possibly a "VOUS" (variant of uncertain significance).[18] Thus, Bassuk et al. (2013) propose that a rare 19p microdeletion worsened the clinical outcome, including causing epilepsy, in a mother and her two children with the well-recognized 16p11.2 microdeletion. Gau et al. (2012) suggested an autistic son of parents, each with minor attention deficit, was affected due to having inherited a CNV from each of them: a 1.8 Mb del5q32 from father and a 4.5 Mb dup 4q12q13.1 from mother. It might be more accurate to speak of two hits "multiplying together," rather than "adding up," to produce a phenotype of combined effect. These concepts are discussed in more detail in Chapter 17.

Rosenfeld et al. (2013) have reviewed a number of the more common microdeletions/duplications ("first-hit" imbalances), establishing penetrance estimates ranging from 10% to 62% (the 62% referring to the 16p11.2 microdeletion just mentioned).

These penetrance data are listed in the appropriate entries in Chapter 14 and in toto in Table 4–1. As more data are collected, we may anticipate a better understanding of the nature of the putative second-hit imbalances.[19]

EPIGENETICS AND GENOMIC IMPRINTING

A formal definition of an epigenetic effect includes these points: The DNA sequence of a particular gene remains unaltered, but the capacity of this gene to be expressed is altered. The expression "genomic imprinting" is applied in the setting of epigenetic effects that are imposed during germline transmission. Some parts of some chromosomes are subject to genomic imprinting as a normal occurrence, and this imprinting is parent-specific; that is, genes in the chromosomal segment are expressed, or not expressed, according to whether the chromosome had been transmitted in the sperm or in the ovum ("parent-of-origin effect"). An imprinted segment takes up an "epigenetic mark," and the gene or genes in this segment are not expressed, leaving it to the corresponding locus or loci on the homologous chromosome from the other parent to be the only source of expression. When the phenomenon was first appreciated in humans, it was naturally suspected that many forms of congenital abnormality might be due to aberrant imprinting. As it has transpired, however, the practical application of genomic imprinting appears to be confined to a rather small number of cytogenetic conditions. Nevertheless, the theoretical interest is considerable.

Most of the autosomal genome is not subject to imprinting, and it is functionally disomic. That is, with each locus having a pair of alleles, each of the pair is functionally active, contributing more or less equally to the genetic output from that locus.[20] This is biallelic gene expression. A minority of the genome is subject to imprinting and requires only one of the pair of alleles to be active, while the other one becomes inactivated ("silent"); in other words, the locus is functionally monosomic, with a genetic output from only one allele. This is monoallelic expression. If the

---

18 A rare and different form of two-hit mechanism concerns the "unmasking" of a recessive allele on a normal homolog, due to a deletion of that segment on the other chromosome (Poot 2012; Paciorkowski et al. 2013).

19 Indeed, as regards the complex traits of human intelligence and behavior, "two hits" may come to be seen as a simplistic explanation, as we learn more about how variation at very many loci may add up to the genetic basis of the observed phenotypes—in other words, the classical concept of polygenic inheritance.

20 But exceptions exist, and approximately 5% of autosomal genes are randomly expressed from only one or other parental allele (Gimelbrant et al. 2007).

allele of maternal origin is inactivated, only the allele of paternal origin is functionally active, and vice versa. Following conception, the imprint remains through cycles of postconceptional somatic mitoses: The chromosome "remembers" the sex of the parent who contributed it (put differently, it retains its epigenetic mark). The imprinting pattern may be specific to a certain tissue or to a certain developmental stage (Ideraabdullah et al. 2008). Thus, in some tissues a gene may express monoallelically, whereas in other tissues biallelic expression is retained; or a gene may express monoallelically in a specific tissue at one stage in embryogenesis and biallelically thereafter. X chromosome inactivation is a special case.

Parent-of-origin imprinting is a normal mechanism of gene regulation. It is mediated through a process taking place during gametogenesis, of which the physical basis includes methylation of cytosine bases within the gene(s), or in controlling sequences upstream of it. This process is reversible, and in the "life" of an autosomal allele or chromosomal segment, as it passes from individual to individual down the generations and across the centuries, imprinting—the epigenetic mark—will be acquired, maintained, lost ("erased"), reacquired ("reset"), and lost again, according to the sexes of the individuals through whom it is transmitted. Throughout, it retains the same DNA sequence.

Mechanisms Whereby Functional Genetic Abnormality Can Arise

In the context of imprinting, we may consider three categories of functional genetic defect. These are as follows: uniparental disomy with overexpression or nonexpression of genes in certain chromosomal segments; deletion with nonexpression; and relaxation of imprinting with overexpression. (1) Uniparental disomy will lead to either biallelic expression or no expression at the locus or loci within the imprintable segment. (2) If a deletion removes a chromosomal segment that would otherwise have been "silenced," all that is lost is a nonfunctioning genetic segment, and there is no untoward consequence. On the other hand, if the deletion removes the segment on the active chromosome, the corresponding part of the other homolog is inactive, and so neither chromosome will be genetically functioning in this segment; in a sense, the silent allele is unmasked. (3) Relaxation of imprinting allows a segment that should be nonexpressed to lose its imprint. The locus or loci contained therein will be operating

biallelically, which will be, theoretically, at double normal capacity. These mechanisms are dealt with in detail in Chapter 18.

Another category of epigenetic effect is that imposed by compromise of controller elements, such that the client gene, which is of itself normal, is inappropriately nonfunctioning or overfunctioning. This may reflect a "position effect" due to a translocation separating the controller and the client, as mentioned above.

CONSEQUENCES OF GENETIC ABNORMALITY

STRUCTURAL IMBALANCE

Our anatomy is due to our chromosomes (Gardner 2016). Chromosome imbalances are harmful because of the fundamental reason that many genes are dosage sensitive; and if megabase amounts of chromatin are involved, it is highly likely dosage-sensitive genes will be included. In duplications, there is 150% of the normal amount of this chromosomal segment; and in the deletion, there is 50% of the normal amount. The imbalance involves a whole chromosome (full aneuploidy) or a part of a chromosome. From classical cytogenetics, the latter state is described as partial or segmental aneuploidy, a deletion or a duplication. In molecular karyotyping, in which the focus is on much smaller segments, the terms used are microdeletion and microduplication. "Copy number variants" typically refer to yet smaller segments, but there can be overlap in size, and in the use of terminology, with microdeletions/microduplications.

An incorrect amount of dosage-sensitive genetic material in every cell of the conceptus distorts its development to a greater or lesser extent. Large losses or gains almost invariably set early anatomical development so awry that natural abortion occurs. Lesser imbalances may be compatible with continued intrauterine survival, but with the eventual production of a phenotypically abnormal child. Very minor partial aneuploidies may cause defects that are not readily detectable in early infancy; and some chromosomal "defects" may be without phenotypic effect. However, as a first principle, anything but 100% of the normal amount of genetic material (in classical, megabase cytogenetic terms) produces a less than 100% normal phenotype. Mental defect is the almost universal consequence of classical autosomal imbalance, and vice versa, much mental defect is due to a chromosome abnormality.

On the other hand, imbalances detectable only by molecular karyotyping (microdeletions/microduplications, copy number variants) may be so small that no dosage-sensitive material is affected, and the phenotype is unaffected; or, the imbalance may only lead to phenotypic abnormality when it exists in the company of another micro-imbalance elsewhere in the genome ("second-hit" effect, as discussed above). The distinction between very small classical and larger molecular imbalances is not as clear-cut as the foregoing might suggest, and indeed some cases could carry either description; but it is useful nevertheless to consider these as two categories. A fuller discussion appears in Chapter 17.

It is generally too simplistic to think of deletions and duplications leading to opposite qualities of phenotype (Neri and Romana Di Raimo 2010). But in some instances the concept of "type and countertype," originally proposed by Lejeune (1966), may be invoked. Deletion of 7p15 may cause the cranial bones to fuse prematurely (craniosynostosis), due to abnormal behavior of osteoblasts at their periphery, whereas duplication leads to underdevelopment of the skull, with a large and confluent fontanelle (Stankiewicz et al. 2001c) (Figure 14–51). Deletion of 15q26.1qter (which removes the growth factor locus *IGFR1*) is associated with intrauterine growth retardation, whereas dup(15) (q26.1qter) may cause a syndrome of postnatal overgrowth (Faivre et al. 2002; Nagai et al. 2002). Similarly, carriers of reciprocal copy number variants at 16p11.2 exhibit mirror phenotypes of obesity/macrocephaly (deletion) and underweight/microcephaly (duplication) (Loviglio et al. 2017).

ASSESSMENT OF IMBALANCE

With respect to classical degrees of cytogenetic imbalance, the blunt quantitative tool of haploid autosomal length (HAL; see Appendix B) measurement can be applied, albeit that this may be becoming of somewhat historic interest in the molecular era. The largest chromosome, no. 1, comprises 8.4% of the HAL, whereas chromosome 21, the smallest, is 1.9%. As a very general rule, if the imbalance consists of less than 1% of HAL (corresponding to 30 Mb), the conceptus is often viable in utero, and live birth frequently results. If the excess is greater than 2%, in utero lethality, with spontaneous abortion, is likely. Imbalance involving autosomal deficiency (partial monosomy) is generally much less survivable than is duplication (partial trisomy).

A firmer assessment is based on the empiric observations of phenotypes. Some large segments (e.g., 9p, all of 21) appear to have a substantial pre- and postnatal survivability in the trisomic state, whereas a lesser number of segments (e.g., distal 4p) are often viable when monosomic. Chromosome 13 provides the most impressive examples of viability for a large autosomal imbalance. Trisomy for the whole of chromosome 13— fully 3.7% of the HAL—frequently goes through to live birth, and in the 13q– deletion syndrome, monosomy occurs for up to 2.5% of HAL. This reflects the low gene density on this chromosome, only 6.5 genes per Mb. The same principle applies to chromosomes 18 and 21.[21] Occasionally, imbalance detectable classically is so "small" that the effect on the child's physical phenotype is only very minor, and intellectual function can remain within the normal range, albeit toward the lower end of that range. Indeed, there are some segments of Mb size which, when duplicated or deleted, appear to cause no abnormality at all (Stumm et al. 2002). The concept of heritable "euchromatic deletions and duplications without phenotypic effect" is discussed in Chapter 17.

Molecular karyotyping has enabled a finer view of the genome, and microdeletions and microduplications of kilobase size are routinely detectable. These imbalances display a phenotype—when it is actually abnormal, which is not always the case (as discussed above)—in which cognitive and behavioral abnormality is the predominant observation. Dysmorphism may be evident, but can be of quite minor degree. This may reflect that these small imbalances affect only a single gene, or a regulatory factor. Since the organ commanding the largest component of a person's genome is the brain, it is plausible to suppose that "brain genes" will be the

---

21 Chromosome 21 has a similar density, at 6.7 genes/Mb, whereas chromosome 18 is the least dense, at 4.3 genes/Mb (Nusbaum et al. 2005). The most gene-rich, chromosome 19, has 20 genes/Mb, and this is presumably the basis of its severe lethality as a trisomy, despite its small size, in early embryogenesis; cf. Figs. 19–3 and 19–6.

most likely type of gene to reside within the micro-deletions/duplications concerned.

Differing lengths of deleted or duplicated segments enable a dissection of the specific segmental contributions to components of an abnormal phenotype. A broad-brush "malformation map" can be produced from documenting the association of certain congenital defects or known syndromes with particular segmental aneusomies (Brewer et al. 1998, 1999; Carey and Viskochil 2007) (Figure 3–10). Specific malformations can be interrogated: van Karnebeek and Hennekam (1999) document imbalances associated with congenital heart disease; Tyshchenko et al. (2009) have assembled a brain list; Marcelis et al. (2011) record chromosomal segments associated with anorectal malformations; and we have undertaken phenotype mapping studies with respect to epilepsy (Singh et al. 2002a) and to kidney defects (Amor et al. 2003). Catelani et al. (2009) have searched for molecular imbalances in children with syndromic deafness. The chromosome regions thus illuminated may serve as candidate regions for the discovery of culprit genes. Note that a one-to-one connection between a deleted/duplicated segment and a specific trait cannot necessarily be drawn; and, for example, we have proposed that the particular nervous system malformation of periventricular nodular heterotopia might be an epiphenomenon accompanying a number of microdeletion syndromes, rather than the direct consequence of specific segmental imbalances (van Kogelenberg et al. 2010).

Looking at segments as a whole is, as mentioned, to take a broad-brush approach. But bear in mind that an aneuploid segment of interest is of course a length of DNA, typically containing a number of protein-coding genes, possibly as few as one, or indeed perhaps none; in the latter case, noncoding DNA may contain regulatory elements that influence activity of genes elsewhere. In those segments in which a single major locus is involved, such as the *PMP22* gene of Charcot-Marie-Tooth disease, a (relatively) simple one-to-one genotype-phenotype relationship may apply, and the other loci resident within the segment are noncontributory. Many imbalances, however, involve a number of phenocontributory loci; or in other words, a number of loci within the segment may be dosage-sensitive. Several authors have collected particular cases from their own experience and from the literature. As the data from cohorts of cases are brought together, we may be able to tease out the individual genes, or regulatory elements, responsible for the different components of an abnormal phenotype. As an example of a multigene pathogenesis, Engels et al. (2012) studied five patients with molecular-defined deletions at 14q32.3, refining the phenotype map, and they hone down to a region containing just seven known genes, which may be assumed, in total, to produce the phenotype as defined by them. The concept of genes acting "in total," or perhaps better said, "in concert," is addressed by Carvalho et al. (2014) in their review of the 17p13 deletion (p. 301). They studied the small number of genes within this segment, and judged the relative roles of these genes in determining one particular aspect of the phenotype of this syndrome (microcephaly); they propose there to be functional interconnections (that is, epistasis) between some of these genes (Figure 3–11). The end result of this interaction may be a "second-level," or higher-level, effect upon the phenotype; in other words, the whole may be different from the sum of the individual parts. Surely, similar scenarios apply rather widely in the generality of the chromosomal syndromes.

For the most part, the clinical states due to chromosomal imbalance are fixed and static. Structural defects such as a cardiac septal defect, or facial dysmorphism, are not progressive (although they may be evolving) conditions: They were established during embryogenesis and fetal development and, in essence, and unless surgically repaired, will stay that way. They may, of course, set the stage for consequential progressive change, such as a urinary tract defect that has back-pressure effects upon a kidney, affecting renal function; but this is a secondary factor. The brain, the most vulnerable organ, is similarly fixed in terms of its underlying anatomy, and chromosome disorders would not, as a general rule, be described as neurodegenerative. The most notable exception to that rule is the long-recognized dementia that typically commences around age 40 years in Down syndrome, and which reflects the effects of a triple dose of the amyloid precursor protein gene on chromosome 21, with a gradual accumulation in the brain of the abnormal protein.

It is an obvious point, but worth restating: The defect in these aneuploid states involves too much or too little of what is *normal* chromosome material. The "third" chromosome in standard trisomy 21 is a perfectly normal chromosome 21, with a perfectly normal complement of chromosome 21 genes. How, therefore, could it be that an additional amount of normal genetic message leads to

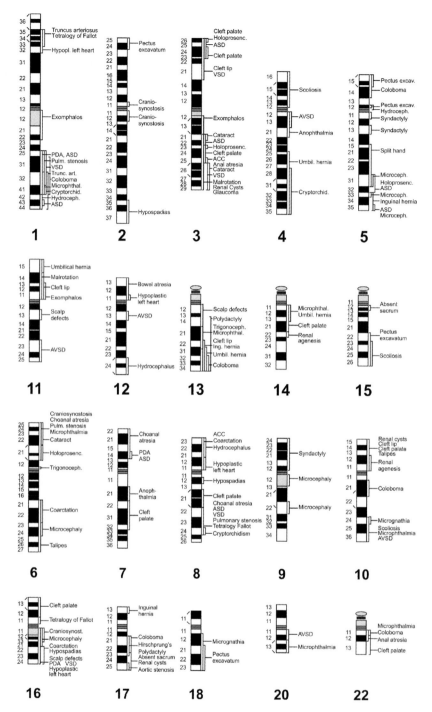

FIGURE 3–10 A duplication-malformation correlation map. Some chromosomal regions, in the duplicated state, are particularly associated with certain types of malformation. Presumably, these regions harbor genes that have roles in the formation of these particular organs. Other regions (including all of chromosome 19) are unrepresented, and some of these may contain "triplo-lethal genes." ACC, agenesis of the corpus callosum; ASD, atrial septal defect; AVSD, atrioventricular septal defect; PDA, patent ductus arteriosus; VSD, ventricular septal defect. A similar map has been drawn for deletions (Brewer et al. 1998). In a somewhat similar vein, autism-susceptible copy number variant loci have been mapped (Menashe et al. 2013; Fig. 17–2).

Source: From Brewer et al. (1999), A chromosomal duplication map of malformations: Regions of suspected haplo- and triplo-lethality—and tolerance of segmental aneuploidy—in humans, *Am J Hum Genet* 64: 1702–1708. Courtesy C. Brewer and D. R. FitzPatrick, and with the permission of the University of Chicago Press.

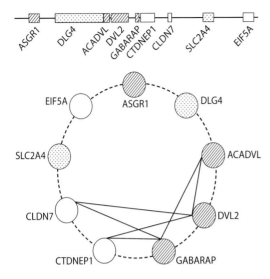

FIGURE 3–11   The17p13 deletion syndrome: effect of individual loci upon head size, and interaction of genes within this region. *Above,* gene map with nine loci within the deletion segment depicted. Cross-hatched locus, severe impact upon phenotype (microcephaly); dotted locus, moderate effect upon phenotype; open locus, no apparent effect. *Below,* proposed interaction between some of these loci, as inferred from zebrafish study.

Source: From Carvalho et al., Dosage changes of a segment at 17p13.1 lead to intellectual disability and microcephaly as a result of complex genetic interaction of multiple genes, *Am J Hum Genet* 95:565–578, 2014. Courtesy C. M. B. Carvalho and J. R. Lupski, and with the permission of Elsevier.

an abnormal interpretation of that message? How is dosage sensitivity mediated? This is one of the great remaining unanswered questions of biology, which we touch upon (no more than that) in Chapter 13.

THE SEX CHROMOSOMES

Sex chromosome imbalances need to be considered separately. Any X chromosomes in excess of one are genetically inactivated. Thus, indicating the inactivated X in lowercase, normal females are 46,Xx; normal males are 46,XY; Turner females are 45,X; Klinefelter males are 47,XxY; and other X aneuploidies are 47,Xxx, 48,Xxxx, 48,XxYY, 49,XxxxY, and 49,Xxxxx. As for the Y chromosome, its active genetic material is confined to only a small segment, these genes being mostly related to sex determination and testicular function. Thus, despite the presence of one or more whole X or Y chromosomes in excess in the 47-, 48-, and 49-chromosome states,

in utero survival remains possible. Indeed, for 47,XXX, 47,XXY, and 47,XYY, survival from conception is apparently uncompromised. Gonadal development in X aneuploid males is particularly affected, and intellectual function is jeopardized to a mild or moderate or severe extent in the $n \geq 47$ states in both sexes. The cognitive compromise may reflect, inter alia, an influence upon normal cortical asymmetries in the brain (Lin et al. 2015). The severe language disorder in one of the polysomic states, 49,XXXXY, may be due at least in part to poor development of the white matter tract from the language area (Broca's area) of the frontal cortex to the premotor cortex (Dhakar et al. 2016). Monosomy X, in contrast, has a high in utero lethality, although the small fraction surviving to term as females with Turner syndrome show, in contrast, a remarkably mild phenotype.

PHENOCOPIES

Similar phenotypes may flow from different genotypes. "Pseudotrisomy 13" may be an autosomal recessive condition (Amor and Woods 2000). The expression "DiGeorge syndrome" refers to an ensemble of signs that characterize the 22q11 deletion. Somewhat similar clinical pictures can be seen in deletions of 10p13 and of 4q34.2. Syndromes resembling Silver-Russell syndrome, Prader-Willi syndrome, and Angelman syndrome, but due to other chromosomal imbalances, are described, and some examples are noted in Chapters 14 and 15.

THE MOSAIC STATE

Whether mosaicism matters depends upon which tissue, and how much of that tissue, is abnormal. If a majority of the soma is chromosomally abnormal, then naturally the phenotype is likely to be abnormal. If only a tiny fraction of some tissue were involved, in which the aneuploidy would have essentially no effect—if, for example, some of the bony tissue of the distal phalanx of the left little toe were trisomic 21, and the rest of the person 46,N— it would never be known. Indeed, as mentioned above, possibly everyone has mosaicism, essentially harmlessly, in certain tissues or organs. However, in regard to disease, a very minor degree of mosaicism could still be important, if a crucial tissue carried the imbalance. An abnormal chromosome confined to tissues of, say, a localized area or cell type in one part of the brain, could theoretically cause neurological dysfunction.[22] Abnormality involving a gonad or part of a gonad ("gonadal mosaicism") could lead to a child being conceived with that aneuploidy, as discussed above. Mosaicism confined to extraembryonic tissue may be without phenotypic effect, although it can certainly cause anxiety if it produces an abnormal test result at prenatal diagnosis: This is confined placental mosaicism (CPM). CPM may exist unbeknownst in pregnancies producing normal infants, as Lestou et al. (2000) showed in a study of 100 placentas, with five revealing CPM for trisomies 2, 4, 12, 13, and 18. Mosaicism may frequently be observed at the IVF laboratory in the early cleavage embryo, and of spectacular degree, with different cells having different aneuploidies—a state of affairs that becomes very relevant in preimplantation genetic diagnosis (Chapter 22).

Mosaicism for a Full Aneuploidy

As a general principle, an individual with an aneuploid line in only some tissues is likely to have a less severe but qualitatively similar phenotype to someone with the nonmosaic aneuploidy. The ascertainment of these individuals is biased: Those with a more obvious phenotypic defect are, naturally, more likely to be detected. Mosaic Down syndrome—47,+21/46,N—can be less obvious than standard trisomy 21, and with a lesser compromise of intellectual function (Papavassiliou et al. 2015). The existence of 46,N cells in some of the brain tissue presumably has a moderating effect. Some aneuploidies can only, or almost only, exist in the mosaic state, the nonmosaic form being lethal in utero. Examples of this are 47,+8/46,N and 47,+9/46,N mosaicism. If the distribution of the aneuploid cell line is asymmetric, body shape may be asymmetric, generally with the hypoplasia present in regions of aneuploidy. De Ravel et al. (2001) described hemifacial microsomia (one side of the face being underdeveloped) and other body asymmetry in two children with autosomal mosaicism, one for trisomy 9 and the other trisomy 22. The child with 47,XY,+22/46,XY had 9/10 cells +22 on skin fibroblasts from the arm on the right (underdeveloped) side, compared with 5/11 on the left arm (the child's blood karyotype was 46,XY). Molecular analysis

supported there having been a postzygotic anaphase lag that had produced the 46,XY line from an initially 47,XY,+22 conception. Niessen et al. (2005) studied in some detail a girl with three shades of skin pigmentation—hypopigmented, normally pigmented, and hyperpigmented ("cutis tricolor")—following the lines of Blaschko (see next section). She karyotyped 45,X on blood, and 47,XX,+7 on skin biopsied from the darker skin. A surprising case is that of Greally et al. (1996): a child with mosaic trisomy 16, a cardiac malformation, and otherwise (barring a unilateral simian crease) not dysmorphic, and her neurodevelopmental progress has been quite normal. One might suppose (but could not prove) that the trisomic cell line was confined in distribution and excluded the brain.

Mosaicism excluding the bone marrow will give a normal blood karyotype, and vice versa, mosaicism confined to marrow would be seen on routine peripheral blood analysis but not on other samplings; mosaic trisomy 8 may provide examples in both directions. Examples of presumed very low-level trisomy mosaicism have come to light through prenatal diagnosis, such as trisomy 13 mosaicism in an apparently normal child with 1 cell out of 400 on cord blood (Delatycki et al. 1998). In sex chromosome mosaicism, fertility can exist when otherwise infertility is the rule—for example, in "formes frustes" of Turner syndrome with 45,X/46,XX and of Klinefelter syndrome with 47,XXY/46,XY.

Mosaicism for a Structural Rearrangement

Mosaicism for a structural rearrangement—a translocation, an inversion, a deletion, or a duplication—is rare, but it may be less rare than generally recognized. Kovaleva and Cotter (2016) reviewed 104 cases from the literature, either balanced or unbalanced. In the experience of one Sydney laboratory, two cases of unbalanced translocation mosaicism were seen among 75,000 karyotypes from 1989 to 2013. One was a normal woman presenting with recurrent miscarriage, with 46,XX,der(6)t(6;8)(q27;q22.1)/46,XX; and the other a globally delayed infant with 46,XY,der(22),t(14;22)(q32.1;q13.3)/46,XY (Dalzell et al. 2013). With an

---

22 Mosaic aneuploidy of the brain arising in prenatal or postnatal life may be a basis of neurological disease, having somewhat of a parallel with the evolution of some cancers (Rosenkrantz and Carbone 2017); but here we are considering mosaicism generated in early embryonic life and established ab initio over the period of intrauterine brain development. Perhaps twenty-first century technology will devise a "functional cytogenomic MRI scan" that could map out brain regions with an aneuploid chromosomal complement!

unbalanced karyotype, the broad (indeed, obvious) rule applies, that the mosaic form is likely to be less severe than the nonmosaic form. Pigmentary skin anomaly is a notable and clinically useful phenotypic trait that can characterize this type of unbalanced mosaicism, the important categories being hypomelanosis of Ito (Figure 3–12), linear and whorled nevoid hypermelanosis, and "phylloid" (leaf-like) pigmentary disturbance (Vreeburg and van Steensel 2012). The distribution of the abnormal cells in hypomelanosis of Ito, and thus of dyspigmentation, follows the lines of Blaschko, and Magenis et al. (1999) use the expression "Blaschkolinear malformation complex." Asymmetry is a further clinical pointer (Woods et al. 1994). "Functional mosaicism" for a structural rearrangement is exemplified by the X-autosome translocation in which different regions of the body have differing ratios of inactivation of the translocation and the normal X, and this, also, can lead to hypomelanosis of Ito (Hatchwell et al. 1996). Martin et al. (2016) studied mosaicism for a del(20p), chr20:80,928-1,659,921, in a child with speech delay and borderline dysmorphology. They proposed a sequence whereby the normal 20 was used as a template to "repair" the deleted chromosome in one cell, the descendants of which then generated a normal cell line, and thus attenuating the del(20p) clinical picture.

An interesting category of mosaicism for a structural rearrangement is that in which two lines

of opposite imbalance coexist, with or without a normal cell line as well. Here, the error must have happened at a very early stage, and quite possibly, in those cases lacking a normal cell line, at the very first mitosis of the zygote. Such a case is described in Morales et al. (2007a), who analyzed a boy with the karyotype at birth of 46,XY,del(7q)/46,XY,dup(7q), although by age 12–14 months, the deletion cell line had disappeared, at least from blood and exfoliated urinary epithelial cells. Presumably, the karyotype at conception was 46,XY, but then the two chromosome 7 homologs underwent an unequal exchange of q21.1q31.3 material, generating, in the two daughter cells from the first mitosis, the deletion and duplication lineages. If, for example, the error occurred one division later, at one of the two second mitotic divisions, a normal cell line might be retained, according to which progeny cells then came to comprise the inner cell mass.

TISSUE SAMPLING IN THE DETECTION OF MOSAICISM

As already noted, mosaicism can, in theory, be very widespread, and the distribution of the different cell lines can vary considerably. Analysis of tissues other than blood can clarify the picture: readily accessible tissues such as buccal mucosal cells and urinary epithelial cells, and infrequently available material from post-termination or postmortem studies. Kingston et al. (1993) described a fetal study in which several tissues taken post-termination had various fractions of mosaicism for an additional abnormal chromosome, including 88% of brain cells, while only 3% of amniotic fluid cells and no cells from a sample of fetal blood had the abnormal chromosome. Reddy et al. (1999) studied an intellectually disabled woman with mosaicism for an "add(3)," whose blood karyotype proved to be 46,XX,der(3)t(3;14)(q29;q31)/46,XX. They showed that 86% of buccal cells contained the der(3), while 14% were normal; this ratio was very similar to that of the peripheral blood, which was 83:17. The issue is no less problematic with microarray. Pal et al. (2014) studied a man with Charcot-Marie-Tooth neuropathy who had presented to the genetic clinic with his pregnant wife. On blood, he had the expected 17p12 microduplication (p. 327), but also two different 12p microduplications, a larger (6.8 Mb) and a smaller (0.5 Mb). The smaller of these duplications was also seen on skin microarray, but not the larger. Finally, FISH on skin showed a single cell out of 35 with the

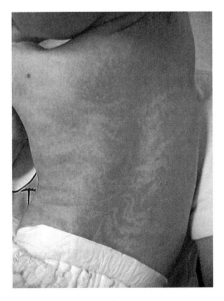

FIGURE 3–12   Hypomelanosis of Ito in a child with mosaicism 46,XX,dup(3)(q26.3qter)/46,XX.

larger 12p duplication. (Incidentally, this case also exemplifies the problem of unexpected microarray discoveries and how one might judge their clinical relevance: p. 383.)

Gonadal (and Somatic-Gonadal) Mosaicism

The classical view is that gametes with a chromosomal abnormality are typically produced by 46,N parents, whose gonads are chromosomally normal. The abnormality is presumed to have arisen at meiosis and to have affected only the gamete(s) arising from that single meiosis. If, however, an abnormality had arisen during formation of a germ cell prior to the onset of meiosis, an abnormal cell line could become established and occupy a part of the gonad or gonads (and as rehearsed above). This is *gonadal mosaicism*. If the abnormality arose in embryogenesis prior to the differentiation of the germ cell line, the soma may also be involved: This is *somatic-gonadal mosaicism*,[23] and in this context, typically a low-level somatic mosaicism, such that the parental phenotype is little, if any, overtly disturbed.

Gonadal mosaicism can also arise due to "correction" of an initially trisomic conception (Figure 3–8c). The classic example is low-level mosaic trisomy 21, in which a 47,+21 embryo at a very early postzygotic stage discards the extra chromosome in a cell, thus giving a 46,N lineage. This 46,N line then contributes to most tissues, and an apparently normal physical phenotype results; but the gonad is not so fortunate, as it were, and may receive a larger fraction of 47,+21 cells (Kovaleva 2010). A clinical observation supporting this conclusion is that the low-level mosaic mothers (who had presented due to their having had a nonmosaic Down syndrome child) are of a typical maternal age range, whereas *their* mothers—the *grand*mothers of the Down syndrome children—were of older maternal age at the time their daughters had been born. This is consistent with their daughters having been conceived as (maternal-age-influenced) trisomy 21.[24]

Gonadal mosaicism is suspected upon the observation of a chromosomally normal couple (on blood testing) having had two children with the same abnormal karyotype. Molecular analysis can allow an inference of who is the carrier parent, such as Tosca et al. (2010) show in the family study of two children with a dup(4)(q22.2q32.3), in which the microsatellite pattern indicated a maternal origin. In Kuroda et al. (2014), even though chromosome studies on the mother were normal, a maternal origin could be assumed in two siblings with Angelman syndrome due to a chromosome 15 inversion, which had deleted (among other genes) the *UBE3A* gene (p. 199). Direct proof is provided by analysis of gametes. For example, in a case that had come to notice through an IVF clinic, Somprasit et al. (2004) report a couple having had a 21q duplication in two embryos subjected to PGD, and then showed the same duplication in 6.6% of 1,002 of the father's sperm. The abnormality was not present in his blood.

The recognition of the same abnormality in somatic tissue of a parent, albeit at low level, naturally allows the inference of somatic-gonadal mosaicism. Sachs et al. (1990) studied a mother who had had one Down syndrome child and three other trisomic 21 pregnancies, and her blood karyotype was 47,+21[3%]/46,N[97%]. Ovarian biopsies showed almost half the cells in each ovary to be 47,XX,+21. Figure 3–13 shows an example of somatic-gonadal mosaicism for a structural rearrangement. The index case was identified with a small intrachromosomal del(1) at routine prenatal diagnosis. The father was mosaic for this deletion, in 20% of lymphocytes. Of his two other children, one had normal chromosomes, and the other had the same deletion. The father is phenotypically normal, and the older child with the deletion has an IQ in the low normal range. A similar circumstance is recorded in Fan et al. (2001): A university-educated man working as a financial planner, having the blood karyotype 46,XY,dup(8)(p21.3p23.1)[6]/46,XY[24], fathered two daughters with 46,XX,dup(8) (p21.3p23.1). These girls had poor language development, clumsy motor abilities, and minor facial dysmorphism. We have seen, as have others, the phenotypically normal parent of a child with

---

23 Gametes may derive from the splanchnopleuric mesoderm, and be identifiable within this tissue in the 23- or 24-day human embryo (Fenu et al. 1993); or, they may arise from the adjacent yolk sac, as discussed above (De Felici 2013). A mutation carried in the gonad and in another or other (somatic) tissues must have arisen prior to this differentiation, and thus presumably as early as within about the first 3 weeks of postzygotic existence.

24 Intriguingly, the female embryo may engage this process of postzygotic correction more efficiently than the male, and this may explain the skewed (male excess) sex ratio in typical nonmosaic Down syndrome.

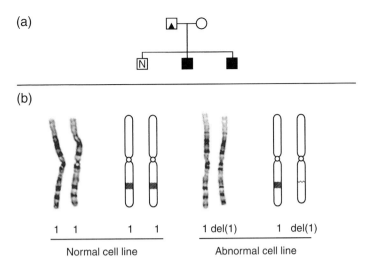

(a)

(b)

Normal cell line				Abnormal cell line			
1	1	1	1	1	del(1)	1	del(1)

FIGURE 3–13   A family exemplifying somatic-gonadal mosaicism. (*a*) Pedigree. The father had the mosaic karyotype 46,XY,del(1)(q25q31.2)[16]/46,XY[4] on lymphocyte study. Two children have the del(1) (q25q31.2) in nonmosaic state. The family was ascertained following routine prenatal diagnosis. The older sibling's development was judged, at age 5 years, to be in the low average range; height, weight, and head circumference were in the range 20–25th centiles. The father worked as an electrician. (*b*) Partial karyotype showing the father's two cell lines: two normal no. 1 chromosomes, and one normal and one deleted chromosome 1. The segment 1q25q31.2 is shown cross-hatched. (Case of G. Dawson.)

Pitt-Hopkins syndrome due to an 18q microdeletion, having him- or herself a low-level mosaicism demonstrable on blood (Figure 14–37) (Doudney et al. 2013; Kousoulidou et al. 2013) or on blood, urinary, and salivary (but not hair) cells (Steinbusch et al. 2013).

If the proportion of abnormal cells in the mosaic parent is higher or differently distributed, that parent may manifest some signs of the partial aneuploid state. The father reported in Kennedy et al. (2001) had a dup(8)(p23.1p23.1) in mosaic state, in the ratio normal:duplication of 17:8 on blood sampling, and he himself had a heart defect, as did his nonmosaic dup(8) daughter. Her defect was, however, rather more severe than her father's defect: She had a fairly complex malformation, including a right-sided aortic arch, whereas he had only a right-sided arch. Notably, the daughter was described as "achieving top grades in school," a very unusual phenotypic commentary in a child with a nonmosaic classical chromosome duplication. A mother and daughter in Freitas et al. (2012) carried a 6.2 Mb deletion at 2q36.1q36.3, mosaic (~15% on blood) in the mother, nonmosaic in the daughter. The intellectually disabled daughter presented an obvious facial dysmorphism, but in the mentally normal mother, this was very mild, and only appreciated in retrospect.

While (somatic-) gonadal mosaicism might be, in theory, common, its actual recognition is not. Nimmakayalu et al. (2013) report a case from molecular karyotyping: two macrocephalic and retarded siblings with a 399 kb 19p13.13 microdeletion, this being the only time gonadal mosaicism was recognized in a cohort of 1,800 patients studied. Campbell et al. (2014) undertook a systematic analysis of parents from a prospectively collected cohort of 100 children with a microdeletion, and they showed four parents to be mosaic for their child's deletion (the mosaicism level, on blood, was from <1 to 9%)—a quite surprising number, but perhaps more widely indicative.

Mosaicism at Prenatal Diagnosis

About 1%–2% of placentas can have a different chromosomal constitution from that of the embryo, with usually the embryo being normal and the placenta trisomic. This is "confined placental mosaicism." Thus, in 1%–2% of *chorionic villus sampling* (which can be considered a placental biopsy) there will be a potentially misleading result. Fortunately, these uncommon instances can, as a rule, be recognized as such, although not without causing some anxiety at the time. In a few confined placental aneuploidies, the function of the placenta may be compromised, and fetal well-being may be affected.

Infrequently, true mosaicism is recognized at *amniocentesis*. Occasional cells with a chromosomal abnormality, if they are solitary or involving a single clone, are generally regarded as having arisen in vitro ("artifactual mosaicism"). At least most of the time, this is probably the correct interpretation. The recognition of mosaicism at *noninvasive prenatal diagnosis* will be dependent upon the fraction of aneuploid cells. We consider mosaicism at prenatal diagnosis in detail in Chapter 21.

QUALITATIVE IMBALANCE

The idea that abnormality could be due to unequal parental contributions of an overall correct amount of chromosome material seemed most remarkable in 1980 when Engel first made the suggestion and coined the expression "uniparental disomy." It came to be accepted fact. The two disorders that, par excellence, exemplify the concept of qualitative imbalance are Prader-Willi syndrome (PWS) and Angelman syndrome (AS). The concept of genomic imprinting, discussed above, is central to an understanding of the etiology. Each syndrome is due to the nonexpression of different (but neighboring) segments within the proximal long arm of chromosome 15. A "PWS critical region" is normally expressed from only one chromosome, in this case the paternally originating chromosome. The maternal-originating region is normally inactive, and alleles in this region are not transcribed. Thus, there is a "functional monoallelism." If the paternal PWS region is absent, the maternal one cannot "fill the gap," and the consequential functional nullisomy is the root cause of PWS. An "AS critical region" exists, lying just a little distal from the PW region. Likewise, it needs only monoallelic expression for normal phenotypic function. In this case, it is the maternal region that is active, and the paternal region, having been imprinted, is inactive. If the maternal region is absent, there can be no genetic activity, and this causes the AS phenotype.

Absence of the paternal PWS region or maternal AS region can flow from two major mechanisms.

First, in UPD, the chromosome 15 from one parent is lacking, and the "correcting" presence of two copies from the other parent cannot restore a proper balance. This can be heterodisomy (the two homologs being different) or isodisomy (they are identical). Second, there can be a deletion within proximal 15q that removes a segment of chromatin containing the PWS and AS regions. These issues are dealt with in some detail in Chapter 18.

As the imprinting story has evolved, it has emerged that most of the genome appears not to be subject to imprinting.[25] For many chromosomes, and with both homologs equally genetically active, regardless of the parent of origin, UPD will have no untoward effect. Only if the UPD contributing parent should happen to be heterozygous for a recessive gene, and if this is the isodisomy category of UPD, will the child be affected, displaying the condition concerned, due to homozygosity ("isohomozygosity") for that recessive gene. Rare instances of this scenario are known.

Similar considerations may apply in the trisomies. Naturally, one parent must have contributed more than one homolog. Considering the example of Down syndrome, does the parent from whom the disomic gamete came contribute two different chromosome 21s? In other words, does the child inherit a chromosome 21 from three of the grandparents—"heterotrisomy"? Or does the parent contribute two identical (isodisomic) chromosome 21s? Whether phenotypic differences may flow from these different possibilities is quite uncertain, although Baptista et al. (2000) suggest that heterotrisomy 21 may, of itself, convey a greater risk for a specific heart malformation, ventricular septal defect, speculatively due to a damaging interaction of three subtly different protein products from a 21q "heart locus."

Uniparental disomy for the entire chromosome set—"uniparental diploidy"—has a devastating effect on development. If a conceptus has lost its maternal complement, and the paternal complement is doubled, embryonic development arrests, leaving only grossly abnormal chorionic villi comprising the pregnancy. This is a hydatidiform mole (p. 440). If a 46,XX ovum at meiosis I attempts a parthenogenetic development, a grossly disorganized mass of embryonic tissue results: an ovarian teratoma. If a triple set of chromosomes (triploidy) is present at conception, there is either a diploid

---

25 Several small segments across the karyotype show an imprinting effect, but a clinical implication of this remains uncertain (Joshi et al. 2016; and see Figure 18–2).

maternal set plus a haploid paternal set or vice versa. These different parental origins determine quite different abnormal fetal and placental phenotypes (p. 239).

SEGMENTAL UNIPARENTAL DISOMY

A mitotic mechanism that can lead to functional imbalance, if the segments exchanged are in a region subject to imprinting, is somatic recombination. The first shown example of this causing a dysmorphic syndrome is the segmental paternal uniparental disomy for 11p that underlies some Beckwith-Wiedemann syndrome, 11p being a segment that is normally maternally imprinted. In the partial UPD(pat) cell line, this segment will now be expressing biallelically at distal 11p, instead of the normal monoallelic expression. The asymmetry of body growth that may be observed in this syndrome reflects the distribution of two cell lineages: the normal biparental disomic line and the functionally imbalanced UPD(pat) line.

SPORADIC AND RECURRENT ABNORMALITIES

Chromosomally normal parents can produce abnormal gametes by nondisjunction, rearrangement, or one of the other mutational mechanisms we have discussed above. The combination of factors that causes these defects in an individual case is unknown. No convincing case has ever been made for the agency of diet, illness, chemical exposure, or "lifestyle factors" in maternal chromosome 21 meiotic nondisjunction (Chapter 24), nor is there much support from epidemiological studies (Chapter 13). Noting the similarity of Down syndrome prevalence rates worldwide, Carothers et al. (1999) comment that "the totality of published data could well be consistent with no real

variation at all, and [this] might explain why a search for environmental factors associated with Down syndrome has been so unproductive." The maternal age effect is of course important, indeed central, and any search for causes of chromosomal aneuploidy must take it into account. A plausible view is that there is a natural degeneration of the oöcyte, as we discussed above, and with reference to Figure 3–7. Simply put, eggs get older, and they show their age.

Chromosomes are plastic, dynamic entities, and cell division is a complex mechanical process; and these qualities alone may suffice to endow the vulnerability that causes human aneuploidy and rearrangement. Given the assumption that all persons with intact gametogenesis are capable of producing an abnormal gamete, one view is that it may simply be that a certain background abnormality rate is intrinsic to the human species, and that it is a chance matter whether this or that couple will have the misfortune to conceive the abnormality which, inevitably, someone has to bear.

PARENTAL PREDISPOSITION TO NONDISJUNCTION OR DELETION/DUPLICATION?

An alternative view is that some 46,XX and 46,XY people are more prone than others to produce chromosomally unbalanced gametes. An intrinsic fault, or at least a vulnerability, in the mechanism of chromosome distribution at cell division could be the basis of the rare examples of recurring defects. The synaptonemal complex gene SYPC3 (mentioned above), and the mismatch repair genes, with particular reference to MLH1 (otherwise familiar to the counselor in Lynch syndrome) and MLH3, and the related meiosis genes MSH4 and MSH5, would all be plausible candidates, in which subtle variation might affect integrity (Baarends et al.

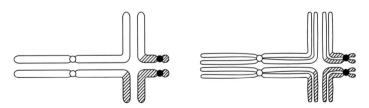

FIGURE 3–14 Chromosomes at synapsis exist as double-chromatid structures (e.g., the reciprocal translocation quadrivalent at *right*). But, for simplicity, we generally represent them with just the one chromatid (*left*).

2001; Lenzi et al. 2005; Terribas et al. 2010). A case for variation at the methyltransferase *DNMT3B* locus is tenuous (Jaiswal et al. 2015). The product of the *PRDM9* gene is a regulator of meiotic recombination, and there is slight evidence that a variant form might predispose to microdeletion, specifically the 7q11.23 of Williams syndrome (Borel et al. 2012). Given the complexity of the apparatus and process of cell division, it is logical that error-causing mutants in the controlling genes (whether or not this might include any of the aforementioned) would exist. Whether there might be milder alleles at postulated cell-division or recombination loci, which could more widely be the cause of occasional nondisjunction or del/dup, remains a matter for speculation. Nevertheless, a geneticist could scarcely ignore that there might exist subtle genetic variation potentially setting the stage for chromosomal aberration.

A Note on the Diagrams. Following the progress of rearranged chromosomes during meiosis is not easy, so we have taken some liberties in simplifying the diagrams. Most of these diagrams depict the synapsing chromosomes at meiosis with just one chromatid; of course, the chromosome has actually replicated at this point and exists as a double chromatid entity (Figure 3–14).

4

DERIVING AND USING
A RISK FIGURE

RISK IS A CENTRAL CONCEPT in genetic counseling. By *risk,* we mean the probability that a particular event will happen. Probability is conventionally measured with a number ranging from 0 to 1. A probability (p) of zero means never, and a probability of 1 means always. For two or more mutually exclusive possible outcomes, the individual probabilities sum to 1.0 (or 100%). Thus, someone who is a heterozygote for a particular rearrangement might, in any given pregnancy, have a probability of 0.10 (10%) of having an abnormal child and a probability of 0.90 (90%) of having a normal child. We may speak in terms of risks of *recurrence* or of *occurrence:* the probability that an event will happen again, or that it will happen for the first time. Risk can also be presented as *odds:* the ratio of two mutually exclusive probabilities. The odds for the hypothetical heterozygote just mentioned would be 9:1 in favor of a normal child.

The work *risk* has two important meanings in the English language. First, there is the scientific sense of probability that we already discussed. Second, as most people use the word, it conveys a sense of exposure to danger. Our hypothetical heterozygote runs the risk that an unfortunate outcome may occur (an abnormal child, or an abnormal result at prenatal diagnosis). In the genetic counseling clinic, these meanings of risk coalesce in some ways, to which the counselor needs to be sensitive. We might instead use such everyday words as *chance* or *likelihood,* which have no negative connotation, to refer to the fortunate outcome of normality. The words *fortunate* and *unfortunate* are also chosen deliberately: The wanted or the unwanted event will occur entirely by chance, analogous to tossing a coin, throwing a dice, or being dealt a card.

Different Types of Risk Figure

Geneticists arrive at risk figures in a number of ways (Harper 2010), two of which, empiric and Mendelian, have particular application to cytogenetics.

1. *Empiric risks.* In the great majority of chromosomal situations, no clear theory exists from which

a risk figure can be derived, and one must observe what has happened previously in (as far as one can judge) the same situation in other families, and make an extrapolation to the family in question. Empiric risks thus appeal to experience, and they only *estimate* the intrinsic, true probability. The data may be available in the literature record or in specific databases; or the counselor may need to derive a "private estimate" from an analysis of the client's family. The risk estimate has a greater or lesser degree of precision, depending on how much data had been accumulated, upon which the estimate is based.

2. *Mendelian risks.* If a clear model of inheritance is known, risk figures derived by reference to that theory may be used. In practice, only Mendel's law of segregation is applied in this context. When a pair of homologous chromosomes segregates at meiosis, it is a random matter which chromosome enters the gamete that will produce the conceptus. Each has an equal chance: a probability of 0.5. Thus, a parent who carries a microdeletion 16p11.2 has a 50/50 likelihood to transmit this chromosome to a child, a 1:1 segregation. This is assumed to be a *true* risk, not an estimate: It is 0.5 exactly.

Consider, for example, the common situation of a young couple having had a child with Down syndrome. Nothing is known about nondisjunction that could provide a theoretical model on which to base a recurrence risk figure. We therefore use empiric data—that is, information obtained from surveying large numbers of other such families. It may be observed, for example, that in these families about 1 pregnancy in 100, subsequent to the index case of Down syndrome, produced another child with Down syndrome. Formally expressed, this is a segregation analysis. From this rate of 1/100 we can derive a risk figure of 1%, which we then have as the basis for advising patients. (Actually, it is not quite as straightforward as this in Down syndrome; see Chapter 13.) Likewise for the circumstance of the parent heterozygous for a chromosomal rearrangement, the counselor can consult data that have been accumulated by workers in the field, foremost among whom, in respect of reciprocal translocations, are Stengel-Rutkowski et al. (1988), Cohen et al. (1992, 1994), and Midro et al. (2000). Since almost all reciprocal translocations are unique to one family, it is not necessarily simple to estimate a figure for a family with a "new" translocation, but an attempt can be made (see Chapter 5). On the other hand, for the Robertsonian translocations, each

type of which can generally be regarded as the same between families, extrapolation of risk figures from historical data to a current family is usually valid.

If a theoretical construct can be applied, this may allow a more precise calibration of the empiric figure. The del 17q21.31 of Koolen-de Vries syndrome (p. 302), which has a population frequency of 1/16,000, offers an example. This particular deletion may have, as a necessary but not sufficient basis for its generation, a 17q inversion encompassing the length of the deleted segment (chr17:45.6-46.1 Mb). The risk is related to the inversion status of the parents, the dimorphism referred to as H1 (normal 17q21.31 sequence, N) and H2 (inverted 17q21.31 sequence, V). Koolen et al. (2012) apply some fundamental genetic concepts, in order to tailor the risk figure according to the parental inversion genotypes, and the counselor may find it an interesting exercise to follow their reasoning. The population frequency ratio of the dimorphic forms H1 and H2 is 0.8:0.2 ($p + q = 1$). Given that a parent can be H1/H1 (NN), H1/H2 (NV), or H2/H2 (VV), the relative proportions of these genotypes will be 64:32:4 (from the classic formula $p^2 + 2pq + q^2 = 1$). Koolen et al. write this slightly differently, /25 rather than %, as

NN	$4/5 \times 4/5$	=	$16/25$
NV	$2 \times 1/5 \times 4/5$	=	$8/25$
VV	$1/5 \times 1/5$	=	$1/25$ Total $25/25$

From this, the six possible parental combinations are NN × NN, NN × NV, NN × VV, NV × NV, NV × VV, and VV × VV, in approximate ratios 41:41:5:10:2.5:0.5. Or, more precisely stated, Koolen et al. continue thus:

1	NN × NN	$16/25 \times 16/25$	=	$256/625$
2	NN × NV	$2 \times 16/25 \times 8/25$	=	$256/625$
3	NN × VV	$2 \times 16/25 \times 1/25$	=	$32/625$
4	NV × NV	$8/25 \times 8/25$	=	$64/625$
5	NV × VV	$2 \times 8/25 \times 1/25$	=	$16/625$
6	VV × VV	$1/25 \times 1/25$	=	$1/625$
			Total	$625/625$

We now ask, What is the risk to have a recurrent child with the 17q21.31 deletion, in each of these six couple circumstances? Let a be the risk if one parent is H1/H2 (NV) heterozygous, and let $2a$ be the risk if one parent is H2/H2 (VV) homozygous, whence the relative risks per couple r are

$$
\begin{array}{llll}
r_1 & \text{NN} \times \text{NN} & \rightarrow & 0 \\
r_2 & \text{NN} \times \text{NV} & \rightarrow & a \\
r_3 & \text{NN} \times \text{VV} & \rightarrow & 2a \\
r_4 & \text{NV} \times \text{NV} & \rightarrow & 2a \\
r_5 & \text{NV} \times \text{VV} & \rightarrow & 3a \\
r_6 & \text{VV} \times \text{VV} & \rightarrow & 4a
\end{array}
$$

Weighting these risks according to the relative frequencies f of each couple combination, and assuming that these several risks add up to the population base of $1/16{,}000$, we have

$$
(0 \times f_1) + (a \times f_2) + (2a \times f_3 \text{ and } f_4) \\
+ (3a \times f_5) + (4a \times f_6) = 1/16{,}000
$$

And thus,

$$
a \times (256/625) + 2a \times (32/625 + 64/625) \\
+ 3a \times (16/625) \\
+ 4a \times (1/625) = 1/16{,}000
$$

whence, $a \times 500/625 = 1/16{,}000$, and $a = 1/12{,}800$.

Substituting for a, we have recurrence risks p for each couple class:

$$
\begin{array}{llll}
p_1 & \text{NN} \times \text{NN} & \rightarrow & 0 \\
p_2 & \text{NN} \times \text{NV} & \rightarrow & 1/12{,}800 \\
p_3 & \text{NN} \times \text{VV} & \rightarrow & 1/6{,}400 \\
p_4 & \text{NV} \times \text{NV} & \rightarrow & 1/6{,}400 \\
p_5 & \text{NV} \times \text{VV} & \rightarrow & 1/4{,}266 \\
p_6 & \text{VV} \times \text{VV} & \rightarrow & 1/3{,}200
\end{array}
$$

Absent a knowledge of H1/H2 status, the weighted average is $1/9{,}446$ (0.01%), about twice the population figure. Albeit that these figures are somewhat academic—differences between 0.03% (VV × VV) and 0.008% (NN × NV), versus the population figure of 0.006%, barely dent the >99.9% chance of nonrecurrence—the principle behind the exercise is to be acknowledged.

A somewhat similar approach may apply to the inverted duplication of 8p (inv dup 8p), as discussed on p. 198. An inversion polymorphism at chr8:7.6-12.3 Mb, which has a high (26%) frequency in the general population, predisposes to a misalignment during meiosis (Giglio et al. 2001). Indeed, generation of the rearrangement may only be possible in the setting of this parental inversion. However,

the absolute risk among this quarter of the (at least European) population must remain extremely low, given the rarity with which the inv dup 8p is seen, and the absence of any report of recurrence. The risk to the noncarrier may be a true 0.0%.

Hook and Cross (1982) note the importance of distinguishing between the *rate* (which may be thought of as "past tense") and the *risk* (which is "future tense"). They emphasize that although geneticists routinely extrapolate from rates in one population at one point in time, and may use these figures as risk estimates in another population and certainly at a later point in time, they should be on their guard for any evidence that a condition varies with time, geography, or ethnicity. But actually, there is little indication that any important variation exists: Chromosomal biology appears to be rather consistent throughout the human race and across the centuries.

Doing a Segregation Analysis

Segregation analysis is essentially a simple exercise. A farmer who surveys a flock of newborn lambs and notes that 3 are black and 97 are white has done a segregation analysis. In human cytogenetic segregation analysis, the exercise involves looking at a (preferably large) number of offspring of a particular category of parent: parents who carry some particular chromosome rearrangement, or those who have had a child with a chromosomal abnormality, they themselves being karyotypically normal. The proportion of these parents' children who are abnormal is noted (say, 3 out of 100), and this datum serves as the point estimate of the recurrence risk (thus, 3%).

Although segregation analysis is simple in principle, there are potential pitfalls in its application, the most important of which is *ascertainment bias*. We will deal with this problem only briefly. It is important that the counselor know of ascertainment bias, and recognize whether it has been accounted for in the published works consulted. But it is not necessary to understand the complex and sophisticated mechanics of segregation analysis in detail. The reader wishing fuller instruction is referred to Murphy and Chase (1975), Emery (1986), and Stene and Stengel-Rutkowski (1988). The classic example of ascertainment bias is that of the analysis of the sex ratio in sibships of military recruits in World War I. Adding up the numbers of brothers and sisters, there was a marked excess of males.

But of course (in 1914–1918) the recruit himself had to be male. Once he was excluded from the total in each sibship, the overall sex ratio was normal, namely 1.0. Likewise, in a cytogenetic segregation analysis, the individual whose abnormality brought the family to attention—the proband—is excluded from the calculation. That person *had* to be abnormal. Furthermore, for very many classical chromosomal scenarios, that individual's carrier parent, grandparent, and so on in a direct vertical line, had to be phenotypically normal to have been a parent. These individuals must also be excluded from an analysis of their own sibship, if that generation is available for study. Other sibships may be included in full.

These manipulations—dropping the proband and the heterozygous direct-line antecedents—are the major steps to be taken to avoid the distorting effects of ascertainment bias. Another potential methodological confounder for the aficionado is *ascertainment probability*. For example, families with more affected members may be more likely to come to medical attention, which would unduly weight the data. There are means to overcome this problem.

Family/population studies on the microdeletions, microduplications, and copy number variants (CNVs) of twenty-first-century chromosomology present a more difficult problem. Nonpenetrance and variable expressivity, and phenotypes confined to intellectual/behavioral traits, in some of mild degree, complicate the picture. Where is the threshold to be taken as affected/unaffected? The pioneers in this field are Vassos et al. (2010) and Rosenfeld et al. (2013), who compared prevalences of CNVs in affected cohorts versus a presumed normal population. The work of Vassos et al. was focused specifically on schizophrenia. Rosenfeld et al. chose 13 of the more frequently seen microdeletion/duplication syndromes and assessed penetrances, as listed in Table 4–1. We discuss these conditions in Chapter 14.

Essential to a good analysis is good data, or at least as good as possible. Some retrospective information may be uncertain. In a family translocation study, did a phenotypically abnormal great uncle who died as a child in 1930 have the "family aneuploidy"? (Old photos may be very helpful in this respect.) Some family skeletons may remain in cupboards unopened to the interviewer. Particularly in the follow-up of prenatal diagnosis results, it is important to know the endpoint of data collection of the child and how the data were collected: at birth, or until school age; by formal examination, or by anecdotal report. The investigative zeal, clinical judgment, and personal qualities of the researcher, are crucial in getting the right information, and getting it all.

Table 4–1. Penetrance Estimates for a Number of Microdeletions, Microduplications, and Copy Number Variants

REGION (LANDMARK GENE WITHIN REGION)	COPY NUMBER	PENETRANCE ESTIMATE % (95% CONFIDENCE LIMITS)
Proximal 1q21.1 (*RBM8A*)	Duplication	17.3 (10.8–27.4)
Distal 1q21.1 (*GJA5*)	Deletion	36.9 (23.0–55.0)
Distal 1q21.1 (*GJA5*)	Duplication	29.1 (16.9–46.8)
15q11.2 (*NIPA1*)	Deletion	10.4 (8.45–12.7)
16p13.11 (*MYH11*)	Deletion	13.1 (7.91–21.3)
16p12.1 (*CDR2*)	Deletion	12.3 (7.91–18.8)
Distal 16p11.2 (*SH2B1*)	Deletion	62.4 (26.8–94.4)
Distal 16p11.2 (*SH2B1*)	Duplication	11.2 (6.26–19.8)
Proximal 16p11.2 (*TBX6*)	Deletion	46.8 (31.5–64.2)
Proximal 16p11.2 (*TBX6*)	Duplication	27.2 (17.4–40.7)
17q12 (*HNF1B*)	Deletion	34.4 (13.7–70.0)
17q12 (*HNF1B*)	Duplication	21.1 (10.6–39.5)
22q11.21 (*TBX1*)	Duplication	21.9 (14.7–31.8)

Source: From Rosenfeld et al. (2013).

THE DERIVATION OF A "PRIVATE" RECURRENCE RISK FIGURE

We will demonstrate some of the previously noted principles in estimating a private recurrence risk figure for the hypothetical family depicted in Figure 4–1 and Table 4–2. Six sibships are available for analysis: one in generation II, two in generation III, and three in generation IV. We determine the segregation ratio in each. It is conventional to form a table with a row for each sibship, noting the numbers of phenotypically normal (carrier, noncarrier, unkaryotyped) and phenotypically abnormal offspring. The figures in parentheses give raw totals in these sibships, but then the proband (IV:4) and his heterozygous antecedents (II:1 and III:1) are excluded from their sibships. Thus, we have the following:

Table 4–2. Data Derived from Family in Figure 4–1

PARENT OF SIBSHIP	PHENOTYPICALLY NORMAL			
	AFFECTED	CARRIER	NON-CARRIER	UNKARYO-TYPED
I:1	0	1 (2)	2	0
II:1	1	1 (2)	0	2
II:2	0	1	0	1
III:1	2 (3)	0	1	0
III:2	0	1	0	0
III:7	0	0	1	0
Total	3	4	4	3

(Note, in passing, I:1's heterozygosity must be inferred from his wife's and children's karyotypes. It is a subtle question whether his offspring should properly be included in the analysis, which we will not pursue here.) We see that the offspring of heterozygous parents total 14, the proband and the heterozygous antecedents having been excluded. The proportion of abnormal children is 3/14 (0.21). This, then, is a point estimate of the risk for recurrence in a future pregnancy of a heterozygote. The reader should know intuitively that an estimate based on just 14 children is not going to be very precise (but not to be discarded). And what of children who died in infancy, before the family cytogenetic study has been done? Let us suppose this was the case with III:4 and 5. If there

was good evidence for their having been chromosomally abnormal, a better estimate would be 5/14 (0.36).

Genetic Heterogeneity and the Use of Empiric Risk Data

It is not necessarily valid to extrapolate from one family's experience to a prediction for another. Different factors may cause an abnormality in different families. As an obvious example, it would be misleading to "lump" all Down syndrome families to determine a recurrence risk figure. We need to "split" into the different karyotypic classes of standard trisomy, familial translocations, and de novo translocations. The standard trisomic category requires further splitting in terms of maternal age. In a unique case, a woman had three trisomy 21 conceptions and displayed a tendency to produce multiple cells with differing ("variegated") aneuploidies in at least skin, blood, and gonad (Fitzgerald et al. 1986). She required unique advice. And in reciprocal translocation families, uniqueness is the rule! It is generally reasonable (and often all that is feasible or possible) to apply a risk figure derived from the study of families with a similar, albeit not exactly identical, chromosomal arrangement. But occasionally a family is large enough for a "private" estimate of the recurrence risk to be made from the family itself. This estimate, if it is precise enough (see the later discussion of confidence limits and standard error), is the most valid to offer that family.

PREGNANCY OUTCOMES TO WHICH THE RISK FIGURES REFER

With particular reference to the situation of a parent heterozygous for a chromosomal rearrangement, risk figures are generally presented in terms of "the risk that a liveborn child would have a chromosome imbalance related to the parental translocation." The numerator is the number of aneuploid babies, and the denominator is the number of all babies. Thus, considering the example of the common t(11;22)(q23;q11) translocation (p. 87), Stengel-Rutkowski et al. (1988) accumulated data on a total of 318 births (the denominator) to carrier parents, of whom, after ascertainment correction, 9 (the numerator) had the 47,+der(22) aneuploidy; and 9/318 gives the

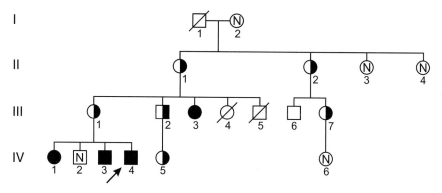

FIGURE 4–1   Hypothetical pedigree in which a chromosomal rearrangement is segregating. Filled symbol, abnormal individual with unbalanced karyotype; half-filled symbol, balanced carrier; N in symbol = 46,N. The proband is, as is conventional, indicated by an arrow.

risk expressed as a percentage, 2.8%. Separating out mothers and fathers, the respective risk figures are 3.7% (9/241) and <0.7% (0/77). For those choosing prenatal diagnosis, the risk figure of interest relates to the timing of the procedure, generally chorionic villus sampling (usually done at 10–12 weeks) and amniocentesis (15–17 weeks). In other words, they want to know how likely it is they will have to face the actuality of a decision about termination. The risk here is likely to be higher (7% in the case of the 11;22 translocation), given that some of the abnormal pregnancies would have spontaneously aborted some time after that period of gestation. Table 4–3 sets out these and other possible ways of considering risk.

Table 4–3. Different Ways of Looking at the Quantum of Reproductive Risk due to a Parent Being a Carrier of a Chromosomal Rearrangement

NUMERATOR	DENOMINATOR
Abnormal liveborn baby	All liveborns
Abnormal liveborn baby	All recognized pregnancies
Abnormal amniocentesis result (early second trimester)	All pregnancies at ~16 weeks
8–14 week miscarriage	All recognized pregnancies
Abnormal embryo on biopsy	All embryos from one in vitro fertilization procedure

Association: Coincidental or Causal?

The counselor not infrequently encounters the problem of a chromosomal "abnormality" discovered in a phenotypically abnormal individual, but in whose family others—who are quite normal—are then shown to have, apparently, exactly the same rearrangement. Does a genetic risk apply, then, to children of the carrier, to whom the same rearranged chromosome may be transmitted? From classical cytogenetics, the familial paracentric inversion is a good example. In a review of 69 probands, Price et al. (1987) list the phenotypic abnormalities that led to these individuals coming to a chromosome study. There was a collection of various clinical indications, with no consistent pattern (other than that mental retardation was frequent), and several ascertained quite by chance at prenatal diagnosis. By definition, one parent carries the same inversion; and if the net is widened, often other relatives do so as well (Groupe de Cytogénéticiens Français 1986a). In this context, and provided of course that the carrier relatives are phenotypically normal, one would reach the conclusion that the chromosome rearrangement was balanced, with no functional compromise of the genome, and that it was coincidence that led to its discovery (Romain et al. 1983).

But when some very unusual clinical picture is associated with a paracentric inversion that is rare or previously undescribed (as many inversions are), some writers are skeptical of coincidence and propose a causal link (Fryns et al. 1994; Urioste et al. 1994). Similarly, Wenger et al. (1995), noting the coincidence of children with an apparently balanced familial translocation, and being phenotypically abnormal, wrote that "the chance that two rare events in the same individual are unrelated seems unlikely to us." Here, there is a risk of deception due to "Kouska's fallacy"—Kouska was a fictional nineteenth-century philosopher who concluded that the combination of unlikely events that led to his parents meeting was too implausible to believe, and that therefore he himself could not exist (Lubinsky 1986). As does Lubinsky, we must insist on the point: The proband *had* to be phenotypically abnormal, and the coexistence of a subsequently discovered different abnormal event (the karyotype) need not be seen as necessarily remarkable. (Having made that point, we cannot, nevertheless, discount the alternative interpretation that these authors may actually have concluded correctly.)

A similar question arises when two rare karyotypes are seen in the same family, or when one individual has more than one aneuploidy. A double aneuploidy such as Klinefelter plus Down syndrome, 48,XXY,+21, could be interpreted as two separately arising nondisjunctions, but each occurring on the basis of the same underlying predisposing factor (such as maternal age). The two conditions occur together more often than the product of the frequency of each singly, which would be consistent with that interpretation. Alternatively, if the XXY component could be shown to reflect a paternal meiotic error, while the trisomy 21 was of maternal origin, then the association could be seen as coincidental. Two different types of abnormality, such as Klinefelter plus Prader-Willi syndrome, a handful of cases of which have been published (Nowaczyk et al. 2004), might also be judged to reflect two unrelated abnormal events, at least for the deletional form of Prader-Willi syndrome, given that the mechanisms leading to nondisjunction and to deletion are quite different. The prior probability of two abnormal karyotypes coinciding might be a very small figure ($1/2000 \times 1/15,000 = 1/30,000,000$ in the foregoing example); but recalling that the range of abnormal karyotypes is very wide, it should not necessarily be seen as reflecting some extraordinary predisposition when two abnormalities are diagnosed in the one individual or family. Coincidences do happen, and interesting coincidences are publishable (Schneider et al. 2004).

In the molecular era, the matter of CNVs brings the question of causality into a sharp focus, albeit that some of the answers may be less than sharp. A small molecular duplication, for example, that might at first sight appear to be a plausible candidate as explanation for a child's abnormal phenotype, may be judged less likely as culpable if the same observation is made on the DNA sample from a parent. And yet, in the complexity that CNVs present, there may yet remain a possibility that such a duplication could contribute to abnormality, when existing on a different genetic background. In other words, and as discussed above, a particular CNV may be nonpenetrant in a parent but penetrant in the child—a concept that hitherto has had little relevance in clinical cytogenetics. We can expect that CNV associations, and their causing, or not, of abnormality, will continue to be an active area of study (see Chapter 17).

Presentation of a Risk Figure

A risk figure is a probability statement, and it should be presented as such to the counselee in everyday language—for example, "There is a 50/50 chance for such and such an event" and "The risk for such and such to happen is around 1 chance in 10." The raw probability figure may not of itself be sufficient, and it is a test of the counselor's skill to interpret figures so as to provide empathic guidance rather than presumptuous direction. Loaded interpretative comments such as "The risk is quite high that . . ." or "There is only a small chance that . . ." should be used with great care. The perception of a risk figure as high or low may vary greatly according to an individual's personality and life experiences, and the way he or she uses the language of numbers; the very act of discussing the risk may help the client see it in a less threatening light (Kessler and Levine 1987). Some counselors use diagrams with cartoons showing a crowd of 100 people, with the risk fraction shown in a different color.

Dealing with risk advice in a pregnancy, in particular, can be anxiety inducing. Nagle et al. (2009) examined the views of 294 Australian mothers in the postpartum period and recorded preferences for how these women felt, in retrospect, that a risk of having a child with Down syndrome might best have been conveyed. The choices were as follows, with the fractions of the women choosing each category shown:

1. As a number in percentage, such as "1%" or "0.05%"	13%
2. In words such as "no increased risk" or "increased risk"	13%
3. As numbers such as "1 in 10" or "1 in 1000"	37%
4. In words such as "high risk" or "low risk"	19%
5. Other (please specify)	0%
A combination of the above	18%

None of these stood out as an obvious best, to help the counselor decide on the most appropriate approach. People are different!

And people can see the same risk from different positions. For example, older women having an increased age-related risk (say, 1 in 100) for a child with Down syndrome may decide against an amniocentesis if a screening test gives a risk (say, 1 in 200) that is above the cut-off for access to amniocentesis (1 in 250) but lower than their "starting figure"; whereas a younger woman with an age-related risk of, for example, 1 in 500 is likely to opt for amniocentesis if she were to have the same 1 in 200 result from the screening test (Beekhuis et al. 1994).

Responses to risk figures might not always be what we, as scientifically trained professionals, would necessarily consider objective. This, Dear Reader, is in the nature of the human condition! Urquhart (2016), a folklorist, gives her own perspective on the counseling she received during the course of prenatal diagnosis (in this case, not for a chromosome condition but, rather, for a Mendelian disorder, albinism). She had

> always had an insatiable urge to know the future. Coupled with a keen interest in the supernatural—as a folklore scholar and as a layperson—this has led me to forms of soothsaying like tarot cards and

runes but also to the people who trade in clairvoyance.

When she was about to hear the results of her amniocentesis test, she writes, "First, she [the counselor] tells me the odds. But the numbers never meant anything to me. I put as much faith in those predictions as I might in a palm reading. This child will either have albinism, or he will not." In the event—to her initial consternation, but then fierce acceptance—he did not.

PRECISION OF THE RISK FIGURE

As noted above, theoretical risk figures are true, and empiric risk figures are estimates; the former are exact, and the latter are not. For an empiric figure we have a point estimate (e.g., 10%) and a likely range (e.g., 5%–15%) of where the risk actually is. The more data that have been gathered, the more accurate the estimate, and the narrower the likely range; and the more confidently, therefore, can the counselor present the figure. The likely range can be measured in different ways. The standard error, which formally measures the precision of the estimate, can be used to give a sense of the region within which the true risk can realistically be considered to lie. The 95% confidence limits define the broad range that very probably ($p = 0.95$) encompasses the true risk. Formulae to determine these parameters are set out in Appendix C.

PART TWO

PARENT OR CHILD WITH A CHROMOSOMAL ABNORMALITY

5

AUTOSOMAL RECIPROCAL TRANSLOCATIONS

RECIPROCAL TRANSLOCATIONS ARE COMMON, and every counselor can expect to see translocation families. The usual form is the simple, or two-way, reciprocal translocation: Only two chromosomes, usually autosomes, are involved, with one breakpoint in each. It is this category we consider in this chapter. The special cases of translocations involving sex chromosomes, and of complex translocations, are dealt with in separate chapters.

The translocation heterozygote (carrier) may have a risk to have a child who would be intellectually and physically abnormal due to a "segmental aneusomy." Typically, the imbalance is due to a segment of one of the participating chromosomes being duplicated, and a segment of the other chromosome being deleted. This confers a partial trisomy and a concomitant partial monosomy. A few translocations are associated with a high risk, as much as 20%, or very rarely up to 50%, to have an abnormal child. Many translocations imply an intermediate level of risk, in the region of 5%–10%. Some carriers have

a low risk, 1% or less; but the woman who is a carrier, or the partner of a male carrier, may have a high miscarriage rate. Others imply, apparently, no risk to have an abnormal child, but the likelihood of miscarriage is high. Yet others, discovered fortuitously, seem to be of no reproductive significance, with carriers having no difficulties in conceiving or carrying pregnancies and having normal children. The counselor needs to distinguish these different functional categories of translocation, in order to provide each family with tailor-made advice.

BIOLOGY

Simple reciprocal translocations arise when a two-way exchange of material takes place between two chromosomes. The process of formation follows the physical apposition of a segment of each chromosome, which may have been promoted by the presence in each segment of a similar DNA sequence. A break occurs in one arm of each chromosome, and the portions of chromosome material distal to

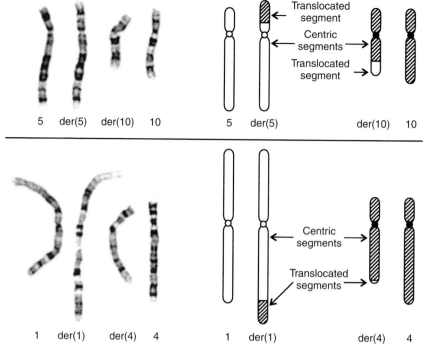

FIGURE 5-1   Reciprocal translocations demonstrating (*above*) double-segment and (*below*) single-segment exchange. The translocations are t(5;10)(p13;q23.3) and t(1;4)(q44;q31.3). (Cases of M. A. Leversha and N. A. Adams.)

the breakpoints switch positions. The distal portions exchanged are the *translocated segments*; the rest of the chromosome (which includes the centromere) is the *centric segment*. The rearranged chromosome is called a *derivative* (der) chromosome. It is identified according to which centromere it possesses, as in the der(5) and der(10) depicted in Figure 5–1. When no loss or perturbation of genetic material occurs—in other words, the translocation is balanced—the phenotype of the heterozygote is normal, other things being equal. On classical cytogenetics, approximately 1 person in 500 is a reciprocal translocation heterozygote (Jacobs et al. 1992). The translocation may have arisen de novo in the person, or it may be widespread throughout a family, with many carriers, and sometimes of centuries-long duration. Koskinen et al. (1993) trace a t(12;21) in western Finland back to a couple born in 1752.

When one of the translocated segments is very small and comprises only the telomeric cap of a chromosome arm—and thus we suppose contains no genes—this is regarded as being, effectively, a *single-segment* exchange. The t(1;4) translocation shown in Figure 5–1, involving a substantial piece of chromosome 4 long arm exchanging positions with the terminal tip of a chromosome 1 long arm, exemplifies single-segment exchange. On the other hand, when both translocated segments are of substantial size, we refer to this as a *double-segment*[1] exchange. The translocation shown in Figure 5–1 between a chromosome 5 and a chromosome 10, with breakpoints in about the mid-short arm of chromosome 5 and a little below the middle of the chromosome 10 long arm, is an example of a double-segment exchange. The translocation involving breakpoints right at, or actually within, the centromere, with an exchange of entire arms, is a particular and rare type

---

1 There is scope for confusion in the use of these terms: Of course, all reciprocal exchanges, by definition, involve two segments. A true single-segment exchange—that is, a one-way translocation—is generally considered not to exist, in that a segment of chromosome cannot attach to an intact telomere, although there are rare exceptions to this rule. The distinction begins to break down when a translocated segment is very small (subtelomeric) but could still contain genes. Be this as it may, the terms double- and single-segment exchange, used knowledgeably, serve a practical purpose.

of double-segment exchange known as a *whole-arm* translocation (Vázquez-Cárdenas et al. 2007).

DETAILS OF MEIOTIC BEHAVIOR

At meiosis I in the primary gametocyte, the four chromosomes with segments in common come together as a foursome: a *quadrivalent*. To match homologous segments, the four chromosomes must form a cross-shaped configuration. This is most clearly seen when the chromosomes are at the pachytene stage (Figure 5–2). As meiosis progresses, the four components of the quadrivalent release their points of attachment except at the tips of the chromosome arms, and they form a ring; if attachment fails, or if one of the terminal pairings release, a chain forms instead of a ring (Oliver-Bonet et al. 2004). With breakdown of the nuclear envelope, spindles forming at each pole of the cell can track to the equator and seek attachment to the centromeres. A cellular motor comes into play, and the chromosome travels to one or other pole. According to which spindle attaches to which centromere—and this may in part be influenced by the configuration of the ring or chain—the distribution of the four homologs to the two daughter gametocytes is determined. Which homologs go to which pole is referred to as *segregation*. The expression *2:2 segregation* describes two chromosomes going to one daughter cell, and two to the other. In *3:1 segregation*, three chromosomes go to one daughter cell, and one to the other. In *4:0 segregation*, all four chromosomes go to one daughter cell, and none to the other.

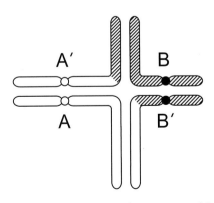

FIGURE 5–2   Pachytene configuration, simplified outline. The two normal (A, B) and the two translocation (A′, B′) homologs align corresponding segments of chromatin during meiosis I.

MODES OF SEGREGATION

Within these three broad categories, we can list the particular modes of segregation, according to which chromosomes actually go where. Referring to the four chromosomes of the quadrivalent as A, B, A′, and B′ (Figure 5–2), the modes of segregation are summarized as follows (Table 5–1):

Table 5–1.

ONE DAUGHTER GAMETOCYTE WITH:	OTHER DAUGHTER GAMETOCYTE WITH:	SEGREGATION MODE
2:2 Segregations		
A and B	A′ and B′	Alternate segregation
A and B′	B and A′	Adjacent-1 segregation
A and A′	B and B′	Adjacent-2 segregation
3:1 Segregations		
A B A′	B′	3:1 segregation with
A B and B′	A′	tertiary trisomy or monosomy
A′ B′ and A	B	3:1 segregation with
A′ B′ and B	A	interchange trisomy or monosomy
4:0 Segregation		
A B A′ B′	None	4:0 segregation with double trisomy or monosomy

Figure 5–3 depicts five of the possible pairs of daughter gametocytes. Other things being equal, the chromosomal combination is conserved through meiosis II, and the mature gamete forms. From one primary gametocyte, four spermatozoa, or one ovum and its polar bodies, are thus produced. Gametes from alternate segregation are normal or balanced. Conceptions from adjacent-1 gametes have trisomy (duplication) for one translocated segment and monosomy (deletion) for the other. Adjacent-2

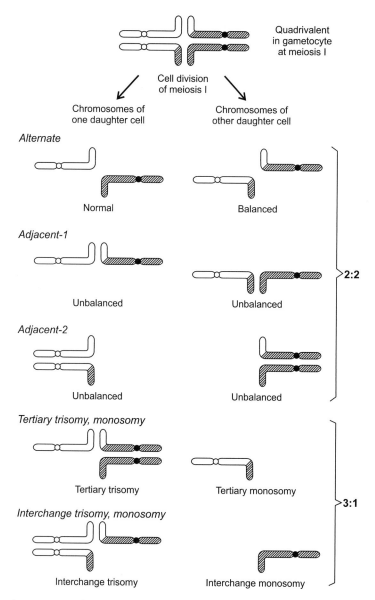

FIGURE 5–3 The categories of 2:2 and 3:1 segregation that may occur in gametogenesis in the translocation heterozygote. In the four 3:1 categories, only one of the two possible combinations in each category is depicted (both of each are shown in Fig. 5–4).

conceptions have trisomy for one centric segment and monosomy for the other. Tertiary aneuploidies have trisomy, or monosomy, with respect to the combined chromosomal content of one of the derivative chromosomes. Interchange aneuploidies have a full autosomal trisomy or a full monosomy. In 4:0 segregation, there is a double trisomy or a double monosomy. Some of the gametes with these unbalanced combinations may be "viable," in the sense of being "capable of giving rise to a conceptus, which would

proceed through to the birth of a child." Mostly, in fact, they are not.

Recombination at meiosis I, and asymmetric segregation at meiosis II, can complicate the story, although not often does this have a practical implication. If recombination occurs in the interstitial segment (between the centromere and the breakpoint), further unbalanced combinations are generated, most of which would not be remotely viable. This phenomenon may possibly have some relevance in preimplantation genetic diagnosis because testing is done at a stage where there has been little opportunity for selective pressure to have applied. Scriven et al. (1998) list various of these recombination possibilities, and Van Hummelen et al. (1997) diagram the process with respect to a particular translocation on which they had undertaken sperm studies (and also illustrate the interesting point that a normal/balanced gamete can be restored following recombination in adjacent-1 segregation). The most telling evidence that recombination can happen, comes from the observation of a meiosis I chromosome having one normal and one derivative chromatid, and polar body analysis has enabled such an observation to be made (Munné et al. 1998). At meiosis II, asymmetric segregation may lead to two copies of a derivative chromosome being transmitted, as noted below in the section "Meiosis II Nondisjunction."

ALTERNATE SEGREGATION

In 2:2 alternate segregation, looking at each centromere in turn around the quadrivalent, one centromere goes to one pole, and the next centromere goes to the other pole. In other words, each centromere goes "alternately"[2] to one or the other pole. Thus, the two daughter cells come to contain, respectively, the two normal homologs in one, and the two derivative chromosomes in the other. Note that alternate segregation is essentially the only mode that leads to gametes with a complete genetic complement—one with a normal karyotype, the other with the reciprocal translocation in the balanced state. All other modes can be classified as *malsegregation*.

ADJACENT SEGREGATION

In 2:2 adjacent segregation, adjacent centromeres travel together ("adjacent" in the sense of centromeres being next to each other, in their positions around the quadrivalent). There are two categories. In *adjacent-1* segregation, adjacent chromosomes with unalike (nonhomologous) centromeres travel to the same daughter cell (an

aide-mémoire: In adjacent-*1*, the daughter cells get *one* of each centromere). Overall, adjacent-1 is the most frequently seen mode of malsegregation in the children of translocation heterozygotes. In *adjacent-2* segregation, which is rather uncommon, adjacent chromosomes with like (homologous) centromeres go to the same daughter cell (another aide-mémoire: In adjacent-2, the *two* homologous centromeres go *together*). Thus, adjacent-2 segregation rather resembles nondisjunction.

3:1 SEGREGATION

This is also referred to as 3:1 nondisjunction. Gametes with 24 chromosomes and 22 chromosomes are formed, and the conceptuses therefore have 47 or 45 chromosomes. Almost always, the 47-chromosome conceptus is the only viable one. Two categories exist: Either the two normal chromosomes of the quadrivalent plus one of the translocation chromosomes go together to one daughter cell (*tertiary trisomy*) or, rarely, the two translocation chromosomes and one of the normal chromosomes segregate (*interchange trisomy*). Tertiary monosomy, with a 45-chromosome conceptus, is extremely rare. Interchange monosomy has never been seen, except at preimplantation genetic diagnosis.

4:0 SEGREGATION

In autosomal translocations, 4:0 segregation has been regarded as being of academic interest only. But it may have some practical relevance in preimplantation genetic diagnosis.

In theory, 16 possible chromosomal combinations could be produced in the gametes of the autosomal translocation heterozygote. Four of these we can, for the most part, ignore (3:1 interchange monosomies and 4:0 segregants), because they are never viable. The two balanced gametes (2:2 alternate segregants) are always viable, other things being equal. Of the remaining 10 possibilities, it is common for none to be viable, with spontaneous abortion the universal outcome. If a translocation heterozygote does have the potential for viable imbalance in an offspring, it is most likely that there will be only one such combination (this was the case in 99% and 100% of translocations, respectively, in the considerable experience of two groups;

---

2 Not "alternatively", as some publications erroneously use.

Scriven et al. 1998). Usually, this sole survivable imbalance will be one that endows a partial trisomy. Infrequently two and, very rarely, more than two may be viable. Figure 5–4 depicts the various combinations that may be considered (using the previously discussed t(1;4) translocation as an example). In a review of 1,159 translocation families, Cohen et al. (1994) found the proportions of chromosomally unbalanced offspring as follows: 71% adjacent-1, 4% adjacent-2, 22% tertiary trisomy/monosomy, and 2.5% interchange trisomy.

Gamete Studies It is, apparently, the norm for the heterozygote to produce gametes in which many of the possible chromosomal combinations occur, albeit the proportions may differ, and very substantially so, for some different translocations. Sperm karyotyping results from 45 men, heterozygous for a translocation, are summarized in Table 5–2, along with öocyte karyotyping data (in most indirectly, via polar body analysis) from nine women: 56% of sperm, and 70% of ova, were chromosomally

unbalanced. The great majority, if not all, of these studied individuals would have presented to the clinic because of reproductive difficulty, and so the data are rather likely to be biased in the direction of unbalanced forms, compared to the whole population of translocation heterozygotes.

On average, alternate and adjacent-1 segregants are the predominant types in spermatogenesis, occurring in fairly similar fractions (44% and 31%, respectively). Adjacent-2 at 13% and 3:1 at 11% are less frequently seen; and barely any 4:0 segregant sperm. The spread of segregant types seems to be rather similar with men having the same translocation, such as the related individuals noted in Table 5–1. Between different translocations, considerable variation occurs: Some male heterozygotes had no 3:1 segregants, and one had 47%; for adjacent-2, the range is 0%–40%. The fractions in ova are derived from very few numbers, and alternate segregations per woman range from 0% to 100%; thus, the reader should not place too great a weight on the average fraction of 30% normal in Table 5–2. The higher

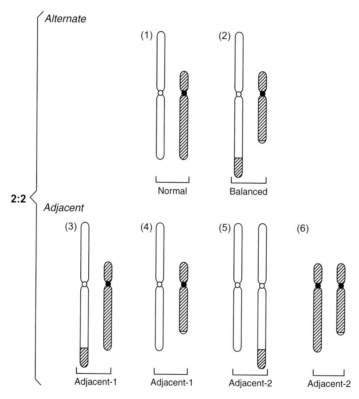

FIGURE 5–4   The full range of segregant gametes that may be produced by the translocation heterozygote, using the t(1;4) depicted in Figure 5–1 as an example. Chromosome 1 chromatin is shown open; chromosome 4 chromatin is cross-hatched.

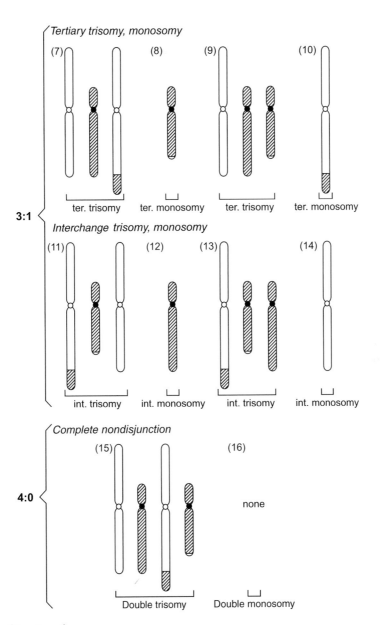

3:1

Tertiary trisomy, monosomy

(7) (8) (9) (10)

ter. trisomy   ter. monosomy   ter. trisomy   ter. monosomy

Interchange trisomy, monosomy

(11) (12) (13) (14)

int. trisomy   int. monosomy   int. trisomy   int. monosomy

4:0

Complete nondisjunction

(15) (16)

Double trisomy   Double monosomy

FIGURE 5-4   (Continued)

fraction of 3:1 segregations in ova (27%) may be an age-related effect.

Conceptions It might be expected that the distribution of normal and abnormal conceptions would reflect the distributions of karyotypes in the gametes. If the reader will allow, we could comment, rather inconclusively, that this may, or may not, be so. Comparing the fluorescence in situ hybridization (FISH) data in Tables 5–2 and 5–3, for female translocation heterozygotes, a modest increase is seen

in the average normal fraction for embryos (45%) cf. gametes (30%). In contrast, for male translocation heterozygotes, the average normal fraction of embryos (41%) is similar to that of gametes (44%). Molecular methodologies return a similar range of findings (Table 22–2) (Tan et al. 2013; Tobler et al. 2014; Idowu et al. 2015).

Acrocentric chromosomes participating in a reciprocal translocation might be expected to influence segregation, due to the very small lengths of their short arms and thus a marked asymmetry

Table 5–2. Chromosome Segregations in Gametes of 9 Female and 45 Male Reciprocal Translocation Heterozygotes, Shown as Percentages in Each Segregant Category

t	ALT	ADJ-1	ADJ-2	3:1	4:0
Female Heterozygotes					
46,XX,t(1;18)(p34.3q12.3)	16%	50	16	16	0
46,XX,t(2;14)(q23;q24)	11	22	22	44	0
46,XX,t(2;14)(q31;q24)	14	57	14	14	0
46,XX,t(4;12)(q22q23)	9	0	36	36	18
46,XX,t(4;14)(p15.3;q24)	27	55	0	18	0
46,XX,t(6;21)(q13;q22.3)	0	50	0	50	0
46,XX,t(7;20)(q22;q11.2)	50	17	0	33	0
46,XX,t(9;11)(p24;q12)	100	0	0	0	0
46,XX,t(14;18)(q22;q11)	40	0	60	0	0
Average fractions (eggs)	30%	24%	16%	27%	2%

Total abnormal = 70%

t	ALT	ADJ-1	ADJ-2	3:1	4:0
Male Heterozygotes					
46,XY,t(1;2)(q32;q36)	41%	42	6	11	0
46,XY,t(1;4)(p36.2;q31.3)[a]	46	38	7	9	0
46,XY,t(1;4)(p36.2;q31.3)[a]	39	50	8	3	0
46,XY,t(1;9)(q22;q31)	46	38	13	4	0
46,XY,t(1;11)(p36.3;q13.1)	33	43	16	8	0
46,XY,t(1;13)(q41;q42)	41	42	15	2	0
46,XY,t(2;3)(q24;p26)	55	36	7	1	0
46,XY,t(2;6)(p12;q24)	50	42	3	4	0
46,XY,t(2;9)(q21;p22)	43	28	24	4	0
46,XY,t(2;17)(q35;p13)	56	33	11	0	0
46,XY,t(2;18)(p21;q11.2)	42	35	14	8	0
46,XY,t(3;7)(q25;q36)	28	46	19	7	0
46,XY,t(3;8)(p13;p21)	34	44	21	1	0
46,XY,t(3;11)(q25.3;q25)	48	46	6	0.8	0
46,XY,t(3;15)(q26.2;q26.1)	48	36	12	12	2
46,XY,t(3;16)(p23;q24)	37	41	16	5	0
46,XY,t(3;19)(p21;p13.3)	39	36	22	3	0
46,XY,t(4;6)(q28;p23)	46	52	2	0.5	0
46,XY,t(4;8)(q28;p23)	35	33	20	11	0
46,XY,t(4;12)(p11;p11)	49	14	28	9	1
46,XY,t(4;17)(q21.3;q23.2)	57	35	7	2	0
46,XY,t(5;7)(q13;p15.1)	40	26	17	17	0
46,XY,t(5;11)(p13;q23.2)[b]	70	26	0	4	0
46,XY,t(7;14)(q11;q24.1)[b]	30	48	0	17	4
46,XY,t(5;13)(q11;q33)	77	21	2	0	0
46,XY,t(5;18)(p15;q21)	81	16	0	3	0
46,XY,t(6;9)(p12;q13)	24	14	40	22	0
46,XY,t(7;8)(q11.21;cen)[a]	57	25	11	7	0.04
46,XY,t(7;8)(q11.21;cen)[a]	63	18	13	7	0.3
46,XY,t(8;9)(q24.2;q32)	44	41	3	9	0.6
46,XY,t(8;22)(q24.22;q11.21)	24	15	19	42	0
46,XY,t(9;10)(q11;p11.1)	56	13	9	21	0
46,XY,t(9;22)(q21;q11.2)	56	26	11	6	0.6

Table 5–2. (Continued)

t	ALT	ADJ-1	ADJ-2	3:1	4:0
46,XY,t(10;14)(q24;q32)	45	39	12	5	0
46,XY,t(11;17)(q13.1;p11.2)	41	26	26	7	0
46,XY,t(11;22)(q23;q11)	22	14	32	30	0
46,XY,t(11;22)(q23;q11)	27	18	13	40	0.5
46,XY,t(11;22)(q25;q12)	29	22	15	35	0
46,XY,t(14;20)(p11.2;p11.1)	51	19	21	4	0
46,XY,t(15;17)(q21;q25)[a]	51	35	9	3	0
46,XY,t(15;17)(q21;q25)[a]	49	38	8	3	0
46,XY,t(15;17)(q21;q25)[a]	48	40	9	2	0
46,XY,t(15;17)(q21;q25)[a]	53	34	11	1.5	0
46,XY,t(15;22)(q22;q13)	19	16	16	43	0
46,XY,t(17;22)(q11;q12)	19	13	6	47	0
Average fractions (sperm)	44%	31%	13%	11%	0.4%

Total abnormal = 56%

Notes: ALT, alternate; ADJ-1, adjacent-1; ADJ-2, adjacent-2. The tested populations were presumably biased toward less fortunate reproductive outcomes. The sperm data are arbitrarily set out according to the methodology used. Those down to the t(5;18) were analyzed using the human-hamster hybrid model; the remainder, from the t(6;9), were based upon FISH analysis of interphase sperm nuclei (the results from the two approaches are quite similar). The t(7;14) is "out of order"; it is placed beneath the t(5;11) also carried by this subject.[b] Some sperm FISH cases were interpreted as showing "other" combinations; these are not listed, and the totals here come to less than 100%. The full data set according to the two methodologies is contained in Benet et al. (2005), with a total of 89 individuals analyzed.

[a]Related individuals; note the quite similar fractions.

[b]Both translocations carried by the same man, as a double heterozygote; note the very different proportions from each translocation.

Sources: Sperm data from Benet et al. (2005). Oöcyte/polar body data, which naturally are based on much smaller numbers (2–11 observations per woman), from Munné et al. (1998b, 1998c), Conn et al. (1999), Escudero et al. (2000), Durban et al. (2001).

of the quadrivalent (Benet et al. 2005). Lim et al. (2008b) were able to demonstrate the truth of this proposition. They observed that those translocations involving an acrocentric chromosome had fewer alternate segregants compared to those that did not (15% cf. 26%), but more 3:1 malsegregants (27% cf. 20%), in 508 embryos analyzed.

Viability In Utero Most unbalanced combinations would produce such enormous genetic imbalance that the conceptus would be lost very early in pregnancy (occult abortion), or even fail to implant. Moderate imbalances would proceed to the stage of recognizable miscarriage, or to later fetal death in utero. Only those conceptuses with lesser imbalances might result in the birth of an abnormal child.

Viability is much more likely in the case of effective single-segment imbalance, with only one segment of substantial size. In the unbalanced state, a partial monosomy/deletion or trisomy/duplication for the other very small terminal segment is likely to contribute minimally, or (if it contains no genes, or

at any rate no dosage-sensitive genes) not at all, to the overall imbalance. This is of particular relevance in adjacent-1 segregation. Consider, for example, gamete (3) in Figure 5–4. The material missing from the telomeric tip of chromosome 1 long arm—the telomeric cap—is so small that its loss is, as far as we can tell, of insignificant phenotypic effect. For practical purposes, we can ignore this partial monosomy. So the significant imbalance reduces to a partial 4q trisomy (dup 4q31.3qter). This, as it happens, is well recognized as being a viable complement (and it is the imbalance in the children whose photograph appears in the frontispiece). On the other hand, in the double-segment exchange, the imbalance contributed by each segment must be taken into account. Thus, adjacent-1 gametes have both a partial trisomy and a partial monosomy to a significant degree and would produce a "phenotypic hybrid." Very frequently, the combination is nonviable.

If very early miscarriages could be karyotyped, one might expect to discover more

Table 5–3. Chromosome Segregations in Embryos of 33 Female and 20 Male Reciprocal Translocation Heterozygotes Studied at Preimplantation Diagnosis Using FISH (Shown as Actual Numbers in Each Segregant Category)

t	ALT	ADJ-1	ADJ-2	3:1	4:0
Female Heterozygotes					
46,XX,t(1;7)(p34.1;p14.3)	1	3	0	0	0
46,XX,t(1;13)(q23;p11)	0	2	0	1	0
46,XX,t(1;19)(q32.1;q13.1)	12	5	2	6	1
46,XX,t(2;4)(p22.2;q33)	4	6	0	0	0
46,XX,t(2;7)(q37.1;q32)	3	1	1	1	0
46,XX,t(2;10)(q37.1;p13)	5	5	1	1	0
46,XX,t(2;11)(q37.1;q23.1)	0	1	0	2	0
46,XX,t(3;5)(p12;q14.2)	0	1	0	0	0
46,XX,t(3;13)(q13.2;q12.1)	6	0	3	2	0
46,XX,t(4;6)(p15.2;q13)	2	3	2	0	0
46,XX,t(4;8)(p16.1;p23.1)	0	1	0	0	0
46,XX,t(4;8)(q21.3;p21.3)	0	3	1	1	0
46,XX,t(4;13)(p15.2;q22)	1	3	0	0	0
46,XX,t(4;15)(q26;q13)	4	3	1	2	0
46,XX,t(4;19)(p16;p13.3)	6	0	0	0	0
46,XX,t(5;14)(p15.1;q32.1)	4	2	0	2	0
46,XX,t(5;16)(p12;q23)	6	1	0	4	0
46,XX,t(7;9)(q21.2;q33)	0	0	1	1	0
46,XX,t(7;13)(q11.21;p13)	5	0	0	2	0
46,XX,t(8;18)(p21.1;q21.1)	2	0	0	0	0
46,XX,t(9;16)(q33.3;p13.11)	5	5	0	0	0
46,XX,t(9;20)(q34.2;q11.2)	5	3	0	0	0
46,XX,t(10;13)(q26.3;q21.2)	0	2	1	0	0
46,XX,t(11;17)(p15.5;p13)	1	3	0	0	0
46,XX,t(11;17)(p15.5;p13)	7	4	0	5	0
46,XX,t(11;22)(q23.3;q11.2)	0	0	0	1	0
46,XX,t(11;22)(q23.3;q11.2)	1	0	0	0	0
46,XX,t(11;22)(q23.3;q11.2)	6	1	1	4	0
46,XX,t(11;22)(q23.3;q11.2)	1	2	0	3	0
46,XX,t(11;22)(q23.3;q11.2)	4	1	1	3	0
46,XX,t(12;17)(p13;p13)	19	13	1	4	0
46,XX,t(14;18)(q11.2;q23)	3	0	2	4	0
46,XX,t(14;22)(q11.2;q13.3)	7	0	3	1	0
Average fractions	45%	28%	8%	19%	0.4%
			Total abnormal = 55%		
Male Heterozygotes					
46,XY,t(1;6)(p13.3;p22.2)	6	4	2	3	0
46,XY,t(1;9)(p13.3;p13)	3	2	2	2	0
46,XY,t(1;15)(q21;p11.2)	5	6	0	0	0
46,XY,t(1;17)(q21.3;p13.3)	3	6	2	0	0
46,XY,t(1;19)(p10;p10)	2	0	0	0	0
46,XY,t(2;14)(q32.2;23)	1	0	1	0	0
46,XY,t(3;6)(q25;q23)	8	10	2	2	0
46,XY,t(3;7)(q23;q36)	3	1	3	0	0

Table 5–3. (Continued)

t	ALT	ADJ-1	ADJ-2	3:1	4:0
46,XY,t(3;7)(q25.3;p22.1)	4	1	3	1	0
46,XY,t(4;5)(p16;q35)	3	2	0	0	0
46,XY,t(4;9)(q31.2;q34.3)	1	4	0	0	0
46,XY,t(5;6)(q35.3;q24.2)	5	6	0	0	0
46,XY,t(6;10)(q23.1;p13)	4	4	1	1	0
46,XY,t(8;20)(p21.1;p13)	2	0	0	0	0
46,XY,t(9;12)(p24;p11.2)	4	3	2	0	0
46,XY,t(9;14)(p22;q22)	1	2	2	1	0
46,XY.t(11;15)(q13.3;q13)	3	1	0	0	0
46,XY,t(11;22)(q23.3;q11.2)	7	3	3	0	0
46,XY,t(11;22)(q23.3;q11.2)	9	6	5	3	1
46,XY,t(14;16)(q32.3;p11.2)	1	3	0	0	0
Average fractions	41%	35%	16%	7%	0.7%
				Total abnormal = 59%	

Notes: ALT, alternate; ADJ-1, adjacent-1; ADJ-2, adjacent-2. Average fractions are derived from pooling the data in each group. The tested populations were presumably biased toward less fortunate reproductive outcomes. Similar studies are reported in Ko et al. (2010).
Source: Scriven et al. (2013); see also Fig. 22–4.

of the imbalanced forms. Fritz et al. (2000) conducted such an exercise, using comparative genomic hybridization as the cytogenetic tool. They had identified a family segregating a subtle t(4;12)(q34;p13), in which two children had been born with 46,der(4),t(4;12)(q34;p13), giving a distal 4q monosomy. There had been five previous abortions, and archival pathology material (paraffin-embedded placental tissue) was available for analysis from three of these. A 12- and a 17-week abortus both showed the same karyotype as the surviving children. An 8-week abortus, described as a hydatidiform mole, karyotyped as a tertiary trisomy for almost the whole of chromosome 4: 47,XY,+der(4),t(4;12)(q34;p13), combination (9) in Figure 5–4.

Predicting Segregant Outcomes

How can we determine, for the individual translocation carrier, which segregant outcomes, if any, might lead to the birth of an abnormal child? What might be the relative roles of an inherent tendency for a particular type of segregation to occur, and of in utero selection against unbalanced forms? A useful approach is to imagine how the chromosomes come to be distributed during meiosis. Following Jalbert et al. (1980, 1988), we may draw, roughly to scale,

a diagram of the presumed pachytene configuration of the quadrivalent, and then deduce which modes of segregation are likely to lead to the formation of gametes, which could then produce a viable conceptus. The following, and with reference to Figure 5–5, are the ground rules:

1. We assume that alternate segregation is (a) frequent and (b) associated with phenotypic normality.

2. The least imbalanced, least monosomic of the imbalanced gametes is the one most likely to produce a viable conceptus.

3. If the translocated segments are small in genetic content, adjacent-1 is the most likely type of malsegregation to be capable of giving rise to viable abnormal offspring (Fig. 5–5a).

4. If the centric segments are small in content, adjacent-2 is the most likely segregation to give a viable abnormal outcome (Fig. 5–5b).

5. If one of the whole chromosomes of the quadrivalent is small in content, 3:1 disjunction is the most likely (Fig. 5–5c). The small chromosome may be a small derivative chromosome or a chromosome 13, 18, or 21.

6. If the quadrivalent has characteristics of both Rules 3 and 5, or of Rules 4 and 5, then both adjacent and 3:1 segregations may give rise to viable offspring.

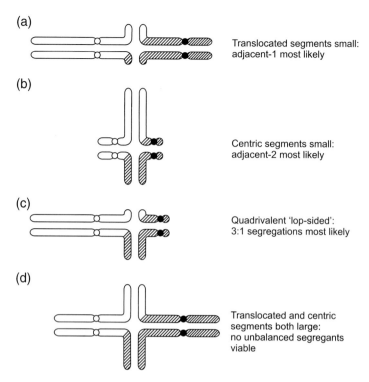

(a)   Translocated segments small:
adjacent-1 most likely

(b)   Centric segments small:
adjacent-2 most likely

(c)   Quadrivalent 'lop-sided':
3:1 segregations most likely

(d)   Translocated and centric
segments both large:
no unbalanced segregants
viable

FIGURE 5–5   Prediction of likely viable segregant outcomes by pachytene diagram drawing and assessment of the configuration of the quadrivalent.

7. If the translocated and centric segments both have large content, no mode of segregation could produce an unbalanced gamete that would lead to a viable offspring (Fig. 5–5d).

8. If the translocated segments are both very small (subtelomeric), the chromosomes may not necessarily form a quadrivalent, and the pairs of homologs might simply join up as bivalents, each pair then segregating independently.

Some examples to illustrate these points follow.[3]

ADJACENT-1 SEGREGATION, SINGLE-SEGMENT EXCHANGE

Many translocations involve an effectively single-segment exchange, with the "single" translocated segment comprising a fairly small amount of chromatin (1%–2% of the haploid autosomal length, or HAL). This is the classical scenario for adjacent-1 segregation to occur, and to produce a phenotype

capable of postnatal survival. The family with the t(1;4) in Figure 5–1, whose children with partial 4q trisomy are shown in the frontispiece and as discussed above, provides an example.

Consider now the family whose pedigree is depicted in Figure 5–6a, in which the individuals shown as heterozygotes have the balanced translocation 46,t(3;11)(p26;q21). A segment of chromatin consisting of almost half of the long arm of chromosome 11, and comprising 1.4% of the HAL, is translocated to the tip of chromosome 3 short arm (Figure 5–6b). The telomeric tip of chromosome 3 short arm, which we imagine to comprise little or no phenotypically important genetic material, has moved reciprocally across to chromosome 11. The presumed pachytene configuration during gametogenesis in the heterozygote would be as drawn in Figure 5–6c. The adjacent-1 segregant gamete with der(3) plus normal 11 (heavy arrows) produces a conceptus that has a partial 11q trisomy, since the der(3) carries the segment 11q21qter. The loss

---

3 The reader wishing to study further worked examples is referred to Midro et al. (1992), who analyze in some detail a series of translocations of differing risk potentials.

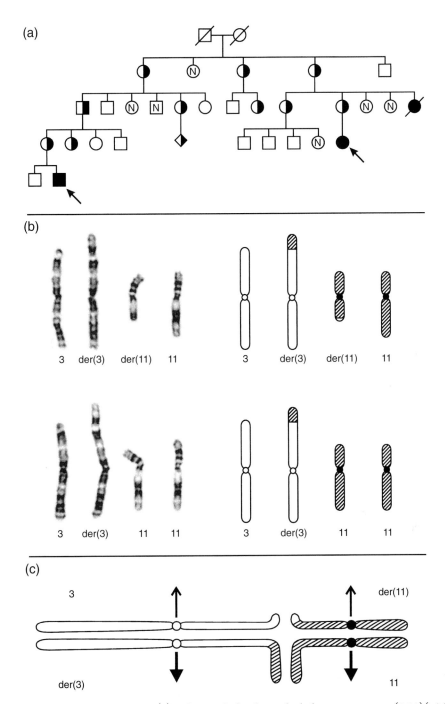

FIGURE 5-6 Adjacent-1 segregation. (*a*) Pedigree of a family in which there segregates a t(3;11)(p26;q21) having the characteristics associated with adjacent-1 malsegregation. Two independently ascertained probands have a partial 11q trisomy, and a deceased relative, who died at age 18 years in an institution for the retarded, had a similar appearance from photographs, and so very probably had the same karyotype. Filled symbol, unbalanced karyotype; half-filled symbol, balanced carrier; N in symbol = 46,N; small diamond, prenatal diagnosis; arrow, proband. (*b*) Partial karyotype of a translocation heterozygote (*above*), showing the 3;11 translocation, and a child with the unbalanced complement (*below*). (Case of A. J. Watt.) (*c*) The presumed pachytene configuration during gametogenesis in the heterozygote (chromosome 3 chromatin, open; chromosome 11 chromatin, cross-hatched). Arrows indicate movements of chromosomes to daughter cells in adjacent-1 segregation; heavy arrows show the combination observed in this family.

of the 3p telomeric tip in this der(3) we suppose to have no effect. Two, probably three children in the family had been born with this karyotype. No individuals are known having the other adjacent-1 combination (Figure 5–6c, light arrows), that is, the 46,+der(11) karyotype, which would endow a partial 11q monosomy. Consulting Schinzel (2001), viability for the segment 11q21qter in monosomic state is recorded in only two cases. We assume, therefore, that it has a very high lethality in utero.

The scenario of a single survivable imbalanced form, due to a partial trisomy from adjacent-1 segregation in a "single-segment" translocation, as in this t(3;11) example, is, as mentioned above, much the most commonly encountered circumstance in translocation families at risk for an abnormal child.

Infrequently, both the partial trisomic and the partial monosomic forms are observed. A good example of this is given by distal 4p translocations: Both deletion and duplication for this segment are well recognized as having substantial in utero viability. Consider the translocation t(4;12)(p14;p13) described in a family study in Mortimer et al. (1980). A number of family members over three or more generations were balanced carriers, and abnormal children had been born with typical Wolf-Hirschhorn syndrome (all dying in infancy), while others presented the syndrome of partial 4p trisomy (all surviving at least well into childhood). The breakpoints of the translocation are in distal 4p and at the very tip of 12p (12pter). The presumed pachytene configuration would be as drawn in Figure 5–5a (imagining the chromosome 4 chromatin open and chromosome 12 chromatin cross-hatched). With such short translocated segments (and very long centric segments), adjacent-1 segregation is the only possibility for viable imbalance. If we ignore the tiny contribution of a duplication or deletion for telomeric 12p—in other words, if we interpret this as an effective single-segment imbalance—the situation reduces to the two possible adjacent-1 outcomes being a partial 4p trisomy and a partial 4p monosomy. Both of these are recognized entities, as noted above, and apparently both have substantial viability in utero. The abnormal karyotypes would be written 46,der(12)t(4;12)(p14;p13) and 46,der(4)t(4;12)(p14;p13).

If the "other segment" can actually be proven not to contain any coding genes, the case for considering the translocation as a single-segment entity is particularly valid, with the resulting imbalances being demonstrably "pure." Martínez-Juárez et al. (2014) allowed such a conclusion to be drawn in the case of two children born from a translocation carrier mother, 46,XX,t(2;12)(p24.2;q24.31). The 12q breakpoint was at chr12:132,960,869, and the 12q translocated segment, which comprised only 300 kb, was beyond the distalmost gene on that chromosome.[4] Thus, the children's abnormal phenotype was due purely to trisomy for the large segment chr2:1-32,745,624 (containing very many genes). Given that the short arms of the acrocentrics contain no protein-coding genes, De Carvalho et al. (2008) could conclude, in a large family segregating a t(5;15)(p13.3;p12) translocation, that the 5p deletions and duplications observed (in an extraordinary total of 21 individuals) would represent, respectively, pure partial monosomies and trisomies, from an effectively single-segment rearrangement.

ADJACENT-1 SEGREGATION, DOUBLE-SEGMENT EXCHANGE

With a double-segment translocation, an adjacent-1 imbalanced conceptus has both a partial trisomy and a partial monosomy (also called a duplication/deficiency, or duplication/deletion, abbreviated to dup/del). The combined effect of the two imbalances is more severe than either separately. Thus, it is infrequent that the carrier of a "double-segment" exchange can ever have a chromosomally unbalanced pregnancy proceeding through to term, or close to term. Multiple miscarriage is the typical observation (e.g., Figure 5–15). But occasionally viability is observed for one, or rarely both, of the dup/del combinations. Nucaro et al. (2008) studied a t(3;10)(p26;p12) family with affected individuals in three generations, and yet all still living, and able to be examined and their karyotypes confirmed as 46,der(3)t(3;10)(p26;p12), conveying a partial 3p monosomy and 10p trisomy; the countertype adjacent-1 karyotype was not observed, but it may well have been the cause of the several miscarriages recorded. The

---

4 The final nucleotide on chromosome 12, at 12qter, is number 133,275,309.

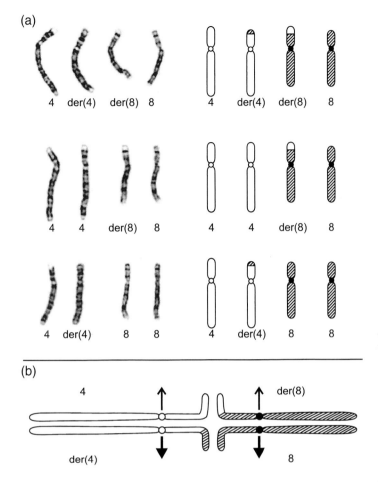

(a)

4 der(4) der(8) 8   4 der(4) der(8) 8

4 4 der(8) 8   4 4 der(8) 8

4 der(4) 8 8   4 der(4) 8 8

(b)

4   der(8)

der(4)   8

FIGURE 5-7   Adjacent-1 segregation, double-segment translocation with very small segments. (*a*) Parent with the translocation t(4;8)(p16.1;p23.1). The index case, his child, has the karyotype 46,+der(4) and so has a del(4p)/dup(8p) imbalance, and an uncle has the countertype dup(4p)/del(8p) imbalance due to the 46,+der(8) karyotype. (Case of C. E. Vaux.) (*b*) The presumed pachytene configuration during gametogenesis in the heterozygote (chromosome 4 chromatin, open; chromosome 8 chromatin, cross-hatched). Arrows indicate movements of chromosomes to daughter cells in adjacent-1 segregation. The upper combination (light arrows) would produce the dup(4p)/del(8p) imbalance, and the lower (heavy arrows) the del(4p)/dup(8p) imbalance.

double-segment t(4;8)(p16.1;p23.1) depicted in Figure 5–7 has very small translocated segments: the tip of chromosome 4 and the tip of chromosome 8 have exchanged positions.[5] In this family, both of the two possible adjacent-1 segregant outcomes were observed: the index case with del(4p)/dup(8p), and his uncle with dup(4p)/ del(8p). In the former, a Wolf-Hirschhorn gestalt was discernible, reflecting

the del(4p) component. A similar example is seen in the family reported in Rogers et al. (1997). They provide in their paper a photograph of six siblings sitting on a sofa in 1958, one with a dup(11q)/del(4q) karyotype, two who since died presumed to have been del(11q)/(dup(4q), and one girl carrying the family t(4;11)(q34.3;q23.1) who went on to have, in the next generation, a del(11q)/(dup(4q) child.

---

5 This same 4;8 translocation has been observed in a small number of unrelated families, and it may be, after the t(11;22) noted below, the most frequent human reciprocal translocation. This recurrence reflects the presence in distal 4p and 8p of "olfactory-receptor clusters," which can act as recombination-predisposing duplicons (Maas et al. 2007). Other recurrent rearrangements are the translocations t(4;18)(q35;q23) and t(8;22)(q24.13;q11.21) (Horbinski et al. 2008; Sheridan et al. 2010). But some apparent recurrences may actually reflect unrecognized identity by descent (Youings et al. 2004).

Very small double-segment imbalances, detectable with clarity (or at all) only upon molecular karyotyping, may be associated with viability in the del/dup circumstance. In the t(7;12)(q36.2;p13.31) family reported in Izumi et al. (2010), the translocated segments were both of small size, and both contained genes. The 5.53 Mb distal 7q segment, at chr7:153,908,498-qter, carried, among others, the *SHH* and *MNX1* genes. Some 80 genes were resident in the 7.27 Mb distal 12p segment, chr12:1-7,272,466. The phenotype in the del(7q)/dup(12p) case presumably reflected the combined effects of a haploinsufficiency of the 7q loci, and triplo-excess of the 12p loci. And likewise, Iype et al. (2015) describe a five-generation kindred segregating a t(3;4)(p26.3;p16.1), in which several individuals had either del(3p)/dup(4p) or del(4p)/dup(3p)—or, to be more precise, del or dup chr3:1-2.1 Mb, and del or dup chr4:1-10.3 Mb. In meiosis of a parent carrying a translocation such as these, it is probable that the normal and the derivative would simply pair up as would a normal bivalent, leaving the tiny nonhomologous segments at the ends unpaired. In that case, the expected segregations at meiosis would be random, with equal probability for each outcome, namely normal:balanced:(dup/del):(del/dup) in the ratio 1:1:1:1.

Exceptionally, both translocated segments can be of substantial size and yet be survivable, if barely, to term. The outlying points in Figure 5–17 reflect such cases. The double-segment t(5;10)(p13;q23.3) exchange illustrated in Figure 5–1 provides an example, this translocation having been identified in a family following the death of a neonate with multiple malformations. The genetic abnormality comprised a deletion of 5p and a duplication of 10q, for a total imbalance of 2.5% HAL (1.1% HAL monosomy plus 1.4% HAL trisomy).

When entire arms of chromosomes are translocated (whole-arm translocation), it is almost always so that the unbalanced segregants would be unviable (Vázquez-Cárdenas et al. 2007). Rare exceptions exist. Czakó et al. (2002) report a t(18;20)(p11.1;p11.1), in which the abnormal child of a carrier father was effectively trisomic for all of 20p and monosomic for all of 18p (1.0% HAL trisomy plus 0.8% HAL monosomy). The woman with a whole-arm 15p;16q translocation described in Chen et al. (2004c) had a history of miscarriage and stillbirth, and two further pregnancy losses proven to have complete 16q trisomy, this imbalance conveying as much as 2.1% HAL trisomy, and associated with

a severe phenotype. (Since the concomitant 15p monosomy presumably did not contribute to the fetal defects, this example has more of the flavor of a single-segment translocation.)

The opportunity occasionally arises to provide direct evidence of early in utero lethality of a particular imbalanced state. In a family study of a t(8;18)(p21.3;p11.23), Cockwell et al. (1996) demonstrated on a severely malformed spontaneously aborted 11-week fetus one of the adjacent-1 conceptions, the dup(8p)/del(18p) state. This chromosomal constitution caused a double-segment imbalance, with a trisomy for 8p21.3pter, and a monosomy for 18p11.23pter, giving a combined 1.2% HAL imbalance (0.8% for trisomy, 0.4% for monosomy). The countertype dup(18p)/del(8p) karyotype had produced, in this family, a child with an abnormal phenotype. Atypically, this viable form had more HAL monosomy than trisomy.

ADJACENT-2 SEGREGATION

This is an uncommonly observed mode of segregation, typically limited to translocations in which each of the two participating chromosomes has a short arm of small genetic content, and small enough that the whole short arm can be viable in the trisomic state. In fact, most cases involve an exchange between chromosome 9 and an acrocentric, or between two acrocentrics (Duckett and Roberts 1981; Stene and Stengel-Rutkowski 1988; Chen et al. 2005c). The breakpoints characteristically occur in the upper long arm of one chromosome and immediately below the centromere in the long arm of the other (an acrocentric). Thus, the centric segments are small.

The t(9;21)(q12;q11) illustrated in Figure 5–8 exemplifies the adjacent-2 scenario. At meiosis I, the form of the quadrivalent would be as drawn in Figure 5–8b. The "least imbalanced, least monosomic" gamete from 2:2 malsegregation is the one receiving chromosome 9 and the der(9) (heavy arrows). The conceptus will have, in consequence, a duplication of 9p (and a small amount of 9q heterochromatin) and a deletion of 21p (and a minuscule amount of subcentromeric 21q). Although comprising a substantial piece of chromatin (1.8% of HAL), 9p is qualitatively "small" in the trisomic state. Monosomy for 21p is without effect, and the 21q loss makes little if any contribution, and thus the picture is practically that of a pure 9p trisomy. This is a known viable aneuploidy. The countertype gamete with the der(21) causes monosomy 9p and

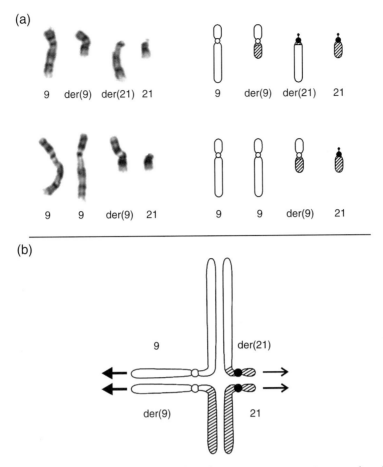

FIGURE 5–8 Adjacent-2 segregation. (*a*) Mother (*above*) has a reciprocal translocation t(9;21)(q12;q11), and her child (*below*) has the adjacent-2 karyotype 46,+der(9)t(9;21)(q12;q11). (Case of C. M. Morris and P. H. Fitzgerald.) (*b*) The presumed pachytene configuration during gametogenesis in the heterozygote (chromosome 9 chromatin, open; chromosome 21 chromatin, cross-hatched). Arrows indicate movements of chromosomes to daughter cells in adjacent-2 segregation; heavy arrows show the viable combination, as observed in this family.

is not viable. A very similar circumstance applies with the t(4;13)(q12;q12) described in Velagaleti et al. (2001); the open and cross-hatched chromosomes in the cartoon karyotype (Figure 5–8) could be regarded, for this example, as chromosomes 4 and 13, respectively. The index case in this family was trisomic for all of 4p, and the small segment 4cen-q12 (and monosomic for the tiny segment 13p-q12), having the karyotype 46,XY,+der(4),–13.

The del(22)(q11) syndrome, so well known otherwise due to microdeletion, can also arise from a familial translocation, and this provides an example of a double-segment imbalance with adjacent-2 segregation. Imagine a t(9;22)(q12;q11.21) with the 22q breakpoint just *below* the DiGeorge critical region

(DGCR; at chr22:19.0-20.0 Mb). Considering the cross-hatched chromosome in Figure 5–8b to be a chromosome 22, then the der(9) will lack the DGCR. A 46,+der(9),–22 child from adjacent-2 segregation (the heavy arrows) will have the 22q deletion syndrome, superadded upon a 9p trisomy. Pivnick et al. (1990) and El-Fouly et al. (1991) describe children in whom these separate-and-together dup(9p) and del(22q) phenotypes could be distinguished.

A double-segment exchange with both adjacent-2 segregants observed, and reflecting a parent-of-origin effect, is shown in the family reported by Abeliovich et al. (1996). The family translocation, carried by the father, was due to breakpoints in the long arms of chromosomes 15 and 21, t(15;21)

(q15;q22.1). Both centric segments, 15pter-q15 and 21pter-q22.1, are of quite substantial size. One child had the karyotype 46,–15,+der(21), with a proximal partial 15q monosomy and a proximal partial 21q trisomy. The phenotype was predominantly that of the Prader-Willi syndrome (PWS), reflecting the lack of a *paternally* contributed PWS critical region, residing in 15q11q13. There was no clearly apparent contribution from the partial trisomy for 21pter-q22.1. The other child, with a dup(15q)/del(21q) combination, 46,+der(15),–21, displayed a combination of features due to monosomy 21pter-q22.1 and trisomy 15pter-q15. An analogous story is that of a mother carrying a translocation t(15;22)(q13;q11.2), and in this case her child with the 46,–15,+der(22) combination presented the clinical picture of Angelman syndrome (AS), due to absence of a *maternally* originating AS critical region in 15q11q13 (Kosaki et al. 2009). Another child of hers had the opposite adjacent-2 imbalance, 46,–22,+der(15), and his phenotype was that of DiGeorge syndrome.

A double-segment case in which the two centric segments were much smaller is exemplified in Chen et al. (2005c). Here, in a 14;21 rearrangement, described as t(14;21)(q11.2;q11.2), both breakpoints were in the first sub-band below the centromere. The der(14) thus comprised almost all chromosome 21 material, with just the short arm, centromere, and a very small amount of proximal

long arm being from chromosome 14; and vice versa, the der(21) consisted largely of chromosome 14 material. Three affected family members, two brothers and their aunt, carried the der(14) in unbalanced state due to adjacent-2 segregation, and they were thus trisomic for the small proximal 14q segment and monosomic for the small proximal 21q segment. The dysmorphology was quite mild, but the functional neurobehavioral phenotype was rather severe. A quite similar scenario is described in Dave et al. (2009): The carriers in this family typed 46,t(14;21)(q21.2;q21.2), and the three affected individuals as 46,XX,+der(14)t(14;21)(q21.2;q21.2),–21. At the molecular level, the imbalances comprised a combination of dup chr14:20.03-42.62 Mb and del chr21:14.80-23.89 Mb. Another example with very proximal q arm breakpoints in acrocentric chromosomes is the t(14;15)(q11.2;q13.3) seen in Koochek et al. (2006). Affected individuals inheriting a duplication of proximal 15q due to a maternal adjacent-2 malsegregation displayed a phenotype of which autism was a prominent feature (presumably due to triplo-excess of chr15:30.38-32.39 Mb at 15q13.3; see p. 324).

The reason so few examples of adjacent-2 segregants are seen is that most convey a lethal imbalance during early embryogenesis. Naturally, if the window of observation were to be shifted to this period of development, more cases would reveal themselves. An example is shown in Figure 5–9, this being the

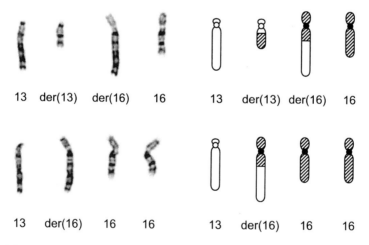

13   der(13)   der(16)   16   13   der(13)   der(16)   16

13   der(16)   16   16   13   der(16)   16   16

FIGURE 5–9   Adjacent-2 segregation, with an imbalance lethal in early pregnancy. The mother (*above*) has the karyotype 46,XX,t(13;16)(q12.3;q13). Tissue from the products of conception of a spontaneous first-trimester abortion was cultured, and the chromosomal complement from these cells (*below*) showed the karyotype 46,XX,–13,+der(16). There is monosomy of proximal 13q for a segment of HAL 0.6%, and partial trisomy 16 for a segment of HAL 2.1%. (Case of M. D. Pertile.)

karyotype from the products of conception obtained at miscarriage in the first trimester from a woman who was herself a translocation carrier, 46,XX,t(13;16)(q12.3;q13). The karyotype of the cultured products, 46,XX,−13,+der(16), displays an overall HAL imbalance of 2.6%. Two previous miscarriages to this couple might possibly also have had this karyotype. Earlier in the piece, at the 3-day embryo stage, selection pressures have not yet come to bear; thus, the finding of three embryos at preimplantation diagnosis, all with an adjacent-2 imbalance, as seen from a 46,XY,t(10;18)(q24.1;p11.2) carrier, is perhaps not too remarkable (Munné et al. 2000b).

3:1 SEGREGATION WITH TERTIARY TRISOMY

Tertiary trisomy is fairly uncommon—or to be precise, fairly uncommonly seen in a term pregnancy—and may arise only when one of the derivative chromosomes is of small content. It exists in the abnormal individual as a supernumerary chromosome, with the karyotype 47,+der. The centric segment will necessarily contain the whole short arm of the derivative chromosome, and it will necessarily be of a chromosome having a small short arm. Almost always, complete long arms (and in fact most complete short arms) contain too much material to allow viability in a supernumerary derivative chromosome, and spontaneous abortion ensues. A rare chance to illustrate this point is given in Fritz et al. (2000), who, as mentioned above, studied archived material from an abortus, the mother carrying a subtle translocation, 46,XX,t(4;12)(q34;p13). They showed a tertiary trisomy, 47,XY,+der(4), with almost the entire chromosome 4, and the tip of 12p, present as an additional chromosome. There is, as noted below, a significant maternal age effect in 3:1 imbalance.

Curiously enough, in the most common, by far, human reciprocal translocation, practically all abnormal offspring of the heterozygote have a tertiary trisomy, due to 3:1 meiosis I malsegregation. This is the t(11;22)(q23;q11) (Figure 5–10a). Carter et al. (2009) review the clinical features associated with this imbalance, known as Emanuel syndrome. The quadrivalent of this 11;22 translocation would have the form outlined in Figure 5–10b. The

content of the smallest chromosome, the der(22), is small (respecting the requirement for the derivative to have a small short arm, chromosome 22 easily qualifies), and its major genetic composition is accounted for by the distal 11q segment. The presence of this 47th chromosome does not necessarily impose a lethal distortion upon intrauterine development, and a pregnancy could continue through to the birth of a child who would have trisomy for the segment 11q23qter (and for the very small segment 22pter-q11), with the karyotype 47,+der(22),t(11;22)(q23;q11). The male t(11;22) heterozygote produces other types of unbalanced gamete, as shown on sperm chromosome study (Table 5–1), but none of these is ever viable[6]; presumably, it is similarly so in the female. Comparing[7] the sperm findings with data from embryos of male t(11;22) heterozygotes, we see a fall from the frequencies of 3:1 sperm (35%) to 3:1 embryos (21%). In the very small data from the female t(11;22) carrier, close to half of embryos, 45%, are due to 3:1 malsegregation, and this compares with 27% observed in the gametes. We should not read too much into these comparisons.

This t(11;22) is the spectacular exception to the rule that, in different families, translocations arise at different sites. The great majority of families have a "private translocation," and many may represent the first and only case in the whole of human evolution. Apparently, few predispositions for specific rearrangement exist; equally apparently, 11q23 and 22q11 show a remarkable predisposition, which may reflect a physical proximity between the two chromosomes during meiosis (Ashley et al. 2006). Kurahashi and Emanuel (2001) studied normal volunteers, and, being able to test very large numbers of sperm, they could show that de novo t(11;22)(q23;q11) translocations must be being generated from time to time; and Ohye et al. (2010), studying eight de novo cases, showed the translocation in each to have been of paternal origin.

Note the point that probands in whom a supernumerary marker chromosome (SMC) is discovered

---

6 Except in the extraordinary setting of postzygotic rescue. Kulharya et al. (2002) report a t(11;22) carrier mother having had a child from presumed adjacent-1 segregation with 46,XY,der(22) at conception, and then mitotic loss of the der(22) in one cell and duplication of the normal 22, leading to 46,XY,der(22)/46,XY mosaicism.

7 Gamete data in Table 5–1; embryo data from Table 5–2.

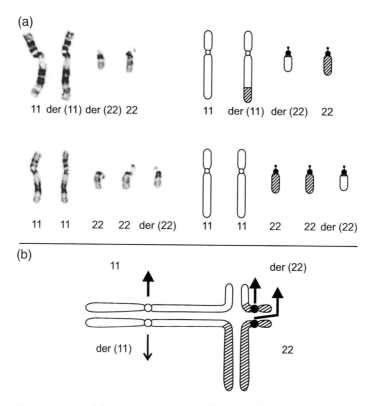

(a)

11 der (11) der (22) 22   11   der (11) der (22) 22

11   11   22   22 der (22)   11   11   22   22 der (22)

(b)

11   der (22)

der (11)   22

FIGURE 5–10   Tertiary trisomy. (*a*) The common t(11;22)(q23;q11) in the heterozygous state (*above*) and in the typical unbalanced state, associated with Emanuel syndrome (*below*). (*b*) The presumed pachytene configuration during gametogenesis in the heterozygote (chromosome 11 chromatin, open; chromosome 22 chromatin, cross-hatched). Arrows indicate movements of chromosomes to daughter cells in a 3:1 tertiary segregation; heavy arrows show the viable trisomic combination.

are often found, on parental study, to have a derivative chromosome reflecting a tertiary trisomy (Stamberg and Thomas 1986). Braddock et al. (2000) describe a family in which an SMC due to 3:1 malsegregation had, initially, escaped recognition as such. A child with "atypical Down syndrome" had been karyotyped as trisomy 21. On attending a Down syndrome clinic at age 9 years, the clinical picture raised doubt and his chromosomes were restudied. He turned out to have a tertiary trisomy for a der(21), which comprised much of chromosome 21 and a small part of distal 5p. His mother and several other relatives carried a t(5;21)(p15.1;q22.1), and a similarly abnormal aunt had the same tertiary trisomy, 47,+der(21). A rather similar account comes from Valetto et al. (2013). A young woman with a mild intellectual deficiency and what looked like 47,XX,+21 on classical karyotyping proved actually to have 47,XX,+der(21) due a maternal 46,XX,t(8;21)

(q24.21;q21.1), and the imbalance precisely defined as dup chr8:128,493,142-145,054,634, dup chr21:13,045,202-22,115,024. These stories have lessons both for cytogeneticists and for genetic counselors.

3:1 SEGREGATION WITH TERTIARY MONOSOMY

If one derivative is very small, and the amount of material that is missing is "monosomically small," the countertype 3:1 22-chromosome gamete may lead to a viable conceptus. Consider the 12;13 translocation t(12;13)(p13.32;q12.11) shown in Figure 5–11a. The large derivative chromosome is not far from being a composite of the two complete chromosomes. It is missing only subterminal 12p and pericentromeric chromosome 13. This is a "small" loss, and thus the 45,der(12) conceptus is viable (Figure 5–11b).

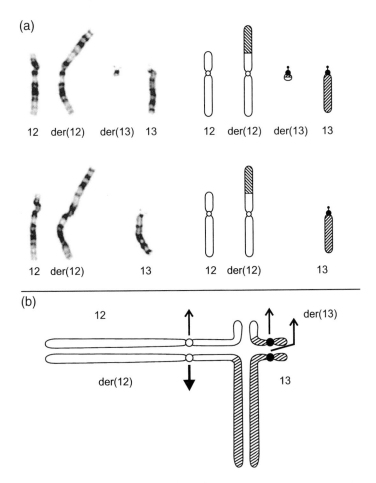

FIGURE 5–11 Tertiary monosomy. (*a*) Mother (*above*) has a reciprocal translocation between nos. 12 and 13, 46,t(12;13)(p13.32;q12.11). Two children (*below*) inherited the derivative 12, but no normal chromosome 12 or 13 from the mother, and have the karyotype 45,der(12). They are thus monosomic for the tip of 12p and pericentromeric 13 (and show only a mildly abnormal phenotype). Chorionic villus sampling in a subsequent pregnancy gave a 46,XX result; an elder sister was a balanced carrier. (Case of M. D. Pertile.) (*b*) The presumed pachytene configuration during gametogenesis in the heterozygote (chromosome 12 chromatin, open; chromosome 13 chromatin, cross-hatched). Arrows indicate movements of chromosomes to daughter cells in a 3:1 tertiary segregation; heavy arrow shows the monosomic complement. Alternatively, the three large chromosomes might form a trivalent, and the tiny der(13), being unattached, might segregate at random.

Any initially 45-count karyotype obliges consideration that there may, in fact, be a tertiary monosomy. For example, Courtens et al. (1994) describe an infant who died at birth with, at first sight cytogenetically, monosomy 21 (45,–21). But on further study, a 45,+der(1) from a maternal 1;21 translocation was discovered.

Sometimes the two phenotypes of the two contributing monosomies can be separately discerned. Thus, Reddy et al. (1996) describe children with a combined Di George (DGS) and Wolf-Hirschhorn (WHS) phenotype, having the karyotype 45,der(4)t(4;22)(p16.3;q11.2) mat. The large derivative chromosome comprised almost all of 4 and almost all of 22q, but it lacked the WHS and DGS critical segments. Similarly, McGoey and Lacassie (2009) give an account of the child of a carrier father who had features of both DGS and subtelomeric 9q deletion, with the karyotype 45,XX,der(9)t(9;22)(q34.3;q11.2)pat. Wenger et al. (1997) report a mother with a t(8;15)(p23.3;q13) whose child had the karyotype

45,der(8) and presented a phenotype with features of Angelman syndrome (due to loss of the maternally originating segment 15q11q13) and of 8p– syndrome. Torisu et al. (2004) describe a severely retarded, epileptic child with tertiary monosomy dictating a combination of Angelman syndrome and the 1p36 deletion syndrome: Her karyotype was 45,XX,der(1)t(1;15)(p36.31;q13.1)mat. An interesting historical example, in that it provided a key observation toward the discovery of the *TSC2* locus, is that of a child with 45,der(16), who had monosomy for the segment 16p13pter, and who had both tuberous sclerosis and polycystic kidney disease, due to loss and disruption, respectively, of the adjacent *TSC2* and *PKD1* loci. The heterozygous 46,t(16;22) family members had polycystic kidney disease, due to the disruption of *PKD1* (European Polycystic Kidney Disease Consortium 1994).

However, the great majority of conceptions with a tertiary monosomy are expected to be lethal in utero. A direct demonstration of this circumstance is illustrated in the case of a 3:1 malsegregation of a maternal t(11;22) in a spontaneous abortus at 7 weeks gestation with 45,der(11), which resulted in monosomy for distal 11q and monosomy for proximal 22q (Jobanputra et al. 2005).

3:1 SEGREGATION WITH INTERCHANGE TRISOMY

This mode of segregation can only produce a liveborn child when a "trisomically viable chromosome" (i.e., 13, 18, or 21, or even 22) participates in the translocation (Figure 5–12a). This chromosome accompanies the two translocation (interchange) elements of the quadrivalent to one daughter cell (Figure 5–12b). Interchange trisomy 21 is rare, interchange trisomies 13 and 18 are extremely rare, and interchange trisomy 22 is barely recorded (Stene and Stengel-Rutkowski 1988; Teshima et al. 1992; Koskinen et al. 1993; Patel and Madon 2004). Concerning other (nonviable) autosomes, interchange trisomy can be seen at PGD (Lim et al. 2008b) or upon analysis of abortus material, such as the trisomy 2 in a pregnancy from a t(2;17) (q32.1;q24.3) carrier discussed in Lorda-Sánchez et al. (2005).

Theoretically, uniparental disomy can be a consequence of interchange trisomy, if one of the "trisomic" chromosomes is subsequently lost postzygotically, and if this chromosome had come from the noncarrier parent. If this chromosome is one that is subject to imprinting according to parent of origin, phenotypic abnormality will be the consequence, notwithstanding the apparently balanced karyotype, the same as the parent's. Thus, for example, a 46,t(8;15) father could have a 46,t(8;15) child with Angelman syndrome, or a mother could have a child with Prader-Willi syndrome. Actual examples of this type of mechanism are extremely rare (Table 18–5).

3:1 SEGREGATION WITH INTERCHANGE MONOSOMY

Autosomal monosomy is typically associated with very early arrested development of the embryo. Only with PGD does a practical relevance of interchange monosomy possibly emerge, since there has not yet been the chance for selection pressure to have operated. In the PGD case reported in Conn et al. (1999) noted earlier, the woman being a t(6;21) heterozygote, a transferred embryo that implanted only transiently may have had an interchange monosomy 6. Sperm capable of giving rise to interchange monosomy can certainly be produced in numbers, as Midro et al. (2006) show in man heterozygous for a t(7;13)(q34;q13), from whom 2.8% of sperm showed interchange nullisomy 7, and 8.0% interchange nullisomy 13; had these sperm fertilized, the corresponding interchange monosomy would have resulted.

Yet to be observed is uniparental disomy following "correction" by duplication of the single normal homolog in the embryo resulting from interchange monosomy. The countertype gamete in Figure 5–12a, for example, would be nullisomic for 21. Replication of the chromosome 21 from the other gamete could restore disomy and with a normal karyotype. Note that this would be uniparental *iso*-disomy, and from the *other* parent.

4:0 SEGREGATION

A total nondisjunction of the quadrivalent complex is rare indeed. In sperm studies, only fractions of a percent of 4:0 gametes are ever seen (Table 5–1).

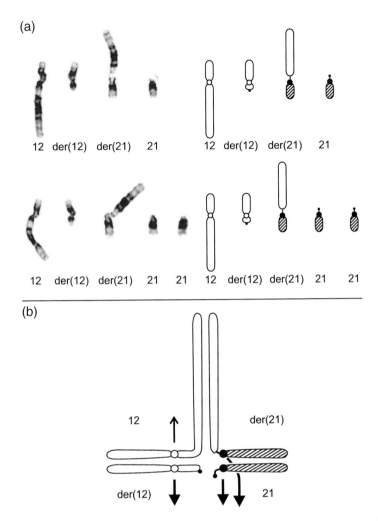

(a)

12   der(12)   der(21)   21   12   der(12)   der(21)   21

12   der(12)   der(21)   21   21   12   der(12)   der(21)   21   21

(b)

12   der(21)

der(12)   21

FIGURE 5-12   Interchange trisomy. (*a*) Mother (*above*) has a reciprocal translocation between nos. 12 and 21; her child (*below*) inherited the maternal translocation chromosomes and a "free" chromosome 21. The breakpoints are 12q13.1 and 21p13; an apparent gap, comprising satellite stalk, can be discerned between the centromere of the der(21) and its 12q component. (Case of R. Oertel.) (*b*) The presumed pachytene configuration during gametogenesis in the heterozygote (chromosome 12 chromatin, open; chromosome 21 chromatin, cross-hatched). Arrows indicate movements of chromosomes to daughter cells in 3:1 interchange segregation; heavy arrows show the trisomic combination.

If 4:0 segregation should happen, and conception follow, preimplantation lethality would, in practically all, supervene. Out of interest, the reader may care to note how a hypothetical double trisomy of 18 plus 21, based on the 4:0 combination in Figure 5–4(15), and potentially associated with some in utero survival (Reddy 1997), could come from the t(18;21) shown in Figure 5–14. The question may not be entirely academic, however, now that PGD has brought the 4:0 gamete out from its former place of practical irrelevance (Ye et al. 2012).

MORE THAN ONE UNBALANCED SEGREGANT TYPE

Sometimes a reciprocal translocation has characteristics associated with more than one type of malsegregation; so each type may be seen in the family (Abeliovich et al. 1982). Consider the 11;18 translocation t(11;18)(p15;q11) shown in Figure 5–13. First, the translocated segments are small: 18q is known to be viable in the trisomic state, and the tip of 11p contributes a minimal/nil imbalance

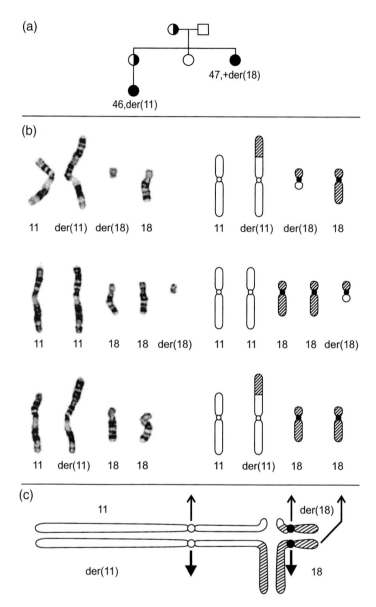

FIGURE 5–13 More than one viable segregant form. (*a*) Pedigree. Filled symbols, unbalanced karyotype, as shown; half-filled symbols, heterozygote. (*b*) Mother and one daughter have a reciprocal translocation of chromosomes 11 and 18, t(11;18)(p15;q11) (*upper*). Each had one unbalanced offspring, one having 47,+der(18) due to 3:1 tertiary trisomy (*middle*), and the other 46,+der(11) from adjacent-1 segregation (*lower*). The former had a complete trisomy 18p and the latter a partial 18q trisomy. (Case of C. Ho and I. Teshima.) (*c*) The presumed pachytene configuration during gametogenesis in the heterozygote (chromosome 11 chromatin, open; chromosome 18 chromatin, cross-hatched). Heavy arrows indicate one adjacent-1 segregant movement of chromosomes, and light arrows indicate movements of chromosomes to daughter cells in a 3:1 tertiary trisomy segregation, each of which occurred in this family.

Source: From Gardner et al., Autosomal imbalance with a near-normal phenotype: The small effect of trisomy for the short arm of chromosome 18, *Birth Defects Orig Artic Ser* 14: 359–363, 1978.

(thus, this is regarded as a single-segment imbalance). Accordingly, one of the adjacent-1 segregants is presumed to be viable. Second, two component chromosomes of the pachytene configuration, the der(18) and chromosome 18, are of small overall genetic content. Thus, 3:1 segregation with either tertiary trisomy or interchange trisomy is possible. In the event, the two unbalanced karyotypes in this family reflected adjacent-1 and 3:1 tertiary trisomy segregation. The t(9;21) discussed above as an example of adjacent-2 segregation could also, in theory, produce a second viable complement, interchange trisomy 21.

Rather more spectacular is the translocation illustrated in Figure 5–14. A mother had the karyotype 46,XX,t(18;21)(q22.1;q11.2): These breakpoints are toward the end of 18q and immediately below

the centromere in 21q. She had a stillborn child with tertiary monosomy, a miscarriage with adjacent-1 malsegregation (and two other unkaryotyped miscarriages), and a surviving child with tertiary trisomy. These three karyotyped pregnancy outcomes were, respectively, 45,der(18), 46,der(18), and 47,+der(18). An uncle said to have had Down syndrome may have had the 46,der(18) karyotype (the der(18) includes the segment of 21 that contributes substantially to the Down syndrome phenotype), or possibly interchange trisomy with 47,+21,t(18;21). Some of the other possible imbalanced segregants could theoretically be viable, and the reader may wish to determine which ones these would be. This is due to the fact that many of these combinations have a genetically "small" imbalance. All partial trisomies and some partial monosomies for segments

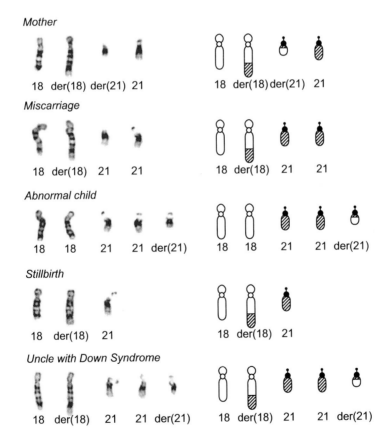

FIGURE 5–14   Several viable unbalanced forms. The karyotype is illustrated (*top*) of a mother carrying the translocation t(18;21)(q22.1;q11.2). She had a miscarriage due to adjacent-1 segregation, an abnormal child with a tertiary trisomy, and a stillborn child with a tertiary monosomy, as depicted in the cartoon karyotypes. An uncle with Down syndrome may have had the same adjacent-1 karyotype as in the second row, or possibly interchange trisomy 21, as depicted in the bottom row. (Case of M. D. Pertile.)

of chromosomes 18 and 21 can be viable as a single imbalance; and when two different imbalances occur in combination, for example, partial trisomy 21 plus partial monosomy 18, a pregnancy may still be capable of proceeding substantially along its course.

NO UNBALANCED MODE POSSIBLE

Finally, for the translocation in which the quadrivalent is characterized by long translocated and long centric segments, no mode of segregation could produce a viable unbalanced outcome. We emphasize the point that many reciprocal translocations (including whole-arm translocations) are in this category. Consider the family depicted in Figure 5–15, in which a 4;6 translocation t(4;6) (q25;p23) was discovered by chance at amniocentesis. The quadrivalent would have the form depicted in Figure 5–5d. It possesses none of the criteria that would allow a viable imbalance to result, by whatever mode of segregation. The translocated segments are both large (leading to double-segment imbalance); the centric segments are very large; and the content of all four chromosomes is large. Miscarriage is as far as any unbalanced conceptus could ever get, and in some instances infertility will be the presenting complaint. The large kindred of Madan and Kleinhout

(1987) graphically illustrates this circumstance: 11 carriers of a t(1;20)(p36;p11) had had two or more miscarriages, and numerous normal children, but none had had an abnormal child. In some such translocations identified fortuitously, for example, at amniocentesis for maternal age, there may be little or no history of apparent reproductive difficulty.

Meiosis II Nondisjunction. The great majority of segregant forms will have been determined at meiosis I. Meiosis II is not to be completely overlooked, however. A balanced complement may have been transmitted at meiosis I, but a nondisjunction at the following second meiotic division could then produce a gamete with an extra copy, or no copy, of one or other of the derivative chromosomes. In consequence, the conception would have either a partial trisomy of the component parts of the additional derivative chromosome, or a partial monosomy (Masuno et al. 1991). Illustrating the former possibility, Wu et al. (2009) document the case of a father who carried a t(9;15)(q34.3;q13), and whose child, who developed severe autism, had the karyotype 47,XY,t(9;15),+der(15). This imparted a duplication of the proximal long arm of chromosome 15 (which contains autism-susceptibility genes), and of an 8 Mb segment on distal 9q. This

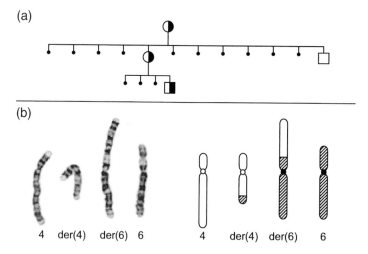

FIGURE 5–15 No unbalanced product viable. (*a*) Pedigree of a kindred in which mother and daughter have had multiple miscarriages, each having (*b*) the karyotype 46,XX,t(4;6)(q25;p23). (Case of A. J. Watt.) The presumed pachytene configuration during gametogenesis in the heterozygote would be as in Figure 5–5d (chromosome 4 chromatin, open; chromosome 6 chromatin, cross-hatched) and, with large centric and translocated segments, the translocation has none of the features that enable viability of any unbalanced segregant combination.

type of "secondary nondisjunction" is very rarely observed.[8]

Meiotic Drive. As well as the effect of in utero survivability discussed above, the nature of the quadrivalent may, of itself, influence segregation. The propensity for a particular segregation outcome may reflect a particular geometry of the quadrivalent, and what sort of ring or chain it forms. Quadrivalents that have translocation chromosomes with short translocated segments more usually form a ring, and have the quality of being more likely to generate adjacent-1 gametes, while those with short centric segments, more often existing as a chain, may have a predisposition to the formation of adjacent-2 and 3:1 gametes (Faraut et al. 2000; Benet et al. 2005). Zhang et al. (2014) analyzed segregations at preimplantation genetic diagnosis (PGD), and determined that increasing asymmetry of the quadrivalent (estimated from increased ratios of the lengths of the two translocated and of the two centric segments) reduced the fraction of embryos due to alternate segregation, by an average of almost one half. This predisposition to form particular classes of segregant gamete may be considered a form of "meiotic drive."

As we have had cause to comment more than once, each translocation is entitled to its individuality, and need not necessarily follow the "rules" set out earlier. Faraut et al. (2000) identified a few translocations that "should" have produced sperm with certain expected proportions of adjacent-1 and adjacent-2, but which did not. We have seen a remarkable family in which, over some 10 years of marriage, the wife had had innumerable very early miscarriages, about eight at 12–14 weeks, one at 16 weeks, and one phenotypically normal son. The husband (and the son) had the translocation 46,XY,t(12;20)(q15;p13). Perhaps, the quadrivalent was configured in such a way that alternate segregation was very difficult to achieve, and so almost all sperm had an unbalanced complement. De Perdigo et al. (1991) report a possibly similar case, in which they propose that heterosynapsis in the quadrivalent permitted spermatogenesis to proceed, but at the cost of producing many unbalanced gametes. In a family reported in Groen et al. (1998) with a mother having the karyotype 46,XX,t(5q;6q)(q35.2;q27), seven sequential

retarded siblings of hers are presumed to have had a dup(5)/del(6) karyotype, and only the two eldest and the youngest were phenotypically normal. Observations from the PGD laboratory are further illustrating the point that translocation carriers with very poor reproductive histories may indeed reflect a very high rate of meiotic malsegregation. The patient in Conn et al. (1999) mentioned earlier, she having the karyotype 46,XX,t(6;21)(q13;q22.3), had had four miscarriages and one child with interchange trisomy 21. She came to PGD, and not one of two oöcytes and nine embryos were chromosomally normal (they were mostly 3:1, some adjacent segregations).

Failure to Form Quadrivalent. Where very small segments are involved, the imperative may lack for the coming together of the four chromosomes with segments in common. This likely applies to the general case of the subtelomeric translocation, such as the t(3;4)(p26.3;p16.1) in Iype et al. (2015) referred to above, in which the der chromosomes comprise almost a complete copy of the normal. The opposite, in which the der consists almost entirely of chromatin of the other chromosome, is exemplified in the t(14;15)(q12;q12) in Burke et al. (1996), in which the derivative chromosomes each comprise near to an entire chromosome 14 and chromosome 15, respectively. In the above examples, the 3 and the der(3) and the 4 and der(4), and the 14 and der(15), and the 15 and der(14), respectively, might simply synapse as bivalent pairs. If that were indeed so, then a segregation ratio of 1:1:1:1 would presumably operate, for normal, balanced, and the two imbalanced outcomes: clearly, a high-risk circumstance.

Different grounds for the nonformation of a quadrivalent may exist if one chromosome is a very small one. While the three other chromosomes could have come together as a trivalent, the fourth very small one might fail to be captured by the meiotic mechanism. That being so, it could then segregate at random. This could imply a high risk, and might be the reason, for example, that the t(12;13) carrier mother in Figure 5–11 had two out of her four children with a tertiary monosomy. But this is speculative. Detaching of the small derivative from the quadrivalent is an alternative possibility, as discussed in the next paragraph.

---

8 Another route to this observation could be a 3:1 disjunction following a crossover in an interstitial segment (Petković et al. 1996).

Parental Origin and Parental Age Effect. There are more women who have been mothers (whether the children are normal or not) than there are men who have been fathers in translocation families. In their review of 1,597 children in 1,271 translocation families, Faraut et al. (2000) found the mother to be the carrier parent in 61% of the adjacent-1 children, 70% of the adjacent-2 children, and in as many as 92% of the unbalanced offspring from 3:1 segregations. This 3:1 association may reflect an actual maternal predisposition. With advancing maternal age, and after some decades of being held in meiosis I prophase, the small supernumerary chromosome may be increasingly likely to detach from the quadrivalent, and then to migrate at random to one or other daughter cell, when meiosis reactivates in that particular menstrual cycle. On the other hand, no maternal age effect applies to adjacent-1 or adjacent-2 offspring. Here, the maternal excess may more accurately be termed a paternal deficiency, due to reduction in fertility of the male heterozygote (discussed below). No paternal age effect is discernible in any segregation mode.

THE PRACTICAL PROBLEM OF THE APPARENTLY BALANCED TRANSLOCATION

The apparently balanced translocation, and particularly when de novo, which has been discovered in the course of investigation of a child with a nonspecific picture of cognitive compromise and sometimes also some dysmorphic signs, raises the question: Is the translocation causative, or simply coincidental (Feenstra et al. 2011)? Families like those reported in Hussain et al. (2000) offer useful illustration: in this example, an apparently balanced translocation that was co-segregating with a phenotype of nonsyndromic mental retardation. Presumably this translocation, a t(1;17) (p36.3;p11.2), had been de novo at some prior point, possibly with the 65-year-old grandmother of their index case. In this family, there were children and grandchildren, seven of them, to bear witness to the apparent harmful role of the translocation. Thus, the point is underlined: Certainly, some apparently balanced translocations are indeed the cause of the nonspecific clinical picture with which they are associated.

The point is further demonstrated, and often convincingly so, on molecular karyotyping, or next-generation sequencing (NGS) (Bertelsen et al.

2016). De Gregori et al. (2007) undertook a systematic search and showed that 40% of 27 apparently balanced de novo translocations in abnormal individuals, originally analyzed on classical karyotyping, in fact were not so, with microdeletion demonstrable at the sites of breakpoint. (In some, they identified coincidental de novo deletions at chromosomal sites other than at the translocation breakpoints.) Baptista et al. (2008) undertook a similar exercise in 31 normal and 14 abnormal cases. Some in the abnormal group had microdeletions (although not all were at the breakpoint sites) that offered a likely explanation for the observed phenotype, but none of the normals did.

A detailed example of gene disruption is provided in Kurahashi et al. (1998). A child with lissencephaly (a severe structural brain abnormality) had a de novo t(8;17)(p11.2;p13.3). The p13.3 breakpoint on the chromosome 17 was sited within intron 1 of the *LIS* gene, with the gene being split between the two derivative chromosomes: its 5′ part on the der(8), and the rest of it on the der(17). The gene could not, in consequence, function. A similar circumstance, but in which the translocation was familial, is given in Luukkonen et al. (2012), who studied a t(10;11)(q23.2;q24.2) in a family with apparently autosomal dominant thoracic aortic aneurysm. They could show that the 11q25 breakpoint was sited in intron 1 of a splicing isoform of *NTM* (chr11:131.3 Mb); in principle, haploinsufficiency of this gene could be the basis of the vascular disease, although the pedigree was not of sufficient size to allow a confident interpretation. In a study of autism patients with apparently balanced rearrangements, most turned out not to have a detectable genomic imbalance (Tabet et al. 2015). But in one case from this series, with an apparently balanced de novo translocation t(5;18)(q12;p11.2), a 4.2 Mb deletion at the 18p11.2 breakpoint, chr18:5,408,998-9,625,752, was found. An apparently balanced familial t(3;5) (q25;q31) in Bertelsen et al. (2016) turned out, on NGS, to be sufficiently complex that it was labeled a "germline chromothripsis" event (p. 226). Finally, Redin et al. (2017) applied whole-genome sequencing in 248 subjects, in whom a spectrum of congenital anomalies and neurobehavioral disability was presented, and each with an apparently balanced rearrangement (Figure 5–16). Most were de novo. The analyses led to a revision of the interpretation, in terms of the cytogenetic band(s) involved, in as many as 93% of karyotypes. In two-thirds, gene disruption at a breakpoint site, or genomic imbalance

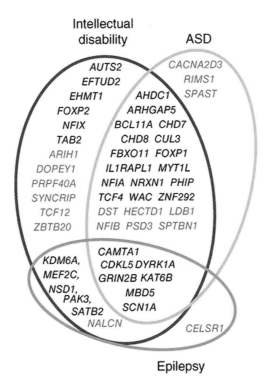

Intellectual disability

ASD

AUTS2
EFTUD2
EHMT1
FOXP2
NFIX
TAB2
ARIH1
DOPEY1
PRPF40A
SYNCRIP
TCF12
ZBTB20

AHDC1
ARHGAP5
BCL11A CHD7
CHD8 CUL3
FBXO11 FOXP1
IL1RAPL1 MYT1L
NFIA NRXN1 PHIP
TCF4 WAC ZNF292
DST HECTD1 LDB1
NFIB PSD3 SPTBN1

CACNA2D3
RIMS1
SPAST

KDM6A,
MEF2C,
NSD1,
PAK3,
SATB2
NALCN

CAMTA1
CDKL5 DYRK1A
GRIN2B KAT6B
MBD5
SCN1A

CELSR1

Epilepsy

FIGURE 5–16   Apparently balanced rearrangements subjected to analysis by whole genome sequencing, from a study of 248 cases. At the molecular level, the loci depicted were compromised, due to their residence at or near a chromosomal breakpoint. Those loci in bold are presumed to have been, by virtue of their structural/functional haploinsufficient state, definitely pathogenic; those in gray are likely pathogenic. The Venn diagram shows phenotypes otherwise associated with these several loci. ASD, autism spectrum disorder.

Source: From Redin et al., The genomic landscape of balanced cytogenetic abnormalities associated with human congenital anomalies, Nat Genet 49: 36–45, 2017. Courtesy M. E. Talkowski, and with the permission of Nature Publishing Group.

consequential thereupon, was likely the basis of the abnormal phenotype.

In the extraordinary coincidence of a recessive mutation being on the intact homolog, a translocation breakpoint that disrupted a gene would lead to the appearance of the recessive syndrome, as Kuechler et al. (2010) exemplify in a teenage girl with gonadal failure, who received an apparently balanced t(2;8)(p21;p23.1) from her mother that removed two exons from the FSHR gene (FSH receptor gene, which is located at 2p21), and a point mutation in that same gene on her paternal chromosome 2.

As for the position-effect scenario, there are numerous examples, in which a specific phenotype is caused due to a close-by intact gene failing to function. We illustrate in Figure 14–2 one of the earliest such cases, due to a chromosome 17q25.1 translocation whose breakpoint is ~50 kb away from the SOX9 locus, leading to campomelic dysplasia (Fonseca et al. 2013). Other cases include a translocation with an 11p13 breakpoint that moves the PAX6 gene into a chromosomal environment which does not permit its normal expression, with consequential abnormal development of the iris (aniridia); a girl with severe speech impairment who had a t(7;10)(q31;p14) influencing the FOXP2 language-acquisition gene at 7q31; a t(12;17)(p13.3;q21.3) affecting the function of the HOXB gene cluster, causing mental retardation and skeletal malformations; and blepharophimosis-ptosis-epicanthus inversus syndrome due to translocation (3;11)(q22.3;q14.1), the 3q22.3 breakpoint of which is located upstream of the FOXL2 gene, and separating the gene from its cis-regulatory elements (Crolla and van Heyningen 2002; Yue et al. 2007; Kosho et al. 2008; Schlade-Bartusiak et al. 2012).

In the study of Redin et al. (2017) mentioned above, a number of patients with a phenotype consistent with the 5q14.3 deletion syndrome (p. 278) had a breakpoint at, or close to, *MEF2C* at 5q14.3. Here, a position effect—a "disrupted long-range regulatory interaction"—is implicated, and may be the consequence of an inappropriate apposition, or otherwise perturbation, of "topologically associating domains"[9] in this part of the chromosome (see also below).

A salutary tale comes from the study of a family with an apparently dominantly inherited syndrome of skeletal anomalies, in which previous cytogenetic tests had given normal results (Stalker et al. 2001). Only after the birth of an infant with severe multiple malformations with an unbalanced karyotype was the fact revealed of a balanced t(13;17)(q22.1;q23.3) co-segregating with the phenotype of the syndrome in the family. There is a fair case for considering that a "bone locus" at 17q23.3 had been disrupted or otherwise influenced by the translocation. Stalker et al. rightly comment that a chromosome test is always worth doing in the investigation of an apparently new familial syndrome, earlier reports of normal cytogenetics notwithstanding, especially if the original laboratory material is not available for review. However, there does always remain the simple possibility that a breakpoint and a disease locus are closely linked, and so the translocation and the disease co-segregate in the family (Hecht and Hecht 1984).

Constitutional translocations might convey a risk for cancer if, for example, a tumor suppressor gene is disabled, or an oncogene is separated from its controlling region. Translocations possibly implying risks for renal cancer, hematological malignancy, and neurofibromatosis type 2, are noted in the section on "Genetic Counseling."

With molecular karyotyping substantially replacing the classical approach, some balanced reciprocal translocations will fail to be detected. This could, in principle, lead to recognition occurring only after a child with an imbalance has been born from a carrier parent. Pasquier et al. (2016) wrote an article "Karyotype Is Not Dead (Yet!)," in which they illustrate that translocations which disrupt a gene but without loss of genetic material, or in which the breakpoint lies within an intron,

may not be seen with current molecular methodology. Yet it would be difficult to justify the cost of routine microscope karyotyping in patients with a previous normal molecular karyotype, based on the very small increase in diagnostic yield. New methodologies may answer the question (and offer further challenge to classical karyotyping), as presented in Redin et al. (2017) above, and as Ordulu et al. (2016) and Liang et al. (2017) exemplify in NGS studies of apparently balanced rearrangements ascertained in the prenatal diagnosis clinic.

Remarkable insight is due to the international breakpoint mapping consortium presented in Tommerup et al. (2017), who have compared NGS findings in phenotypically normal and abnormal carriers of apparently balanced rearrangements. Breakpoints in the abnormal cases are more likely to occur within known autosomal dominant genes, or genes that are susceptible to loss of function; or, within 'topologically associating domains' (TADs; footnote 9). The long-range position effect that we noted above may inhere in perturbation of 'conserved non-exonic elements' residing within these TADs (cneTADs). Such cneTADs are enriched for control factors bearing upon developmental genes; we could thus imagine, in the example of the 17q25.1 campomelic dysplasia above, that a non-exonic element acting as a transcription factor within a TAD that would normally influence activity of SOX9, would be rendered impotent by a translocation breakpoint at that site, and insufficient SOX9 production would then lead to the anatomic defects characterizing the syndrome.

INFERTILITY

Infrequently, the process of gamete formation in the male translocation heterozygote is disturbed to the extent that gametogenic arrest results. In the analysis of reproductive outcomes in the translocation families of Faraut et al. (2000), looking at prenatal diagnoses in order to avoid bias, 61% of all fetuses came from a carrier mother, versus only 39% from a carrier father; this ratio presumably reflects male infertility associated with the carrier state (and as also mentioned above). This infertility is generally not something that is predictable from the nature of the translocation, and indeed the same translocation

---

9 A topologically associating domain is a segment of chromatin, the DNA of kb to Mb size, within which physical interactions can take place: a spatial folding brings enhancers into closer proximity to their client genes (which might otherwise be quite apart in linear genomic distance), and thus enabling a long-range regulatory control. A 3-D genome browser enables interrogation apropos: http://promoter.bx.psu.edu/hi-c/ (Wang et al. 2018).

may compromise fertility in only some men in the family. Presumably there is, in addition, an effect of the genetic background otherwise (Rumpler 2001).

The detrimental effect upon fertility is considered to be a consequence of failure of pairing (asynapsis or heterosynapsis) of homologous elements in the translocation chromosomes during meiosis I, which promotes association of the quadrivalent with the X-Y bivalent, also known as the sex chromosome vesicle (Paoloni-Giacobino et al. 2000b). The more frequently this association occurs, the more marked the effect upon sperm count. The semen profiles of translocation carriers may not always predict fertility outcomes. In the two cases reported by Oliver-Bonet et al. (2005), one male carried a t(10;14), was normozoöspermic, but had 30% of spermatocytes showing synaptic pairing abnormalities; the other was a t(13;20) man, who was azoöspermic, and showed synaptic pairing abnormalities in 71% of meiotic spreads. This latter carrier also showed decreased recombination frequencies. In carrier men with intact fertility, the spatial organization of chromosomes within the sperm nucleus differs from normal controls (Wiland et al. 2008). Rearranged chromosomes are not able to be packaged as neatly as they should, so to speak; and this might, in some men, be an additional contributory factor compromising spermatogenesis.

The sex difference in susceptibility is striking in the family of Paoloni-Giacobino et al. (2000b). A mother was a t(6;21)(p21.1;p13) heterozygote, and she had eight children, four sons and four daughters (and two miscarriages). The four sons, each one 46,XY,t(6;21), were all married, one three times, and none had any children. Each had severe oligospermia or oligoasthenoteratospermia, and the two having testicular biopsies manifested spermatogenic arrest at meiosis I prophase, with extensive asynapsis of several chromosomes. Two sisters were 46,XX,t(6;21), and the one who was married had had two children (and two miscarriages).

Oögenesis may not, however, always be immune to the translocation obstacle. Tupler et al. (1994) report two women, one with primary and the other with secondary amenorrhea, who each had a balanced reciprocal translocation. Ovarian biopsy in the former, whose translocation was a de novo one, showed absence of the follicle structures in the cortex. D'Ippolito et al. (2011) describe a woman in her thirties presenting

with infertility, and of karyotype 46,XX,t(1;11)(q23;p11.2), whose hormonal markers were normal, but who responded very poorly to follicle-stimulating hormone (FSH) stimulation. On the first stimulation cycle, only two mature follicles resulted, and intracytoplasmic sperm injection (ICSI) was unsuccessful. On a second cycle, with an increased FSH dose, just one oöcyte was retrieved, and again ICSI failed. More widely, Chen et al. (2005d) studied a number of "translocation couples" and compared ovarian responses between those where the male or the female partner was the heterozygote. The 28 female rcp carriers did worse than the women whose male partner was the heterozygote, as measured by estradiol levels following human chorionic gonadotrophin (HCG)[10] stimulation: 23% were "very low responders," compared with 7% where the female was not the carrier. It remains true, however, that oögenesis in most female carriers is apparently unscathed.

Assisted Reproduction. Assisted conception may enable infertile men with a translocation to become fathers. But of course the translocation will, in any event, convey a genetic risk. Meschede et al. (1997) report a man with a t(1;9)(q44;p11.2) having ICSI, and two embryos were successfully transferred. At prenatal diagnosis, one twin had an adjacent-1 imbalance conferring a 9p trisomy, the other being 46,XX, and the parents chose selective abortion. Belin et al. (1999) describe a triplet pregnancy achieved via ICSI, the father being a t(20;22) heterozygote. Two normal babies were born (one karyotypically normal, one with the translocation), but the third, with a dup(20p)/del(22q) imbalance, was severely malformed and died in the neonatal period.

RARE COMPLEXITIES

Double Translocation Carrier. The double two-way rcp translocation comprises, essentially, two coincidental simple rcps (Phelan et al. 1990; Yardin et al. 1997). Presumably, two separate and independently operating quadrivalents can form. Burns et al. (1986) record sperm karyotypes in a man with a double two-way 46,XY,rcp(5;11)(p13;q23.2),rcp(7;14)(q11.23;q24.1), whose wife had had four miscarriages, a child with cri du chat syndrome, and a normal son carrying the rcp(7;14). Only four of 23 sperm analyzed had an overall balanced complement,

---

10 HCG is very similar functionally to luteinizing hormone (LH). FSH and LH promote egg production and estrogen output.

and the majority (13) had adjacent-1 segregants for one or the other translocation. Another five showed 3:1 and one sperm showed 4:0 segregation.[11]

Bowser-Riley et al. (1988) review the specific case of the double two-way translocation, and propose that the risk to have an abnormal child would be approximately the sum of the figures derived separately for each rcp. They acknowledge that might be an overestimate due to nonviability of doubly imbalanced combinations, albeit that each on its own might be viable. We have seen a couple, the husband having a double two-way translocation 46,XY,t(2;20)(p25.1;p11.23),t(4;8)(q27;p21.1), who had presented following four first-trimester miscarriages, although their first pregnancy having produced a normal (but unkaryotyped) son. Of 320 theoretically possible karyotypes, only four (1.25%) would be balanced (and thus raising a glimmer of hope that their first fortunate pregnancy might reflect a tendency toward a balanced combination). Following ovulation stimulation with the collection of 25 eggs, of which 23 were subjected to ICSI and 18 embryos resulting, biopsy was achieved in 15 embryos; but none had a balanced constitution.

Carrier Couple. Since reciprocal translocation heterozygotes are not uncommon in the population, on rare occasions both members of a couple will, by chance, carry a translocation (Neu et al. 1988b). We have seen, for example, a couple who had had several miscarriages, from 5 to 9 weeks gestation. The husband's karyotype was 46,XY,t(7;11)(q22;q23) and the wife's 46,XX,t(7;22)(p13;q11.2). Presumably, their history of miscarriage reflected at least one parent transmitting, with each pregnancy, an unbalanced gamete: Rather many unbalanced karyotypes, as the reader can determine, are possible! A normal child is possible if each contributes a normal or a balanced gamete to the same conceptus. It should, in theory, be reasonably likely in a given conception for the two contemporaneous gametes to have arisen from alternate segregation—as an educated guess, the chance might be about 20%—although at the time of our seeing this family, only miscarriage had occurred. A child of theirs having each parental translocation would qualify as having a "double two-way translocation."

If a translocation is in a family, and a couple are related, the possibility is open that they might both be carriers. Such a scenario is illustrated in Kupchik et al. (2005), who report a husband and wife with the karyotypes 46,XY,t(16;18)(p13.3;p11.2) and 46,XX,t(16;18)(p13.3;p11.2). Their child received two copies of the der(18) and one of the der(16), due to alternate segregation in one parent and adjacent-1 in the other. As the reader may determine, the end result was a duplication of distal 16p and a deletion of 18p. In Martinet et al. (2006), a first cousin couple each carried a t(17;20)(q21.1;p11.21), and their severely malformed fetus was homozygous for the translocation. The phenotype may have been due to a recessive gene or genes. Similar histories with respect to a Robertsonian translocation, and to an inversion, are noted in Chapters 7 and 9, respectively.

Mosaicism. Almost all balanced reciprocal translocations are seen in the nonmosaic state. This reflects either that the translocation had been inherited from a carrier parent, or that the rearrangement had arisen preconceptually, in one or other gamete. Rarely, a balanced translocation can be generated as a postzygotic event, and the person is a 46,t/46,N mosaic. In a literature review, Leegte et al. (1998) recorded 29 such cases. One of their subjects, for example, was a man who had presented with infertility, and he had the balanced karyotype 46,XY,t(9;15)(q12;p11.2). His mother had this translocation in a minority of cells on peripheral blood analysis, with the karyotype 46,XX,t(9;15)(q12;p11.2)/46,XX; thus, she was revealed as a somatic-gonadal mosaic. Wang et al. (1998) report a mother mosaic for a whole-arm translocation, 46,XX,t(10q;16q)/46,XX, who had a child with a presumed uniparental disomy 16 phenotype from postzygotic "correction" of interchange trisomy 16. The grandmother in Dupont et al. (2008) had 46,XX,t(9;22)(q34.3;q13.3)[10]/46,XX[10] mosaicism; her normal daughter was a nonmosaic translocation carrier; and her abnormal grandson (since deceased) and her abnormal daughter were both 46,der(22)t(9;22)(q34.3;q13.3). The translocated segments were very small, but the 22q segment, for which the affected individuals were deleted, included the *SHANK3* locus (cf. Phelan-McDermid syndrome, p. 309). (Mosaicism for an *un*balanced translocation

---

11 This case is instructive in illustrating the point that different rcps can have different meiotic behavior, as also is the man in Table 5–1 with 46,XY,t(5;11)(p13;q23.2),t(7;14)(q11;q24.1). In the latter, 70% of the rcp(5;11) segregants but only 30% of the rcp(7;14) showed alternate segregation, any environmental effect accounted for by both translocations acting in the same gonad.

is well recorded (e.g., Choi et al. 2015), but our concern here is with the balanced state.)

Unstable Familial Translocation. Tomkins (1981) documents a family in which a mother with 46,XX,t(11;22)(p11;p12) had one daughter with the same translocation, and another daughter with 46,XX,t(11;15)(p11;p12), and a very few other similar cases are on record. Typically, the translocation breakpoints are at telomeres, centromeres, or in nucleolar organizing regions. There is some sequence similarity in these regions between different chromosomes, and this may set the stage for these very rare "second translocation" events (and see "Jumping Translocation," p. 226).

GENETIC COUNSELING

The counselor may have to deal with these questions:

1. Is there a risk of having an abnormal child?
2. If so, what is the magnitude of the risk?
3. What would be the abnormality, and would the child survive?
4. What if the same translocation that I have is found at prenatal diagnosis?
5. What is the risk for pregnancy loss through abortion? Is pregnancy possible?
6. Anything else I should know?

DOES A RISK EXIST OF HAVING AN ABNORMAL CHILD?

If a family is ascertained through a liveborn aneuploid child, that very fact demonstrates viability for that particular aneuploid combination. It could happen again.

If, on the other hand, the family was ascertained by miscarriage or infertility, or fortuitously, and there is no known family history of an abnormal child, the picture is less clear. Most likely, no aneuploid combination is viable. Alternatively, a viable imbalance may be possible, but it has not yet happened; or an imbalance could occasionally be viable, but usually it is not, and (so far) has led only to abortion. The approach, here, is to determine the potentially unbalanced segregant outcomes, according to the favored mode of segregation—adjacent-1, adjacent-2, or 3:1—and check to see whether any is on record in a pregnancy that produced an abnormal child. Valuable sources of information include Schinzel's (2001) catalog and the European

Cytogeneticists Association register of unbalanced chromosome aberrations (ECARUCA).

Where a single-segment imbalance is a potential outcome in a conceptus, from adjacent segregation, and if the potential imbalance comprises an aneuploidy equal to, or less than, one of these segments on record, viability must be assumed to be possible. If the potential imbalance comprised an aneuploidy greater than any on record, viability would be unlikely, especially if the aneuploidy is much greater. The great majority of double-segment imbalances from adjacent segregation due to a translocation, ascertained other than by a liveborn aneuploid child, would be expected to lead to lethality in utero. Nearly always, a new double-segment exchange presenting at the clinic will truly be new, and there will be no literature record of exactly the same thing to which the counselor may appeal. In many instances one has to make an educated guess, erring on the side of caution, whether the combination of imbalances from a derivative chromosome might, in sum, be viable.

The Magnitude of Risk

If, in a family, it is judged that there does exist a risk to have an abnormal child, a broad estimate of the level of risk may be derived from a consideration of these factors: the assessed imbalance of potentially viable gametes; the predicted type of segregation leading to potentially viable gametes; the mode of ascertainment of the family; and in 3:1, the sex of the transmitting parent. Most risk figures fall in a range from 0% to 30%; higher risks are rare. These percentages are expressed in terms of abnormal live births as a proportion of all live births, although there are other ways of looking at the risk (see section on "Risk at the Time of Prenatal Diagnosis" and also Table 4–3). Overall, the risk is higher in cases ascertained through an abnormal child, versus those identified through other routes; in the review of Youings et al. (2004), the respective pooled figures were 19% and 3%.

A precise risk estimate needs to be based on the actual cytogenetic imbalance. Different chromosomal segments contain, of course, different genomic information. It is scarcely possible to come up with a unifying format, given that chromatin is not uniform; as Cohen et al. (1994) comment, "it would be hazardous to suggest a simple mathematical relationship between unbalance length and viability." Some segments, in the trisomic state, impose a lesser degree of compromise on the process of embryonic development; such as, for example, 18p, and distal 5p. The family of De Carvalho et al. (2008) with a single-segment rcp(5p;21p), mentioned above, had a risk of essentially 50% for 5p monosomy or trisomy, supposing that no prenatal losses happened, and that segregation occurred evenly between alternate and adjacent-1. Other segments, although they may be of shorter length, are lethal during early pregnancy and lead to miscarriage. Some translocations can have their own peculiar segregation characteristics, which a priori were quite unpredictable.

Nonetheless, it is interesting to attempt a correlation of quantitative chromatin imbalance with risk to have a liveborn affected child. Daniel et al. (1989), Cans et al. (1993), and Cohen et al. (1994) have compared the haploid autosomal length (HAL) with viability in translocation families. Most (96%) viable imbalances comprise up to 2% monosomy, and up to 4% trisomy, with combinations of monosomy/trisomy viable only when the additive effect of x% monosomy plus y% trisomy falls within a triangular area defined by joining the 2% and 4% points on the x and y axes of a graph (Figure 5–17).

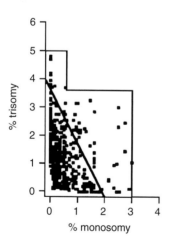

FIGURE 5–17   Viability of combined duplication/deletion states, according to amount of imbalance, measured as % HAL. Most (96%) fall within the triangular area whose hypotenuse lies between 4% duplication/0% deletion and 2% deletion/0% duplication, and a few outliers define an envelope of viable imbalances.

Source: From Cohen et al. 1994, Viability thresholds for partial trisomies and monosomies. A study of 1,159 viable unbalanced reciprocal translocations, *Hum Genet* 93: 188–194. Courtesy O. Cohen, and with the permission of Springer-Verlag.

A few (4%) fall outside of this area, and these cases define the boundaries of a "surface of viable unbalances," reflecting the effects of qualitative differences in different segments of chromatin.

For routine practice in the genetic clinic, and if the counselee wishes to have a good idea of the level of risk, we suggest starting off with the unvarnished empiric data for individual chromosome segments collected by Stengel-Rutkowski and colleagues, as set out in their invaluable monograph (Stengel-Rutkowski et al. 1988), and discussed in a review and further illustrated in practice (Stene and Stengel-Rutkowski 1988; Midro et al. 1992), and to which we have already referred several times above. The figures set out in Tables 5–4, 5–6, and 5–7, for the three major categories of malsegregation, are summarized from their monograph and from additional subsequent data. It would give a false sense of precision to use decimal points; a rounded figure will suffice. The paucity of information for some chromosomes has necessitated lumping of data for considerable lengths of a chromosome arm; the risk figures derived in this way are, naturally, composites, and indicative rather than definitive. We assume that, in different families with (apparently) the same translocation, the genetic risks will likely be the same, regardless of what may have been the mode of ascertainment. And of course, the principle always applies: If the counselee's family is large enough, do a segregation analysis to derive a "private" recurrence risk.

The figure given for a segment, say, q31/q34qter—in other words, a lumped figure applying to a segment extending anywhere from q31qter to q34qter—might be given as, say, <0.8%: in other words, a very small risk. (The "less than" sign in the risk data tables is used for estimates in those translocations where no additional aneuploid child has been born apart from probands.) But this figure might have been based mostly on data from families having a q31 breakpoint. A breakpoint at q34 might happen to exclude a dosage-sensitive region of major effect within q33, and thus imbalance for the slightly smaller segment q34qter might be of considerably greater viability. The risk figure needs to be interpreted intelligently in the light of what is otherwise known from the literature and web resources about the segments in question, and naturally from observation within the same family.

The reader consulting and using these figures, imperfect though they may be, will gain a good sense of the practical principles of estimating

Table 5–4. Specific Risk Figures, Based upon Empiric Data, for Having a Liveborn Aneuploid Child, or a Child Stillborn or Dying as a Neonate,[a] Because of Single-Segment Imbalance from 2:2 Adjacent-1 Segregation[b]

TRANSLOCATED SEGMENT THAT WOULD BE IMBALANCED[c]		RISK		
		% LIVEBORN	S.D.	+ % STILLBORN, NEONATAL DEATH[E]
1.	1pter→1p11–p34	0		
	1p35	?		
	1qter→q11–q22	0		
	q23–q32	<1.3		+ 5.1
	q42	13.6	5.2	
2.	2pter→p11–p12	0		
	p13–p16	<2.5		+ 15.0
	p21–p23	5.7	3.9	+ 14.3
	2qter→q11–q23	0		
	q31–q32	<1.7		+ 6.7
	q33	20.0	8.9	
	q34–q35	22.9	7.1	+ 11.4
3.	3pter→p13–p14	0		
	p21	<2.3		+ 13.6
	p22–p25	28.6	17.1	
	3qter→q12–q13.2	0		
	q21–q27	<1.1		
4.	4pter→p11	7.7	5.2	+ 38.5
	p14	15.4	4.5	+ 7.7
	p15	28.6	12	+ 7.1
	4qter→q11–q13	?0		
	q21–34	0.8	0.8	+ 14.1
5.	5pter→p11–p12	3.3	2.3	+ 13.1
	p13	7.0[d]	2.6	+ 4.0
	p14	29.4	11.1	
	5qter→q13–q21	?		
	q22–q33	7.7	7.4	+ 7.7
	q34	25.0	7.2	
6.	6pter→p11–p12	?		
	p21.2–24	1.3	1.3	+ 11.8
	6qter→q11–q16	?0		
	q21–q24	20.0	17.9	
	q25–q26	33.3	15.7	+ 33.3
7.	7pter→p11–p13	4.4	3.0	+ 4.4
	p15–p21	19.1	8.6	+ 4.8
	7qter→q11–q21	?0		
	q22–q35	<0.8		+ 7.9
8.	8pter→p11–p23	9.1	3.5	
	p23.1	40[e]	12.6	+20
	8qter→q11–q13	2.0	2.0	
	q21.2–q24.2	11.1	6.1	
9.	9pter→p11.2	11.8	3.7	+9.2
	p13	25	8.8	+4.2
	p22	21.2	4.4	+2.4
	9qter→q11–q13	0		
	q21–33	<0.8		+ 8.3

(*continued*)

Table 5–4. (Continued)

TRANSLOCATED SEGMENT THAT WOULD BE IMBALANCED[c]		RISK		
		% LIVEBORN	S.D.	+ % STILLBORN, NEONATAL DEATH[e]
10.	10pter→p11.1	4.7	2.6	+ 4.7
	p12–p14	18.8	9.7	+ 18.8
	10qter→q11–q21	?0		
	q22–q23	<1.4		+ 5.7
	q24	5.9	2.6	+ 9.4
	q25–q26	14.0	4.9	+ 12.0
11.	11pter→p11–p13	?0		
	p14	<3.1		+ 6.3
	11qter→q13–q22	<2.6		
	q23	7.0	3.9	+ 18.6
12.	12pter→p11.1	9.4	5.2	+ 3.1
	p12	9.1	8.7	+ 18.2
	12qter→q11–q15	0		
	q21–q24.3	<1.5		+ 3.8
13.	13qter→q11–q33	1.6	1.1	
14.	14qter→q11.1–q31	1.0	1.0	
15.	15qter→q11–q15	0		
	q21–25	2.7	2.7	
16.	16pter→p11.11	8.3	3.6	
	16qter→q11–q13	6.2	6	+ <3.1
	q21–q23	<5.4		+ <5.4
17.	17pter→p13.3	18.9	3.5	+ 7.1
	p11.1	<2.7		
	17qter→q11–12	?0		
	q21–23	10.0	6.7	
18.	18pter→p11.1–p11.2	? (probably high)		
	18qter→q11.1–q12	2.5	2.5	
	q21	2.9	2.8	+ 6.7
	q22	15.0	7.8	+ 15.0
19.	19pter→p11–p13.2	?0		
	19qter→q11–q12	?0		
	q13.2–q13.3	11.1	6.1	
20.	20pter→p11.1–p11.2	20.0	8.0	
	20qter→q11.1	?0		
21.	21qter→q11.1–q22	13.8	6.4	
22.	22qter→q11.1–q13	<2.6		

[a]Figures are expressed as a percentage of all karyotyped liveborn infants, typically considered as a baby of >28 weeks gestation, with survival at least beyond the neonatal period. Where there are data relating to unkaryotyped stillbirths or neonatal deaths, the figures for these are indicated with a + sign in the third column under "Risk," as a probable additional component of the overall risk, on the assumption that many, at least, of these cases would have been karyotypically abnormal. The maximum estimate of risk will thus be given by the sum of the two percentage figures. This combined figure may be an overestimate, but if so, likely of small degree; and this may be the more useful figure to consider.

[b]One specific translocated segment is of substantial genetic content (the one shown here), and the other is judged to be of minimal content. For adjacent-1 segregation, the risk does not differ between male and female heterozygotes. For segments not listed here, no specific data are recorded in Stengel-Rutkowski et al. (1988).

[c]Some segments are noted precisely (e.g., 1pter→1p35). Most are given as a pair of breakpoints encompassing a range (e.g., 1pter→1p11–34), extending from a maximum length of terminal-to-proximal breakpoint to a minimum length of terminal-to-distal breakpoint. Thus, 1pter→1p11–p34 refers to an imbalanced segment comprising anywhere from a maximum of 1pter→1p11 (the whole of the short arm) to a minimum of 1pter→1p34 (about one-third of the short arm).

[d]In one reported large family with several cases of "pure" deletion or duplication of this segment (the other segment being derived from acrocentric short arm), the risk was very high: 54% (De Carvalho et al. 2008; and see text).

[e]When the combined live birth + neonatal death figure approximates 50%, this may suggest that the single-segment imbalance is fully viable in utero in either the duplicated or deleted state, with approximately equal numbers of offspring due to alternate and to adjacent-1 segregation.

S.D., standard deviation; ?, rare cases have occurred, but data too few to derive a figure; ?0, probably no risk; <, no additional aneuploid child has been born apart from the proband, figure is estimate of upper limit of risk interval.

Sources: From Stengel-Rutkowski et al. 1988, with further entries/amendments from Pollin et al. 1999 (17p13.3), Stasiewicz-Jarocka et al. 2000 and 2004 (1q42, 2q33, 16q), and Panasiuk et al. 2007 and 2009 (4p, 9p), and personal communications A. Midro (8p23.1) and M. Ozaki (5p14).

risk. New data may come to hand. For example, Stasiewicz-Jarocka et al. (2004) assembled data from 65 new pedigrees involving 16q, to add to the original 35 pedigrees from Stengel-Rutkowski et al., and their new risk calculations are included in Tables 5–4 and 5–5. As expected, the new data continue to be consistent with the notion that the risk for unbalanced offspring increases with decreasing length of the segments. In another study, the methods of Stengel-Rutkowski et al. were applied to a large pedigree segregating a double-segment t(7;13)(q34;q13), together with a sperm karyotype analysis. Midro and colleagues (2006) were able to predict the chance of a miscarriage or stillbirth from carriers in this family to be 13% and 30%, respectively, whereas direct examination of sperm karyotypes indicated 60% abnormal sperm. The high rate of selection against abnormal karyotypes, applying in particular in the latter part of pregnancy with this particular translocation, resulted in a very low presumed risk (0.3%) of the abnormal outcome of a surviving liveborn (and see Table 5–5).

Only in the case of recurrent rearrangements does the potential exist for direct extrapolation between families. The representatives of this tiny group are the t(11;22)(q23;q11), of worldwide distribution, mentioned numerous times in this chapter, and common enough that its typical unbalanced form acquired an eponymous nomenclature, Emanuel syndrome (Carter et al. 2009). Of orders of magnitude less frequent are the t(4;8)(p16;p23), the t(5;11)(p15;p15) associated with Beckwith-Wiedemann syndrome, the t(4;11)(p16.2;p15.4), and the t(8;22)(q24.13;q11.21) (Slavotinek et al. 1997; Giglio et al. 2002; Thomas et al. 2009; Sheridan et al. 2010). The t(6;20)(p21;p13), reported in three European kindreds, may also represent a rare recurrent translocation (Berner et al. 2012), although we note the suggestion of Youings et al. (2004) that identity by descent is another possibility in this sort of observation.

Individual circumstances for different types of predisposing translocations are discussed below. The lowest risk for a surviving abnormal child, namely zero, applies in the case of imbalances of large genetic content, in which in utero lethality would be seen as inevitable; and in families interpreted as being in this category, invasive prenatal diagnosis could be seen as inappropriate (Vauhkonen et al. 1985). This essentially no-risk circumstance may apply to a considerable fraction, perhaps the great majority of "translocation couples."

RISK AT THE TIME OF PRENATAL DIAGNOSIS

The likelihood of detecting an abnormality is higher at prenatal diagnosis than it is at the birth of a live baby, reflecting the differential survival throughout pregnancy. Very unbalanced conceptions will abort before the time of prenatal diagnosis. Daniel et al. (1988) derived an overall figure of about 25% for carriers to have an unbalanced fetal karyotype detected at early second trimester (the time at which amniocentesis would usually be done) when ascertainment was through a previous aneuploid child, and about 5% when it was through recurrent miscarriage. The amniocentesis-time figure is at its highest, 35%, in the carrier whose risk otherwise to have an aneuploid live birth lies in the "medium" range (5%–10%) (Stengel-Rutkowski et al. 1988). To give an example from a specific chromosomal segment, Stengel-Rutkowski et al. record a 6% risk for an imbalance in the liveborn from translocations with a proximal 9p breakpoint, versus a 33% risk to detect an imbalance at amniocentesis. In a series of 57 pregnancies in 40 translocation couples, Barišić et al. (1996) determined an overall risk of 16% to discover an unbalanced karyotype at second-trimester amniocentesis, confirming a higher risk (32%) for couples who had previously had an abnormal child, versus a lower figure (12%) where ascertainment had been because of miscarriage.

RISK AT THE TIME OF PREIMPLANTATION GENETIC DIAGNOSIS

PGD requires a very different viewpoint, since in utero lethality has scarcely had the chance to operate, and the denominator of the risk figure is quite different: This now refers to the rate of abnormalities in the day 3–5 embryo. The data in Tables 5–2 and 22–2 list PGD outcomes from a considerable number of "reciprocal translocation couples." Unbalanced segregants were seen in about half of all embryos tested (range 31%–59%); but the proportion of embryos available for transfer was further reduced in some embryos, despite their being of alternate segregation, by the presence of other aneuploidies unrelated to the translocation (Scriven et al. 2013; Tan et al. 2013; Tobler et al. 2014; Idowu et al. 2015).

Risks According to Likely Segregation Mode

ADJACENT-1 SEGREGATION, SINGLE SEGMENT

Specific risk figures for individual single-segment imbalances are set out in Table 5–4. A notable point is the number of risk figures that are very small, less than 1%. This most likely reflects that many imbalances are almost always lethal in utero, and survival through to term is the exception. In fact, we can say that, in order of frequency, there are imbalances which are (1) invariably lethal; (2) almost always lethal; (3) often lethal; and (4) the least frequent category, usually survivable. These risk figures are likely to be valid irrespective of the mode of ascertainment of the family or of the identity of the other chromosome contributing the telomeric tip, at least in the majority of translocations.

By way of example, imagine that a carrier in the t(4;12)(p14;p13) family of Mortimer et al. (1980) noted above had sought advice about their own risk to have an abnormal baby. The single-segment involved is 4p14pter. According to the rules set out earlier, adjacent-1 segregation is the category that implies risk for viable imbalance in this family translocation. Consulting Table 5–4, therefore, we see that the risk for imbalance (whether deletion or duplication) is given as 15.4%. The standard deviation (± 4.5) is quite small, indicating that the estimate is based on a good number of cases. But we also pay attention to the datum "+ 7.7" with reference to unkaryotyped stillbirths and neonatal deaths, many of which will have been, surely, chromosomally abnormal (probably Wolf-Hirschhorn syndrome). So the true figure to have an abnormal baby at term, who might or might not live, could well be 15.4 + 7.7 = 23.1%. A "private estimate" in this family had come up with a figure of 25%, which is sufficiently close to 23.1% to provide reassurance as to its accuracy.

ADJACENT-1 SEGREGATION, DOUBLE SEGMENT

Every double-segment translocation is likely to be a unique case (or at least no other described family is known), and risk assessment is less precise. One known recurrent double-segment translocation, the t(4;8)(p16;p23), has been seen in sufficient numbers for a useful risk estimate to be derived (Table 5–5). Of course, if the family is large enough, a private segregation analysis will provide the best estimate; and some other examples are listed in Table 5–5. Otherwise, Stengel-Rutkowski et al. (1988) recommend considering each segment separately. They propose the rule of thumb that the risk will be half that of the smaller of the two risk figures. Even this may be an overestimate. Consider the t(4;9)(p15.2;p13) family listed in Table 5–5. The smaller of the risks is that applying to 9p13, as a single-segment, and which is given at 25% (from Table 5–4); this halves to 12.5%. But from an actual family study, the empiric figure was only 3.2% (Midro et al. 2000). And in many cases, the duplication/deficiency from a double-segment imbalance will be invariably lethal in utero—a risk of 0%—notwithstanding that each segment separately is on record with viability in the single-segment state.

When the translocated segments are very small, one or possibly both of the dup/del and del/dup combinations could well be viable. Segregation may be due to the adjacent-1 format, or possibly simply an independent 1:1 segregation of each normal homolog and its derivative chromosome, as discussed above. The family history may well be informative, as illustrated by the t(1q;3p) family reported in Kozma et al. (2004). In one PGD case reported, relating to a couple one of whom carried a t(2;17)(qter;qter), 13 of 18 embryos showed 2:2 segregation for the translocation (six alternate, seven adjacent-1), consistent with either two independent 1:1 events or 2:2 disjunction from a quadrivalent (McKenzie et al. 2003). But the fact that the remaining five malsegregants displayed 3:1 disjunction suggests that a quadrivalent may indeed have formed, even if, considering the nature of this translocation, 3:1 is contrary to the "rules" of malsegregation set out earlier.

The different scenario implied by preimplantation analysis is seen, by way of example, in a double-segment translocation t(3;11)(q27.3;q24.3) carried by a brother and sister (Coonen et al. 2000). At least 15 out of 18 embryos of the brother were karyotypically unbalanced, and only one was normal or balanced. This one embryo was transferred, amniocentesis showed 46,XX,t(3;11), and a healthy carrier daughter was in due course born. His sister, a carrier of the same translocation, underwent two treatment cycles, with two out of six embryos apparently normal, but neither transferred successfully.

ADJACENT-2 SEGREGATION

Very few translocations are capable of producing viable adjacent-2 segregant products, and the data on

Table 5–5. Empiric Risk Figures for Having a Liveborn Aneuploid Child, or a Child Stillborn or Dying as a Neonate,[a] Because of Double-Segment Imbalance from 2:2 Adjacent-1 Segregation, in 13 Specific Translocations[b]

TRANSLOCATION	RISK[c]		
	% LIVEBORN	S.D.	+ % STILLBORN, NEONATAL DEATH
t(1;2)(q42;q33)	6.8		
t(1;3)(q42.3;p25)	63.6	14.5	
t(2;13)(p25.1;q32.3)	14.5	7.6	+ 4.8
t(3;10)(p26; p12)	24.0	8.5	
t(3;15)(q21.3;q26.1)	?0		+ 17
t(4;5)(p15.1;p12)	1.6		
t(4;8)(p16.1;p23.1)	15		
t(4;9)(p15.2;p13)	3.2	3.2	+ 6.5
t(4;19)(p15.32;p13.3)	3.7	3.6	+ 7.4
t(7;9)(q36.2;p21.2)	30	14.5	+ 10
t(7;13)(q34;q13)	0.3*		+ 29.0
t(12;14)(q15;q13)	?0		+ ?0
t(16;19)(q13;q13.3)	1.2		
t(16;20)(q11.1;q12)	1.1		

*Plus another 0.2% to account for a theoretical risk for interchange trisomy 13. The considerable gap to the next risk figure, 29%, reflects the several instances in this family of unkaryotyped stillbirths and early neonatal deaths.

[a]Figures are expressed as a percentage of all karyotyped liveborn infants, as described in the legend in Table 5–4. ?0 indicates probably no risk, albeit that the 17% risk figure above for stillbirth/neonatal death in the t(3;15)(q21.3;q26.1) indicates viability of the unbalanced state through to the end of pregnancy.

[b]Families published in Kozma et al. (2004), Midro et al. (2000, 2006), Nucaro et al. (2008), Stasiewicz-Jarocka et al. (2000, 2004), Tranebjaerg et al. (1984), Wiland et al. (2007), and Šumanović-Glamuzina et al. (2017), and personal communication, A. Midro.

[c]Some figures come from direct segregation analysis, and in others, from applying this rule: halving the risk for the lesser of the two risks, which would otherwise have applied to each translocated segment when viewed as a single-segment imbalance (and see text).

specific risk levels are limited (Table 5–6). Where the potential imbalance has considerable viability, for example, trisomy 9p and trisomy 21q, the risk is likely to be substantial and may be in the range of 20%–30%. The carrier mother in Figure 5–8 would have, from Table 5–6, an 18% risk for the recurrence of trisomy 9p.

3:1 SEGREGATION, TERTIARY ANEUPLOIDY

In contrast to 2:2 segregation, the probabilities for unbalanced 3:1 outcomes differ between the sexes, with the female having the greater risk. For translocations other than the common t(11;22) (q23;q11), the risk is generally small and less than 2%. Nevertheless, each translocation is entitled to its individuality, and atypically higher risks are possible, as may be exemplified in the t(12;13) noted

earlier and shown in Figure 5–11, in which two out of four children had a tertiary monosomy. In this case, it could be that the tiny derivative segregated independently, at random.

The Common t(11;22). Practically the only segregation mode to produce a viable abnormal baby in the common t(11;22)(q23;q11) is 3:1 with tertiary trisomy (Emanuel syndrome) (Figure 5–10). Different figures have been proposed for the level of risk. From the data of Stengel-Rutkowski et al. (1988), as listed in Table 5–7, the risk is 3.7% and <0.7%, respectively, for the female and the male carrier. In a very large collaboration, with data from 110 families seen in 15 countries (there being some overlap with the material in Stengel-Rutkowski et al.), Iselius et al. (1983) arrived at risk figures for the female and male heterozygote, respectively, of 2.1% and 1.8%. Notably, in most of these families

Table 5–6. Specific Risk Figures for Liveborn Aneuploid Child due to Imbalance from 2:2 Adjacent-2 Segregation

CENTRIC SEGMENT THAT WOULD BE IMBALANCED	RISK	
	%	S.D.
4pter→q11–q13	?0	
8pter→q12–q13	?	
9pter→q11–q13	18.4	4.5
10pter→q11–q21	?	
12pter→q11–q13	?	
13pter→q14–q21	?	
14pter→q21–q22	?	
15pter→q13–q24	11.8	7.8
20pter→q11.1	27.3	13.4
21pter→q11.1–q22	?.	

Note: Figures are expressed as a percentage of all live births. No obvious difference exists according to sex of parent. For the very many segments not listed, no specific data are recorded in Stengel-Rutkowski et al. (1988). ?, rare cases have occurred, but data are too few to derive a figure; ?0, probably no risk.

Source: From Stengel-Rutkowski et al. (1988).

the index case was the only one known definitely to have the unbalanced karyotype. However, it could be supposed that reported malformed still-born infants in these families were rather likely also to have had the unbalanced karyotype, and if this assumption is accepted, the risk figures for a live- or stillborn affected infant would increase to 5.7% and 5%, respectively. A rather higher risk figure for the female carrier, namely, ~10%, is due to Zackai and Emanuel (1980). These authors also observed that the chance of transmitting the translocation in balanced state is significantly greater than the theoretical 50%, with a probability of >70% in the families studied (a form of meiotic drive). An earlier concern about a breast cancer risk to the heterozygote has since been dismissed (Carter et al. 2010).

3:1 SEGREGATION, INTERCHANGE ANEUPLOIDY

The risk to have a child with Patau, Edwards, or Down syndrome from an interchange trisomy is remarkably small. It may be in the vicinity of 0.5% in the female, and less than this in the male (Stengel-Rutkowski et al. 1988). Upper limits of the estimated

Table 5–7. Specific Risk Figures for Liveborn Aneuploid Child due to Imbalance from 3:1 Single-Segment Segregation

A. Tertiary Trisomy or Monosomy

SEGMENT THAT WOULD BE IMBALANCED	RISK	
	%	S.D.
4pter→q12–q13	?	
8pter→q12–q13	?	
9pter→q11–q32	1.7 (mat)	1.7
	?0 (pat)	
10pter→q11.1–q21	?	
11qter→q23*	3.7% (mat)	
	<0.7% (pat)	
12pter→q11–q13	?	
13pter→q12–q33	2.6 (mat)	1.8
	0 (pat)	
14pter→q11.1–q24	2.6 (mat)	2.6
	<0.8 (pat)	
15pter→q11.1–q24	<0.9	
16pter→q11.1	<1.8 (mat)	
	0 (pat)	
18pter→q11.1–q21	<1.3 (mat)	
	0 (pat)	
20pter→q11.1	<4.4 (mat)	
	?0 (pat)	
21pter→q11.1–q22	6.9 (mat)	4.7
22pter→q11.1–q13	<3.5 (mat)	
	? (pat)	

B. Interchange Trisomy

CHROMOSOME THAT WOULD BE TRISOMIC	RISK	
	%	S.D.
13	<0.2 (mat)	
	0 (pat)	
18	<0.2 (mat)	
	<0.3 (pat)	
21	0.5 (mat)	0.5
	<0.6 (pat)	

Notes. Figures are expressed as a percentage of all live births. Risks for maternal transmission (mat) are typically greater than for paternal (pat) in 3:1 segregations. For segments not listed, no specific data recorded in Stengel-Rutkowski et al. (1988). ?, rare cases have occurred, but data are too few to derive a figure; ?0, probably no risk.

*The common t(11;22)(q23;q11).

Source: From Stengel-Rutkowski et al. (1988).

risks are given in Table 5–7. The figures for PGD can be much higher, as shown in Table 5–3, and as illustrated by the case of Conn et al. (1999) noted above, in which a woman with the karyotype 46,XX,t(6;21)(q13;q22.3) had 9/9 embryos with chromosome imbalance, including two with interchange trisomy 21, and one with probable interchange monosomy 6.

MORE THAN ONE UNBALANCED SEGREGANT TYPE

It is prudent to assume that where more than one mode of segregation can lead to a viable outcome, the overall risk will be cumulative and will be given by the sum of the individual risks. Thus, the carrier mother of the t(11;18)(p15;q11) shown in Figure 5–13 would have a risk comprising three components: duplication 18q11qter due to adjacent-1; tertiary trisomy 18pter-q11 due to 3:1; and trisomy 18 due to 3:1 interchange. From Tables 5–4 and 5–7, and choosing the closest listed segments, these risks are 2.5%, <1.3%, and <0.2%, respectively, for a total of up to 4.0%.

IMPRINTABLE CHROMOSOMES AND UNIPARENTAL DISOMY

Any translocation, of which a participating chromosome has an imprintable segment, is to be considered from this specific perspective. Here, the gender of the transmitting parent becomes of relevance. But in practice, this is a very rarely observed circumstance. Liehr (2014) recorded only 10 examples of uniparental disomy (UPD) for chromosome 7, 15, 16, and 20, in the setting of reciprocal (not Robertsonian) translocations. For example, Silver-Russell syndrome due to UPD7 has been reported just twice in association with a maternal translocation involving chromosome 7 (Behnecke et al. 2012).

A potential risk for UPD following postzygotic "correction" was noted above. What looks like alternate segregation in the fetus could actually have been 3:1 interchange trisomy, with a post-conceptual loss of the homolog in question. In practice, this appears to be an exceedingly rare outcome (Dupont et al. 2002; Kotzot 2008a; Heidemann et al. 2010). An example is the case in Calounova et al. (2006): A

child with PWS had the same 46,XX,t(8;15)(q24.1;q21.2) karyotype as her mother, with absence of a paternal chromosome 15, and thus with UPD15mat. This much is certain: Any translocation involving chromosome 15 in particular is to be approached very circumspectly.

Phenotype and Survivability

A major degree of dysmorphogenesis, involving several body systems, and globally disordered brain function, is the typical picture in classical viable autosomal imbalance resulting from a parental reciprocal translocation. The physical phenotype is usually less markedly abnormal in those imbalances detectable only on molecular karyotyping, and indeed sometimes essentially unscathed, although neurocognitive and behavioral difficulty is often of important degree. Many patients will come with the knowledge of the particular phenotype of at least one of the viable segregant outcomes—the proband in their own family. The same imbalance in a future pregnancy would be expected to lead to a similar physical and mental phenotype.[12] Survivability is less predictable because, for many conditions, there is a fine line between relative robustness and a fragile hold on existence, intrapartum and postnatally. Whether there is a heart defect (a frequent malformation in many chromosomal disorders) may be a major factor in this. As for the phenotype of potentially survivable outcomes other than those already exemplified in the family, reference to the chromosomal catalogs and databases and to the journal literature provides a guide. For imprintable chromosomes, there may be an influence of the parental origin of the aneuploid segment, as noted above.

PRENATAL DIAGNOSIS

Aspects of prenatal diagnosis are discussed in detail in Chapters 20 and 21. In a "translocation pregnancy," ultrasonography can be used as an adjunctive diagnostic procedure, with normal nuchal translucency in the first trimester and absence of structural anomalies in the second trimester predicting a normal/balanced karyotype (Sepulveda et al. 2001). Noninvasive prenatal testing of cell-free DNA in

---

12 Similar may only mean "quite similar, but a little different." Just as trisomy 21 presents quite a range in intellectual capacity, variation may be observed with the identical segment, duplicated or deleted, in different family members. The rest of the (balanced) genome, which will of course differ, may, in (usually) small degree, dictate a relative vulnerability, or resistance, to the damaging effects of the imbalance.

maternal blood may enable testing for unbalanced segregants of a translocation, provided that a 24-chromosome sequencing approach is used.

THE PARENTAL BALANCED TRANSLOCATION IN A FETUS

The conventional wisdom is that if the same (balanced) karyotype found in the carrier parent is detected at prenatal diagnosis, there is no increased risk for phenotypic abnormality in the child: Like parent, like child. Some have doubted this, and Fryns et al. (1992) measured a 6.4% risk of mental and/or physical defects in the heterozygous children of translocation carriers (this figure including the background risk of 2%–3%). Others remained skeptical and imputed ascertainment bias as the confounding factor (Steinbach 1986). Theoretical mechanisms whereby an apparently balanced translocation could have a deleterious consequence, the parental normality notwithstanding, include the following four: a cryptic unbalanced defect beyond the resolution of routine cytogenetics (but nowadays potentially detectable on molecular karyotyping); the postzygotic loss of a derivative chromosome in one cell line, converting an unbalanced to a mosaic balanced/unbalanced state; a position effect; and uniparental disomy.

Concerning the cryptic unbalanced defect, Wagstaff and Hemann (1995) provide a disconcerting example: an apparently balanced parental reciprocal translocation which turned out to be a complex chromosome rearrangement, with a tiny segment from the breakpoint of one of the translocation chromosomes inserted into a third chromosome (Figure 10–5). In families in which the balanced translocation has been transmitted to numerous phenotypically normal individuals, such a scenario is most unlikely, since consistent co-segregation of the "cryptic chromosome" to give an overall balanced complement in all these persons would be improbable. Where the translocation is of more recent origin, perhaps de novo in the parent, the possibility may be more real; if prenatal diagnosis is undertaken, molecular karyotyping would offer a clear advantage over conventional karyotyping.

The case reported by Dufke et al. (2001) illustrates the possible scenario of mosaicism. An abnormal child with the same balanced t(17;22)(q24.2;q11.23) as his mother on peripheral blood analysis, showed, on skin fibroblast culture, a 47,t(17;22),+der(22) karyotype. This mosaic picture may reflect there having been an interchange tertiary trisomy complement in the conceptus, with postzygotic loss of one of the two der(22)s in blood-forming tissue. A similar scenario is documented in Prontera et al. (2006): A mother carrying a t(1;15)(q10;p11) had an abnormal child, in whom the same apparently balanced karyotype had been shown at prenatal diagnosis. In view of the abnormal phenotype, a stringent postnatal analysis was done, which revealed a small fraction of cells, 4% (on blood), with trisomy 15; the conclusion is thus drawn that the initial conception had been from a 3:1 malsegregation with interchange trisomy 15, and a mitotic "correction" thereafter resulted in loss of the additional chromosome 15 in a substantial fraction of cells, but obviously not all. These reports raise the question: Could the excess noted by Fryns et al. (1992) in a postnatal population be accounted for, in part at least, by this process? And, if so, could this be the basis of a misleading prenatal diagnosis? In fact, it could be imagined that, if the mother in Dufke et al. had had an amniocentesis, the unbalanced 47,t(17;22),+der(22) state would have been seen, since the sampling of amniocytes is somewhat equivalent to taking several skin biopsies. On that premise, it could be argued that a good number of normal cells/colonies from amniocentesis might indicate an unlikelihood of any such mosaicism. A chorionic villus sampling, or a maternal blood test for fetal DNA (a "liquid placental biopsy", p. 472), would be less reliable in this respect.

If an important additional risk due to one or other of the aforementioned scenarios really does exist, it is surely very small, perhaps no more than "a fraction of a percent" that a child with the "balanced" parental karyotype might have a defect of mostly unpredictable severity and extent. In the meantime, it remains true that in the great majority the balanced translocation really is balanced, structurally and functionally, and will have, of itself, no detrimental effect (beyond an eventual influence upon the child's reproductive health). Thus, in practical terms, it would be appropriate to advise continuing a pregnancy when the fetal karyotype is the same as that of the carrier parent, and with very considerable (if not absolute) confidence of a normal physical and mental outcome.

Infertility and Pregnancy Loss

INFERTILITY

Occasionally, some male translocation carriers are infertile with a spermatogenic arrest, as discussed above. Fertility is infrequently affected in the female rcp heterozygote, oögenesis being, apparently, a much more robust process (at least from this aspect).

MISCARRIAGE

Conceptions with large imbalances will abort. Against the background population risk of 15% for a recognized pregnancy to miscarry,[13] the risk for the translocation carrier is rather greater, and is in the range of 20%–30% (Stengel-Rutkowski et al. 1988). For a few, the risk is very high, well over 50%. An increasing viability of conceptuses implies a corresponding declining likelihood of pregnancy loss by miscarriage. Not to diminish the distress felt at the loss of a welcomed and wanted pregnancy, patients can perhaps be heartened that miscarriage, in this setting, is the natural elimination of a severe abnormality, which provides the opportunity to make a fresh, and hopefully, a more fortunate start. For a couple having lost all pregnancies to miscarriage, karyotyping in the previous generation may be helpful. The consultand would, in him- or herself, embody the proof that the heterozygote *can* have a normal child, should one of his or her parents also be a carrier. Optimism has to be muted, however, in the setting of a family history of many miscarriages, which may indicate a propensity for the production of unbalanced gametes.

Preimplantation Genetic Diagnosis. PGD has obvious theoretical attraction as a means to avoid a pregnancy with an imbalance, by choosing only embryos with a balanced complement, following embryo biopsy; and we discuss this question at some length in Chapter 22. As we have commented a number of times above, the risk figures for malsegregation at PGD will be specific to this developmental stage. A chromosomally abnormal embryo at day 3–5 (when PGD is applied) has not been subject to selection pressure, and so a wide range of imbalances may be seen, the very great majority of which could never survive to term, and many of which would fail even before implantation. The data in Tables 5–2 and 22–2 might suggest a chance in the range 40%–70% for a normal/balanced embryo, although as noted above, a proportion of these embryos will have other aneuploidies unrelated to

the translocation. Obviously, couples in this situation will hope that their in vitro fertilization team can produce a good number of embryos.

Other Issues

OTHER FAMILY MEMBERS WITH THE SAME TRANSLOCATION

It appears to be the case that a translocation studied in one family member will typically display similar meiotic behavior in other carriers in the family; at least, this applies to the male, in whom gametic analysis is more readily pursued (Benet et al. 2005; Wiland et al. 2007). Thus, genetic advice can be, in practice, the same, for one and all.

ASSOCIATED MENDELIAN CONDITION

Rare translocations are associated with a Mendelian disorder due either to the breakpoint disrupting or influencing a locus, or with coincidental linkage to a mutation near the breakpoint. We note some examples in the earlier section on "Biology." We may here mention another, a father and daughter with an apparently balanced t(1;22)(p36.1;q12), both having neurofibromatosis type 2, due to the *NF2* gene having been disrupted (Tsilchorozidou et al. 2004). In such families, over and above any risk associated with unbalanced segregants, one should discuss the risk of transmitting the abnormality peculiar to that chromosome.

CANCER RISK

In rare familial translocations, the rearrangement may promote mitotic malsegregation, or disrupt a tumor suppressor gene, and thus comprise a "hit" in the cascade of events leading to the cellular phenotype of cancer. A well-recognized case is that of chromosome 3 translocations implicated in familial renal cancer, of which a number of examples have been published (Haas and Nathanson 2014). According to one construction, a three-hit sequence is envisaged, the first hit being the actual inheritance of the balanced translocation. Then, the mechanism is a mitotic malsegregation in an embryonic kidney cell. The derivative chromosome containing the 3p segment is lost (the second hit),

---

13 This figure applies with respect to clinically diagnosable miscarriage, mostly occurring in the period 8 to 16 weeks of gestation. Severely imbalanced forms may be lost as very early, even occult, abortions.

and in consequence one daughter cell, and thus the lineage from it, has only one copy of distal 3p, on the normal homolog. Thereafter, on this remaining normal chromosome, a somatic mutation occurs in postnatal life at a tumor suppressor gene on 3p (such as *VHL*) in a kidney cell within this lineage (the third hit); and now the stage is set for a renal cancer to come into being. Other examples include familial adenomatous polyposis, of which rare reports document a constitutional reciprocal translocation having a breakpoint at 5q22, wherein lies the *APC* tumor suppressor gene (Sahnane et al. 2016). An excess of constitutional rearrangements, some inherited, in a series of children with various tumors, suggests the possibility of a causative role for some of them, and whole exome sequencing has been capable of pinning down an actual genetic disruption in some (de novo) cases (Betts et al. 2001; Ritter et al. 2015). Where the cytogenetic-cancer associations are firm, heterozygotes should receive appropriate counseling, and entry into a cancer surveillance program is appropriate. Often, the associations appear to be no more than fortuitous (given that rearrangements are not uncommon, and cancer is very common).

INTERCHROMOSOMAL EFFECT

There had originally been concern that a reciprocal translocation heterozygote might be prone to produce gametes aneuploid for a chromosome not involved in the translocation, specifically, in this context, chromosomes 13, 18, 21, or X, and there has been the occasional report of a translocation carrier having offspring with chromosomal imbalance not related to the family's translocation (Couzin et al. 1987). Warburton (1985) reviewed the associations of reciprocal translocations and trisomy 21 from unbiased (amniocentesis) data and found no evidence to support the contention. Uchida and Freeman (1986) and Schinzel et al. (1992) studied families in which a child with trisomy 21 also had

a balanced translocation, and while in several the translocation was of paternal origin, in fact the extra chromosome 21 came from the mother.

More directly, numerous sperm karyotyping studies have, for the most part, shown no increase in disomies unrelated to the translocation, although some workers have raised doubts (Estop et al. 2000; Oliver-Bonet et al. 2004; Machev et al. 2005). Pellestor et al. (2001) suggest that carrier males with poor semen indices are the only ones in whom any such effect might exist; in which case, it might be the altered testicular environment, rather than the translocation of itself, that is the cause (Kirkpatrick et al. 2008). Analysis of embryos at preimplantation diagnosis had initially seemed against any such effect (Gianaroli et al. 2002); but more recently, Anton et al. (2011) adduced rather firmer evidence in favor of the phenomenon, and Kovaleva (2013) and Li et al. (2015) provide tenuous support. It may well be that some specific translocations do have a *very* small individual risk, but there seems little reason to withdraw from the generality of Jacobs's assessment from 1979, and in practical terms we expect her view to prevail, albeit that we add cautionary comments in brackets:

> There is no [definite] indication that parents with a structural abnormality are at a [discernibly] increased risk of producing a child with a chromosomal abnormality independent of the parental rearrangement . . . and their recurrence risk for such an event is [practically] the same as the incidence rate in the population.

Only with infertile men (needing ICSI for conception) might there really be a "less indiscernible" risk, and as noted above, this may be due more to the infertility per se. Interestingly, there is stronger evidence for the existence of an interchromosomal effect in the setting of Robertsonian translocations (see Chapter 7).

6

SEX CHROMOSOME
TRANSLOCATIONS

THE SEX CHROMOSOMES (gonosomes) are different,[1] and sex chromosome translocations need to be considered separately from translocations between autosomes. A sex chromosome can engage in translocation with an autosome, with the other sex chromosome, or even with its homolog. The unique qualities of the sex chromosomes have unique implications in terms of the genetic functioning of gonosome-autosome translocations. Unlike any other chromosome, the X chromosome is capable of undergoing "transcriptional silencing" or, as more usually spoken, facultative inactivation, of almost all of its genetic content. This fact has crucial consequences for those who carry an X-autosome translocation, in both the balanced and the unbalanced states. And unlike any other chromosome, the Y is composed of chromatin which is, in large part, permanently inert. Some

translocations of this inert material can thus be of no clinical significance.

BIOLOGY

THE X-AUTOSOME TRANSLOCATION

Both females and males can carry, as heterozygotes or hemizygotes, an X-autosome translocation, in balanced or unbalanced state. But the implications for the two sexes are rather different, and we therefore need to treat the two cases separately. First, we need to review the concept of X-inactivation.

X-INACTIVATION

The normal female has two X chromosomes, and yet the possession of only a single X is sufficient to

---

1 But about 200 million years ago in mammalian evolution, they were the same, and functioning as autosomes. The sex chromosomes as they are now, comprise an older X-conserved region, shared across marsupial and placental mammals; and a more recent X- and Y-added region (an autosomal sequence translocated to the X and Y chromosomes) evolving only in placental mammals, and which happened about 100 million years ago (Cotter et al. 2016).

produce normality in the 46,XY male. Are the sexes really so genetically different? Does the female really need a second X? The second X is largely surplus to requirement, and it is subject to transcriptional silencing. Very early in embryonic existence, around the period of the morula and blastocyst stages, a process is initiated whereby one of the X chromosomes in every cell of the female conceptus is randomly[2] genetically inactivated (van den Berg et al. 2009). This process is called (after Dr. Mary Lyon) *lyonization*. In all descendant progeny cells thereafter, the same X chromosomes remain inactive or active, respectively. This "dosage compensation" allows for a functional monosomy of most of the X chromosome.

Transcriptional silencing is initiated at an X-inactivation center (XIC) in Xq13 (Figure 6–1), and it spreads in both directions along the chromosome. Within the XIC is a gene *XIST* that is cis-acting (that is, it can influence only the chromosome that it is actually on), and that is transcribed only from the *in*activated X. This transcript, named "XIST," for X (inactive) specific transcript, is not translated into protein, but functions as a long-noncoding RNA molecule (lncRNA). The XIST RNA "coats" the X chromatin and may act first by influencing the degree of acetylation and other modification of the histones, and this then prevents the DNA from being transcribed.[3] This inactive state is then "locked in" by methylation of CpG islands, and this methylation status remains in place in the descendant daughter cells. The reader wishing full detail is referred to Migeon's *Females Are Mosaics* (2007) and to Yang et al. (2011). Normal women can have quite skewed ratios of active X^m and inactive X^p chromosomes[4] and vice versa, even more than 90:10, and there can be differences in ratios between different tissues in a woman (Sharp et al. 2000). The inactive X replicates late during the cell cycle; the active X replicates early, along with the autosomes.

But this is not to say that the female's second X chromosome is unnecessary (a rather obvious statement, considering the difference between 46,XX and 45,X women). Not all genes on the X chromosome are inactivated, and thus some loci are, in the normal female, functionally disomic. There is a block to the spread of transcriptional silencing into the primary pseudoautosomal region (PAR1), which comprises the terminal 2.6 Mb of Xp in band p22.3, and which carries about 24 genes; this segment has an homologous region on distal Yp (Figure 6–1). There is a secondary PAR (PAR2), which extends over 320 kb within distal Xq, holding only four genes, and having homology with distal Yq (Mangs and Morris 2007). An obligate recombination event occurs in the PAR1 of the X and the Y chromosome at male meiosis; recombination between the secondary PARs, if it occurs at all, is infrequent. Certain other loci elsewhere on the X than in the PARs (some of which have homologs on the Y) are not subject to inactivation, and disomic expression of these genes in the female (and, for some, in the male) is normal (Disteche 1995). One such is the non-pseudoautosomal X-Y homologous region, at Xq21.3 and Yp11.2, respectively, and in fact this is the largest region, some 4 Mb in length, of shared sequence between the sex chromosomes (Wilson et al. 2007).

Transcriptional silencing can spread into the autosomal component of an X-autosome translocation. The molecular basis of this process is reviewed in Cotton et al. (2014). The phenomenon can act to prevent, or equally to exacerbate, an abnormal phenotype, as we discuss further below. An interesting example is the child in Sakazume et al. (2012) who had Prader-Willi syndrome with hypopigmentation, with a de novo 46,XY,der(X)t(X;15)(p21.1;q11.2),–15, and in whom the particular 15q13 autosomal region[5] of the der(X) was inactivated. (On the other hand, as a very rare observation, transcriptional silencing may originate in autosomal heterochromatin, and spread into a translocated X segment, as Genesio et al. (2011) propose in a girl with 46,XX,t(X;2)(Xpter→Xq23::2q35→2qter;2pter→2q34::Xq24→Xqter)dn, who had presented with a clinical picture including incontinentia pigmenti. One scenario is that inactivation may have started at the heterochromatic band 2q34.[6])

---

2 Renault et al. (2013) consider that actually there may be a genetic influence upon the pattern of inactivation, rather than its being a purely random process. They suggest a system possibly analogous to the mouse *Xce* (cis-acting X controlling element) paradigm, through which a choice is imposed upon which X is inactivated.

3 At the molecular level, the process involves the interaction of XIST with the protein SHARP, which recruits SMRT, activating HDAC3 which deacetylates histones, which then leads to Pol II being excluded across the X chromosome (McHugh et al. 2015).

4 Denoting the one from her mother as X^m, and the one from her father as X^p.

5 15q13 contains the PWS-critical region and the pigmentation gene *OCA2*.

6 The gene for incontinentia pigmenti, *NEMO*, lies at very distal Xq28, about 34 Mb distant from the Xq24 translocation breakpoint. The chromosome 2q34 originating inactivation may have spread this considerable distance, affecting some, but not all, Xq loci, en route; or, as Cotton et al. (2014) write, there was a "variegated silencing through epigenetic modifications."

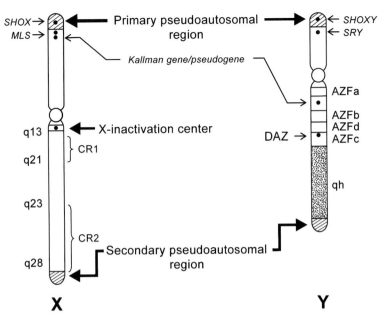

FIGURE 6–1   Notable regions of the sex chromosomes. AZF, azoöspermia factor regions a–d. Dots show specific loci: *DAZ*, deleted in azoöspermia locus; *MLS*, microöphthalmia with linear skin lesion gene; *SHOX*, short stature homeobox gene (X chromosome); *SHOXY*, short stature homeobox gene (Y chromosome); *SRY*, testis-determining locus. CR1, 2 show critical regions 1 and 2 (p. 117). (A more nuanced view of the Y is offered in Mann et al. 2017.)

The Female X-Autosomal Heterozygote

The phenotypically normal balanced X-autosome female translocation carrier has two translocation chromosomes, the der(X) and the der(autosome). The X segment in one of these, most commonly the der(X), contains the XIC, and the X segment in the other, usually on the der(autosome), lacks the XIC. The latter segment, having no XIC of its own and being beyond the influence of the XIC on the other derivative, is always active. The only way, then, for the karyotypically balanced female X-autosome heterozygote to achieve a functionally balanced genome is to use, as her active X complement, the two parts of the X in the two translocation chromosomes: Together, they add up to an equivalent whole, and functioning, X chromosome. The other chromosome, the *normal* X, is inactive. The cartoon karyotype in the 46,X,t(X;12) carrier mother in Figure 6–2 shows the normal X as inactive (dotted outline), and the X-segments of the der(X) and der(12) as active (solid outline).

Probably, the mechanism to bring about this asymmetric inactivation is as follows. Inactivation is initiated at random in each cell, at either one of the XICs. Some cells will be functionally balanced, with the intact X inactive, as described above. Others, in which the intact X is active, will have a functional disomy for the X chromosome segment that is translocated to the der(autosome), due to this X segment not being subject to transcriptional silencing, and thus genetically active. According to this theory, cell selection then eliminates the functionally partially disomic X lines (Figure 6–3, sequence a→b→c). This mechanism is successful in a fraction of translocation heterozygotes, and aside from a possible gonadal effect or rare position effect (see below), such individuals are phenotypically normal.

This mechanism, as it would seem, may not infrequently fail, and phenotypic abnormality is the consequence. "Not infrequently" may translate to as much as 25%, with reference to the literature study of Schmidt and Du Sart (1992). If some functionally disomic cells survive and come to comprise part of the soma (Figure 6–3, sequence a→b→d), this would, presumably, have some deleterious effect. The natural prediction is that only cells with small partial disomies would be capable of survival. Thus, we might more commonly expect to observe, in these affected carrier females, translocation breakpoints in distal Xp or distal Xq (Xp22 and Xq28),

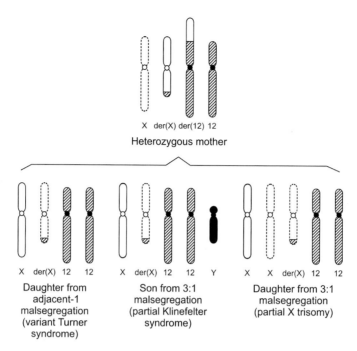

X   der(X) der(12) 12

Heterozygous mother

X   der(X) 12   12   X   der(X) 12   12   Y   X   X   der(X) 12   12

Daughter from   Son from 3:1   Daughter from 3:1
adjacent-1   malsegregation   malsegregation
malsegregation   (partial Klinefelter   (partial X trisomy)
(variant Turner   syndrome)
syndrome)

FIGURE 6–2   Inactivation patterns. Mother with a *balanced* X-autosome translocation, showing patterns of inactivation in herself and in her two chromosomally *unbalanced* children with partial Turner and partial Klinefelter syndrome, respectively. Dashed outline indicates inactivated chromosome. The inactivation pattern of a theoretical third child with a partial X trisomy is shown at right. Note that the balanced carrier inactivates her normal X chromosome, while it is the abnormal X which is inactivated in the unbalanced offspring (and, in the third child, one of the additional normal X chromosomes as well). Based on family in Figure 6–4.

which would impart disomy for only a very small segment of either distal X short arm or distal X long arm. But while this is sometimes so, the pattern is not consistent (Du Sart et al. 1992; Schmidt and Du Sart 1992; Waters et al. 2001). More such data would be useful.

Otherwise, the phenotypically abnormal apparently balanced carrier may reflect, just as with autosomal rearrangements, disruption of loci at the site of breakpoint (Moysés-Oliveira et al. 2015b). Such a scenario, in the severely affected 46,X,t(X;6)(p22.1;q27) patient of Podolska et al. (2017), may have been due to disruption of lethal effect in a key DNA replication gene (*POLA1*) at Xp22.1, and paradoxically the only cells surviving were those with the *normal* X active; thus, she suffered a functional 6q27qter monosomy and an Xp22.1pter disomy.

Measuring Inactivation Status. Inactivation status can be assessed cytogenetically (replication-banding, or R-banding), which enables, in principle, distinction of the early replicating (active) and the late replicating (inactivated) X chromosomes, and allows a precise estimate of the ratio of normal-X^{active} to translocation-X^{active} cells. Mostly, however, the analysis is done using molecular methodologies. The androgen receptor locus, at Xq13 (quite close to the XIC), is often used as the basis of this test. In the phenotypically normal heterozygote, the observation of a complete skew of translocation-X^{active} and normal-X^{active}, in the representative tissue analyzed, would indicate that the same 100:0 proportion applied elsewhere in the soma. Since it is impossible ever to test the entire soma (and in particular the brain), it would have to remain an open question, in a phenotypically abnormal but structurally balanced X-autosome heterozygote, that a more random skewing pattern might apply in some tissues, notwithstanding a complete skew in the peripheral tissue(s) tested. Abnormal individuals may show incomplete inter-tissue concordance of inactivation status, with sometimes quite different ratios in different tissues—for example, 80:20 in blood and 30:70 in skin (Schmidt and Du Sart 1992).

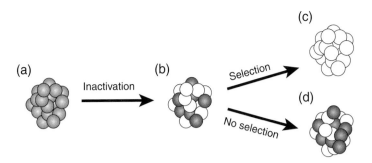

FIGURE 6–3   Skewing or nonskewing of X chromosome inactivation, as a theoretical explanation for the X-autosome carrier being of either normal or abnormal phenotype (and see text). (*a*) Before X-inactivation occurs, both the normal and the der(X) are active in all cells (shown in light gray). (*b*) X-inactivation occurs as a random, cell-autonomous process. Cells shown in white have the der(X) as the active chromosome, and thus the genetic activity of these cells is balanced with respect to X chromosomal output. The cells shown in dark gray have the normal X-active, and in consequence their X chromosomal activity is imbalanced, due to the additional output from the X-segment of the der(autosome). Subsequently in embryonic development: *Either* (*c*) the cells with the normal X-active (dark gray) die out, due to their functional genetic imbalance, leaving only the cells with the der(X) active (white). These latter cells functionally are genetically balanced, and the phenotype is normal. The individual has a skewed X-inactivation pattern.[7] *Or* (*d*) the dark gray cells persist, despite their functional genetic imbalance (the defect is not severe enough to be lethal), and the individual is a mosaic of functionally balanced tissue (white cells) and imbalanced tissue (dark gray cells). In consequence, the phenotype is abnormal.

Source: Adapted from Lanasa and Hogge (2000).

OVARIAN FUNCTION AND THE X "CRITICAL REGIONS"

Breakpoints at certain locations in the X, in the balanced female carrier, may affect ovarian function (Table 6–1). A breakage and reunion within either of two "critical regions," CR1 and CR2, is characteristically associated with premature ovarian failure (these regions are also called POF2 and POF1, respectively). CR1 is located in Xq13.3q21, and CR2 in Xq23q28 (Figure 6–1), although there is some disagreement concerning the exact position of CR2 (Fusco et al. 2011). Some breakpoints could affect X-borne genes in the vicinity that normally require disomic expression, while others might lead to an epigenetic downregulation of "ovarian genes" located on the translocated autosomal segment (Rizzolio et al. 2009). In one series of 30 women presenting with premature ovarian failure, in whom the cytogenetic findings were reviewed, Devi and Benn (1999) recorded just one to be an X-autosome translocation heterozygote; thus, it is an infrequent cause of this problem.

Table 6–1. Occurrence of Gonadal Dysgenesis (Primary or Secondary) in 118 t(X-Autosome) Women According to X Chromosome Breakpoint

BREAKPOINT	GONADAL DYSGENESIS	NORMAL GONADAL FUNCTION
Xpter-q12	5	37
q13	4	8
q13-q22	20	1
q22	11	6
q22-q25	7	1
q26	3	5
q27-qter	1	9

Source: From Therman et al. (1990).

An unusual case is that of a daughter and mother reported in Fusco et al. (2011), who were both heterozygous for an *unbalanced* X;18 translocation, (X;18)(q27;q22).

---

7 An actual example of this sort of process, although occurring at a postnatal rather than an early embryonic stage of life, confined to one tissue (hematogenous), and at a Mendelian rather than a chromosomal level, is given in Martinez-Pomar et al. (2005). These workers studied a girl with the syndrome of incontinentia pigmenti and immunodeficiency, due to the *NEMO* locus on the X chromosome. From age 2 to 4 years, her X-inactivation status in peripheral blood progressed from random to completely skewed in favor of the X with the normal *NEMO* gene, and in parallel there was correction of her immune function.

The only manifestation in the daughter was a diminished ovarian reserve. Her healthy mother had had menopause at age 47 years (she had also had another daughter, 46,XX, and monozygous male twins). The X deletion segment, of 13.97 Mb, included the POF1 region. In addition, a 13.52 Mb segment of 18q was duplicated; this was apparently without phenotypic effect.

The Male X-Autosomal Hemizygote

Almost invariably, the cytogenetically balanced male hemizygote is, without intervention, infertile, due to spermatogenic arrest; disruption of the sex vesicle (see below) is the presumed proximate cause of the obstruction (Hwang et al. 2007). In two men subject to testicular biopsy, Quack et al. (1988) showed germ cell maturation arrest mostly at the pachytene stage of meiosis I, although a few cells managed to make the first and some even the second meiotic metaphase, and thus might have become spermatozoa. This outcome of a very modest success might more likely be achieved in those men in whom the breakpoints are more centromerically placed. A man reported in Perrin et al. (2008), hemizygous for a whole-arm translocation (X;18)(q11;p11.1), was subject to sperm chromosomal fluorescence in situ hybridization (FISH) analysis; he had presented with infertility and "very severe oligoasthenoteratozoöspermia." Analysis showed a range of segregant types in the small number of 447 cells able to be studied: alternate segregation in just over 50% (with half of these normal 23,Y), and adjacent-1, adjacent-2, 3:1, and 4:0 in 8%, 5%, 22%, and 2%, respectively. If sperm could be retrieved, intracytoplasmic sperm injection may be attempted in the carrier male in order to enable fertility.

Patterns of Inactivation in the Unbalanced Offspring

FEMALE OFFSPRING OF THE X-AUTOSOMAL HETEROZYGOTE OR HEMIZYGOTE

As a rule (but one that can be broken), the pattern of inactivation that is observed, following selection, will be the one that allows the least amount of functional imbalance, as discussed above. This is typically arrived at in the karyotypically unbalanced daughter by inactivation of the *abnormal* chromosome, always supposing that the choice exists (and the choice can exist only if the abnormal chromosome contains an XIC).

If the abnormal chromosome is a der(X) from a single-segment exchange, containing no autosomal material other than a telomeric tip, it comprises, essentially, a deleted Xp or Xq chromosome. In a girl with the 46,X,der(X) karyotype, preferential inactivation of this deleted X leads simply to a phenotype of partial Turner syndrome. Consider the family segregating a t(X;12) shown in Figures 6–2 and 6–4. The segregation shown in Figure 6–2 (daughter from adjacent-1) and Figure 6–4a (daughter) illustrates the case for an Xq deletion. Here, the normal X is active (shown as solid outline in Figure 6–2), and the der(X) is inactivated (dotted outline). Leichtman et al. (1978) provide an example of the Xp deletion circumstance in a three-generation family with seven persons having an Xp– Turner syndrome variant on the basis of a segregating t(X;1).

If the der(X) carries a larger translocated autosomal segment—conferring, therefore, a partial autosomal trisomy in the 46,X,der(X) subject—the effects of this imbalance may be mitigated by selective inactivation of the abnormal chromosome. Transcriptional silencing can spread, albeit patchily, into the autosomal chromatin on the der(X), converting, at least partially, a structural autosomal trisomy into a functional autosomal disomy. Figure 6–9 shows an example of blocked spread of inactivation into the autosomal (16p) segment of an inherited X;16 translocation: Observe the der(X) in the lower row, with pale (inactivated) long arm and dark (active) short arm. (This case is mentioned further below.) Consider these two cases following in which a practically complete trisomy 15—which typically causes first-trimester abortion—produced, in comparison, a very much attenuated phenotype. Garcia-Heras et al. (1997) reported on the terminated pregnancy of a t(X;15)(p22.2;q11.2) carrier mother, from whom the 19-week fetus with the der(X) was trisomic for 15q11.2qter, but only rather mild abnormalities of fetal morphology were to be noted. A t(X;15)(q22;q11.2) involving the same 15q11.2 breakpoint (in this case de novo) and diagnosed in a mildly dysmorphic and moderately developmentally delayed 3-year-old child, is described in Stankiewicz et al. (2006).

The converse, whereby the process of spreading autosomal inactivation may be detrimental to the

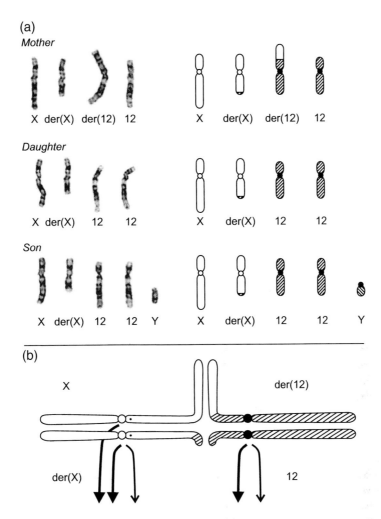

(a)
Mother

X der(X) der(12) 12   X der(X) der(12) 12

Daughter

X der(X) 12 12   X der(X) 12 12

Son

X der(X) 12 12 Y   X der(X) 12 12 Y

(b)

X   der(12)

der(X)   12

FIGURE 6–4   (a) Mother with balanced X;12 translocation, showing two different segregant outcomes. Her daughter had presented with clinical Turner syndrome, in whom the karyotype was initially interpreted as del(X)(q22). Her son was subsequently studied, and he had a partial Klinefelter syndrome. (Case of J. A. Sullivan.) (b) The presumed pachytene configuration during gametogenesis in the mother (X chromatin, open; chromosome 12 chromatin, cross-hatched; dot indicates X-inactivation center). Light arrows indicate movements of chromosomes to daughter cells in adjacent-1 segregation, as observed in the daughter with partial Turner syndrome. Heavy arrows show the tertiary trisomy combination seen in the son with partial Klinefelter syndrome. These two segregations are represented in b and c in Figure 6–7.

phenotype, by converting a functional disomy (or near disomy) into a functional monosomy, is rarely observed. The family illustrated in Figure 6–11 provides a possible example. At first sight, one might have expected only a Turner syndrome phenotype in the daughter with a 45,X,der(X),–22 karyotype, since the essential defect appeared to comprise an Xp deletion, with her total complement of 22q material being intact, or nearly so. However, a more severe clinical picture evolved, and this may have reflected, speculatively, a transcriptional silencing of some crucial 22q loci, notwithstanding the apparent block to inactivation at the breakpoint on cytogenetic study. This case is mentioned further below.

If, in the female with a 46,XX,der(autosome) karyotype, the derivative chromosome has no XIC in its translocated X-segment, this cannot be inactivated, and a functional partial X disomy is the consequence (Sivak et al. 1994). Figure 6–5 demonstrates

(a)

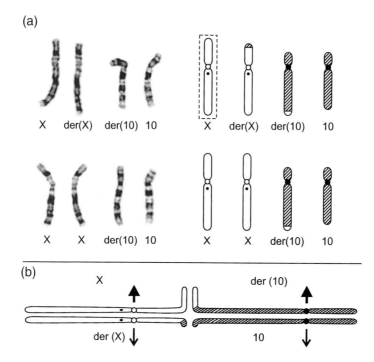

(b)

FIGURE 6–5   Functional X disomy. (*a*) Mother with balanced X;10 translocation (*above*), and her daughter with a 46,XX,der(10) karyotype from adjacent-1 segregation (*below*). The translocation is t(X;10)(p22.31;q26.3). Dashed box on cartoon karyotype indicates preferentially inactivated chromosome; dot indicates X-inactivation center. The der(10) contains Xp material in the translocated segment, which cannot be inactivated, and so the daughter has functional X disomy. Since the 10q breakpoint is in the terminal band, we may regard this as an effectively single-segment exchange, with the phenotype of severe mental deficit and minor dysmorphism due entirely to disomy for the small Xp22.31→pter segment. (Case of A. Ma and H. R. Slater.) (*b*) The presumed pachytene configuration during gametogenesis in the mother (X chromatin, open; chromosome 10 chromatin, cross-hatched; dot indicates X-inactivation center). Arrows indicate movements of chromosomes to daughter cells in adjacent-1 segregation; heavy arrows show the combination observed in this family. This is essentially the segregation *a* shown in Figure 6–7.

a functional disomy[8] for a part of Xp (Xp22.31pter) in a chromosomally unbalanced daughter; in this instance, since the autosomal breakpoint is at the telomere, we assume there to be little or no effect from a 10q monosomy. Functional disomy of distal Xq, Xq28qter, has been reported sufficiently often that a clear core phenotype can be described, and the Rett syndrome *MECP2* locus at chrX:154.0-154.1 Mb is a key pheno-contributory factor (Sanlaville et al. 2005; Shimada et al. 2013).

De Novo Apparently Balanced X-Autosome Translocations in the Female. We may usefully consider de novo balanced translocations some of which could be, in principle, the same as if they had

been transmitted from a carrier parent, in order to illustrate some aspects of inactivation behavior, as per the following examples. Giorda et al. (2008) analyzed cells from a girl with mild dysmorphology, arthritis, obesity, microcephaly, and mental and behavioral disability, who had the karyotype 46,X,der(X)t(X;5)(q22.1;q31)dn, and was thus partially trisomic for the large segment 5q31qter. They were able to show that of 17 interpretable genes tested in this translocated segment, nine had been inactivated, while another eight were active (as measured by methylation status). This inactivation did not "weaken" as it spread further into 5q31qter segment, and indeed the autosomal gene closest to the Xq-5q breakpoint remained active; thus, some

---

8 And presumably a functional trisomy for the pseudoautosomal region within this segment.

autosomal genes were susceptible, and some were resistant, to the spreading influence from the XIST of the der(X).

Another instance of aberrant inactivation is illustrated in the child reported in Genesio et al. (2015b), with a Turner-like clinical picture, and heterozygous for t(X;1)(q21;q41)dn. The normal X showed, as expected, 100% inactivation; but the Xq translocated segment was also, in part, inactivated, despite its having no connection with the *XIST* locus. This "illegitimate" inactivation may well have been a contributory factor in her phenotype. An intriguing example is that of a de novo X-autosome translocation 46,X,der(X)t(X;17)(p22.1;p11.2) in a mildly retarded female who had Charcot-Marie-Tooth neuropathy (CMT) (King et al. 1998). The extra segment of 17p attached to Xp produced an attenuated picture of partial 17p trisomy, presumably reflecting an extension of inactivation into the 17p segment from the X-inactivation center of the der(X). The "supernumerary" *PMP22* gene on the 17p segment was apparently fully functioning, however, since the neuropathy was typical for CMT. The inactivation process could be supposed to have "hopped over" the *PMP22* region. Gustashaw et al. (1994) describe a case of a de novo 46,XX,−13,+der(13)t(X;13)(p21.2;p11.1), in which they could be sure the distal Xp structural trisomy/functional disomy was the sole cause of the abnormal phenotype, since the autosomal breakpoint was in 13p and the loss of one acrocentric short arm has, of itself, no effect.

An informative study comes from Yeung et al. (2014), whose patient had the karyotype 46,XX,der(15)t(X;15)(q13.1;p10)dn, giving the structural imbalance chrX:71,874,142-155,998,655×3, equating to a partial Xq trisomy. Xq trisomy is typically, like full 47,XXX trisomy, a mild phenotype; but this infant had multiple malformations and died at 83 days. This was the result of a functional autosomal imbalance, effectively a partial 15q monosomy, due to spreading inactivation from the XIC of the der(15). This mechanism was proven on a genome-wide DNA methylation microarray, which showed that several CpG islands on the 15q component of the der(15) were hypermethylated.

The de novo apparently balanced X-autosome translocation in the female provided the door to discovery of the chromosomal location of some X-linked disorders, concerning which affected girls had been seen. Duchenne muscular dystrophy is a classic example (Figure 6–6). Quite a number of loci were initially mapped by study of rare/unique female patients with the particular Mendelian condition (Schlessinger et al. 1993). If a girl presents with an X-linked disease, a chromosome study may be revealing. Zenker et al. (2005) studied twin girls with a de novo t(Xp;5q), who had ornithine transcarbamylase (OTC) deficiency, due to disruption of the OTC gene on the der(X), and skewed inactivation of the normal X chromosome. Lonardo et al. (2014) report on a case of Hunter syndrome; the child had a de novo t(X;9), and the combined effects of inactivation of her (normal) maternal X, and influence of 9qh heterochromatin on the nearby Hunter locus of the paternal-originating rea(X), reduced production of the "Hunter enzyme."

A most remarkable scenario is that of an "incorrect" inactivation of the der(X) comprising the "first hit" in a tumor cascade. A mentally handicapped woman in her twenties developed schwannomas, and she was found to carry a de novo t(X;22)

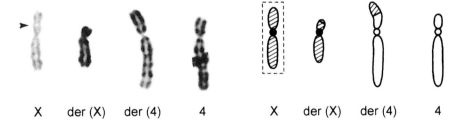

FIGURE 6–6   A de novo X-autosome translocation 46,X,t(X;4)(p21;p16) in which the *dystrophin* locus at the Xp21 breakpoint is presumed to be disrupted, in a 7-year-old girl. In consequence, very little dystrophin is produced, and the girl has a Becker-like muscular dystrophy. The approximate position of the dystrophin locus is indicated (arrowhead) on the intact X. The intact X is preferentially inactivated, as shown here with replication-banding and indicated in dashed outline on the cartoon karyotype. Early replicating (active) chromatin and the late replicating (inactivated) chromatin stain dark and light, respectively. (Case of J. A. Sullivan.)

(p21.3;q11.21); these breakpoints are very close to the t(X;22) discussed elsewhere and shown in Figure 6–11. Although the X-inactivation pattern on blood was appropriate, in tumor tissue the der(X) was inactivated (Bovie et al. 2003). This inactivation may have spread through to the 22q segment, which contains two loci (*NF2* and *SMARCB1*) associated with schwannoma susceptibility.

MALE OFFSPRING OF THE FEMALE X-AUTOSOME HETEROZYGOTE

Analogous to the female, the male inheriting a der(autosome) is affected according to whether the X translocated segment does or does not contain an XIC. If the X-segment lacks an XIC (Figure 6–7a), X disomy ensues, with a severe phenotypic effect. If the X-segment contains an XIC, the X-segment is inactivated and, other things being equal, a Klinefelter-like phenotype might be expected. But this expectation might not be met, and a more severe clinical picture, whether due to incomplete inactivation or to the effect of a concomitant autosomal deletion, could result. Balcı et al. (2007) report a three-generation family with a t(X;19)(q11;p13.3): a normal grandmother and mother with the balanced translocation, and a severely retarded boy, physically somewhat resembling Prader-Willi syndrome, whose karyotype was 46,XY,der(19)t(X;19). Virtually the entire Xq—including the XIC—was present in disomic dose on the der(19). Its otherwise lethal effect was considerably mitigated by transcriptional silencing, but nevertheless the phenotype was a great deal more severe than "Klinefelter-like."

Origin of the X-Autosome Translocation. All de novo balanced X-autosomal translocations so far studied have been of paternal origin, which may reflect the availability in male meiosis of the X chromosome for exchange with other chromosomes; the X pairs with the Y only at the PAR1, and the rest of the chromosome is unsynapsed (Turner 2007). In one well-analyzed example, Giacalone and Francke (1992) did a molecular dissection on a de novo t(X;4)(p21.2;q31.22) in a girl with Duchenne muscular dystrophy, and they proposed a format in which two GAAT sequences 5 kb apart in Xp, and one GAAT in 4q, came together during meiosis in spermatogenesis, deleted the 5 kb length in Xp (which comprised a small part of the *dystrophin* gene), and re-formed as a der(X) and a der(4). Similar mechanisms likely underlie the formation

of most X-autosome translocations. Once a balanced translocation is established in a family, and if the (female) heterozygous state is associated with phenotypic normality, male infertility dictates that transmission thereafter will only be matrilineal.

The X and the Brain. The X chromosome may have a particular load of "brain genes" (Turner 1996), and it is of interest that a number of pure brain-related phenotypes, without dysmorphism or malformation, have been associated with these translocations. A girl with lissencephaly and an X;2 translocation pointed the way to the discovery of the *doublecortin* gene at Xq22.3 (Gleeson et al. 1998). The disruption of an X-linked neuronal gene, *oligophrenin-1*, caused isolated mental defect in a female with an X-autosome translocation 46,X,t(X;12)(q11;q15). The breakpoint was in the second intron, and thus the first two exons of the gene were on the der(12), and the remaining 23 exons on the der(X). No transcript could be produced, due to this disruption of the allele, and with the other allele on the normal X having been inactivated (Billuart et al. 1998). Another gene at Xq11, with effects in a number of compartments of the neural substrate (but not outside it), is *collybistin*, which influences a specific type of neuronal receptor. A woman with an X;18 translocation that disrupted *collybistin* (the breakpoint of the 18 was in a region devoid of genes) presented a syndrome of mental retardation, aggressive behavior, epilepsy, anxiety, and a disturbed sleep pattern (Kalscheuer et al. 2009). And rare patients with an X-linked dominant infantile spasm syndrome, reminiscent of the Rett syndrome phenotype, and having its basis in the gene *CDKL5*, have had translocations in which the X breakpoint is within the *CDKL5* locus at p22.1 (Córdova-Fletes et al. 2010).

DETAILS OF MEIOTIC BEHAVIOR: FEMALE MEIOSIS

In oögenesis, a quadrivalent presumably forms, just as in the two-way translocation between autosomes. 2:2 alternate segregation with the intact X and intact autosome can lead to 46,XX or 46,XY conceptions, while transmission of the translocation in balanced state produces heterozygous or hemizygous conceptions. As for malsegregation, Figures 6–7 and 6–8 set out certain outcomes that may be viable, for various categories of single-segment and double-segment translocation, as discussed below. Given the greater survivability of X imbalances due

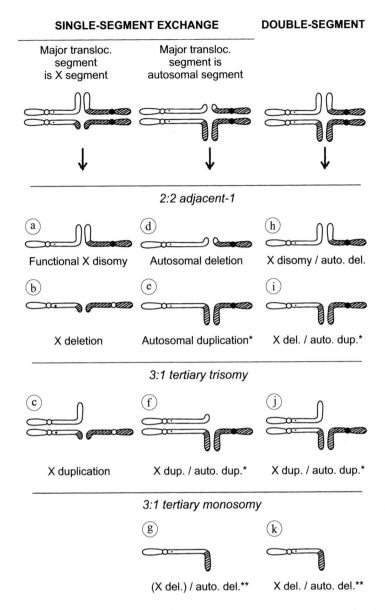

SINGLE-SEGMENT EXCHANGE **DOUBLE-SEGMENT**

Major transloc. segment is X segment

Major transloc. segment is autosomal segment

2:2 adjacent-1

(a) Functional X disomy

(d) Autosomal deletion

(h) X disomy / auto. del.

(b) X deletion

(e) Autosomal duplication*

(i) X del. / auto. dup.*

3:1 tertiary trisomy

(c) X duplication

(f) X dup. / auto. dup.*

(j) X dup. / auto. dup.*

3:1 tertiary monosomy

(g) (X del.) / auto. del.**

(k) X del. / auto. del.**

FIGURE 6–7   Major categories of adjacent-1 and 3:1 malsegregation in the X-autosome female carrier. The top row shows quadrivalents at maternal meiosis, and the following rows various combinations of segregant products. Open, X chromatin; cross-hatched, autosomal chromatin; dot indicates X-inactivation center. "Single-segment" and "double-segment" are defined in the text. X exchanges can occur in either Xp or Xq; only Xq exchanges are shown here. Circled letters provide reference points for text comments.

*Effect of autosomal duplication may be lessened by spreading of transcriptional silencing into the autosomal segment of the der(X).

**Blocking of spread of inactivation into the autosomal segment of the der(X) may avoid further functional autosomal monosomic effect.

to inactivation, and likewise a possible lessened effect of autosomal imbalance, a greater number of conceptuses are potentially viable than from the autosome-autosome translocation. The "rules" of segregation (p. 79) may not apply; for example, a viable adjacent-2 malsegregation can occur with a derivative chromosome having a large centric segment. The coexistence of tertiary monosomy and adjacent-2 aneuploidy in

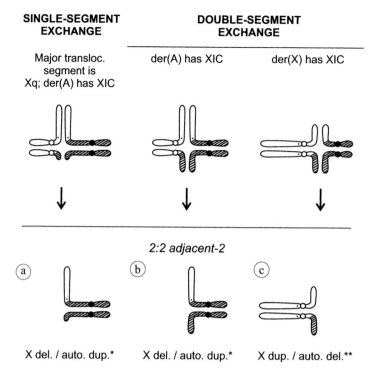

SINGLE-SEGMENT EXCHANGE

Major transloc. segment is Xq; der(A) has XIC

DOUBLE-SEGMENT EXCHANGE

der(A) has XIC   der(X) has XIC

2:2 adjacent-2

(a)   (b)   (c)

X del. / auto. dup.*   X del. / auto. dup.*   X dup. / auto. del.**

FIGURE 6–8   Three categories of adjacent-2 malsegregation in the X-autosome female carrier. The top row shows quadrivalents at maternal meiosis, and the next row various combinations of adjacent-2 segregant products. Note that these potentially viable outcomes occur only in the setting of the transmitted derivative chromosome, be it the der(X) or the der(autosome), having an X-inactivation center (XIC). In the first two columns, the der(autosome) has the XIC; here, the X breakpoint must be in proximal Xq, above the XIC, as depicted. In the third column, in which the der(X) has the XIC, X exchanges can occur either in Xp or in Xq distal to the XIC; only an Xp exchange is shown here. Open, X chromatin; cross-hatched, autosomal chromatin; dot indicates XIC; der(A), der(autosome). Circled letters provide reference points for text comments.

*Effect of autosomal duplication may be lessened by spreading of transcriptional silencing into the autosomal segment of the der(A).
**Blocking of spread of inactivation into the autosomal segment of the der(X) may avoid further functional autosomal monosomic effect.

the family described in Figure 6–11, two otherwise very uncommon segregations, reflects the unique characteristics of the X-autosome translocation.

Categories of Translocation and Modes of Malsegregation

We consider here various chromosomal scenarios, which ought to cover the majority of clinical circumstances. Concerning terminology with respect to the size of translocated segments: If one of the translocation breakpoints is at the telomeric tip of either the autosome or the X chromosome, and thus only one of the translocated segments (X or autosomal) comprises an important amount of chromatin, this may be considered an effective "single-segment exchange." If both translocated segments are of significant size, this is a "double-segment exchange."

SINGLE-SEGMENT EXCHANGE, X-TRANSLOCATED SEGMENT

The first two columns in Figure 6–7 and the first column in Figure 6–8, segregations *a–c* and segregation *a*, respectively, depict the general form of a translocation in which the single important exchanged segment comprises X chromatin. A particular example is shown in Figure 6–4, in which the derivative X chromosome is deleted for a large segment of Xq and has only the telomeric tip of 12p in exchange. A child receiving this abnormal "Xq–" in place of a normal X, or as an additional chromosome, could present with a partial form of a sex chromosome aneuploidy syndrome. Thus, a daughter with 46,X,der(X) from adjacent-1 malsegregation (*b* in Figure 6–7) would have a variant form of Turner syndrome. From tertiary trisomy (*c* in Figure 6–7), a son with 47,XY,+der(X) would have incomplete Klinefelter syndrome; and a 47,XX,+der(X) daughter might show the 47,XXX phenotype to a diminished degree.

More severe consequences follow the countertype adjacent-1 segregation, *a* in Figure 6–7. Conceptions with 46,der(12) from adjacent-1 segregation would, in the family in Figure 6–4, be functionally disomic for a large, unsurvivable amount of Xq, and they would abort. However, if the translocated X segment is small, the functionally disomic X state may be viable. This is shown in Figure 6–5, in which the mentally retarded and dysmorphic daughter has a 46,XX,der(10) karyotype and is functionally disomic for the small amount of Xp22.31pter.

As for adjacent-2 segregation (Figure 6–8a), such a gamete would, in theory, have viability only if it is the der(autosome) that is transmitted, along with the intact autosome, *and* if the X segment of the der(autosome) includes the XIC. In that case, inactivation could spread through the autosomal material, converting, at least partially, a structural autosomal trisomy into a functional autosomal disomy. Of course, there would be a partial X monosomy as well. This scenario is discussed in more detail in the section on "Double-Segment Exchange, Adjacent-2."

A truly single-segment X-autosome translocation, the translocated segment comprising X material, is recorded in de Vries et al. (1999). A mother had a submicroscopic segment of the PAR1 in distal Xp (p22.31pter) translocated across to the short arm of a chromosome 14, but, as far as could be seen, there was no reciprocal movement back to the X of any 14p material. She transmitted the der(X) to a son, who presented signs interpreted as consistent with nullisomy for certain genes in the distal PAR1: the *SHOX*, *MRX*, *CDPX*, and *STS* genes, their absences responsible respectively and collectively for short stature, developmental delay, short limbs, and ichthyosis.

SINGLE-SEGMENT EXCHANGE, AUTOSOMAL TRANSLOCATED SEGMENT

The single segment being of autosomal origin, with only the telomeric tip of Xp or Xq translocated in exchange, is shown in the middle column of Figure 6–7, segregations *d–g*. The imbalanced conceptions from 2:2 adjacent-1 malsegregation would be partially monosomic or partially trisomic for the autosomal segment: 46,der(autosome) and 46,der(X), respectively (segregations *d* and *e* in Figure 6–7). The partial autosomal trisomic state may, in the 46 X,der(X) female, have an attenuated phenotype due to spreading of transcriptional silencing from the XIC of the der(X) into the autosomal segment. The 46,Y,der(X) male conceptus, in which no X-inactivation occurs, would show the undiluted effect of the partial autosomal trisomy. The partially monosomic state, 46,XX,der(autosome) or 46,XY,der(autosome), would be no different than if the other chromosome participating in the translocation had been an autosome, instead of an X, and the typical clinical consequence associated with that autosomal deletion would be expected.

DOUBLE-SEGMENT EXCHANGE, ADJACENT-1

In a double-segment exchange with adjacent-1 segregation (right column, Figure 6–7, segregations *h–i*), there may be, in the unbalanced conceptus, effects of a combined X functional disomy and autosomal monosomy, or of X monosomy (or nullisomy) and autosomal trisomy. Such combinations would often be lethal in utero. But in the 46,X,der(X) female (segregation *i*), the effects may be very considerably modified by spreading of inactivation. Consider the t(X;16) illustrated in Figure 6–9. The 46,X,der(X) daughter has both a monosomy for most of Xp, giving a Turner-like phenotype, and a structural trisomy for most of 16p. Following spread of inactivation in the der(X) into its autosomal segment in a fraction of cells, the 16p trisomy has been converted, in these cells, into a functional 16p disomy. In 76% of cells (at least in blood), however, and in the cell illustrated, the inactivation has not extended into the 16p segment. Thus, she has, effectively, a functional mosaic 16p trisomy/16p disomy. This same combination with a Y replacing the X as the intact sex chromosome, 46,Y,der(X), with nullisomy Xp/trisomy 16p, would not be viable. The other adjacent-1 conceptions with 46,XX,der(16) and 46,XY,der(16) (light arrows in Figure 6–9; *h* in Figure 6–7) would not be similarly "modifiable" and would have a very large functional imbalance, and they would also be expected to abort early in the pregnancy.

If the translocated segments are small, survival may be possible, notwithstanding the inactivation status. Ben-Abdallah-Bouhjar et al. (2012) describe

(a)

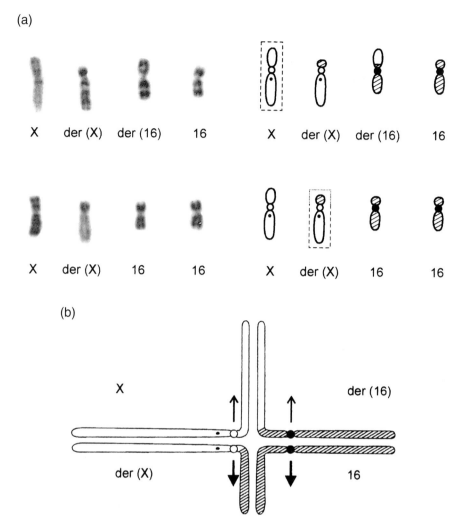

(b)

FIGURE 6–9   Spread of inactivation into autosomal segment. (*a*) Mother with balanced X;16 translocation (*above*), and her daughter with a 46,X,der(X) karyotype from adjacent-1 segregation (*below*). The translocation is t(X;16) (p11;p12). Replication-banding shows active (darker-staining) and inactive (lighter-staining) chromosome segments. The normal X is inactivated in all cells analyzed in the mother (dashed box on cartoon karyotype; dot indicates X-inactivation center). The daughter's abnormal X lacks Xp and contains distal 16p material. This chromosome is preferentially inactivated (dashed outline of box), but in 76% of cells analyzed (lymphocytes) the inactivation has not continued through the translocated 16p segment (dotted outline of box). The phenotype is the combined result of the Xp monosomy and a "partial" 16p trisomy. The child is short and has a developmental age of about 2½ at a chronological age of 4 years. (Case of C. E. Vaux.) One other daughter had the same balanced translocation as the mother and showed consistent inactivation of the normal X chromosome in blood lymphocytes, but she suffered intellectual deficit. (*b*) The presumed pachytene configuration during gametogenesis in the mother (X chromatin, open; chromosome 16 chromatin, cross-hatched; dot indicates X-inactivation center). Arrows indicate movements of chromosomes to daughter cells in adjacent-1 segregation; heavy arrows show the combination observed in this family. This is essentially the segregation *i* in Figure 6–7, with an Xp breakpoint in this case.

a mother with 46,X,t(X;3)(q27.3;p26.3), whose son, with severe psychomotor delay and a somewhat Prader-Willi-like phenotype, inherited the der(3) in unbalanced, adjacent-1 state. The imbalance conveyed a dupX:147.42 Mb-qter (this includes the region of the dup Xq28 syndrome; p. 357), and superimposed upon this, a distal 3p monosomy, del chr3:pter-1.42 Mb.

DOUBLE-SEGMENT EXCHANGE, ADJACENT-2

Adjacent-2 segregation typically produces trisomy for much of one chromosome along with monosomy for much of the other, and this is not, in the usual autosome-autosome translocation, remotely viable (e.g., segregation (5) in Figure 5–4). But such an enormous degree of structural imbalance can be accommodated in some X-autosome translocations, in a female conceptus. First, consider the case of the intact autosome and the derivative autosome being transmitted together: 46,X,–X,+der(autosome). Provided the X segment of the der(autosome) includes the XIC (segregation *b* in Figure 6–8), inactivation can spread from the XIC in both directions and into the autosomal segment, counteracting the effect of the autosomal duplication, at least partially. The concomitant partial X monosomy is, of itself, a viable state. The child would be expected to display a partial Turner phenotype, upon which the effect of a variably inactivated partial autosomal trisomy would be added. This is illustrated in Leisti et al. (1975), who record a mother carrying a t(X;9)(q11;q32) and her daughter being 46,X,–X,+der(9). In the daughter, transcriptional silencing spread through much of the autosomal segment, which very substantially, although not completely, neutralized the effect of the partial trisomy 9: She had a Turner picture with superadded microcephaly and mental defect. The case in Williams and Dear (1987) is similar, with a retarded and dysmorphic child having the karyotype 46,X,–X,+der(10),t(X;10)(q11;q25)mat, but in this instance inactivation into the autosomal segment was apparently blocked at the centromere of the der(10). This left the child with an effective duplication of 10p, along with the X deletion (Figure 6–10). Concerning a male conception in this setting, of course an adjacent-2 conceptus could not survive.

Second, viability is also possible in one very rare circumstance of an intact X and the der(X) being transmitted together, with the adjacent-2 karyotype 46,XX,–(autosome),+der(X), segregation *c* in Figure 6–8. The der(X) must contain an XIC; its autosomal segment must comprise a very substantial amount of the chromatin of that autosome; and there must be little or no spread of inactivation beyond the X segment of the translocation chromosome into the autosomal segment. In this way, the autosomal component can maintain sufficient disomic genetic activity to produce a viable phenotype. Only autosomes with "genetically small" short arms

could enable these criteria to be met. An example from a maternal t(X;22)(p21.3;q11.21) is shown in Figure 6–11 (daughter with adjacent-2, bottom row). The der(X) comprises most of an X and all, or almost all, of 22q. If its 22q segment were blocked from inactivation, there would be, in effect, a near-normal functional disomy 22, along with a partial XXX syndrome. In fact, this woman had a mild intellectual disability and attended a special school; the relative contributions to her phenotype of the two components of the cytogenetic abnormality are open to speculation.

DOUBLE-SEGMENT EXCHANGE, 3:1 SEGREGATION WITH TERTIARY MONOSOMY

The same criteria noted in the paragraph above may also obtain in the rare situation of tertiary monosomy being viable (in essence, this is segregation *k* in Figure 6–7). The t(X;22) in Figure 6–11 again provides an example. In the index case in this family having the tertiary monosomy state 45,X,–X,+der(X),–22 (middle row, Figure 6–11), the der(X) chromosome is preferentially inactivated, but inactivation has not (at least on blood lymphocytes) spread through to the 22q component of the der(X). Thus, a functional 22 disomy is maintained, or nearly so. The important structural imbalance, one might have predicted, could have been limited to the Xp21.3pter deletion (loss of 22p being without effect), with the phenotype confined to a Turner-like picture. In the event, however, there were minor congenital anomalies, and she was assessed as being intellectually disabled. This does suggest that the pattern of inactivation elsewhere in the soma may have differed from that observed on peripheral blood, and there might have been a degree of functional 22q monosomy in other tissues, including brain.

3:1 SEGREGATION, INTERCHANGE TRISOMY/MONOSOMY

From each of the categories of single- and double-segment exchange, 3:1 interchange trisomy could theoretically produce Klinefelter syndrome or XXX syndrome along with the balanced translocation; and interchange monosomy could produce standard 45,X Turner syndrome. We are aware of only one such outcome, an infertile woman with 47,XX,t(X;12) from a 46,X,t(X;12)(q22;p12)

(a)

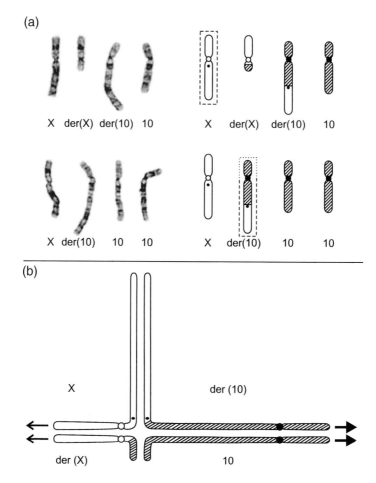

X der(X) der(10) 10   X der(X) der(10) 10

X der(10) 10 10   X der(10) 10 10

(b)

X   der (10)

der (X)   10

FIGURE 6–10 Adjacent-2 segregation. (*a*) Mother with balanced X;10 translocation (*above*), and her daughter with a 46,X,–X,+der(10) karyotype (*below*), on G-banding. The translocation is t(X;10)(q11;q25). Replication-banding showed the normal X to be inactivated in all 30 lymphocytes analyzed in the mother (dashed box on cartoon karyotype; dot indicates X-inactivation center). The daughter's der(10) was preferentially inactivated (dashed outline of box) in 50/50 cells, but the inactivation did not continue through to the 10p segment (dotted outline of box). The phenotype is the combined result of the 10p duplication and Xp monosomy. (Case of J. Williams; Williams and Dear 1987.) (*b*) The presumed pachytene configuration during gametogenesis in the mother (X chromatin, open; chromosome 10 chromatin, cross-hatched; dot indicates X-inactivation center). Arrows indicate movements of chromosomes to daughter cells in adjacent-2 segregation; heavy arrows show the combination observed in this family. This is segregation *b* in Figure 6–8.

mother, the imbalance being equivalent to 47,XXX (Madan et al. 1981).

4:0 SEGREGATION

With a trisomically viable autosome, say chromosome 21, a 48,XX,+der(X),+der(21) karyotype might be equivalent to the potentially viable 48,XXX,+21 state, a combined Down syndrome plus XXX syndrome. But we know of no such report.

DETAILS OF MEIOTIC BEHAVIOR: MALE MEIOSIS

Meiosis in the X-autosome hemizygote is typically compromised, due to failure of formation of the sex vesicle, and spermatogenesis arrests. Infrequently, some sperm may be made, albeit in small numbers. Perrin et al. (2008) propose formation of a quadrivalent, in which the Y chromosome participates with apposition of its PAR1 and PAR2 to the

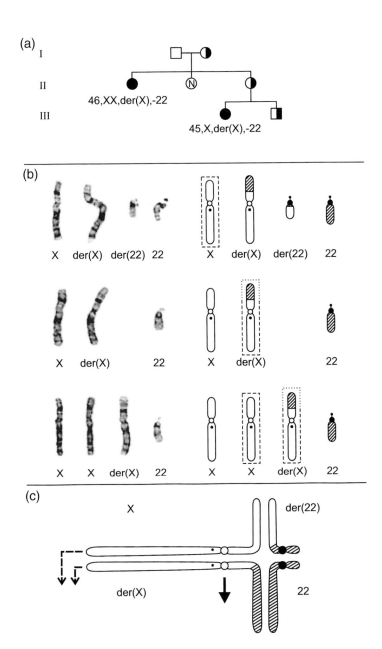

FIGURE 6–11   3:1 tertiary monosomy and adjacent-2 segregation both occurring in the same family (and see text). (*a*) Pedigree of family segregating a t(X;22)(p21.3;q11.21). Filled symbol, imbalanced state; half-filled symbol, heterozygote/hemizygote; N = 46,XX. (*b*) Partial karyotypes of heterozygotes (*top*) and of the two unbalanced states (*lower*). On replication-banding, the normal X is inactivated in all cells analyzed in the heterozygotes, whereas the der(X) is inactivated in the two affected persons (dashed box on cartoon karyotype; dot indicates X-inactivation center). In the affected child in generation III with a 45,X,–X,+der(X),–22 karyotype (middle karyotype), the der(X) was positive for a probe recognizing a sequence in the DiGeorge critical region. The der(X) chromosome showed, in 50/50 cells, apparently no inactivation going through to its 22 component (dotted outline of box), but the clinical picture might suggest otherwise (see text). The affected woman II:1 has the adjacent-2 karyotype 46,XX,+der(X),–22. (Case of T. Burgess.) (*c*) The presumed pachytene configuration during gametogenesis in the heterozygote (X chromatin, open; chromosome 22 chromatin, cross-hatched). Heavy arrow indicates movement of the der(X) chromosome to one daughter cell in 3:1 segregation (essentially segregation *k*, Fig. 6–7). Dashed arrows show the movement of chromosomes in the adjacent-2 combination (segregation *c*, Fig. 6–8).

(a)

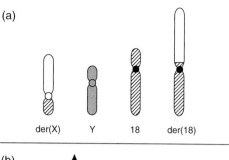

der(X)   Y   18   der(18)

(b)

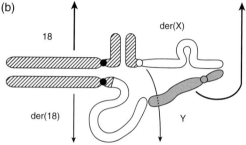

18

der(X)

der(18)

Y

FIGURE 6–12   The X-autosome translocation in the carrier male, if meiosis is able to proceed. (*a*) Father with balanced X;18 translocation, from whom pregnancy was achieved following in vitro fertilization with intracytoplasmic sperm injection. (*b*) The presumed pachytene configuration during gametogenesis in the father (X chromatin, open; Y chromatin, gray; chromosome 18 chromatin, cross-hatched). According to this construction, the X segments and the Y align only at the respective pseudoautosomal regions (PARs), and otherwise lie free. Heavy arrows indicate movement of chromosomes to daughter cells in one of the 2:2 alternate segregations, to produce a normal gamete, as observed in the 46,XY son. Light arrows show the other alternate combination, which could lead to a carrier daughter. (Drawn after the case in Perrin et al., 2008.)

homologous regions on the der(X) and the der(A) (Figure 6–12). As with the female, some malsegregant forms would have potential viability, due to the potential lesser effects of X imbalance. Similarly according to the principles as set out above for the female, but with the additional factor of a Y chromosome to be considered, the reader can determine the range of possibilities in a particular case, for this rarely encountered circumstance.

Y-AUTOSOME TRANSLOCATIONS

Y-autosome translocations fall into two major Yq-breakpoint categories, one of which has important

clinical implications, and the other of which does not. Certain other rare forms exist. First, some brief comments on the nature of the Y chromosome are in order.

THE ROLE AND BEHAVIOR OF THE Y CHROMOSOME

The particular raison d'être of the Y chromosome is to bring about male development. The testis-determining gene, *SRY*, lies in the euchromatic region on the short arm, just 5 kb proximal to the pseudoautosomal boundary. As noted above, and see Figure 6–1, the primary pseudoautosomal regions (PAR1) of the Y and X short arm contain homologous loci, and certain other loci elsewhere in the Y have homologs on the X. The secondary pseudoautosomal region (PAR2) is located at distal Yq and distal Xq; its loss from Yq seems to be without phenotypic consequence (Kühl et al. 2001). From the point of view of reproductive health, three "azoöspermia factor regions" on Yq are of importance, named AZFa, b, and c. Besides sex determination, the Y has certain other, including immune-related loci (Maan et al. 2017). Otherwise, about half the Y—the amount is variable—comprises the genetically inert heterochromatic region of the long arm (Yq12), which contains highly repetitive DNA sequences.

MEIOSIS

During normal meiosis in the male, the X and Y chromosomes recombine, synapsing at the PAR1 at the tips of Xp and Yp. The two sex chromosomes joined together in this way, but otherwise unsynapsed, comprise the "sex vesicle" (or sex-body, or XY-body), which can be considered as a peripheral nuclear subdomain within which the X and Y chromosomes lie, genetically inactivated, during the pachytene stage of meiosis (Turner 2007). A properly formed sex vesicle is necessary for normal spermatogenesis, and anything that interferes with its normal formation—such as the presence of a translocation chromosome—will compromise the process of sperm development. We have seen above that an X-autosome translocation in the male practically always causes spermatogenic arrest. And fairly infrequently, some autosomal translocations, and more especially those involving an acrocentric chromosome, can cause interference with the sex vesicle, with consequential infertility.

Similar considerations apply to the balanced Y-autosome translocation (other than the Y-acrocentric translocation) (Maraschio et al. 1994). The autosomal components of the quadrivalent, "dragged into" the sex vesicle, as it were, can have a disruptive effect, possibly due to their being inactivated, and preventing any further progress of meiosis (Turner 2007). Delobel et al. (1998) illustrate this circumstance in their study of a phenotypically normal infertile man with a translocation t(Y;6)(q12;p11.1). They analyzed meiotic preparations from a testicular biopsy, noting the configuration of the quadrivalent, this comprising the X,der(Y),der(6), and normal chromosome 6. The autosomal elements of the quadrivalent were seen to have been drawn into the sex vesicle and to be hypercondensed. The result was spermatogenic arrest at the pachytene stage, with subsequent degeneration of spermatocytes. In a similar case, Sun et al. (2005) analyzed testicular tissue from an azoöspermic man with a Yq;1q translocation, and showed (using MLH1 staining) a reduced level of meiotic recombination, with only a small fraction of cells progressing through to pachytene, and again the autosomal translocated segment drawn into the sex vesicle. Yet (and in contradistinction to the X-autosome story in the male) the Y-autosome carrier may occasionally retain natural fertility. Otherwise, fertility may be "rescueable" by means of assisted reproduction, as discussed further below.

Y-Autosome Translocation Types

BALANCED RECIPROCAL YQ AND AUTOSOME TRANSLOCATION

Reciprocal exchange between the Y long arm and an autosome (other than an acrocentric short arm) produces a balanced Y-autosome translocation. In the form being considered here, the Y breakpoint is usually given as q11.2 or q12, and the autosomal breakpoint is anywhere on the autosomal karyotype (Braun-Falco et al. 2007). There are associated phenotypic abnormalities in a few individuals, and this may be due to a disruptive effect at the breakpoints, or a deletion of autosomal material distal to the breakpoint (Erickson et al. 1995). In most, the rearrangement may be truly balanced, with the physical and intellectual phenotype being normal, and infertility is the usual presenting factor. Given this latter fact, it follows logically enough that the

translocation would typically arise as a de novo event, and this is indeed the observation (Pinho et al. 2005). The infertility may be a result of disruption of the sex vesicle, as discussed above. In other cases, loss of the AZF region may explain the infertility (Brisset et al. 2005).

Azoöspermia is typical (Kim et al. 2012). But if spermatogenesis is able to proceed, there is a risk for the generation of unbalanced forms, and a few examples are on record. Mademont-Soler et al. (2009) describe a fertile couple, the father having the karyotype 46,X,t(Y;12)(q12;q24.33). The der(12) was deleted for a very small distal segment of chromosome 12 (12q24.33qter), whereas the der(Y) carried this material. In two pregnancies, the two different adjacent-1 segregations were observed: 46,der(12) in one, and 46,der(Y) in the other. Both pregnancies, with thus an autosomal deletion and a duplication respectively, were terminated.

A very few familial cases have been reported, with father and son having the same balanced rearrangement. Teyssier et al. (1993) document a man with severe oligoasthenospermia who had a t(Y;1)(q11;q11), and whose father proved to carry the same translocation. Intact fertility is well illustrated in the family described by Sklower Brooks et al. (1998), depicted in Figure 6–13. One son in a sibship of five males and two females, he himself a university graduate, had presented for genetic counseling when his wife had a third miscarriage (they also had a normal daughter). The deceased father must have carried a t(Y;8)(q12;p21.3), with three sons showing the balanced state and two sons having inherited an unbalanced complement, 46,X,der(Y). The unbalanced state conferred a partial trisomy for 8p22pter, which was associated with a mild learning difficulty.

With access to intractyoplasmic sperm injection (ICSI), biological paternity becomes possible for some carriers. The man we had seen with the 46,X,t(Y;18)(q11.2q21) translocation shown in Figure 6–14 had been karyotyped in the course of investigation for infertility with severe oligospermia, he being an otherwise normal person. In this Y;18 case, of the 16 possible embryos, more than half, including one of the 4:0 segregants, would in theory be viable; the reader may wish to work out which ones these might be. Only one sperm, the 23,X, is capable of producing a phenotypically and karyotypically normal child; the other gamete from

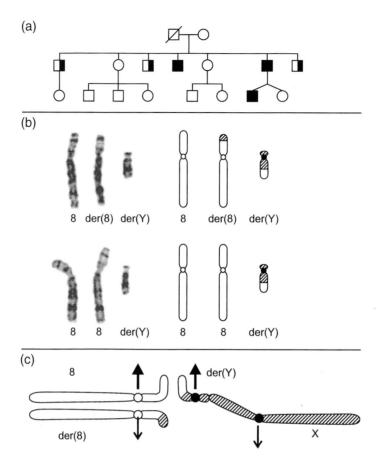

(a)

(b)

8   der(8)   der(Y)   8   der(8)   der(Y)

8   8   der(Y)   8   8   der(Y)

(c)
8

der(Y)

der(8)   X

FIGURE 6–13   A Y-autosome translocation, not involving an acrocentric short arm. In this particular example, and somewhat unusually, fertility is apparently normal. The autosomal translocated segment is of small size, structurally and functionally, and the aneuploid state with a dup(8p) is not only viable but also associated with only a mildly abnormal intellectual phenotype and an essentially normal physical appearance. (*a*) Family tree. Filled symbol, unbalanced karyotype; half-filled symbol, balanced carrier. The deceased grandfather is presumed to have been a translocation heterozygote. (*b*) Partial karyotype of a translocation heterozygote (*above*), showing the Y;8 translocation, and one of the individuals with the unbalanced complement (*below*). (*c*) The presumed pachytene configuration during gametogenesis in the heterozygote (chromosome 8 chromatin, open; Y and X chromatin, cross-hatched). Arrows indicate movements of chromosomes to daughter cells in "adjacent-1" segregation; heavy arrows show the combination observed in this family. (Case of S. Sklower Brooks et al. 1998.)

alternate segregation, 23,t(Y;18), would produce a son who would likely have similar infertility. At preimplantation genetic diagnosis, the chromosomally unbalanced embryos could be discarded. With a small number of eggs retrieved on each stimulation cycle, a normal combination might well not happen, given that there are 14 unbalanced possibilities, *if* each outcome were equally likely. But in fact the observations of Sklower Brooks et al. (1998; see above) and Giltay et al. (1999; see below) provide some encouragement that the odds for the Y-autosome carrier (in other words, the meiotic predisposition) may be tipped in favor of the normal and balanced forms. As it turned out in this Y;18 case, one embryo was indeed 46,XX, and this was successfully implanted.

This question is more directly answered in Giltay et al. (1999), these workers undertaking a sperm analysis in a man with a t(Y;16)(q11.21;q24). Sperm were present, but few in number, with many abnormal forms (oligoasthenoteratozoöspermia). Although alternate segregation accounts for only

Father

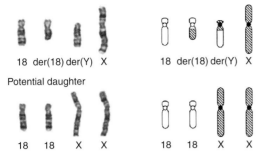

18 der(18) der(Y) X   18 der(18) der(Y) X

Potential daughter

18   18   X   X   18   18   X   X

FIGURE 6–14 The Y-autosome translocation and infertility. This t(Y;18)(q11;2q21) was identified in a man presenting with oligospermia during investigation for infertility. The fact that some sperm are still being produced allows the option of in vitro fertilization with intracytoplasmic sperm injection. A considerable number of these unbalanced gametes could, in theory, be viable. Only a 46,XX daughter could be both karyotypically and phenotypically normal. (Case of L. Harris and L. Wilton.)

2 out of the 16 segregation possibilities, in fact in this case half of all morphologically normal spermatozoa were normal or balanced, with about 40% showing adjacent segregation, and about 10% with 3:1. But the fractions were less favorable if abnormal sperm were included. With reference to assisted conception and using ICSI, Giltay et al. speak of in vitro and in vivo selection (the former artificial, the latter natural) combining to effect a considerable reduction in the risk for an unbalanced offspring. In fact, this man had had

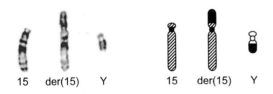

15   der(15)   Y   15   der(15)   Y

FIGURE 6–15 An example of the Y-autosome translocation involving an acrocentric autosome, the der(15) depicted here, with the breakpoint in the acrocentric short arm. Normal chromosome 15 and normal Y shown alongside for comparison (chromosome 15 chromatin, cross-hatched; Y heterochromatin, filled; Y euchromatin, open). The translocation chromosome can be carried equally by males and females. The karyotype appears unbalanced, but the phenotype is normal.

three children by ICSI, two normal daughters and a carrier son.

Y LONG-ARM AND ACROCENTRIC SHORT-ARM TRANSLOCATIONS

This is the most common form of Y-autosome translocation, accounting for some 70% of cases. The autosome is one of the acrocentrics, most commonly chromosome 15, der(15)t(Y;15)(q12;p12), which may be particularly prevalent in an Israeli Ethiopian community (Chen-Shtoyerman et al. 2012), followed by chromosome 22. There is no loss or gain of euchromatin; the result is that one acrocentric carries some phenotypically irrelevant Y heterochromatin, looking rather like (and sometimes mistaken for) a very long short arm (Neumann et al. 1992). The breakpoints are sited in the acrocentric short arm (p11p13) and in the heterochromatin of the Y long arm (Yq12) (Figure 6–15). Males and females can equally be carriers. Neither phenotypic abnormality nor infertility appears to be associated (Hsu 1994). Rare disquieting reports need to be viewed cautiously, such as that of Rajcan-Separovic et al. (2001), who raise the possibility of a secondary chromosomal abnormality, in documenting the remarkable instance of a woman with the karyotype 46,XX,der(15)t(Y;15)(q12;p13)mat, of older childbearing age, who had had two trisomic 15 pregnancies.

Rare Forms

Y MATERIAL-TO-AUTOSOME TRANSLOCATION, 45-CHROMOSOME COUNT, INCLUDING "45,X MALE"

The testis-determining region of the Y, containing the SRY gene, can be translocated onto an autosome, usually an acrocentric (Farah et al. 1994). The individual, phenotypically male, has 45 chromosomes, including the Y + autosome fusion product. The translocated Y segment may be beyond the level of cytogenetic resolution, and the classic karyotype can appear as 45,X ("45,X male") until further studies cast light (Chen et al. 2008) (the 45,X male due to t(X;Y) is mentioned below). The translocation may be of no phenotypic or reproductive effect, as Callen et al. (1987) record in a family identified quite by chance, in the course of a research study, in which a man and two sons had the karyotype 45,X,dic(Y;22)(q11.23;p11.2).

A similar story is presented in Morales et al. (2007b), in this case the karyotype being 45,X,psu dic(Y;22) (qter;p11.2), with the Y + 22 chromosome comprising almost an entire Y and almost an entire 22. The chromosome very evidently did not affect fertility in 10 carrier fathers in this large family; this may have reflected that recombination of the PAR1 of the Y with that of the X was not obstructed, due to the chromosome 22 component being well "out of the way" of the sex vesicle, so to speak. The active centromere of the Y + 22 chromosome was from the chromosome 22, the Y centromere being inactivated, and thus it was segregation of the 22 chromosomes that was the sex-determining mechanism in the offspring of these men. It was interesting that only normal children were born, whereas, in theory, segregation might also have led to 45,X Turner syndrome and 46,XX,psu dic (Y;22) Klinefelter syndrome.

More often, the reproductive and sometimes the physical phenotype is affected. Azoöspermia is a frequent finding, as documented in a review of 31 cases of "45,X male" (Chen et al. 2008). The Y component may be translocated insertionally, as Yenamandra et al. (1997) demonstrated in a phenotypically abnormal "45,X" boy, in one of whose chromosomes 4, at 4p15.3, the SRY-bearing segment was accommodated. Rather more obvious cytogenetically was the de novo dicentric Y;13 translocation, 45,X,dic(Y;13)(p11.3;p11.2), described in Shanske et al. (1999): The translocation comprised almost a complete 13 + Y composite. Their patient was a very short and otherwise normal 10-year-old boy, in whom the SHOX growth control gene, normally located in the PAR1, was absent. A patient with a very similar karyotype reported in Alves et al. (2002) was a man, 170 cm (5 feet 7 inches) tall, with severe oligospermia.

Yqh MATERIAL ON A NON-ACROCENTRIC CHROMOSOME, 46-CHROMSOME COUNT

If Yq heterochromatin is translocated to the tip of an autosome, other than to an acrocentric short arm, there may or may not be reproductive implications. A der(1)t(Y;1)(q12;p36) in a French family could be traced back to a common couple married in 1773, with self-evident fertility, male and female, for more than two centuries (Morel et al. 2002a); and Vozdova et al. (2011) showed normal seminal indices in a man with a familial der(4)t(Y;4) (q11.23;p16.3).

Y MATERIAL-PLUS-ACROCENTRIC SHORT ARM TIP, 46-CHROMOSOME COUNT

This is essentially the countertype of the common case exemplified by the Y;15 described earlier, in which the other reciprocal product, the der(Y), replaces a normal Y. Hoshi et al. (1998) identified a perfectly normal man, the father of three, who had a 46,X,–Y,t(Y;15)(q12;p13) karyotype. The der(Y) contained the necessary male-determining and fertility regions. He was only investigated because his sister had a gonadal tumor of testicular origin, she having the mosaic karyotype 46,X,Y,t(Y;15)/45,X.

Specific Very Rare Cases

FAMILIAL t(Y;15) WITH PRADER-WILLI SYNDROME

A very few cases of Prader-Willi syndrome (PWS) have been due to a fusion between a Y and a chromosome 15, having the karyotype 45,X,t(Y;15) with varying breakpoints, either de novo or familial (Vickers et al. 1994; Puvabanditsin et al. 2007). A remarkable example concerns a familial t(Y;15) (p11.2;q12), described in Gole et al. (2004). The father with the balanced translocation had a daughter with presumed PWS, she having inherited his X chromosome and the der(Y) which comprised almost all of 15q but lacking the PWS region, and most of the Y but lacking SRY. Her karyotype 46,XX,–15,+der(Y) reflected what might be called a "version" of adjacent-2 segregation. The absence of a paternally originating PWS region led to the development of that syndrome, while the absence of SRY was the basis of female sex. Her brother had the countertype "standard" adjacent-2 combination, 46,X,–Y,+der(15): He was of below-average intelligence, presumably due to duplication of the proximal 15q region, 15cen→q12, and had required treatment for hypogonadism.

DE NOVO t(Yq;1q) WITH 1q TRISOMY

A few cases are on record of a de novo unbalanced translocation t(Y;1)(q12;q21), seen in mosaic state, with the abnormal cell line imposing an essentially complete 1q trisomy (Scheuerle et al. 2005; Li 2010). Presumably, similar sequences on 1q21 and Yq21 predispose to this recurring rearrangement. The phenotype, unsurprisingly, is very severe.

TELOMERIC ASSOCIATION

A girl with gonadal dysgenesis but no other sign of Turner syndrome had 45,X diagnosed prenatally, but as a child a t(Y;7) was identified, in mosaic state (Beneteau et al. 2013). This was due to "telomeric association," without any loss of genetic material (and including retention of *SRY*), and thus the more accurate karyotype is written 45,X/46,X,tas(Y;7) (p11.32;q36.3).

X-Y TRANSLOCATIONS

The Classical X-Y Translocation

Of the major types of X-Y translocation, the classical form is the most frequently seen (Figure 6–16a, b). The X and Y breakpoints are constant, at the cytogenetic level, involving Xp22.3 in the distal X short arm, and Yq11/q12 in the proximal Y long arm (Bukvic et al. 2010). It is, certainly, readily recognized cytogenetically, and has the karyotypic notation 46,X or Y,der(X),t(X;Y)(p22.3;q11). The important genotypic defect is deletion of the distal Xp segment, with the loss including PAR1. At the molecular level, there is variation in the amount of Xp deleted, and the phenotype depends in part at least upon which of the following distal Xp genes may be lost: *ARSE* (arylsulfatase E, for chondrodysplasia punctata), *SHOX* (short

stature homeobox, for Leri-Weill dyschondrosteosis), *STS* (steroid sulfatase, for ichthyosis), *KAL* (Kallmann syndrome), *MRX49* and *NLGN4* (mental retardation), and *OA1* (ocular albinism). The Y-originating segment does not contain *SRY*. The (female) person who is 46,X,der(X)t(X;Y) has a partial monosomy for this Xp segment, and the (male) individual with 46,Y,der(X)t(X;Y) is partially nullisomic.

The *female* t(X;Y) heterozygote is characteristically fertile and of normal intelligence, but intellectual disability, uterine anomaly (Figure 6–17), facial dysmorphism, and eye abnormalities are associated in a minority (Dobek et al. (2015). If *SHOX* is deleted, the monosomic state for this gene determines a particular form of short stature and wrist deformity (Leri-Weill dyschondrosteosis). The pattern of X-inactivation tends toward preferential inactivation of the der(X)t(X;Y), but this is variable and unpredictable (Gabriel-Robez et al. 1990).

The *male* t(X;Y) hemizygote is typically the son of a t(X;Y) mother (Hsu 1994). Some may be cognitively normal, in those in whom the breakpoint is more distal. If the male has Leri-Weill dyschondrosteosis, it is no more marked than in the female, reflecting the fact that the *SHOX* locus is in the PAR1, and that each sex still retains one copy of the gene, on their normal X or Y, respectively. Infertility is almost invariable, due to spermatogenic arrest (Gabriel-Robez et al. 1990). Sperm production has,

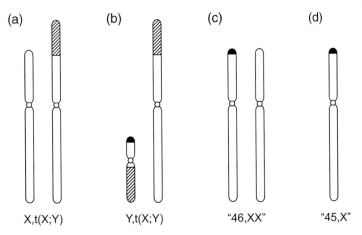

FIGURE 6–16   The four more frequent ways in which X-Y translocations are seen. (*a*) The classical t(X;Y) (p22.3;q11) together with a normal X (in a female). (*b*) The classical t(X;Y) together with a normal Y (in a male). (*c*) The cryptic t(Xp;Yp), with the Yp segment containing the *SRY* gene, in a "46,XX male." (*d*) The cryptic t(Xp;Yp) as the sole gonosome, in a "45,X male." Y chromatin: White indicates Y euchromatin, black indicates that part of distal Yp euchromatin encompassing the pseudoautosomal region and the SRY locus, and cross-hatching indicates Yq heterochromatin. Note that gonadal sex accords with the absence (*a*) or presence (*b–d*) of the SRY gene.

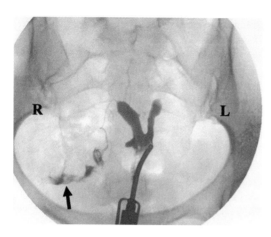

FIGURE 6–17   Bicornuate (or possibly septate) uterus in a woman with a classic 46,X,der(X),t(X;Y)(p22.3;q11) translocation. The arrow points to free spill of the contrast medium, due to patency of the right fallopian tube.

Source: From Dobek et al., Long-term follow-up of females with unbalanced X;Y translocations—Reproductive and nonreproductive consequences, *Molec Cytogenet* 8: 13, 2015. Courtesy L. C. Layman, and with the permission of Elsevier, per the Creative Commons Attribution License.

however, been documented in one case, albeit at a very low level (125,000 per ml), in a man with the typical 46,Y,der(X),t(X;Y)(p22.3;q11) karyotype (Morel et al. 2001). He was of normal intelligence, height 165 cm (5 feet 5 inches), with normal external genitalia and normal endocrine indices, and he had presented with infertility. There were equal numbers of 23,der(X) and normal 23,Y sperm, but about 20% of sperm were otherwise abnormal, the most common defect being 24,Y,der(X). Should a more proximal molecular breakpoint expose a Mendelian "brain gene," such as *MRX49* and *NLGN4* mentioned earlier, mental impairment results. A greater degree of nullisomy may suffice to determine stillbirth (Dobek et al. 2015).

The majority of cases are familial. Presumably, the X-Y chromosome arose following a reciprocal exchange between the X and Y during spermatogenesis in the man fathering the originating (female) translocation carrier in the family. This event is facilitated by the apposition of X and Y segments having a high degree of homology; for example, a crossover between the Kallmann locus on the X chromosome and a Kallmann-like nonfunctional pseudogene on the Y chromosome long arm (Guioli et al. 1992).

Some X-Y translocations cytogenetically apparently identical to the classical type are associated with the rare syndrome of microöphthalmia with linear skin defects (MLS). This phenotype results from aberrant expression of certain genes coding for components of the mitochondrial respiratory chain, *HCCS, COX7B,* and *NDUFB11* (van Rahden et al. 2015). One of these, *HCCS,* at Xp22.2, has been linked to X-Y translocations with an Xp22 breakpoint, presenting as MLS (Kotzot et al. 2002).

THE CRYPTIC Xp-Yp TRANSLOCATION ("XX MALE" AND "45,X MALE")

This form of the X-Y translocation is usually not visible (or barely visible) to the cytogeneticist without the use of FISH using Yp sequences as probe. Again, the X breakpoint is within Xp22.3; but the Y breakpoint is in the short arm, proximal to the *SRY* testis-determining gene. The genotypic consequences are loss of the distal region of the X chromosome and the transfer of the *SRY* gene onto an almost intact X chromosome. Thus, the person is male. The karyotype would initially appear to the classical cytogeneticist either as 46,XX or as 45,X (Figure 6–16c, d). In truth, it is 46,X,der(X)t(X;Y)(p22.3;p11) or 45,der(X)t(X;Y)(p22.3;p11). This translocation accounts for most supposed XX males and some 45,X males (Y-autosomal forms of 45,X male are discussed above). If there is loss of one copy of the *SHOX* gene, Leri-Weill dyschondrosteosis is the expected consequence (Stuppia et al. 1999). The MLS syndrome, mentioned above, has been observed (Anguiano et al. 2003). The translocation arises from an abnormal X-Y recombination during paternal meiosis (Weil et al. 1994). Almost always, it occurs sporadically, and the affected males are infertile, although an extraordinary familial exception is recorded in Sharp et al. (2004). Two individuals, likely distantly related, presented with an ovotesticular disorder of sex development. It may be that *SRY* in these two was partially operating, due to a variably penetrant position effect.

46,X,DEL(Yq) WITH CRYPTIC Xq-Yq EXCHANGE

A third category is the X-Y translocation arising de novo from an exchange during paternal spermatogenesis between Yq and distal Xq, producing an apparent del(Yq) chromosome that actually contains a very small segment of distal Xq (Lahn et al.

1994). The karyotype could be written 46,X,der(Y) t(X;Y)(q28;q11.2). The functional distal Xq disomy produces a characteristic severe phenotype (Sanlaville et al. 2009). In the female, the reciprocal 46,X,der(X) karyotype might hypothetically imply a mild phenotype, essentially reflecting a very small distal del(Xq), and assuming that the abnormal X would be preferentially inactivated. Cheng et al. (2009) provide a rare example of an Xq;Yq female, a 33-year-old woman who presented with premature ovarian failure, and whose karyotype was 46,X,der(X)t(X;Y)(q26.3;q11.223). The X chromosome could be appreciated as subtly abnormal on classical cytogenetics; it took comparative genomic hybridization to discover the Yq material, and then FISH to reveal the true nature of the rearrangement.

Other Variant Forms

Other forms of t(X;Y), typically but not always arising de novo, are often associated with infertility, and in some with intellectual deficit. The possibilities are listed and illustrated in Hsu (1994), and include der(X) chromosomes from translocations of varying lengths of Yq to a breakpoint at various levels on Xp or Xq, and der(Y) chromosomes from translocations of varying small lengths of Xp to a breakpoint at various levels on Yq. The dicentric X-Y translocation comprises an almost complete Y attached at a distal Yp breakpoint to an X chromosome, at either an Xp or an Xq breakpoint. For example, Baralle et al. (2000) describe a girl with a Yp-to-Xp rearrangement, the karyotype 46,X,dic(X;Y)(p22.3;p11.2), who presented with Leri-Weill dyschondrosteosis. Her pubertal development was regarded as being normal, although she had yet (at age 14 years) to undergo menarche. Her femaleness was due to absence of the SRY gene, the breakpoint on Yp being proximal to its locus.

Other rare examples include the following: (1) A girl who presented at age 10 years with an ovarian cancer, and in whom the X breakpoint was in the proximal long arm, her karyotype 46,X,der(Y)t(X;Y)(q13.1;q11.223), is reported in Lissoni et al. (2009); her female gender may have reflected inactivation of SRY from the influence of the XIC upon the der(Y). (2) A girl presenting with developmental delay and hyptonia, and with normal female external genitalia, had the karyotype 46,X,der(Y)t(X;Y) (p21.1;p11.3)dn (Ashton et al. 2010). She was thus monosomic for proximal Xp and all of Xq; the Y chromosome was almost entirely present, including the SRY gene. These authors review the handful of similar cases. (3) A notable familial case is described in Portnoï et al. (2012): A 46,X,der(X)t(X;Y)(p11.4;p11.2)/45,X mother with clinical features of Turner syndrome had a child with a different mosaic picture, 47,X,der(X)t(X;Y)x2/46,X,der(X)t(X;Y). As a baby, this girl was below average length (−1 standard deviation), and otherwise normal. The Y component of the translocation lacked the PAR1 and the SRY gene. (4) Searle et al. (2013) had offered noninvasive prenatal screening to a mother with familial 46,X,del(X)(p22.1p22.3). An anomalous readout for SRY, in the setting of a subsequent 46,XX CVS result, led to a reinterpretation of her karyotype as 46,X,der(X) t(X;Y)(p22.33p21.1;p11.2).

X-X TRANSLOCATIONS

The general karyotype is written 46,X,der(X), t(Xp;Xq), and the resultant imbalance is a dup/ del of Xp/Xq, or vice versa. The translocation could have arisen following unequal recombination between the two X chromosomes in the oöcyte. Or, the rearrangement could have occurred within the one X chromosome, folding in upon itself, in which case the origin is more likely paternal (Giglio et al. 2000). Xp11.23 and Xq21.3 are favored as breakpoints, and the translocated del/dup segments may therefore be large.

Pubertal and/or menstrual abnormality is the usual presentation, and infertility is the rule (Letterie 1995). Maternal transmission is, however, recorded in Reinehr et al. (2001), concerning a mother and daughter with short stature both having a t(X;X)(p22;q26) chromosome. These breakpoints are distal, and thus the del/dup segments in this case are small. The monosomic Xp segment included the SHOX gene, and this presumably was the cause of the short stature. The mother had had a normal menstrual history, and she had two other healthy children of normal heights. Grams et al. (2016) record a three-generation family segregating a t(X;X)(q21.2;p11.21p11.22), the male proband having presented with developmental delay, mild dysmorphism, and hypotonia. He had the karyotype 46,Y,der(X)ins(X;X)(q21.2;p11.21p11.22), determining a functional disomy for a relatively small segment[9] within Xp11.21p11.22. The rea(X) in the four-generation family in Magini et al. (2015; p. 357) could be seen in a similar light.

Y-Y TRANSLOCATIONS

For the sake of completeness, the presumed existence of the very rare Y-Y translocation is noted. Some may in fact have been isodicentric Yq chromosomes (p. 349) (Hsu 1994; Hernando et al. 2002).

GENETIC COUNSELING

THE X-AUTOSOME TRANSLOCATION

Fertility is affected in the X-autosome heterozygote and hemizygote. Approximately half of the female carriers, and practically all males, are likely to be infertile.

The Female Heterozygote

If fertile, the female heterozygote has a substantial risk for having abnormal offspring due to an imbalanced chromosomal constitution. At one end of the scale, the abnormality might be mild (e.g., partial Klinefelter syndrome) or barely discernible (e.g., partial X trisomy). At the other end, it could be severe (e.g., partial X disomy or autosomal aneuploidy, not modified by inactivation). The counselor should determine the theoretical gametic combinations from the particular category of translocation, with reference to the examples described in the section on *Biology*. Adjacent-1 and 3:1 tertiary trisomy are the major malsegregation modes to be considered. Figures 6–7 and 6–8 provide a guide; but each translocation needs to be assessed on its own merits. General comments follow.

1. A single-segment translocation with an X segment of *large* size would imply risks for partial Turner, partial Klinefelter, and partial XXX syndromes (Figs. 6–2 and 6–4; Fig. 6–7b, c).

2. A single-segment translocation with an X segment of *small* size would imply a risk not only for one of these three partial gonosomal aneuploidies, but also for functional disomy or nullisomy for a small distal Xp or Xq segment. A functional disomy would have a severe outcome (Fig. 6–5b, segregation as per heavy arrows; Fig. 6–7a). Nullisomy in the male, for all but the smallest segments, would be lethal in utero (Fig. 6–5b, segregation as per light arrows; Fig. 6–7b). The borderline between viable (but severe) and nonviable Xp deletion in the male may be at Xp22.2, in which about 10 Mb of DNA is removed (Melichar et al. 2007).

3. A single-segment translocation with an autosomal translocated segment of "viable size" (Fig. 6–7d–f) implies a risk for partial autosomal monosomy or trisomy from adjacent-1 segregations. In the female conceptus, the trisomy may be modified by spreading of inactivation, but this is unpredictable.

4. Any 2:2 unbalanced segregant from a double-segment translocation (Fig. 6–7h–j) has a combined duplication/deficiency, and spontaneous abortion is probable. But spreading of inactivation in a female conception may attenuate a partial autosomal trisomy and allow for survival, albeit with phenotypic defect.

5. Adjacent-2 possibilities need individual assessment (Fig. 6–8).

THE LEVEL OF RISK

The risk for many female heterozygotes, who are fertile, will be "substantial." An otherwise nonviable unbalanced conception may survive because inactivation tempers the imbalance; and some conceptions with the structurally balanced complement may be functionally unbalanced due to aberrant inactivation patterns. The counselor should go through the exercise of determining possible malsegregant outcomes, as depicted in Figures 6–7 and 6–8. The risks to have a liveborn child with a structural and/or functional aneuploidy may be in the range 20% or higher. In Stene and Stengel-Rutkowski (1988), and with specific reference to single-segmental translocations involving Xp, the risk for adjacent-1 malsegregants was 24%, although interestingly the risk associated with 3:1 segregation leading to interchange trisomy X was very low, less than 0.8%. As we discussed above, the components making up the total risk may comprise a very mild abnormality through to severe mental and physical defect. There is the difficulty of knowing what risk might apply to a child with the

---

9 ChrX:50,350,047-54,964,018, on build hg19.

same balanced translocation (see below). Only with the 46,XX and 46,XY karyotype can one be confident of normality, other things being equal.

Even more so than with the common autosomal translocation, the risks relating to each X-autosome translocation will be specific to that particular rearrangement, and extrapolation from other translocations will be fraught. Panasiuk et al. (2004) have made a start, in deriving specific risk figures for four different translocations, in each case the X breakpoint involving the short arm (Table 6–2). The one circumstance in which they consider data pooling to be permissible is in rearrangements in which the autosomal breakpoint is in the short arm of an acrocentric.

Table 6–2. Estimated Risk Figures for Having a Liveborn Aneuploid Child, or a Child Stillborn or Dying as a Neonate[a] Because of Imbalance due to X-Autosome Malsegregation (Adjacent and/or 3:1), in Four Specific Translocations, Three Double Segment, and One, the X;22, Effectively Single Segment[b]

TRANSLOCATIONS	RISK[c] (%)
t(X;5)(p22.2;q32)	4.2
t(X;6)(p11.2;q21)	3.3[d]
t(X;7)(p22.2;p11.1)	2.1
t(X;22)(p22.1;p11.1)[e]	17

[a]Figures may be considered as expressing the percentage risk to have an aneuploid liveborn or stillborn infant, from a pregnancy which had proceeded to at least 28 weeks gestation.

[b]Families published or cited in Panasiuk et al. (2004).

[c]The figure in one family (X;22), in which the autosomal breakpoint is in the p arm of an acrocentric chromosome, comes from direct segregation analysis, and combining with literature cases of another X;acrocentric p arm translocation (of chromosome 15). In the remaining three, the figure is indirect and derived from applying this rule: halving the risk for the lesser of the two risks, which would otherwise have applied to each translocated segment when viewed as a single-segment imbalance.

[d]This carrier mother had presented having had an unkaryotyped malformed stillbirth at 42 weeks gestation, suggesting that at least one of the malsegregant combinations might be compatible with survival to term. The figure of 3.3% might thus be an underestimate, if the risk figure were taken to include stillbirth.

[e]This translocation is very close to, and might possibly be the same as, the t(X;22) in Figure 6–11.

The Male Hemizygote

Infertility is almost inevitable, barring the possibility of medical intervention (Ma et al. 2003). If sperm can be accessed, from an ejaculate or via testicular sperm extraction, in vitro fertilization (IVF) using ICSI may be attempted; greater spermatogenic success may attend translocations with pericentromeric or centromeric breakpoints (Perrin et al. 2008). The outcomes from which normality could be expected, other things being equal, are the two alternate segregations leading to 46,XY and to 46,X,t(X;A), respectively. The segregant fractions can vary quite considerably between men, and may suggest optimism for IVF, or pessimism, accordingly (Perrin et al. 2009b). Normality in a (necessarily heterozygous) daughter would require inactivation to have been skewed in favor of the normal X; the likelihood for this to have happened may be greater, but could not be assumed as certain, in the case of larger translocated segments. Phenotypic normality in the hemizygous father would allow the inference of a truly balanced rearrangement, and thus no question should arise about a cryptic deletion/duplication.

The presumption of an approximately 50% risk was, for example, brought to the attention of the man with an (X;18)(q11;p11.1) translocation noted earlier (see *Biology* and Figure 6–12); nevertheless, and given the practical matter of a long wait for preimplantation genetic diagnosis (PGD), the couple went ahead with IVF and ICSI, having prenatal diagnosis in the pregnancy, and they had a normal 46,XY son (Perrin et al. 2008). Ma et al. (2003) describe a successful outcome in a man with a whole-arm translocation, t(X;20)(q10;q10), maternally inherited, and from whose ejaculate only about 50 sperm were able to be retrieved; an embryo created at IVF went on to become a carrier daughter, who was normal physically and developmentally on assessment at age 12 months. The child, and her heterozygous paternal grandmother, both displayed skewed X-inactivation. Interestingly, the man's brother, also an X;20 hemizygote, had had 7 years of infertility, but then had two normal daughters. These girls' karyotypes, and paternity status, had not been evaluated.

The Balanced Inherited X-Autosome Detected Prenatally. This is a vexed question. Consider the circumstance of a phenotypically normal carrier mother, who has prenatal diagnosis, or PGD. A balanced X-autosome karyotype identified in a female fetus, or in a female embryo (the balanced translocation, and normal states not routinely distinguishable), might eventually lead to a normal daughter, but by no means can this be made as a firm statement (Scriven 2013). Indeed, Ferfouri et al. (2016), writing about the detection of a balanced X-autosome at PGD, speak of "the resulting phenotype remaining a mystery." As yet, we lack a good understanding of the relative roles of aberrant X-inactivation, versus gene disruption at a breakpoint, in causing phenotypic abnormality. If it were the former mechanism, then a normal carrier mother (and she having a "perfect" 100:0 normal:derivative X-activation ratio) could have an abnormal carrier daughter, if the daughter's inactivation ratio were "imperfect." The case in Figure 6–9 might possibly exemplify this scenario. But if the latter, then the mother's normality would, of itself, indicate absence of gene disruption; and presumably her daughter would inherit the same intact translocation, and herself be normal, other things being equal. There is a need for a large study, with unbiased ascertainment, of the carrier daughter offspring of the (normal) carrier mother, in order to address this issue. As for the de novo circumstance, phenotypic abnormality is well recorded (see above).

Too little information exists concerning the phenotype of the male hemizygote born to a female X-autosome heterozygote for any firm advice to be offered. Normality has been recorded in this setting, but so has major genital defect, which in one case was the consequence of compromised function of the androgen receptor gene (Buckton et al. 1981; Kleczkowska et al. 1985; Callen and Sutherland 1986; Ma et al. 2003). Fetal ultrasonography may be useful to check for normal male genital development. This approach was offered to the mother whose karyotype appears in Figure 6–11, and who had a 46,Y,t(X;22) result at amniocentesis in her second pregnancy. A normal baby boy was subsequently born, whose infant development was quite normal. Otherwise normal male carriers would almost certainly be infertile.

Y-AUTOSOME TRANSLOCATIONS

The Apparently Balanced Y-Autosome Translocation

It is notable that the same balanced Y-autosome translocation can behave differently in different male members of a family in terms of fertility, this presumably reflecting the importance of the background genetic contribution to the control of the mechanics of spermatogenesis (Teyssier et al. 1993; Rumpler 2001). For those who are fertile, risk data are too few to form a secure base for genetic counseling. From first principles, unbalanced forms are probable, several of which will often be viable (according to the autosome in question, and the site of the autosomal breakpoint), and the option of prenatal diagnosis is appropriately offered or, and especially if IVF is needed, PGD.

As discussed in the *Biology* section, despite there being several more imbalanced than balanced possibilities, there are tentative grounds for supposing that alternate segregations (normal and balanced forms) may be favored. The t(Y;8) family of Sklower Brooks et al. (1998) noted above and shown in Figure 6–13 demonstrated three of the four predicted alternate and "adjacent-1" karyotypic outcomes: 46,XX, the 46,X,t(Y;8) balanced carrier, and 46,X,der(Y), the former two outnumbering the latter. The 46,X,der(Y) karyotype produced sons with an 8p duplication; the other unbalanced karyotype, 46,XX,der(8), would have produced a daughter with an 8p deletion. Manifestly, the carrier male, while he could have a normal daughter, could never conceive a 46,XY child. Sperm karyotyping, if available, may be a helpful investigation. In the man with the rare 13p;Yp fusion mentioned earlier (Alves et al. 2002), having demonstrated that most sperm had a balanced complement, reassurance could be offered, in this particular case, that if pregnancy were achievable there would be a good chance of producing a normal child.

For the infertile man, assisted reproduction may offer the possibility of paternity (Mackie Ogilvie et al. 2010). A sperm count way below the level needed for natural conception may yet allow retrieval of sperm for ICSI. Testicular aspiration may provide sperm even when they are completely absent in the ejaculate. With the need for IVF, PGD becomes attractive because of the probable substantial genetic risk, in most cases, for unbalanced forms, and considering the practical point that the embryo is nicely accessible. Taking the example of the oligospermic man with a 46,X,t(Y;18)(q11.2;q21) karyotype, shown in Figure 6–14, he could, in theory, and through IVF, have a 46,XX daughter, and a 46,X,t(Y;18) son like himself. The substantial fraction of unbalanced forms that could be viable in this case, out of the 16 total possible conceptions, does becomes a relevant matter at PGD. These issues of IVF and PGD are discussed in more detail in Chapter 22.

THE Yqh-ACROCENTRIC TRANSLOCATION

Probably, these translocations can be regarded as being no more than interesting variant chromosomes, and of no clinical significance. In the case of the t(Yq;15p), a theoretical risk for trisomy 15 with correction to uniparental disomy (White et al. 1998; Rajcan-Separovic et al. 2001) is neither to be completely ignored nor to be overstated.

The "45,X" Yp-Acrocentric Translocation. These chromosomes are probably stable, and not (if fertility is achievable) implying a risk for phenotypically abnormal offspring (Callen et al. 1987).

THE CLASSICAL X-Y TRANSLOCATION

The female with an X-Y translocation is usually fertile and of normal intelligence. She has a 50% risk for having a child, whether a son or daughter, who would have the translocation. An X-Y translocation son may be abnormal, according to the extent of distal Xp nullisomy and the loci involved (Seidel et al. 2001). If the mother is short, an X-Y translocation daughter would also be short, likely because of deletion of the *SHOX* locus. As with Turner syndrome, growth hormone treatment may be appropriate for such a child. She would probably be, like her mother, fertile. A child receiving the mother's normal X would of course be normal, 46,XX or 46,XY. Prenatal diagnosis is appropriately offered.

The male X-Y translocation carrier is almost invariably infertile. A sperm chromosome study has been undertaken in only one 46,Y,der(X)t(X;Y) man, referred to in the *Biology* section above (Morel et al. 2001). He had severe oligozoöspermia, and notably sex chromosome aneuploidy was recorded in 20% of sperm. Otherwise, 40% of sperm were normal 23,Y, and 40% had the t(X;Y). Conception in such a case could only ever be achieved via IVF. If preimplantation diagnosis were to be attempted, the choice of a 46,XY embryo (the only normal gonosomal possibility) would allow avoiding the genetic risk for the next generation.

X-X TRANSLOCATIONS

Infertility is the expectation, and a theoretical question of genetic risk will usually be academic. In a small imbalance, fertility may be retained, as in the exceptional examples of Reinehr et al. (2001) and Grams et al. (2016) discussed above. A daughter receiving the X-X translocation would be expected to have a phenotype similar to that of her mother. A male pregnancy would be very likely to miscarry at any early stage, due to an X nullisomy/disomy. If the del/dup segments were very small, viability might be possible, but with probable major phenotypic defect. Children receiving the mother's normal X chromosome would of course be normal, other things being equal.

7

ROBERTSONIAN TRANSLOCATIONS

THE AMERICAN INSECT CYTOGENETI-CIST W. R. B. Robertson first described translocations of chromosomes resulting from the fusion of two acrocentrics in his study of insect speciation in 1916, and this type of translocation is named Robertsonian (abbreviation *rob*) in his honor. There are five human acrocentric autosomes—chromosomes 13, 14, 15, 21, and 22 (the 13, 14, and 15 are the D group chromosomes, and the 21 and 22 comprise the G group)—and all are capable of participating in this type of translocation. The composite chromosome produced includes the complete long arm chromatin of the two fusing chromosomes, although it lacks at least some of the short arm chromatin. Robertsonian translocations are among the most common balanced structural rearrangements seen in the general population, with a frequency in newborn surveys of about 1 in 1,000 (Blouin et al. 1994). Historically, the most important Robertsonian translocations are the D;21 and G;21, which are the basis of most familial translocation Down syndrome. Uniparental disomy

is of relevance, with respect to the two imprintable acrocentrics, chromosomes 14 and 15.

In this chapter, we consider the case of the phenotypically normal person who carries, in balanced form, a Robertsonian translocation. We generally use a short cytogenetic description for the carrier state, thus, 45,XX,rob(14q21q) or simply rob(14q21q). The formally correct ICSN designation for a short arm to short arm fusion Robertsonian translocation is, for example, 45,XX,der(14;21)(q10;q10) or 45,XX,rob(14;21)(q10;q10).

BIOLOGY

The great majority of balanced Robertsonian translocations involve two different chromosomes (a *heterologous* or *nonhomologous* translocation); those involving the fusion of homologs (*homologous* translocation) are rare. Heterologous translocations can be transmitted through many generations of phenotypically normal heterozygotes, whereas the homologous translocation is

Table 7–1. The Frequency of Robertsonian Translocations

TRANSLOCATION	LITERATURE REVIEW	UNBIASED ASCERTAINMENT
13q13q	3%	2%
13q14q	33%	74%
13q15q	2%	2%
13q21q	2%	1%
13q22q	1%	2%
14q14q	½%	–
14q15q	2%	5%
14q21q	30%	8%
14q22q	1%	2%
15q15q	2%	–
15q21q	3%	½%
15q22q	½%	1%
21q21q*	17%	3%
21q22q	2%	½%
22q22q	1%	–

Note: Relative frequencies in literature review (most cases being of biased ascertainment), and in studies in which ascertainment was unbiased.

*Most are i(21q) Down syndrome; the figure for true rob(21q21q) is probably nearer ½%.

Source: From Hook and Cross (1987a) and Therman et al. (1989).

almost always seen as a de novo event in the consultand. As Table 7–1 attests, the rob(13q14q) and the rob(14q21q) are predominant. If we exclude the rob(21q21q)—most of which are actually isochromosomes for 21q—the rob(13q14q) accounts for around 75% of all Robertsonian translocations in unbiased studies, and indeed it is the most common single chromosome translocation in the human race. Since 1 in 1,000 persons is a rob heterozygote, the prevalence of the rob(13q14q) carrier is about 1 in 1,300. Karyotypes of the 13q14q and 14q21q carrier states, and of the unbalanced 14q21q state leading to translocation Down syndrome, are shown in Figures 7–1through 7–3. Balanced carriers for any of the five homologous translocations are of about equal rarity.

Formation of the Translocation

There are three possible mechanisms of formation of the balanced *heterologous* translocation (Figure 7–4): union following breaks in both short arms; fusion at the centromere (centric fusion); and union following breakage in one short arm and one long arm (essentially, a whole-arm reciprocal translocation) (Guichaoua et al. 1986). The first mechanism results in a chromosome with two centromeres (dicentric), and this is much the most common. The other two mechanisms are rare (if ever, in

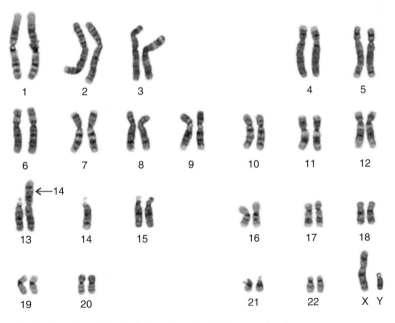

FIGURE 7–1   The balanced rob(13q14q) in a phenotypically normal male.

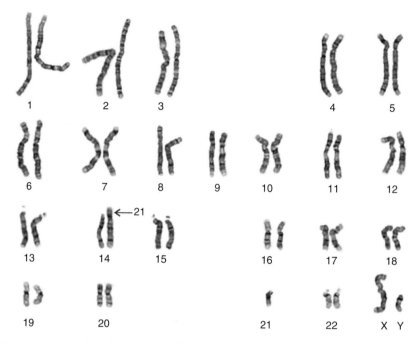

FIGURE 7-2 The balanced rob(14q21q) in a phenotypically normal male.

the case of centric fusion) and would produce a translocation chromosome with one centromere (monocentric). The common rob(13q14q) and rob(14q21q) translocations are practically always dicentric, and they are formed predominantly during female meiosis, with consistent breakpoints at the molecular level (Bandyopadhyay et al. 2002). In some dicentrics, one centromere is "suppressed," and the chromosome appears monocentric. This heterogeneity of formation is not of any clinical

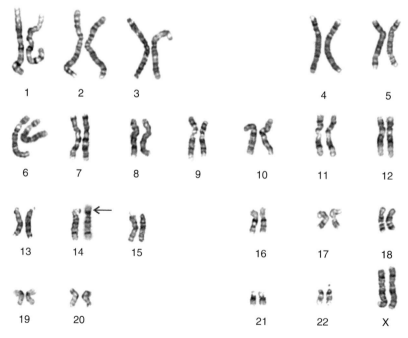

FIGURE 7-3 The unbalanced rob(14q21q) in a girl with translocation Down syndrome.

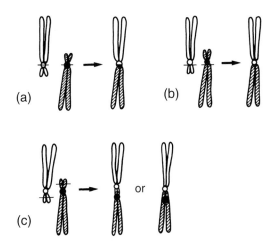

(a)

(b)

(c)

or

FIGURE 7–4   Mechanisms of formation of Robertsonian translocations. (*a*) Centric fusion, giving a monocentric chromosome; (*b*) breakage in one short arm and one long arm, giving a monocentric; and (*c*) breakage in both short arms, giving a dicentric or, after suppression of one centromere, a monocentric.

significance that can presently be discerned. In the reciprocal type, the other product may rarely survive as a stable small bisatellited marker (Schmutz and Pinno 1986).

The propensity to recombine may be the consequence of recombination between similar sequences shared by acrocentric chromosomes. The predominance of the rob(13q14q) and the rob(14q21q) may be due to specific homologous but inverted segments in these pairs of chromosomes that encourage crossover, while the variable breakpoints in the uncommon translocations point to a more random process (Bandyopadhyay et al. 2001a, 2001b, 2002). Rare cases are due to postzygotic joining together, a point that can be proven when the two component chromosomes can be shown to have come one from one parent, and one from the other (Bandyopadhyay et al. 2003). Just as a Robertsonian translocation can form de novo from the fusion of chromosomes, so can it (very rarely) revert to two separate chromosomes by a "back-mutational" fission (Pflueger et al. 1991) (p. 222).

The balanced *homologous* Robertsonian chromosome may arise from fusion in the zygote of the paternal and maternal homologs, in which case it is a true translocation. The site of formation may be at the first mitosis, a conclusion we drew from

studying a woman with 45,XX,rob(13q13q), who showed no mosaicism on biopsy samples from a number of different tissues taken during surgery for tubal ligation (Gardner et al. 1974). Alternatively, it may be an isochromosome, with the stage having been set in meiosis: A nullisomic egg due to a maternal nondisjunction leads to a monosomic conceptus, which is then "rescued" by reduplication of the paternal homolog as an isochromosome, and thus with uniparental disomy for the chromosome in question (discussed below). Berend et al. (1999) showed a de novo 45,i(13q),upd(13)pat in a normal infant to have complete isozygosity for chromosome 13 markers, indicative of this scenario of postzygotic monosomy rescue. In another instance, they could show a paternal meiotic origin of the i(13q) in a normal adolescent with 45,i(13q),upd(13)pat. This individual would have had trisomy 13, had it not been for gametic complementation: The mother contributed a nullisomic 13 ovum (she being, by extraordinary coincidence, a 13q14q heterozygote). These two cases came to attention only through fortuitous discovery at prenatal diagnosis.

NUCLEOLAR ORGANIZING REGIONS AND THE ROBERTSONIAN TRANSLOCATION

The nucleolar organizing regions (NORs) are located in the "stalks" of the short arms of the acrocentric chromosomes, in the p12 regions, and comprise multiple copies of genes coding for ribosomal RNA. Not all NORs are active: As judged by silver (Ag-NOR) staining, most individuals have four to seven per cell that are functioning (Varley 1977). Presumably, there is a minimum requirement for normal cellular function. When a Robertsonian translocation forms, the NORs of two of the fusing chromosomes are lost, at least with the rob(13q14q) and rob(14q21q). Thus, an individual with a Robertsonian translocation has only eight acrocentric short arms and therefore eight NORs. But this is a more than sufficient number, as witness the several reported normal individuals who carry *two* Robertsonian translocations, most commonly homozygosity for the rob(13q14q) (Miryounesi et al. 2016). The lesser NOR load has been exploited as a means to identify rob carriers by molecular methodology at noninvasive prenatal testing (Huang et al. 2016).

THE HETEROLOGOUS ROBERTSONIAN TRANSLOCATION

DETAILS OF MEIOTIC BEHAVIOR

This type of Robertsonian translocation chromosome comprises the long arm elements of two *different* acrocentric chromosomes. At meiosis in the heterozygote, the translocation chromosome and the two normal acrocentric homologs synapse as a trivalent. Following 2:1 segregation, six types of gamete are produced (Figure 7–5). "Alternate" segregation leads to the production of normal and balanced gametes, and adjacent segregation produces two types of disomic and two types of nullisomic gamete. 3:0 segregation occurs, but it is rare. In obvious contrast to what happens with the reciprocal translocation, the chromosomally abnormal conceptuses have a complete aneuploidy. Only unbalanced conceptuses that are effectively trisomic for chromosome 13 or 21 can survive substantially through the course of the pregnancy (whether to fetal death in utero, stillbirth, or live birth). Fetal trisomy 14, 15, and 22 are expected to end in miscarriage in the first or early second trimester, and the monosomies would typically abort in early embryogenesis.

Of these six possible outcomes (eight if we include 3:0 segregants), some are more likely to occur than others. Judging from the outcomes at birth, one might conclude that alternate segregation is favored. From the male heterozygote, translocation Down syndrome (DS) and translocation trisomy 13 are scarcely ever seen in the offspring, and in a minority for DS, 10%–15% of children, from the female (Table 7–2). But of course, as just mentioned, there has been the complete prenatal selection against some unbalanced forms, and a variable prenatal selection against the two potentially viable imbalances, trisomy 13 and trisomy 21.

Segregation at the level of the gamete is a different story. Sperm and oöcyte studies show considerable fractions of unbalanced forms. (Naturally, most if not all of the individuals proceeding to gamete testing in these reported studies will have experienced reproductive difficulty, and thus the data from their gametes may not necessarily be applicable to the larger number of carriers with apparently normal fertility.) Ogur et al. (2006) have reviewed the literature on sperm analysis and contributed their own cases, and their findings are set out in Table 7–3. Across all types of translocation (and it is likely that no important differences exist), 81%–92% of sperm are normal/balanced due to alternate segregation, and 7%–19% unbalanced due to adjacent segregation. Rounding these figures, 10%–20% of sperm are unbalanced, and 80%–90% are balanced. Spermatogenic factors may have an influence: Translocation malsegregants

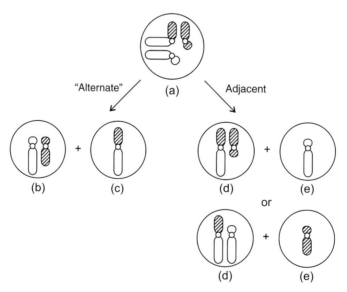

FIGURE 7–5   Meiotic behavior of the Robertsonian translocation. (*a*) Trivalent at synapsis. (*b*) Normal and (*c*) carrier gametes from "*alternate*" segregation. (*d*) Disomic and (*e*) nullisomic gametes from *adjacent* segregation. Note that there are six possible combinations (ignoring 3:0 segregation), of which two are normal/balanced, and four are unbalanced.

Table 7–2. Estimates of Risks to Have a Child with Aneuploidy or with a Uniparental Disomy Syndrome, for the Heterologous rob Carrier

| | CARRIER PARENT | | | |
| | MOTHER | | FATHER | |
rob	UNBAL.	UPD*	UNBAL.	UPD*
13q14q	1%	<½%	<1%	<½%
13q15q	1%	<½%	<1%	<½%
13q21q	10%–15%	–	<1%	–
13q22q	1%	–	<1%	–
14q15q	–	½%	–	<½%
14q21q	10%–15%	<½%	<1%	<½%
14q22q	–	<½%	–	<½%
15q21q	10%–15%	<½%	<1%	<½%
15q22q	–	<½%	–	<½%
21q22q	10%–15%	–	<1%	–

Note: Estimates for the uncommon rob translocations are extrapolated from data for the common robs.

Unbal., unbalanced, with a full aneuploidy for chromosome 13 or 21; UPD, uniparental disomy; UPD*, abnormal child with syndrome of UPD 14 or UPD 15.

are seen more often in men with oligospermia (Ferfouri et al. 2011).

Ova are more prone to error. On oöcyte analysis, using the ingenious approach of fluorescence in situ hybridization (FISH) analysis on polar bodies, Munné et al. (2000a) determined in four 45,XX,rob(14q21q) carriers an average 42% of unbalanced forms, and seven 45,XX,rob(13q14q) carriers with an average 32%; others have provided similar data (Table 7–3), and Bint et al. (2011) assemble a review. In the important 14q21q group, about 20% of ova may be disomic 21, and evidently half or more of these are able to survive through to term, to give the 10%–15% risk figure for a child with DS, mentioned above.

Comparable results have been obtained from in vitro fertilization (IVF) embryos, analyzed using preimplantation genetic diagnosis (PGD) and single nucleotide polymorphism (SNP) microarray. Combining data from maternally and paternally inherited Robertsonian translocations, it is not surprising that the figures from one study are intermediate between the sperm and ova data. Of 218 day-5 embryos of translocation carriers, 23% had a translocation-related imbalance (Tan et al. 2013). However, a rather lower figure was seen in Idowu et al. (2015): Of 201 embryos at either day 3 or day 5, there was a translocation-related imbalance in only 8% (see also Chapter 22).

Meiotic Drive. Meiotic drive is an influence whereby one of the products at meiosis may be favored and have a better-than-even chance of coming to be in the successful gamete. The Robertsonian translocation provides an apparent example. At the level of the offspring produced, de Villena and Sapienza (2001) demonstrated that children of female carriers of rob translocations have a ratio close to 60:40 for the balanced rob compared to normal karyotypes. No such effect could be confirmed for the male rob carrier. Daniel (2002) has confirmed these interpretations in a retrospective analysis of prenatal diagnosis data, with rigorous attention to the need to avoid bias, showing a 116:81 ratio in favor of balanced carrier offspring compared to normal karyotypes where the mother is the carrier parent, compared to a 42:41 ratio for carrier fathers.

POSTZYGOTIC "CORRECTION" AND ASSOCIATED UNIPARENTAL DISOMY

Trisomic Correction. An initial translocation trisomy may be "corrected" by mitotic loss of one of the free homologs and lead to uniparental disomy (UPD) in the embryo. For example, a presumed mechanism whereby UPD 15 could arise from a rob(13q15q) parent is outlined in Figure 7–6. Essentially, adjacent segregation

Table 7–3. Segregation Patterns in Gamete Studies upon Heterologous Robertsonian Heterozygotes (Several of Whom Had Presented with Infertility)

TRANSLOCATION	SEGREGATION PATTERN	
	2:1 ALTERNATE	2:1 ADJACENT (fractions with the viable disomy)
SPERM		
t(13q;14q)	74–92% (85%)	8%–26% (14%)
t(13q;15q)	76–93% (82%)	7%–23% (17%)
t(13q;21q)	87–88% (88%)	11%–12% (11%)
t(13q;22q)	86%	14%
t(14q;15q)	91–93% (92%)	7%–8% (7%)
t(14q;21q)	72–93% (87%)	7%–13% (10%)
t(14q;22q)	79–81% (80%)	19%–20% (19%)
t(15q;22q)	90%	10%
t(21q;22q)	60%–97% (81%)	3%–40% (19%)
Range of the means	81%–92%	7%–19%
OÖCYTES		
t(13q;14q)[a]	68%	32% (10%)
t(13q;14q)[b]	26%	68% (16%)
t(13q;14q)[c]	60%	20%*
t(13q;14q)[c]	40%	50%*
t(14q;21q)[a]	58%	42% (20%)
t(14q;21q)[b]	43%	57% (0%)
Range	40%–68%	32%–68%

Notes: The numbers of male subjects range from 25 (the common 13;14) to one per translocation type (the 13;22 and 15;22 cases). Each female subject is listed individually, six in all. Just over 24,000 sperm were studied, but only 200 analyzable eggs. Only 2:1 segregants are listed: 3:0 segregants are very rare, in sperm at least (three 3:0 egg segregants are footnoted below*). 2:1 alternate segregants would produce a normal or balanced karyotype in the conceptus; 2:1 adjacent segregants would produce trisomy or monosomy. Figures in parentheses are average ranges (sperm data), and fractions of gametes (oöcyte data), that could have produced the relevant viable aneuploidy, trisomy 13 or trisomy 21, accordingly. See also the review of Bint et al. (2011).

Sperm data: From the review in Ogur et al. (2006), plus 13;15 and 14;22 cases from Moradkhani et al. (2006a, 2006b), and with these other entries: 13;21 (Hatakeyama et al. 2006; Chen et al. 2007b), 13;22 (Anahory et al. 2005), 14;15 (Moradkhani et al. 2006a), 14;22 (Chen et al. 2005d), and 15;22 (Martin et al. 1992).

Oöcyte (polar body) data: From [a]Munné et al. (2000a), [b]Durban et al. (2001), and [c]Pujol et al. (2003). *Shortfall from 100% totals due to three 3:0 forms.

produces a trisomic 15 conception, and then loss of the chromosome 15 contributed from the other parent,[1] at an early postzygotic stage, "corrects" the karyotype. UPD has no untoward effect if the chromosome is not subject to imprinting (except for the question of isozygosity for a recessive gene; see below), and chromosomes 13, 21, and 22 are in this category. If there is UPD for an imprintable chromosome—in this context, chromosome 14 or 15—a UPD syndrome would result. Liehr (2016a) assembled a total of 36 cases in which a UPD syndrome had been associated

with a Robertsonian translocation, comprising 20 cases of upd(14)mat (Temple syndrome), four of upd(14)pat (Kagami-Ogata syndrome), six of upd(15)mat (Prader-Willi syndrome), and six of upd(15)pat (Angelman syndrome). In most, the Robertsonian translocation was inherited from a parent, but a handful of de novo translocations are also recorded. Nonetheless, UPD due to a parental rob is extremely rare; the overall risk to have a child with a UPD syndrome, as determined from prenatal diagnosis data where one parent is a heterologous rob carrier, is <½%.

---

1 Note that with one or other chromosome 15 being the candidate to be lost, the risk for UPD to be generated is 50%. This is in contrast with correction in standard trisomy, in which, with three candidate chromosomes, the chances are 1 in 3 for the "wrong" one to be lost.

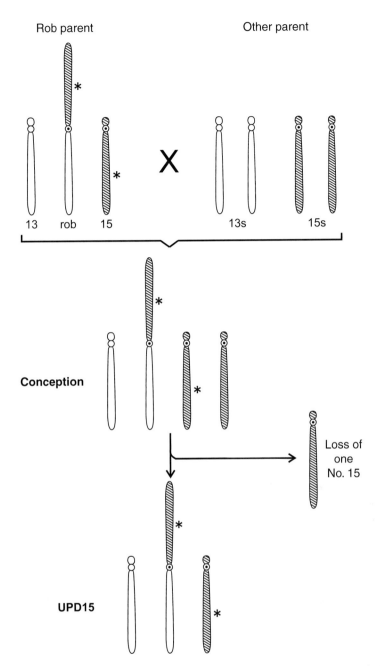

Rob parent

Other parent

X

13   rob   15   13s   15s

Conception

Loss of
one
No. 15

UPD15

FIGURE 7–6   Uniparental disomy 15 from a rob(13q15q) parent, due to "trisomy rescue." The heterozygous parent produces a malsegregant gamete with the translocation, and with a free chromosome 15. The conception thus has trisomy 15. Subsequently, as a postzygotic event, the chromosome 15 from the other parent is lost. Since most malsegregations will have been of maternal origin, the uniparental disomy (UPD) in this setting will usually be a maternal heterodisomy. (Chromosome 13 elements, white; chromosome 15 elements, cross-hatched. The two chromosome 15 elements from the carrier parent are asterisked.)

Residual Low-Level Trisomy. If the "correcting" mitosis occurs too late to include every cell that will contribute to the embryo proper, a translocation trisomic cell line may persist. The only example in the survey of Berend et al. (2000) was that of a child with upd(13)mat from a rob(13q14q) mother, in whom a low level (4%) of trisomy 13 was shown on prenatal diagnosis, 45,XX,rob(13q14q)[48]/

46,XX,+13,rob(13q14q)[2]. Bruyère et al. (2001) record in an abstract three such cases detected in a series of 281 prenatal diagnoses. Jenderny et al. (2010) showed 4%–8% translocation trisomy 13 mosaicism on blood, and 11% on buccal cells, in an abnormal boy whose karyotype could be written 45,XY,rob(13q14q)/46,XY,+13,rob(13q14q)mat; UPD was excluded.

Monosomic Correction. Hypothetically, correction may also go the other way—that is, the conversion of a monosomic conceptus, due to a nullisomic gamete from 2:1 adjacent segregation in the rob parent, into a disomic conceptus. This conversion to disomy, or "correction," would be achieved by the replication of the homolog contributed in the (normal) gamete of the other parent. A replicate "free" chromosome might be produced, in which case the karyotype would appear normal. Or the homolog could replicate as an isochromosome, which would produce the intriguing circumstance of a de novo Robertsonian-like chromosome in the setting of a true Robertsonian parent. This event, whichever one, would take place at a very early postzygotic stage and would necessarily lead to uniparental isodisomy (Berend et al. 2000). It is, apparently, very rare and might usually fail unless it occurred by about the blastocyst stage, since monosomy becomes a lethal impediment thereafter (Figure 19–3).

Association with Infertility

There is an approximately 7-fold excess of Robertsonian heterozygotes among couples who are infertile, and a 13-fold excess among oligospermic men (Tharapel et al. 1985; Ogur et al. 2006). A minority of rob carriers may have an individual predisposition, not necessarily shared by their heterozygous relatives, for a high frequency of unbalanced segregations—an insight that has been afforded by IVF studies. Alternatively, or additionally, the rob translocation may, of itself, compromise the fidelity of the first few mitoses, affecting mitotic segregation of the other chromosomes (Emiliani et al. 2003). By way of example, Conn et al. (1998) treated two couples with a Robertsonian translocation, who had been unable to achieve a normal pregnancy: a man with 45,rob(13q14q) and a woman with 45,rob(13q21q). They were able to karyotype

a total of 33 day-3 embryos from the two couples. A considerable majority of embryos, almost 90%, were chromosomally abnormal. Of these, 40% were trisomic or monosomic for 13, 14, or 21 (some mosaic, and some double monosomic), and this might have been expected. Notably, 60% had a "chaotic karyotype," in which the chromosome constitution varied randomly from cell to cell, and indeed the karyotype of the original zygote could not usually be determined.

MALE INFERTILITY

As just mentioned, there is a 13-fold excess of rob heterozygotes among oligospermic men. A case has been made that, in this setting, synapsis is incomplete in the trivalent, and the heterochromatic regions of the short arms remain unpaired; these "exposed" regions then interfere with pairing in the X-Y bivalent so that spermatogenesis is blocked from further progression (Johannisson et al. 1987; Luciani et al. 1987). Guichaoua et al. (1990) have directly observed the asynapsed short arms of the trivalent associating with the X-Y bivalent in testicular tissue from an oligospermic man heterozygous for a rob(14q22q), and Navarro et al. (1991) have similarly studied a rob(13q14q) man, and Sobotka et al. (2015) a rob(14q22q) man. Electron microscopic sperm analysis in a rob(14q22q) man with oligoasthenospermia showed marked ultrastructural defects in the great majority of spermatozoa, and attempted IVF was unsuccessful (Baccetti et al. 2002). Mice with several Robertsonian translocations show spermatogenic arrest if the translocations form a chain and associate with the sex chromosomes (Johannisson and Winking 1994). But it is notable that with some infertile 45,XY,rob(13;14) men, their brothers, fathers, or other male relatives may have unimpaired fertility (Rosenmann et al. 1985).

RARE COMPLEXITIES

Robertsonian Fission. The Robertsonian translocation arises through a "fusion" of the short arm sequences. Equally, it can, in somatic tissues, revert to "normality" by fission (Perry et al. 2005). Although the resulting two acrocentric chromosomes would have somewhat truncated short arms that lacked NORs, this appears to be without any clinical consequence (and see also Chapter 12).

Mosaicism for Two Robertsonian Translocations. A few examples are known of individuals with a 21-containing rob, such as 14q21q or 21q22q, plus an isochromosome of 21q, and presenting as a normal parent of a Down syndrome child, or with mosaic Down syndrome (Gross et al. 1996; Berend et al. 1998; Bandyopadhyay et al. 2003). Iwarsson et al. (2009) undertook sperm analysis in their patient with two Robertsonian translocations, a man whose karyotype of 45,XY,rob(13;13)(q10;q10)/45,XY,rob(13;15)(q10;q10)dn had originally been identified in fetal life, at amniocentesis. Presenting some 22 years later for genetic counseling, a semen analysis revealed oligoasthenoteratozoöspermia, and on FISH study about 40% had disomy or nullisomy 13. These abnormal sperm were presumably due to that fraction of the gonadal tissue bearing the rob(13;13).

Couple Both Heterozygous. An interesting curiosity is the rare case of a union between Robertsonian heterozygotes. For example, Martinez-Castro et al. (1984) describe two parents both with a 45,rob(13q14q) karyotype, whose three phenotypically normal children had a diploid number of 44, with their chromosomes 13 and 14 existing as a matching pair of rob(13q14q) translocations. Two rob(13q14q) × rob(13q14q) couples, being first cousin pairs and all four having the same rob(13q14q) by descent, each presented with three first-trimester abortions in Bahçe et al. (1996). A couple both carrying a rob(14q21q) are recorded having had a child with Down syndrome, with the unique karyotype 45,XY,rob(14q21q)pat,rob(14q21q)mat,+21mat (Rajangam et al. 1997). Similarly, Mori et al. (1985) reported a couple both of whom were 45,rob(13q15q), and who had had a child with translocation trisomy 13. Due to a founder effect, this otherwise rare Robertsonian translocation was rather common in their small village in the province of Cuidad Real, in Spain, and this couple were surely distantly related, even though they were unaware of any link. The reader may care to construct a hypothetical balanced karyotype with $2n = 41$ and five Robertsonian translocation chromosomes.

Interchromosomal Effect. The concept of an interchromosomal effect (ICE) has been invoked in the setting of the balanced Robertsonian heterozygote. Could a translocation somehow influence the distribution of another chromosome not involved

in the rearrangement, with the production of a gamete aneuploid for a chromosome not involved in the translocation? Anecdotal reports of DS children born to 14q22q and 13q14q rob carriers (Farag et al. 1987; Sikkema-Raddatz et al. 1997b) seemed to support this notion. However, formal segregation studies in large numbers of families with a rob(13q14q) or with trisomy 21 showed no excess of trisomic offspring or of parental Robertsonian translocations, respectively (Harris et al. 1979; Lindenbaum et al. 1985). Therman et al. (1989) ascertained no Robertsonian translocation through a trisomic child other than one that included the trisomic chromosome.

Sperm FISH studies in male heterozygotes have produced inconsistent results. From the literature, Anton et al. (2010) summarized data from 33 Robertsonian translocation males, and added three new cases of their own: ICE was detected in the sperm of slightly more than half (20/36) of males studied. The failure of sperm studies to resolve the question of whether ICE exists may be attributed to two factors. First, sperm FISH technology is limited to analyzing only a handful of chromosomes, and therefore many aneuploidies will be missed. Second, the presence of compromised spermatogenesis in heterozygous males is an important confounding factor, because oligospermia is independently associated with increased levels of aneuploidy in sperm. Ferfouri et al. (2011) found that rates of aneuploidy in the sperm of oligospermic males with a Robertsonian translocation were not elevated compared to 46,XY oligospermic males. However, Godo et al. (2015) observed, in 10 rob(13;14) carriers and one rob(13;22) carrier, that sperm aneuploidy for another chromosome (15/22, 18, 21, X, Y) correlated with malsegregants of the rob chromosome, suggesting that ICE might take place only in rob-malsegregant sperm.

More precise data might be derived from the study of PGD embryos, which provide an opportunity to analyze segregation of all 24 chromosomes, irrespective of whether the aneuploidy arises in ova, sperm, or during a postfertilization mitosis. Alfarawati et al. (2012) analyzed oöcytes and early embryos of Robertsonian translocation carriers and compared them to age-matched chromosomally normal controls. Malsegregation of structurally normal chromosomes (that is, chromosomes not involved in the translocation) was seen in 70% of the embryos of Robertsonian translocation carriers, compared to 64% of controls. Thus, the relative risk of a Robertsonian translocation carrier producing an abnormal cleavage-stage embryo, due to an error unrelated to their constitutional rearrangement, was 1.10, a small but statistically significant difference[2] that was not influenced by maternal age. At the level of the chromosome (rather than the embryo), the relative risk of aneuploidy in embryos of Robertsonian translocation carriers compared to controls was 1.41, the higher risk accounted for by the fact that many abnormal embryos had multiple aneuploidies. Alfarawati et al. conclude that ICE exists, and that it may contribute, in small degree, to the subfertility and increased miscarriage risk in some Robertsonian heterozygotes. An additional and unexpected finding was that ICE was detected in cleavage-stage embryos, but not in oöcytes, suggesting that the origin of ICE may be mitotic rather than meiotic. The rearranged chromosomes in an early embryonic mitosis might either (1) disturb the arrangement of chromosomes on the spindle or (2) alter the normal pattern of chromosome positioning in interphase nuclei, with consequences for attachment to the mitotic spindle during metaphase. Alternatively, Solé et al. (2017) propose spermatogenesis as a site wherein ICE may operate, with the geography of the chromosomes within the nucleus perturbed by the presence of a rob.

The apparent existence of an ICE, albeit one of very small effect, strengthens the rationale for using 24-chromosome PGD in couples with a Robertsonian translocation.

THE HOMOLOGOUS ROBERTSONIAN TRANSLOCATION (OR ACROCENTRIC-DERIVED ISOCHROMOSOME)

This Robertsonian translocation chromosome comprises the long arm elements of two acrocentric chromosomes that are the *same*. The site of formation is typically postmeiotic (Robinson et al. 1994). If the translocation forms from the fusion of the two parental homologs, then manifestly there is biparental inheritance (Abrams et al. 2001). If, on the other hand, the rearrangement is actually an isochromosome, each long arm is an exact copy of the other, and there will be uniparental isodisomy. Such an isochromosome may have arisen as a "correction"

of monosomy in the one-cell zygote, or at a postzygotic stage (Riegel et al. 2006). Isochromosomes of chromosomes 14 and 15 will result in an imprinting syndrome, and Liehr (2016a) has collated a total of 26 cases, comprising 13 of upd(14)mat, two of upd(14)pat, four of upd(15)mat, and seven of upd(15)pat. The rarity of isochromosome-related upd(14)pat may reflect the higher in utero lethality for this syndrome.

Rare cases of mosaicism for a "Robertsonian isochromosome" offer insights into causative mechanisms, albeit that these may not reflect the typical scenario. Bartsch et al. (1993) note some recorded cases of parental mosaicism for 47,+i(21q) and describe their own unique case of a woman with mos47,+i(21p)/47,+i(21q)—some hundreds of cells from blood, gonad, marrow, skin were 47,+i(21p), and one single blood cell was 47,+i(21q)—who had had two children with Down syndrome due to the karyotype 46,i(21q). In herself, apparently, the isochromosomes arose as a postzygotic event from a 47,+21 conception, with classic centromere misdivision at the pre-embryo stage. The i(21p) line came to be the predominant in most tissues, but the i(21q) line had at least some representation in gonad and blood.

DETAILS OF MEIOTIC BEHAVIOR

Only two segregant outcomes are possible at meiosis in the homologous 45,rob heterozygote. Either the gamete will receive the translocation chromosome, and be effectively disomic, or it will not, and be nullisomic. Essentially, this is 1:0 segregation (or "1+1":0 segregation). No balanced gamete is possible. Thus, if the other gamete is normal, only trisomic or monosomic conceptions are possible. Occasionally, conceptuses with translocation trisomy 13 are viable, and translocation trisomy 21 not infrequently survives to term. None of the other unbalanced possibilities (trisomies 14, 15, and 22,[3] nor any of the monosomies) are viable.

Postzygotic "trisomic correction" is a mechanism that could, rarely, enable the carrier to have a phenotypically normal child. If, for example, in the case of an unbalanced 46,–22,rob(22q22q) conception, the free chromosome 22 were lost at a very early mitosis, genetic balance in this cell line would

---

2 Interestingly, in this study ICE was detected only in the setting of Robertsonian translocations. No evidence for ICE was seen with reciprocal translocations (but cf. p. 112) or inversions.

3 In other settings, trisomy 22, extremely rarely, has gone through to stillbirth, or very short postnatal survival.

be restored, with a 45,rob(22q22q) karyotype. Provided the unbalanced cell line contributed negligibly or not at all to the embryo, and provided there were no effect due to uniparental disomy (and in the case of chromosome 22, there is not), the child would be normal. Very few such cases are recorded, with the 13q13q and 22q22q thus represented (Slater et al. 1994, 1995; Engel and Antonarakis 2002; Ouldim et al. 2008).

"Monosomic rescue" is another theoretical, and as yet unobserved mechanism in this context, whereby the homolog from the other parent could be duplicated postzygotically, as two separate homologs, or as an isochromosome, to produce a pregnancy with either a normal karyotype or 45,iso. Finally, for completeness (but almost never in reality), gametic complementation is to be mentioned, whereby the non-rob parent contributes a gamete that happens to lack the homolog for which the rob parent's gamete is disomic (Berend et al. 1999). For the rob(14q14q) and rob(15q15q) carrier, even if one of these rescuing mechanisms did happen, the child would in any event be abnormal, since these UPDs lead, of themselves, to an abnormal phenotype.

GENETIC COUNSELING

THE HETEROLOGOUS ROBERTSONIAN TRANSLOCATION CARRIER

INFERTILITY AND MISCARRIAGE

The Robertsonian translocation involving nonhomologs is occasionally associated with repeated spontaneous abortion and with male infertility. The risks for miscarriage are set out in Table 7–4. It may be unclear, in an individual case, whether the association is causal or fortuitous. We can theorize that, in some miscarrying couples, there may have been a majority of zygotes with nonviable adjacent segregants; and in some infertile males, the translocation may have disrupted spermatogenesis. Cytogenetic analysis of products of conception, and of testicular tissue, respectively, may cast some light. It remains possible that some other cause could underlie the problem. The infertile male usually produces some sperm and may thus be a candidate for IVF using intracytoplasmic sperm injection (ICSI) and possibly PGD (Lee and Munné 2000) (and see Table 7–4 and Chapter 22).

Risks of Having Abnormal Offspring from Individual Translocations

Figures for the risks to have an abnormal child, or for the probability of detecting an unbalanced form at prenatal diagnosis, are taken (making a few assumptions about extrapolating to the rare translocations) from data of a number of North American and European collaborative studies (Harris et al. 1979; Ferguson-Smith 1983; Daniel et al. 1989) and set out in Table 7–2. These data relate essentially to the risk for a full trisomy. Risks for UPD are drawn from the review of Shaffer (2006), again allowing for figures from the more common translocations being applicable to the rarer ones. Detailed comments on each individual translocation follow, with general comments thereafter on the theoretical risks of uniparental disomy (14- and 15-containing translocations), "isozygosity" for a recessive gene, residual low-level trisomy mosaicism, and interchromosomal effect.

Table 7–4. Risk of Miscarriage, and Proportions due to Trisomy, for the 13q14q and 14q21q Robertsonian Translocations, According to Gender of the Carrier

	rob(13q14q)		rob(14q21q)	
	MISCARRIAGE	TRISOMIC	MISCARRIAGE	TRISOMIC
Mother	22%–27%	1%–7%*	24%	10%–14%
Father	13%	1%	33%	1%

Note: It is apparent that translocation-related trisomy accounts for only a minority of the miscarriages.
*Data depend on the gestational age at the time of ascertainment.
Source: Table adapted from Kim and Shaffer (2002) and Engels et al. (2008).

THE MORE COMMON TRANSLOCATIONS

rob(13q14q). The karyotype of the balanced rob(13q14q) is shown in Figure 7–1. Translocation trisomy 13 can result from adjacent-1 segregation, with a typical Patau syndrome phenotype. The risk for this is very small. Almost all instances are index cases in families, not secondary cases. A review of several pedigrees in Harris et al. (1979), well subjected to statistical rigor, identified *no* apparent increased risk for a malformed infant (they noted that a risk of up to 2% could have been missed, due to the sample size). In a European collaborative study, none of 230 prenatal diagnoses had an unbalanced karyotype (Boué and Gallano 1984), suggesting a risk of less than 0.4%. An incidence in Daniel et al.'s (1989) North American data of 3/204 (1.5%) may have been influenced by ascertainment bias, but in any event, combining the two data sets gives a figure of only 0.7%.

A study from this century, based upon the impressive total of 101 pedigrees, provides support for these historic reports. Engels et al. (2008) identified no cases of translocation trisomy 13, after correction for bias, in live births, albeit that a number of their families had come to attention through an index case with translocation trisomy 13. These authors propose risk estimates of <0.4% for female carriers to have a liveborn child with translocation trisomy 13, and <0.6% for the male; and if the genders are combined, one arrives at a lower figure of <0.23%. They did, however, document a 7% (3/42) incidence in amniocenteses. Further, one translocation trisomy infant had been stillborn; and it is a fine point, in undertaking this sort of analysis, to make a distinction between a stillborn baby versus one that survives only a few days (the usual in Patau syndrome). A risk estimate of ¼% to ½%, or more conservatively <1%, may be a practical figure to offer.

If there is male infertility, needing IVF with ICSI to achieve pregnancy, the additional exercise of PGD would be reasonable, to improve the chances of producing a normal/balanced conception; PGD may also be an appropriate choice for some female heterozygotes. Otherwise, an offer of prenatal diagnosis remains a discretionary matter. A focused ultrasound should be capable of detecting the great majority of trisomy 13, and any residual risk could be virtually eliminated by a normal noninvasive prenatal test (NIPT). Exclusion of the small risk of UPD 14 would require invasive testing.

rob(14q21q). The rob(14q21q) is the most important Robertsonian translocation in terms of its frequency and genetic risk, and it shows a marked difference according to the sex of the parent. Most familial translocation DS is due to the rob(14q21q) (Figure 7–2). Adjacent segregation may lead to the conception of translocation trisomy 21 (Figure 7–3). At amniocentesis, the *female* heterozygote has a risk for translocation trisomy 21 of about 15% (Ferguson-Smith 1983; Boué and Gallano 1984; Stene and Stengel-Rutkowski 1988; Daniel et al. 1989). The risk of having a liveborn child with translocation DS is a little less (in the range 10%–15%): This likely reflects the loss, through spontaneous abortion, of a fraction of DS fetuses after the time during gestation when prenatal diagnosis is done. The risk for the *male* heterozygote is very different, and a figure of <1% is appropriate to offer. The matter of UPD 14 is noted below.

THE RARE TRANSLOCATIONS

rob(13q15q). Few data are available concerning genetic risks to the carrier (Mori et al. 1985; Daniel et al. 1989). We would expect these individuals are no more likely to produce adjacent segregants than the rob(13q14q) carrier, and a similar risk of <1% for translocation trisomy 13 may therefore apply. The risk for UPD 15 is noted below.

rob(13q21q). In Boué and Gallano's (1984) study, the risk for translocation DS, in terms of the likelihood of detection at amniocentesis, was 10% for the female; and in Daniel et al.'s (1989) study, the figure was 17%. This 10%–17% range suggests there may be no real difference from the 10%–15% that applies to the common rob(14q21q). The risk for the male heterozygote is low, and probably similar to the <1% proposed for the male rob(14q21q) carrier. A 1% or less risk for translocation trisomy 13 may apply, for either sex.

rob(13q22q). We presume the risk for translocation trisomy 13 would be "small," and perhaps similar to that for the rob(13q14q); a risk for trisomy 22 would presumably be minuscule.[3] In Boué and Gallano's (1984) study of 262 Robertsonian prenatal diagnoses not involving chromosome 21, there were only three rob(13q22q) cases, and in fact one of these showed trisomy 13; no unbalanced karyotypes were diagnosed in Daniel et al.'s (1989) seven cases. The man subjected to a sperm study in

Anahory et al. (2005; see Table 7–3) had presented with infertility, and oligospermia was shown.

rob(14q15q). Adjacent segregants (translocation trisomy 14, translocation trisomy 15) are invariably lethal in utero. UPD 14 or UPD 15 are possible outcomes, as noted below.

rob(14q22q) and rob (15q22q). The potentially trisomic states from these translocations (trisomy 14, 15, or 22) would all be anticipated to abort spontaneously.[3] Neu et al. (1975) record the segregation of a rob(14q22q) chromosome in a large family, in which some carriers had an increased miscarriage rate. We comment below on UPD.

rob(15q21q). From Boué and Gallano's (1984) small series of nine carrier mothers, one (11%) had translocation trisomy 21 detected at amniocentesis; and in Daniel et al.'s (1989) data, the fraction was 0/9. These figures derive from too small a body of data to be sure, as yet, that the risk is really any different from the more solidly based 10%–15%, which applies to the rob(14q21q) female carrier. Again, we suppose a low risk (<1%) for the male carrier in terms of DS. The possibility of UPD is noted below.

rob(21q22q). For a rob(21q22q) carrier parent, the risks for translocation trisomy 21 are about the same as for the rob(14q21q), according to the sex of the parent. UPD need not be a concern, and neither, practically speaking, trisomy 22.[3]

Homozygosity Since some Robertsonian translocations are, relatively, not uncommon, it is not surprising that a few instances are known where both of a couple are carriers (see above, "Couple Both Heterozygous"). It is possible then for these couples to have children who are homozygous and phenotypically normal, and also fertile—for example, the 44,rob(13q14q)×2 mother in Miryounesi et al. (2016), who had a healthy 45,XY,rob(13q14q) son, albeit also four other pregnancies ending in first-trimester loss. The 44,XY,rob(14q15q)×2 son of carrier parents in Song et al. (2016) had a very high proportion (99.7%) of chromosomally balanced sperm.

UNIPARENTAL DISOMY

UPD in a setting of parental Robertsonian heterozygosity is rare. We need consider only those acrocentric chromosomes subject to imprinting: chromosomes 14 and 15. The four syndromes that can arise, as mentioned above and as described in detail in Chapter 18, are maternal UPD 14 (Temple syndrome), paternal UPD 14 (Kagami-Ogata syndrome), maternal UPD 15 (Prader-Willi syndrome), and paternal UPD15 (Angelman syndrome). The potential mechanisms are, as discussed above, adjacent segregation followed by "correction" of trisomy with loss of a homolog, or (hypothetically) by "correction" of monosomy with replication of a homolog. In the review of Shaffer (2006), combining prenatal diagnostic data from seven groups, and including both familial and de novo cases, four instances of UPD were identified out of 482 prenatal diagnoses, for a point risk estimate, therefore, of 0.8%. The two familial cases were upd(13)mat due to a rob(13q14q)mat, and upd(14)mat due to a rob(14q22q)mat; for the record, the de novo cases were upd(14)mat with a rob(13q14q), and upd(14)mat with a rob(14q21q).

This pooled figure of 0.8% may possibly be slightly less in the case of the father being the heterozygous parent (and possibly slightly greater in the de novo case), but the numbers are too small to make that call, and it remains quite possible that no such differences exist. For practical purposes, the figure of 0.8% should be seen as applicable across the three parental classes (maternal, paternal, de novo) and across all types of rob. This risk is small, but not negligible. Thus, with respect to the "relevant" robs (those involving chromosome 14 or 15), it may be reasonable to consider adding UPD analysis to karyotyping, if the same 45,rob karyotype as the parent's is observed. Trisomy 13 and trisomy 21 can be virtually excluded by a normal ultrasound and NIPT result, although exclusion of UPD 14 and 15 would still require invasive testing. As for maternal and paternal UPD 13, 21, and 22, these are, apparently, without phenotypic effect, and need not be a cause for concern.

"Isozygosity" for a Recessive Gene. Monosomic rescue, whether producing an isochromosome or a 46,N karyotype, theoretically has the potential to cause an autosomal recessive disorder, should the non-rob parent happen to be heterozygous for a Mendelian condition the locus for which was on the chromosome in question. But the risk is likely to be very low. In one small series in which a specific search was made for UPD due to monosomic rescue, from a rob parent, no such case came to light (Ruggeri et al. 2004). Barring knowledge of such a condition (e.g., Bloom syndrome, locus on chromosome 15) elsewhere in the family, molecular testing is not practicable. Of the more common recessive genes that might in some jurisdictions be suitable for population screening (cystic fibrosis, thalassemia, Tay-Sachs disease), none has its locus on an acrocentric chromosome.

PREIMPLANTATION GENETIC DIAGNOSIS

Tan et al. (2013) analyzed 218 embryos of Robertsonian translocation patients using SNP array, and found that 23% had a translocation-related imbalance, and an additional 19% had other aneuploidy, leaving 58% of embryos suitable for transfer. When these embryos were transferred, 52% resulted in a pregnancy, and the miscarriage rate was only 12%. A median of two transferrable embryos were obtained from each IVF cycle. In a similar study, Idowu et al. (2015) analyzed 201 embryos, of which only 8% had a translocation-associated imbalance; however, the rate of other aneuploidy was higher, at 55%, leaving 37% of embryos suitable for transfer. A transferrable embryo was identified in 81% of cycles; 56% of transferred embryos resulted in pregnancy, and 52% resulted in a live birth. The apparent existence of an interchromosomal effect, albeit one of very small influence (discussed above), strengthens the rationale for using 24-chromosome PGD in couples with a Robertsonian translocation.

Polar body biopsy ("preconception diagnosis") is another approach available through a few IVF clinics, and obviously applicable only to the female heterozygote. Molina Gomes et al. (2009), in a pilot study, describe the procedure in seven women, six with 45,rob(13q14q) and one 45,rob(14q21q).[4] From 32 embryos transferred, three successful pregnancies resulted.

THE HOMOLOGOUS ROBERTSONIAN TRANSLOCATION CARRIER

We refer to these rearrangements as "rob" recognizing, as discussed above, that most such cases do actually involve an acrocentric-derived

isochromosome ("rob-iso"). Virtually all conceptions of the heterozygote result in either trisomy or monosomy. Monosomy results in occult abortion. Trisomy 14 and 15 always, and trisomy 22 virtually always, miscarry. Most trisomic 13 pregnancies miscarry, although some survive until the third trimester; while of course many trisomic 21 pregnancies will proceed through to the birth of a child with Down syndrome. Practically speaking, no normal child could be produced from homologous rob or isochromosome carrier individuals (the scenario of postzygotic correction, discussed earlier, can scarcely be raised as a realistic hope). Appropriate advice for these carriers is to consider sterilization. Alternatively, the use of donor gametes may allow the couple to have a normal child.

SPECIFIC TRANSLOCATIONS

Specific comments relating to the risk for abnormal offspring in each type of rob follow.

rob(13q13q). The carrier parent can produce only monosomic or trisomic 13 conceptions, and these would either miscarry or, in the case of trisomy, produce a very abnormal child (Patau syndrome). Three recorded exceptions to this statement are given in Slater et al. (1994, 1995) and Stallard et al. (1995), of a normal parent having a normal child with rob(13q13q). The translocations were probably dicentric 13q isochromosomes, arising from postzygotic correction, and thus the children had uniparental isodisomy.

rob(14q14q), rob(15q15q). Trisomies and monosomies for chromosomes 14 and 15 are not viable, and thus, all pregnancies of these heterozygotes would be expected to terminate in occult abortion or miscarriage. Even if postzygotic correction did happen, the child would have a UPD syndrome, according to the translocation and the sex of the transmitting parent. Thus, it is, in theory and in reality, impossible to have a normal child from any gamete of the heterozygote.

rob(21q21q). Although the rob(21q21q) is extremely rare, every counselor knows about this famous translocation. It is a classic example of a

---

4 It was of interest that in five women where the infertility was due to the male partner, the imbalance rate was 30%, whereas in the two in whom a previous aneuploidy had been documented, the rate was 84%. Further studies will be necessary to confirm whether this finding might be more generally applicable.

genetic risk of (essentially) 100%. All pregnancies continuing to term can be expected to produce a child with DS. Sudha and Gopinath (1990), for example, report a couple who had 13 pregnancies, with four children proven or presumed to have had DS, and nine miscarriages. The mother was 45,rob(21q21q). No case of postzygotic correction for this translocation has ever been reported.

rob(22q22q). All conceptions would be monosomic or trisomic 22, other things being equal. For example, one carrier woman had 24 miscarriages, but no normal child (Farah et al. 1975). Two cases are mentioned above of postzygotic correction, with the birth of a normal child, but this is not a realistic hope to offer in the individual case.

PRENATAL DIAGNOSIS OF THE DE NOVO HOMOLOGOUS ROBERTSONIAN TRANSLOCATION

The de novo homologous Robertsonian translocation (or isochromosome) has a high risk for UPD; this entity is commented upon in Chapter 21.

8

INSERTIONS

INSERTIONS ARE A TYPE OF TRANSLOCA-TION: Sometimes the expressions "insertional translocation," "interstitial translocation," or "non-reciprocal translocation" are used. In the common, simple insertion, three breaks are required. The first two breaks release an interstitial segment of chromatin, which is then inserted into the gap created by the third break. In the simple one-way *inter*chromosomal insertion, a segment from one chromosome is intercalated into another chromosome. A more complicated four-break rearrangement is the reciprocal insertion, whereby two nonhomologous chromosomes exchange intercalary segments. In the *intra*chromosomal insertion, a segment is intercalated into another part of the same chromosome. The segment may be inserted "right way around"—that is, with the same orientation to the centromere as before; this is a direct insertion (dir ins). Or it may be reversed—an inverted insertion (inv ins). More complicated scenarios, which may involve both insertional and terminal translocated segments, are more appropriately dealt with in Chapter 10 (Complex Chromosomal Rearrangements). In this

chapter, we consider the case of the phenotypically normal heterozygote, in whom the rearrangement is assumed to be balanced.

Insertions are rare rearrangements, at the level of detection according to classical cytogenetics. With molecular technology, previously undetectable insertions of very small size are coming to light, de novo and familial, and it is proving that "uncommon" is a more accurate adjective to describe frequency than is "rare." Kang et al. (2010) found a 20-fold increased discovery of insertions, compared with earlier studies, in a large series of cases presenting with typical chromosomal clinical pictures. Many of these turned out to be (probably) harmless polymorphisms (copy number variants [CNVs]), upon the recognition of a parent carrying the same insertion. But a fraction were, in all probability, truly pathogenic. Further to this work, Nowakowska et al. (2012) identified 477 cases of interstitial CNVs from a large pool of patients with CNVs, in whom the parents had also been tested. They showed 10 of these to be, in fact, pathogenic interstitial insertions, of sizes ranging from 0.78 to 12.3 Mb, and due to one parent being an insertional translocation carrier. Eight of these were interchromosomal, and two intrachromosomal insertions. A detailed literature review is given in Domínguez et al. (2017).

THE INTERCHROMOSOMAL INSERTION

BIOLOGY

The simple *one-way* interchromosomal insertion is the most common form of this uncommon rearrangement. The formation of the rearrangement is depicted in Figure 8–1. The recipient chromosome now carries the insertional segment, and the donor chromosome lacks it. Van Hemel and Eussen (2000) estimate a prevalence, on classical cytogenetics, on the order of 1 in 80,000; with molecular methodology, the true figure may actually be sixfold this estimate (Nowakowska et al. 2012).

DETAILS OF MEIOTIC BEHAVIOR

In theory, two categories of meiotic behavior are possible, according to whether the homologs pair independently or as a quadrivalent.

INDEPENDENT SYNAPSING OF HOMOLOGOUS PAIRS

Meiosis could proceed in the usual fashion, with homologs pairing independently as bivalents. In essence, we can suppose that the insertional

segment is disregarded and that the homologs synapse, with segments matching for as much of their length as they are able. In theory, and perhaps only with larger insertions, the insertional segment could fold out[1] to accommodate this requirement (Figure 8–2, upper). (Some crossing-over will presumably occur between synapsed regions, but this would not alter segregation outcomes.) Alternatively, homologs may pair along their full lengths, which would bring some nonmatching segments "incorrectly" alongside each other ("heterosynapsis").

Then, with normal segregation of the two bivalents, independently of each other, two alternative pairs of gametes are possible. Overall, there would be gametes of four possible segregant types, in the ratio 1:1:1:1. Two of these would have a correct amount of genetic material, and two would not. The former two combinations are 46,N and the balanced insertion carrier. The two unbalanced combinations would produce conceptuses one with a partial trisomy

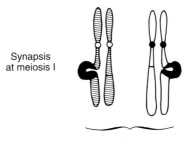

Synapsis at meiosis I

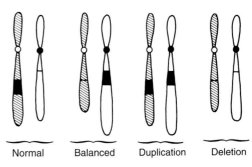

Normal Balanced Duplication Deletion

FIGURE 8–2   Gamete production following independent pairing of the two sets of homologs. The insertional segment is shown in black, both in its original and in its translocated positions. The horizontal line marks the site whence came the segment from the donor (cross-hatched) chromosome, and the site of its destination on the recipient (white) chromosome.

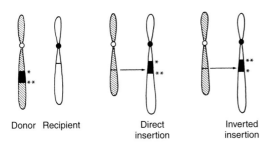

Donor Recipient   Direct   Inverted
                       insertion   insertion

FIGURE 8–1   The formation of an interchromosomal insertion. Single and double asterisks indicate orientation of the insertion segment. The *direct* insertion has the same orientation to the centromere; the *inverted* insertion has the opposite orientation.

---

1 Described also as ballooning out, looping out, or as translocation loops.

(duplication) and the other with a partial monosomy (deletion), for the insertional segment (Figure 8–2, lower). As discussed below, studies of testicular biopsies and sperm have shown that (at least with smaller insertions) the homologs can pair normally as bivalents, and that the expected ratios hold true. It makes no difference whether the insertion is direct or inverted. The foregoing scenario of independent synapsing is more likely to apply when the insertional segment is of small size. The case illustrated in Figure 8–3 exemplifies this: a small (0.4% of haploid autosomal length [HAL]) segment from 8q inserted into 10q, with the duplication and deletion outcomes depicted (this case discussed further below).

FORMATION OF A QUADRIVALENT

Probably only in exceptional cases, with larger insertional segments, a quadrivalent forms, and this would enable recombination within the insertional segments. In the review of Van Hemel and Eussen (2000), the mean size of the inserted segment in recombining cases was 1.5% HAL, compared with 1.0% and 0.5% HAL in nonrecombining families

in which the imbalances were due, respectively, to duplication and to deletion. With the *direct* insertion, a recombinant chromosome would be monocentric, and therefore functional. *Inverted* insertions, on the other hand, could produce dicentric or acentric recombinant chromosomes, with the resulting gametes presumably nonviable.

Consider the large *direct* insertion depicted in Figures 8–4 and 8–5. Most of the material within the chromosome 5 long arm (q11q22) has been removed and inserted within the distal long arm of chromosome 1 (Jalbert et al. 1975). A pachytene configuration at meiosis I such as that depicted, with the insertional segments thrown into an overlapping loop, would allow for complete synapsis of homologous segments. If no crossover occurred in the insertional loop (and assuming 2:2 disjunction with symmetric segregation of centromeres), the same four outcomes noted in the preceding section would eventuate. The gametic combination [a,c] would produce a del(5)(q11q22), and the combination [b,d] would produce a duplication for this same segment. But if a crossover did occur, two recombinant chromosomes would be formed, and

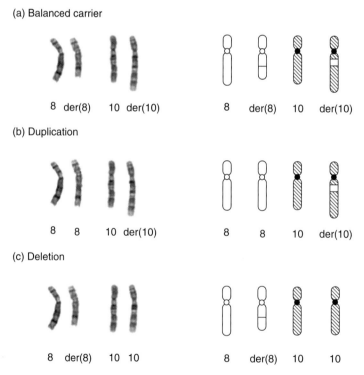

FIGURE 8–3 An insertion from chromosome 8 to chromosome 10, ins(10;8)(q21;q21.2q22), showing (*a*) the balanced carrier, (*b*) the duplication, and (*c*) the deletion states. In this family, the duplication was the only unbalanced form to be observed. (Case of P. A. Bowen; Bowen et al. 1983.)

now three further unbalanced outcomes from symmetric 2:2 disjunction would be possible: gametes [b',d'], [b',c], and [a,d'] in Figure 8–4. The duplication/deletion combinations, [b',c] and [a,d'], are judged to be nonviable, although they might cause miscarriage. The "least imbalanced, least monosomic" combination is the "dup ins" [b',d'], which leads to a partial trisomy for the insertional segment, 5q11q22. This was, in fact, the karyotype of the proposita in this family (Figure 8–5). Actually, this karyotype endows the same genetic imbalance as would the nonrecombinant [b,d] gamete; so in practical terms, it made no difference that this recombination did happen.

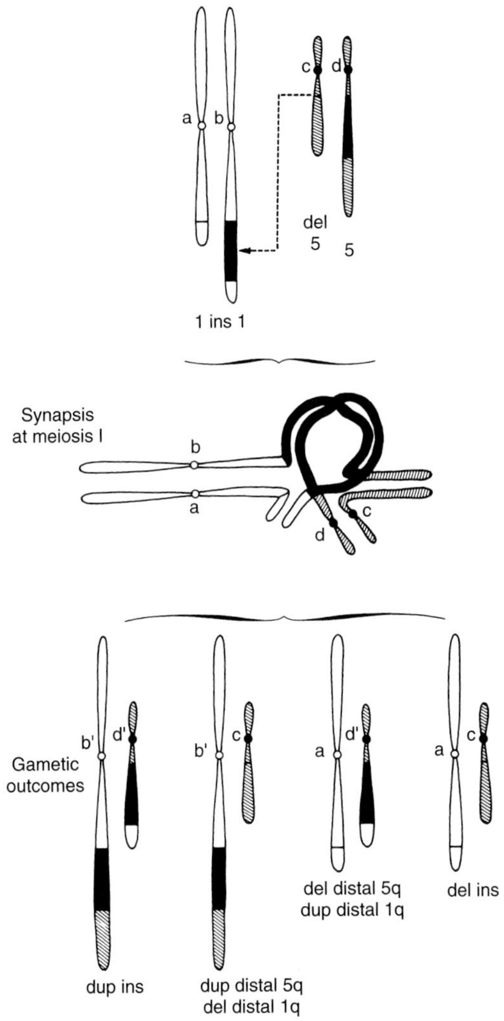

SEGMENT CONTENT AND VIABILITY

The viability of the conceptuses—in other words, the level of risk to the heterozygote of having an abnormal child—depends on the degree of the aneuploid states. Consider the example illustrated in Figure 8–3. A small segment from the middle of chromosome 8 long arm, 8q21.2q22, has been removed and is inserted within the chromosome 10 long arm. This segment comprises about 0.4% of HAL. The heterozygote for this rearrangement could produce two types of unbalanced conceptus: one with a duplication of the segment 8q21.2q22 (Figure 8–3b), and one with this segment deleted (Figure 8–3c). In this family (Figure 8–6), only the duplication was observed. These individuals had mild to moderate mental retardation and minor physical anomalies (Bowen et al. 1983). A segregation analysis of the family was done, and the segregation ratio was close to 1:1:1:0 for normal:balanced:partial trisomy:partial monosomy. This implies a normal viability for the partially trisomic conceptus, and nonviability for the partially monosomic state. Thus, in this family, the risk for having an aneuploid child is estimated to be $1/1 + 1 + 1 + 0$, or 33%. (This assessment is an example of a "private" segregation analysis.)

A genetically smaller insertional segment has the potential to be viable in both the duplicated and deleted states. For example, Doheny et al. (1997) describe two first cousins, one with a duplication of a segment of 10q, the other with a deletion. The connecting relatives carried an insertion, 46,ins(12;10)(q15;q21.2q22.1).[2] The insertional segment, 10q21.2q22.1, was small, comprising about 0.5% HAL. The child with the duplication was identified with learning difficulty in first grade, and her IQ measured at 74; the physical phenotype was rather mild. Her cousin with the deletion had, as an infant, considerable lag in neurodevelopmental progress, which would lead one to anticipate a more serious mental defect at older age, and she had a more obviously dysmorphic appearance. A similar circumstance is illustrated in Arens et al.

FIGURE 8–4   Gamete production following formation of a quadrivalent in the interchromosomal insertion, with a single crossover having occurred in the insertion loop. Only one of each sister chromatid is shown. Recombinant chromosomes noted as b' and d'. (Based on the case shown in Figure 8–5.)

2 In the ISCN nomenclature, the recipient chromosome is noted first, followed by the donor chromosome.

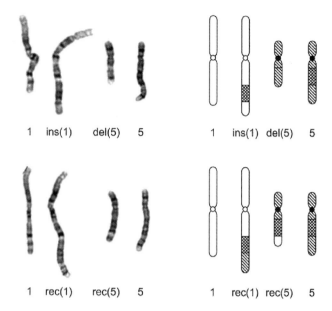

FIGURE 8–5   Interchromosomal insertion with recombinant chromosomes in phenotypically abnormal offspring. Partial karyotypes of 46,ins(1;5)(q32;q11q22) carrier parent (*above*) and her recombinant child with 46,rec(1)rec(5)dup(5q)ins(1;5)(q32;q11q22) (*below*). The latter is the [b′,d′] combination in Figure 8–4. The child is trisomic for the segment 5q11q22. Cartoon karyotype: white, chromosome 1; criss-cross-hatched, 5q11q22; cross-hatched, remainder of 5. (Case of P. Jalbert; Jalbert et al. 1975.)

(2004), who describe a family in which an ins(3;5)(q25.3;q22.1q31.3) is segregating in four generations, with 10 persons having inherited the del or dup state for the 5(q22.1q31.3) segment: those with the deletion were more markedly affected than those inheriting the duplication state.

An insertion of a very small segment may, on classical cytogenetics, be difficult to detect, although with increasing use of microarray analysis, more such cases are coming to light. Löffler et al. (2000) were presented with an adult male thought possibly to have fragile X syndrome. In the event, he had an

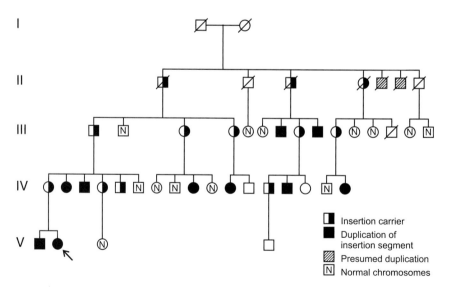

FIGURE 8–6   The pedigree of the family in which the insertion illustrated in Figure 8–3 was segregating.

abnormal chromosome 14, with additional material at band 14q13. His retarded brother and normal mother had the same chromosome. Was this an insertion, an inversion, or what? Fluorescence in situ hybridization (FISH) using microdissection from the abnormal 14 showed a very small hybridizing segment on chromosome 7. Both no. 7 chromosomes in the brothers showed this spot of hybridization, but just one of the mother's. Going back to the G-banded preparations, and now knowing exactly where to look, a deletion at 7q32q34 could be discerned on the mother's other chromosome 7, and the definitive interpretation could be made. She had the karyotype 46,XX,ins(14;7)(q13;q32q34), and the two sons were 46,XY,der(14)ins(14;7)(q13;q32q34)mat.

In similar vein, consider the insertion in Figure 8–7, in which two small subbands from 2q (2q33.2 and q33.3) and adjoining parts of 2q33.1 and 2q34 are inserted into chromosome 4. This is only about 0.3% of HAL. This rearrangement was at the limit of detection of high-resolution G-banding.

In this family, three of five children had a duplication of the insertion, inheriting from the carrier parent the normal chromosome 2 along with the derivative chromosome 4 containing the insertional segment, 2q33.1q34. The children with this very short duplication had a clinical picture of poor speech development, distractable and aggressive behavior, and subtle facial dysmorphism. The insertion in Dolan et al. (2011) comprised a segment of no more than 5.8 Mb; the 46,XY,ins(18;11)(q23;p14.1p13) carrier father had had children, one with the deletion, and the other the duplication, of this segment. At the molecular level, the imbalance comprised chr11:29.3-35.2 Mb, and included the *WT1* Wilms tumor gene. The child with the deletion was born in poor condition and died after a few days; his brother with dup(11)(p14.1p13) had been slightly delayed as an infant, but with age-appropriate development by age 4 years.

Insertional segments of yet smaller size, shading into the measurement lengths associated with copy number variants, may present the remarkable

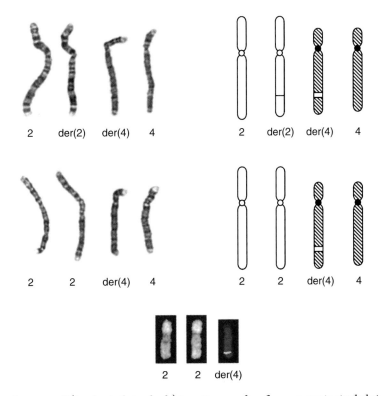

| 2 | der(2) | der(4) | 4 | | 2 | der(2) | der(4) | 4 |

| 2 | 2 | der(4) | 4 | | 2 | 2 | der(4) | 4 |

| 2 | 2 | der(4) |

FIGURE 8–7   A very small (by classical standards) insertion, needing fluorescence in situ hybridization (FISH) to be seen clearly. The karyotype of the carrier parent (*upper*) is 46,inv ins(4;2)(q32;q34q33.1). The child is duplicated for the segment 2q33.1q34, but this is difficult to appreciate on the G-banded karyotype (*middle*). FISH with chromosome 2-specific paint (*lower*) shows the small insertion segment from chromosome 2 present in the der(4). (Case of M. Curtis.)

circumstance of pathogenicity due to deletion, but normality with the duplication. Such a story is seen in Nowakowska et al. (2012), who describe a family segregating an ins(1;2)(p13q36.3q37.1), the inserted segment of size 2.1 Mb. Six family members presented severe intellectual disability and minor dysmorphism, and they each had deletion for the 2q36.3q37.1 segment. But one family member with the duplication was normal, and this observation informed prenatal advice for her carrier nephew.

If an insertional segment coincides with that of a known segmental aneuploidy, the particular syndrome may be observed in the family. Consider the story in Fernández et al. (2016): Two family members, related as uncle and nephew, presented some aspects of the HDR syndrome of hypoparathyroidism, deafness, and renal disease, which is due to monosomy 10p14 (p. 286). In this instance, the deletion comprised the segment chr10:2,471,915-14,544,442. The heterozygotes in the family carried a balanced insertion, ins(16;10)(q22;p13p15.2).

We may include here mention of insertions which are present in *un*balanced state in the transmitting parent, with the parent's (the mother's) phenotype presumably protected, partially or fully, by X-inactivation. An ins(X;5)(p22.1p13.2p13.2) is described in the family of Walters-Sen et al. (2015). Two brothers had autistic features and mild dysmorphism, and their two sisters had poor language development, one with a major unilateral limb defect. Their mother was of mild physical phenotype and normal development. All five had duplication of the 5p13.2 segment; the mother showed skewed X-inactivation (the X with the 5p segment being preferentially inactivated), while her daughters had random skewing. The inserted segment is chr5:36,669,467-37,010,647, containing only two genes, and indeed, only parts of these genes, *SLC1A3* and *NIPBL*; an abbreviated form of the NIPBL protein might plausibly have been the pathogenic factor. A somewhat similar case is reported in Haines et al. (2015); but here the pathogenic effect was due to the insertional segment (which consisted of ~700 kb from 1q25) compromising the activity of a nearby locus, *SOX3*, at the site wherein it was inserted on the X chromosome; we describe this case in Chapter 23 (Chromosomal Disorders of Sex Development).

The Two-Way Insertion. A two-way reciprocal insertion (a rare observation) has the potential for two different imbalances: a partial monosomy from the segment of one chromosome with the reciprocal partial trisomy of the segment from the other chromosome; or the opposite, with a partial trisomy of one chromosome and a partial monosomy of the other (Figure 8–8).

Gametogenesis Studies. Gametic analysis has been reported in two insertion heterozygotes. Goldman and Hultén (1992) examined testicular material from an ins(6;7) heterozygote and demonstrated independent synapsis of the chromosome 6 and chromosome 7 homologous pairs at diakinesis, with the two bivalents occupying quite separate parts of the nucleus. This is a direct demonstration that the segregation scenario set out in Figure 8–2 does happen. Testicular tissue and sperm were studied from one ins(3;10) carrier in whom a very small segment of chromosome 10 (p13p14) was inserted into chromosome 3 at q13.2 (Goldman et al. 1992). In meiosis I, the pairing chromosomes did not loop out the nonhomologous segments; but in fact the normal chromosome 3 appeared to pair fully with the der(3), and likewise the chromosome 10 and the der(10). This may be heterosynapsis. Sperm karyotyping showed, as expected from the theoretical considerations noted earlier, similar proportions of gametes with normal, balanced, duplication, and deletion chromosomes: The actual figures were 22%, 32%, 24%, and 22%, respectively. No recombinant forms were seen. Possibly, small insertions may show similar meiotic behavior, with absence of looping out, and no quadrivalent formation. Spermatogenesis may be compromised in some carriers, a conclusion drawn from the observation that only half as many index cases have carrier fathers as they do carrier mothers (Van Hemel and Eussen 2000).

Instructive Cases. Because nonreciprocal insertional translocations lead to "pure" single segmental imbalances, they can be helpful in delineating genes or phenotypes. Such is the case of an ins(13;11) (q14.1p11.2p12) segregating in a family, in which the deletion individuals had biparietal foramina (skull bone deficiencies), multiple exostoses (bone growths), and developmental delay (Shaffer et al. 1993). The description of this family led to the recognition of other deletion individuals, and eventually to the discovery of genes involved in multiple exostoses and biparietal foramina (Wakui et al. 2005; and see Potocki-Shaffer syndrome, p. 287).

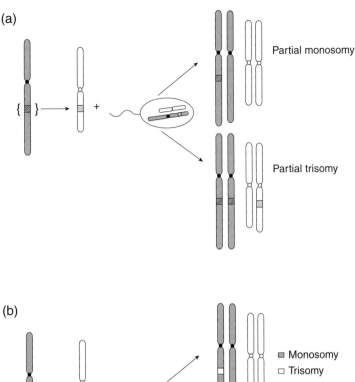

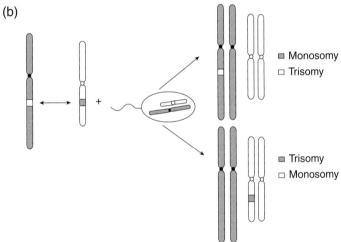

FIGURE 8–8   Insertional translocations and abnormal segregation. (*a*) One-way, single-segment, or nonreciprocal insertion. The hatched bar represents the portion of the chromosome inserted from the gray chromosome to the white chromosome. Upon fertilization by a normal sperm (region of interest from the gray chromosome is shown), there are two possible outcomes (arrows). The upper set of chromosomes shows the outcome after fertilization of an oöcyte carrying a deleted gray chromosome and a normal white chromosome; this leads to a partial monosomy (deletion). The lower set shows the outcome after fertilization of an oöcyte carrying two normal gray chromosomes and a white chromosome with the insertion; this leads to a partial trisomy (duplication). (*b*) Two-way, double-segment, or reciprocal insertion. Upon fertilization by a normal sperm, the upper set of chromosomes shows the outcome after fertilization of an oöcyte carrying only the insertion from the white chromosome. The result is trisomy for the white segment and monosomy for the gray segment. The lower set shows the reciprocal product, with trisomy for the gray segment and monosomy for the white segment.

An insertional translocation involving the critical region for Down syndrome provides an interesting illustration that this small segment is indeed sufficient to produce the phenotype. Lee et al. (2005) describe a father with 46,XY,ins(4;21) (q21q22.13q22.2), who had a child with typical Down syndrome, having inherited the paternal ins(4) with the small 21q segment, along with two normal chromosomes 21. This case had actually been diagnosed at amniocentesis, when a FISH probe recognizing 21q22 showed three signals; interpretation of the karyotype was a rather more subtle exercise, since 4q21 and 21q22 have similar staining properties, and the small inserted segment thus did not stand out.

RARE COMPLEXITIES

An insertion may not be "clean," and might undergo rearrangement, before being inserted into the recipient chromosome. Such a case is exemplified in Wentzel et al. (2014). A mother carried a de novo insertion from 6q13q16 into 15q11, but within the 6q13q16 segment, a 2.3 Mb piece, chr6:80.9-83.2, was "missing." Thus, she—a healthy woman—was deleted for this region: 46,XX,ins(15;6)(q11;q13q16.1),del(6)(q14.1). Her two daughters had presented, the elder with developmental delay and autism, the younger with a more complicated picture. The elder inherited the ins(15;6), along with normal no. 6 homologs, and was thus duplicated for 6q13q16 (except for the 2.3 Mb piece in the middle). The younger received the deleted chromosome, as 46,XX,del(6)(q13q16).

Most nucleolar organizing region (NOR) translocations are thought harmless. But a NOR insertion into the X chromosome associated with a familial X-linked spastic paraplegia (a condition in which there is stiffness and weakness of the lower limbs, due to neurological deficit at the level of motor neurons in the spinal cord) was apparently pathogenic (Tamagaki et al. 2000). NOR material comprises DNA coding for ribosomal RNA. Two brothers and their maternal uncle had the disease, and the carrier mother was unaffected. Plausibly, the inserted material disrupted a "spinal motor neuron gene" in this region, at Xq11.2, and the male hemizygote, with no gene product being made, thus developed the disorder. It cannot yet be excluded that there is an X-linked Mendelian disorder whose locus resides in Xq11.2, co-segregating in the family by chance, and the NOR insertion is simply serving as a cytogenetic marker. The discovery of the gene would prove the point.

There can be a link with cancer if a tumor suppressor gene is located in the insertional segment (Barber et al. 1994). An extraordinary case is seen in a father who had had Wilms tumor as a child, and whose daughter had retinoblastoma, due to an insertion that was apparently balanced in him, and unbalanced in his child. A segment from 13q14 including the retinoblastoma (*RB*) gene was inserted into 11p13, this being the site on chromosome 11 of the *WT1* Wilms tumor locus (Punnett et al. 2003).

GENETIC COUNSELING

Insertions are among rearrangements implying the highest reproductive risk. Pooled data from a number of insertion families (Van Hemel and Eussen, 2000) indicate an average risk of having an abnormal child of 32% for the male carrier and 36% for the female. It may reach 50%. Broadly speaking, the risk is greater in the small-segment insertion, and smaller in the large-segment insertion. Offering prenatal testing should, in most cases, be the rule. Of the phenotypically normal offspring, approximately half will have normal chromosomes, and half will be insertion heterozygotes. A more detailed discussion follows.

SHORT INSERTION SEGMENT

For the *short* insertion (<1% HAL), the segregation ratio at conception would be expected to be 1:1:1:1 for normal:balanced:duplication:deletion (as discussed above). If the insertional segment is not only short but also genetically "small," both trisomically and monosomically, the maximum risk of having a liveborn aneuploid child would approach 50% (1+1/1+1+1+1). The segment 18q11q21 (HAL = 0.8%), for example, meets these criteria, as seen in the insertion family presented in Chudley et al. (1974). Carriers for this insertion had all four karyotypic classes of offspring—insertion heterozygotes, karyotypically normal individuals, individuals with a duplication of a small segment of 18q, and individuals with the same segment deleted—in approximately equal numbers. A similar scenario is seen in Marinescu et al. (1999), with a family segregating an insertion ins(16;5)(q22p14p15.3). Here, the "small" segment comprised 5p14p15.3. In two generations from a heterozygous grandparent, there were two children with 5p−, two with 5p+, four normals, and three carriers. The same level of risk, with a 1:1:1:1 segregation as above, is also likely to apply to the very small insertion that requires molecular karyotyping for its recognition.

If viability is reduced or impossible for the trisomic or monosomic conceptuses, the risk would be correspondingly less. Trisomic lethality presumably increases with an increasing fraction of HAL, with monosomic imbalances being more lethal.

It may not be possible to make a clear judgment, based on the literature, about the qualitative content of the imbalance, because the insertion involves an interstitial segment of chromosome, whereas most data on record relate to distal segments.

A review of the insertional data on record up to 2000, taken from nearly 90 families, is provided in Van Hemel and Eussen (2000), and Figure 8–9 is taken from their paper. Any insertion involving the same open bar (deletion) or filled bar (duplication) segment, or part thereof, will have a significant risk. Schinzel's (2001) cytogenetic database and the Internet sources ECARUCA and DECIPHER may also be consulted. Of course, any unbalanced child in the counselee's family will provide proof of viability, and an illustration of that particular phenotype. A study of the wider family may provide a guide to the recurrence risk—a "private" segregation analysis, as illustrated above in the "Biology" section. But in any case, the starting point with a patient having a short insertion is that the risk for an abnormal child is high, by which we mean in the range 10%–50%.

LONGER INSERTION SEGMENT

For the direct insertion involving a *longer* segment (>1.5% HAL), there is theoretically an additional risk for the formation of recombinant duplication and deletion chromosomes. But in fact the deletion for a long segment (whether the result of a nonrecombinant or recombinant chromosome) would usually impose a nonviable degree of partial monosomy. The dup/del combinations (see Figure 8–4) are even more unbalanced, leading to spontaneous abortion. Thus, only the duplication (whether nonrecombinant or recombinant) is likely to allow for viability. In the great majority of cases, therefore, the segregation ratio for pregnancies going to term is 1:1:*x*:0 for normal:balanced:partial trisomy:other imbalances, where *x* is less than 1, and probably very much less than 1.

In the family of Jalbert et al. (1975) discussed above (Figure 8–5), the insertional segment (5q11q22) comprised 2.2% HAL, and this duplication did allow survival, although the child was dysmorphic and severely mentally retarded. This case is the sole example of dup(5)(q11q22) in Schinzel's (2001) database. The risk for recurrence in this family, or occurrence in another family, must surely be small, and perhaps *x* is only a low single-digit number. In a family such as that in Abuelo et al. (1988), with an insertional segment comprising most of 3p (3p26p13, 2.5% HAL), one could be rather confident that any imbalanced conception would

miscarry. The closest viable segment in Schinzel's database is 3p14pter, and there are only two cases of this listed; no cases in ECARUCA were close to matching. A risk of "close to 0%" for an abnormal child could be offered. Prenatal diagnosis in cases judged to be of this very low risk category would be discretionary; a normal ultrasonographic fetal anatomy scan would likely be considerably reassuring of itself.

INTERMEDIATE LENGTH SEGMENT

Intermediate length segments (1%–1.5% HAL) might imply a risk in the range 5%–10%. But each segment needs to be judged on its merits, both according to the reproductive history in the family and with reference to the cytogenetic databases.

THE INTRACHROMOSOMAL INSERTION

BIOLOGY

Intrachromosomal insertions are very rare, with only about 70 cases published (Domínguez et al. 2017). The cytogenetic recognition can be difficult, with some having originally been interpreted as paracentric inversions with unbalanced meiotic products (Madan and Nieuwint 2002). The formation of the intrachromosomal insertion is outlined in Figure 8–10. These insertions can be within-arm or between-arm, and direct or inverted, and they may undergo incomplete or complete synapsis. These differences may (but not necessarily) have practical reproductive consequences, and it is useful to consider each in turn.

Details of Meiotic Behavior

Meiosis perforce proceeds in a modified fashion.

BETWEEN-ARM INSERTION

The between-arm[3] insertion has a segment of chromatin from one arm inserted into a point in the other arm (Figure 8–11). If we consider the part of the chromosome containing the centromere as the fixed reference point of a chromosome, we can regard

---

3 Also called inter-arm, centromere shift, and pericentric insertion.

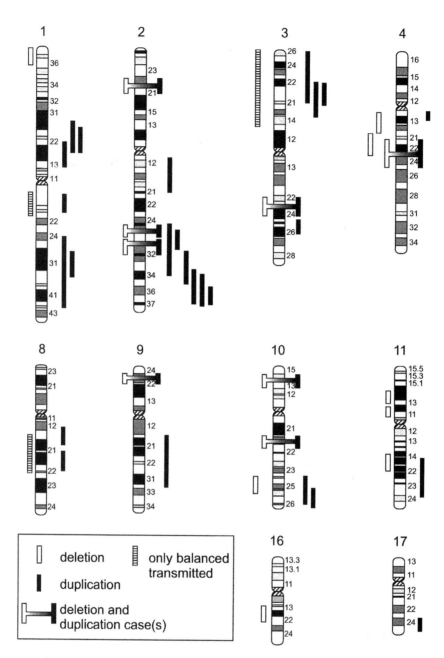

FIGURE 8–9 (*Above and opposite*) Presentation of chromosome segments in which recombinant imbalances have been recorded (on classical cytogenetics), in the child of a parent heterozygous for an interchromosomal insertion. Segments seen only as duplications are shown in filled bars, those seen only as deletions in open bars, and filled and open bars connected show segments observed in either state. Insertions seen only in the balanced state are identified with striped bars.

Source: From Van Hemel and Eussen, Interchromosomal insertions: Identification of five cases and a review, *Hum Genet* 107: 415–432, 2000. Courtesy J. O. Van Hemel, and with the permission of Springer-Verlag.

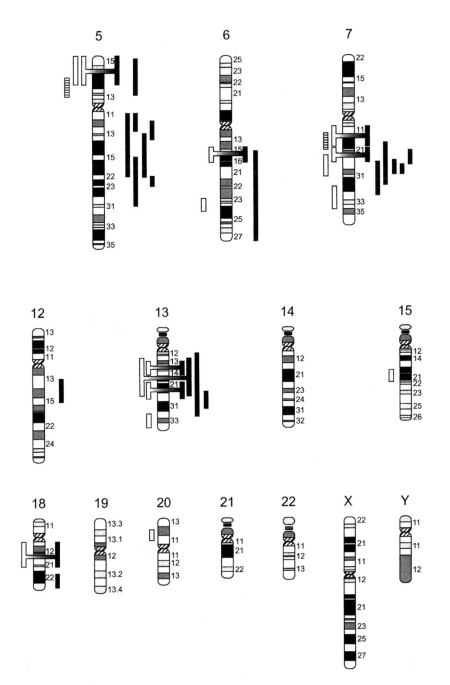

FIGURE 8–9 (Continued)

the centromeric segment as "staying still," while the insertion segment shifts from one arm to the other. This somewhat arbitrary point of view allows us to use the term "inserted segment" unambiguously, in the context of the between-arm insertion. Thus, in Figure 8–11, the segment shown in black has moved "up" from the long arm and is inserted into the short arm (rather than the segment containing the centromere moving "down" into the long arm).

WITHIN-ARM INSERTION

A shift of chromatin within the same arm is called, logically enough, a within-arm[4] insertion. Since both

---

4 Also called intra-arm, and paracentric insertion.

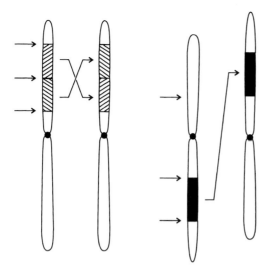

FIGURE 8–10   The formation of the intrachromosomal insertion. *Left*, the within-arm insertion, with the inserted segments cross-hatched. The normal chromosome is on the left, and the insertion chromosome on the right. *Right*, the between-arm insertion, with the inserted segment in black. The normal chromosome is on the left, and the insertion chromosome on the right. Compare with the ins(5) shown in Figure 8–15 and the ins(5) in Figure 8–16, respectively.

segments shift, essentially switching positions, each could be called an "inserted segment." If both segments maintain the same orientation toward the centromere, it is a *direct* insertion. If the orientation of one segment is reversed, it is an *inverted* insertion. In the case of the inverted inversion, we can distinguish one segment from the other by referring to respective inverted and noninverted segments. In the direct insertion, the shorter of the two segments can be arbitrarily labeled as the inserted segment, and the longer as the "noninserted" or "interstitial" segment (Madan and Menko 1992; Barber et al. 1994); since they are both really insertion segments, we can also speak of the "shorter inserted" and the "longer inserted" segments.

INCOMPLETE SYNAPSIS, DIRECT BETWEEN-ARM INSERTION

Perhaps in most cases of the direct between-arm insertion, the inserted segments fold out so as to allow a good degree of synapsis of the bivalent. This synapsis would include that part of the chromosome between the two inserted segments—that is, the centromeric segment. There would be no

difference, at least in theory, if the insertion is direct or inverted. One (or any odd number) crossover within the centromeric segment will produce recombinant chromosomes: one with a duplication of the insertion segment, and the other with a deletion (Figure 8–11). The centromeric segment may be quite long, as a proportion of the whole chromosome, and provide considerable opportunity for crossover. Thus, the genetic risk is expected to be high, and in theory could approach 50%. In other words, the segregation ratio for the four possible segregant outcomes of normal:balanced insertion:duplication:deletion would be close to 1:1:1:1.

According to the level of in utero genetic compromise imposed by the duplicated and deleted states, respectively, the risk for an abnormal outcome in a liveborn child may be correspondingly less. Siblings in Xanthopoulou et al. (2010) with ins(7) (p22q32q31.1) had had two liveborn children, and one prenatal diagnosis, with the duplication, but no recorded pregnancy from the deletion (this family is also mentioned below in the section "Gametogenesis Studies"). Contrariwise, in the family illustrated in

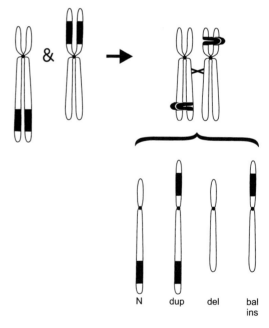

| N | dup | del | bal ins |

FIGURE 8–11   Gamete production following a recombination *between* the sites of rearrangement in the between-arm intrachromosomal insertion. At the top of the figure, the normal chromosome is on the left, and the insertion chromosome on the right. There is incomplete synapsis, with ballooning out. (Based on the ins(5) shown in Figure 8–16.)

Figure 8–12, with a between-arm insertion involving the small Potocki-Shaffer segment (11p11.2), both imbalanced outcomes are observed. Here, it may be the case that, with no reduced viability of either imbalanced state in utero, the risk to the carrier is indeed in the region of the theoretical 50%.

The interpretation can be difficult with a smaller insertion, as Lybæk et al. (2009) discuss in their case of a "19p13-into-19q" insertion, an ins(19) (q13.3p13.2p13.3). A profoundly retarded infant girl with precocious puberty had a distal 19p duplication of 8.9 Mb, and her mother had a rea(19), initially assessed as a pericentric inversion. It took FISH to reveal the true nature of the abnormal chromosome as being due to a between-arm shift.

INCOMPLETE SYNAPSIS, DIRECT WITHIN-ARM INSERTION

The within-arm shift, in the case of the direct insertion, can have a similar folding out of one inserted segment,

and its homolog on the normal chromosome, to enable synapsis of the other inserted segment and its homologous region. In Figure 8–13, we depict the shorter insertion segment folded out, with synapsis of the larger inserted segment; equally, it could have been drawn the other way around, with synapsis involving the smaller inserted segment. Recombination within the *larger* segment will lead, respectively, to duplication, or to deletion, of the shorter segment, in the recombinant products thus giving rise to the gametocytes. Or, if there is synapsis of the *shorter* inserted segments, followed by recombination, there would be duplication of the larger inserted segment in one gametocyte, and deletion of this segment in the other.

In theory, the longer the larger segment is, the more likely it is that recombination will happen; but nevertheless, cases are on record of crossing-over taking place in very short inserted segments (Webb et al. 1988; Barber et al. 1994). A molecular example is the following. A girl with a severe intellectual disability, autism, and minor facial dysmorphism, had a

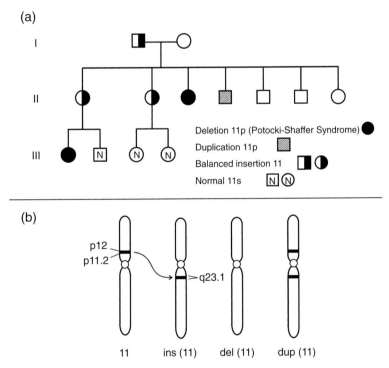

FIGURE 8–12   Family tree (*a*) showing segregation of an intrachromosomal insertion ins(11) (q23.1p11.2p12), with both deletion and duplication observed in the family, and (*b*) cartoon karyotype to show the nature of the rearrangement. The insertional segment is of approximately 2 Mb in length. Half-filled symbol, balanced carrier; filled symbol, 11p deletion (Potocki-Shaffer syndrome); cross-hatched symbol, 11p duplication. The formal karyotypes of the deletion and duplication states are rec(11)del *or* dup(11)(p11.2p12) ins(11)(q23.1p11.2p12). (Case of J. Gastier-Foster and C. Astbury.)

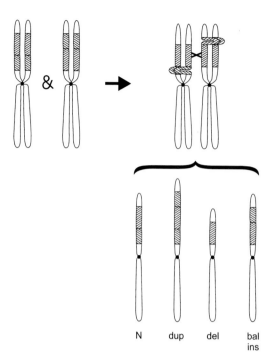

N   dup   del   bal
                    ins

FIGURE 8–13   Gamete production following a recombination *within* one of the insertion segments (the longer segments) of a direct within-arm intrachromosomal insertion. There is incomplete synapsis. There are four possible gametic outcomes. Compare with the ins(5) shown in Figure 8–15, although note the subtle difference that in the latter the recombination took place between the shorter inserted segments.

3.4 Mb microdeletion at 14q11.2, chr14:19,663,407-23,061,615, and interpreted initially as a de novo rearrangement, as a FISH probe for the deleted region hybridized to 14q11.2 in both parents. The family requested that the girl's uncle, a jovial man with mild intellectual deficiency, be tested; and he proved to have the countertype duplication. It then needed further three-color FISH analysis to reveal the subtlety of the insertion of the 3.4 Mb segment into a more distal position in one homolog, but still within the same band, in the connecting relatives, and in whom the rea is described broadly (but inadequately) as ins(14)(q11.2q11.2q11.2) (R. Beddow and K. Gibson, personal communication, 2016).

COMPLETE SYNAPSIS, DIRECT BETWEEN-ARM INSERTION

If complete synapsis can be achieved, the insertion and the centromeric segments (between-arm

shift) or the two insertion segments (within-arm shift), and their matching segments on the normal homolog, would need to loop back and forth into each other, forming a double loop (Figure 8–14). Various outcomes are possible from crossing-overs within one or other loop. Considering the direct between-arm shift, crossing-over within the *centromeric* segment will lead to recombinant chromosomes deficient or duplicated for the inserted segment (Figure 8–14a, b). If, however, following complete synapsis, there is crossing-over within the *inserted* segment, this will lead to the generation of new recombinant forms: chromosomes that are duplicated for terminal p and deleted for terminal q, or vice versa (Figure 8–14c, d). A notable such example is illustrated in Ardalan et al. (2005), concerning a mother who carried a dir ins(20)(p13q11.21q13.33) (initially thought to be a pericentric inversion). The "shifted" segment was relatively large, about half the length of the chromosome, and the del qter/dup pter recombinant karyotype conveyed a survivable imbalance.

COMPLETE SYNAPSIS, DIRECT WITHIN-ARM INSERTION

If complete synapsis is achieved in the direct within-arm shift, there is no new category of recombinant form beyond the four that could be generated from incomplete synapsis with folding out of one of the segments (as in Figure 8–13); indeed, distinction between the two processes is not possible. Crossing-over within the longer inserted segment will lead to recombinant chromosomes deficient or duplicated for the shorter inserted segment (Figure 8–14i, j). Vice versa, crossing-over within the shorter inserted segment will lead to recombinant chromosomes deficient or duplicated for the longer inserted segment (Figure 8–14k, l). We illustrate such a case from Webb et al. (1988) in Figure 8–15, from the G-banding era. Of more recent attribution, Quinonez et al. (2012) describe an insertion of 6.33 Mb at 1q21.3q23.3 into 1q42.12, in the mother of two children with multiple malformations, severe intellectual deficit, and anatomic brain abnormalities on imaging. The children were deleted for this 1q21.3q23.3 segment, chr1:154,796,145-161,130,692. A meiotic crossover within the intervening region (or, within the longer insertion segment) led to gametes deleted for 1q21.3q23.3 (the shorter insertion segment), as per the scenarios depicted in Figure 8–13 (del), or Figure 8–14

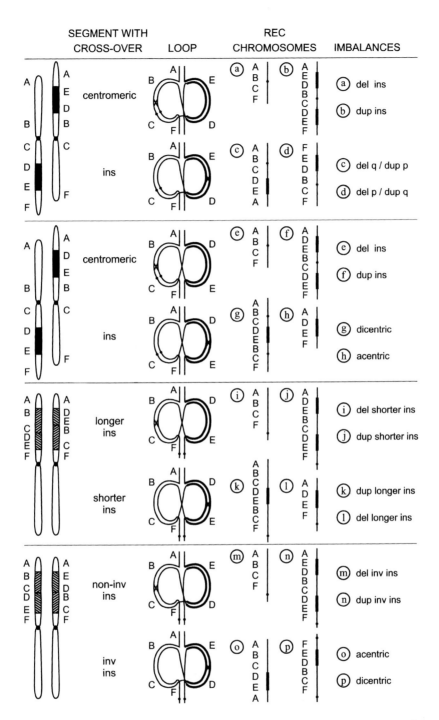

FIGURE 8–14 The range of possible recombinants from crossing-over in one or other insertion loop following complete synapsis of the intrachromosomal insertion. The four panels show, from above down, the direct between-arm insertion, the inverted between-arm insertion, the direct within-arm insertion, and the inverted within-arm insertion. In the loop diagrams, the dots signify the centromere, and the × shows the point of crossover. The insertion segment DE is shown in thick line in the loop and in the recombinant chromosomes. Circled letters provide reference points for text comments.

Source: Adapted from Madan and Menko (1992).

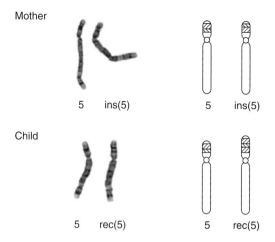

Mother

5   ins(5)   5   ins(5)

Child

5   rec(5)   5   rec(5)

FIGURE 8–15   Recombination from a direct intrachromosomal insertion (within-arm shift). Partial karyotypes of an insertion heterozygote mother, and her recombinant child. The karyotypes are 46, dir ins(5)(p14.1p14.3p15.1), and 46, rec(5),dup(5p)dir ins(5)(p14.1p14.3p15.1)mat.[5] The child is duplicated for 5p14.3p15.1, shown as the larger cross-hatched segment. The recombination may have arisen from crossing-over within band p14.1 (smaller cross-hatched segment) at either partial synapsis with ballooning out of segments p14.3-p15.1, as in Figure 8–13, or from complete synapsis following double-loop formation, as in Figure 8–14k. (Case of L. E. Voullaire; Webb et al. 1988.)

(imbalance *i*), and as shown in Figure 8–16. FISH was necessary to clarify the picture. (Of interest, this rearrangement had previously been interpreted as a harmless paracentric inversion, and the two affected children's karyotypes as normal.)

COMPLETE SYNAPSIS, INVERTED BETWEEN-ARM INSERTION

Recombination in the inverted between-arm insertion, in the setting of complete synapsis, has the same consequences as for the direct insertion as discussed above, when crossovers take place within the *centromeric* segment (Figure 8–14e, f). The family illustrated in Figure 8–17 demonstrates this. The recombinant child with a dup(5) could equally have arisen from recombination in a partial synapsis (Figure 8–11) or in a complete synapsis (Figure 8–14f), but in either event, the crossover is

within the centromeric segment. The duplication comprises the inverted insertion segment. If, however, the crossover is within the *inserted* segment, dicentric and acentric products will result, and, if a zygote were to result from such a gamete, the compromised conceptus will likely degenerate very early and may not even implant (Figure 8–14g, h).

COMPLETE SYNAPSIS, INVERTED WITHIN-ARM INSERTION

Nonviability is the fate of conceptions from crossovers in the inverted within-arm shift, if crossing-over happens within the *inverted* segment (Figure 8–14o, p). But if crossing-over is in the *noninverted* segment, we see the same imbalances (Figure 8–14m, n) as in the direct within-arm shift (Figure 8–14i, j). Thus, Rethoré et al. (1989) describe a child with a duplication for the very short segment 5p13.32p14.2 due to a parental inv ins(5)(p13.31p14.3p15.12) with recombination in the even shorter segment p14.3p15.11, reflecting the scenario set out in either Figure 8–14n or Figure 8–13.

A notable example of a three-generational inverted within-arm insertion is the inv ins(15)(q15q13q11.2) family described in Collinson et al. (2004). The grandmother, her son and her daughter, and one grandchild were heterozygous for the insertion, with the detailed karyotype written inv ins(15)(pter→q11.2::q13→q15::q13→q11.2::q15→qter). Three grandchildren were abnormal: one with Prader-Willi syndrome (PWS), one with the dup(15)(q11q13) syndrome (p. 323), and the third with Angelman syndrome (AS). As the reader may already have guessed, the AS grandchild was born to the carrier daughter, while the PWS grandchild was fathered by her son: These two grandchildren had each inherited a deletional rearrangement. The grandchild with the dup(15)(q11q13) syndrome, 46,XX,rec(15),dup(15)(q13q11.2) ins(15)(q15q13q11.2)mat, was the carrier daughter's child, having inherited a duplicational rearrangement. The rearrangements would have arisen following either the scenario set out in Figure 8–13 or Figure 8–14m (the deletion) or Figure 8–14n (the duplication).

The reader may have discerned a pattern in the various aforementioned constructions. Whichever segment recombination takes place in (the active

---

5   This karyotype stretches the limits of the short nomenclature, since "dup p" could refer to either 5p14.1 or 5p14.3p15.1. The full nomenclature describes the rearrangement: 46,XX,–5,+rec(5)(pter-p14.1::p15.1p14.3::p13.3qter),dir ins(5)(p14.1p14.3p15.1)mat.

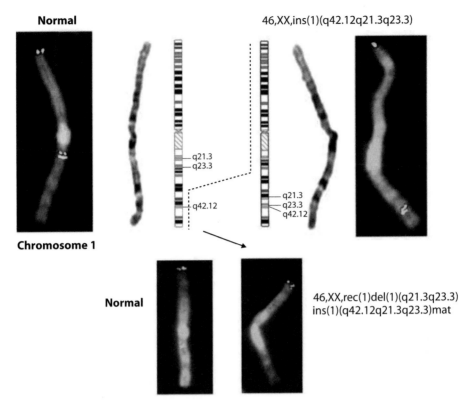

Normal

46,XX,ins(1)(q42.12q21.3q23.3)

q21.3
q23.3

q42.12

q21.3
q23.3
q42.12

Chromosome 1

Normal

46,XX,rec(1)del(1)(q21.3q23.3)
ins(1)(q42.12q21.3q23.3)mat

FIGURE 8–16   Meiotic recombination from a direct intrachromosomal insertion (within-arm shift). *Above,* chromosomes 1 of a carrier mother, 46,XX,ins(1)(q42.12q21.3q23.3), normal on left, insertion chromosome on right. The segment at 1q21.3q23.3 is inserted into 1q42.12. The zigzag line shows the region of crossover between the normal and the ins(1), in the gametes giving rise to her affected children. *Below,* chromosomes 1 in her affected daughter. FISH with probes for 1q21.3q23.3 shows a normal signal in the normal position on the paternal chromosome 1 (below left), and absence of this signal on the deleted, maternal rec(1) (below right).

Source: From Quinonez et al., Maternal intrachromosomal insertional translocation leads to recurrent 1q21.3q23.3 deletion in two siblings, *Am J Med Genet* 158A: 2591–2601, 2012. Courtesy J. W. Innes, and with the permission of John Wiley & Sons.

segment, so to say), it is the *other* (passive) segment that comes to be duplicated or deleted. This is logical. A crossover will create a new version of the active segment that contains a portion from each contributing chromosome—but it will be the same length as it was before. The other, non-crossing-over segments follow, as it were, passively along.

If the insertional segment is itself rearranged, such that one part is in direct orientation, and the other inverted, this is an "intrasegmental double inversion," and represents a four-break rather than a three-break rearrangement (Wang et al. 2010a). In this (not uncomplicated!) case, Figure 8–14c would need to be redrawn, following Figure 2 in Wang et al. This reinterpreted crossing-over

configuration might allow a closer coming together of the two segments in the normal and the insertional homologs, and possibly be the basis of a particularly high risk of producing imbalanced gametes.

Embryogenesis Studies. An insight into meiotic behavior of the direct between-arm insertion is offered in Xanthopoulou et al. (2010), who studied embryos created at preimplantation diagnosis from a sister and brother, who were both heterozygous for ins(7)(p22q32q31.1). The sister had 13/17 analyzable embryos which were normal or balanced, three with dup 7q31 and one with del 7q31, and thus with an imbalanced fraction of 24%. Her brother had a majority, nine out of 14 (64%) imbalanced, five deleted for 7q31 and four duplicated, and only five

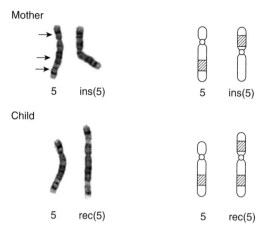

Mother

5   ins(5)   5   ins(5)

Child

5   rec(5)   5   rec(5)

FIGURE 8–17   Recombination from an inverted between-arm shift. Partial karyotypes of an insertion heterozygote mother and her recombinant child. The karyotypes are 46,inv ins(5)(p13q22q33), and 46,rec(5)dup(5q)inv ins(5)(p13q22q33)mat. The child is duplicated for 5q22q33 (indicated by the cross-hatched segment). The recombination may have arisen from crossing-over anywhere between 5p13 and 5q22 at either partial synapsis with ballooning out of segments 5q22q33, as in Figure 8–13, or from complete synapsis following double loop formation, as in Figure 8–14*f*. (Case of N. J. Martin; Martin et al. 1985.)

normal/balanced. The combined fractions from the two siblings are normal/balanced, 58%; duplicated, 39%; and deleted, 19%—from a total of 31 embryos.

GENETIC COUNSELING

The risk to have an abnormal recombinant child from an intrachromosomal insertion carrier parent, in the 27 families reviewed by Madan and Menko (1992), was 15%, although they considered this quite possibly to be an underestimate. This is an average figure, and it was derived from families studied with classical cytogenetics. We may presume a range from near 50% to zero in the individual case. A high risk is likely if one of the segments is small, and the other long, so that (*1*) there is a high

survivability in both the duplicated and deleted state for the small segment, and (*2*) with one long segment, recombination may be more likely to take place. In this situation, a figure of 30%–40% may be the appropriate one to offer. Given that the partial aneuploid states will involve interstitial regions of the chromosome, very little data, quite possibly none, may be on record for the viability and phenotype of the particular segment (but of course the appropriate databases should be checked); and an educated assessment will have to be made. In the case of very small insertions, detectable at the level of molecular karyotyping, the risk is likely to be at the upper end of the range.

Risks are presumably less, and possibly zero, if both segments are long (that is, no recombinants are viable). The risks *may* also be less—say, below 10%—if both segments are short, which might weigh against recombination; but we have no firm data with which to buttress this suggestion. As always, a "private" segregation analysis, if the family offers that opportunity, may provide the best estimate of risk. For one specific insertion, Allderdice et al. (1983) calculated a risk of 31% for female inv ins(9)(q22q34.3q34.1) heterozygotes. But prediction is imprecise. One short-segment between-arm shift, 46,dir ins(7)(p22.1p21.4q36.1), with a long centromeric segment for which, from the foregoing, a high risk might have been predicted, in fact produced no liveborn recombinant child in a three-generation family, although some first- and second-trimester pregnancy losses may have been due to unbalanced forms (Farrell and Chow 1992).

The ins(14)(q11.2q11.2q11.2) described above (in the section "Incomplete Synapsis, Direct Within-Arm Insertion") conveys an important message. The presenting child with a deletion was interpreted, following parental analysis, as having a de novo rearrangement; thus, a low recurrence risk for others in the family was assumed. But the discovery of her uncle with the countertype duplication demanded reappraisal; and with the identification then of the (very subtle) insertion in the connecting relatives, in fact a high-risk scenario was recognized. To state the obvious, family histories can be very revealing.

9

INVERSIONS

INVERSIONS ARE INTRACHROMOSOMAL STRUCTURAL rearrangements. The commonest is the simple (or single) inversion. If the inversion coexists with another rearrangement in the same chromosome, it is a complex inversion. The simple inversion comprises a two-break event involving just one chromosome. The intercalary segment rotates 180°, reinserts, and the breaks unite (Figure 9–1). The rearranged chromosome consists of a central inverted segment, and flanking distal, or noninverted segments. If the inverted segment includes the centromere, the inversion is *peri*centric; if it does not, it is *para*centric. Figure 9–2 depicts two different pericentric inversions of chromosome 3. Note that the pericentric inversion has one break in the short arm and one in the long arm, whereas in the paracentric inversion both breaks occur in the same arm. Thus, when reading cytogenetic nomenclature, one can readily tell which is which: For example, 46,XX,inv(3)(p25q21) is pericentric and 46,XY,inv(11)(q21q23) is paracentric (inv = inversion). The particular clinical relevance of inversion chromosomes is that they can set the stage for the generation of recombinant (rec) gametes that may lead to abnormal pregnancy. In this chapter, we pay attention largely to the circumstance of the familial balanced and phenotypically normal carrier, and that carrier's risk for abnormal offspring; but we also refer to inversions, familial or (most often) de novo, that are unbalanced or which disrupt genes, and with an associated phenotypic abnormality.

The heterozygote is, other things being equal, a phenotypically normal person. The reorientation of a sequence of genetic material apparently does not influence its function, and breakage and reunion at most sites do not perturb the smooth running of the genome. Some inversions of the X may be an exception to this rule: A breakpoint involving the X long arm within the "critical region" can cause gonadal insufficiency. Some pericentric breakpoints occur at preferential sites, including 2p13, 2q21, 5q13, 5q31, 6q21, 10q22, and 12q13 (Kleczkowska et al. 1987); and certain paracentric breakpoints are likewise overrepresented (Madan 1995).

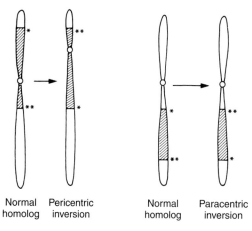

Normal | Pericentric | Normal | Paracentric
homolog | inversion | homolog | inversion

FIGURE 9–1   The structure of the pericentric (*left*) and paracentric (*right*) inversions. The inverted segment is cross-hatched. Asterisks provide landmarks at each end of the inversion segment.

FREQUENCY OF INVERSIONS

Excluding variant forms (see below), classical inversions are a fairly uncommonly recognized rearrangement. Estimates of frequency range from about 0.12% to 0.7% (pericentric) and about 0.1% to 0.5% (paracentric) of individuals (Van Dyke et al. 1983; Kleczkowska et al. 1987; Worsham et al. 1989; Pettenati et al. 1995). With respect to the paracentric inversion, Madan (1995) suspects that many small examples remain undetected, and comments

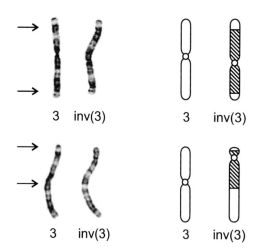

3   inv(3)   3   inv(3)

3   inv(3)   3   inv(3)

FIGURE 9–2   Two pericentric inversions of chromosome 3. Both of the noninverted segments are small in one (*a*) and one is large in the other (*b*). (Cases of N. A. Adams and L. M. Columbano-Green.)

that these are "the most common form of chromosomal polymorphism found in nature."

MOLECULAR KARYOTYPING

As with other balanced chromosome rearrangements, inversions will not be detected by chromosome microarray, the exception being when there is a copy number loss or gain or loss at one of the breakpoints (that is, when the inversions is not truly balanced). When a balanced rearrangement is suspected—for example, due to family history of an inversion or a history of recurrent miscarriage—a classical microscope karyotype is required. In contrast, imbalance due to recombination within an inverted segment should be readily detected by microarray.

CRYPTIC INVERSIONS

An inversion may not necessarily be detected on routine study, and knowing when to mount a directed search requires clinical acumen. Thus, Yokoyama et al. (1997) discovered an inv(17)(p13.1q25.1) in a father whose child had lissencephaly, a particular type of severe brain malformation. At first sight, the inverted chromosome looked normal. They noted a family history of similarly affected children, suspected a diagnosis of Miller-Dieker syndrome (which is due to 17p13.3 deletion), and went on to demonstrate the cytogenetic abnormality using fluorescence in situ hybridization (FISH) with a probe recognizing the Miller-Dieker sequence.

Chia et al. (2001) studied a girl with an apparent del(2)(q37) on high-resolution analysis. Using subtelomeric probes to clarify the nature of the deletion, they were surprised to see a 2p signal at each end of the chromosome. Thus, the "deletion chromosome" could be seen for what it really was: a recombinant inversion chromosome, the essential genetic consequence of which was a deficiency of distal 2q. Since the short arm breakpoint was right at the tip of the chromosome at 2p25.3, there may have been little or no duplication of functional 2p genetic material.

Molecular methodology was needed to clarify in detail the nature of a chromosome 20 inversion, in which classical karyotyping had been interpreted as normal, but with multiplex ligation-dependent amplification and FISH then revealing a del/dup of distal 20p/20q, respectively, in three adult siblings (Stevens et al. 2009). The mother's karyotype was 46,XX,inv(20)(p13q13.33), and the siblings each had the identical rec(20)dup(20q) inv(20)(p13q13.33)mat. The imbalances were molecularly very small, the duplication being 2.5 Mb, and the deletion, 1.1 Mb. Dysmorphology was subtle, but the cognitive/behavioral phenotypes were quite abnormal.

A rather different type of inversion is the small (40 kb to 4 Mb) inversion flanked by short (~600 kb) duplications (termed dupINVdup), and in which the generation had been facilitated by interaction between the two duplicated segments (Brand et al. 2015). The functional impact of a dupINVdup is likely to be variant-specific and locus-specific. Presumably it is too small to engage in recombination with its non-inverted fellow on the other homolog.

DELETION OR DUPLICATION AT INVERSION BREAKPOINT

A "clean" break and rejoin may not necessarily happen, and the rearrangement may, rarely, comprise, or give rise to, an associated deletion or duplication. This is a "complex inversion." Langer-Giedion syndrome (LGS) is due to a deletion at 8q24.11q24.13 (p. 284), and Sasaki et al. (1997) studied a child with LGS who had a de novo inv(8)(q13.1q24.11). Molecular analysis revealed a 4 Mb deletion encompassing the LGS region; presumably this segment had been deleted as part of the process that generated the inversion. A familial inv(18)(q21.1q23), in which a gene for brain myelination and likely some adjacent genes were deleted, led to some features of the 18q− syndrome in a mother and daughter (Keppler-Noreuil et al. 1998). A familial inv(15) (p11q13), when transmitted from mother to child, underwent loss of the region that contains the Angelman syndrome (AS) locus (Webb et al. 1992). The loss was not detectable cytogenetically—the child appeared to have the same inversion that his mother and grandfather carried—but it was revealed on molecular analysis. The child had AS. Kähkönen et al. (1990) likewise describe a child with Prader-Willi syndrome and a 15q11 deletion, whose father and grandmother were 46,inv(15)(p11q12) carriers.

BREAKPOINTS WITHIN GENES

In the event that a breakpoint occurs actually within a gene, the inversion could be directly pathogenic. Rare de novo examples include an inv(16) (p13.3q13) disrupting the Rubinstein-Taybi

syndrome locus; an inv(17)(q12q25) disrupting SOX9 and causing campomelic syndrome; an inv(20)(p12.2p13) with one breakpoint occurring between exons 5 and 6 of the JAG1 gene, causing Alagille syndrome; an inv(X)(p21.2;q28) disrupting the dystrophin gene at Xp21.2 and a long non-coding RNA at Xq28 in a mentally retarded boy with Duchenne muscular dystrophy; and an inv(X) (p22.1q28) leading to dysregulation of the MECP2 gene in a girl with a Rett-like syndrome (Maraia et al. 1991; Lacombe et al. 1992; Stankiewicz et al. 2001b; Tran et al. 2013; Vieira et al 2015). A de novo inv(2)(q35q27.3) provided, in fact, the entrée to the mapping of a Waardenburg syndrome locus to 2q35 (Ishikiryama et al. 1989). A paracentric inversion on one homolog 21 "exposed" a mutation in the HLCS gene on the other, leading to metabolic disease of the newborn, in the case of Quinonez et al. (2017b).

That a role for classical cytogenetics remains in the molecular age is illustrated in a study by Schmidt et al. (2014). A child with branchio-oto-renal syndrome had been studied for mutation within one of the three known BOR loci, but no abnormality was seen. Finally, on cytogenetics, the discovery of a de novo inv(8)(p22q13) led to the answer: a "clean break" in the EYA1 gene at 8q13.3.

Familial examples of inversions with gene disruption include an inv(15)(q11.2q24.3) transmitted from a normal mother to her Angelman syndrome daughter, and which actually led to the cloning of the causative UBE3A gene (Greger et al. 1997). In a family with a number of members suffering from attention deficit disorder, and the affected persons also carrying an inv(3)(p14q21), a locus at each breakpoint was disrupted, these being in an intron of a solute carrier gene (SLC9A9) at the q arm and in an intron of the DOCK3 gene at the p arm breakpoint (de Silva et al. 2003). One or other of these genes is a fair candidate for having a role in the genesis of this neurobehavioral disorder, and a mouse model has since implicated SLC9A9 (Yang et al. 2016).

On the X chromosome, a familial inv(X) (p11.4q22) damaging the Norrie syndrome gene is described in Pettenati et al. (1993). Xu et al. (2003) report a family with congenital androgen insensitivity segregating an inv(X)(q11.2q27); presumably, the break at Xq11.2 compromised the integrity of the androgen receptor locus. An inversion chromosome with gene damage at both breakpoints was reported in Saito-Ohara et al. (2002): A mother with the karyotype 46,X,inv(X)(p21.2q22.2) had a severely retarded 46,Y,inv(X) (p21.2q22.2) son with Duchenne muscular dystrophy, these effects being due to disruption of the *dystrophin* gene at Xp21.1, and of the *RLGP* gene at Xq22.2.

A somewhat different scenario is described in Gray et al. (2006), concerning a child presenting with obesity and hyperphagia but also, atypically in this setting, with hyperactivity. She had a de novo paracentric inversion inv(11)(p13p15.3), in which the 11p13 breakpoint was not within the brain-derived neurotrophic factor (*BDNF*) gene, but 850 kb 5′ of it. Plausibly, this led to downregulation of the copy of this gene on the inversion chromosome, and the resultant functional haploinsufficiency was the basis of the clinical phenotype.

INVERSIONS IN ACROCENTRIC CHROMOSOMES

Additional complexities may arise when the pericentric inversion involves an acrocentric chromosome, because the nucleolar organizing regions (NORs) become located on the long arm. Leach et al. (2005) describe a de novo case, 46,XX,inv(14) (p12q11.2). The first clue, on classical cytogenetics, that a pericentric inversion is present is the finding of a nonstaining gap in the long arm.

"Normal Variant" Inversions. "Inversions" having a breakpoint within the heterochromatic regions of chromosomes 1, 9, 16, and Y are frequently seen, and they are to be thought of as normal variants, not abnormal chromosomes. In "the world's largest epidemiological study" of the inv(9), Šípek et al.

(2015) found no significant differences in frequencies between the inv(9)(p12q13) and the normal 9 in populations ascertained for various clinical reasons. A single case is recorded of a rearrangement leading to a possibly pathogenic duplication of 9p, from a father with the typical inv(9) (Malinverni et al. 2017). The most common inversion in humans not involving centromeric heterochromatin is the inv(2)(p11.2q13); here, just two recorded cases in the world are known of a possibly related pathogenic recombination (see p. 192). De novo cases are rarely seen (Yakut et al. 2015a). Other presumed harmless inversion variants include the following: inv(3)(p11q11) and inv(3)(p11q12), inv(3)(p13q12), inv(5)(p13q13), and inv(10)(p11.2q21.2). The inv(10) has been rather extensively studied by a collaborative group of five laboratories in the United Kingdom that had, between them, 33 families available for investigation (Collinson et al. 1997). They found no excess of infertility or spontaneous abortion among carriers; of interest, all carriers of the inv(10) may be descendant from the same ancient northern European heterozygote (Gilling et al. 2006). A similarly large collaborative Canadian study came to a similar conclusion with respect to the inv(2) (Hysert et al. 2006).

THE PERICENTRIC INVERSION

BIOLOGY

The Autosomal Pericentric Inversion

DETAILS OF MEIOTIC BEHAVIOR

The inversion heterozygote may produce chromosomally unbalanced gametes, and in consequence

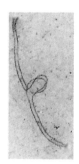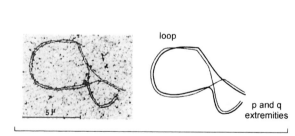

loop

p and q
extremities

FIGURE 9–3   Inversion loop in meiosis, direct observation. *Left*, inversion loop in a mouse study. *Right*, spermatocyte study of a man with inv(6)(p22q22.2).

Source: From de Perdigo et al., Correlation between chromosomal breakpoint positions and synaptic behavior in human males heterozygous for a pericentric inversion, *Hum Genet* 83: 274–276, 1989. Courtesy Y. Rumpler, and with the permission of Springer-Verlag.

suffer reproductive pathology. The chromosomal imbalance is a result of the formation of a recombinant (rec) chromosome. This is *"aneusomie de recombinaison"*—aneusomy due to recombination. Recombination occurs if there is, within the inverted segment, a crossover between the inversion chromosome and the normal homolog.

Synapsis and Recombination. Classically, crossing-over follows the reversed loop model (Figures 9–3 and 9–4) (Anton et al. 2005). This configuration of the bivalent at meiosis allows as complete as possible alignment and pairing of matching segments of the inversion chromosome and its normal homolog (homosynapsis). One (or an uneven number of) crossover(s) within the inversion loop, between a chromatid of the normal homolog and a chromatid of the inversion chromosome, leads to the production of two complementary recombinant chromosomes. One of these has a duplication of the distal segment of the short arm, and a deletion of the distal segment of the long arm (chromosome c-c′ in Figure 9–4); and the other way around in the other rec chromosome (d-d′ in Figure 9–4). Thus, the conceptuses that result would have both a partial trisomy for one distal segment and a partial monosomy for the other, or vice versa. Typically, only one of these—the least monosomic—is ever viable. Consider the recombinant 7 due to a paternal inversion illustrated in Figure 9–5. There is a duplication of the substantial segment 7p14.2pter, and a deletion of only the tiny segment comprising the distalmost subband of 7q (7q36.3qter), the combination being survivable. The countertype form, having a monosomy for 7p14.2pter (and trisomy 7q36.3qter), would, we suppose, cause a miscarriage.

The cytogenetic nomenclature to describe the recombinant karyotype is straightforward. In the above case, for example, we have

- Parent: 46,XY,inv(7)(p14.2q36.3)
- Recombinant offspring (c-c′): 46,XY,rec(7) dup(7p) inv(7)(p14.2q36.3)

It is not necessary to put "dup(7p)del(7q)"—the complementary deletion is taken as read. More fully, the nomenclature is 46,XY,rec(7)dup(7p)inv(7)(pter→p14.2::q36.3→p14.2::q36.3→qter)pat.

This complex twisting of the chromosomes to form a loop may not necessarily take place. In an inversion with a short inverted segment

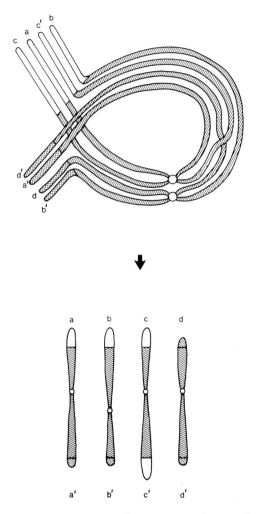

FIGURE 9–4   Inversion loop in meiosis, theoretical recombinant outcomes (based on the inv(3) shown in Fig. 9–2a). Both sister chromatids are shown. The inversion (centromeric) segment is cross-hatched, the long arm noninverted segment is stippled, and the short arm noninverted segment is open. The four possible gametic outcomes following one crossover within the inversion loop are depicted. Chromosomes a-a′ and b-b′ are the intact homolog and the inversion, respectively; chromosomes c-c′ and d-d′ are the dup p and dup q recombinant chromosomes. Compare with the actual observation in Figure 9–3, right.

(Figure 9–6a), a partial pairing may occur. Both distal segments, or sometimes just one, align in homosynapsis. The inverted segment and the corresponding part of the normal homolog either "balloon out" (asynapsis of the inversion segment) or lie adjacent but unmatched (heterosynapsis) (Gabriel-Robez and Rumpler 1994; Anton et al.

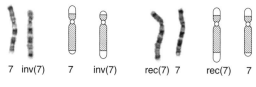

7 inv(7)   7   inv(7)   rec(7) 7   rec(7)   7

FIGURE 9–5   Pericentric inversion 7 in the father (*left*) of an abnormal child with a recombinant 7 (*right*). The recombinant chromosome has a duplication of just over half of 7p, and a minuscule deletion involving the distal-most subband of 7q. The child has a triple amount of the segment 7p14.2pter. The karyotypes are 46,inv(7)(p14.2q36.3) and 46,rec(7)dup(7p) inv(7)(p14.2q36.3)pat. (Case of S. M. White.)

2005). Thus, no crossing-over can happen within the inverted segment, and recombinant products do not form. Conversely, some inversions with long inverted and very short distal segments may undergo synapsis of the inverted segment only, with the distal segments at each end remaining unpaired (Figure 9–6b). Recombination can occur in this setting. The quality of the chromatin may of itself have an influence. If both breakpoints are in G-light bands, the lack of homology is detected at synapsis, and the chromosomes respond by formation of a loop, achieving a complete homosynapsis.

(a)   (b)

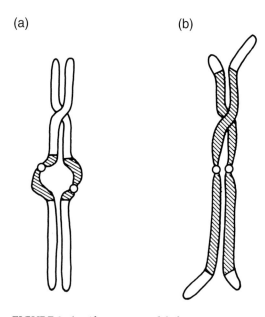

FIGURE 9–6   Alternative models for meiotic pairing, in which only a partial synapsis is achieved. Synapsis of (*a*) both distal segments; (*b*) the inverted segment. One crossover is shown in each.

If, however, one or both breakpoints are in a G-dark band, nonhomology may not be recognized, and heterosynapsis is not prevented (de Perdigo et al. 1989; Ashley 1990). In this latter state, recombination is suppressed (Jaarola et al. 1998). With specific reference to some X inversions, it may be that they have a lesser propensity to engage in recombination within the inverted segment (Shashi et al. 1996).

Sperm Studies. Sperm studies in a small number of inversion heterozygotes give an indication of the frequency with which recombination happens, at least in male gametogenesis (Anton et al. 2005; Morel et al. 2007; Luo et al. 2014). Table 9–1 sets out the findings from a number of such studies, and the data are shown graphically in Figure 9–7. Initially, this work was done using the sperm-hamster methodology; in the late 1990s and 2000s, FISH came to be used, and this approach allowed very large numbers of sperm to be analyzed. Dual-color FISH methodology, with one color (e.g., green) for the p arm and another (e.g., orange) for the q arm of the inversion chromosome, can show whether a sperm is recombinant. Sperm with nonrecombinant chromosomes would show one orange spot and one green spot. A recombinant chromosome with two orange spots would reveal the dup(q)/del(p) state, while vice versa, the dup(p)/del(q) chromosome would have two green spots.

These several studies show that the longer the inverted segment, the more likely is recombination to happen. Presumably, a longer inverted segment allows a more ready formation of an inversion loop. We can separate the studied cases into those with a long inversion segment (over 50% of the length of the whole chromosome) and those in which it is short. In six examples from Table 9–1 with longer inversion segments, inv(1)(p36.3q43), inv(3)(p25q21), inv(6)(p23q25), inv(7)(p13q36), inv(8)(p12q24.1), and inv(8)(p23q22), the proportions of dup(p)/del(q) and dup(q)/del(p) recombinant chromosomes were substantial: 32%, 31%, 38%, 24%, 38%, and 13%, respectively. No recombinants at all were seen in inversions with a short (or a very short) inversion segment: three "normal variant" pericentromeric inversions of chromosomes 2, 3, and 9, and an inv(20)(p13q11.2). Morel et al. (2007) offer this rule: A high risk of recombination applies when the inversion segment is over

Table 9–1. Sperm Analysis of 22 Autosomal Pericentric Inversion Heterozygotes

	INV SEGMENT SIZE (%)	NONRECOMBINANT* (%)	REC	
			DUP(P)/DEL(Q)	DUP(Q)/DEL(P)
inv(1)(p11q12)	9	100	0	0
inv(1)(p22q42)	60	80	7	7
inv(1)(p31q12)**	30	100	0	0
inv(1)(p31q12)**	30	99.6	0.25	0.13
inv(1)(p32q21)	37	91	4	5
inv(1)(p32q32)	62	83	9	8
inv(1)(p36.3q21)	60	85	7	9
inv(1)(p36q32)	81	83	9	7
inv(1)(p36.2q42	92	59	20	21
inv(1)(p36.3q43)	95	68	12	19
inv(2)(p11q13)	10	99.4	0	0
inv(2)(p11.2q13)	10	100	0	0
inv(2)(p23q33)	71	61	20	18
inv(3)(p11q11)	5	100	0	0
inv(3)(p25q21)	60	69	14	17
inv(4)(p16q21)	42	99.2	0.8	
inv(6)(p23q25)	80	46	19	19
inv(7)(p13q36)	65	75	7	17
inv(8)(p12q21)	31	97	1	0.4
inv(8)(p12q24.1)	61	61	20	18
inv(8)(p23q22)**	62	88	6	6
inv(8)(p23q22)**	62	87	6	7
inv(9)(p11q13)	16	100	0	0
inv(10)(p13q22.3)	47	97	3	
inv(12)(p11q23)	51	91	4	4
inv(17)(p13.1q25.3)	89	73	0.8	0.6
inv(20)(p12.3q13.33)	84	80	10	8
inv(20)(p13q11.2)	51	100	0	0

Notes: Frequencies of recombinant (rec) and nonrecombinant chromosomes are shown as percentages. The size of the inversion segment, as a fraction (%) of the whole chromosome, is noted. Note that, as a rule, the larger the inversion size (especially >50%), the greater the fraction of recombinant forms. The proportions of the two recombinant forms from each inversion chromosome, dup(p)/del(q) and dup(q)/del(p), are very similar.

*Whether normal or the inversion.

**These two pairs represent the same inversion initially studied by the sperm-hamster test, and subsequently by FISH. Note how close the findings are.

Sources: From the review of Morel et al. (2007), and including also the inv(1)(p22q42) case of Chantot-Bastaraud et al. (2009) and five inv(1) cases of Luo et al. (2014).

50% in length; the risk is small when the length is between 30% and 50%; and no recombination appears to take place when the inversion segment comprises less than 30% of the chromosome. Figure 9–7 in essence bears this out. And in any event, even if recombination occurred in a small inversion segment, the recombinant chromosome would have such a large duplication and deletion that the risk of an abnormal live birth would, very probably, be negligible.

The fractions of each vice versa recombinant type are essentially the same. In the inv(8)(p23q22) listed in Table 9–1, for example, about equal numbers of sperm showed the del(p)/dup(q)

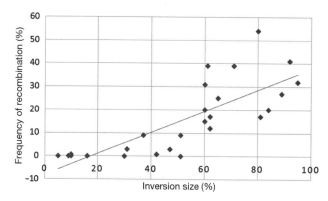

FIGURE 9–7   The proportion of gametes that are recombinant, compared with the relative size of the inversion. Graphical representation of the data from Table 9–1; individual data points and the regression line are shown. The clear trend is that the larger the inversion size, the more frequently recombinants are seen.

Source: Adapted from Luo et al. (2014).

state (which is viable) and the dup(p)/del(q) state (which is not), 7% and 6%, respectively. The other inversions in this listing show, for the most part, similar ratios.

An exception to the rule about recombination is given in the long-segment inv(17)(p13.1q25.3) carrier reported in Mikhaail-Philips et al. (2005). Of the 2,000 sperm scored, 73% showed balanced segregants, and only 1.4% showed the classical dup/del recombinants; 15% had deletion only of 17p, which is the basis of Miller-Dieker syndrome (and this was the diagnosis in two pregnancies fathered by this man). Similarly, recombination was rare in another inversion with a large inverted segment, inv(1)(p31q12): only 23 recombinants seen in 5,966 sperm, a fraction of 0.4% (Jaarola et al. 1998). This reflected a near-complete suppression of recombination.

Different inversions in the same chromosome can have quite different recombinant fractions. Caer et al. (2008) examined sperm from three men, with three different chromosome 8 inversions: p12q21, p12q24.1, and p23q24, respectively. With the p12q21 inversion, almost all sperm, 97%, were nonrecombinant, whereas the other two (with larger inverted segments) had 60% nonrecombinant. Concerning the common inv(2)(p11q13), Ferfouri et al. (2009) studied seven men presenting either with infertility or during the course of a family study. Of just over 7,000 sperm, 99.7% were nonrecombinant; the rate of aneuploidy otherwise did not differ from a control group. This work is interesting in proving that recombination can occur, even with this

very short inverted segment; equally, the very tiny fraction manifesting recombination is to be noted.

Segment Content and Viability. While a long inversion segment can set the stage for recombination, what determines the viability of the recombinant conceptus is the functional content of the *noninverted* (distal) segments. We speak of a "genetically small" content, if the combined effect of a duplication and deletion does not cause lethality during the earlier part of pregnancy, but allows development to proceed well through the pregnancy and possibly to live birth. Thus, only those heterozygotes who have inversions with genetically small distal segments will ever have a chromosomally unbalanced, phenotypically abnormal, liveborn child. The inversion shown in Figures 9–2a and 9–5 illustrates this case. Inversion heterozygotes in whom one or both distal segments are genetically large (e.g., Figure 9–2b) cannot have an abnormal recombinant child, although they may well have an increased risk for miscarriage. Any recombinants produced by such a person would impart a degree of imbalance that would be lethal in utero.

Genetic content corresponds fairly well to chromosome length. In inversion families in which recombinant children have been born, the distal (noninverted) segments together comprise, on average, only 35% of the total chromosome length; whereas in families having no known recombinant offspring, the figure is 62% (Kaiser 1988). Nevertheless, if the distal segments comprise "genetically small" material, a larger fraction would not necessarily preclude a reproductive risk. Consider the inv(13)(p11q14) and inv(13)(p12q13), in which the distal segments comprise as much as 75% of the chromosome length. Although the imbalance in the recombinant is large in terms of haploid autosomal length, the result in the dup(q) form is, in effect, a partial trisomy 13 (the partial monosomy for 13p being without phenotypic influence). This is, of course, well known to allow intrauterine and postnatal survival. Similarly, an inversion in chromosome 18 can have distal segments that may be long relative to a short inversion segment, but they are still small genetically, and the dup+del combination can be viable (Schmutz and Pinno 1986; Ayukawa et al. 1994). With specific reference to chromosome 4, Stipoljev et al. (2002) reviewed 20 reported familial cases and showed that recombinant forms have never been seen in those with smaller inversions, but frequently in the larger ones.

If the deletion of one segment and the duplication of the other are each associated, on their own, with a clinical phenotype, a combination of both may be seen in the recombinant child. Thus, Putoux et al. (2013) describe a child in whom they saw features of both Beckwith-Wiedemann syndrome (which can be due to duplication of paternal 11p) and Jacobsen syndrome (which is due to 11q deletion). The father was heterozygous for an inv(11)(p15.3q24.1), and the child had a rec(11)dup(11p)inv(11)(p15.3q24.1)pat.

As noted above, it is typically the case that only one recombinant form is ever viable. This is rather impressively illustrated in Allderdice et al. (1975) in a kindred with the inv(3)(p25q21). Numerous cases of known or suspected dup(3q) children have been born, but none with the countertype del(3q). There is not even an increase in the miscarriage rate, suggesting that the del(3q) is lethal very early in pregnancy and causes "occult abortion." Viability with both recombinant forms from the same inversion, the dup/del and the reciprocal del/dup, is infrequently seen, and includes these reported examples: inv(4)(p15.1q35.1), inv(4)(p15.32q35),

inv(4)(p16.2q35.1), inv(5)(p13q35), inv(10) (p15.1q26.12), inv(13)(p11q22), inv(18) (p11q21), and inv(20)(p13q13.3) (Kaiser 1984; Hirsch and Baldinger 1993; Dufke et al. 2000; Maurin et al. 2009; DeScipio et al. 2010a,b; Ciuladaite et al. 2014). These instances have this quality in common: The noninverted segments are very short.

It is instructive to consider the inv(4)(p15.32q35) in Hirsch and Baldinger (1993), in which recombinant offspring could be del(4p)/dup(4q) or dup(4p)/del(4q) (Figure 9–8). The four separate segmental imbalances are all well known individually to be viable. Distal 4p is, of course, the basis of the Wolf-Hirschhorn syndrome; and distal 4p trisomy has syndromic, if not eponymic, status. The distal 4q segment is small cytogenetically (0.25% haploid autosomal length [HAL]) and functionally, and duplication[1] and deletion are quite well tolerated. So the respective imbalances in the combined states—the del(4p)+dup(4q), and the dup(4p)+del(4q)—remain sufficiently small to be viable, at least much of the time. The index case, with the former imbalance, is a severely retarded child with a Wolf-Hirschhorn phenotype; and an aunt, having the latter combination, had rather minor dysmorphism and mental retardation. The inverted segment is very long: 87% of the total length of chromosome 4. Therefore, crossing-over within the inverted segment is, we assume, very likely to take place. Thus, the genetic risk to heterozygotes for this inv(4) is high. Two other reported families, with slightly different breakpoints (4p16.2/4q35.1 and 4p15.1/4q35.1, respectively), also demonstrate a high risk for imbalanced offspring, with both recombinant products observed (Dufke et al. 2000; Maurin et al. 2009).

Likewise, an inversion such as the inv(9) (p24.3q34.1) in Mundhofir et al. (2012) implies a high risk: The 9p segment is very small (450 kb), and the genetic load due to the 8.9 Mb from 9q34.1qter, at least in the duplicated state, has little or no in utero lethality. An even higher risk might apply to the inv(13)(p11q22) described in Williamson et al. (1980), in a family with several documented, suspected, or possible recombinant abnormal offspring. Here, the contribution of 13p imbalance to the two recombinant states—the del(13p)+dup(13q) and the dup(13p)+del(13q)—has no phenotypic

---

1 Duplication for a considerably longer segment, 4q31.3→qter, comprising 1.15% of HAL, is viable, as the children in the frontispiece photograph illustrate.

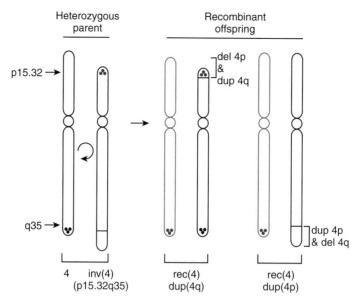

Heterozygous parent

Recombinant offspring

p15.32 →

del 4p
&
dup 4q

q35 →

dup 4p
& del 4q

4   inv(4)
(p15.32q35)

rec(4)
dup(4q)

rec(4)
dup(4p)

FIGURE 9–8   An inversion inv(4)(p15.32q35) with small noninverted segments, in which each of the two recombinant possibilities is viable. The del(4p)/dup(4q) karyotype (left recombinant offspring) produces a Wolf-Hirschhorn-like picture, and in the dup(4p)/del(4q) case (right recombinant offspring) the phenotype resembles the partial 4p trisomy syndrome. The normal chromosome 4 contributed by the other parent is shown grayed out. The 4q segment is so small (indicated by the dots) that it might not make a major contribution, whether duplicated or deleted, to the phenotypes. (Case of Hirsch and Baldinger 1993.)

effect, and the effective "single-segment" imbalances of dup(13)(q22qter) and del(13)(q22qter) are each well known to be viable. Applying the principles of "private segregation analysis" as set out in Chapter 4, the risk for a recombinant form in this family comes to a high 50%. We emphasize again the point that, while the length of the inverted segment may influence the likelihood of recombination happening, it is actually the combined genetic content of the *distal* segments that is the direct determinant of viability of the recombinant form.

During the period 1981–1995, more than 50 papers were published which reported the birth (or prenatal diagnosis) of offspring having a recombinant chromosome that derived from a parental pericentric inversion. In their review of this body of literature, and adding a family of their own, Ishii et al. (1997) determined the involvement of specific chromosomal segments. Figure 9–9, which is taken from their paper, depicts the combinations of dup+del genotypes that have been associated with viability. A few of these, which are shown asterisked, were identified at prenatal diagnosis, and in those with no known postnatal case, viability through to term remains unproven. A glance at the figure is enough to see that the gaps—that is, the inverted

segments—are generally longer, and usually a lot longer, than the sum of the lengths of the two noninverted segments. This serves to illustrate again the point that inversions with large inverted segments are, as a rule, the ones with the greatest genetic risk. It is also to be observed that the thick bars (representing duplications) are mostly longer than the thin bars (deletions), a reflection of the preferential viability of the least monosomic combination. The individual autosomal inversions from this review are recorded in Table 9–2.

Inversions with very small distal segments may stretch the limits of classical cytogenetic detection. Biesecker et al. (1995) describe an inv(22) with the long arm breakpoint in subtelomeric 22q, with the terminal 23–30 centimorgans of 22q now attached to 22p, which required molecular analysis and FISH for its identification. Due to the relative lack of G-band landmarks in 22q, and the normal variation that occurs with 22p, the defect was not recognized on a 450-band cytogenetic study. The mother carrying this inversion would have had, presumably, a risk approaching 50% to have a further abnormal recombinant child. Another inv(22) of interest is that described in Boyd et al. (2005), 46,XX,inv(22)(p13q13.1). This rearrangement,

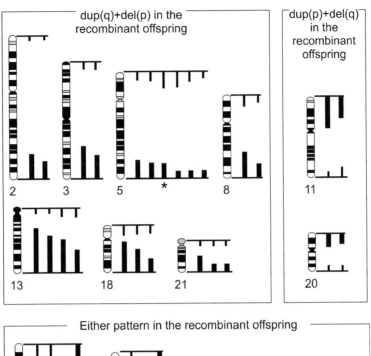

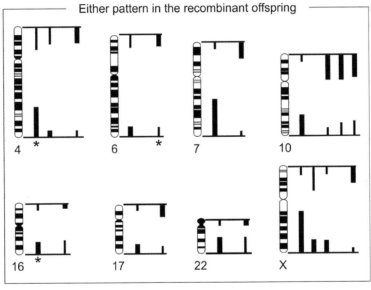

| deleted segments | ▮ duplicated segments |

FIGURE 9–9   Viable recombinants from 55 recorded parental pericentric inversion chromosomes. The pairs of bars alongside each chromosome ideogram, one thick and one thin, show the noninverted segments. The thick bars indicate which is the duplicated segment, and the thin bars the deleted segment, in the recombinant offspring. The detail of the actual breakpoints is set out in Table 9–2. The inversions are grouped according to those chromosomes in which a dup(q) + del(p) is consistently seen in the recombinant offspring (*above left*), those in which a dup(p) + del(q) is consistently seen (*above right*), and those in which either pattern may be observed (*below*). Most of these recombinants had been reported in only one or a few cases, with the notable exception of the inv(8)(p23q22), observed on 54 occasions. Asterisks indicate that a case had been diagnosed prenatally; the inv(4)(p13q28) and the inv(5)(p13q33) had been seen only at prenatal diagnosis, so viability to term is not proven in these cases.

Source: From Ishii et al., Case report of rec(7)dup(7q)inv(7)(p22q22) and a review of the recombinants resulting from parental pericentric inversions on any chromosomes, *Am J Med Genet* 73:290–295, 1997. Courtesy F. Ishii, and with the permission of Wiley-Liss.

Table 9–2. Autosomal Pericentric Inversions Associated with the Birth of a Recombinant Offspring, Listed in "Numerical" Order

CHROMOSOME	INVERSIONS		
1	p36.21q42.13		
2	p25q35	p25.3q33.3	
3	p25q23	p25q25[a]	
4	p13q28	p15.32q35	
5	p13q33	p13q35	p14q35
	p15q32	p15.1q33.3	p15.1q35.1[a]
	p15.3q35		
6	p23q27	p23.07q25.13	
7	p14.2q36.3	p15q36	p15.1q36
	p22q22		
8	p23q22[a,b]	p23.3q24.1	
9	p24.3q34.1		
10	p11q26	p11.2q25.2[a]	p12q25
	p15q24		
11	p11q25	p13q23.3	p15.3q24.1
12	p13q24.3		
13	p11q21	p11q22	p12q13
	p12q14	p13q21[a]	p13q31
14	p12q31		
16	p13q22	p13.1q22	
17	p11q25	p13.3q25.1	
18	p11q11	p11.2q12.2	p11.2q21.3
19	p13.3q13.33		
20	p11.2q13.3	p12q13.3	p13q13.1
	p13q13.33		
21	p11q21.09	p11.2q22.1	p12q22
22	p11q21	p11.2q13.31	p13q12[a]
	p13q12.2		

Notes: Inversions listed here are from 55 families, published over the period 1981–2012. These comprise the cases reviewed in Ishii et al. (1997); the case illustrated in Figure 9–5; and more recent cases in Lagier-Tourenne et al. (2004), Mehra et al. (2005), Grange et al. (2005), Schluth-Bolard et al. (2008), Tagaya et al. (2008), Stevens et al. (2009), Honeywell et al. (2012), Mundhofir et al. (2012), Putoux et al. (2013), and Sgardioli et al. (2013).

[a]Reported in more than one family.

[b]Associated with San Luis Valley syndrome.

in contrast, was very easy to detect, in that the inverted segment involved about half of the long arm and was attached to the particularly long stalk region of the short arm. The stalk region was probably the site of the meiotic recombination which

gave rise to her abnormal child with 46,XX,rec(22) dup(22q)inv(22)mat.

Effect upon Fertility. Uncommonly, the inversion heterozygote can be infertile (Groupe de Cytogénéticiens Français 1986b; De Braekeleer and Dao 1991). Abnormal synapsis of the chromosome pair can affect cellular mechanics at meiosis in the male, more likely if the inversion involves a larger chromosome, in consequence arresting spermatogenesis (Gabriel-Robez and Rumpler 1994). Meschede et al. (1994), for example, describe azoöspermic brothers, one with histologically documented arrest at the level of the primary spermatocyte, and each heterozygous for an inv(1)(p34q23) inherited from their female parent. The counselor may be intrigued to learn of the role of a gene familiar in a different setting, namely, *BRCA1*: The BRCA1 protein may co-locate on the unsynapsed regions of meiotic chromosomes, and this is associated with maturation arrest. Kirkpatrick et al. (2012) showed BRCA1 staining on the inversion segment of an inv(1)(p21q31) in a man who had presented with azoöspermia.

Parental Mosaicism. Mosaicism for a (balanced) inversion is rarely recognized. Lazzaro et al. (2001) describe a mother with 46,XX,inv(21)(p12q21.1)[19]/ 46,XX[11] on blood karyotyping, who had a child with a partial form of Down syndrome. The child's karyotype was nonmosaic 46,XX,rec(21)dup(21q) inv(21)(p12q21.1)mat. Given the mother's karyotype was from a peripheral blood sample, and she having had a recombinant child, clearly enough this is a case of somatic-gonadal mosaicism.

Pericentric Inversions Frequently Innocuous. Many pericentric inversions are not associated with any discernible reproductive problems. The families of Voiculescu et al. (1986) and Rivas et al. (1987) are not atypical: an inversion chromosome transmitted through several generations, with numerous carriers identified, and no difference between the offspring of carriers, and those of noncarriers, in the incidences of abortion and neonatal death.

Interchromosomal Effect. Some pericentric inversions have been discovered in the setting of a child with an aneuploidy such as trisomy 21, and "interchromosomal effect" has been invoked (Groupe de Cytogénéticiens Français 1985b). More likely, these associations are fortuitous: Sperm studies endorse this inference (Anton et al. 2002; Mikhaail-Philips et al. 2004).

RARE COMPLEXITIES

The range within the rubric "complex inversion" is wide indeed, and we cannot do justice here. We may consider the case in Manolakos et al. (2013) as just one representative example. A father carried a rearranged chromosome 2, in which (*1*) there was a paracentric inversion, inv(2)(p13p23), and adjacent to this, (*2*) a between-arm insertion, ins(2)(2p23;2q14.1q21.2). His child, in whom the phenotype was severe, inherited a rec(2), conveying a 20 Mb deletion of 2q14.1q21.2, and a 5.6 Mb duplication of 2p22.3p22.2.

Collectors of remarkable cases will find fascinating the report of Alderdice et al. (1991). They studied a kindred (mentioned also above) with a segregating inv(3)(p25q21), which originated from a couple marrying in 1817, and which was quite widely spread over the maritime provinces of Canada and other parts of eastern Canada and the northeastern United States. In the course of the study, a normal man was found to have two recombinant 3 chromosomes: one with a dup(q)+del(p), and the other with a complementary dup(p)+del(q), such that his karyotype was balanced. Presumably, both of his (distantly consanguineous) parents were inv(3)(p25q21) heterozygotes, and one produced one recombinant gamete, and the other the other. Similarly, Kariminejad et al. (2011) document a consanguineous couple each heterozygous for inv(18)(p11.31q21.33), who produced a child with a complementary recombinant karyotype—dup(18p)/del(18q) from one parent, dup(18q)/del(18p) from the other—of normal phenotype, and in whom analysis showed segmental upd(mat) for 18p and segmental upd(pat) for 18q.[2]

Consanguinity may lead to homozygosity for the (nonrecombined) inversion chromosome. This might be without harm, unless there has been genetic mischief at an inversion breakpoint. Jones et al. (2013) report a couple 46,XY,inv(5)(p15.1q14.1) and 46,XX,inv(5)(p15.1q14.1), whose homozygous inv(5) child had the blood disorder Hermansky-Pudlak syndrome, due to homozygosity for disruption of the relevant gene (*AP3B1*) at the 5q14.1 breakpoint. In the inversion inv(7)(p15q21) studied in Watson et al. (2016), the 7p15 breakpoint is close to (523 kb upstream of) the *HOXA13* gene. Consanguineous parents produced a homozygous inv(7) child with the hand-foot-uterus syndrome, typically an autosomal dominant disorder. It may be that a displaced enhancer of *HOXA13*, in the homozygous state in the child, sufficed to compromise gene activity, while having been without effect in the heterozygous parents.

The Pericentric Inversion X

Pericentric inversions of the X are rare indeed, and of 23 examples reviewed in Ramírez-Velasco and Rivera (2014), only seven were known to be familial; a further familial case is in Chen et al. (2016b). The inv(X) can be transmitted both by the male and by the female carrier. Baumann et al. (1984) and Schorderet et al. (1991), for example, describe families with an inv(X) transmitted through four generations, with all carriers—female heterozygotes and male hemizygotes—being phenotypically normal. Demonstrably unimpaired fertility is evidenced in the carrier matriarch of the family of Madariaga and Rivera (1997) (Figure 9–10). The X inversion forms in the same way as an autosomal inversion, but the implications may differ. This is because (*1*) breakpoints in certain parts of the X (its critical region) may have an influence on the phenotype of the female; (*2*) X chromosomal imbalance in the 46,X,rec(X) female may be mitigated by selective inactivation of the abnormal X; and (*3*) the 46,Y,rec(X) conceptus will have a partial X nullisomy and functional X disomy. The female and male inv(X) carrier need to be discussed separately.

THE FEMALE INV(X) HETEROZYGOTE

Outwardly, the female heterozygote is normal, and not infrequently may be of normal fertility. The concept of "position effect" is of practical importance in the context of X rearrangement. If the long arm breakpoint lies within the segment Xq13q22 or Xq22q26, gonadal dysfunction may occur, but by no means invariably (Therman et al. 1990), as Figure 9–10 illustrates. There may be primary amenorrhea; or, after a fertile period in early adulthood, a premature menopause. Meiosis in the fertile carrier

---

2 These authors raise the intriguing theoretical point that continuing inbreeding in a region with a high prevalence of such a rearrangement could lead to several homozygous individuals being the beginning of a "new" species.

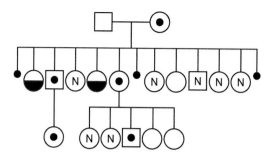

FIGURE 9–10   Pedigree of a kindred segregating an inv(X)(p22q22). Carriers have bull's-eye symbol; two women with gonadal dysgenesis and 46,X,rec(X)dup(Xp)inv(X)(p22q22) have half-filled symbol; normal karyotype shown as N; no annotation, not tested; black dot, miscarriage. The fertility of the heterozygous matriarch is very evident.

Source: From Madariaga and Rivera (1997).

would be expected to proceed according to one of the preceding scenarios (Figures 9–4 and 9–6), with recombination within the inverted segment a possibility.

Prima facie, we presume that an ovum with a normal X or the intact (nonrecombinant) inv(X) would produce a normal child, whether male or female. In the case of the male, this would require there to have been no compromise of loci at the breakpoints, and evidence of normality in the male in another family member would be reassuring. A hemizygous son would typically be of normal fertility. If, in the family, the balanced inversion is associated with normal gonadal function in the female, a heterozygous daughter would be expected to have, likewise, normal puberty, fertility, and menopause at the usual time. This family information may not be accessible (or may not exist). In the family of Soler et al. (1981), for example, a hemizygous father, 46,Y,inv(X)(p22q13), had three sons and three daughters—each daughter, of course, an obligate heterozygote. He, apparently, had no gonadal deficiency, but his two older daughters had menopause at ages 37 and 34 years (the youngest was only 30 years old). There was no family history recorded antecedent to him.

An ovum carrying a recombinant X would have two very different results, depending on whether it is fertilized by an X- or a Y-bearing sperm, as follows.

The 46,X,rec(X) Conceptus. In their review, Madariaga and Rivera (1997) record outcomes in recombinant cases in 10 families. The del(Xq)/dup(Xp) combination is, in female offspring, characterized by normal or tall stature, and ovarian dysgenesis. The countertype, del(Xp)/

dup(Xq), is associated with short stature and, in some, intact ovarian function. These phenotypes presumably reflect the loss of stature genes (in particular *SHOX*) located on Xp, and ovarian genes located on Xq, respectively. Any effect of the concomitant duplication is, presumably, mitigated by selective inactivation of the recombinant X chromosome. There is no obvious effect upon intellect.

Consider the case presented by Buckton et al. (1981) (Figure 9–11). One of the breakpoints is at the tip of the short arm, and the other is in proximal Xq. The recombinant chromosome, with a deficiency of the tip of Xp and a duplication of distal Xq (Figure 9–11, lower right), was, in this family, associated only with shortness of stature. The partial Xq trisomy made no discernible contribution to the phenotype. A 26-year-old mother with the rec(X) herself had a rec(X) daughter—unarguable evidence that oögenesis had not (at least by age 26 years) been compromised. A more recent case, with the countertype Xp/Xq imbalance, and having molecular study, is reported in Kim et al. (2014): a woman with premature ovarian failure who had the karyotype 46,XX,rec(X)dup(Xp)inv(X)(p22.3q27.3) from a maternal inv(X), the Xp duplication involving chrX:pter-8.9 Mb, and the Xq deletion, chrX: 145.9-qter Mb.

The 46,Y,rec(X) Conceptus. There will be a nullisomy for the deficient X segment. If this segment constitutes any but the tiniest length of chromatin, the conceptus would not be viable. Nullisomy for a tiny telomeric segment may be viable, but with major dysmorphogenesis and severe neurodevelopmental compromise. Furthermore, the concomitant

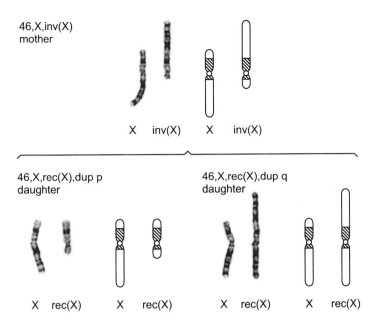

46,X,inv(X)
mother

X   inv(X)   X   inv(X)

46,X,rec(X),dup p
daughter

46,X,rec(X),dup q
daughter

X   rec(X)   X   rec(X)   X   rec(X)   X   rec(X)

FIGURE 9–11 X chromosome inversion. The mother (*above*) has the karyotype 46,X,inv(X)(p22q13). *Below*, The two possible unbalanced reproductive outcomes in daughters, following recombination within the inverted segment; the normal X on the left in each has been contributed by the father. Each type of daughter would have a variant form of Turner syndrome. Male recombinant conceptuses are not shown: The combination of X nullisomy and functional X disomy in the 46,Y,rec(X) conceptus would in this instance be lethal in utero. (Case of Buckton et al. 1981.)

disomy X is functional, not being subject to inactivation, and therefore of itself produces a major deleterious effect. For example, the carrier mother in Chen et al. (2016b), 46,X,inv(X)(p22.3q26.3), had an abnormal ultrasound, and amniocentesis showed 46,Y,rec(X)dup(Xq)inv(X)(p22.3q26.3); at 24-week termination, fetal defects were observed. She had a second pregnancy, amniocentesis showing the inversion in a male, 46,Y,inv(X) (p22.3q26.3); the baby boy was born prematurely but did well.

THE MALE INV(X) HEMIZYGOTE

In the male carrier (as the baby boy just mentioned, in the fullness of time), the rearrangement apparently has no effect on phenotype or on reproduction. Meiosis proceeds unperturbed (rather obviously, there can be no recombination within the inverted segment). All his daughters will be heterozygotes. Many will have normal gonadal function, although a family history of premature ovarian failure might predict the same problem. Sons receive his normal Y and their mother's (normal) X chromosome, to become 46,XY.

The Pericentric Inversion Y

A pericentric inversion of the Y, inv(Y) (p11.2q11.23), is not uncommon in the general population (Verma et al. 1982; Tóth et al. 1984). Three major forms are recognized, types I–III, with differing Yq breakpoints, the Yp site being constant (Knebel et al. 2011). Types I and II, inv(Y) (p11.2q11.23) as noted above, typically have no phenotypic effect, and imply no risk for having an abnormal child; these may be regarded as normal variants. The type III, inv(Y)(p11.2q11.223), which splits the DAZ and CDY fertility gene cluster in AZFc, may be associated with infertility.

UNBALANCED DE NOVO APPARENT RECOMBINANT FROM AN INV

Rivera et al. (2013) studied a number of cases, ascertained either pre- or postnatally, in which a rec-like chromosome—that is, deleted for a p segment and duplicated for a q segment, or vice versa—was found. This might have raised a question of a gonadal mosaicism for an inversion in the mother, and thus have implied an important genetic risk. But in fact, they could show that the typical mechanism was that of a nonallelic homologous recombination, which spoke for a sporadic, one-off, meiotic generation.

GENETIC COUNSELING

The Autosomal Pericentric Inversion

Variant Forms. The not uncommon inv(2) (p11.2q13), a very small pericentric inversion, is practically always innocuous (Hysert et al. 2006; Ferfouri et al. 2009). Two possible exceptions are on record to belie its reputation: two abnormal children, one with a 2p duplication and the other a 2p deletion, the proximal boundary at or adjacent to 2p11.2, and the fathers being inversion heterozygotes, described as inv(2)(p11.2q12.2) and inv(2)(p11.2q13), respectively (Magee et al. 1998a; Lacbawan et al. 1999). It may be that the configurations adopted by the chromosome 2 homologs led to an unequal crossing-over, and hence the duplication or deletion. With only two such observations of recombination in the decades of history of clinical cytogenetics, some circumspection is required, and Lacbawan et al.'s comment that "at this point, it seems premature to recommend prenatal diagnosis of all couples in this situation" is perfectly reasonable.

No genetic risks are known to be associated with the other inversion variants noted in the "Biology" section: "inversions" of 1, 9, 16, and Y heterochromatin, and inv(3)(p11-13q11-12), inv(5) (p13q13), and inv(10)(p11.2q21.2). Concerning the inv(10)(p11.2q21.1), Collinson et al. (1997) offer the practical advice that "family investigation of carrier status is not warranted in view of the unnecessary concern this may cause family members." We exclude these inversion variants from the discussion below.

RISKS OF HAVING AN ABNORMAL CHILD

Ascertainment via Recombinant Child. Identification of a family through a recombinant individual proves the viability of at least one of the two recombinant chromosomes. Table 9–2 lists a large number of different inversions for which a carrier is known to have had a recombinant child. There have been various empiric estimates of the overall level of risk to the heterozygote in families ascertained through an abnormal child. From a number of studies, a consensus range for the usual risk to have a liveborn abnormal child due to recombination is 5%–15% (Groupe de Cytogénéticiens Français 1986b; Sherman et al. 1986; Stene 1986; Daniel et al. 1989). As a general rule, the longer the inversion segment—and, consequently, the shorter the distal segments—the greater the risk to produce a viable recombinant gamete. Very long inversions, such as that in Roberts et al. (1989), an inv(10) that comprised 80% of the whole chromosome, or the inv(20) in Stevens et al. (2009) comprising 94%, would imply the highest risks: in these particular cases, two out of the inv(10) carrier father's three children were recombinant, and all three of the inv(20) carrier mother's children were recombinant. At least in theory, as the inverted segment approaches maximum size, the risk of a viable recombinant gamete will approach 50% (Luo et al. 2014). For the majority of families, there is probably no risk difference depending on sex of heterozygote (Kaiser 1984; Stene 1986); but in some families, the female heterozygote may run a greater genetic risk (Sutherland et al. 1976; Pai et al. 1987). Indeed, for the inv(21)(p12q21.1), recombinant children (with dup(21q), and thus a partial form of Down syndrome) have been seen only where it is the mother who is the carrier parent (Lazzaro et al. 2001).

Each individual inversion carries its own individual risk. This may be arrived at by analyzing the patient's family, studying the literature, and assessing the degrees of imbalance potentially arising in the recombinant conceptuses.

A specific figure has been derived for one relatively common inversion, inv(8)(p23q22), from which the rec(8)dup(8q)inv(8)(p23.1q22.1) form leads to the "San Luis Valley syndrome." This reflects a presumed founder effect[3] in an Hispanic population in southern Colorado and northern New Mexico, albeit that the same condition is also seen elsewhere (Graw et al. 2000; Vera-Carbonell et al. 2013). The risk for liveborn recombinant offspring, all of whom would have this del(p)/dup(q) form, is 6.2%, for both maternal and paternal transmission (Smith et al. 1987). This compares closely with the figure of 6%–7% of sperm with the del(p)/dup(q) form (Table 9–1), attesting to an essentially

---

3 Another example of founder effect is reported from the Guadalajara region of Mexico, from whence there have been reported a number of cases of rec(22)dup(22q) due to a parental inv(22)(p13q12.2) (Tonk et al. 2004).

uncompromised viability of the unbalanced embryo. In contrast, the countertype dup(p)/del(q) recombinant, which is seen in 6% of sperm, is never seen in liveborn offspring, reflecting zero viability.

Concerning chromosome 18, Lustosa-Mendes et al. (2017) reviewed the literature: a heterogeneous material, with inversion breakpoints variously at p11.2 or p11.3, and at q11, q12, q21, q22, or q23. A total of 37% of offspring in 18 families had either the del/dup or the dup/del combination; but adjusting for ascertainment bias (a little bluntly, by removing one proband in each family), the overall risk figure is 19%. This is still a high figure, presumably reflecting the viability of many of the recombinant forms. In due course, figures may be determined for other inversions seen in more than one family, such as the inv(3)(p25q21), inv(4)(p14q35), inv(10)(p11q25), inv(13)(p13q21), and inv(21)(p12q21.1). The precision that molecular analysis allows will enable subtler distinctions to be drawn, such as Starr et al. (2014) illustrate in comparing with earlier reports their patient with a rec(20) due to a parental inv(20)(p13q13.12).

The risks to produce abnormal offspring from pericentric inversions in an acrocentric chromosome are again dependent on the size of the inversion, but in this case only the long arm segment needs to be considered; and rather than a composite del/dup imbalance, a recombinant chromosome would simply convey, in functional essence, either a dup(q), for a partial trisomy, or a del(q), for a partial monosomy. A loss or gain of the p arm material would be without phenotypic consequence. The risk associated with a large inversion, with the q arm breakpoint sited distally, may therefore be particularly high; whereas a small inversion would, as typically, convey the least, and, for chromosomes 14 and 15, a practically zero risk (Leach et al. 2005).

No Family History of Recombinant Form. For families identified by means other than through the birth of an abnormal child (e.g., discovered fortuitously at prenatal diagnosis), the overall risk is—for what this figure is worth—about 1%. The individual risk, which is what really matters, depends on the actual inversion. Is the inversion chromosome on record (Table 9–2) as being associated with viable imbalance? Or does the inversion segment include and extend beyond the inversion segment of one of these recorded cases? In that circumstance, a significant risk surely does apply. Is the inversion segment much shorter in length than

any of those listed in Table 9-2? Here, the risk may be as low as zero. The level of risk can be assessed from a study of the family, noting the reproductive histories of other heterozygotes, and from a consideration of the degrees of potential imbalance in a conceptus. As a rule, any chromosome with a short inversion segment (less than one-third of the chromosome's length) is most unlikely ever to lead to a viable recombinant product (Kaiser 1988; Morel et al. 2007).

Nevertheless, one should determine the composition of the theoretically possible recombinant gametes and gauge whether the resulting partial trisomy and partial monosomy might be viable. This applies in particular to inversions of chromosomes 13, 18, and 21, partial trisomies and partial monosomies of these chromosomes being well recognized as viable. If, in any inversion chromosome, one breakpoint is very close to the telomere, one recombinant form will impose very little partial monosomy. The contribution of the duplication can then be assessed essentially on its own, and reference to the viability of this segment in other cytogenetic contexts (translocation, de novo rearrangement) will likely provide a valid comparison. For example, had the father in Figure 9–5 been identified before he had had children, we could have deduced that the rec(7)dup(7p) genotype might survive to term, knowing that the databases of Stene and Stengel-Rutkowski (1988) and Schinzel (2001) record a viable phenotype for trisomy 7p14pter.

Prenatal or preimplantation diagnosis should be offered to the following people:

1. Any heterozygote in whose family a recombinant child has been born.
2. A heterozygote for any of the inversions listed in Table 9–2.
3. A heterozygote for an inversion involving a segment longer than, but including, a region listed in Table 9–2.
4. Any other heterozygote for whom the theoretical recombinant product(s) might be viable. Many inversions of chromosomes 13, 18, and 21 will fall into this category.
5. Molecular analysis to exclude deletion in the Prader-Willi/Angelman region of 15q11q13 may be appropriate in an inversion having a breakpoint within or adjacent to this segment.

Of the phenotypically normal offspring, approximately half will have normal chromosomes, and half will be inversion heterozygotes (Groupe de Cytogénéticiens Français 1986b). A question of "transmission distortion," whereby the 50/50 ratio is skewed, has been proposed in some inversions (Honeywell et al. 2012; Lustosa-Mendes et al. 2017).

A risk to the child for some other rearrangement than the classic recombination (see above, "Deletion or Duplication at Inversion Breakpoint") we presume to be very small, likely well under ½%, and prenatal molecular analysis targeted to the breakpoint regions would not normally be warranted. A question of interchromosomal effect appears not to be an issue.

The Inversion X

The female heterozygote could have a premature menopause, if the long arm breakpoint is in the critical region, and if there is a family history of early ovarian failure; and pragmatic advice might be to have children sooner rather than later. But normal reproductive function is perfectly possible. Recombination may be less likely than for an autosomal inversion (Pinto Leite and Pinto 2001), although a risk to produce an abnormal daughter with a recombinant X does, certainly, exist. The abnormality is, to some extent, predictable according to the deleted segment, Xp or Xq: Short stature is typically seen in del(Xp), and ovarian failure in del(Xq). Hemizygous sons would be expected to be normal, and reassurance in this respect may be drawn from the observation, if it can be made, of normality in a male relative. For the most part, no practical risk exists for having an abnormal son, because recombinant male conceptuses, having partial X nullisomy and disomy, would be nonviable. Only when the breakpoints are very close to the telomere is male viability possible, and such a child would have major physical abnormalities and mental retardation, probably severe. Due to this male lethality, the sex ratio of the offspring would, in theory, be 1 male:2 females.

All daughters of the male heterozygote would be inv(X) heterozygotes. Other things being equal, they will be phenotypically normal. If the long arm breakpoint is in the "critical region," and if heterozygous female relatives have had ovarian deficiency (e.g., primary amenorrhea, premature menopause), they may develop the same problem. All sons would have a 46,XY karyotype.

The Inversion Y

This inversion is generally considered a normal population variant of no clinical significance. It is self-evident that all the sons of the inv(Y) carrier will be, themselves, inv(Y) carriers. They are all normal and, other things being equal, have normal gonadal function. All the daughters would be 46,XX.

THE PARACENTRIC INVERSION

BIOLOGY

DETAILS OF MEIOTIC BEHAVIOR

According to classical theory, the phenotypically normal heterozygote for an *autosomal* paracentric inversion will only have children who are karyotypically normal, or with the same balanced inversion. They cannot have viable unbalanced progeny. If a recombinant gamete is formed following a crossover in the inverted segment, the chromosome would be either acentric (lacking a centromere) or dicentric (Figure 9–12). An acentric chromosome is never viable, since it lacks a point of attachment to the spindle fibers. The dicentric is generally considered a lethal impediment, being attached to spindle fibers pulling in opposite directions, with the chromosome thus suspended between the daughter nuclei at telophase, and excluded from either cell. If the dicentric were to rupture, however, the possibility theoretically exists for a product (this might be, effectively, a dup+del chromosome) to enter the

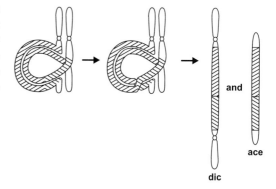

and

ace

dic

FIGURE 9–12   Theoretical recombinant products from classical crossover in paracentric inversion. One is acentric (ace), and the other dicentric (dic). The inversion segment is shown cross-hatched, and the different directions of cross-hatching indicate the parts proximal and distal to the crossover point.

zygote and to be viable. Alternatively, if the dicentric were to be included in the nucleus of a gamete, McClintock's classical breakage-fusion-bridge cycle might impose an eventually insuperable obstacle to continuing cell division, as the chromosome is tugged in two directions by its two centromeres in succeeding mitoses after formation of the zygote. The possible scenarios are more fully dealt with in Madan (1995).

What are the findings on direct observation of gametes? In brief, recombination is scarcely ever seen. Anton et al. (2005) review the small total of five sperm studies, with inversion segments ranging from 6% to 32%. The fractions of recombinant sperm ranged from zero to 0.81%. The study with the largest number of cells analyzed (8,158) had a recombinant rate of 0.03%, with this particular rearrangement described as inv(4)(p14p15.3). The inversion with the largest inverted segment in this series, inv(14)(q24.1q32.1), was analyzed by karyotyping in 120 sperm, and none of them showed a recombinant (Martin 1999). Exceptionally, however, an inv(2)(q21.2q37.3), the largest (103 Mb) paracentric inversion on record, was associated with a much higher fraction of abnormal sperm, 28%, in a man who had presented with infertility and repeated failure of implantation at in vitro fertilization (Yapan et al. 2014). Presumably, the large size of the inversion, comprising about three-quarters of 2q, meant that formation of an inversion loop was not hindered, and recombination possible.

Brown et al. (1998) analyzed 282 sperm from a man with a paracentric inversion, 46,inv(9)(q32q34.3), whose wife had had a number of miscarriages (they had also had two children). Recombination was suppressed in the inversion segment; but, notably, of the five recombination events within the segment that were observed, each involved at least two crossovers. Brown et al. suggested the following mechanism. Synapsis, which starts at the telomere, advances along the chromatids, and then encounters a region of heterosynapsis and "stalls." This stalling allows an increase in recombination in the chromatid regions that are already synapsed. Synapsis eventually advances past the inversion segment and continues toward the centromere. But within the inversion segment itself, an "active search" for homology goes on, which may require the chromatids to take on a particular configuration (such as a microloop), and this may set up a hot spot for recombination. Only rare double recombinants from this setting would be able to form morphologically normal chromosomes, with sperm that would then be able to continue along their process of maturation; sperm with a single recombination would be acentric or dicentric.

Meiosis in oögenesis commences during fetal life, and its study therefore requires access to fetal tissue. Cheng et al. (1999) analyzed ovarian tissue from a 19-week termination of pregnancy, in which a de novo inv(7)(q11.23q21.2) had been shown at amniocentesis. By using a FISH probe for the Williams syndrome critical region (WSCR), which is at 7q11.23, they could determine whether the inverted segments were aligned alongside each other (homosynapsis) or not (heterosynapsis). Most cells showed the chromosome 7 homologs lined up side by side, but with the WSCR signals off from each other: Thus, the inversion segment was unaligned. A classical inversion loop was seen in only 10% of cells. This example, concerning a small inversion segment, offers an explanation for the rarity with which recombinant forms are seen: The necessary prerequisite of homosynapsis may often not be attained.

RECOMBINATION/REUNION WITH VIABLE PRODUCTS

Classical theory remains valid in essence, some exceptions notwithstanding. The abnormal process of "U-loop recombination" (Feldman et al. 1993; Mitchell et al. 1994) is a mutational event, not a predictable consequence of a "normal" meiotic process (albeit in a chromosome that is abnormal). *Reunitant* may be a better word than *recombinant*. The crossover within the inversion loop, instead of continuing on in the same direction along the chromatid, reverses upon itself as a "U-loop." The mechanism is illustrated in Figure 9–13. According to this construction, the resulting reunitant chromosomes would have either a duplication of that part of the inversion loop proximal to the crossover, and a deletion of that part distal to it, or vice versa. A crossover (or, rather, chromatid breakage with abnormal reunion) at one of the entry points to the loop would produce a duplication alone, or a deletion alone.

Feldman et al. (1993) review the inversion duplication (inv dup) chromosome, and notably, of the

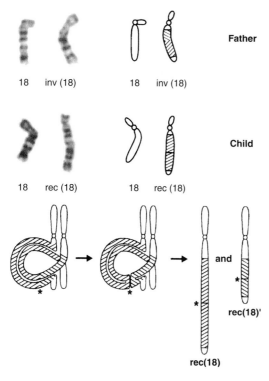

Father

Child

rec(18)'

and

rec(18)

FIGURE 9–13 *Above*, parent with paracentric inversion and child with recombinant ("reunitant") chromosome. Father has paracentric inversion of 18q, inv(18)(q12.1q23). The inverted segment is shown cross-hatched (cross-hatching changes slope at q21.3). Child has duplication of the segment q12.1q21.3 on the reuniting chromosome (shown cross-hatched) and deletion q21.3q23. (Case of N. L. Chia and L. R. Bousfield.) *Below*, Proposed mechanism of U-loop exchange depicted; asterisk indicates point of U-loop. The position of the point of exchange within the inversion loop (in this case, q21.3) determines the nature of the imbalance. There is duplication of chromatin proximal to the crossover point (q12.1q21.3), and deletion of distal chromatin (q21.3q23), as in the child's rec(18); and vice versa in the complementary product, rec(18)'. (An alternative interpretation is that the father's rearrangement is a within-arm insertion of 18q, rather than an inversion, in which case the karyotype of the child would have been derived from recombination in the inserted segment.)

six familial cases on record, five may have been due to presumed U-type reunitant from a maternal paracentric inversion. Chia et al. (1992) describe a case that quite probably reflected the same mechanism, a man with 46,inv(18)(q12.1q23) who had a child with

a duplication/deletion 18q syndrome due to a presumed rec(18)(pter→q21.3::q21.3→q12.1::q23→qter) chromosome, as shown in Figure 9–13. Another very similar inv(18) case is noted in Hani et al. (1995). In their exhaustive review, Pettenati et al. (1995) collected about a dozen similar cases. These cases represented offspring in 3.8% of their series of 446 paracentric inversions; but since all of these offspring were probands, and some we actually doubt were truly paracentric "reunitants," we presume the actual reproductive risk due to U-loop reunion or other abnormal process would be a much smaller figure (Sutherland et al. 1995). Madan and Nieuwint (2002) pursue this question, and show that indeed most "paracentric inversions" found through a recombinant child were really insertions.

Classical theory needs also to accommodate the phenomenon of centromere suppression, which, extremely rarely, can allow the basically dicentric recombinant to function stably as, in effect, a monocentric (or "pseudodicentric"). The chromosome attaches to the spindle fiber at only one centromere, the other being nonfunctional or suppressed; thus, no fusion-bridge cycle is initiated. "Extremely rarely" could, at this writing, be defined as four recorded cases from an autosomal paracentric inversion. Mules and Stamberg (1984) describe an infant dying as a neonate with a rec(14) whose mother had an inv(14)(q24.2q32.3); Worsham et al. (1989) studied in considerable detail a child with a rec(9) from a maternal inv(9)(q22.1q34.3); Whiteford et al. (2000) report a dysmorphic infant with growth and neurodevelopmental retardation and having a major heart defect, with the karyotype 46,XY,rec(15)(pter→q26.3::q11.2→pter)inv(15) (q11.2q26.3)mat; and Lefort et al. (2002) describe an abnormal child in whose dicentric rec(14) chromosome one centromere could be demonstrated to have been inactivated, the mother's karyotype being 46,XX,inv(14)(q13q32.2). These four cases share the features of a large inversion involving most or almost all of a long arm, and with the short arms (14p, 9p, 15p, and 13p, respectively) being genetically "small": In other words, the dup p+q/del q combination might not impose a lethal imbalance. Only in this setting, and if the chromosome were stable, could recombination cause an imbalance due to a dicentric chromosome, that would be viable and allow the birth of an abnormal child.

A mechanism reminiscent of paracentric inversion U-loop reunion may be the cause of some isochromosome Xq Turner syndrome (Wolff et al. 1996). Two zinc-finger genes (*ZXDA* and *ZXDB*) in proximal Xp, just above the centromere, have about 98% homology and transcribe in opposite directions. In X-to-X synapsis in some meioses, a small inversion loop in proximal Xp might enable *ZXDA* (the more centromeric locus) in one Xp to match up with *ZXDB* on the other Xp, and vice versa. Then, a breakage and U-loop reunion between the two ZXD loci would generate an isodicentric chromosome Xqter→cen→*ZXDA*::*ZXDA*→cen→Xqter. Similar events at other loci may underlie other Xq isochromosomes (Giglio et al. 2000).

A minuscule number of cases of other sorts of viable recombinant offspring are known (Worsham et al. 1989). A dicentric recombinant chromosome, pulled in two directions, may rupture and yield a deletion. This may be the mechanism in the case in Courtens et al. (1998), in which a mother with 46,XX,inv(18)(q21.1q22.3) had monozygotic twins with a deletion of the segment distal to the inversion (q22.3qter), and duplication of a small part proximal to it (q12.1q21.1). In Figure 9–13, although the scale is not right for this example, it could be imagined that a break occurred in the dicentric recombinant chromosome just above the lower centromere. South et al. (2006) describe a 46,XX,inv(5)(p13.3p15.3) parent who had a child with del(5)(p14.3) cri-du-chat syndrome, which was likely due to a dicentric recombinant chromosome having ruptured in the middle of the inversion segment.

A different mechanism is that the abnormal synapsis could set up a milieu that enables an unequal crossing-over at the base of an inversion loop due to an imperfect alignment of homologous segments, a format initially proposed by Hoo et al. (1982). The rearranged chromosome would be monocentric. Yang et al. (1997) propose such a scenario in a family in which the index child had the deletion 46,XY,del(17)(p11.2p11.2), while the father and two aunts carried the paracentric inversion 46,inv(17)(p11.2p13). The deletion removed the Smith-Magenis region. This was "the first unequivocal demonstration by molecular analysis that a parent who carries a paracentric inversion is capable of having a

viable child with an unbalanced monocentric recombinant chromosome." Paskulin et al. (2011) relate a similar story: a child with a deletion in 7q31.32q33 (chr7:113.1-136.3 Mb) at the base of the presumed meiotic inversion loop, from a maternal 46,XX,inv(7) (q11.23q33), this being quite a large inversion segment, about two-thirds of the q arm. Phelan et al. (1993) report the unique case of a father with an inv(9)(p13p24) having a child with a rec(9) containing a tandem duplication, which they propose came from breakage and reunion between sister chromatids within the inversion loop. Another unique case is that described in McClarren et al. (2006), in which an inv parent had a child with a deleted ring 22, leading to DiGeorge syndrome. An inversion with a breakpoint in the vicinity of 15q12 may lead to a rearrangement that would cause Prader-Willi syndrome or Angelman syndrome, as mentioned above in the pericentric case. Two cases, each the child of a mother with a paracentric inversion, in which microarray with FISH gave the interpretation, are cases of L. G. Shaffer. First, in a child with developmental delay and dysmorphic features, analysis showed a single copy gain at 7q31.1q31.31 and a single copy loss at 7q31.33q32.3, while the intervening sequence was present in two normal copies. In the second case, a child had a single copy gain at 18q21.32q23 and an additional proximal signal on one chromosome 18.

Some inversion carriers have been ascertained through their having had many miscarriages (Madan 1995). In most of these, surely, the discovery was fortuitous. One family with an inv(10) was widely studied, and 19 carriers in three generations had only one miscarriage out of 36 pregnancies (Venter et al. 1984). The report in Devine et al. (2000) mentioned above of two brothers with 46,XY,inv(2) (q14.2q24.3) presenting with reproductive pathology may be suggestive, but other causes are quite possible. One brother's wife had had three miscarriages, and at in vitro fertilization in the partner of the other brother, five of 10 fertilized eggs failed to cleave, and progression in the remaining five failed at the blastocyst stage. No karyotyping was done of any of these several products of conception. In a very few cases, theoretical dicentric recombinant products might convey a genetic imbalance that could allow at least some weeks of in utero growth before miscarrying (Bocian et al. 1990; Bell et al. 1991). The nine miscarriages suffered by the carrier grandmother in the family in Worsham et al. (1989) we might more reasonably imagine to have been due (some of them at least) to recombinant gametes, the dicentric state having been proven in her index grandchild.

A Special Case, inv(8)(p23). A subtle paracentric inversion of 8p23 is a very common "abnormality," and indeed should be described as a polymorphism, since it occurs in approximately a quarter to a third of European and Japanese populations, respectively. From the millions, perhaps billions of people who carry this inversion, the tiniest number of abnormal infants have been born, 50 or so known worldwide. In these very rare cases, the inversion has led to a classic recombination with production of a dicentric chromosome, essentially as outlined in Figure 9–12, in which a segment including one centromere is then "clipped off" to produce a monocentric inv dup del(8p) (8qter→8p23::8p23→proximal 8p). The recombinant chromosome is typically generated (unusually for a structural rearrangement) in maternal meiosis (Shimokawa et al. 2004).

X Chromosome. If a paracentric inv(X) is associated elsewhere in the family with normality, no defect would be anticipated in future heterozygotes or hemizygotes (Neu et al. 1988a). Breakpoints in the critical regions in Xq might, however, compromise gonadal integrity. For example, Dar et al. (1988) report a woman with a de novo inv(X)(q13q24) who had ovarian dysgenesis with primary amenorrhea and no spontaneous pubertal development, and Németh et al. (2002) describe an infertile man with a Klinefelter-like phenotype having an X inversion with rather similar breakpoints, 46,Y,inv(X)(q12q25). A woman with a somatotype of Turner syndrome having an Xp inversion (p11.2p22.1) is described in Dahoun (1990).

Y Chromosome. A paracentric inv(Yq) is a rare observation (Madan 1995; Liou et al. 1997; Aiello et al. 2007). In Liou et al.'s three-generation family, the normal grandfather and father were 46,X,inv(Y)

(q11q21), and the child with the same karyotype had ambiguous external genitalia with Müllerian structures internally and intra-abdominal testes. The inversion Y may have been coincidental; alternatively, there may have been, in the child, a position effect whereby the expression of a gonadogenesis gene had been compromised. The father and son with 46,X,inv(Y)(q11.2q12) in Aiello et al. were normal (the chromosome having been an incidental observation at prenatal diagnosis).

Coincidental Abnormality. In some instances, the finding of a chromosome abnormality in a child from a paracentric inversion parent may be coincidence, even if the same chromosome is implicated, as seen in the case reported by Bourthoumieu et al. (2003) of a child with cri-du-chat syndrome and a del(5)(p14pter) karyotype, the deletion on the paternal chromosome. Parental chromosome studies revealed that the *mother* carried an apparently balanced paracentric inversion of the *long* arm of one chromosome 5.

Other Mechanisms Causing Abnormality. Mendelian loci can be vulnerable when chromosomal rearrangement happens, due to "position effect," epigenetic influence, or direct disruption. We have seen, for example, a family in which a chromosome 7 inversion, inv(7)(p22.2p21.2), has been associated with Saethre-Chotzen syndrome, this being a Mendelian disorder due to the *TWIST* gene. Two heterozygous children showed major craniosynostosis, but the father and grandfather had only the subtlest facial, auricular, and digital signs. It may be that Saethre-Chotzen syndrome due to position effect has a milder phenotype than when it is due to point mutation (Rose et al. 1997). On chromosome 7, at 7q21q22, an inversion has been described in association with the split hand/foot malformation, and again it is proposed that "position effect," with compromised expression of a putative hand/foot morphogenesis gene(s) in neighboring chromatin, might be the underlying causal mechanism (van Silfhout et al. 2009).[4]

An epigenetic mechanism may apply in the case of imprintable chromosomes. Norman et al. (1992) described a family in which a mother had one child with Beckwith-Wiedemann syndrome

---

4 A paracentric inversion of molecular scale, a "microinversion" segment of only 20 kb in 2p21 within the *MSH2* gene and causing Lynch syndrome, is of interest, but not a matter for this document (Liu et al. 2016); although we do mention (p. 258) the paracentric microinversions in low copy repeats that can predispose to nonallelic homologous recombination.

and a presumably affected fetus, all three carrying an apparently balanced inv(11)(p11.2p15.5). The normal imprinting state of the Beckwith region on distal 11p was likely perturbed. Parental gonadal mosaicism is the probable explanation for the observation of Angelman syndrome in two siblings, each with an inv(15)(q11.2q26.1), but the mother karyotyping normal, in Kuroda et al. (2014). The q11.2 breakpoint deleted the *UBE3A* locus. Presumably, given the parent of origin effect, the inv(15) would necessarily have been of maternal origin (since one cause of Angelman syndrome is deletion of *UBE3A* on the maternal chromosome). A small (11.7 Mb) familial paracentric inversion (1)(q42.13q43) in Rigola et al. (2015) may have compromised the functioning of genes in this region, leading to intellectual deficiency in heterozygous family members.

PARACENTRIC INVERSIONS USUALLY INNOCUOUS

The above rather extensive compendium notwithstanding, the observed facts attest to the general innocuousness of the autosomal paracentric inversion, concerning either the heterozygous state per se, or a risk for chromosomally unbalanced offspring. Madan (1995) reviewed 184 cases of autosomal paracentric heterozygosity. Many were ascertained fortuitously, and including those discovered during the course of investigation for recurrent miscarriage, 58% were identified in a normal person. Several had an abnormal phenotype, but this was, of course, the reason they had had the chromosome test done in the first place: By definition, they had to be abnormal. No clear consistent pattern among phenotypes of presenting cases is apparent. As Madan comments, there may have been a bias in choosing cases for publication, and editors of journals might not find compelling a paper describing an "uninteresting" inversion discovered incidentally in a normal individual (a series of a dozen or more cases might stand a better chance). In their review, Pettenati et al. (1995) could be confident about a causal association with a specific phenotype only in the paracentric inv(X), and not with any of the autosomal inversions.

The Groupe de Cytogénéticiens Français (1986a) note that the reproductive fitness of heterozygotes in 32 French families was normal. Two quite common inversions seen in a number of families in more than one part of the world are the inv(3)(p13p25) and the inv(11)(q21q23) (Madan

1995). No abnormalities directly attributable to these inversions have been documented. It may be founder effect, or recurring mutation, that is the basis for their frequency. In the one sperm study of a paracentric inversion heterozygote, having the relatively common inv(7)(q11q22), as mentioned above, Martin (1986) found no recombinants. The smallness of the inversion segment may have been a factor militating against formation of a synaptic loop. (It is not without interest to note that a similar inversion is the norm in the gorilla chromosome 7, and so this human form could be thought of as a "back mutation" to that of the ancestral primate.)

Interchromosomal Effect. Watt et al. (1986) raised the possibility that the paracentric inversion might have an "interchromosomal effect." They noted an apparently high level of reported associations, within families, of an inversion plus some other chromosomal defect. We suspect this is artifactual; as these authors noted, ascertainment and publication biases are potential confounders in this setting. Pettenati et al. (1995) reached a similar conclusion. But an open mind is to be kept.

Technical Comment. Paracentric inversions are not detected by microarray and can be technically difficult to detect on classical cytogenetics. Gross chromosome morphology is not altered, and unless major landmark bands are shifted, the rearrangement may go unnoticed. Only with the use of good-quality, high-resolution banding are paracentric inversions likely to be detected regularly. These cytogenetic difficulties may be why relatively few cases of this type of inversion have been published. Also, for technical reasons, reported cases of recombination in the literature should be regarded with caution; as mentioned above and noted below, some "inversions" are likely actually to be intrachromosomal insertions ("paracentric/within-arm shifts"). The cytogenetic distinction can be difficult to make, especially so for chromosomal regions without distinctive banding patterns, or where the inverted segments are very small (Callen et al. 1985; Madan 1995). For example, the inverted insertion of chromosome 15 described in Collinson et al. (2004), associated with recombinant offspring having Prader-Willi and Angelman syndrome (and see p. 174), had originally been reported, some 10 years prior, as a paracentric inversion. We have seen a family in which the index case seemed to have an unbalanced translocation at distal 4p, but the normal mother and grandfather had the same anomaly, which could then be reinterpreted as the minimum inversion detectable on routine cytogenetics, a one-band paracentric inversion, in this case inv(4)(p15.3p16.3) (Smith et al. 1992).

GENETIC COUNSELING

On practical grounds, the reassuring point to note is that practically all paracentric inversion heterozygotes identified have been discovered incidentally, and not through the birth of a child with an abnormality attributable to the parental inversion (Madan 1995). We agree with Madan: "The vast majority of paracentric inversions are likely to be harmless." Apparently, the genetic risks to offspring are extremely small. In the U.S. collaborative study described in Daniel et al. (1988), there were no unbalanced karyotypes in 30 prenatal diagnoses. The sex chromosomes warrant separate attention, and it may be that some X and Y paracentric inversions have an effect upon gonadal development in the intact (that is, unrecombined) state.

However, a tiny handful of abnormal offspring, and as reviewed at length above, refute a complete harmlessness in the parental paracentric inversion, whether due to classic recombination or to other forms of rearrangement. Whether this would warrant prenatal diagnosis, when a parent is a carrier of one of these implicated inversions, is a matter for debate. Even where the new chromosome from a classic recombinant or U-loop reunion might on theoretical grounds be viable, the risk for one to be generated, while its exact magnitude is unknown, is surely "extremely small." "Better than 99.9%" might be a fair estimate that there will be no untoward reproductive outcome due to behavior of the inversion. Albeit that molecular karyotyping offers the potential to screen, at prenatal diagnosis, for submicroscopic molecular damage associated with a particular apparently balanced inversion, the case for so doing is very modest. Caution—but in realistic perspective—should be exercised during genetic counseling, in that it is prudent never to say "never."

Thus, we suggest that, in practice, an offer of prenatal diagnosis be discretionary, in the case of a fortuitously discovered inversion in the family; and we would regard it as not inappropriate if the offer were declined (or not made). A firmer stance may be appropriate if there has been a previous history of an apparently associated reproductive abnormality. Inversions on record with a demonstrated recombinant would oblige the offer of prenatal diagnosis. These include those noted above: inv(7)(q31.31q31.33), inv(9)(p13p24), inv(9)(q22.1q34.3), inv(14)(q24.2q32.3), inv(17)(p11.2p13), inv(18)(q12.1q23), inv(18)(q21.1q22.3), and inv(18)(q21.32q23). But again, we return to the expressions used above: "vast majority," and "better than 99.9%," in respect of favorable behavior of the inversion.

As mentioned above, a diagnosis of a paracentric inversion might be incorrect, and the rearrangement is actually a within-arm insertion, which carries a high genetic risk (p. 169). Since the distinction in the routine laboratory can be difficult, a practical view might be to risk overinterpreting subtle paracentric inversions as potential insertions, in those cases in which the cytogeneticist is not absolutely certain. The true picture may emerge by determining the order of a number of FISH probes across the relevant region.

The Special Case of the inv dup del(8p)

The inv dup del(8p), noted in the "Biology" section earlier, arises from a maternal cryptic (on classical cytogenetics) paracentric inversion. Yet for a couple who have had this happen, the risk of recurrence is still, in all likelihood, extremely small. Nevertheless, it would be understandable for a couple having had that experience to seek the reassurance of prenatal diagnosis in a subsequent pregnancy.

THE PARACENTRIC INVERSION DETECTED PRENATALLY

If an apparently balanced paracentric inversion is discovered at prenatal diagnosis, and if the parental karyotypes are normal, there yet remains a possibility that the rearrangement is not truly balanced, and a risk for abnormality exists. This question is dealt with in detail in Chapter 21 (p. 500).

10

COMPLEX CHROMOSOMAL
REARRANGEMENTS

COMPLEX CHROMOSOMAL REARRANGE-MENTS (CCRs) occurring in phenotypically normal persons are rare. In her exhaustive review at the time, Madan (2012) recorded 103 published cases. Three or more chromosomes are involved, and a considerable variety of rearrangements are possible. Translocation may involve distal segments, as in the usual reciprocal translocation, or interstitial segments, as in the insertion. All the chromosomes except for no. 19 are listed as participating in a CCR. Molecular methodology is revealing more complexity among some "simple" rearrangements than previously appreciated, and the definition of what actually is a "CCR" could become unwieldy (Poot and Haaf 2015). We here largely limit our discussion to those CCRs that may be seen in balanced

form in heterozygotes who are themselves of normal physical health, and who may be at risk of producing abnormal pregnancies.[1]

BIOLOGY

Four Major Categories of Complex Chromosome Rearrangement

Madan (2012) defines CCRs as those involving three or more chromosomes, in which there are three or more breaks. This definition excludes the double two-way reciprocal exchange (p. 99). He proposes four major categories of CCR, types I–IV, based essentially upon the number of chromosomes versus the number of breaks, and whether there are insertions

---

1 Most (~90%) apparently balanced CCRs in abnormal individuals prove in fact to be imbalanced on molecular methodology (Feenstra et al. 2011). Some de novo imbalanced CCRs are proposed to have undergone gene disruption at the breakpoints due to "chromothripsis," a word coined this century to mean "shattering of a chromosome." The concept may actually be more applicable in cancer cytogenetics: A chromosome may indeed break into very many fragments, and reassemble, as a single event. In the constitutional CCR, the number of breaks is merely a single digit, or low double-digit number. Poot and Haaf (2015) review in detail mechanisms of the formation of CCRs (as more widely defined).

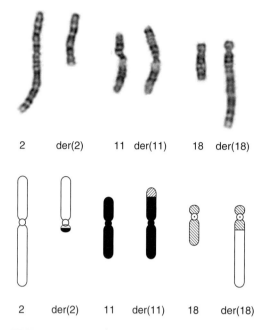

2   der(2)   11   der(11)   18   der(18)

2   der(2)   11   der(11)   18   der(18)

FIGURE 10–1   A three-way complex chromosome rearrangement. Most of 2q is translocated onto 18q; part of 18q is translocated onto 11p; and the tip of 11p is translocated onto 2q. The woman had presented with multiple miscarriages.

Source: From Gardner et al. 1986a, A three-way translocation in mother and daughter, *J Med Genet* 23: 90, and with the permission of the British Medical Association.

or inversions. In type I, there is the same number of breaks as there are chromosomes, and much the most common is the three-way exchange, in which three segments from three different chromosomes break off, translocate, and unite (Fig. 10–1). There are a very few examples of type I CCRs with four chromosomes and four breaks. In type II, there is one more break than the number of involved chromosomes, and this is due to one chromosome having an inversion. Similarly in type III, there are more breaks than involved chromosomes, but this time there is an insertion (or insertions).[2] The most complex scenario is seen in type IV, in which one (or more) of the derivative chromosomes comprises segments from three, or even more, chromosomes. In the discussion below, we group types II–IV as "exceptional CCRs."

The original CCR in a family typically arises as a single complex event, rather than sequential changes, at a meiosis during male gametogenesis (Grossmann et al. 2010). In the familial CCR, transmission thereafter is much more often seen through the mother, and this is a reflection of the infertility to which the male is often susceptible (although in one of the largest kindreds on record, showing five-generation transmission, three (great)grandfathers must have been CCR heterozygotes; Farrell et al. 1994). CCRs with up to four breakpoints are more typically familial, and ascertained through the female; those with more breakpoints are usually de novo, and discovered through male infertility (Poot and Haaf 2015).

Nomenclature of the CCR, as per the ISCN (2016), is straightforward with the type I CCR, although it can become rather complicated with exceptional CCRs. In principle, the involved chromosomes and breakpoints are listed in the following order: first, the lowest numbered (or X) chromosome; second, the chromosome that receives a segment from the first; and last, the chromosome donating a segment to the first listed chromosome. Thus, in the simplest type I case, for example, the karyotype of the CCR shown in Figure 10–1 would be written 46,XX,t(2;18;11)(q13;q21.1;p15.3).

DETAILS OF MEIOTIC BEHAVIOR

The carrier of a CCR has a risk for an abnormal conception due either to malsegregation of the derivative chromosomes or, rarely, to the generation of a recombinant chromosome. Malsegregation follows the general principles as set forth for the simple translocation, but naturally the range of unbalanced combinations is greater. The broad categories of malsegregation are 3:3 (alternate and adjacent), 4:2, and hypothetically 5:1 and 6:0 (the distinction between adjacent-1 and -2 is mentioned below). The windows of observation are at gamete formation; at embryo testing following in vitro fertilization (IVF); or at prenatal diagnosis or birth. At prenatal diagnosis, from the review of Madan (2012), adjacent-1 is overall the most frequently observed malsegregant mode (72%), 4:2 in 25%, and adjacent-2 in only 3%. There is a difference with respect to CCR type. For the type I three-way CCR, in fact, 3:3 adjacent and 4:2 were seen in approximately equal numbers. In contrast, adjacent-1 accounted for approximately 90% of malsegregation from exceptional CCRs (types II–IV). Recombination, whether producing a balanced or unbalanced karyotype, is

---

2 The inversion or insertion chromosomes have also undergone exchange with one of the other chromosomes of the CCR. Thus, a reciprocal translocation between two chromosomes, coincidentally accompanied by an inversion in some other chromosome, would not qualify as a CCR. A chromosome cannot be an outsider; each has to be a CCR participant.

rare indeed, and only eight such familial CCRs were recorded in the review of Berend et al. (2002b). In the exceptional CCR, scarcely ever are meiotic recombinants observed, and the family in Gruchy et al. (2010), in which a CCR with five insertional translocations with eight breakpoints was transmitted over three generations without recombinant offspring, is typical in this respect.

At gametogenesis and at preimplantation diagnosis, natural selection, at least in the "simpler" three-way CCR, has not come into play. Sperm studies have shown varying fractions of the different segregant forms, but with normal/balanced always in a minority: 14% in the t(2;22;11) in Cifuentes et al. (1998); 15% in the t(1;19;13) in Loup et al. (2010); and 27% in the t(5;13;14) in Pellestor et al. (2011). The sperm study in the case in Loup et al., of karyotype 46,XY,t(1;19;13)(p31;q13.2;q31)mat, showed the following proportions among the 76% unbalanced sperm: 34% from 3:3 malsegregations, 38% from 4:2, and even 5:1 (3.5%) and 6:0 (0.05%, representing 1 sperm out of 1,822).[3] As is well understood in the simple translocation, wide variation in segregation ratio is to be expected. Scriven et al. (2014) examined embryos from three male carriers of a type I three-way CCR. Slightly more than one-fourth (28%) of embryos had a normal/balanced constitution, due to 3:3 alternate segregation. Two-thirds were abnormal, reflecting either 3:3 adjacent (41%) or 4:2 (24%) segregation. Interestingly, in adjacent malsegregation, adjacent-2 (35%) was considerably more common than adjacent-1 (7%). A further one-fourth reflected 4:2 malsegregation; no instances of 5:1 or 6:0 were seen. The remainder (7%) were not analyzable. No real conclusion could be drawn from the data of the single female carrier in this report.

With increasing numbers of chromosomes involved in the translocation, as with CCR types II–IV, meiosis is increasingly compromised. If meiosis can proceed, the odds for a balanced segregation becomes very low. More often, especially in the male, the process may arrest, with a consequential azoöspermia, as we discuss below.

THREE-WAY COMPLEX CHROMOSOME REARRANGEMENT (TYPE I CCR)

At meiosis in the three-way CCR heterozygote, the expectation is that the chromosomes involved

in the rearrangement will come together and form a multivalent (Saadallah and Hultén 1985; Fig. 10–2). Consider how meiosis would proceed in the rcp(2;18;11) translocation illustrated in Figure 10–1. In theory, a hexavalent configuration would allow full synapsis of homologous segments (Fig. 10–3). If disjunction were then 3:3, up to 20 possible gametic combinations could occur. The two arising from alternate segregation (arrows in Fig. 10–3) would be the only ones to be balanced; the remaining 18 from adjacent segregation would be unbalanced to a greater or lesser degree. Were 4:2, 5:1, or 6:0 segregation to occur, a great number of extremely unbalanced gametes would result. However, it may be that, in some families at least, a tendency to favor symmetric alternate segregation, and a combination of very early lethality of severely unbalanced conceptuses, imply a modest, or even fair, prospect for achieving a normal pregnancy (Walker and Bocian 1987).

Adjacent segregation can be classified as adjacent-1 and adjacent-2, similarly to the principles set forth in the simple reciprocal translocation. Thus, the segregant gamete shown at left in Figure 10–4, having one of each chromosome pair represented (one of each centromere), would reflect adjacent-1 segregation. An example of 3:3 adjacent-2 segregation is given in Xu et al. (1997). A mother had the karyotype 46,XX,t(5;16;22), and cytogenetic analysis of her morphologically abnormal fetus following intrauterine death at 16 weeks gestation showed 46,XY,der(5),der(16),–22,t(5;16;22). In this case, the abnormal ovum would have had one chromosome 5, two chromosome 16s (one normal, one the derivative), and lacked a chromosome 22.

4:2 segregation particularly characterizes CCRs in which chromosomes with "small content" short arms (9, the acrocentrics) are a component. Schwinger et al. (1975) reported a mother of two children with typical Down syndrome, who herself had a three-way t(7;21;11) CCR. The affected children had an interchange trisomy 21, in that they had, in addition to the maternal translocation pattern, a second intact chromosome 21. Fuster et al. (1997) give an example of a 4:2 malsegregant, diagnosed at chorionic villus sampling, from a three-way paternal t(2;22;11)

---

3 The total falls short of 100% due to the interpretation in 9% of sperm being ambiguous.

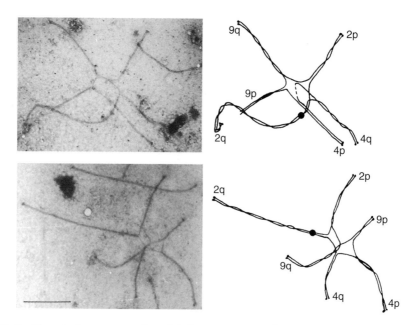

FIGURE 10-2   The actual appearance of a multivalent at meiosis I. Electron micrograph of a spermatocyte from a testicular biopsy of a man with a type I three-way complex chromosome rearrangement 46,XY,rcp(2;4;9)(p12;q25;p12); line drawing shows component parts of the hexavalent.

Source: From Saadallah and Hultén, A complex three breakpoint translocation involving chromosomes 2, 4, and 9 identified by meiotic investigations of a human male ascertained for subfertility, *Hum Genet* 71: 312–320,1985. Courtesy M. A. Hultén, and with the permission of Springer-Verlag.

CCR. The fetal karyotype was interpreted as 47,−2,der(2),der(22)t(2;22;11)(q13;q11.2;q23). The parents continued the pregnancy, and the retarded and abnormal child had a double partial

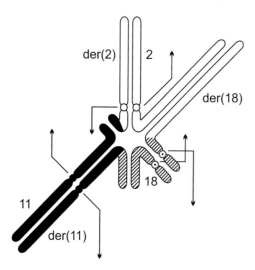

FIGURE 10-3   Diagrammatic representation of the formation of a hexavalent at meiosis in the three-way 2;18;11 translocation depicted in Figure 10-1. The arrows indicate 3:3 alternate segregation.

trisomy: a duplication of the segments 11q23qter and 22pter-q11.2. The couple had previously had one normal child and three miscarriages.

The risk of having a pregnancy that would go to term, but then produce an abnormal child, reflects the nature of the rearrangement—that is, the familiar question of whether there are possible chromosomal combinations that would lead to aneuploidy for a survivable amount of genetic material. Thus, considering the preceding rcp(2;18;11) example, three unbalanced combinations, one 3:3 and two 4:2, might be expected to be viable (Fig. 10-4). Madan (2012) determined that the criteria applying to simple translocations (Chapter 5) are broadly appropriate for the CCR: If the translocated segments are short, adjacent-1 segregation may lead to liveborn abnormal offspring; and if chromosomes with "small content" short arms (9, the acrocentrics) are involved, 4:2 segregation is usual. Large translocated segments are typically associated only with nonviable products, and consequent pregnancy loss. Recombination would add yet further possibility of imbalance, but this is, as mentioned above, very rarely seen.

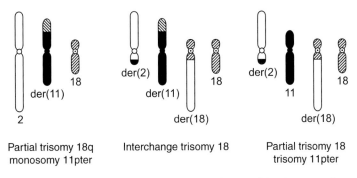

der(11)	der(2)	der(2)
18	der(11) 18	11 18
2	der(18)	der(18)

Partial trisomy 18q   Interchange trisomy 18   Partial trisomy 18
monosomy 11pter   trisomy 11pter

FIGURE 10–4   Three segregant outcomes of meiosis in the rcp(2;18;11) heterozygote shown in Figure 10–1, that might be expected to produce viable but unbalanced offspring. The 3:3 adjacent-1 gamete on the left may be the one most likely to be observed.

EXCEPTIONAL COMPLEX CHROMOSOME REARRANGEMENT

More complex rearrangements imply an even greater potential range of abnormal gametes. Kausch et al. (1988) calculated a minimum of 70 possible unbalanced gametes due to 4:4, 5:3, 6:2, and 7:1 segregations from an octavalent, in the case of a woman with a five-breakpoint CCR, with translocations of chromosomes 1, 2, 5, and 11 and an inversion of chromosome 1, who had presented with three first-trimester miscarriages. Van der Burgt et al. (1992) report a similarly complex de novo balanced CCR (chromosomes 5, 11, 12, 16; five breakpoints in all) in a mother who had had one miscarriage, one 46,XY child, the index abnormal child, and, as a quite unexpected outcome, a de novo 45,rob(13q14q) at prenatal diagnosis in her fourth pregnancy.

One of the most complicated familial CCR scenarios described is the case in Röthlisberger et al. (1999). A father carried a de novo CCR, with eight breakpoints altogether, two in chromosomes 6 and 18, three in 7, and one in 21, with the following wonderfully complex nomenclature:

46,XY,t(6;7;18;21)(6pter → 6q22 ::
6q25 → 6qter;7pter → 7q21.3 ::
21q21.3 → 21qter;7qter → 7q32.1 ::
18p11.21 → 18q21.3 ::
7q31.3 → 7q32.1 :: 6q22 → 6q25 ::
18q21.3 → 18qter;21pter → 21q21.3 ::
7q21.3 → 7q31.3 :: 18p11.21 → 18pter)dn.

Fluorescence in situ hybridization (FISH) and spectral karyotyping were needed to clarify the detail of the rearrangement. Most remarkably, among his three children, three different recombinant forms were passed on: a rec(7), a rec(21), and a rec(18). The child with the rec(21) had a balanced karyotype, and he has become a balanced carrier for a simple translocation, 46,t(7;21)(q21.3;q21.3): a "rebuilt" translocation (see below). The other two have partial trisomies for 6q and 7q.

An unbalanced CCR could be "corrected" by having the countertype imbalance in another rearrangement. Thus, the mother in Zou et al. (2010) had a three-way CCR t(5;15;7)(q13;q24;p15), which was missing the segment 5q13.1q14.1. But this segment was otherwise present, as an insertion into a chromosome 4, as der(4)ins(4;5)(q31.3;q13.1q14.1), thus qualifying as an exceptional, type III, CCR. She was phenotypically normal and (unsurprisingly, therefore) balanced on microarray analysis. However, she transmitted this der(4) to her son, whose karyotype was 46,XY,der(4)ins(4;5)(q31.3;q13.1q14.1)mat, and he presented an abnormal clinical picture, due to this segmental duplication. In molecular nomenclature, the imbalance is chr5:66,783,672-77,559,998)×3mat, representing a 10.8 Mb duplication.

"CRYPTIC" COMPLEX CHROMOSOME REARRANGEMENT

A CCR may be shown, upon detailed cytomolecular study, to have a greater number of breakpoints or a more complex imbalance than had originally been appreciated (Ballarati et al. 2009; Feenstra et al. 2011). Now that molecular methodology is so widely used, "cryptic" may not be the appropriate word: Rather, we might speak simply of CCRs requiring modern analysis for their full delineation. It may be instructive to consider a case from the days of classical cytogenetics, in which Wagstaff and Hemann (1995) describe a phenotypically normal father and his two abnormal children, the father and son having—on classical cytogenetics—an apparently balanced 46,XY,rcp(3;9)(p11;p23) and the daughter apparently 46,XX. On FISH and DNA studies, they could show that the father had a tiny segment of chromatin from the breakpoint in 9p23 removed and inserted into the long arm of a chromosome 8 (Fig. 10–5). At meiosis, it may have been that a quadrivalent formed from the chromosome 3 and chromosome 9 elements, while the two chromosome 8 homologs synapsed independently as a bivalent. On this interpretation, the two children reflect alternate segregation of the chromosome 3 and 9 elements; with respect to the homologs of chromosome 8, the rcp(3;9) son inherited his father's normal homolog, and so the lack of the 9p23 segment was not corrected, while the "46,XX" daughter received the chromosome 8 with the 9p23

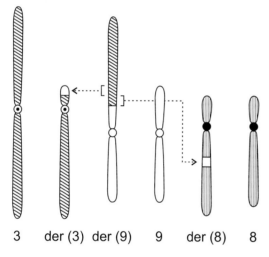

3   der (3) der (9)   9   der (8)   8

FIGURE 10–5   A cryptic complex chromosome rearrangement (and see text). On the original cytogenetic study, father and son appeared to have the same simple balanced translocation, 46,XY,rcp(3;9)(p11;p23), and the daughter seemed to be 46,XX. Molecular and FISH study showed a complex chromosome rearrangement, in which a tiny segment within 9p23 had been insertionally translocated into 8q in the father. Brackets and dotted lines show translocation of two separate segments from distal 9p across to 3p and to 8q, respectively. Thus, both the son and the daughter had an unbalanced complement, the son with a deletion, and the daughter with a duplication, for the 9p23 segment. (From the family reported in Wagstaff and Hemann 1995.)

insertion. Thus, the father carried a type III CCR; the son had a del(9)(p23), and the daughter a dup(9)(p23). A microarray study would easily have seen the "tiny segment" from 9p23.

A familial case in which a supposed simple translocation was shown to be a CCR, and then with a microdeletion coming to light on molecular analysis, is presented in Aboura et al. (2003). A mother and her infant son, the latter with minor dysmorphism and abnormal functional neurology, appeared at first to have the same simple t(3q;22q) translocation. FISH analysis showed this to be a CCR t(3;22;9)(q22;q12;q34.1). Yet finer analysis using a probe to the *ABL* locus on 9q34.1 revealed a very small deletion at this site on the der(9) of the proband, but not in his mother or in a carrier sister. The deletion was thus presumed to have arisen de novo, during maternal meiosis. These scenarios raise pressing questions: How often might other apparently balanced simple reciprocal translocations have a cryptic complex rearrangement; and how often does a de novo deletion occur on the background of a parental balanced rearrangement?

Numerous examples are on record of cases of de novo CCRs in which the initial report had been of a normal karyotype, a simple rearrangement, or a rearrangement of more complexity than at first appreciated (Burnside et al. 2014; Guilherme et al. 2013a; Oegema et al. 2012). Cases such as these are, of course, of considerable interest, but we are here limiting discussion to familial CCRs.

"Rebuilding" of Chromosomes from a Parental Complex Chromosomal Rearrangement. The coming together of several translocation chromosomes during meiosis may set the stage for recombination that Soler et al. (2005) describe as "rebuilding." The CCR shown in Figure 10–6 with six breakpoints in five chromosomes offers useful illustration (Bass et al. 1985). The woman who carried this rearrangement had four pregnancies, only one of which miscarried, and two produced offspring with a balanced constitution, though different in each child and different from their mother! Recombination involving the centric segment of chromosome 1 led to a daughter receiving a rebuilt der(1), with just the 6p segment being translocated, and a son with a different rebuilt der(1) having just the 7q segment. A son and a grandson had unbalanced karyotypes, which were different, but each led to partial 7q trisomy. Readers who relish esoteric puzzles may wish to refer to the original paper.

Rebuilding can lead to a simpler rearrangement. Madan (2012) describes a mother with a familial

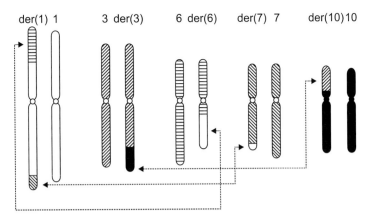

der(1) 1   3 der(3)   6 der(6)   der(7) 7   der(10)10

FIGURE 10–6 An extraordinarily complex rearrangement involving three two-way exchanges, with six breakpoints in five chromosomes (see text). (From the family reported in Bass et al. 1985.)

four-breakpoint t(2;3;8) type IV CCR, in which the 2q translocated segment had split, with 2q23q33 going to the der(3), and 2q33-qter to the der(8). Her child's karyotype was a simple 46,t(2;3) with a rebuilt der(3); the simplification resulted from recombination at maternal meiosis between her der(3) and normal chromosome 2. A similar story is told in Tihy et al. (2005).

A unique case of rebuilding in sequential generations is given in Zahed et al. (1998). A grandfather had two separate translocations: a simple translocation rcp(1;8)(p31;q21.1) and an insertional translocation ins(9;8)(q34;p23.1pter). Thus, he had two abnormal no. 8 chromosomes, one having a segment from distal 1p attached at 8q21.1, and the other having a deletion at 8p23.1. He had a daughter and a son, to each of whom he transmitted a rec(8), the same rec(8) to each, in balanced state. This rec(8) had a deletion at its p extremity, and a 1p translocated segment on its q extremity. Presumably, his two abnormal no. 8 chromosomes had recombined in meiosis, at a point somewhere between the p23.1 and q21.1 breakpoints. His daughter in turn had two children, and in each of them she restored, by recombination again in this generation—a rebuilt rebuilding!—the grandpaternal chromosomes: the del(8p) in one child, and the der(8)t(1p;8q) in the other. Both children had an unbalanced state, but different in each. One had a straightforward del(8) (p23.1) karyotype, and thus a partial 8p monosomy. The other had the grandpaternal simple rcp(1;8) and would otherwise have been normal; but in addition she inherited the ins(9), which conferred a partial 8p trisomy. The reader may care to draw the chromosomes of the three generations from

this description, and check back to Figure 2 in the original paper.

Rather evidently, the detailed structure of a CCR could not be discerned on a molecular methodology; and as mentioned above, classical karyotyping remains very necessary here.

Effect upon Fertility. In several complex rearrangements, gametogenesis can accommodate itself to the complexity thrust upon it, and the heterozygote may be fertile and have pregnancies that produce phenotypically normal children (Cai et al. 2001; Madan 2012). However, the rule of the greater vulnerability of spermatogenesis to chromosomal complexity seems to apply particularly in the situation of the CCR, and the male heterozygote is often sterile due to spermatogenic arrest, or subfertile (Bartels et al. 2007; Kim et al. 2011b). Indeed, in Madan's review, of 19 patients presenting with infertility, only one was a woman (and in her case, one of the breakpoints in the CCR being at Xq24, a critical ovarigenesis region, was the likely culprit). Fertility treatment with intracytoplasmic sperm injection (ICSI) may enable fatherhood (Joly-Helas et al. 2007), provided, of course, that sperm are being produced. Wang et al. (2015) undertook testicular biopsy in a man presenting with azoöspermia, whose karyotype was 46,XY,t(5;7;9;13) (5q11;7p11;7p15;9q12;13p12). Germ cells were reduced in number, some undergoing apoptosis; but no sperm or spermatids were present. Meiosis had proceeded part way, and octavalents were identifiable in all pachytene cells, albeit that several of the homologous segments had failed to synapse (Fig. 10–7).

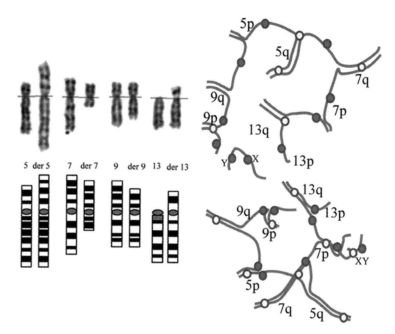

FIGURE 10-7   Meiosis in a man with a complex chromosome rearrangement, who had presented with azoöspermia. The karyotype is 46,XY,t(5;7;9;13)(5q11;7p11;7p15;9q12;13p12). Diagrams drawn from immunofluorescence directed to the centromeres of the participating chromosomes showed octavalents forming in most testicular spreads. Note that synapsis is incomplete, with some segments unaligned. In most cells, the X-Y body, which should normally lie separately, associates with the octavalent (*lower diagram, right*).

Source: From Wang et al., Abnormal meiotic recombination with complex chromosomal rearrangement in an azoospermic man, *Reprod Biomed Online* 30: 651–658, 2015. Courtesy Q. Shi, and with the permission of Elsevier.

GENETIC COUNSELING

The male CCR heterozygote who is not otherwise known to be fertile should have a semen analysis to check whether sperm are being produced. If there is oligospermia, IVF will have to be considered, and preimplantation genetic diagnosis may be appropriate. For the heterozygote (male or female) who is fertile, or for whom fertility can be achieved, a conceptus having either a normal chromosome constitution or the same balanced CCR as the parent would be expected to produce a normal child. But a high proportion of conceptions have an unbalanced karyotype.

An assessment of possible viable imbalances will be helpful, along the lines of the discussion above about the rcp(2;18;11), and as illustrated in Figure 10–3. Madan (2012) refers to the overall figures from Gorski et al. (1988) of an approximately 50% risk for spontaneous abortion, and 20% for a liveborn abnormal child, but he emphasizes the fact of each CCR being unique, and carrying its own particular risk profile. In the type III

CCR, the risk for a liveborn abnormal child with deletion or duplication of the inserted segment may be as high as 35%. The level of risk is related to the mode of ascertainment—whether through the birth of abnormal infants, multiple miscarriage, male infertility with abnormal spermatogenesis, or fortuitously—and to the family history. The risk for a liveborn abnormal child may be considerably less for the male carrier, and Scriven et al. (2014) suggest a figure of 3%. If multiple miscarriages have been the pattern in the family in the past, it is likely to continue to be so. In such cases, it may be that all unbalanced forms would lead to miscarriage (Creasy 1989). If abnormal infants have been born, carriers are likely to have a high risk for the same unfortunate event to happen again.

For the three-way CCR, it is generally justifiable to advise that, sooner or later, a normal outcome could possibly be expected. Thus, the couple may be willing to make continued attempts until a successful pregnancy is achieved. As always, the pedigree should be studied, in order to understand what might be the particular pattern of meiotic behavior with that CCR. If the reproductive history is very unpromising, optimism may need to be guarded, and the reality faced of a low chance for a normal child (Evans et al. 1984). As for the exceptional CCR, the likelihood for a successful pregnancy would be less, and possibly very small.

PRENATAL DIAGNOSIS

Once a pregnancy from a CCR carrier parent is actually achieved, some may prefer initially to rely on first-trimester ultrasonography, declining invasive diagnosis, and leaving early abortion to happen naturally if that would be the case, as an unfortunate previous miscarriage history might well cause a heightened sensitivity to the small risk associated with a prenatal diagnostic procedure. Others may prefer the early information that a chorionic villus sampling could provide. If the pregnancy continues normally by ultrasound criteria into the second trimester, a judgment can be made whether this of itself would be sufficiently reassuring (perhaps in the setting of all unbalanced forms being very unbalanced), or whether amniocentesis would in fact be desirable. On several levels, each case will have to be assessed on its merits. The CCR will need to be very carefully characterized cytogenetically in the parent and the fetus to ensure accurate prenatal diagnosis.

A noninvasive methodology would, naturally, be preferable. Srinivasan et al. (2013) have shown that massively parallel sequencing applied to samples of cell-free DNA from maternal plasma can pick up a microdeletion as small as 300 kb, and they propose that this methodology in prenatal diagnosis is as good as microarray. Such an approach may become feasible in the context of a CCR, targeting the potential imbalances due to a particular rearrangement.

The same balanced state identified at prenatal diagnosis raises the same questions, but more pointedly, as in the simple reciprocal translocation. By way of example is the CCR 46,XX,t(5;16;10;18)(q13;q22;q11.2;q21) identified at routine prenatal diagnosis in a woman having a history of recurrent miscarriage, reported in Lee et al. (2002),

with the same karyotype then being shown in herself. Normal ultrasonography was encouraging, and the pregnancy was continued; at age 2 years, the child was normal. But this fortunate outcome could not have been taken for granted. Molecular methodologies might allow a more precise determination, and specifically, addressing the question of possible cryptic (at the level of classical cytogenetics) imbalances arising de novo during generation of the gametes from the carrier parent. Such a case is exemplified in Malvestiti et al. (2010), who identified a CCR at amniocentesis, following the discovery of multiple fetal malformations at ultrasonography (which naturally gave a strong indication that the karyotype would be unbalanced). The fetal karyotype was interpreted to be 46,XY,der(4)ins(1;4)(q25;q25q31.1), due to a maternal CCR 46,XX, der(1)ins(1;4)(q25;q25q31.1)t(1;5)(q41;q35),der4)ins(1;4),der(5)t(1;5). Proceeding to array comparative genomic hybridization, the (normal) mother's genome was balanced, but a fetal deletion at 4q27q31.23, a gene-rich region of about 30 Mb, could clearly be appreciated.

Prenatal detection of a de novo CCR is discussed on p. 500.

PREIMPLANTATION GENETIC DIAGNOSIS

Given the very high fraction of embryos expected to be chromosomally unbalanced, preimplantation genetic diagnosis (PGD) would have an obvious attraction, in order to select in favor of the few embryos, if such there be, that might be normal or balanced. The PGD research of Scriven et al. (2014) noted above demonstrates the reality of this high risk. Escudero et al. (2008) and Lim et al. (2008a) provided PGD to some eight couples carrying a range of types of CCR: three-way, double two-way, reciprocal plus insertion, reciprocal plus Robertsonian, and others. Four of the couples eventually had a take-home baby. However, these babies were outnumbered by the created embryos 50 to 1, attesting to the very high genetic risk conveyed by the CCR.

11

AUTOSOMAL RING CHROMOSOMES

RING CHROMOSOMES ARE UNCOMMON, and it is even more uncommon for a person with a ring (or someone on his or her behalf) to seek genetic advice about reproductive possibilities. The typical physical phenotype comprises major dysmorphogenesis and intellectual deficiency, and procreation is not usually a relevant issue. But exceptions exist. Indeed, some persons with a ring chromosome appear to be of entirely normal phenotype. Only mild mental incapacity, or short stature with minor dysmorphism, characterizes some other cases. The ring 20 has a unique association with epilepsy. It is these categories of normal or mildly abnormal phenotype—in other words, of possible reproductive potential—we particularly consider in this chapter, although at the outset we can state that only a few examples of parental transmission of ring chromosomes are known. About 99% of rings arise sporadically (Kosztolányi et al.

1991). The ring X Turner syndrome variant and the "tiny ring X syndrome" are noted on p. 348, and the ring Y on p. 350.

BIOLOGY

There are two major types of ring chromosome that can be associated with either a normal phenotype or a clinical picture of relatively mild mental compromise, growth restriction, and absence of major malformation. First is the full-length or nearly full-length ring that replaces one of the normal homologs with the karyotype 46,(r).[1] Second is the very small ring typically comprising pericentromeric chromatin, which exists as a supernumerary chromosome, with the karyotype 47,+(r). On classical cytogenetics, a ring was very obvious to see. With microarray, recognition of a ring is indirect. The observation of p and q telomere deletions on the

---

1 A formal report might include the format such as ::p11→q21:: to show the breakpoints :: at p and q, book-ending the chromosomal segment that is retained.

same chromosome would point to the likelihood of 46,(r), but a classical karyotype would be needed for definitive confirmation. A 46(r) with deletion of just one arm would not be distinguishable from a simple linear deletion, while 46(r) rings in which the telomeres are retained would typically return a normal microarray result. 47,+(r) rings could be suspected on the basis of a duplication containing a centromere, but again final proof would require classical karyotyping. If, on next-generation sequencing, a DNA fragment containing sequences from both p and q arms were seen, this would allow the inference of a probable ring structure (Ji et al. 2015). A telomere-to-telomere fusion could only be discovered on classical cytogenetics (Burgemeister et al. 2017).

Individuals with either of these types of ring, 46(r) or 47,+(r), may have intact fertility, and they may present with questions about risks to their offspring. A third type of ring, in which the phenotype would always be abnormal, may have a complex structure at the breakpoint junctions with terminal deletions and duplications (Rossi et al. 2008b; Guilherme et al. 2011, 2013b); we do not further discuss this category. We deal with the first two categories separately, and list representative reported cases of individual ring chromosomes.

The Apparently Balanced, or Nearly Balanced, Ring Chromosome, 46,(r)

We may list these theoretical mechanisms that could lead to the generation of a ring that might appear, at least on classical cytogenetics, to be balanced:

1. Fusion of telomeres, without loss of other chromosomal material; thus, truly balanced, in terms of the amount of chromatin
2. Deletion of subtelomeric material at terminal p and/or q arms, with fusion of the exposed ends, with only the repetitive subtelomeric segments lost (telomere healing)
3. Deletion of "small" amounts of euchromatin at p and/or q arms, with fusion of the exposed ends

In the first scenario, no genes are lost, and thus no haploinsufficiency is imposed; and at least some telomeric capacity may be retained. In the second, again no genes are lost, but the absence of telomeres might (at least in some rings) have an epigenetic influence upon nearby gene function. In the third case, and if the deletions include actual genes, and

if these genes are dosage-sensitive, then there would be a phenotypic effect.

In each scenario, the circular structure of the ring may, of itself, compromise postzygotic mitotic cell division. The rings can become entangled, broken, doubled, or otherwise disrupted, following sister chromatid exchange during the cell cycle (Fig. 11–1). Thus, daughter cells arise that could be partially or totally aneuploid (whether trisomic or monosomic) for the chromosome in question—"dynamic mosaicism." These cells might die; some, however, could survive in the mosaic state, and presumably make an unfavorable contribution to the phenotype. This continuous generation and loss of cells could undermine the growth rate, although it might not greatly influence the quality of growth. The result would be the "general ring syndrome"—whichever autosome is concerned—of growth retardation, mild to moderate cognitive impairment, minor dysmorphogenesis, and, perhaps, intact fertility (Kosztolányi 1987; Guilherme et al. 2011). Intriguingly, the trivial but perhaps diagnostically helpful sign of café-au-lait macules is quite often seen, although this may be diagnostically confusing if neurofibromatosis is suspected (Denayer et al. 2009; Sodré et al. 2010).

A contrary view is that, in some cases at least, genomic imbalance suffices, of itself, to lead to phenotypic abnormality; and that being so, that there is no need to invoke a general ring syndrome (Rossi et al. 2008a). Or, the alternative mechanism of an epigenetic influence may be called upon: The ring configuration per se may lead to silencing, or possibly upregulation, of some genes, with particular reference, from preliminary research, to r(14), r(17), and r(22) (Zollino et al. 2010b; Surace et al. 2014; Guilherme et al. 2016).

MEIOSIS

At gametogenesis in the 46,(r) heterozygote, the expectation is, other things being equal, for symmetric disjunction, with 1:1 segregation of the ring and the normal homolog (Fig. 11–2). Thus, half of the conceptuses would be entirely normal karyotypically, and half would carry the ring. If "dynamic mosaicism" then occurs, these latter may be lethal in utero, or those surviving to term might have phenotypic abnormality.

There are tentative grounds for considering that the ring heterozygote might have an increased risk for nondisjunction, resulting in 2:0 segregation. In this event, with respect to chromosomes 13, 18,

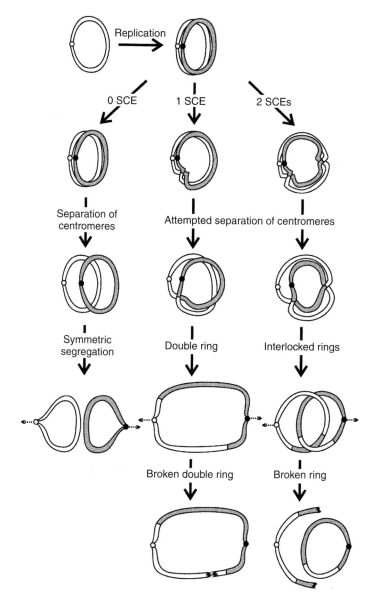

Replication

0 SCE   1 SCE   2 SCEs

Separation of centromeres   Attempted separation of centromeres

Symmetric segregation   Double ring   Interlocked rings

Broken double ring   Broken ring

FIGURE 11–1   Dynamic mosaicism. The single-chromatid ring chromosome replicates during interphase. Sister chromatid exchanges (SCEs) may, or may not, take place. At meiosis, if there are no SCEs (*left*), segregation is symmetric (dotted arrows represent spindles drawing homologs to opposite poles). If there is one SCE, a double-sized ring is generated (*middle*). With each centromere being tugged to opposite poles at anaphase (dotted arrows), the chromosome may break. If there are two SCEs, in the same "direction of rotation" (*right*), the two rings become interlocked. Breakage, or other mechanical compromise, is the consequence. A second SCE in the opposite direction of rotation would restore the situation.

or 21, a child with the respective trisomy might be born. Almost all instances of parent-to-child ring transmission involve the mother as the carrier parent (MacDermot et al. 1990). This likely reflects that spermatogenesis is compromised in the presence of a ring chromosome, and infertility is the consequence for most male heterozygotes. Every autosome is represented in the list of rings having the form 46,r(A). In a few, there has been an association with phenotypic normality and parenthood, and we provide commentaries below. (As noted above, there is sometimes mosaicism, more usually

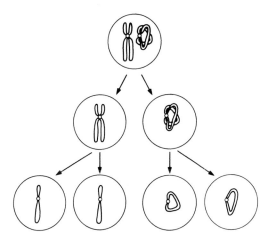

FIGURE 11–2   Meiosis with symmetric segregation in the ring heterozygote.

with one cell line monosomic for the chromosome concerned, and occasionally a minor cell line with two copies of the ring.)

Ring 1, 46,r(1). Few reports exist (Gardner et al. 1984; Cutenese et al. 2000). Growth retardation is typical.

Ring 2, 46,r(2). Prenatal and postnatal growth retardation and microcephaly are consistent features. Lacassie et al. (1999) summarize eight published cases and provide a photographic record of their own patient from birth to age 10 years, a microcephalic child with some mild cognitive and behavioral compromise, and profoundly growth retarded. Dee et al. (2001) showed a subtle distal 2p deletion in a ring 2 child with a similar phenotype, and they suggest that some other cases of r(2) may also have very small deletions. This thought was taken further in Severino et al. (2015), whose severely affected patient had, on microarray, a loss at distal 2p of only chr2:1-0.469 Mb, as well as a substantial 2qter deletion comprising chr2:238.7 Mb-qter. The phenotype in these cases may be, in part, a manifestation of the general ring syndrome, but likely more important, the direct consequence of distal deletion. No parent-to-child transmission has been recorded.

Ring 3, 46,r(3). The mechanism of deletion of one arm, and fusion with the intact other arm, is exemplified in the case in Guilherme et al. (2011), in which there was a 5.7 Mb loss at distal 3p (3p26). The 10-year-old boy was growth retarded, had a

mildly dysmorphic facies, and had a degree of intellectual deficiency. Barely double figures of this ring are recorded in the review of Zhang et al. (2016b); these authors describe their own r(3) case with a 10 Mb deletion at 3p.

Ring 4, 46,r(4). Sigurdardottir et al. (1999) describe a growth-retarded infant with normal developmental progress and whorled skin areas of hyperpigmentation and hypopigmentation. The r(4) was a true telomere-to-telomere fusion, as demonstrated with fluorescence in situ hybridization (FISH) using subtelomeric probes. A similar story is told in Burgemeister et al. (2017), who conclude that the concept of the "general ring syndrome" is supported by such cases in which no genetic material is lost. We have seen a man with 46,XY,r(4) manifesting the presumed general ring syndrome: He was considerably shorter than his brothers, and his occupation of warehouse manager compared with the professional qualifications of his siblings. Nevertheless, he could fully appreciate the genetic implications of his condition, and he and his wife chose to have donor insemination.

If the ring formed following terminal deletions, the individual might or might not present a Wolf-Hirschhorn syndrome phenotype, according to the extent of the deletion into 4p (Balci et al. 2006; Kim et al. 2009). The case in Guilherme et al. (2011), in which one "Wolf-Hirschhorn locus," namely the *LETM1* gene, was included in the 1.3 Mb deleted segment, could be considered to show some features of the syndrome.

Ring 5, 46,r(5). Molecular methodology allows a precise delineation of the extent of the pter and qter deletions in the ring, and the r(5) child described in Basinko et al. (2012) provides an example. At 5pter→5p13.2, the deletion comprised 34.61 Mb; and at 5q33.3→5qter, 2.44 Mb. The 5p deletion dictated a partial cri du chat clinical picture, while the 5q deletion may have been the basis of a congenital heart defect.

Ring 6, 46,r(6). Urban et al. (2002) reviewed 23 cases. Hydrocephalus was a common observation. At one end of the spectrum, malformations and microcephaly with severe retardation are typical. Kara et al. (2008) describe epilepsy as part of the phenotype in a patient whose r(6) included a 6q deletion. With the greater precision afforded by next-generation sequencing, Zhang et al. (2016c) could see, in their patient with a severe phenotype, 6p and 6q subtelomeric deletions of 1.78 Mb and 0.56 Mb, and they could point to probable pheno-contributory genes in these regions (*FOXC1, FOXF2, IRF4,* and *GMDS*). At the other end of the spectrum, a much milder phenotype of growth retardation evokes the general ring syndrome. An example is provided by the case of a young woman with mild dysmorphism and short stature, but normal psychomotor development and intact fertility (her son had a normal karyotype), reported in Höckner et al. (2008). The r(6) had approximately 200 kb deleted from each arm of the chromosome. No instance is known of parent-to-child transmission of a r(6).

Ring 7, 46,r(7). In a review of 16 cases of r(7), most had presented with microcephaly and intellectual deficit (Kaur et al. 2008). Salas-Labadía et al. (2014) studied an r(7) child with additional monosomic and duplicated cell lines, in whom the roles of several deleted genes could be postulated.

Ring 8, 46,r(8). Variable cognitive capacity, including normality, was observed in the family described in Le Caignec et al. (2004), in which the ring 8 chromosome, transmitted from mother to son and likely also carried by grandmother and uncle, was determined to have no loss of euchromatin. A man having a ring 8 with megabase-size deletions at 8pter and 8qter, and whose intellectual deficit was less marked than in most r(8) cases, proved to be mosaic, with a upd(8)pat 46,XY cell line (Gradek et al. 2006). The probable sequence was as follows: 46,r(8) at conception, the ring of maternal origin; mitotic loss of the ring to give a 45,–8 cell; and subsequent "rescue" of the monosomic line by duplication of the normal (paternal) homolog. This mechanism may have operated in some other ring cases in which there is a concomitant normal cell line.

Ring 9, 46,r(9). The phenotype in the r(9) is comparable to that of deletion 9pter and 9qter cases, according to the extent of the deleted segments (Purandare et al. 2005; Sheth et al. 2007; la Cour Sibbesen et al. 2013). Common elements include dysmorphism, microcephaly, cardiac malformations, growth and psychomotor retardation, and skeletal anomalies. A particular feature may be ambiguous genitalia or, sometimes, sex reversal, caused by deletion of *DMRT1* on 9p. 9q deletions

including the *EHMT1* locus contribute a component due to Kleefstra syndrome (p. 285) to the overall picture.

Molecular analysis can offer a precise insight, such as, for example, shown by Penacho et al. (2014) in 46,r(9)(p24.2q34.3) diagnosed prenatally, with 2.57 Mb deleted at 9p, and 2.60 Mb at 9q (as well as an interstitial deletion of 0.15 Mb at 9p24.1). Each of these distal segments contained a number of genes, whose loss was presumably the basis of the abnormal fetal phenotype observed.

Ring 10, 46,r(10). Gunnarsson et al. (2009) report a girl with growth and psychomotor retardation, microcephaly, congenital heart defects, and dysmorphic features. The nonmosaic ring showed, on microarray, terminal deletions of 285 kb at 10p15.3, and 12.5 Mb at 10q26.12. The subjects in Guilherme et al. (2011, 2013b), one with a 7.4 Mb deletion at 10q and the other with deletions at 10p (820 kb) and 10q (8.6 Mb), were both intellectually affected, and the latter also microcephalic.

Ring 11, 46,r(11). The mosaic complexity that can characterize the ring is well illustrated by the case in Galvão Gomes et al. (2017), with the karyotype 45,XY,-11[18]/46,XY,r(11)[78]/ 46,XY,dic r(11;11)[4]dn. Loss of an 8.6 Mb segment in 11q24.2qter in the major cell line led to a Jacobsen syndrome phenotype (p. 288). A notable example of familial transmission of a ring chromosome is given in Hansson et al. (2012), who report a child, her mother, and her aunt all with a r(11), all three short and microcephalic, but only the child with a mild developmental (language) delay. All three had café-au-lait macules. The grandmother presumably carried the same chromosome. A deletion at 11p, chr11:1-565,839, encompassed 20 genes; there was no loss at 11q.

Ring 12, 46,r(12). Parmar et al. (2003) review the findings in six cases of 46,r(12). Growth retardation and intellectual compromise of varying degree were consistent features. In one 46,XY,r(12) (p13q24.3)[85%]/46,XY[15%] mosaic case, a man in his twenties presented with infertility associated with severe oligospermia; the diagnosis led to retrospective review, and it was noted that he had been assessed as a child for delayed learning and microcephaly (Martin et al. 2008). He also had a number of café-au-lait skin macules, misleadingly the basis of a previous diagnosis of neurofibromatosis; but as noted above, this sign is observed in a number of ring chromosome syndromes.

Ring 13, 46,r(13). The typical phenotype, due to the distal 13q deletion component of the ring, presents microcephaly and poor psychomotor development, and genital malformation (Walczak-Sztulpa et al. 2008). Bedoyan et al. (2004) report mother-to-daughter transmission of a ring 13 chromosome, in which there had been loss only of subtelomeric material. The mother attended a special school; at age 21 years, she "showed no difficulties with speech, could read a newspaper, and worked as an assistant in a day-care center." Her daughter had presented with delayed language development. A molecular view may reveal further complexity, such as Kaylor et al. (2014) describe in a malformed newborn with a 46,XY,r(13)(p13q34) karyotype, but single nucleotide polymorphism (SNP) study then showing a cell line with an 87 Mb partial 13q trisomy. This line was lost on further study, presumably a reflection of instability due to "dynamic mosaicism."

Ring 14, 46,r(14). This chromosome is somewhat prone to ring formation, with over 60 cases reported (Zollino et al. 2012). About a quarter of cases are shown on microarray to have no loss of genetic material, and in the remainder, 14q deletions vary in length from 0.3 Mb to 5 Mb. A degree of genotype-phenotype distinction, with respect to 14q deletion/nondeletion, can be drawn: The characteristic facies, and poor behavior, are more prevalent with larger deletions. There is a distinctive facies; intellectual deficiency is practically universal; epilepsy is common; and eye defects of various kinds are frequent. When no genes are lost, the latter two traits may inhere in silencing of (structurally intact) loci in the proximal long arm, possibly due to a spread of inactivation from nearby 14p material. As direct evidence of an epigenetic effect, Guilherme et al. (2016) showed downregulation at two of eight studied loci in one patient. Given the fact of chromosome 14 being subject to a parent-of-origin effect, it is notable that uniparental disomy is not observed.

As for transmission of the ring, Bowser-Riley et al. (1981) described a 46,XX,r(14) mother "at the lower end of the normal range" of intelligence, who had two retarded 46,XX,r(14) daughters (and a third 46,r(14) pregnancy which was terminated). In the review of Zollino et al. (2012), one patient had a healthy parent, the father, who had an r(14) in 1% of cells on blood analysis.

Ring 15, 46,r(15). The range of clinical phenotype is recorded in Eid et al. (2013), with mild intellectual disability and short stature typical; the latter trait is prominent if the deletion includes the *IGFR1* locus at distal 15q (Guilherme et al. 2011, 2012). We have seen a young woman in whom a suspicion of Turner syndrome was the grounds for karyotyping (Gardner et al. 1980), as also have Glass et al. (2006) and probably, we imagine, several other observers. Parent-to-child transmission of 46,r(15) is recorded (Horigome et al. 1992).

Ring 16, 46,r(16). In a child with autism but no physical anomalies, Conte et al. (1997) found an r(16) with apparently no loss of genetic material, and in mosaic company with a normal 46,XY cell line. Six other cases reviewed by these authors had different karyotypes, some with 45,–16 mosaicism, and the phenotypes of these, and of a subsequent case reported in He et al. (2002), were more severe.

Ring 17, 46,r(17). Ring 17 may present with the severe neurological picture of Miller-Dieker syndrome (p. 302), if the deletion extends to the *LIS1* locus, or a not quite so severe phenotype with epilepsy, microcephaly, and mental retardation (and café-au-lait macules), if only subtelomeric 17p sequence is removed (Ricard-Mousnier et al. 2007). Surace et al. (2014) discuss the intriguing concept that retention of telomeres may be associated with a milder phenotype, while loss of telomeres, albeit that no genes are removed, could lead to an epigenetic ill-effect. In a child with a severe clinical picture, these workers showed downregulation of a number of distal 17p and 17q genes. Somatic loss of the normal homolog with consequential mosaic hemizygosity for the NF1 gene could be a "first hit" leading to neurofibromatosis type 1 (Havlovicova et al. 2007).

A mother with r(17) mosaicism, 46,XX,r(17)(p13q25)[22]/46,XX[28], cognitively normal but with the skin sign of multiple café-au-lait macules, and the ring with retained telomeric sequences, had a child who was mildly delayed as an infant, but who went on to develop intractable epilepsy. The child was also mosaic: 46,XX,r(17)[36]/46,XX[14] on blood, while on fibroblast study, almost all cells were normal, and just 2% had a double ring. The relative roles of tissue distribution and epigenesis, and even de novo ring generation, in the differing phenotypes of mother and daughter, are open to speculation.

Ring 18, 46,r(18). As Carter et al. (2015) note in their extensive review, this was one of the first ring syndromes to have been discovered, in the early 1960s. They record the interesting historic point that pioneer French cytogeneticist Jean de Grouchy's prediction, that the gene for aural atresia would lie at 18q, was vindicated a half century later. Consistent features include microcephaly, mental retardation, seizures, maxillofacial dysmorphism, and clefting (Koç et al. 2008; Ono et al. 2010). Stankiewicz et al. (2001a) studied seven phenotypically abnormal cases in some detail. Loss of 18q material was consistent, and thus a picture reminiscent of 18q– resulted, while loss of 18p was variable. Of the three cases reported in Guilherme et al. (2011), two had deletions of both arms (1.3 Mb and 15.3 Mb of 18p; 11.1 Mb and 1.7 Mb of 18q), and one had just an 18.6 Mb deletion of 18q. The abnormal child in Miller et al. (2003) had two rings, one derived from 18p and the other from 18q. Loss of the *TCF4* gene at 18q21.2 may contribute a Pitt-Hopkins (p. 304) picture to the *tout ensemble*, as Takenouchi et al. (2012) describe in a mosaic case. Ji et al. (2015) illustrate the application of next-generation sequencing, in order to define with complete (i.e., base-pair) precision the extent of the loss and the breakpoint sites, in their analysis of two r(18) cases, one prenatal and the other in an abnormal infant.

Parental transmission is rarely reported (Balci et al. 2014). Yardin et al. (2001) document the history of a woman with the ring 18 syndrome, her karyotype 46,XX,r(18)(p11.3q23)[32]/45,XX,–18[4] on peripheral blood analysis. Of six pregnancies, chromosome analysis, which in fact showed the r(18), was done in three, two being children, one similar to herself and the other apparently normal, as well as a terminated pregnancy following amniocentesis; a child dying as a neonate and two miscarriages were not karyotyped.

Ring 19, 46,r(19). Flejter et al. (1996) describe a normal mother having ring 19 mosaicism, 46,XX,r(19)/46,XX, with only 4% of cells (lymphocytes) having the ring, while her abnormal daughter was 46,XX,r(19) in 98% of cells. A telomeric probe hybridized to the ring on FISH, suggesting a telomere-to-telomere fusion format. A small ring, such as this, would be less likely to undergo dynamic mosaicism. Speevak et al. (2003) report a very similar case.

Ring 20, 46,r(20). Two main forms exist: a mosaic karyotype of mitotic origin, with end-to-end fusion of one chromosome 20; and a nonmosaic type, the ring having deletions of p arm or q arm, or of both arms, and having arisen at meiosis (Conlin et al. 2011; Daber et al. 2012). The nonmosaic form presents the more severe picture. Epilepsy is the notable clinical feature, with the onset of seizures typically at a younger age in the nonmosaic form (Mefford et al. 2012; Vignoli et al. 2016). The electroencephalogram (EEG) has a characteristic pattern, with trains of "theta waves." Any patient with epilepsy who has long runs of epileptiform activity on the EEG in the nonseizing state, which may or may not be associated with confusion or diminished consciousness, should have cytogenetic analysis with this ring chromosome in mind. A clinical pointer may be, in childhood onset, an association with terrifying hallucinations as part of the seizure. There may be an earlier period of normal mental development, which slows following the onset of epilepsy. The location at distal 20q of the neuronal channel genes *KCNQ2* and *CHRNA4*, and their loss in the deletion, had offered an attractive explanation for the genesis of the epilepsy; but in fact the story may be rather more complicated (Daber et al. 2012).

An otherwise unaffected parent with a lower level of mosaicism can have affected children with the ring chromosome in higher proportion (Canevini et al. 1998). Herrgård et al. (2007) document a mother with 10% r(20) mosaicism, who had an onset of seizures in her mid-twenties, and who was intellectually normal. Her daughter had epilepsy from age 7 years, and cognitive capacity fell away in subsequent years; her son was always behind in development, showed poor behavior, and had seizures from age 5 years. These children both had 40% of their cells with the r(20).

Ring 21, 46,r(21). The cognitive phenotypes can vary from normal to mild retardation. A child we followed up into adulthood achieved tertiary education and was a skilled musician; but he was, as can often be the case with the male r(21) heterozygote, infertile, with azoöspermia (Dallapiccola et al. 1986; Gardner et al. 1986b). A sperm study on a ring 21 infertile man with an extremely low sperm count, karyotyping 45,XY,–21[3]/46,XY,r(21)[95]/46,XY[2] on blood and with fairly similar proportions on buccal cells, came up with an interesting result: FISH showed most (92%) of 169 spermatozoa to be normal, 7% with the ring, and 1% disomic with the normal 21 and the ring 21. These authors suggested that the (presumed) small fraction in the gonad of normal spermatogonia were selectively favored at meiosis, leading to the majority of gametes being normal (Hammoud et al. 2009).

Parent-child transmission, and indeed grand parent-parent-child transmission, is known. An example of mother-daughter transmission is recorded in Bertini et al. (2008b), with each having the same karyotype on blood, 46,XX,r(21)/45,XX,−21, the ring being the majority species in each (98% and 94%, respectively). In this instance, the rearrangement was due to a subtelomeric 21q deletion of 3.4 Mb, and apparently no critical dosage-sensitive genes had been lost. A transmitting father in Papoulidis et al. (2010) had just one cell out of 100 with the ring (discovered after the birth of his child), likely reflecting a somatic-gonadal mosaicism; the ring 21 child was normal on assessment at 10 months.

Three-generation kindreds are described in Falik-Borenstein et al. (1992) and Melnyk et al. (1995). In one family, a 46,XX,r(21) heterozygote had had seven pregnancies with four early miscarriages, one normal son, one son with Down syndrome, and one 46,XX,r(21) daughter, the latter herself having a 46,XX,r(21) daughter. Most karyotyped cells in these individuals were 46,r(21), but a few were 45,−21, and some had a double-size or multi-size rings. Short stature, but normal IQ/development, accompanied the abnormal karyotype in these females; one male heterozygote may have had a low-normal intelligence. In another family, a 46,XX,r(21) mother had a prenatal diagnosis that showed one 46,XY twin and the other with 46,XX,r(21)/45,XX,−21 mosaicism. Both babies were normal, and the girl's postnatal karyotype was nonmosaic 46,XX,r(21).

The ring 21 might, of itself, predispose to the generation of a trisomy 21 karyotype: either 47,+r(21) or a recombinant 21 (Howell et al. 1984; Fryns and Kleczkowska 1987; Miller et al. 1987; Kosztolányi et al. 1991). In their review of this circumstance, Muroya et al. (2002) illustrate a reverse picture: a normal mother with a rather complex der(21) who had a mildly mentally retarded son with 46,XY,r(21), and 4/100 cells 45,XY,−21.

Ring 22, 46,r(22). A handful of inherited cases are on record (Teyssier and Moreau 1985; Crusi and Engel 1986; Wenger et al. 2000). In some, the ring was inherited from a phenotypically normal parent to phenotypically normal offspring, and presumably in these, no crucial genetic material had been deleted. In other cases, one or more of the family members with the ring have had mental retardation or other clinical features. A r(22) with no loss of genetic material may yet be associated with phenotypic abnormality (Guilherme et al. 2011). In some cases, the parent is mosaic and the child has inherited the ring in a nonmosaic state, which may substantially explain parent-offspring differences in phenotype (Jobanputra et al. 2009). The r(22) mother in Wenger et al. had required special education in high school. Her son had bowel and heart defects, with very little language development by age 20 months. By a strange coincidence he had, on his other chromosome 22, a de novo del(22)(q11.2).

Some ring 22s have a more proximal q arm breakpoint and are deleted for the 22q13.33 region, which is the basis of the Phelan-McDermid syndrome (p. 309); haploinsufficiency for the *SHANK3* gene is the key pathogenetic factor (Koç et al. 2009; McGaughran et al. 2010; Hannachi et al. 2013). The severity of the phenotype is proportional to the length of the deleted segment.

A ring 22 may, of itself, function as a "first hit" in the generation of certain tumors. The gene for neurofibromatosis type 2 (NF2) is located at 22q12. The neural crest is the embryonic tissue that gives rise to the investing membranes of nervous system structures. Due to its mitotic instability, a cell line in this tissue might lose the ring and thus become monosomic for 22. Subsequently, a mutation occurring in the *NF2* gene on the remaining intact homolog would be "exposed" and allow the development of a classic tumor, a schwannoma of the eighth cranial nerve, or a meningioma of the cranial or spinal meninges (Zirn et al. 2012). A similar scenario has been shown with respect to the *SMARCB1* gene, in a child (who also had Phelan-McDermid syndrome) presenting with an atypical teratoid rhabdoid tumor of the brain (Byers et al. 2017).

The Supernumerary Small Ring, 47,+(r)

The small ring as a 47th chromosome could as well be dealt with under the category "small supernumerary marker chromosome" (sSMC), but we nevertheless record them here, acknowledging their particular ring identity. These rings may have formed as in the 46,(r) story above, with (large) distal deletions and end-to-end fusion; or, the "Barbara McClintock mechanism" involving breaks at the centromere and in one arm, with material from only that arm then represented in the ring, may in some be invoked (Baldwin et al. 2008). A supernumerary chromosome implies, naturally, a partial trisomy. Daniel and Malafiej (2003) presented six cases of their own and reviewed the literature. Generally, it is only when the ring chromosome is very small, or when there is mosaicism with a substantial fraction of normal cells—in other words, where the overall load of genetic imbalance is small—that a question of genetic risk for offspring of the heterozygote will be relevant. Postnatally ascertained cases have naturally presented with an abnormal phenotype, but a fraction of cases come to attention fortuitously, some being phenotypically normal. Mosaicism complicates the interpretation. These very small rings are mitotically unstable, and this is likely the basis of the frequently observed mosaicism (Spittel et al. 2014). A few cases are known in which a parent with low-level mosaicism has had an abnormal child with a higher proportion of the cells with the ring. The levels of mosaicism as determined from a peripheral blood sample may not necessarily reflect the levels in other tissues, and including brain; and in a number of rings, little correlation is recognized between the degree of mosaicism and the severity of phenotype.

Small supernumerary rings have been reported for almost every autosome. Brief sketches of some of these follow, with particular reference to recorded cases in which a parent with the ring has had offspring. For several of the chromosomes, the genetic content of the rings may vary quite considerably, and thus it is not surprising that often no clearly consistent phenotype is observed between cases due to the same chromosome (and the factor of variable mosaicism, as just mentioned above, also influencing the picture).

Ring 1, 47,+r(1). Callen et al. (1999) and Bernardini et al. (2007) presented series of patients with very small supernumerary r(1) chromosomes, ranging in phenotype from normal to abnormal, and showed that the size of the ring was correlated with phenotype. Further cases are listed in Liehr (2016b), several being of normal individuals, discovered incidentally. Chen et al. (2013b) record 24 prenatal diagnoses, just one of which was due to

parental (maternal) transmission. Several had fetal anatomical abnormalities; but in some proceeding to birth, and followed up at least into infancy, the child developed apparently normally. A remarkable familial example is given in Kosztolányi et al. (2011), concerning a ring 1 chromosome of 28 Mb size. Two children were of distinctly abnormal appearance, and one requiring special education; their mother was of slightly similar appearance, but having developed normally; and the grandfather was normal. Ring 1 mosaicism was present in 75% in one child and 55% in the other, in 16% of the mother, and in 2.6% of the grandfather.

Ring 2, 47,+r(2). A 47,XX,+r(2)/46,XX mother with minor facial dysmorphology and apparently otherwise normal had a son with mosaicism for the same tiny ring chromosome, who presented with mental retardation and a psychotic disorder (Giardino et al. 2002). The ring was present in 54% of cells (peripheral blood) in the mother, and 80% in the son. A mosaic case in Liehr et al. (2007), a child with an r(2) comprising distal 2q elements with a neocentromere, had severe psychomotor retardation and dysmorphic features.

Ring 3, 47,+r(3). A normal mother and her normal infant son had the karyotype 47,+r(3)/46, at frequencies of 33% (mother's lymphocytes) and 41% (prenatal diagnosis in the son, amniocyte analysis) (Anderlid et al. 2001).

Ring 4, 47,+r(4). Bonnet et al. (2006) review the ring 4 and describe their own case of a child of low-normal intellect, in whom they demonstrated up to three copies of a very small ring chromosome, about 20 Mb in size, in 82% of cells. Three recorded diagnoses were from amniocentesis; all three pregnancies were terminated, with the very severe brain defect of alobar holoprosencephaly identified in one.

Ring 5, 47,+r(5). Masuno et al. (1999) reported a child with minor dysmorphisms and no speech at age 3 years. A molecular dissection of a ring 5 allowed Hadzsiev et al. (2014) to propose that trisomy for the 21 Mb segment 5p14.1-cen, of which the ring was comprised, was the basis of the Binder maxillonasal malformation seen in their patient.

Ring 6, 47,+r(6). James et al. (1995) report a child with paternal uniparental isodisomy 6, in whom an r(6) of maternal origin was also observed.

Ring 7, 47,+r(7). Tan-Sindhunata et al. (2000) describe a family in which the mother of low-normal intelligence, and two of her three children, had mosaicism for a very small supernumerary ring, 47,+r(7)/46,N. Although the fractions of mosaicism were similar in the three (~50%), the children were more severely affected, at least with respect to language acquisition, than their mother. Speculatively, this could reflect, in the mother, a lesser "ring load" in the brain. Her other child was normal. Similar 47,+r(7) cases are recorded in the reviews of Lichtenbelt et al. (2005) and Bertini et al. (2008a); in two, Silver-Russell syndrome was due to uniparental disomy (UPD) 7. The additional copies of the *STX1A* and *LIMK1* genes in 7q11.23 (chr7:73.7 and 74.1 Mb, respectively), common to many r(7) cases, may contribute importantly to the developmental deficits. Of entirely different origin is the mosaic small r(7) in Louvrier et al. (2015), in which the 7 material was derived from the distal long arm, at 7q22.1q31.1, and in which mitotic stability was enabled due to the generation of a neocentromere.

Ring 8, 47,+r(8). The ring 8 may impose, compared with other rings, a lesser degree of functional genetic imbalance, and indeed normality is recorded. Daniel and Malafiej (2003) report a normal woman karyotyped incidentally (because she had had a child with Wolf-Hirschhorn syndrome) and who turned out to have a very small r(8) in 27% of lymphocytes. A phenotype suggestive of the MURCS (Müllerian and renal aplasia, cervicothoracic somite dysplasia) association was seen in the patient of Loeffler et al. (2003), a mildly retarded teenage girl, in whom 70% of cells contained a tiny r(8) chromosome. Filges et al. (2008) studied a developmentally delayed girl mosaic for a small ring 8 of 43.8 Mb size. Bettio et al. (2008) document a prenatally diagnosed de novo very small ring comprising about 5 Mb of proximal 8p and 8q euchromatin, in mosaic state (50% of cells with the ring on chorion villus sampling, 90% at amniocentesis, and 96% at postnatal blood sampling). Although early infant development was within the normal range, by age 3 years it was clear that language acquisition was poor, and that behavior was affected.

Familial transmission is known. A normal father, a university graduate, with low-level mosaicism for a very small supernumerary r(8), had two nonmosaic 47,XX,+r(8) daughters (Rothenmund et al. 1997). They were intellectually handicapped and displayed emotional immaturity, although their physical growth was normal.

Ring 9, 47,+r(9). Rings derived from the pericentromeric heterochromatin are likely harmless (Callen et al. 1991). In their review of ring chromosomes and a possible association with uniparental disomy, Anderlid et al. (2001) note a moderately retarded, nondysmorphic girl with 36% mosaicism for a supernumerary ring 9. This, rather than the maternal UPD, was presumed to be the basis of her abnormal phenotype.

Ring 10, 47,+r(10). A young woman with mosaicism (14% in blood, 16% in buccal mucosa) presenting only with short stature is reported in Trimborn et al. (2005). Sung et al. (2009) review three prenatal reports, and they describe their own case of mosaic 47,XX,+r(10)/46,XX detected at amniocentesis and confirmed in the newborn. The child was apparently normal on assessment at age 1 year.

Ring 12, 47,+r(12). No clear clinical phenotype has emerged, other than abnormality in all (Davidsson et al. 2008). Yeung et al. (2009) and Lloveras et al. (2013) document cases in which the ring 12 included two copies of 12p, thus determining a Pallister-Killian phenotype (p. 505).

Ring 14, 47,+r(14). Infertility was the only presenting complaint in a man with a ring 14 reported in Stahl et al. (2007).

Ring 15, 47,+r(15). A very small ring 15 can be compared to the relatively common small bisatellited supernumerary chromosome (sSMC) 15 (p. 324). An exceptional case is that of a sSMC derived from chromosome 15 in grandparent (mosaic) and parent (nonmosaic), evolving into a very small ring 15 in the grandchild. All three, and two other siblings with the sSMC, were normal (Adhvaryu et al. 1998).

Ring 16, 47,+r(16). In a prenatal case, Cignini et al. (2011) note major fetal abnormalities in association with nonmosaic 47,XY,+r(16).

Ring 17, 47,+r(17). A mildly retarded boy with a ring 17 is described in Dupont et al. (2003).

Ring 18, 47,+r(18). Jenderny et al. (1993) describe a phenotypically normal mother with 47,XX,+r(18) in only 2/100 cells on blood analysis, the remainder being 46,XX, and who had a daughter with nonmosaic 47,+r(18). Balci et al. (2014) record another normal mother with ring 18 mosaicism, in her case 47,XX,+r(18)(::p11→q21::)[10]/46,XX[90], who had a handicapped son with 46,XY,r(18)[75]/46,XY[25] mosaicism; these authors showed more underlying complexity in the structure and formation of the rings than at first appreciated, in undertaking a SNP-array family study. A man with a VACTERL-like (vertebral, anal, cardiac, trachea-esophageal, renal, limb association) clinical picture, and with a normal intellect, carried at low-level mosaicism an r(18) that endowed "octasomy" for an ~5 Mb segment of pericentromeric chromosome 18 (van der Veken et al. 2010).

Ring 19, 47,+r(19). A few cases are on record, with phenotypes from mild (possibly reflecting mosaicism) through severe (Shahwan et al. 2004; Vaz et al. 1999). A normal mother with r(19) mosaicism came to attention only because she had had a child with defects probably due to a different, coincidental chromosomal imbalance (Argiropoulos et al. 2011).

Ring 20, 47,+r(20). Guediche et al. (2010) provide a review of 13 cases, eight ascertained postnatally and five prenatally, with psychomotor and growth retardation as frequent but not universal observations. Kitsiou-Tzeli et al. (2009) document prenatal diagnosis, following which the child, at age 3 months, was judged to be essentially normal; in contrast, Callier et al. (2009) describe dysmorphic features in an aborted fetus. The only example of parental transmission is in Pinto et al. (2005).

Ring 21, 47,+r(21). A ring may result from a more complicated process than end-to-end fusions, as Villa et al. (2011) analyze in a child with minor dysmorphism and delay in language development: An initial trisomy 21 at conception gave rise to a large ring, which subsequently "deleted out" a segment, leaving a small ring comprising two noncontiguous regions.

Ring 22, 47,+r(22). Mears et al. (1995) document a family in which a phenotypically normal grandfather and father were mosaic for a tiny ring 22 chromosome, 47,XY,+r(22)/48,XY,+r(22),+r(22). A grandchild, also 47,+r(22)/48,+r(22),+r(22) but whose ring chromosomes had increased in size, had cat-eye syndrome (p. 333).

RARE COMPLEXITIES

Supernumerary Ring with a Balancing Deletion. If a ring chromosome is derived from a segment of chromosome that has been deleted interstitially from an autosome, and if this newly generated ring contains the centromere, it can, in some cases, be transmitted stably at mitosis; and, if so, the karyotype is balanced. But the carrier can be at high risk to produce unbalanced gametes. The ring might be transmitted as a supernumerary chromosome, to give a partial trisomy; or, the deleted chromosome, for a partial monosomy. And, even if it is the balanced combination that is present at conception, a substantial risk exists for postzygotic mosaicism, which might well generate an abnormal phenotype.

If the ring is very small, the balancing deletion may be missed on classical cytogenetics, as Baldwin et al. (2008) describe in a mother whose karyotype, at first sight, was 47,XX,+r(4)/46,XX; but the small r(4) was in fact derived from a deleted segment of 4p on one of her chromosome 4 homologs. She was described as intellectually normal but with unilateral ear anomalies and minor visual deficiencies; this mild phenotype may have reflected a partial 4p monosomy in body tissue with the "46,XX" (but actually del 4p12-cen, chr4:45-50 Mb) karyotype. Her child, who inherited the small ring, but not the balancing deleted 4, and thus with dup chr4:45-50 Mb, had a "mild speech delay." Mantzouratou et al. (2009) studied embryos from a couple, the wife being 47,XX,del(22),+r(22), and herself normal. They had had two natural pregnancies, both mosaic 47,+r(22)/46, the first producing an abnormal child, and the second terminated after prenatal diagnosis. Unfortunately, following two preimplantation genetic diagnosis (PGD) cycles, none of the embryos had received the normal, intact maternal chromosome 22, and thus none were transferred.

Formation of a Neocentromere. A fragment of a chromosome not containing a centromere would not normally be able to be transmitted during cell division. But if a "neocentromere" is generated on this fragment, its survival may be assured, as a "small supernumerary marker chromosome." If the supernumerary ring balances a deletion, the physical phenotype may be normal, such as Slater et al. (1999) show in an infertile but otherwise normal man. A segment was deleted from one chromosome 1, and this same segment (1p32p36.1) existed as a tiny supernumerary ring chromosome. This man thus has the karyotype 47,XY,del(1)(p32p26.1)+r(1) (p32p36.1). The ring chromosome was able to activate the formation of certain centromere binding proteins, which presumably enabled its stable transmission. A similar circumstance is recorded in Knegt et al. (2003), in this case a phenotypically normal woman who had presented with recurrent miscarriage, and in whom a tiny ring 13 chromosome was derived from an interstitial deletion of the segment 13q21.31q22.2. Amniocenteses in her fourth and fifth pregnancies demonstrated normal karyotypes. If, however, a gene is disrupted in the process of ring formation, the phenotype may be impacted upon, such as Quinonez et al. (2017a) propose in an infertile man with Marfan syndrome, who had an apparently balancing neocentromeric supernumerary ring 15 (the fibrillin-1 gene being located at 15q21).

GENETIC COUNSELING

Parental Karyotype 46,(r), Mosaic or Nonmosaic

In the person who is mosaic on somatic (blood) analysis, with a 46,N/46,(r) karyotype, the mosaicism might extend also into the gonad. This would convey an important risk to have a nonmosaic 46,(r) child; and, even if this might overstate the case, this risk would need to be assumed to exist. Quantifying the risk would be most imprecise: as high as 50%, as low as (essentially) zero, but anywhere between.

The great majority of transmitting parents are 46,XX,(r) mothers, presumably reflecting that most male heterozygotes are infertile. Those offspring inheriting the ring could be expected to present the similar clinical picture as, and indeed quite probably more severely than, their heterozygous parent. In the review of Kosztolányi et al. (1991), about one-third of 46,(r) children were more severely affected mentally than their parent. The 46,(r) parent may be an atypical ring carrier, perhaps having had a fortunate pattern of mitotic disruption, to have reached the level of social phenotype that procreation would be likely.

In the particular case of the 46,r(21) heterozygote, who is often phenotypically normal, there is a small but as yet unquantified risk of having a child with Down syndrome due to an uncommon karyotype: 47,+r(21), 46,rob(21q;21q) or 46,tan dup(21q;21q) (Kosztolányi et al. 1991). If, in prenatal diagnosis for a pregnancy of a r(21) heterozygote parent, the same r(21) karyotype were demonstrated in the fetus, based on the slender evidence thus far available, the chance for phenotypic normality would seem to be "substantial," but a (probably mild) degree of abnormality could by no means be excluded. As noted above (Hammoud et al. 2009), gametogenesis (if fertility is retained) in the mosaic 46,N/46,(r) male, at least with respect to the r(21), may favor the production of chromosomally normal spermatogonia.

Rings of chromosomes 11, 17, and 22 may predispose to cancer, due to sequential events in susceptible tissue of (1) loss of the ring to produce a cell line with monosomy, and (2) a gene mutation on the remaining homolog within that cell line. For the three chromosomes mentioned, the genes are, respectively, WT1 (Wilms tumor), NF1, and, as discussed above, NF2 (Carella et al. 2010; Zirn et al. 2012). Tumor surveillance may be considered in persons carrying these rings.

Parental Karyotype 47,+(r)

Each ring needs to be assessed individually, and careful cytogenetic analysis is needed. Reference to the brief outlines earlier will give a sense of the range of outcomes. A nonmosaic parent with a very small ring might be expected to transmit the abnormal chromosome with up to 50% probability, assuming (and this may not necessarily be the case) meiotic and mitotic stability. The parental phenotype would, in principle, predict that of a potential 47,+r child. Mosaicism in the parent, and potential mosaicism in the child, considerably complicate prediction. A higher-grade mosaicism in the child than in the parent, or complete nonmosaicism in the child, would be expected to produce a more severe phenotype, and quite possibly cause lethality in utero. Molecular analysis of sperm would be a means, in principle, to assess the degree of mosaicism in a male heterozygote, although not practicable as a routine. Prenatal diagnosis by PGD or amniocentesis is appropriately offered.

Parental Karyotype 47,del(A),+r(A). In the ring with a balancing deletion, normality in an offspring can only be regarded as secure (other things being equal) in the context of the normal homolog (A) having been transmitted from the 47,del(A),+r(A) parent. Even though the carrier parent may be normal, the risk is high that the same balanced karyotype in a conceptus could be followed by postzygotic misdivision, with the eventual generation of offspring who would be partially trisomic, or partially monosomic, for the autosome concerned, and thus abnormal. A detailed discussion is offered in Mantzouratou et al. (2009).

12

CENTROMERE FISSIONS, COMPLEMENTARY ISOCHROMOSOMES, TELOMERIC FUSIONS, BALANCING SUPERNUMERARY CHROMOSOMES, NEOCENTROMERES, JUMPING TRANSLOCATIONS, AND CHROMOTHRIPSIS

THIS CHAPTER provides a setting for certain very rare abnormalities that cannot easily be accommodated elsewhere. Barely double-digit numbers, if that, for most of these are known. *Centromere fission* results when a metacentric or submetacentric chromosome splits at the centromere, giving rise to two stable telocentric products. In a sense, this is the reverse of what happens in whole arm translocations. The heterozygote, a phenotypically normal individual, thus has 47 chromosomes. The *Robertsonian fission* reverses the fusion that had originally generated it. *Telomeric fusion* leads to a 45-chromosome count, due to the joining up of two chromosomes, tip-to-tip, not unlike the Robertsonian mechanism. The fusion chromosome has two centromeres, but one of these becomes inactivated. With the balanced *complementary isochromosome* carrier, two stable exactly metacentric products are generated. A *balancing small supernumerary marker chromosome* contains material deleted from the normal homolog. A supernumerary chromosome lacking a normal centromere can

become stable and functional due to the generation of a *neocentromere*. In *jumping translocations*, a segment can move from one chromosome to two or more recipient chromosomes. *Chromothripsis* ("chromosome shattering") takes complex rearrangement to a yet more complex level.

BIOLOGY

Centromere Fission

In simple terms, a nonacrocentric chromosome undergoes a horizontal splitting at the centromere (Fig. 12–1a), although the true basis may be more complex than this (Rivera and Cantú 1986; Perry et al. 2004). Two new telocentric chromosomes result (Fig. 12–2). One comprises the short arm of the original, and the other its long arm. It is as though the cell ignores the fact that the split happened and continues on normally, treating each part as a properly functioning whole. The other normal homolog remains intact. The heterozygous person

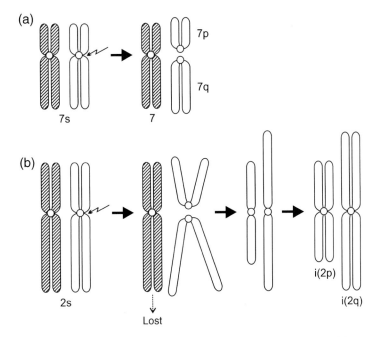

FIGURE 12–1 Comparing the processes of (*a*) centric fission of chromosome 7 and (*b*) complementary isochromosomes of chromosome 2. The chromosome pairs are to be imagined as existing in the zygote (*left*); they have replicated to give the double-chromatid state. The lightning arrow indicates misdivision of the centromere in one homolog. By the time the cell enters the first mitotic division (*right*), the abnormal states have been generated. Note that according to the proposed mechanisms in (*b*), uniparental disomy would necessarily result. Cross-hatching indicates original homolog from one parent; open indicates original homolog from the other.

(47,cen fis) may have a balanced complement of genetic material and thus be phenotypically normal. Among the very few families on record, just seven chromosomes—4, 7, 9, 10, 11, 12, and 21— have been involved (Shim et al. 2007; Cetin et al. 2011). The karyotype may be written, for example, 47,XX,–4,+fis(4)(p10),+fis(4)(q10).

At meiosis in the heterozygote, the centric fission products presumably form a trivalent with the intact homolog, and 2:1 segregation, essentially as in the

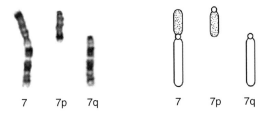

FIGURE 12–2 Partial karyotype from a case of 47,cen fis(7). One chromosome 7 exists as a normal homolog, and the other homolog is represented by the 7p and the 7q chromosomes.

Robertsonian carrier, then follows. "Alternate" 2:1 segregation produces normal and balanced centric fission gametes, while adjacent 2:1 segregation leads to gametes disomic or nullisomic for either of the fission products (Fig. 12–3). Monosomy would probably be associated with occult abortion and trisomy with miscarriage or, in exceptional cases, with the live birth of an abnormal child. Thus far, trisomies only for 4p, 9p, and 12p are on record.

The paucity of data does not allow for a precise assessment of the genetic risk run by the centric fission carrier, other than to suggest it could, in some, be quite high. Dallapiccola et al. (1976) report a chromosome 4 centric fission in a woman who had had two children with trisomy 4p and one normal child. Fryns et al. (1980) describe a man and his normal daughter having a centric fission of chromosome 10. Recurrent miscarriage in the families of Janke (1982) and Shim et al. (2007) may well have been a result of asymmetric segregation of a chromosome 7, and a chromosome 11 centric fission, respectively; in the latter case, the cen fis(11) heterozygous woman then went on to have a normal

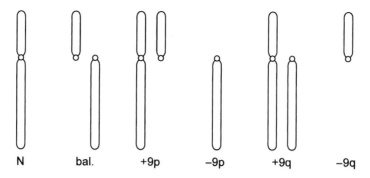

FIGURE 12–3   The six possible gametes arising from 2:1 segregation in a 47,cen fis(9) heterozygote. Two of these would lead to a normal phenotype, the 46,N and the balanced 47,cen fis(9) states. Of the unbalanced states, only the 48,cen fis(9),+9p, in which the imbalance would be a 9p trisomy, might possibly be viable.

46,XX child. Miscarriages and childhood deaths in the family of Del Porto et al. (1984) might have been due to a cen fis 4, which was shown to have been transmitted, in balanced state, from a mother to her son.

Robertsonian Fission

The Robertsonian translocation is capable of reversing its evolutionary development, and the fused component chromosomes can separate. Perry et al. (2005) studied two families coming to attention due to a known family history of a segregating rob(13;15). They observed fission products in samplings of somatic tissues (chorionic villus, amniocytes, and blood) in 11 individuals or pregnancies, although mostly at single-digit percentage levels. These "new" acrocentric chromosomes were actually telocentric chromosomes 13 and 15, having no visible short arm material. This phenomenon appeared to be without any clinical consequence.

Telomeric Fusion

This is the tip-to-tip fusion of two complete, or practically complete, chromosomes, and the person thus has a 45-chromosome count (Engelen et al. 2000; Lemyre et al. 2001). The fusion occurs at the level of the telomere or the subtelomeric region. All the necessary functional genetic material is "present and correct" (if there is a missing bit, it contains no crucial genes), and the phenotype is normal, other things being equal. The composite chromosome has two centromeres (hence an alternative name of "stable non-Robertsonian dicentric chromosome"), but one of the two centromeres becomes functionally

suppressed. The karyotype is written 45,t(A;B), 45,dic(A;B), or 45,tas(A;B), where A and B denote the two chromosomes. The short arm of an acrocentric chromosome is very frequently involved, and chromosome 18 is often one of the participating chromosomes. Ascertainment is typically fortuitous, or through reproductive difficulty (recurrent miscarriage, gonadal dysgenesis, oligoteratospermia). Familial transmission is recorded. The attachment of an essentially complete long arm of an acrocentric chromosome to the telomeric region of another autosome is a very similar circumstance (Fig. 12–4).

A normal child could be produced following symmetric, essentially 2:1 segregation: That is,

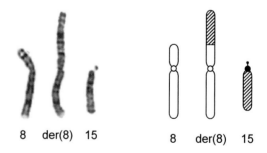

8   der(8)   15   8   der(8)   15

FIGURE 12–4   A telomeric fusion translocation, 45,XY,t(8;15)(p23.3;q11). The normal father with this karyotype has all the functionally necessary part of chromosome 15 attached to the telomere of a chromosome 8. His child with Angelman syndrome has the same karyotype, but haplotyping with DNA markers showed that both chromosome 15 elements derived from the father, with no chromosome 15 contributed from the mother. Probably, this reflected a "corrected" interchange trisomy. (Case of A. Smith; Smith et al. 1994.)

either the two normal homologs are transmitted or the composite chromosome. Asymmetric segregation, were it to happen, would lead to trisomy or monosomy of one of the component chromosomes, and, according to the nature of the chromosome, in utero viability would be compromised. For example, Lemyre et al. (2001) document a 45,XX,dic(14;18)(p11.2;p11.3) mother in whose pregnancy was diagnosed, at 32 weeks gestation, intrauterine fetal death. The fetal pathology examination was consistent with trisomy 18, and the karyotype, 46,XY,+18,dic(14;18)(p11.2;p11.3), confirmed this diagnosis. If the trisomic state were to be "corrected" by loss of the normal homolog from the other parent, a uniparental disomy would result. The case shown in Figure 12–4 is an example of this.

Complementary Isochromosomes

The individual has a full complement of the chromosomal material—and may thus be phenotypically normal—but with the two p arms combined in one chromosome, and the two q arms in the other (Fig. 12–5). A formal karyotype might be written, for example, as 46,XX,i(2)(p10),i(2)(q10). Chromosomes 1, 2, 4, 7, and 9 have been reported with this picture, and at least four instances are known for chromosome 2 (Bernasconi et al. 1996; Shaffer et al. 1997; Albrecht et al. 2001; Baumer et al. 2007; Guvendag Guven et al. 2011).

The usual mechanism of formation may be that, in the zygote, horizontal fission at the centromere of one homologous chromosome produces not two telocentric products (as happened in the fission, discussed above), but two mirror-image metacentric

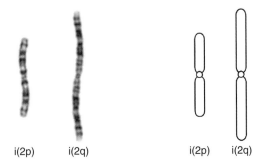

i(2p)   i(2q)   i(2p)   i(2q)

FIGURE 12–5   Chromosomes from a woman with complementary isochromosomes i(2p) and i(2q) (and see Fig. 12–1b). (Case of A. A. Schinzel; in Bernasconi et al. 1996.)

chromosomes: an i(p) and an i(q) chromosome (Fig. 12–1b). This is followed by segregation of both isochromosomes into one daughter cell. There is loss (if it had ever been there) of the homologous normal chromosome contributed by the other parent (unlike the centric fission, in which the normal homolog is necessarily retained); thus, this is a form of monosomy rescue, which engenders a uniparental disomy, usually maternal (Bernasconi et al. 1996; Shaffer et al. 1997; Björck et al. 1999). In other cases, one isochromosome may be of paternal origin, and the other maternally derived, and this may reflect an initial trisomy rescue followed by postzygotic isochromosome formation (Albrecht et al. 2001; Kotzot 2001; Baumer et al. 2007).

A typical clinical presentation has been multiple miscarriage, in phenotypically normal women. Rather analogous to the rob(21q21q) carrier, it is practically impossible for such a person to have a normal child. Any pregnancies from "symmetric" segregation would be either dup(p)/del(q) or dup(q)/del(p), and thus hugely imbalanced. In the male, infertility may be the presenting feature (Guvendag Guven et al. 2011).

Balancing Supernumerary Chromosomes

If deleted material from a chromosome is then accommodated in a newly formed small supernumerary marker chromosome (sSMC), and if this extra chromosome can be stably transmitted, then the carrier individual can be of normal phenotype but may have a risk to have a child with a deletion, or a duplication, of the material in question (Baldwin et al. 2008).

The most remarkable example is that of a four-generation family, in which several persons carried a chromosome 22 with an atypical q11.2 deletion, but this in company with a small supernumerary ring chromosome that comprised the deleted 22q11 material (Nevado et al. 2009). These people had, therefore, a balanced karyotype, and they were phenotypically normal: 47,del(22)(q11.2),+sSMC. On classical karyotyping, the two chromosome 22 homologs had appeared normal, and it required fluorescence in situ hybridization (FISH) to reveal the deletion on one homolog; thus, the initial impression in this scenario may simply be 47,+sSMC, and the sSMC interpreted as "harmless." In fact, two of these family members had had a child with atypical deletion 22q11.2 syndrome. The deletion had a different proximal breakpoint to the common 22q11.2 deletion, such that the ring chromosome included some alpha satellite from the chromosome 22 centromere. The other potential imbalance, that of dup(22q11) due to a 47,+sSMC karyotype, had not been observed in the family.

A prenatal case of mosaicism for a balancing small ring(4) in the setting of an interstitial 4q deletion and probable centromere misdivision is recorded in Capalbo et al. (2013). Other cases of a balancing small ring are noted in Chapter 11.

Neocentromeres

Neocentromeres are ectopic centromeres that originate occasionally from noncentromeric regions of chromosomes (Amor and Choo 2002). Neocentromeres are determined epigenetically, and lack normal centromeric alpha-satellite DNA. The formation of a neocentromere is nearly always associated with a chromosomal rearrangement that generates a chromosome fragment lacking a conventional centromere, and provides a useful reminder of the absolute requirement for chromosomes to have both a centromere and a means of capping the chromosome ends, either with telomeres or by the formation of a ring chromosome. Chromosome rearrangements that are most commonly associated with neocentromere formation include inverted duplications of distal chromosome segments, ring chromosomes derived from deletions within chromosome arms, and, less commonly, deletions of the endogenous centromere. "Centromere repositioning," the formation of a neocentromere in the absence of any chromosome rearrangement, is exceedingly rare (Amor et al. 2004).

Almost all neocentromeres arise de novo, but familial examples are recorded. The mother in Chuang et al. (2005) had the karyotype 46,XX,del(11)(p11.12p11.2), with the deficit corrected by a neocentromere-containing r(11) (p11.12p11.2). Her child inherited only the del(11), and presented with the Potocki-Shaffer syndrome. Other examples, in which the neocentromeric chromosome formed as a ring, are noted in Chapter 11.

Jumping Translocation ("Translocation Sauteuse")

This evocative expression describes a mitotic rearrangement whereby the same piece of one chromosome breaks off, on more than one occasion, and attaches to the tips of other chromosomes. The site of breakage in the donor chromosome is characterized by the presence of an interstitial (internal) telomere, and this region offers the possibility of fusion with the recipient chromosomes (Vermeesch et al. 1997). Only 26 constitutional cases were listed in the review of Iwarsson et al. (2009).

Levy et al. (2000) identified the phenomenon in two couples, themselves karyotypically normal, presenting with recurrent miscarriage and showing evolving "jumping" cell lines in the cultured products of conception. In one of these, for example, the conceptus was initially 46,XX,der(15)t(1;15) (q10;q10). A second line arose, with the 1q part of the der(15) replaced by an additional chromosome 15, which then generated an i(15q), along with (presumably independently) trisomy 7. Five further lines then budded off, all with considerable degrees of imbalance; the pregnancy eventually terminated in first-trimester abortion. Lefort et al. (2001) describe in some detail their own case, an otherwise normal boy with a (possibly coincidental) structural cerebellar defect. He had four separate cell lines, on blood and skin biopsy samples, with the segment 2p12pter attached to 1pter, 5qter, 6qter, and 12qter, respectively. In each, the rearrangement appeared to be balanced. These authors proposed that these translocations were truly one-way—that is, having no reciprocal exchange, and with healing of the 2p12 stump by the formation of new telomeric sequences.

A vulnerable site might already have been expressed as comprising one breakpoint in a translocation. A "jump" might then follow at the same site, such as Carey et al. (2014b) show in a man with the (functionally balanced) karyotype 45,XY,der(4) t(4;22)(q35;q11.2),–22. Albeit that an implanted embryo from this man had typed as balanced on FISH with chromosome 4 and 22 probes at preimplantation genetic diagnosis, at amniocentesis the fetal chromosomes were 45,XY,der(12)t(12;22) (q24.2;q11.2),–22. In other words, a segment of 12q had replaced the 4q segment in the father's translocation, at the same 22q11.2 site. The child was normal.

Chromothripsis

Chromothripsis is a word of recent vintage, meaning "chromosome shattering" (sometimes also called *chromoplexy*). It is mostly a concept applicable in cancer cytogenetics, in which there may be very many chromosomal breaks occurring as a single somatic event, sometimes described as catastrophic, and leading to a jumbled remodeling of the chromosome, which can, of itself, due to inappropriate juxtapositions of certain genes, initiate a cancer. But it can also, very rarely, be seen as a constitutional abnormality, and in this setting may be described as "germline chromothripsis." The imbalances resulting are typically deletions. The paternal gonad is the predominant site of de novo generation. De Pagter et al. (2015) describe three mother-child pairs, the mothers with karyotypes that would certainly qualify as complex chromosome rearrangements (Fig. 12–6). Further complexity was then visited upon their children, due to de novo change within the maternally inherited homologs, with associated severely abnormal phenotypes. As another example, the three-generation familial rcp(3;5)(q25;q31) in Bertelsen et al. (2016), at first sight seeming to be simple two-way reciprocal translocation, proved to be very complicated on analysis by next-generation sequencing, with six different "microrearrangements" at the breakpoint regions. The proposed mechanisms whereby chromothripsis arises are reviewed in Fukami et al. (2017).

Chromothripsis is to be distinguished from the "multiple de novo CNV (MdnCNV) phenotype" (p. 382), a phenomenon in which several independent de novo copy number variants are generated during the perizygotic period—that is, in late gametogenesis, fertilization, and during the first few mitoses (Liu et al. 2017).

GENETIC COUNSELING

Centromere Fission

The centric fission heterozygote has a significant risk of having a phenotypically abnormal child in those cases in which a whole arm aneuploidy is viable. The 4p, 9p, and 12p trisomies are the only examples known so far. In any other combination, spontaneous abortion would be inevitable. Five percent to 25% is an educated guess, where viability is a possibility, of the likely risk range. Prenatal testing is certainly advisable. Of the phenotypically normal offspring of the heterozygote, half would be expected to have the centric fission and half to have normal chromosomes. For the heterozygote in whom neither whole arm imbalance is viable—an obvious example would be a 47,cen fis(1)—no risk for a liveborn abnormal child exists, but the likelihood of abortion may be high.

Robertsonian Fission

This appears to be a phenomenon of academic interest, seen only in somatic tissues, and of no clinical consequence.

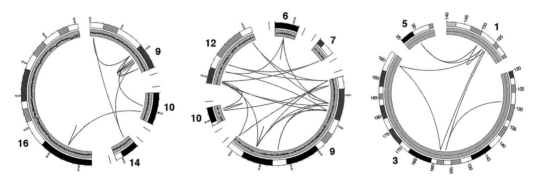

FIGURE 12–6   Chromothripsis. "Circos plots" depict the complexity of the several interconnected breakpoints in the karyotypes of three phenotypically normal mothers, whose abnormal children manifested yet more complicated, and unbalanced, rearrangements.

Source: From de Pagter et al., Chromothripsis in healthy individuals affects multiple protein-coding genes and can result in severe congenital abnormalities in offspring, *Am J Hum Genet* 96: 651–656, 2015. Courtesy W. P. Kloosterman, and with the permission of the American Society of Human Genetics and Elsevier.

Complementary Isochromosomes

The carrier of the complementary p/q isochromosome carrier, essentially with certainty (that is, barring an extraordinary rescue event), cannot have a normal child.

Balancing Small Supernumerary Marker Chromosome

The genetic risk is high, and it may approach 50%, if the del or dup imbalance implied by the material contained in the sSMC is "genetically small." Nevado et al. (2009) emphasize the need to seek a cryptic deletion in persons found to carry an sSMC; if the true state of a cryptic deletion is not recognized, genetic advice would be gravely misplaced.

Telomeric Fusion

Infertility may be frequent. If conception is possible, there is likely to be a substantial risk for aneuploidy of one or other of the chromosomes involved in the translocation, but equally, a normal child could be conceived. Uniparental disomy will need to be considered at least in the case of a chromosome 15 being one of the chromosomes.

Jumping Translocation

These cases are typically de novo, and the reason for the chromosome suddenly becoming susceptible in the individual is unknown. The genetic implications for the next generation remain uncertain. Yet, normality is on record, in the quite extraordinary case of parental transmission described in Hu et al. (2014). A normal father and daughter had translocations involving the same breakpoints at two chromosomes, 16 and 22, but different chromosomes otherwise: t(16;22), t(1;22), and t(22;22) in the father, while the daughter's translocations were t(16;22), t(9;22), and t(5;22).

Chromothripsis

If transmission from parent to child is possible, and indeed cases are on record, the risk for generating further complexity, with an associated phenotypic abnormality, is likely high. The distinction between a particularly complicated complex rearrangement and a less complicated chromothripsis may be rather subtle.

13

DOWN SYNDROME, OTHER FULL ANEUPLOIDIES, POLYPLOIDY, AND THE INFLUENCE OF PARENTAL AGE

IN THIS CHAPTER we consider the circumstances in which there may be an increased risk to have a child, or a pregnancy, with an aneuploidy. First, we review the case of parents, themselves karyotypically normal, who have had a child, or a pregnancy that aborted, with a full aneuploidy or a polyploidy. Thus, we include the major trisomies (13, 18, 21) and sex chromosome aneuploidies (XXX, XXY, XYY, and 45,X) as well as less commonly seen autosomal aneuploidies and sex chromosome polysomies. The category of polyploidy is substantially devoted to triploidy. In the great majority, these defects arise from an abnormal event during meiosis or (in some triploidy) at conception. In a few, there is postzygotic generation of aneuploidy. Only in the case of parental gonadal mosaicism, or in the hypothetical setting of an apparent predisposition to meiotic error, will there apply an increased risk of recurrence of aneuploidy, over and above that associated with any parental age effect. Triploidy needs separate consideration.

Second, we touch briefly on the uncommonly encountered circumstance of possible parenthood in (classically cytogenetic) aneuploid persons. Finally, we rehearse the ways in which parental age may influence the risk to conceive a pregnancy, and potentially to have a child, with an aneuploidy.

BIOLOGY

Full aneuploidy is presumed in the great majority to be the result of meiotic nondisjunction. A diminished degree of meiotic recombination is typically observed in aneuploid offspring, and this led Hassold and Sherman (2000) to propose a two-hit sequence, the first hit being a less well-tethered bivalent at meiosis I, and the second hit being a consequential aberrant distribution at meiotic metaphase. Meiotic nondisjunction can happen at any parental age, but it is more frequent in older mothers, as we discuss in detail below. Alternatively, an abnormality has arisen in a premeiotic gametocyte, with the parent thus having a "wedge" of gonad that carries the abnormality (gonadal mosaicism). Such a parent would, of course, have an increased risk for only the one karyotypic defect. Finally, a small fraction of apparent full aneuploidy may be due to early mitotic nondisjunction in an initially 46,N conceptus with loss, or restriction to extra-embryonic tissue, of the normal cell line.

AUTOSOMAL TRISOMY

Trisomy 21 (Down Syndrome)

Down syndrome (DS) is the archetypal chromosome disorder. It was, along with Klinefelter syndrome, the first medical condition shown to result from a chromosome abnormality, in 1959. It has for many years been recognized as the most common single known cause of intellectual disability, and it has the highest incidence at birth of any chromosome abnormality. Every counselor can expect frequently to deal with problems relating to DS, and thus should be familiar with its genetics. (For convenience, we note here also those forms of DS that are due to translocations.)

The Genotype to the Phenotype. The DS phenotype—the characteristic facial appearance, body build, and mental condition—is, in a sense, a "contiguous gene syndrome," in which there is an additional dose of an en bloc set of genes. The entire chromosome 21 was sequenced by 2000, and the gene complement turned out to be surprisingly low, only 225 protein-coding loci in all (Hattori et al. 2000). This gene sparseness is plausibly a factor in the survivability of the trisomic state; it may also be that only a minority of the duplicated loci are dosage-sensitive, and thus phenocontributory (Pritchard and Kola 1999). Along with the brain phenotype, certain organ systems are particularly vulnerable, and Torfs and Christianson (1998) identified characteristic malformations in a population study of nearly 3,000 affected infants (Table 13–1). At the top of the list is the heart abnormality, atrioventricular canal defect, which Kurnit et al. (1985) propose may reflect an increased adhesiveness of cardiomyocytes, during the processes of tissue migration as the chambers of the heart are forming.

It was logical that attempts be made to define those regions of the chromosome that might contribute predominantly to the DS phenotype—that is, to identify a "DS critical region" (DSCR), which might

Table 13–1. Some Malformations Frequently Observed in Down Syndrome

MALFORMATION	RELATIVE RISK
Atrioventricular canal defect*	1,009
Annular pancreas	430
Duodenal atresia	265
Patent ductus arteriosus*	152
Small intestinal atresia/stenosis	142
Ventricular septal defect*	95
Tricuspid valve defect*	84
Hypoplastic aorta*	77
Tetralogy of Fallot*	77
Atrial septal defect*	71
Ectopic anus	67
Cataract	54
Intestinal malrotation	45
Anal atresia/stenosis	34
Tracheo-esophageal fistula	26
Syndactyly	26

*Cardiovascular defect.

Source: Data from a population study in California 1983–1993, involving 2,894 infants with Down syndrome (Torfs and Christianson 1998).

contain particular "DS genes." The study of cases with informative incomplete trisomies pointed to the key importance of region 21q22.1q22.3. Within this segment, a major gene of import is *DYRK1A*[1] (chr21:37.42-37.51 Mb), this gene having a role in neurite formation (Park and Chung 2013; Van Bon et al. 2016). Other loci contributing to neurogenesis and neuritogenesis, and which have also been implicated in influencing the DS brain phenotype, are the neural cell adhesion *DSCAM* gene (chr21:40.01-40.84 Mb) and *DSCR1* (also known as *RCAN1*) at chr21:34.51-34.61 Mb.

Shapiro (1997) puts a somewhat different viewpoint, championing the "amplified developmental instability" hypothesis, and comments that "the search for a minimal region on chromosome 21 (the so-called DS critical region) responsible for producing DS has come full circle back to almost the entire chromosome." In his view, a direct role for one or a few single loci with a

---

1 Hypothetically, treatment to inhibit *DYRK1A* activity might ameliorate some DS features (Kim et al. 2016; McElyea et al. 2016).

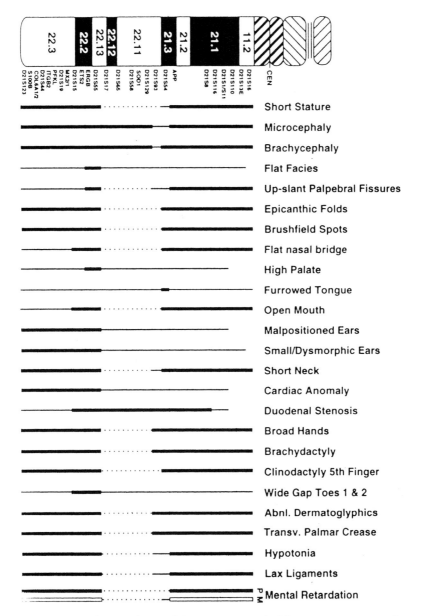

FIGURE 13–1   Phenotypic (trisomic) map of chromosome 21. Thick lines represent regions that must be trisomic to produce the particular trait. Thin-line regions may also contribute to that trait; the contribution of dotted-line regions is less clear. M, mild; P, profound.

Source: From Korenberg et al., Down syndrome phenotypes: The consequences of chromosomal imbalance, *Proc Natl Acad Sci USA* 91: 4997–5001, 1994. Courtesy J. R. Korenberg, and with the permission of the National Academy of Sciences.

one-on-one gene-to-phenotype relationship is simplistic: "Traits that characterize DS are complex, and should be viewed and analyzed accordingly." His general proposition is not unreasonable: That an excess of chromosome 21 encoded gene products perturbs the functioning of the products of many loci, from *all* chromosomes, in all manner of developmental and physiological pathways. An inkling of this concept is put forth in Yu et al. (2015), who, in a study of trisomic 21 fetal cardiac tissue, proposed an interlacing network of gene interaction impacting upon heart development, with a few "hub" genes acting as nodes.

Attempting to draw together the two viewpoints, the gene dosage theory and the amplified developmental instability theory, as do Neri and Opitz[2] (2009), we could suppose that the important genetic segments—the "DS loci"—may have their pathogenic role in the modulation, direct or epigenetic (Aït Yahya-Graison et al. 2007), of layer upon layer upon layer of cellular interactions that leads, as the end result, to a phenotypic *range* that is clinically recognizable as DS. "Complex" may be too simple a word to describe this.

What about the characteristic DS facies? Simply to observe one's fellows is enough to convince one that development of the human face must be the most subtle and complex and precise process. How is it that the DS face is different, and recognizably so? Two proposed contributory factors are the development of the craniofacial skeleton, which might be susceptible to the effects of *DYRK1A* overexpression, and a failure of the facial musculature to divide into its proper various components during fetal development (Bersu 1980; McElyea et al. 2016). A sophisticated 3D imaging analysis of the facies in 55 DS children, compared to their euploid siblings and unrelated euploid children, is offered in Starbuck et al. (2017).

One component of the DS phenotype, an early onset dementia, evolves in adult life and is readily explicable. Duplication of the *APP* locus at 21q21 is the cause, the consequence of a continuing *APP* overexpression, and hence an overproduction of β-amyloid, which, over time, accumulates in the brain (Head et al. 2016). This interpretation is well supported by the observations in the rare form of familial Alzheimer disease due to 21q21 duplication[3] as an isolated genomic rearrangement (Cabrejo et al. 2006).

DIFFERENT CYTOGENETIC FORMS

The usual basis of DS is standard trisomy 21 (Fig. 13–2).The disorder has a number of other cytogenetic forms, and Figure 13–3 depicts the proportions graphically. Differences in the source and nature of the genetic errors underlying these various forms require each to be considered separately.

STANDARD TRISOMY 21 DOWN SYNDROME

The great majority (~95%) of DS is due to simple trisomy of chromosome 21. A little over 90% of these are assumed to reflect a maternal meiotic error, with the rest accounted for by a paternal error, or a (postzygotic) mitotic origin (Yoon et al. 1996; Vranekovic et al. 2012). Approximately 80% of these maternal errors occur at meiosis I, and the remainder apparently at meiosis II, albeit that the latter may actually have been set up at meiosis I. Meiotic I errors are associated with reduced or actual absence of recombination between the chromatids of the chromosome 21 tetrad. Particularly an absence of recombination (with no chiasma forming, thus an "achiasmate" tetrad) may lead to each homolog being able to segregate without reference to the other, and thus without the imperative to move symmetrically.

Among the small fraction (~5%) due to paternal errors, the proportions due to meiotic I and meiotic II errors are nearly equal. As in the female, a reduced frequency of recombination observed in the meiotic I cases may underlie the cause of this male nondisjunction (Savage et al. 1998). Two as yet unexplained observations concerning trisomy 21 due to paternal meiotic errors are these: This fraction is a little greater among prenatally (11%) than postnatally (7%) diagnosed cases; and there is an excess of males among the DS offspring (Muller et al. 2000).

Standard trisomy DS typically occurs as a sporadic, de novo event, and recurrences are rare. These categories of cause of recurrence can be listed: a parental predisposition to nondisjunction, gonadal mosaicism, and chance.

Recurrence due to Nondisjunctional Tendency. Do some (nonmosaic) individuals, for a certain biological or environmental reason, run an increased risk of producing a trisomic 21 conception? Could a specific sequence within chromosome 21 influence its disjunction (Gair et al. 2005)? Are some people susceptible to a dietary deficiency

---

2 Their review celebrates the fiftieth anniversary of the discovery of the chromosomal cause of DS, and it provides a fascinating discussion of nineteenth- and twentieth-century thinking leading up to this event.

3 Such a duplication is on record as having led to a false-positive finding at noninvasive prenatal testing (Meschino et al. 2016).

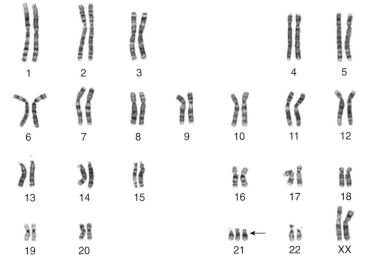

FIGURE 13–2   Karyotype of a child with standard trisomy 21.

affecting meiotic integrity? Is there a range of "meiotic robustness" in the population? These are perfectly respectable concepts, albeit that they remain quite hypothetical. If so, what possibilities might there be? Several theories for a general predisposition to aneuploidy have been put forward, and some of these are discussed on p. 57. While some of these various possibilities may be more plausible than others,

they are all speculative, and we conclude that there is at present no routinely practicable basis enabling the counselor to identify, ahead of time, those parents whose risk is high, and those whose risk is low, to have a second pregnancy with trisomy 21.

Recurrence due to Mosaicism. A trisomy 21 cell population in a parent (gonadal, or

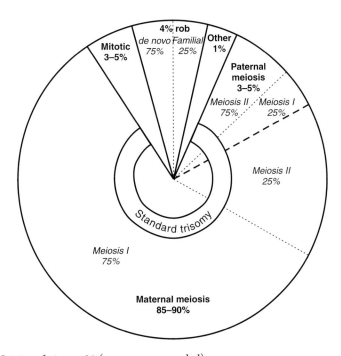

FIGURE 13–3   Origins of trisomy 21 (percentages rounded).

somatic-gonadal mosaicism) is presumed to be an uncommon cause of the production of disomic 21 gametes, although perhaps less rare than originally thought (see below) (Bruyère et al. 2000; Mahmood et al. 2000; Kuo 2002). Pangalos et al. (1992b) studied 22 families in which trisomy 21 had occurred more than once (in siblings, in second- and in third-degree relatives), applying DNA polymorphism analysis. Parental gonadal mosaicism was proposed as the cause of sibling recurrence in five of 13 families (~40%); but other than these, chance alone was enough to explain the recurrences.

Sachs et al. (1990) followed 1,211 pregnancies at prenatal diagnosis, subsequent to the occurrence of trisomy 21 in a previous pregnancy, and observed six recurrences (for a rate of 0.5%). In two of these instances, mosaicism was shown. One father karyotyped as 47,+21/46,N on skin analysis; and one mother showed trisomic cells in 3%, 14%, 44%, and 47% on culture of, respectively, blood and skin, and—in a more direct observation—of each ovary. James et al. (1998) studied four women, each of whom had had three trisomy 21 conceptions. Two of the mothers were under age 35 years at the time of the trisomic conceptions, and they both showed a very low-level mosaicism (0.5% and 4% on blood karyotyping). Neither had a DS phenotype. In their collaborative series from six Japanese clinics, Uehara et al. (1999b) record the exceptional case of a couple having had five successive pregnancies with trisomy 21 (one DS child, four diagnoses at amniocentesis). Both parents had normal karyotypes on blood and skin analysis. It would seem rather probable that one parent may have had fully trisomic gonadal tissue.

Ovarian biopsy proved the point in a mother of three DS children (and one normal child) who typed 46,XX on peripheral blood, but in whom eight out of 20 ovarian cells showed trisomy 21 (Tseng et al. 1994). Other similar examples are on record. We noted Sachs et al. above. Nielsen et al. (1988) report a couple having had six documented pregnancies with standard trisomy 21, and five other unkaryotyped pregnancies ending in neonatal death or abortion. The mother typed 46,XX on peripheral blood, and 47,XX,+21/46,XX in ovarian somatic cells. (Even if the oöcytes were all or nearly all 47,+21, it remains perplexing that no known 46,N conception occurred.) An in vitro fertilization (IVF) setting enabled analysis of the gametes themselves in a woman studied by Cozzi et al. (1999). She had had a normal and a DS child at ages 29 and 32 years, and then had prenatal diagnoses of trisomy 21 at 32 and 36 years. No trisomic mosaicism was detected on peripheral lymphocyte analysis. At IVF, of seven embryos, four were trisomy 21 and one tetrasomy 21, with only two showing normal disomy 21. Four unfertilized oöcytes were analyzed, and three had a supernumerary chromosome 21.[4] A rather elegant demonstration of maternal gonadal mosaicism is described in Cupisti et al. (2003), who, in the study of a woman presenting for fertility treatment, identified three oöcyte-polar body pairs having one copy of chromosome 21 in the egg, and two copies in the first polar body. As for the male parent, Hixon et al. (1998) analyzed sperm samples from 10 men who had fathered a DS child, the additional chromosome 21 having been demonstrated to be of paternal origin. None showed any increase in the fraction of sperm with disomy 21.

The concept that parental gonadal mosaicism may be a substantial contributor to the occurrence (and recurrence) of aneuploidy, and not merely a matter of small-print interest, is latterly due in particular to Kovaleva (2010), Delhanty (2011), and Hultén et al. (2013). Kovaleva assembled data from the literature and from local records, from 80 families in which one parent was gonadal/gonadal-somatic mosaic for trisomy 21. Where the origin of the trisomy in the mosaic parent could be determined, three-quarters had been due to postzygotic rescue of a meiosis I error, and one-quarter came from either rescue of a meiosis II error or a postzygotic mitotic nondisjunction. Interestingly, the sex of the mosaic parent was usually female (61/80 cases), a paucity of mosaic fathers possibly reflecting an impaired spermatogenesis in such men. Kovaleva also proposed a female-specific tendency toward chromosome loss in early embryogenesis (thus allowing trisomy rescue), and suggested that these mosaic females might be not uncommon in the general population. This hypothesis may be supported by observations in the offspring of the mosaic parents. When these parents had nonmosaic DS offspring, the sex ratio was 1.3:1 in favor of males, as observed for DS in the general population. But in the nine instances in which a mosaic DS parent had mosaic DS offspring, in all but one the child was female. The explanation is complex (and unproven), but there may be,

---

4 Two of the no. 21 chromosomes had identical haplotypes, indicating that the mother's mosaicism was due to postzygotic error in an initially normal 46,XX conception (Fig. 3–8a).

first, an intrauterine selection against nonmosaic DS females, and second, a sex-specific tendency for female DS embryos to be converted to the mosaic state by trisomy rescue.

Recurrence Risk Estimates After One Affected Child or Pregnancy. The earliest estimates of risk are due to Penrose (1956),[5] prior to the discovery of the chromosomal basis of DS, and to Stene (1970). Penrose proposed the risk of recurrence to be "doubled, or perhaps nearly trebled" compared to the general population risk, irrespective of maternal age; while Stene derived a figure of 1% for mothers under age 30 years, with no increase in the age-specific risk for those over 30 years, at the time of birth of their DS child. More sophisticated analyses were subsequently enabled by the collection of amniocentesis data, and from population studies, as we present in the sections on parental age and genetic counseling below. It does remain true that for younger mothers the recurrence risk is, in absolute terms, small.

Recurrence Risk Estimates After Two Affected Children/Pregnancies. When a couple have had two (or more) trisomic 21 conceptions, one has to assume an increased risk applies to a subsequent pregnancy, quite possibly a "substantial" risk. The recurrence may well have been due to gonadal mosaicism, but unfortunate chance always remains a possibility, more particularly if the mother is of older age.

Occurrence Risk Estimates with Down Syndrome in a Second- or Third-Degree Relative. More widely in the family, it appears that a history of standard trisomy DS in second- or third-degree relatives does not, in the main, imply an increased risk (Hook 1992; Pangalos et al. 1992b). Berr et al. (1990) assessed 188 families in which a DS child had been born, and there were comparable numbers of DS cases among the second- and third-degree relatives, and in the relatives of 185 control families.

MOSAIC DOWN SYNDROME

47,+21/46,N mosaicism accounts for about 2% of individuals with clinically diagnosed DS. With very low-grade mosaicism, an abnormal phenotype may escape recognition. Papavassiliou et al. (2015) provide an exhaustive literature review, from 1961 to 2014, and offer illustrative examples of the milder phenotype. These authors propose that detection of mosaicism can be achieved when present in as little as 1.6%–1.8% of cells, using fluorescence in situ hybridization (FISH) analysis of peripheral blood (1,000 cells scored) and buccal mucosa (500 cells scored).

Mosaicism results from a malsegregation of homologs, or an anaphase lag of one homolog, occurring postzygotically. Probably the majority of individuals with mosaic DS arise from initially trisomic 21 zygotes, losing one of the chromosomes 21 by anaphase lag, as a form of "trisomy rescue" (Fig. 3–8c in Chapter 3). Others may arise from normal conceptuses, with nondisjunction producing 45,–21/46,N/47,+21 mosaicism, with the 45,–21 line thereafter lost (Fig. 3–8a). Whatever the basis, for practical purposes, counseling needs to proceed as though the child has standard trisomy 21, recognizing that this will overestimate the risk in some. Genetic counseling for the mosaic individuals themselves is covered on p. 237.

Isochromosome 21 Down Syndrome. After standard trisomy 21, this is the most common chromosomal category of DS. It has often been called a "21q21q Robertsonian translocation," but in fact it is almost always the case that the two 21q components are identical, from the same parent, and thus isochromosome is the more accurate term, and the karyotype is more accurately 46,i(21q) (Kovaleva and Shaffer 2003). An agnostic nomenclature is rea(21;21). In one series of 112 de novo rea(21q;21q) DS probands, none of 130 full sibs and 34 half-sibs had DS (Steinberg et al. 1984). Nevertheless, three of the parents actually showed a low-grade mosaicism, and presumably their having had an affected child reflected that the 21q21q cell line was included in the gonad. Indeed, a few examples of recurrence in subsequently born siblings are recorded, and parental gonadal mosaicism is the presumed or proven basis of such recurrence (Hervé et al. 2015). For example, Mark et al. (1977) studied a woman having had sequential pregnancies with the karyotype 46,i(21q), and she herself typed 46,XX,i(21q)/46,XX on ovarian fibroblast analysis (but 46,XX on blood). Hall (1985) offers

---

5 His paper was titled "Some Notes on Heredity Counseling," and he also referred to "genetical counseling," one of the first uses of this expression.

the cautionary story of a mother given a low risk of recurrence, who went on to have a second affected child from a second marriage (on resampling of her, a single 46,XX,i(21q) cell was found in 100 cells analyzed).

ROBERTSONIAN TRANSLOCATION DOWN SYNDROME

Almost all translocation DS concerns a Robertsonian translocation (Chapter 7). About one-quarter of Robertsonian translocation DS is familial and three-quarters is de novo (1% and 3% of all DS, respectively).

De Novo Robertsonian Translocation Down Syndrome. Both parents, by definition, have normal chromosomes. The abnormal chromosome may usually arise as a sporadic event in maternal meiosis I, from a chromatid translocation (Petersen et al. 1991). Such mutational events are rare and, in the great majority of families, recurrences are not seen. But gonadal mosaicism remains a possibility. The so-called rob(21q21q) is, in most cases at least, actually an isochromosome (see above).

Familial Robertsonian Translocation Down Syndrome. One or the other parent (almost always the mother) is a translocation heterozygote and has transmitted the translocation, in an unbalanced state, to the DS offspring. We discuss this in detail in Chapter 7.

DOWN SYNDROME WITH RECIPROCAL TRANSLOCATION

The DS phenotype is substantially due, as we noted above, to a duplication of the chromosome segment 21q22.2q22.3. A reciprocal translocation involving chromosome 21 has the potential to produce, in a gamete from the heterozygote, a duplication of the DS critical region, whether from 2:2 or 3:1 meiotic segregation. The unbalanced adjacent-1 karyotype from the t(18q;21q) illustrated in Figure 5–14 (second row) is an example. Or, interchange trisomy 21 may result (Fig. 5–12). These translocation scenarios are extraordinarily rare, the cause of less than 0.1% of DS. Scott et al. (1995) describe a child with DS from a maternal t(12;21)(p13.1;q22.2), and Nadal et al. (1997) and Lee et al. (2005) describe similar cases from a paternal translocation and insertion, respectively. (It is from studies of cases

of partial trisomy 21, comparing those with typical DS and those with different phenotypes, that phenotypic maps, as in Fig. 13–1, can be drawn; Kondo et al. 2006.) Interchange trisomy 21 was reviewed by Dominguez et al. (2001), with a total of only 23 published families being accumulated.

OTHER CHROMOSOMAL FORMS OF DOWN SYNDROME

A number of chromosomally distinct forms of DS result from specific structural changes to chromosome 21. The least rare of these is the terminal rearrangement that produces a mirror-image chromosome around the telomeric region (Pfeiffer and Loidl 1982). The chromosome has two centromeres, one of which is usually inactive, and satellites on both ends. Such chromosomes are always the result of sporadic mutational events, possibly the result of a translocation between sister chromatids (Pangalos et al. 1992a). DS is seen occasionally in association with other aneuploidies, almost always a sex chromosome aneuploidy, such as 48,XYY,+21 and 46,X,+21; this is known as double aneuploidy. It is usually the result of a double event of nondisjunction resulting in one abnormal gamete. Rather less likely is a scenario of separate events in gametogenesis in both parents.

Interchromosomal effect has been invoked when standard trisomy DS occurs in the setting of a parental karyotypic abnormality not involving chromosome 21 (e.g., a 13;14 Robertsonian translocation, or a reciprocal translocation). It is plausible to imagine that a different "geography" of the chromosomes within the nucleus, imposed by the complicated synapsis of the translocation chromosomes, could perturb the distribution of other "bystander" normal chromosomes at meiosis, and including chromosome 21. The question is controversial; if an effect truly exists, it is apparently of infrequent practical consequence; see also Chapter 5 (Anton et al. 2011; Kovaleva 2013; Li et al. 2015).

PARENT WITH DOWN SYNDROME

Maternal Trisomy 21. At female meiosis, the classical scenario is that the three homologs form either a bivalent and a univalent, or a trivalent (Fig. 13–4; Wallace and Hultén 1983). If the former, the bivalent may disjoin and segregate symmetrically, but the univalent passes at random to either daughter cell (1:1 + 1 segregation). If the latter, a

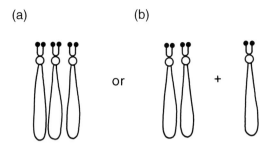

FIGURE 13–4   Possible synapsis of three no. 21 chromosomes: (*a*) as a trivalent and (*b*) as a bivalent and a univalent.

trivalent would of itself set the stage for aberrant segregation (2:1 segregation). Speed (1984) has observed trivalents in about 40% of meiotic cells and a bivalent plus a univalent in the remaining 60%. In either case, the result is disomic (24,+21) and normal (23,N) gametes in equal proportions. An alternative scenario is that the "third" chromosome 21 separates prematurely into chromatids, and each chromatid then passes to a daughter cell (the oöcyte, and the first polar body). Cozzi et al. (1999) provide direct evidence for this mechanism in the FISH study of unfertilized oöcytes from a woman who was presumed to be a 46/47,+21 gonadal mosaic.

In a review of the literature, Shobha Rani et al. (1990) list 30 reports of pregnancy in DS women. The ratio of DS to normal offspring was 10:17 (there were three abortions), not significantly different from a 1:1 ratio, but suggestive of a deficit in trisomic offspring. A reasonable interpretation is that 46,N and 47,+21 conceptions occur with equal frequency, but loss of pregnancy is greater with the trisomic fetuses. About one-third of the 46,N offspring were nevertheless abnormal, which may have reflected paternal factors. Cunniff et al. (1991) noted a diminution in the number of oöcytes in the ovaries of DS girls at the time of birth, which could be the cause subsequently of subfertility.

Paternal Trisomy 21. Spermatogenesis is reduced in the male with nonmosaic DS, but it does not necessarily fail; and a tiny number of examples of proven or suspected fatherhood in DS males have been documented (Pradhan et al. 2006). One notable case concerns the use of IVF with preimplantation genetic screening, with all but one of 10 embryos being eupolid; a phenotypically normal child was born (Aghajanova et al. 2015).

Parental Trisomy 21 Mosaicism. In practice, it is usually only those recognized mosaic individuals with a low percentage of +21 cells who seek genetic advice. These people typically come to notice because they are studied as apparently normal parents of more than one DS child. The important factor, if it could only be known, is the degree to which the gonad comprises 46,N and 47,+21 cells. The trisomic cells produce disomic and normal gametes in equal proportion; of course, normal cells, other things being equal, give rise only to normal gametes. Thus, the proportion of abnormal gametes produced depends on the proportion of germ cells that are trisomic. In the limit, the gonad might be fully 47,+21. Any level of correlation between the degree of mosaicism in lymphocytes and gametes is not readily amenable to study. Familial trisomy 21 mosaicism is on record but is exceptional (Kovaleva 2010).

Trisomies 13 and 18 (Patau Syndrome and Edwards Syndrome)

These syndromes are much less frequent than DS (about 1 in 12,000 and 1 in 6,000 live births for trisomies 13 and 18, respectively), and both show a maternal age effect. As with trisomy 21, correlative phenotypic mapping allows certain segments of chromosomes 13 and 18 to be implicated in the genesis of certain phenotypic traits observed in these syndromes (Tharapel et al. 1986; Epstein 1993; Boghosian-Sell et al. 1994). On molecular studies in trisomy 18, more than 90% reflect a maternal meiotic nondisjunction. Uniquely, nondisjunction is considered to happen most frequently at the second meiotic division, this division not taking place until the short period of time surrounding the process of fertilization (Bugge et al. 1998), although there was a contrary view from Verlinsky's group. From the direct analysis of polar bodies, chromosome 18 meiosis I errors outnumbered those in meiosis II (Verlinsky et al. 2001a). In about 90% of trisomy 13, the additional chromosome is of maternal origin, with meiosis I and II equally susceptible (Bugge et al. 2007); in at least some mosaic cases, the causes may be similar (Jinawath et al. 2011).

Recurrence of trisomy 18 had been recorded in one or two single case reports, and one or two instances of recurrence, or none at all, had been seen in earlier prenatal diagnostic series or retrospective surveys (Pauli et al. 1978; Ferguson-Smith 1983; Stene et al. 1984; Baty et al. 1994; Uehara et al. 1999c). Baty et al. noted a 39-year-old mother having had prenatal diagnosis of trisomy 18 at age 39 years, and a liveborn trisomic 13 infant at age 40 years. No case of trisomy 13 recurrence had been recorded. It had originally seemed that no discernible increased recurrence risk existed, with chance and maternal age the main factors. However, very thorough studies in this century have pointed to an effect, albeit a very subtle one; and this is dealt with in more detail in the section below on "Genetic Counseling."

PARENTAL TRISOMY 18 MOSAICISM

This is extremely rarely recorded in adulthood, and Tucker et al. (2007) review in detail the range of phenotypes. Some had presented with a history of miscarriage, and some due to having had a child with trisomy 18. Because of the usual high rate of lethality of trisomy 18 in utero, the reproductive risks obtaining in such persons would apply substantially to miscarriage. The risk will relate to the gonadal load of trisomic cells; this is not usually known, but some gametic studies are recorded. Bettio et al. (2003) report a woman of normal intelligence with 70% trisomic 18 cells on blood but none on fibroblast karyotyping, presenting with infertility. Ovarian biopsy showed 90% trisomic cells from right ovarian biopsies, and a normal karyotype in left ovarian tissue. A man of normal intelligence and appearance, presenting with severe oligospermia, had approximately 50% trisomy 18 mosaicism on blood and buccal mucosal cell analysis, although only 3% in skin fibroblasts: On sperm study, there was a 10-fold increase in disomy 18, compared with control data, although the absolute fraction was small, 0.68% (Perrin et al. 2009a). Both testes may be free of the trisomic line, as apparently in the father of a normal daughter described in Lim and Su (1998). He was of normal intelligence and worked as a sales representative, and had "slightly unusual facial features." The trisomic line was found only in blood (76%) and not in skin fibroblasts, and the disomic 18 rate in sperm was similar to that of a control.

Other Autosomal Trisomy

It is extremely rare for any other autosomal trisomy to survive through to (or near to) term. About two dozen examples of each of trisomy 9 and 22 are known, and nonmosaic trisomies 7, 8, 10, 14, and 16 are represented by only one or two reports (Brizot et al. 2001; Schinzel 2001; Tinkle et al. 2003; Póvoa et al. 2008; Su et al. 2013). The mosaic state would allow otherwise universally lethal trisomies to survive, such as mosaic trisomy 2, 3, 12, and 17 (Prontera et al. 2011; Baltensperger et al. 2016; Yang et al. 2016; Hong et al. 2017). Some such mosaic cases may have reflected a postzygotic "trisomy rescue."

In contrast, trisomies are very common in miscarrying pregnancies, a matter dwelt upon in detail in Chapter 19. A risk of recurrence, for the same ("homotrisomy") or a different trisomy ("heterotrisomy"), is very slightly increased, and this is discussed in the "Genetic Counseling" section.

PARENTAL TRISOMY 8 MOSAICISM (WARKANY SYNDROME)

Mosaic trisomy 8 arises postzygotically, from an initially normal conceptus (Robinson et al. 1999). Habecker-Green et al. (1998) review reports of reproductive status in 47,+8/46 individuals, and there is only a tiny number of cases, usually in persons in whom the diagnosis would not have been suspected clinically. They describe a woman with mosaic trisomy 8 having a history of four spontaneous losses, including a 46,XX fetal death at 27 weeks; her next pregnancy produced an apparently normal 46,XX daughter. Rauen et al. (2003) report a woman who presented a more typical clinical picture of trisomy 8 mosaicism having a 46,XX child (phenotypic abnormality in the child probably reflected paternal characteristics). Mercier and Bresson (1997) studied an otherwise healthy man, whose partner's recurrent miscarriage was the presenting problem, and in whom the peripheral blood karyotype was 47,XY,+8[8]/46,XY[92]. On FISH analysis of 25,000 spermatozoa, 398 (1.6%) showed disomy 8, which compared with a rate in control sperm of 0.2%. It is perhaps surprising that such a low level of disomic 8 sperm should be associated with a high miscarriage rate (always assuming that the link is causal and not coincidental). We have seen a somewhat similar case, a man of above-average intelligence and excellent physical health, with infertility due to oligospermia, in whom low-level trisomy 8 mosaicism was shown on two separate blood samplings; in his case, one could not exclude that the abnormal cell line was confined to hematological tissue, and the oligospermia coincidental.

Autosomal Monosomy

Many nonmosaic autosomal monosomies are presumed to end in arrested growth in the first few mitoses, at the morula phase, prior even to the time of implantation, with a few possibly proceeding to the stage of "occult abortion." The existence of monosomies would have been unproven, had it not been for the window of observation afforded by pre-implantation diagnosis. The single exception may be monosomy 21, albeit that most earlier reports of monosomy 21 have since been reinterpreted as being due, for the most part, to an unbalanced translocation involving chromosome 21 (Cardoso et al. 2008). One presumed case was identified at 17 weeks of pregnancy, going on to fetal death in utero early in the third trimester, although again the cytogenetic diagnosis was not beyond doubt (Chang et al. 2001; Phelan 2002).

Mosaicism can allow for survival, and for example Hochstenbach et al. (2014) report monosomy 20, in low mosaic state, in a boy with an IQ of 54, poor muscular development, but not dysmorphic, and whose brain MRI was normal. Multiple samples (blood, skin, buccal mucosa) showed monosomy 20 in ½%–4% of cells. As these authors note, this low level of mosaicism would have escaped detection at molecular karyotyping. A clinical index of suspicion should be piqued especially when asymmetry or Blaschko-linear hyperpigmentation (Fig. 3–12) is seen, and that being so, classical karyotyping is the necessary methodology.

POLYPLOIDY

Triploidy

The chromosome count in triploidy is $3n = 69$, with a double ($2n$) chromosomal contribution to the conceptus from one or other parent (Fig. 13–5). Triploidy can reflect di-*andry* or di-*gyny*, with the double contribution coming from the father or mother, respectively (Fig. 13–6). The very great majority of triploid conceptions abort during the first or early second trimester.

The Two Distinct Forms of Triploidy. *Diandry* is usually the consequence of dispermy—that is, two sperm simultaneously fertilizing the ovum (Zaragoza et al. 2000; McFadden et al. 2002).[6] A shorthand description is P1P2M. The fundamental problem in this instance may lie in the "zona reaction," which is the response of the investing shell of the ovum, the zona pellucida, to prevent further sperm entering after the first has penetrated.

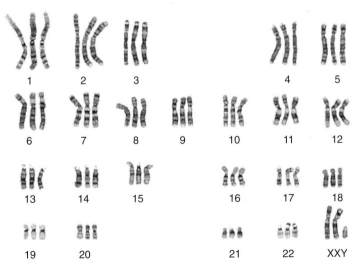

FIGURE 13–5   Karyotype of a 69,XXY triploid fetus (see also Fig. 19–7 in Chapter 19).

---

6 Dispermy could be deduced simply from the cytogenetic analysis in the case reported in Lim et al. (2003), the man carrying a translocation 46,XY,t(2;6)(p12; q24). The 69,XXY mole had both the balanced translocation and one unbalanced form, reflecting fertilization with one sperm from alternate segregation, and the other from adjacent-1. A dispermic mole, at the center of a criminal case, posed a challenge to the assigning of paternity (Budowle et al. 2017).

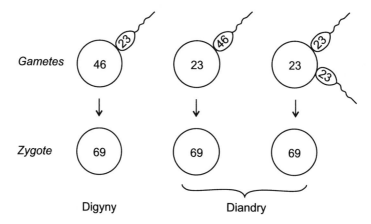

Gametes

Zygote

Digyny   Diandry

FIGURE 13–6   The three major routes whereby triploidy may arise. A complete failure of a meiotic division produces a diploid egg (*left*) or sperm (*middle*). Simultaneous fertilization by two sperm is dispermy (*right*).

Digyny is most commonly due to a diploid egg, which may be the result of nondisjunction of the entire chromosome set at either the first or the second meiotic division in oögenesis, meiosis II being the more vulnerable; or, a polar body may fail to be extruded (Filges et al. 2015). An individual susceptibility may exist, as discussed below. A very rare cause may be the fusion of two eggs (whimsically called "dieggy"). Diploidy can be presumed to exist in the "giant binucleate oöcyte," and these visibly abnormal gametes have actually been shown at IVF to lead to a triploid embryo (Balakier et al. 2002; Rosenbusch et al. 2002).

Natural History. Triploidy is not uncommon in early pregnancy (~1% of recognized conceptions, and 10% of recognized miscarriages), but about 99.99% are lost as first-trimester miscarriage or second-trimester fetal death in utero. Of those aborting at the embryonic stage, most are digynic, while in contrast, most fetal losses reflect a diandric state (McFadden and Robinson 2006). The appearances on morphological examination at the stage of the embryo do not differ according to a digynic versus diandric origin, whereas the clinical presentations are readily distinguishable by the time of the fetal stage of development.

Diandric triploids mostly abort in the first or early second trimester, presenting as hydatidiform mole (Scholz et al. 2015). The very few diandric triploid pregnancies that survive to the second trimester typically show partial hydatidiform mole; growth retardation of the fetus is usual but not invariable (Daniel et al. 2001).

Dygynic triploids are nonmolar, and mostly abort early (mean 10 weeks), although those exceptional few that remain are able to continue through to the third trimester. These surviving digynic triploids develop as a severely growth retarded fetus with marked head-body disproportion, the head being relatively large, and with an abnormally small and nonmolar placenta (McFadden and Langlois 2000; Daniel et al. 2001). In one case of a digynic 69,XXX triploid coexisting with a normal 46,XY twin, survival to 20 weeks (when selective feticide was done) may have been supported by the normal fetus (Gassner et al. 2003). Intrauterine survival may also be promoted if there is fetal-placental karyotypic discordance, with the placenta being diploid (Kennerknecht et al. 1993a). Survival to the third trimester is associated almost invariably with perinatal death. Of those liveborn, hardly any digynic triploids survive for more than a month; there is one extraordinary instance of death not until 312 days (Sherard et al. 1986; Hasegawa et al. 1999).

From Hawaiian data, of 38 recognized triploid pregnancies over the period 1986-1999, approximately 40% were XXX, 60% XXY, and a single case of XYY. Most (80%) aborted early, a few (10%) presented as fetal deaths in utero, and 10% were electively terminated (Forrester and Merz 2003a). In a large Danish series, 84% of triploids were diandric. Of the diandric cases, 69,XXX, 69,XXY, and 69,XYY karyotypes were seen in the proportions 7:8½:1. Of the digynic cases, XXX and XXY cases were of similar frequency (Joergensen et al. 2014). Of all 16-week pregnancies, only 1 in 30,000 are estimated to be triploid, and at 20 weeks, only 1 in 250,000 (Snijders et al. 1995).

RECURRENCE

While most triploidy occurs sporadically, a genetic predisposition does exist, and recurrences are well described. Filges et al. (2015) make the case for a failure of maternal meiosis II as a common basis for this predisposition. In the study of an extraordinary mother-daughter pair, both of whom had had multiple miscarriages, known or likely due to recurrent triploidy, they analyzed a number of candidate genes. One was *PLCD4*, for which mother and daughter were both heterozygous for a predicted pathogenic mutation; and this gene may have a role in the extrusion of the second polar body. Might variation at this, or at some of the other candidate loci, be contributory to digynic triploid recurrence? More difficult to explain is the occurrence of triploidy of both digynic and diandric etiologies to the one couple, and the occurrence of both partial hydatidiform mole (due to diandric triploidy) and complete mole (the rare type associated with biparental disomy) to the same couple (Kircheisen et al. 1991; Deveault et al. 2009). A role for the *NLRP7* gene is proposed (Ulker et al. 2013). These aspects are discussed in more detail in Chapter 19.

> The prevention of chromosomal pathology, as a direct exercise, largely involves secondary prevention: in essence, the selective termination of pregnancies in which a chromosomal abnormality has been identified, or the discarding of abnormal embryos following PGD. Primary prevention is indirect, and encouraging a younger maternal age may be the only feasible approach, absent any clear understanding of environmental factors that might compromise the chromosomal integrity of gamete or zygote. But one remarkable exception to this state of affairs concerns the actual correction of a chromosomally abnormal zygote; and this involves the diandric triploid zygote, otherwise destined to undergo implantation failure or, in the minority that actually implant, to proceed to a severe fetal defect. A triploid zygote due to dispermy will possess three pronuclei. In vitro removal of one pronucleus, at IVF, would restore normality. This would have to be, in the case of

dispermy, one of the paternal pronuclei, thus leaving one maternal and one paternal pronucleus. Escribá et al. (2006) applied this approach to tripronuclear embryos in the research laboratory, removing the pronucleus farthest from the second polar body (the one closest to the polar body being very likely maternal), and followed the embryo through to the blastocyst stage. They were able to confirm restoration of diploidy, and could also observe that these corrected embryos showed normal development at day 5, unlike the uncorrected embryos, in which no inner cell mass was seen to form. And in the first ever example of "chromosomal cure" of a child-to-be, Kattera and Chen (2003) corrected a tripronuclear zygote, implanted the embryo, and a normal 46,XY boy was subsequently born. These authors comment, cautiously, that this approach should be used "only as a last resort." In contrast, Pergament (2010) boldly predicted that, by 2020, we will fully understand the mechanisms of meiosis, and we will be able to "treat oöcytes, sperms and preimplantation embryos to ensure that the euploid state will be obtained at conception and then maintained during early embryonic development," initially doing this in vitro, but eventually in vivo. We shall see.

Diploid/Triploid Mosaicism. Van de Laar et al. (2002) accumulated 25 cases from the literature, and reported three of their own. These three came from a population catchment of 15 million over a 20-year period, attesting to the rarity of the condition. The triploid line typically reflects digyny, and the basic mechanism may be inclusion of the second polar body at a very early stage after conception of a diploid zygote. Similarly in diandric cases, the mechanism may be dispermy, but with one sperm pronucleus sequestered in the cytoplasm for a few divisions before being incorporated into the nucleus (Daniel et al. 2003b; Wegner et al. 2009). Daniel et al. refer to "delayed digyny" and "delayed dispermy," respectively, as the course of events whereby the extra pronucleus sits to one side, so to speak, while the diploid lineage is in the process of being established, and the pronucleus then being taken up into the nucleus of one blastomere to give rise to the triploid cell line. Survival of the affected fetus in utero is presumably promoted by the diploid cell line. In most cases the triploid line is not seen on a blood analysis, and fibroblast culture is necessary (Boonen et al. 2011).

A single instance of a false-negative amniocentesis due to diploid/triploid mosaicism is to be noted (Flori et al. 2003). Controversially, Esfandiari et al. (2016) propose that an embryo diagnosed as triploid at preimplantation trophoblast biopsy might yet be transferred to the uterus, in couples who have otherwise had no normal embryos at PGD. This is done in the hope that the inner cell mass might be diploid, and capable of developing normally, and given that this may be the only hope that they could ever have a baby.

Rare Complexities. "Hypotriploidy" describes the circumstance of a 68-chromosome constitution. The usual mode of formation may be fertilization of a diploid egg with a 22,–X sperm, leading to a 68,XX karyotype; the phenotype resembles that of digynic triploidy (Pasquini et al. 2010).

45,X/69,XXY mosaicism is recorded in a single case, an infant presenting with genital ambiguity, and who displayed complete soft tissue syndactyly of the index and middle fingers of one hand (this being a feature of triploidy) (Quigley et al. 2005). On blood, the karyotype was nonmosaic 45,X, and on skin fibroblast culture, 45,X[3]/69,XXY[77]. The authors propose an initial 46,XY zygote, which lost an X in one cell at possibly the first cell division, giving rise to the 45,X lineage, followed by delayed dispermy of a (or the) 46,XY cell, to give the 69,XXY cell line.

TETRAPLOIDY

A number of mechanisms may lead to a conceptus with 92 chromosomes, four of each homolog ($4n = 92$). The simplest is a reduplication of the diploid set in the zygote: At the first mitosis, the chromosomes replicate, but the cell fails to divide. These would karyotype as either 92,XXXX or 92,XXYY. In the case of a 92,XXXY karyotype, a different mechanism would need to be supposed. In a review of Danish cases having presented as hydatidiform mole, Sundvall et al. (2013) showed two-thirds to reflect the former scenario. In a minority, it is necessary to invoke such processes as trispermy, retention of a polar body with concomitant dispermy, or dispermy with a haploid and a diploid sperm; Sundvall et al. rehearse these and other (rather complicated) possibilities, and propose very early mitotic events that could further modify the

karyotype, with consequential mosaicism. Two examples are on record of women having had a previous digynic triploid, and subsequently a 92,XXXX and 92,XXXY conception, respectively, the latter case proven to reflect an extraordinary coincident maternal and paternal gametic diploidy (Check et al. 2009; Soler et al. 2016).

The typical phenotype is that of miscarriage with complete hydatidiform mole, or "hydropic abortion" (Fukunaga 2004).Tetraploidy in a term pregnancy is exceedingly rare, and survival in one apparently nonmosaic case to 26 months unprecedented (Teyssier et al. 1997; Guc-Scekic et al. 2002). Mosaic diploidy/tetraploidy in a person has been described in association with severe mental defect, and it may only be detectable on skin fibroblast study (Edwards et al. 1994). A complex case is that reported in Leonard and Tomkins (2002) of a retarded woman with body asymmetry and hypomelanosis of Ito, in whom some fibroblasts cultured from hypopigmented skin showed 92,XXXX, others being 46,XX and 46,XX,t(1;6)(p32;q13), and 46,XX on blood.

True diploid/tetraploid mosaicism may be quite frequent at the blastocyst stage of development, but either the abnormal embryo is cast off shortly thereafter or, especially if the proportion of tetraploid cells is small and the blastocyst is otherwise of good quality, the polyploid component may be confined to the trophoblast and in due course come to comprise a minor fraction of placenta (Bielanska et al. 2002b; Clouston et al. 2002). Possibly for this reason, tetraploidy can occasionally be seen at chorionic villus sampling (CVS) and at amniocentesis, reflecting a "normal" tetraploidy of part of the placenta, with the remaining extrafetal and fetal tissues being karyotypically normal (Benkhalifa et al. 1993). Alternatively, tetraploidy at prenatal diagnosis may be artifactual.

THE INFLUENCE OF PARENTAL AGE IN PREDISPOSING TO ANEUPLOIDY

The maternal age association in DownSyndrome was known long before its chromosomal basis. In 1909, Shuttleworth wrote that

> with regard to parentage . . . the outstanding point is the advanced age of the mother at the birth of the child. . . . The next point that strikes one is the large proportion of Mongol children that are lastborn, often of a long family.

He considered that either age or parity could be an etiologic factor. Subsequently, Penrose (1933, 1934) demonstrated that it was the mother's age that was the key factor. A powerful insight into the actual nature of the maternal age effect has been afforded by Battaglia et al.'s (1996) study in normal women, showing that the oöcyte's meiotic apparatus deteriorates with age (Fig. 3–7, and see also color insert).

Sherman et al. (1994) stated that "increasing maternal age is one of the most important factors in human reproductive failure, as well as being a leading contributor to mental retardation among live-borns." Hassold et al. (1993) commented that "the association between increasing maternal age and trisomy is arguably the most important etiologic factor in human genetic disease. Nevertheless, we know almost nothing about its basis"; and likewise, Wolstenholme and Angell (2000) observed, "There is still no consensus of opinion as to how aneuploidy arises in man, and there is a surprising lack of understanding of the basic mechanism(s) of the well-established links to maternal age." Some suggested factors are outlined in Chapter 3. Comparing "ovarian age" (as measured by anti-Müllerian hormone and antral follicle count) with chronological age, in a pregnant population subject to first-trimester screening, showed a subtly more precise, but not materially useful, distinction (Grande et al. 2016).

The maternal age effect in DS—whatever it may be—has been considered to operate upon oögenesis, predisposing to nondisjunction of chromosome 21 predominantly at the first meiotic division. In more general terms, segregation of some other chromosomes is vulnerable to the maternal age effect; and, thus, "older women" who are pregnant run an increased risk for having a pregnancy with trisomies 13, 16, and 18, 47,XXX and 47,XXY, as well as trisomy 21. There is also a slight maternal age association with disorders due to maternal uniparental disomy with trisomy rescue (Ginsburg et al. 2000), this point being discussed in more detail in Chapter 18.

Paternal age generally does not usefully enter the equation, at least with respect to the numerical full aneuploidies (Donate et al. 2016).[7] Fathers of DS children are older than average, but simply because couples are usually of similar ages, a point determined by Penrose in 1934. Nevertheless, albeit that Allen et al. (2009), in a study from the Atlanta and National Down Syndrome Projects, had identified no association with paternal age per se, Steiner et al (2015) made the surprising observation of a subtle but definite effect of younger age of the father (Fig. 13–7). Concerning gametic studies in older men, numerous sperm analyses have been done, with somewhat conflicting findings (Robbins et al. 1997; Shi and Martin 2000b; Eskenazi et al. 2002;

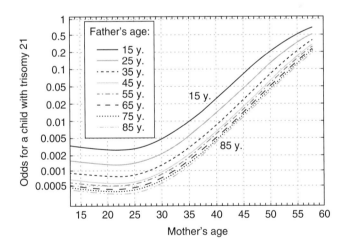

FIGURE 13–7   Parental ages compared to risk to have a child with Down syndrome. Note that *younger* paternal age is a slight risk factor, against the well-known and marked older maternal age effect.

Source: From Steiner et al., An unexpected finding: Younger fathers have a higher risk for offspring with chromosomal aneuploidies, *Eur J Hum Genet* 23: 466–472, 2015. Courtesy B. Steiner and A. Schinzel, and with the permission of Nature Publishing Group.

7 As for structural rearrangements, a true paternal age effect is considered to exist, albeit at an order of magnitude less than the maternal/aneuploidy association (Sloter et al. 2004).

Shi et al. 2002; Iwarsson et al. 2015). Some have shown slight increases in some autosomal disomies, and some have shown increases in sex chromosome disomies, with XY disomy being more consistently noted. Other studies report no significant differences in at least autosomal abnormalities comparing older and younger men (one group even using testicular sperm from men in their eighties; Guttenbach et al. 2000).

Risk Figures According to Maternal Age

How old is "older," and what is "advanced" maternal age at childbearing? Conventionally, the mid- to late thirties is taken as the boundary. The risk curve for DS, the major condition of concern, begins to steepen during this period, although there is no sudden jump. Risk figures for individual ages with respect to this and other aneuploidies have been collected in various jurisdictions, and estimates refined according to certain statistical assumptions, and the information from these studies has long been used as the basis of preconceptional and prenatal genetic counseling. These data are also useful in screening programs for fetal trisomy (Chapter 20), the woman's age-related risk being an important datum to be included, along with the various laboratory test results, in order to derive her overall risk estimate.

For trisomies 13, 18, and 21, spontaneous abortion is more likely than for a normal conceptus. Thus, the prevalence of chromosome abnormality is greater at the time of prenatal diagnosis than at term, and we need access to stage-specific figures. Looking through these different windows of observation—at chorion villus sampling and noninvasive prenatal testing (10 or 11 weeks), at amniocentesis (about 15–17 weeks), at screen-triggered amniocentesis (may be closer to 20 weeks), and at term—the frequency of chromosomal abnormality, for a particular maternal age, progressively reduces. For trisomy 21, it is estimated that about one-third of all pregnancies existing at the time of CVS spontaneously abort between then and term, and one-quarter abort during the period from amniocentesis to term (Table 13–2 and Fig. 13–8). Trisomies 13 and 18 (and monosomy X) have high rates of fetal lethality, with the majority of pregnancies aborting. For XXX and XXY, in contrast, there appears to be very little, if any, selective loss in the latter part of pregnancy.

These matters may be of particular importance to those women who, having had an abnormal result, nevertheless decide to continue a pregnancy. How

Table 13–2. Natural Fetal Loss Rates from Early Pregnancy Through to Term, Estimated for the Three Major Autosomal Trisomies and X Monosomy

ESTIMATED AVERAGE NATURAL PREGNANCY LOSS RATE (%)

CHROMOSOME ABNORMALITY	FROM 9–14 WEEKS TO BIRTH	FROM 15–20 WEEKS TO BIRTH	FROM >20 WEEKS TO BIRTH
Trisomy 13	50	44	40
Trisomy 18	70	65	64
Trisomy 21	32	25	10
Monosomy X	65	52	

Note: 9-15 and 15-20 weeks approximate to the stages at which CVS and amniocentesis are performed.
Sources: From Snijders et al. (1995), Won et al. (2005), Savva et al. (2006), and Cavadino and Morris (2017).

likely is it that they will have a liveborn baby with the trisomy in question, or that fetal death in utero will supervene ? Won et al. (2005) reviewed 392 women who had continued a trisomy 21 pregnancy, and 106 with trisomy 18; the diagnoses had been given somewhat later than might be usual, because these women had entered a public maternal serum screening program at gestations ranging from 15 to 20 weeks, with amniocentesis then offered to those who returned an increased risk result. For trisomy 21, fetal demise occurred in 10%, and for trisomy 18, 32%. About one-third of the trisomy 21 losses happened before the stage of viability (i.e., 24 weeks), the comparable figure in trisomy 18 being 15%. In those pregnancies proceeding beyond 24 weeks, the losses were evenly spread according to duration. More recent figures for trisomies 13 and 18 are due to Cavadino and Morris (2017), derived from a whole population study in England and Wales. From their work, for trisomy 13, a surprisingly high 50% of fetuses diagnosed at 12 weeks will survive to term, and for trisomy 18, the figure is 30%; these authors discuss possible reasons for the very considerable differences between studies. It is their more recent data that we use in Table 13–2.

DOWN SYNDROME

The largest body of data to be collated for the age-related risk of trisomy 21 is that of Morris et al.

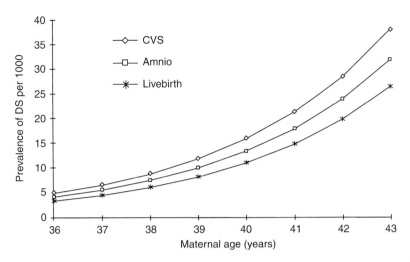

FIGURE 13-8   Prevalence of Down syndrome for maternal ages 36–43 years, at three "windows of observation": the time at which CVS is done (~10 weeks), amniocentesis (15–17 weeks), and at live birth.

Source: From Halliday et al., New estimates of Down syndrome risks at chorionic villus sampling, amniocentesis, and livebirth in women of advanced maternal age from a uniquely defined population, *Prenat Diagn* 15: 455–465, 1995. Courtesy J. L. Halliday.

(2002), who examined records from a 10-year period, 1989–1998, in England and Wales. We have used their material as the basis of the age-related live-birth figures to age 44 years presented in Table 13–3, as probably the best available, although in fact the estimates for younger women (up to age 34 years) have been very similar in all studies, and quite similar in the 35- to 44-year age bracket (Morris et al. 2003). However, and contrary to earlier interpretations, the risk of having a baby with trisomy 21 does not increase from age 45 years and older (Morris et al. 2005a). This might reflect a greater tendency to miscarry an abnormal fetus in women into their forties and early fifties (Stern et al. 2016); or hypothetically a "meiotic robustness" in some women of this age who are yet able to achieve pregnancy. Estimates for the likelihoods of detection of trisomy 21 at prenatal diagnosis, at the maternal ages at which the procedures would be done, are given in Table 13–4.

Subtly different data are due to Hartwig et al. (2016), who analyzed directly prenatal first-trimester diagnoses made over the period 2005–2014 in a whole country population in Denmark, with practically 100% ascertainment. They concluded that the risks from previous indirect studies (Snijders et al. 1995, 1999; Morris et al. 2002) had been slightly overstated. Figure 13–9 shows a graphical comparison. These workers derived similar data for trisomies 13 and 18, again showing very subtle differences compared with earlier material. Hartwig et al. propose that these more accurate data, when incorporated into prenatal risk assessment algorithms, might usefully adjust thresholds at which interventions would be advised.

OTHER ANEUPLOIDY

The figures for DS are of most interest because this condition (1) produces a major mental handicap, (2) implies a major burden for parents in that survival well into adult life is now the norm, and (3) is the most common single chromosome defect in newborns. But the data for other aneuploidies are important. Women seeking advice on their age-related risk, and considering prenatal diagnosis, should know also that some other rather uncommon trisomies of severe effect (13 and 18) might be detected; and that, on the other hand, there are some age-related sex chromosome aneuploidies (XXX, XXY) that have much milder, but not trivial, effects. Tables 13–5 and 13–6 set out age-related risk estimates for these other categories of aneuploidy. There is also the possibility, irrespective of maternal age, that some other type of chromosome defect might exist. Table 13–7 sets out the risk for any chromosomal defect, whether maternal-age associated or not, to be detected at prenatal diagnosis. To put these figures into some perspective, we remind the reader that the prevalence of unbalanced chromosomal abnormality in the whole newborn population is approximately 0.5%, or 1 in 200 (Table 1–1). Another window of observation is

Table 13–3. Maternal Age-Specific Risks for Trisomy 21 at Live Birth

MATERNAL AGE (YEARS)	PREVALENCE AT LIVE BIRTH		MATERNAL AGE (YEARS)	PREVALENCE AT LIVE BIRTH	
	%	1 IN		%	1 IN
14	0.09	1,108	34	0.23	430
15	0.04	2,434	35	0.30	338
16	0.05	2,013	36	0.39	259
17	0.06	1,599	37	0.50	201
18	0.06	1,789	38	0.62	162
19	0.07	1,440	39	0.88	113
20	0.07	1,441	40	1.2	84
21	0.07	1,409	41	1.5	69
22	0.07	1,465	42	1.9	52
23	0.07	1,346	43	2.7	37
24	0.07	1,396	44	2.6	38
25	0.07	1,383	45 or older	3.4	30
26	0.08	1,187			
27	0.08	1,235			
28	0.09	1,147			
29	0.10	1,002			
30	0.10	959			
31	0.12	837			
32	0.14	695			
33	0.17	589			

Note: The figures to age 44 years are based on data from just over 6 million births in England and Wales 1989–1998; the figures for 45 years or older come from a review of several sources internationally. Prenatal diagnostic data were included in this material, weighted according to the probability of survival to term. No trisomy 21 pregnancies were recorded at ages 11–13 years (274 births) or at ages 53–55 years (169 births). The percentage figures are rounded.*Source:* From Table 2 in Morris et al. (2002), the data up to age 44 years; and from Morris et al. (2005a), for age 45 years or older.

afforded at preimplantation diagnosis; rates of aneuploidy increase, according to the mother's age, in biopsied embryos (Table 13–8).

NO PARENTAL AGE EFFECT IN SOME DEFECTS

There is no discernible increasing risk with increasing maternal age for the following chromosomal abnormalities: de novo rearrangement, XYY, triploidy, and unbalanced karyotype due to transmission of parental translocation. For monosomy X, the risk actually lessens with increasing maternal age. With only the barest paternal age association (Fig. 13–7), advanced paternal age is not of itself a particular indication for chromosomal prenatal diagnosis, although a case might hypothetically be made for a much older (sixties

and older) father, in respect of de novo structural rearrangement.

SECULAR CHANGES IN MATERNAL AGE DISTRIBUTION AND DOWN SYNDROME PREVALENCE

Changing maternal age profiles in a population will influence the birth prevalence of DS. In the England of Shakespeare's time, few women lived long enough to bear children in older age, and along with the effects of poor survival in DS, perhaps no more than 100 individuals with trisomy 21 then existed in that country, in a total population of 4 million (Berg and Korossy 2001); a similar situation exists in some developing countries today. (Nevertheless, Levitas and Reid (2003) were able to record a number of probable and possible depictions in art

Table 13–4. Maternal Age-Specific Risks for Trisomy 21 Calculated at 10 Weeks Gestation (the Usual Time for CVS) and at 16 Weeks (Amniocentesis)

MATERNAL AGE* (YEARS)		GESTATION 10 WEEKS	16 WEEKS
20	1 in	800	1050
25		710	930
30		470	620
31		410	540
32		350	460
33		290	380
34		235	310
35		185	245
36		150	195
37		115	150
38		90	115
39		65	90
40		50	70
41		40	50
42		30	40
43		20	30
44		15	20

*Age at the indicated gestation.
Source: From Table 2 in Snijders et al. (1995). Figures are rounded.

from centuries past, and indeed Martínez-Frías (2005) has presented a photograph of a terracotta head, made in about 500 AD in Mexico, that convincingly captures the essence of the DS facies.) In New Zealand in the 1920s, maternal mortality was much less of an issue, but family planning was rudimentary, and about 45% of all mothers were aged 30 years or older. The great majority (~90%) of all DS babies from that period, at least those surviving to the 1960s to have a chromosome study, were born to mothers in this age group. Over the next four decades, family planning practices became gradually more widespread. By the late 1960s, most women were completing their families while still in their twenties, and "older mothers" made much less contribution to the overall birth rate. Only 20% of all mothers were aged 30 years or older; and the proportion of all DS babies born to this age group had fallen to 53% (Gardner et al. 1973a). We presume, therefore, that the birth prevalence of DS in New Zealand progressively fell over the period 1920–1970.

Hook (1992) reviewed the prevalences of DS in various areas of the world during the early 1980s, in relation to the proportions of mothers aged 35 years or older. The former Czechoslovakia had the lowest proportion, 3.6%, of older mothers, and Northern Ireland, at 11.1%, the highest. As expected, the observed rates of DS births showed a relationship, with 0.106% in Czechoslovakia, and 0.16% in Northern Ireland. In the 1980s and 1990s, there was

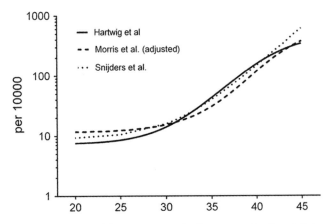

FIGURE 13–9   The maternal age-related first trimester risks for trisomy 21, 18 and 13 based on Danish first trimester data from 2005 to 2014, Prenat Diagn 36: 643-649, 2016. Similar graphs for trisomies 13 and 18 are also in Hartwig et al. (2016).

Source: From Hartwig et al., The maternal age-related first trimester risks for trisomy 21, 18 and 13 based on Danish first trimester data from 2005 to 2014, *Prenat Diagn* 36: 643–649, 2016. Courtesy T.S. Hartwig, and with the permission of John Wiley & Sons.

Table 13–5. Maternal Age-Specific Risks for Trisomies 13 and 18 Calculated at 10 Weeks Gestation (the Usual Time for CVS), 16 Weeks (Amniocentesis), and at Live Birth

MATERNAL AGE* (YEARS)		TRISOMY 13				TRISOMY 18		
		10 WEEKS	16 WEEKS	LIVE BIRTH		10 WEEKS	16 WEEKS	LIVE BIRTH
20	1 in	6,500	11,000	14,300	1 in	2,000	3,600	10,000
25		5,600	9,800	12,500		1,750	3,200	8,300
30		3,700	6,500	11,100		1,200	2,100	7,200
35		1,500	2,600	5,300		470	840	3,600
36		1,200	2,000	4,000		370	660	2,700
37		900	1,600	3,100		280	510	2,000
38		700	1,200	2,400		220	390	1,500
39		530	920	1,800		170	300	1,000
40		400	700	1,400		130	230	740
41		300	530	1,200		95	170	530
42		230	400	970		70	130	400
43		170	300	840		55	95	310
44		130	220	750		40	70	250

*Age at the indicated gestation or at birth, respectively.

Source: Prenatal data from Tables 3 and 4 in Snijders et al. (1995), and modeled livebirth estimates from Appendix A in Savva et al. (2010). Figures are rounded.

Table 13–6. Maternal Age-Specific Risks for 47,XXX and 47,XXY at Amniocentesis and at Live Birth

MATERNAL AGE (YEARS)	XXX			XXY		
	AMNIO (%)	LIVE BIRTH (%)	1 IN	AMNIO (%)	LIVE BIRTH (%)	1 IN
33		0.04	2,500		0.04	2,500
34		0.05	2,000		0.04	2,500
35	0.04	0.05	2,000	0.05	0.06	1,650
36	0.05	0.06	1,650	0.06	0.07	1,450
37	0.07	0.08	1,250	0.08	0.09	1,100
38	0.09	0.09	1,100	0.11	0.11	900
39	0.11	0.11	900	0.14	0.14	700
40	0.14	0.13	770	0.18	0.17	600
41	0.18	0.16	630	0.24	0.22	450
42	0.22	0.19	530	0.31	0.27	370
43	0.28	0.22	450	0.41	0.34	300
44	0.36	0.27	370	0.54	0.43	230
45	0.45	0.32	310	0.70	0.54	180
46	0.57	0.38	260	0.90	0.68	150
47	0.70	0.45	220	1.2	0.85	120
48	0.90	0.55	180	1.5	1.1	95
49	1.1	0.65	150	2.0	1.3	75

Source: From data in Tables 20.4 and 20.7 in Hook (1992). Figures are rounded.

Table 13–7. Maternal Age-Specific Risks for All Unbalanced Chromosomal Abnormalities at Chorionic Villus Sampling[a] and at Amniocentesis,[b] for the Age Range 33–45 Years

	CHORIONIC VILLUS SAMPLING		AMNIOCENTESIS	
MATERNAL AGE[c] (YEARS)	%	1 IN	%	1 IN
33			0.5	200
34			0.6	160
35	0.9	115	0.8	120
36	1.2	85	1.0	100
37	1.5	65	1.2	80
38	2.0	50	1.5	65
39	2.5	40	2.0	50
40	3.5	30	2.5	40
41	4.5	22	3	33
42	6.0	17	4	25
43	7.5	13	5	20
44	10	10	6	17
45	13	8	7	14

[a]Including invariably lethal defects.
[b]Including those for which there is no maternal age effect.
[c]Age at time of procedure.
Source: Taken from "averaging" data for ages 33–45 years in Tables 20–7 and 20–8 (amniocentesis) and for ages 35–45 years from Table 20–10 (CVS) in Hook (1992). Figures are rounded.

a reversal of the maternal age trend in several areas of the world, with older mothers closing the gap on their younger counterparts. In South Australia, for example, after falling to a trough around 1975–1978,

the fraction of mothers older than age 35 years progressively rose, and the birth prevalence of DS was anticipated to rise from a low point of about 0.09% in the late 1970s to greater than 0.15% in 1990–1994 (Staples et al. 1991). In Israel, maternal age dipped in 1978 to a low of 8% of Jewish mothers being age 35 years or older, and rose to 17% by 1992; and in Alberta, Canada, the comparable figures are 4% in 1980, to 16% in 2007 (Shohat et al. 1995; Lowry et al. 2009). These trends are similar in most affluent countries.

Trisomies 13 and 18 have a maternal age association, and so it is not surprising that similar changes in prevalence are observed. From UK and Australian data (and adjusting for prenatal diagnosis and termination), the live birth rates increased by 13% and 25% for the two trisomies, respectively, from 1989–1996 to 1997–2004 (Savva et al. 2010).

The DS birth prevalence is considerably influenced by the use of prenatal diagnosis and selective pregnancy termination, these options becoming widely available in many countries from the 1970s and 1980s, and then with serum screening becoming adopted into the 1990s. In England and Wales over the period 1974–1987, 14% of potential DS births were avoided by selective abortion, reducing the birth prevalence from 0.126% to 0.108% (Cuckle et al. 1991). In Belgium, Verloes et al. (2001) calculated a theoretical halving in the incidence of DS, from 1/800 to 1/1,600, from the 1980s to the 1990s, with at least 90% of trisomic 21 pregnancies terminated. The South Australian figures noted above are estimates of the birth prevalences had termination not been used; in fact, the actual prevalences were correspondingly less (Cheffins et al. 2000). More recent data have come from large studies from England and Wales (Morris and Alberman 2009) and the United States (Egan et al. 2011), and these reflect the increasing

Table 13–8. Aneuploidy Rates in 591 Embryos Tested by FISH at Preimplantation Genetic Diagnosis in the Course of In Vitro Fertilization, with Respect to Chromosomes 13, 15, 16, 18, 21, 22, X and Y, According to Maternal Age

MATERNAL AGE (YEARS)	25–34	35–37	38–39	40–41	42–44
% Aneuploid	8	10	18	26	30
% Other abnormal	31	30	35	31	31
% Normal	61	60	47	43	39

Source: From Munné et al. (2002b).

access to noninvasive screening. In England and Wales from 1989 to 2008, while the number of DS diagnoses overall rose very substantially, by 71%, concomitant with a changing maternal age profile, the number of actual DS births fell marginally, from 755 to 743. The proportion choosing termination over this period remained constant, at 92%.

A similar "evening-out" was seen in 15 countries of the European Union over the period 1980–1999, with both the highest rise in maternal age and the highest use of termination seen in Paris, and the DS prevalence in that city remaining stable at 0.076% (Dolk et al. 2005). Similarly in Switzerland, the mean maternal age rose from 26 years in 1980 to 30 years in 1996, but the incidence of DS remained practically unchanged (Mutter et al. 2002). In the United States over the period 1989–2006, the reduction in DS births has varied according to region, with the observed births 44% of expectation in the West, compared with 68% in the Midwest; in the Northeast and the South, the figures fell between, but tending more toward those of the West. From their analysis, Egan et al. (2011) conclude that "a Down syndrome fetus is more likely to be prenatally diagnosed and terminated in the West and least likely to be diagnosed and terminated in the Midwest." In China, residence in a rural or urban setting has a strong influence upon the prevalence of DS. Deng et al. (2015) surveyed findings over the period 1996–2011 and showed a birth rate rising, by 2003, to 0.199%, and falling thereafter. An increasing utilization of prenatal diagnosis and termination, over 2003–2011, led to substantial reductions in birth prevalence, by 62% in an urban population and 36% in a rural population, over that time frame. In Hawaii, the birth rate has been fluctuating, but is overall static, at about 0.08%, over the period 1997–2005 (McDermott and Johnson 2011). The influence of termination may be more noticeable among older women: In Alberta, Canada, in 2007, the birth rate of DS to mothers in their forties was 1.32%, but it would have been 2.15% had not termination been available, whereas the comparable rates for 20- to 24-year-olds were 0.055% and a not much greater 0.076% (Lowry et al. 2009). A somewhat different picture is reported from Japan, where recourse to termination is less frequently sought; the DS birth incidence has been rising, as the maternal age spectrum moved to the right (Takeuchi et al. 2008).

Prevalence is also influenced by the greater survival of children and adults with DS in recent decades. The survival figure to age 1 year for Western Australia rose from 83% in those born during 1966–1975 to 94% for the period 1991–1996, and survival to age 10 years rose to 85% (Leonard et al. 2000). In Sweden, Englund et al. (2013) reviewed mortality in a DS population over the period 1969–2003 and determined that the median age at death was rising by 1.8 years per year, and approaching 60 years. Dementia (a well-recognized and understood concomitant of DS) was a main or contributing cause of death in one-third.

ETHNICITY

Systematic calculations from other than Caucasian ethnic groups have come from Nigeria, China, Japan, South America, and Hawaii. Adeyokunnu (1982) showed, in Nigeria, no difference in incidence of trisomy 21 compared with Europeans; and in a study encompassing nine South American countries, Carothers et al. (2001) demonstrated incidence data and maternal age correlations very similar to those recorded from other jurisdictions. In Japan, Yaegashi et al. (1998) collected data from four clinics, comprising, in all, 5,484 pregnancies of women aged 35 years or older. The risks for trisomy 21 (and for aneuploidies) overall were, on the face of it, somewhat less than in a European population. The raw figures did, however, fluctuate somewhat, with rather small numbers of affected fetuses at each age category. A question might be raised whether some cases could have escaped ascertainment by earlier screening and not otherwise recorded. It may be premature to suppose that aneuploidy rates could differ to any important degree between Japanese and other ethnic groups, a view that is supported by the observation otherwise of no significant differences in a Hong Kong population (Lau et al. 1998); but bearing in mind also data from Hawaii suggesting that, at older maternal ages, the DS rate *may* be somewhat less in a Pacific Island population (Forrester and Merz 2003b). Taking a more fundamental viewpoint, Ghosh et al. (2009) demonstrated that rates of meiotic recombination in families with a DS child in India were essentially the same as in a U.S. population, pointing to a basic identity of nondisjunctional mechanism across these populations. And taking a refined view of ethnicity (genotyping of "ancestry informative markers"), Franasiak et al. (2016) saw no differences among patients attending an IVF clinic, and whose embryos had been tested for aneuploidy, among those of European, African, East Asian, or Central/South Asian ancestry.

GENETIC COUNSELING

Down Syndrome

The central requirement for accurate genetic advice in DS is knowledge of the chromosomal form in the affected family member. If a child diagnosed as having DS has died and no chromosome studies were performed, and more so if a case of younger maternal age, it may be reasonable to check for the possibility of a familial translocation in the consultand.

PREVIOUS CHILD WITH STANDARD TRISOMY 21 (INCLUDING MOSAICISM)

If the child has standard trisomy 21, or is a 47,+21/46 mosaic, it is unnecessary routinely to study the parents' chromosomes.[8] One can assume, with considerable confidence, that they will type as 46,XX and 46,XY. The risk of recurrence of trisomy 21 (homotrisomy), or occurrence of a different aneuploidy (heterotrisomy), is typically small, but above that of a same-age maternal population. Broad-brush estimates of increased risk are listed in Table 13–9. More precise data are shown in Table 13–10. Small differences between these estimates may relate to simple statistical variation, but note also that Table 13–9 refers to risk for the birth of an affected child, whereas Table 13–10 relates to the risk at the time of amniocentesis.

In any event, regardless of the exact figure, the practical point is that the risk for a recurrence of DS is comfortingly low, only approaching the 1% mark by the mid-thirties. Nevertheless, most couples seek the reassurance of prenatal diagnosis in pregnancies after having had a child with DS. Many may choose the option of noninvasive prenatal diagnosis, which relieves the couple of having to balance the risk of recurrence against the risk of a procedure-related

Table 13–9. Increases in Recurrence Risk, Given as Multiples Compared with the Maternal Age-Related Baseline, for Women Who Have Had a Previous Trisomic Pregnancy

PREVIOUS ABNORMAL PREGNANCY	FOLD INCREASED RISK OF RECURRENCE FOR:	
	SAME TRISOMY	OTHER VIABLE TRISOMY
Trisomy 21 at maternal age <30, current maternal age <30	8.2×	2.4×
Trisomy 21 at maternal age <30, current maternal age ≥30	2.2×	2.4×
Trisomy 21 at maternal age <35	3.5×	1.3×
Trisomy 21 at maternal age ≥30	1.6×	1.7×
Trisomy 21 at maternal age ≥35	1.7×	1.5×
Trisomy 13 overall	8.6–9.5×	1.5×
Trisomy 18 overall	1.7–3.1×	1×
Trisomy 13 or 18 at maternal age <35	7.8×	1.6×
Trisomy 13 or 18 at maternal age ≥35	2.2×	1×
Trisomies 13, 18, XXX and XXY	2.3×	1.6×
Nonviable trisomy in spontaneous abortion*		1.8×

Notes: The above figures relate to the *probability of trisomy at livebirth*. Separate figures are given for the risk of recurrence of the same trisomy (homotrisomy) or of a different trisomy (heterotrisomy). If wished, the appropriate multiple for a particular case can be applied to the woman's current age-related risk, as listed in Tables 13–3 to 13–6, in order to generate an adjusted recurrence risk figure. Figures are from the prenatal data of Warburton et al. (2004) and pre- and postnatal data of De Souza et al. (2009), and they are grouped in various ways, according to the formats of these papers. Specific age-related figures for previous trisomy 21 are also given in Table 13–10, column B. The best data may be those of Hartwig et al. (2016); see above.

*But cf. Robinson et al. (2001), who discerned no increased risk following an aneuploid miscarriage.

---

8 But parental chromosome studies should be considered following the prenatal diagnosis of trisomy 21 by microarray, since microarray cannot distinguish translocation DS from standard trisomy 21.

Table 13–10. Estimates of Recurrence Risk for Trisomy 21, According to the Mother's Current Age (Column A) and According to Her Age at the Birth of the Affected Child (Column B)

A. BASIC AGE-SPECIFIC RISK		B. ADDITIONAL RISK DUE TO PREVIOUS DS	
MATERNAL AGE AT THIS CURRENT PREGNANCY (YEARS)	RISK (%)	AGE AT THE EARLIER DS PREGNANCY (YEARS)	RISK (%)
20	0.09	20	0.62
21	0.09	21	0.62
22	0.09	22	0.61
23	0.09	23	0.60
24	0.09	24	0.58
25	0.10	25	0.57
26	0.10	26	0.54
27	0.11	27	0.52
28	0.11	28	0.48
29	0.12	29	0.44
30	0.14	30	0.40
31	0.16	31	0.35
32	0.19	32	0.29
33	0.23	33	0.24
34	0.29	34	0.19
35	0.37	35	0.15
36	0.49	36	0.11
37	0.66	37	0.08
38	0.88	38	0.06
39	1.17	39	0.05
40	1.52	40	0.04
41	1.92	41	0.03
42	2.35	42	0.02
43	2.78	43	0.02
44	3.20	44	0.02
45	3.58	45	0.02
46	3.92	46	0.01
47	4.21	47	0.01
48	4.45	48	0.01
49	4.64	49	0.01
50	4.80	50	0.01

Notes: Risks A and B are then to be summed. This combined risk figure relates to the *probability of detection of trisomy 21 at early second-trimester amniocentesis*. For example, a woman who is now pregnant and due to deliver at age 30 years (risk = 0.14% from column A), and who had had a DS pregnancy when she was 25 years old (additional risk = 0.57% from column B), has an overall risk for trisomy 21 in the current pregnancy of 0.14 + 0.57 = 0.71%, or 1 in 141. Note how, with advancing maternal age at the current pregnancy (A), the additional risk component due to having had a previously affected child (B) progressively diminishes; in other words, at these older ages, the maternal age factor becomes the overwhelming contributor to the risk.

DS, Down syndrome.

Source: From Morris et al. (2005b).

pregnancy loss. Elkins et al. (1986b) observe that some of these parents declare they would not abort a trisomy 21 fetus, and the counselor needs to be sensitive to possible ambivalent feelings of the parents in this setting.

TWO PREVIOUS TRISOMIC 21 CONCEPTIONS

One can only offer an educated guess that the risk for a third trisomic conception will be "substantial." A skin biopsy study would be largely academic. If gonadal mosaicism (rather than de novo recurrence) is the cause, a considerable fraction of whichever gonad it is must be involved, since two separate samplings have already come from this fraction. A risk in the range of 10%–20% may be a fair figure to offer. Preimplantation genetic diagnosis would have an obvious attraction.

ISOCHROMOSOME 21 DOWN SYNDROME

From the 0/164 fraction among siblings of de novo isochromosome 21q DS in Steinberg et al.'s (1984) series, the risk for recurrence was originally presumed to be small. Nevertheless, three parents (3%) in this series were demonstrably mosaic; and subsequently Hervé et al. (2015) listed 10 cases of recurrence due to known or suspected parental gonadal mosaicism. A concerted search for parental mosaicism (more than one tissue, high cell count) could reasonably be proposed. While the overall risk figure may be low, perhaps in the region of 1%–2%, a cautious approach is certainly prudent. If parental mosaicism is actually detected, a considerably higher risk figure would apply, likely approaching a double-figure percentage.

PREVIOUS CHILD WITH ROBERTSONIAN TRANSLOCATION DOWN SYNDROME

Obviously, distinction between de novo and familial forms of translocation DS is crucial; this distinction is made by chromosomal studies of the parents. For the de novo translocation, a recurrence risk figure of <1% is applicable (Gardner and Veale 1974). In the case of *familial* Robertsonian translocation DS, the genetic risk for the female carrier is substantial. The risk to have a liveborn child with translocation DS is about 10%, while the likelihood to detect translocation trisomy 21 at amniocentesis is about 15%. For

the male carrier, the risk to have a child with translocation DS is small, about 1% (and see Chapter 7).

PREVIOUS CHILD WITH NON-ROBERTSONIAN TRANSLOCATION DOWN SYNDROME

In the rare instance that translocation DS is associated with a familial reciprocal translocation, the principles presented in Chapter 5 are to be followed.

PREVIOUS CHILD WITH OTHER CHROMOSOMAL CATEGORY OF DOWN SYNDROME

For sporadic structural changes such as the terminal rearrangements, the risks are presumed to be very low (<0.5%). For the double aneuploidies, there is no evidence to suggest the risks are any different from the recurrence risks for standard trisomic DS.

WIDER FAMILY HISTORY OF DOWN SYNDROME

There is no conclusive evidence of an increased risk for second- and third-degree relatives of individuals with standard trisomic DS themselves to have offspring with the condition. The appropriate action in the setting of "a family history of DS" is to determine whether the affected member has standard trisomy 21. If this is so, the family may be reassured that there is no discernibly increased risk, which advice could also reasonably be offered if a single case was associated with older maternal age. If the karyotype of the index case is unknown, and the mother had been younger, the small possibility of a familial translocation may be checked by chromosome study of the counselee.

TRISOMY 21 IN PRODUCTS OF CONCEPTION

The finding of trisomy 21 in products of conception after spontaneous abortion (in those centers where this testing may be done) presents a problem. Should this, for genetic counseling risk assessment, be regarded as equivalent to having had a child with DS? From about 10 weeks gestation through to term, about one-third of trisomic 21 conceptions are lost, and it may be stochastic events in utero, in part correlating with maternal age, rather than intrinsic genetic differences, that distinguish those that abort and those that survive. It may be prudent to err on the side of caution and provide a risk figure as though the abortion had been a liveborn child.

PARENT WITH DOWN SYNDROME

The risk to the female with DS is clearly high, as discussed above, although nearer a one-third figure (reflecting natural trisomy 21 miscarriage) rather than a theoretical one-half. It is almost, but not absolutely, unknown for a male with DS to achieve fatherhood. A genetic risk may in fact be small, due to selection against disomic sperm. Ethical issues arising in these circumstances are discussed in Chapter 1.

Previous Pregnancy with Trisomy 13, Trisomy 18, or Other Autosomal Trisomy

Recurrence of trisomy 13 or 18 is a very rare observation. The recurrence risk is, in fact, very small, as displayed in Table 13–9. As for an increased risk for a different potentially viable trisomy, such as trisomy 21 ("heterotrisomy"), again in absolute terms it is very small, but does exist. Warburton et al. (2004) derived an overall 1.6-fold increased risk factor. In their large study of a U.K. population, Alberman et al. (2012) recorded two heterotrisomic recurrences (both trisomy 13) from mothers of a previous child with trisomy 18, but no recurrences (hetereo- or homotrisomic) following a pregnancy with trisomy 13.[9] They commented that these mothers were "relatively elderly," and perhaps this may have been the basis of the recurrences. In the case of a previous pregnancy with some other type of autosomal trisomy (typically identified in products of conception following spontaneous abortion), from Warburton there is an overall increased risk (1.8-fold), which Grande et al. (2017) refine in terms of maternal age (Table 13–11). As Table 13–11 shows, the additional increased risk, over and above that due to maternal age per se, lowers as age increases, from 0.37% at age 20 years, and by the late forties is barely perceptible, at 0.01%.

Table 13–11. Maternal Age-Dependent Excess Risks of Trisomy 21 in a Subsequent Pregnancy, Over and Above that Due to Maternal Age per se, after a Trisomy Other than Trisomy 21 (Heterotrisomy)

MATERNAL AGE AT INDEX PREGNANCY	EXCESS RISK	
	PER 1000 PREGNANCIES	EXCESS RISK 1 IN
20	3.7	272
21	3.7	272
22	3.6	278
23	3.5	284
24	3.5	290
25	3.4	296
26	3.2	310
27	3.1	325
28	2.9	351
29	2.6	381
30	2.4	417
31	2.1	476
32	1.7	580
33	1.4	702
34	1.1	889
35	0.9	1111
36	0.7	1481
37	0.5	2222
38	0.4	2667
39	0.3	3333
40	0.2	4444
41	0.2	6667
42	0.2	6667
43	0.2	6667
44	0.2	6667
45	0.2	6667
46	0.1	13,333
47	0.1	13,333
48	0.1	13,333
49	0.1	13,333
50	0.1	13,333

Source: From Grande et al. (2017).

---

9 They also mention one unfortunate mother who had had three trisomic pregnancies, of 21, 18, and 13.

PARENT WITH MOSAIC TRISOMY 18 OR TRISOMY 13

In those in whom a genetic risk is a realistic question, the trisomic component of the soma is likely to be low. This may well reflect a similar low fraction in the gonad, and the theoretical risk may thus be low, but not dismissible. Wei et al. (2000) describe a man, presumably otherwise normal, presenting with severe oligoasthenozoöspermia, zero to one sperm per high-power field, and with trisomy 18 in 20% (on blood) a surprising finding. With intracytoplasmic sperm injection and IVF, he was able to father a normal daughter. We may recount the case of a child with a 1/150 cell count on umbilical blood, following prenatal diagnosis of a trisomy 13 mosaicism (Delatycki et al. 1998). The child has developed very normally; however, genetic counseling in his case, as an adult, would need to acknowledge a theoretical gonadal mosaicism.

PARENT WITH MOSAICISM FOR OTHER AUTOSOMAL ANEUPLOIDY

An adult with a low-level mosaicism for some other autosomal trisomy, and presenting for genetic advice, will likely have a low or very low trisomic load in tested somatic tissues. The likelihood of a gonadal mosaicism will also probably be very low. Should there be a conception due to a disomic gamete, this, being nonmosaic, and if remaining nonmosaic, would inevitably miscarry.

Triploidy

Diandric triploidy associated with partial hydatidiform mole has an overall 1% risk of recurrence; we discuss this in more detail on p. 445. As noted in the "Biology" section, some women may have a predisposition for digynic triploidy, and recurrence is on record (Pergament et al. 2000). However, the level of risk for recurrence of triploidy, or occurrence of an aneuploidy, must usually be small, since in the series of Robinson et al. (2001) no increased risk was discernible, for women having had more than one previous spontaneous abortion due to triploidy (or aneuploidy), to have yet another chromosomally abnormal pregnancy. Prenatal karyotyping and/or early pregnancy ultrasonography may reasonably be offered.

Tetraploidy

Tetraploidy is too rare for a clear picture to have emerged. Sporadic occurrence, in almost all, would seem very probable.

14

AUTOSOMAL STRUCTURAL
REARRANGEMENTS

DELETIONS AND DUPLICATIONS

IN THIS CHAPTER we consider the circumstance of parents who have had a child in whom a structural chromosome rearrangement, a deletion or a duplication, has been identified. Here, only a segment of a chromosome exists in an imbalanced state. We frequently use the respective abbreviations *del* and *dup*. Older expressions, not necessarily to be discarded, include "partial aneuploidies," "segmental aneusomies," and "contiguous gene disorders." The earliest structural rearrangements to be identified were those large enough to be seen on "solid-stain" cytogenetics, and cri du chat syndrome, a deletion of up to 30 Mb, is the example par excellence. With increasing resolution due to banding and other differential staining methodologies, imbalances comprising a single-digit number of megabases could be detected.

A number—but not a great number—of new del/dup syndromes came to recognition, and the expressions *microdeletion* and *microduplication* syndrome were often applied. Williams syndrome (a 1.6 Mb deletion) and Smith-Magenis syndrome (deletion of 3.5 Mb) are good representatives in this category. These disorders of cytogenetic definition are the classical deletions and duplications (del/dups).

As molecular methodology entered the field, many new del/dup "syndromes" came to light: If we accept Cohen's (1997) view that a single case can, of itself, comprise a syndrome, then some hundreds of such syndromes exist. Here, the imbalance may be small enough to be measured in kilobases, and is usually described in terms of the nucleotide numbering of the chromosome.[1] Chromosome reports

---

1 In this book, the nucleotide numbering is mostly according to the hg38 "build" or "assembly," also known as GRCh38 and NCBI38, established December 2013. It can be important, when reviewing previous reports, to check which "build" was cited, the two main previous builds being hg18/GRCh36 (2006) and hg19/GRCh37 (2009). The numbering does not change greatly (the human genome has scarcely evolved over the past decade!), but recalibrations of sequencing data have led to minor reviews. Chromosome 9, for example, has gone from a length of chr9:1-140,273,252 in hg18, to chr9:1-141,213,431 in hg19, and chr9:1-138,394,717 in hg38. Online tools (e.g., "LiftOver" on the University of California, Santa Cruz [UCSC] browser) exist through which older numberings can be updated.

often show a screenshot of the relevant region from one of the publicly available or commercial genome browsers, and pathogenic roles for individual genes depicted therein can sometimes be proposed. The familial form is hardly ever seen in the classical cytogenetic rearrangement syndrome; but in contrast, familial transmission is frequently the norm in molecular-demonstrable imbalances, and parental normality, or near-normality, often complicates interpretation of the imbalance.

Classical Cytogenetic Rearrangement

If the rearrangement occurs during meiosis, or at a postzygotic mitosis—and the parental karyotypes normal—we generally assume a recurrence risk no different from the general population. These cases arise anew—"de novo"—with the affected child. If, however, the rearrangement arises at a premeiotic mitosis, the parent would be a gonadal mosaic, and an increased risk for recurrence, for a second child with the same abnormality, could in theory apply. Usually, no prior distinction between these two possibilities can be made, although how often a rearrangement is observed (unique/nonrecurrent versus commonly seen/recurrent) may suggest the site of generation, as we discuss below.

Molecular Cytogenomic Rearrangement

The majority of these del/dups of small size, for which the expression copy number variant[2] (CNV) is often applied, are inherited from a parent, and the transmission is simple Mendelian (McCarroll 2008). The considerably more difficult question relates to penetrance (Table 4–1) and expressivity of the particular imbalance. Some of these molecular rearrangements arise de novo, and the similar question of meiotic generation (negligible recurrence risk) versus premeiotic generation (potential recurrence risk) applies, as with the classical rearrangement.

Phenotypes

Some of these deletions and duplications occur sufficiently frequently and/or present a sufficiently distinctive phenotype that they have acquired eponymic

status, and the reader will be familiar with such names as Wolf, Hirschhorn, Williams, and cri du chat. The classical route whereby a chromosomal syndrome came to be established followed the recognition of a group of patients with a very similar clinical picture, often with a characteristic dysmorphology: the "phenotype-first" approach. Subsequent cytogenetic studies revealed the underlying chromosomal basis in common. Williams syndrome is a typical example: The facies and the cardiovascular malformation added up to a distinctive picture, recognized in 1961, but it was not until several years later, 1993, that the chromosomal basis was discovered.

Nowadays, taking the molecular approach, the typical path is "genotype-first," or "reverse dysmorphology." Subtle deletions and duplications may not present a distinctive enough phenotype that would allow the clinician to "call" a syndrome. But in the laboratory, data on recurrent rearrangements, whether seen in-house or often in collaboration with other cytogenetic services, nationally or internationally, can be collected. It is then up to the clinicians to draw together the observations from the patients thus identified and to construct the core features of the new syndrome. This approach of identifying the chromosomal abnormality first can reveal the natural clinical variation of the genomic rearrangements, which might scarcely have been possible with the traditional phenotype-first approach. Concerning the small-size deletions and duplications detectable on molecular karyotyping, in some of these the "natural clinical variation" may include a phenotype well within the range of essential normality. The affected phenotype is often confined to a neurocognitive disability. Many of the del/dups listed below include "autism" as a, or indeed the, clinical manifestation; this broad-brush description may come to admit of more subtle distinction as the complexities within the genetics and phenotypes are teased out (Duyzend and Eichler 2015; Sztainberg and Zoghbi 2016). A del/dup might not, of itself, suffice to produce autism; but should it lie within a susceptible polygenic background, the abnormal phenotype could emerge (Weiner et al. 2017). A growing awareness of previously undiagnosed autism in an adult population (Pilling et al. 2012) may see a wider application of genetic testing.

A rearrangement might be more complicated than a simple del or dup. Molecular methodology might not have the capacity to delineate the actual

---

2 Since many of the conditions we discuss here typically present an abnormal phenotype, the usual CNV nomenclature would be "known pathogenic CNV". It may be less confusing to use the alternative nomenclature of microdeletion and microduplication, in which the inference of phenotypic abnormality is a given. See also the discussion in Chapter 17.

structure of a rearrangement, albeit that the genomic imbalance(s) will be very precisely demonstrable. Classical cytogenetics, or at least the application of fluorescence in situ hybridization (FISH), is likely to have a role for some time yet.

Some patients, indeed quite a number, previously testing normal on classical karyotyping, have since been revealed on molecular testing as having a chromosomal imbalance. This belated discovery may make no real difference to management, but it is often a source of considerable relief to the parents to have, finally, a definite explanation for the problem. And of course, precise genetic advice can now be offered to others in the family.

BIOLOGY

Mechanisms of Formation of Structural Rearrangement

The human karyotype is hostage to the fine detail of its structure. Molecular analysis of structural chromosome rearrangements and their breakpoints has shed light on the underlying generative mechanisms. In particular, it is clear that different mutational mechanisms apply for recurrent versus nonrecurrent rearrangements. Recurrent rearrangements share essentially the same size and genomic content in unrelated individuals, the breakpoints being fixed by the presence of highly homologous long flanking repeats. In contrast, nonrecurrent rearrangements have a size and genomic content that is unique to the individual. Carvalho and Lupski (2016) provide a comprehensive review.

RECURRENT REARRANGEMENTS

The common basis for recurrent del/dup rearrangements lies in the existence of multiple DNA sequences, generally of some thousands of base pairs (bp), known as low copy repeats[3] (LCRs). These LCRs are seen throughout the genome, and

are sufficiently similar ("paralogous," rather than exactly homologous) that they enable the erroneous coming-together of different chromosome regions. The two sequences (inter- or intrachromosomal) involved in a particular exchange have a length of near-perfect homology, and this is the site of the actual strand exchange. In other words, "ectopic synapsis" sets the scene for a subsequent "ectopic homologous recombination." This is nonallelic homologous recombination (NAHR), and meiosis is the usual setting.[4] Studies on the Charcot-Marie-Tooth region of 17p12, and the Smith-Magenis syndrome region in 17p11.2 (Fig. 14–1), in particular, informed this understanding (Lupski 2009).

The reciprocal nature of NAHR dictates that cross-over between chromatids or homologous chromosomes will concomitantly generate a deletion and a duplication of the same interval; thus it is that many genomic disorders that arise from a deletion have a counterpart disorder resulting from the reciprocal duplication.[5] NAHR can also take place within a chromatid, although when this happens, only a deletion is generated; and so overall, NAHR generates more de novo deletions than duplications. Some paralogous sequences run in opposite directions; and in that case, paracentric microinversions, which exist as normal polymorphisms, make it possible for a recombination event to take place. Most NAHR is intrachromosomal, but the same process can also take place between nonhomologous chromosomes, and this is the main mutational mechanism underlying de novo unbalanced translocations (Robberecht et al. 2013).

NONRECURRENT REARRANGEMENTS

As noted above, nonrecurrent structural rearrangements are characterized by the widespread locations of breakpoints,[6] leading to del/dups of

---

3 Other names are duplicons and segmental duplications (Gu et al. 2008). The *Segmental dups* track on the UCSC genome browser gives a nice illustration of their distribution. Color coding shows the degree of homology: gray for 90%–98%, yellow for 98%–99%, and dramatic orange for >99%, as exemplified in color Figure 14–60.

4 MacArthur et al. (2014) studied NAHR in the sperm of 34 males, and identified a sevenfold variation in the rate of NAHR across individuals. The rate of NAHR did not increase with age, nor did it correlate with body mass index, smoking, or alcohol intake, but it did correlate between monozygotic co-twins, indicating a significant genetic contribution.

5 A number of reciprocal deletion and duplication syndromes manifest mirror-image phenotypic traits (Lejeune 1966; Carvalho and Lupski 2016).

6 Although breakpoints of nonrecurrent rearrangement are, by definition, not recurrent, they are nonrandomly distributed across the genome, indicating that local genomic architecture plays a role in their generation.

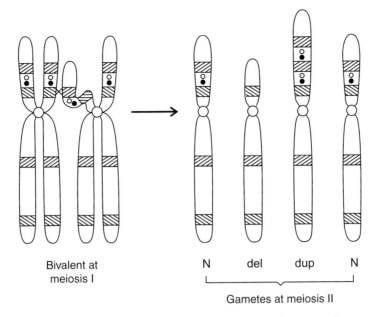

Bivalent at
meiosis I

N   del   dup   N

Gametes at meiosis II

FIGURE 14-1   One mechanism to produce a duplication and a deletion (and see text) is based upon the promiscuous activity of similar DNA sequences, "duplicons," that exist at numerous places along the chromosome (shown as cross-hatched segments). Consider a segment between two such duplicons, indicated here by the black and white spots (imagine these to be two FISH probes). Misalignment of the two duplicons, followed by nonallelic homologous recombination within them (×), produces recombinant products that are reciprocally imbalanced: one with a deficiency of the chromatin between the two duplicons, and the other with a duplication. The deletion chromosome is shown with no black or white spot, while the duplication chromosome has a double set of black and white spots in tandem. The general case is drawn after Chandley (1989). The genotype in the child (normal, deletion, duplication) resulting from such meiotic recombination will depend upon which of the chromatids ends up as the homolog in the gamete. The two classic examples both reside in chromosome 17: Smith-Magenis syndrome and Potocki-Lupski syndrome are due to deletion and duplication, respectively, for the segment 17p11.2p11.2. A little further up the 17 short arm, a 1.7 Mb segment within 17p12, including the *PMP22* gene, is deleted in hereditary pressure-sensitive neuropathy, and duplicated in Charcot-Marie-Tooth neuropathy.

unique size and genomic content. Analysis of the breakpoints, at a sequence level, has provided insight into mechanisms of formation. The absence of any sequence homology ("blunt ends"), or of only 1–3 bp of sequence homology, is indicative of nonhomologous end joining (NHEJ). During mitotic cell division (and including in the pre-meiotic gametocyte), different chromosomal segments may happen to be in close proximity, due to their "geographical space" within the nucleus; or upstream or downstream sequences with similarity (e.g., *Alu* repeats) may have predisposed to their coming together. Then, in the simple case, if breaks occur during replication, instead of the correct ends being brought back together, the broken ends of different segments may inappropriately be ligated.

More commonly, breakpoints of nonrecurrent structural variants are complex, characterized by short (2–33 bp) "microhomologies" between breakpoint junctions, and often with an insertion of a short (<100 bp) length of DNA from an adjacent region. These observations are explained by a replication-based mechanism, in which the error occurs during DNA synthesis. The suggested model is as follows. During DNA replication, the replication fork "stalls," or collapses, for example due to a double-strand DNA break. The broken chromosome 3′ end then seeks out and invades a homologous DNA template, and reinitiates DNA replication. This is break-induced replication (BIR); and provided the correct DNA template is acquired on the homologous chromosome, accurate repair occurs (although with segmental uniparental disomy). But if a long tract of homology is not located, an alternative DNA template, with only a short stretch of "microhomology," may be selected. This is microhomology-mediated break-induced replication (MMBIR). When MMBIR proceeds normally, it allows accurate DNA repair and replication; but its reliance on short homologies means there is a risk that an incorrect template will be selected, and so the process is inherently error-prone. Microhomology mediates "template switching," the change of the single-stranded DNA template during replication within the same replication fork. Template switching can occur over short or long distances, and can be intrachromosomal or interchromosomal, generating a range of complex structural rearrangements. MMBIR is the main mechanism underlying nonrecurrent structural rearrangements in genomic disorders, including simple deletions and duplications, as well as some more complex rearrangements, such as triplications, and deletion/duplication combinations (Zhang et al. 2009).

ORIGIN INTRA-, PRE-, OR POSTMEIOSIS

As just noted, the "recurrent" category of de novo deletion or duplication is considered typically to reflect an origin during *meiosis*. Thus, for a number of deletion syndromes involving a recurrent segment, such as Williams, Prader-Willi, and Smith-Magenis syndromes, and several others, a risk of recurrence is very low, because only the gamete from that particular meiosis carried the defect (Giglio et al. 2001; Saitta et al. 2004). On the other hand, imbalances which are either single cases or which are of a group involving a cytoband or bands in common, but with distinctly different breakpoints, are "nonrecurrent." Some may have been of meiotic origin, and therefore without increased risk of recurrence. Alternatively, the imbalance originated in a *premeiotic mitosis*. In that case, the abnormal cell line is confined to a "wedge" of the parental gonad (gonadal mosaicism), and the parent will have a normal phenotype and normal chromosome analysis. If, however, the abnormal cell line is present in the parental gonad and in nongonadal tissues (somatic mosaicism), the parent may have an (often very subtly) abnormal phenotype, and the imbalance may be detectable, in a mosaic form, in parental blood. In either scenario, there is risk of the imbalance, in a nonmosaic form, being passed to a child. In actual fact, a second affected child of such a parent is only rarely seen.

Nevertheless, it is usually appropriate to check the parental karyotypes, in order to test the possibilities that one parent may be either a carrier of a balanced rearrangement or a low-grade mosaic for the abnormal chromosome (the normal cell line in a phenotypically normal parent being, presumably, predominant in the soma, and prevailing over any effect due to the imbalanced cell line). When the imbalance is submicroscopic, parental microarray studies should be performed; this may essentially exclude mosaicism involving the soma, although it would not identify a balanced rearrangement. An example is illustrated in Figure 3–13 of an interstitial deletion del(1)(q25q31.2) which was identified at amniocentesis, and which led to the discovery of 46,XY,del(1)[80%]/46,XY[20%] mosaicism on blood karyotyping of the father, thus revealing him to be a somatic-gonadal mosaic. Normal parental karyotypes do not exclude absolutely the possibility of mosaicism, as exemplified in two sisters with a chromosome 16 deletion whose parents' karyotypes on blood were normal (Hoo et al. 1985), nor in a case of recurrent, interstitial 1p36 deletion in two sisters from a gonadal mosaic mother, who did not have any evidence of the deletion on blood FISH analysis (Gajecka et al. 2010).

Finally, a rearrangement arising at a *postzygotic mitosis*, from an initially normal conceptus, would lead to mosaicism in the child, typically for a normal and for the abnormal cell line, both with a 46-chromosome count. In a sense, this is a similar scenario as with the parent having a premeiotic mitosis, just discussed, except that the abnormal event took place much earlier in embryonic life, such that development of the soma was overtly compromised. Typically, no increased risk of recurrence would apply for potential future siblings of this child. Somatic mosaicism for a structural rearrangement of this sort is discussed in the comprehensive review of Kovaleva and Cotter (2016); these authors examine the intriguing observation of an excess of females with unbalanced 46,XX,rea/46,XX, and propose a "male-specific selection," during embryonic life, against abnormal cells.

SIMPLE AND COMPLEX DELETIONS

The simple scenario of a "clean-cut" deletion may in some, indeed many instances, be an oversimplification. Davies et al. (2003) restudied a group of 16 deletion patients, and in three the supposed deletion proved to be a rearrangement, involving subtelomeric regions. Gunn et al. (2003) studied a child initially karyotyped as 46,XY, but whose clinical features suggested an 18q deletion. This was indeed proved, but the deletion seemed rather small given the severity of the phenotype. Using FISH and microarray analysis, they could show that a segment from distal 4q had been inserted into the site of the 18q deletion, giving a partial 4q trisomy along with the partial 18q monosomy. And many examples now exist whereby terminal deletions, apparently simple on light microscopy, prove to be complex rearrangements upon molecular investigation, with submicroscopic duplications, triplications, and inversions, in addition to the deletions. Zuffardi et al. (2009) propose that many "deletions," according to cytogenetic analysis, are actually inverted duplications contiguous with terminal deletions. These result from dicentric chromosomes (which can form through either NAHR or NHEJ), which then undergo a breakage-fusion-bridge cycle, with formation of a telomere at the site of rupture (Ballif et al. 2003; Rowe et al. 2009).

Respecting the requirement that integrity of the telomere be maintained, some mechanisms of terminal deletion need to include a process to restore the telomere (Ballif et al. 2000; Daniel et al. 2008). If the terminal deletion is interstitial (thus, actually subterminal), then the original telomere simply remains intact. If, however, the telomere is lost in the deletion process, a neotelomere can be generated ("telomere healing"). If another chromosome is involved in the process, its telomere can be "captured" to fulfill the requirement. Ballif et al. (2003) made particular study of the 1p36 deletion, and showed that all three mechanisms were involved, the commonest being the acquisition of a telomere from another chromosome.

COMPLEMENTARY DELETION/DUPLICATION

The rare complementary deletion/duplication offers insight into the likely site of generation of this particular rearrangement. If the del/dup should arise at the very first somatic replication following conception—in other words, the zygote entering mitosis no. 1—two countertype cell lines will be produced at the two-cell stage, with no normal cell line. In the event that extrafetal tissues can be studied, and still no normal cell line seen, the interpretation of a first-mitosis scenario is strengthened; thus, Rodriguez-Revenga et al. (2005) could draw such a conclusion from their prenatal diagnostic case of dup(18q)/del(18q) mosaicism, the chorionic villi showing both karyotypes, although on amniocentesis and fetal blood, only the del(18q) was present. If one of the cell lines is of lesser viability, a child might show the complementary karyotypes at birth, but later in childhood, only one cell line. Morales et al. (2007a) report an example, an abnormal infant who as a newborn had dup(7)(q21.1q31.3)[90]/del(7)(q21.1q31.3)[10] mosaicism, but upon restudy at age 12 and 14 months, only the dup(7) cell line was seen, looking at blood and exfoliated urinary tract epithelial cells.

If the del/dup arises at the second, or subsequent, mitosis, there will be a normal cell line as well; and Tharapel et al. (1999) illustrate this circumstance in a child initially identified at amniocentesis, undertaken upon the basis of a choroid plexus cyst and echogenic bowel. In this child, the normal cell line was present in about half of cells, with the remaining cells containing either a deletion for 7p11.2p13, or a duplication for this segment. The normal cell line was presumably predominant in the normal mother described in Qi et al. (2015), with a 46,XX,del(6p25.1p24.3)/46,XX,dup(6p25.1p24.3)/46,XX karyotype (her abnormal children leading to the ascertainment; see chromosome 6p below).

INFLUENCE OF SEX OF PARENT

Certain duplication/deletion rearrangements may have a predilection for happening in the parent of one or other sex. Chromosome 17p11.2 rearrangements are more often of paternal origin, and they may be intrachromosomal or interchromosomal in their generation. The nearby 17p12 region is also more susceptible to rearrangement in the paternal gonad, although in contrast to 17p11.2, paternal duplications/deletions are always interchromosomal, and the uncommon maternal cases are all intrachromosomal (Potocki et al. 2000). The X chromosome has a particular vulnerability in the male, likely because it is largely unpaired at meiosis, and it can refold up and down its length (Giglio et al. 2000). The 1p36 deletion varies in size, and the larger deletions are more often of paternal generation (Gajecka et al. 2007). We may also note that de novo Robertsonian translocations are almost always maternal in origin (Bandyopadhyay et al. 2002), while on the other hand, the great majority of de novo apparently balanced translocations and complex rearrangements arise in the fathers (Grossmann et al. 2010; Thomas et al. 2010). The frequency of paternal deletions and duplications shows a small increased age effect, and with some chromosomes being more susceptible than others (Templado et al. 2011). Most rearranged chromosomes that have the del/dup structure resembling that of a recombinant from a parental inversion are of maternal derivation (Rivera et al. 2013).

Deletion

We have traveled a distance from the earliest days of cytogenetics when the first deletion was published, which was large enough to be seen on a solid-stained "B-group chromosome," and associated with cri du chat syndrome (Lejeune et al. 1963). We have, now, a spectrum from large deletions ("classical cytogenetic deletion syndromes"), through microdeletions detectable on high-resolution banding, to deletions beyond the range of banding but detected on combined molecular/cytogenetic (FISH) or purely molecular methodology (array comparative genomic hybridization [CGH], single nucleotide polymorphism [SNP] array, or next-generation sequencing [NGS]). Examples of the general karyotypic form of an interstitial deletion, in any chromosome A, are 46,del(A)(p21p23) or 46,del(A)(q12q12).

CONTIGUOUS GENE SYNDROME

Recollect that loci are arranged in linear order along a chromosome. Some neighboring loci may be functionally related, but in others, the contiguity is mere happenstance: The nonsignificance of two loci being adjacent has been likened to the unimportance one would attach to "Appalachian Mountains" being next to "apple" in an encyclopedia. Our genome differs from an encyclopedia in that about one-third of all the entries relate to one topic: the development and functioning of the brain; unsurprisingly so, this organ being, as it is said, the most complex

structure in the known universe. Many of the other entries (loci) relate to the control of morphogenesis during embryonic life. If a length of chromosome is deleted, a sequence of adjacent (contiguous) genes will be lost. The phenotype resulting from this can be described as a contiguous gene deletion syndrome (Schmickel 1986; Tommerup 1993). In almost any deletion detectable cytogenetically, some of the deleted loci will be brain loci, while others could be for anything, but likely including some morphogenesis loci. Thus, we have the classic clinical picture in deletion syndromes of intellectual deficit of some degree, dysmorphism, and in some, organ malformation. The deletion produces a monosomy—or "haploinsufficiency"—for the region of the chromosome that has been removed, and loci in this segment are underexpressed. Proof that genetic expression is reduced by half, for example, in the case of the 18q– syndrome, was adduced by Wang et al. (1999), in measuring mRNA from a number of 18q loci.

Some of the loci whose haploinsufficiency contributes to the phenotype in the various deletion syndromes are being defined, as noted in individual entries in the "Genetic Counseling" section. It seems likely that many such genes will have their untoward outcome not in a simple one-to-one relationship with a single gene product but, rather, in a complex layering and interlacing of consequential effects (Fig. 3–11). As yet, however, it is mostly just the simple case that we can begin to understand: such as, for example, the brain white matter abnormality of the 18q– syndrome just mentioned, that is presumably a direct consequence of the loss of one structural myelin gene on 18q. As molecular karyotyping defines deletions/duplications of very small extent, only a few genes may be located within the particular segment, and the counselor blessed with a scientific curiosity has the opportunity to check which genes these are, and perhaps to make an informed speculation (which some parents might find helpful) as to which of these might have contributed to a child's phenotype.

If two or more Mendelian disorders coexist in the one person, a contiguous gene deletion is a strong possibility. In order to prove the point, molecular methodology can be brought to bear; or a direct chromosomal test using FISH offers an immediate visual demonstration of the deletion. We have, for example, seen a young woman presenting with a history of recurrent bacterial infections since childhood, and night blindness and diminishing peripheral vision since teenage, leading to diagnoses of chronic granulomatous disease and retinitis pigmentosa (Coman et al. 2010b). The X-linked forms of these conditions being very closely linked, a contiguous gene deletion suggested itself, and a FISH probe targeted to a DNA sequence between the two loci was generated. Its nonhybridization to one X chromosome confirmed the supposition of a deletion. Furthermore, this led the way to another diagnosis, that of a partial protein intolerance, due to deletion of the *OTC* (ornithine transcarbamylase) gene, which lies in the same Xp region.

Deletions and Mendelian Disorders. A Mendelian disorder due to autosomal dominant or X-linked inheritance, and typically the result of a gene mutation, may also result if the particular chromosomal locus is deleted. Thus, only one functional allele remains, and a state of haploinsufficiency is the consequence. Rubenstein-Taybi syndrome was one of the earliest to exemplify this scenario (the gene *CREBBP*); and Charcot-Marie-Tooth disease type 1A and hereditary pressure-sensitive palsy provide an instance of both duplications and deletions concerning a single gene (*PMP22*), and indeed this genomic mechanism being more frequent than classical mutation at this locus. Other cases, several of which are also noted below, include Pitt-Hopkins syndrome (the gene *TCF4*), Sotos syndrome (*NSD1*), Alagille syndrome (*JAG1*), Saethre-Chotzen syndrome (*TWIST*), Greig syndrome (*GLI3*), one type of holoprosencephaly (*SHH*), CHARGE syndrome (*CDH7*), one type of lissencephaly (*LIS1*); and X-linked ichthyosis (*STS*) in a 46,Y,del(X) individual. If neighboring genes are also deleted, this may contribute to a wider phenotype; or, these other genes might not be dosage-sensitive,[7] and the clinical picture is essentially the same as in the Mendelian case.

A deletion that removes an autosomal recessive gene would not normally, of itself, influence the phenotype. But if, coincidentally, a mutation lies on the other, otherwise intact chromosome, there may result further damage due to an "unmasking heterozygosity" at this locus (Coman and Gardner 2007). Flipsen-ten Berg et al. (2007) reported an infant with Wolf-Hirschhorn syndrome (WHS) due to a deletion on one chromosome 4p, and who then went on to develop, over and above the WHS, signs of Wolfram syndrome.[8] The *WFS1* locus for Wolfram syndrome is on chromosome 4 short arm, which led these workers to examine the gene on the "normal" chromosome 4. A point mutation in *WFS1* was discovered. The 4p deletion on the other chromosome allowed this mutation to be "exposed"; and the child, being essentially hemizygous, got the syndrome: WHS + WFS, one could say. Similarly, a child with a 22q13 deletion (Phelan-McDermid syndrome), and having an *ARSA* mutation on the other chromosome 22, would develop the fatal recessive brain disease, metachromatic leukodystrophy (Bisgaard et al. 2009). McDonald-McGinn et al. (2013) review a number of cases with the 22q11.2 deletion syndrome, but having an atypical clinical picture, in whom an "exposed" mutation on the other 22 led to a more severe phenotype.

Gene Discovery. Taking a broader view, deletions/duplications can point the way to discovery of novel genes coding for particular organs and tissues. A deletion that, from clinical observations, has a particular clinical association with clefting, may remove, for example, contiguous genes *w, x, y,* and *z.* It could reasonably be imagined that haploinsufficiency of one of these genes (perhaps gene *x*, if its product had a theoretical role in cell-cell interaction) could contribute to the cause of cleft lip; and then it could further be assumed that the normal role of gene *x* is in contributing to the process of lip formation during early embryogenesis. Brewer et al. (1998, 1999) reviewed some hundreds of deletions and duplications listed in the Oxford Cytogenetic Database, correlating the malformations with which these deletions have been associated (p. 49). Patterns have emerged: Some deletions seem

---

7 Many loci are "haplosufficient"; that is, a single dose of an allele suffices to enable normal functioning. Huang et al. (2010) have analyzed differences between haplosufficient and haploinsufficient loci; among other factors, haploinsufficient loci are more highly expressed during embryonic development, and they have a greater degree of interaction with other loci.

8 Wolfram syndrome = diabetes mellitus, diabetes insipidus, deafness, optic atrophy.

particularly likely to lead to a heart defect, while others may be prone to cause clefting. The component parts of a deletion syndrome can be sheeted back to specific segments, such as Kirchhoff et al. (2009) show with the 13q– syndrome.

With the increased subtlety that molecular karyotyping allows, a finer focus is brought to bear. The DECIPHER database is a marvelous collaborative resource through which to judge the candidacy of loci within the del/dup, and the title of a review paper from this group is worth quoting here: "Facilitating Collaboration in Rare Genetic Disorders Through Effective Matchmaking in DECIPHER" (Chatzimichali et al. 2015). Looking in the direction of phenotype back to genotype, Sajan et al. (2013) identified CNVs at numerous loci associated with agenesis of the corpus callosum. It is of interest that those genes within a del/dup segment that are ohnologs[9] are more likely to be dosage-sensitive, and thus more promising phenocritical candidates (McLysaght et al. 2014).

Researchers hoping to find genes directing development of the heart, or genes controlling lip formation, could focus their searches in these chromosomal regions. Similarly, nephrogenesis genes and neurogenesis genes may come to light in the analysis of deletions associated with renal maldevelopment and epilepsy, respectively (Singh et al. 2002a; Amor et al. 2003; Sajan et al. 2013). Different syndromes with a phenotypic trait in common can clarify the nature of the genetic heterogeneity. Thus, multiple exostoses are a component of the Langer-Giedion syndrome, due to deletion at 8q24, and the Potocki-Shaffer syndrome, due to 11p11.2 deletion, consequent upon haploinsufficiency of different bone-growth genes at these two segments. However, the blunt but very effective procedure of whole exome analysis may now be making such clues seem an old-fashioned, if elegant approach to the question (Amor 2015).

Rare Complexity. A rare (or rarely recognized) complexity is a change in size, from parent to child, of a subtelomeric deletion. Faravelli et al. (2007) observed a mother having a 1.5 Mb 4p deletion, which expanded in size to produce a 2.8 Mb deletion in her child with typical Wolf-Hirschhorn

syndrome; in retrospect, the mother had subtle signs to suggest a *forme fruste*. Similarly, South et al. (2008) describe a normal mother with a de novo 18q subtelomeric deletion of 0.4 Mb, which increased in size nearly 10-fold, to 3.7 Mb, in her abnormal daughter, who had presented with a clinical picture consistent with 18q deletion syndrome. This parent-to-child "expansion" is likely due to a recombination mechanism.

Duplication

Duplicated segments may arise from within the same chromatid, from the sister chromatid, from the same arm, from the other arm, or from a different chromosome, through similar mechanisms as described above. As with the deletion, the association of different duplicated segments with particular phenotypes offers an insight into which regions of the genome may harbor specific critical genes (Brewer et al. 1999). In a few cases, the duplication (or sometimes triplication) of a locus manifests, to some extent, as the "opposite" phenotype as that found in the deletion. Thus, triplication of the *MMP23* gene on 1p36 results in craniosynostosis, while the deletion is associated with a large, late-closing anterior fontanel (Gajecka et al. 2005). Deletion of the *P* gene in the Prader-Willi/Angelman region causes lighter complexion (and when mutated causes oculocutaneous albinism type 2); an increased copy number of this gene leads to hyperpigmentation (Akahoshi et al. 2004). Shinawi et al. (2010) refer to these opposite scenarios as "sister genomic disorders"; Lejeune, in the 1960s, spoke of type and countertype.

Direct and Inverted Intrachromosomal (Tandem) Duplication. The duplication comprises chromatin of the same chromosome, the original and the duplicated segments being ordered in tandem fashion. If the linear orientation of a chromosome A is maintained, the rearrangement is a direct duplication, 46,dir dup(A); if it is reversed, it is an inverted duplication, 46,inv dup(A). As noted earlier, many apparent inverted duplications may in fact exist along with a terminal deletion; the causative mechanism may be either NAHR or NHEJ, and, apart from the inv dup 8p, most often occurring at a

---

9 This expression harks back to the time of the vertebrate lineage, about 500 mya, when tetraploidization (whole genome duplication) set in train this new evolutionary path. Those duplicated loci subsequently retained are ohnologs; the loci lost by natural selection are those for which duplication was deleterious, and a single copy sufficed (Singh et al. 2015). The word honors Dr Susumu Ohno, who first proposed this evolutionary mechanism.

premeiotic mitosis (Giglio et al. 2001; Rowe et al. 2009; Zuffardi et al. 2009). An alternative explanation, based on an analysis of many cases of complex rearrangements of 1p36, is that successive breakage-fusion-bridge cycles result in deletion/duplication chromosomes, particularly near to the telomeres (Ballif et al. 2003).

Additional Material from Another Chromosome. In some rearrangements, the duplicated material has come from another chromosome. For example, Su et al. (2012) report a child with multiple anomalies due to duplication of 6p22, with this segment being attached to the tip of 1p: 46,XX,der(1) t(1;6)(p36.3;p22). An example of the karyotype nomenclature, which would have been used (in classical cytogenetics) before the nature of the additional material had been established, is 46,add(1) (q36.3). Pairing between nonhomologs, followed by crossing-over (due to NAHR or NHEJ), produces reciprocal products that are two derivative chromosomes. In a "single-segment" exchange, one of these will have a duplication (as the der(1) just mentioned in Su et al.), and the other a deletion. If this occurred during meiosis, and if segregation were then asymmetric, contemporaneous gametes with a duplication or with a deficiency would be produced (of course, only one could ever fertilize). Other scenarios, with more complex mechanisms, may be imagined. Coles et al. (1992), for example, studied a child with Wolf-Hirschhorn syndrome who had two separate de novo rearrangements of the X chromosome with a chromosome 4 and the Y, respectively, and they propose that simultaneous or sequential crossovers happened in a meiotic "octad" of four synapsing chromosomes.

If a de novo unbalanced rearrangement could be shown to have its component parts originating from both a maternal and a paternal chromosome, the fact of its postzygotic origin would be thereby demonstrated. Sarri et al. (1997) offer an example of this scenario in a malformed child with 46,X,der(X),t(X;17)(q27;q22) whose der(X) originated from the paternal X and the maternal 17 chromosomes. Eggermann et al. (1997) report a similar case, an abnormal child with a de novo der(18)t(13;18)(q14.3;q23). The chromosome 18 component of the translocation came from the paternal homolog, and the chromosome 13 component from the maternal homolog. In this type of biparental rearrangement, even the very small theoretical risk otherwise associated with parental gonadal mosaicism could confidently be excluded.

Similarly, mosaicism in the presence of a normal cell line would typically allow the presumption of a mitotic origin. Zaslav et al. (1999) report a child with a severe brain malformation who had the karyotype 46,XX,der(4)t(4;15)(q35;q22)/46,XX. They propose that the chromosome constitution at conception was 46,XX. At an early cell division, a reciprocal exchange occurred between chromatids of chromosomes 4 and 15. Then, at anaphase, there was an unfortunate segregation. The newly generated der(4) passed to one daughter cell, along with the normal chromosome 15; and, vice versa, the der(15) and the chromosome 4 passed to the other. The former produced a cell line with a del(4)/dup(15) imbalance, and the presence of this cell line in the developing nervous system presumably caused the brain maldevelopment. The other cell line was not seen (on a peripheral blood karyotype), and it may have been selected against. (If the segregation of the chromosomes at that crucial mitosis had been balanced, then the child would likely have been a phenotypically normal mosaic balanced translocation carrier.) Reddy and Mak (2001) could demonstrate mosaicism in both blood (conventional karyotyping) and on buccal mucosal cells (FISH) in two patients with additional material from another chromosome. For example, one patient had mosaicism for an add(5), the additional material coming from 3p26-pter, in 32% of lymphocytes. Using a 3p-subtelomere probe, a very similar level of mosaicism (40%) was shown in buccal epithelial cells.

Triplication. A very few cases are known, at the level of classical cytogenetic analysis, of a segment of chromosome replicating twice over, being in threefold amount on that homolog. The segment is thus present, in total, in fourfold dose. Triplications observed on classic cytogenetics are reported for chromosomes 2, 4, 5, 7, 9, 10, 12, 13, 15, and 16. In a triplication 12p case, the phenotypically normal mother was a low-level (12%) mosaic for the same rearrangement (Eckel et al. 2006). With molecular karyotyping, we are now seeing several more cases of triplication, and it seems likely that this "rare" complexity may be less rare than initially supposed (Xu et al. 2014). Familial transmission is recorded: The 46,XX,trp(4)(q32.1q32.2) mother in Wang et al. (2009a) had three sons with the same imbalance, 46,XY,trp(4)(q32.1q32.2), this being clearly visible on classical karyotyping.

Apparently Balanced But Actually Unbalanced Rearrangement

It had long been a problem, in classical cytogenetics, to interpret a rearrangement seeming balanced on karyotype but associated with an abnormal phenotype. Was the rearrangement related to the phenotype as cause and effect, or was the association merely coincidental? The molecular approach now enables, in most cases, a clear distinction (Gijsbers et al. 2010). Loss or gain of DNA at the site(s) of rearrangement provides strong supporting evidence in favor of a pathogenic effect, and particularly so if specific genes can be implicated. Conversely, a normal quantitative result would point to the rearrangement being truly balanced, although the possibility of disruption of a gene at the actual site of a breakpoint could yet be the explanation for an abnormal clinical picture (Cacciagli et al. 2010). Note that if the rearrangement that disrupts the gene is a "clean" break, with practically no loss of DNA, then a microarray would not detect it.

Next-generation sequencing may provide precision of analysis down to base-pair level (Utami et al. 2014). Bertelsen et al. (2016) studied a family in which there was segregating an apparently balanced rcp(3;5)(q25;q31), but which turned out to be sufficiently complex that these authors referred to it as chromothripsis (p. 226). Ordulu et al. (2016) present a "nucleotide-level resolution" which enabled definitive interpretation of 10 de novo rearrangements (four reciprocal translocations, five inversions, one complex rearrangement) identified at prenatal diagnosis; some classically interpreted cytogenetic bands were shown to have been inaccurately called by quite significant amounts, up to double-digit numbers of megabases. Occasionally, the result is surprising: There may be no DNA imbalance at the site of breakpoints, but a deletion and/or duplication is seen at some other place in the genome. Here, the rearrangement can presumably be exonerated, as a coincidental event; the real cause lies elsewhere.

Position effect is another mechanism whereby a "balanced" rearrangement can lead to phenotypic abnormality. The *SOX9* gene on chromosome 17 at band q25.1, the basis of campomelic syndrome, provides an example with respect to both a translocation and an inversion. The de novo translocation t(5;17)(q15;q25.1) in Figure 14–2 was seen in a child with this syndrome, as was the de novo paracentric inversion inv(17)(q24.3q25.1) reported in Maraia et al. (1991). Other such examples are mentioned below: see del(7)(q21.3), del(11)(p11.3). This type of rearrangement would probably not be detectable on molecular karyotyping.

GENETIC COUNSELING

Deletions and Duplications

In most children with deletions or duplications, the parents type as 46,XX and 46,XY on routine blood analysis, and the defect is "de novo." The risk for recurrence is very small. Röthlisberger and Kotzot (2007) undertook a review and were surprised at how few actual cases of recurrence had been published. The rare recurrences are likely due to an occult parental mosaicism, which the routine blood chromosome study could not

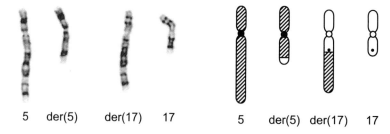

5   der(5)   der(17)   17   5   der(5)   der(17)   17

FIGURE 14–2   An apparently balanced translocation causing the syndrome of campomelic dysplasia (which includes skeletal, genital, and brain defects). One breakpoint is at 17q25.1, on or close to the *SOX9* locus (shown as dot on the cartoon karyotype), where the basis of the syndrome lies. One possibility is that the gene is disrupted. Or, an influence of adjacent chromosome 5 chromatin ("position effect") leads to inactivation of the *SOX9* gene on the der(17), the functional *SOX9* haploinsufficiency then being responsible for the phenotype. (Case of R. Savarirayan; Savarirayan and Bankier 1998.)

detect.[10] The abnormal line in the parent may be gonadal (confined to gametic tissue) or somatic-gonadal (some somatic tissues involved as well—but not, apparently, blood). We refer below to certain known susceptibility polymorphisms in a parent (e.g., 1q21.1, 8p, 17q21.31, 22q), but these factors notwithstanding, the absolute risk scarcely differs from background.

The observation of rarity of recurrence allows us to propose the empiric advice that, in the individual de novo case, recurrence is most unlikely. Röthlisberger and Kotzot (2007) offer a figure of "less than 0.3%"; the counselor should note the converse "greater than 99.7%" for a child without the chromosome defect. If the typical mechanism is a meiotic error (as discussed above), the risk might, in principle, fall to the population baseline. Some couples may find "greater than 99.7%" sufficiently encouraging that they would not request invasive prenatal diagnosis in a subsequent pregnancy, or would be satisfied with a normal ultrasound report.

In those deletions/duplications where a parent is shown to carry a balanced rearrangement, a substantial recurrence risk is probable, and the appropriate chapter should be consulted. Rarely, the same deletion/duplication might be seen, rather unexpectedly, in a parent, an observation that underpins the advice that parental karyotyping does need to be undertaken (Sparkes et al. 2009). Extremely rarely, an inverted duplication may, in fact, be due to recombination within a parental paracentric inversion. Paracentric inversions can be difficult to detect, and a careful and directed search may be appropriate.

Thumbnail sketches of the major deletion syndromes follow, as well as many (but certainly not all) of the lesser well-known ones, in numerical order of chromosomes, and numerical order[11] of p and q segments. Quite a few syndromes are of 2000s–2010s definition, reflecting the widespread application of molecular karyotyping is the twenty-first century. Nucleotide numbers are expressed in build hg38 (data from literature cases having been converted[12]). Each chromosomal section is seen with a banded ideogram, taken from Chia (2009), with particular segments subject to recurrent deletion/duplication indicated, along with a selected relevant gene (or other identifier) located within that segment, as a useful "landmark." Longer or "busier" chromosomes have of necessity been divided into p and q arms. Only "pure" imbalances are considered; it is not feasible to include here those due to combination del/dups of different chromosomes. The ones from classical cytogenetics are depicted in the composite karyotype in Figure 14–3. We comment in greater or lesser length upon the genetics of each and, to the extent that knowledge allows, on recurrence risks. Clinical comments are mostly synoptic and selective, and "intellectual deficiency and facial dysmorphism" very frequently mentioned. The essays in Cassidy and Allanson's *Management of Genetic Syndromes* (2010) offer detailed commentaries for some of the more common of these syndromes. The UNIQUE website has excellent quite detailed descriptions for some of the more common (or less rare) conditions.

DELETIONS

Chromosome 1 Deletions

del 1p21.3 This microdeletion is rare (case reports barely in double figures: Willemsen et al. 2011; D'Angelo et al. 2015), but it is of particular interest in that the reduced amount of a microRNA may be a key factor in determining the clinical picture of intellectual deficit of borderline/mild/moderate degree and abnormal behavior. For the most part, deletions are nonrecurrent and of variable sizes. The smallest region of overlap, of 1 Mb in extent, runs from chr1:97.5-98.5 Mb, and including the sequence coding for *MIR137* (Fig. 14–4). This microRNA is particularly expressed in certain brain regions, and it

---

10 Campbell et al. (2014) set out to test this hypothesis by using a highly sensitive technique, individual breakpoint-specific polymerase chain reaction, to test parental blood in a cohort of 100 patients with nonrecurrent deletion CNVs. Low-level somatic mosaicism was detected in four parents, and presumably these parents would have an elevated risk of recurrence.

11 Thus, reading *upwards* (or to the left) from the centromere in the p arm, and *downwards* (or to the right) in the q arm. Note that in formal cytogenetic nomenclature, when two p arm bands are listed, the correct ordering is from telomere to centromere (anti-numerical order), such as del 2p16.1p15.

12 As previously mentioned, conversion from an earlier genome assembly ("build") to hg38 is straightforward, using the "liftover" tool in the Utilities listing of the UCSC genome browser, and as demonstrated on a YouTube video (search: ucsc genome browser "how to convert from different genomes"). Trap for young players: The system requires a hyphen (-) between nucleotide numbers; it will not accept an en dash (–) or em dash (—). Note that if you refer to the original papers cited herein, almost all of these will have been in hg18 or hg19, and the nucleotide numbers will be slightly, or sometimes not so slightly, different.

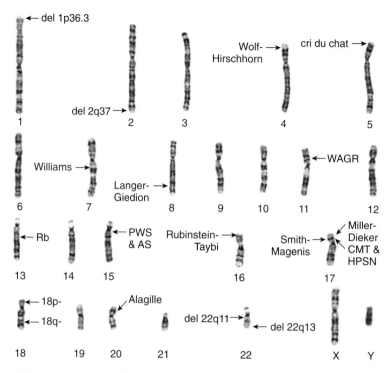

FIGURE 14–3 "Composite karyotype" showing the site of the cytogenetic defect in some of the classic deletion syndromes. AS, Angelman syndrome; CMT, Charcot-Marie-Tooth neuropathy (a duplication); HPSN, hereditary pressure-sensitive neuropathy; PWS, Prader-Willi syndrome; Rb, retinoblastoma plus other features; WAGR, Wilms tumor, aniridia, genital defects, retardation syndrome.

influences the functioning of client genes; its reduced activity has been correlated with psychiatric disease (Strazisar et al. 2015). Other loci within the microdeletion may be responsible for minor dysmorphism and obesity. Three of the cases in Willemsen et al. were siblings; their deceased parents were known to have been of low cognitive ability, and rather probably, one of them had the same 1p21.3 deletion.

del 1p31.3p32.2 This syndrome includes a functional neurocognitive and epileptic phenotype associated with brain malformation, commonly

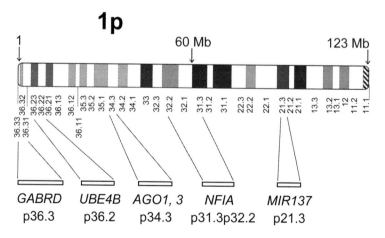

FIGURE 14–4

including agenesis of the corpus callosum, along with limb and urinary tract defects. Labonne et al. (2016) provide a review, and describe in detail their case of a young woman, first diagnosed on classical karyotyping as a ten year-old. Deletions range in extent from 2.2 to 22.9 Mb. Most arise de novo, but familial cases are on record. Revah-Politi et al. (2017) propose *NFIA* at chr1:61.2 Mb as a critical gene, which leads to a similar clinical picture in the deleted (haplo-insufficient) state and as a Mendelian mutation.

del 1p34.3 Deletions in this cytoband, similarly to del 1p21.3 above, may also have their pathogenic effect through a perturbation of the microRNA system. Tokita et al. (2015) describe deletions of sizes 1.1–3.1 Mb, with *AGO1* and *AGO3* (at chr1:36.3 Mb) resident in the 290 kb segment in common. These are "argonaute" genes, whose products direct the process of post-transcriptional gene silencing (that is, RNA interference); their removal may be the basis of the observed phenotype of hypotonia, moderate intellectual disability, and subtle facial dysmorphism. De novo inheritance has been observed in all tested cases.

del 1p36.3 The tip of chromosome 1 short arm is particularly vulnerable to rearrangement, and different del(1)(p36) deletion syndromes exist. We may speak of a distal "classical" deletion; a more proximal deletion; and larger deletions that include both of the foregoing, plus the intervening chromatin.

The most common is the *distal "classical"* chr1:pter-6.3 Mb deletion, del 1p36.3, and in fact this is the most frequently observed of all terminal deletions, seen in about 1 in 5,000 births. Within this segment, smaller deletions may be seen, accommodated within the subbands 1q36.32q36.33, or within 1q36.33 alone; and indeed there is considerable heterogeneity of deletion extent, albeit that phenotypic severity does not correlate well with deletion size (Ōiglane-Shlik et al. 2014). *GABRD* at chr1:1.95 Mb, in 1q36.33, is proposed to be an important pheno-critical locus. The facies is variably dysmorphic, with deep-set eyes and midface retrusion a particular observation, and several minor physical anomalies may be observed (Shimada et al. 2014; Jordan et al. 2015). The mental defect is usually severe; an unsurprising observation, given that a major brain malformation, perisylvian polymicrogyria, is seen in some, and it is plausible that in others anatomic defect might be beyond MRI

resolution; and also, defects in white matter are common (Dobyns et al. 2008; Ōiglane-Shlik et al. 2014). A milder phenotype is seen in the mosaic case (Shimada et al. 2014). A phenotypic overlap with Angelman syndrome and Rett syndrome has been noted. Jordan et al. assess the case for the agency of certain genes whose haploinsufficiency may contribute to the phenotype, and these are listed in Figure 14–5, taken from their work.

del 1q21.1 Two recurrent deletions reside within this segment, each flanked by segmental duplications that dictate a susceptibility to rearrangement (Rosenfeld et al. 2012b). The smaller *proximal* deletion (chr1:145.6-146.1 Mb) includes the *RBM8A* gene (Fig. 14–6), and it has the particular interest of being a susceptibility factor for thrombocytopenia-absent radius (TAR) syndrome. The majority of TAR, 90% or more, is due to having a 1q21.1 deletion on one chromosome, and a low-frequency variant of the *RBM8A* gene on the other. This variant is most often an SNP within the 5′ untranslated region, and less often so, an intron 1 SNP (Albers et al. 2013). The deletion is usually (75%) familial, but may be de novo. Where one parent is heterozygous for the deletion, and the other carries one or other of the *RBM8A* SNPs, the pattern of inheritance of TAR mimics that of autosomal recessive disease.

The *distal* 1q21.1 microdeletion (chr1:147.1-148.0) includes the *GJA5* locus, and is one of the more common CNVs observed in clinical cohorts. The clinical picture includes mental retardation, autism, seizures, cardiac defects, cataract, and minor dysmorphic features (Mefford et al. 2008; Rosenfeld et al. 2012b). Some are de novo cases, some familial with a (usually mildly) affected parent, and some familial from an apparently unaffected parent. A detailed study in Bernier et al. (2016) documents the phenotypic range, with a particular focus on neurocognitive/psychological/behavioral traits. They note that while IQ might "officially" be in a normal range—that is, above 70—the average was about 1 standard deviation below the mean. Phonological processing, the ability to distinguish the meanings of words, is notably impaired. Digilio et al. (2013) describe a family in which a brother had had pulmonary valve stenosis, and an IQ of 87; his sister had had learning difficulties, with an IQ of 58; and the daughter of this sister had moderate mental retardation (IQ = 48) and difficult behavior, absence seizures, a complex heart defect, and

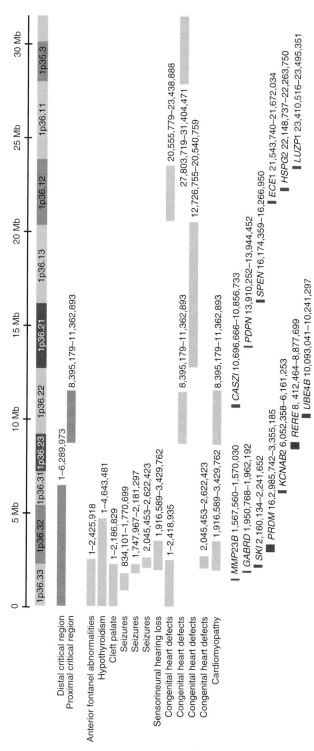

FIGURE 14-5   A genotype-phenotype correlation display for 1p36 deletions. There are two critical regions, a more common "classic" distal, and a proximal region. The distal deletion is shown as encompassing chr1:1–6,289,973, and the proximal deletion resides within segment chr1:8,395,179–11,362,893 (dark bars, *upper*). Different deletions, showing associations with various clinical defects, are shown (*middle*, light gray bars), as are proposed pheno-critical loci (*lower*). (*Top*) 1p36 subbands and (in hg19) molecular marker.

Source: From Jordan et al., 1p36 deletion syndrome: An update, *Appl Clin Genet* 2015;8:189–200. Courtesy D. A. Scott, and with the permission of Dove Press.

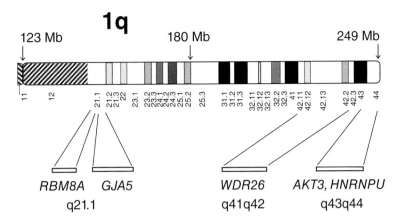

FIGURE 14–6

some dysmorphic features. Each had the deletion chr1:147,093,177-148,262,736. As can apply in the generality of microimbalances, loci elsewhere, if mutated, may exacerbate the clinical phenotype (and indeed bring to medical attention a family that might otherwise have escaped notice), such as Qiao et al. (2017) identified in the whole-exome analysis of a child with microcephaly and a severe articulation disorder.

del 1q41q42 This syndrome is to be numbered among those with an Angelman resemblance, and may prove to be one of the more common of the microdeletion syndromes. Au et al. (2014) had initially proposed the *FBXO28* locus as being of central importance, but Skraban et al. (2017) were drawn rather to the role of the *WDR26* gene (chr1:224.1 Mb). They studied 15 cases of point mutation in this gene, and were struck by the similarity of the facies between those with mutation of the gene, and those with the microdeletion. All cases have been de novo.

del 1q43q44 There is considerable variation in the extent of these deletions, of size ranging from 120 kb through 5.9 Mb, and falling within the region chr1:239.8-246.6 Mb. Ballif et al. (2012) have identified certain genes which, when haploinsufficient, could be responsible for particular components of the phenotype of this severe disorder. Microcephaly may be due to the *AKT3* gene, agenesis of the corpus callosum might be consequential upon haploinsufficiency of the regulatory factor *ZNF238*, while seizures could inhere in the *HNRNPU* gene; an interpretation largely supported in Depienne et al. (2017). The ways in which these and other genes within the segment may interact, and impact upon head size, are rehearsed in Raun

et al. (2017). We have seen a young woman originally, and not unreasonably, diagnosed as Rett syndrome, with severe epilepsy, but normal on *MECP2* mutation study in the early 1990s; microarray some 20 years later showed a microdeletion chr1:244.4-245.3 Mb (R. Beddow, personal communication, 2012). *HNRNPU* was the only one of the above-mentioned three genes included in this segment; very similar deletions are reported in Thierry et al. (2012). De novo inheritance is the norm, but very rare familial cases are recognized (Ballif et al. 2012). Gai et al. (2015) describe a normal father and his microcephalic son, both carrying a 1q44 deletion removing just the *AKT3* gene. Parental very low-level (3.4% on blood) somatic, and inferentially gonadal mosaicism, has been demonstrated (Campbell et al. 2014).

Chromosome 2 Deletions

del 2p15p16.1 Deletions within this region, chr2:53.6-66.4 Mb, are nonrecurrent, of up to 6.9 Mb in extent. Fannemel et al. (2014) provide a review of 14 patients reported since 2007, and describe their own case having the smallest recorded deletion (230 kb, chr2:61.27-61.50 Mb): a mildly dysmorphic and intellectually affected man, who was able to have sheltered employment. Lévy et al. (2017) propose two distinct, albeit very close, critical regions, at 2p15 (*XPO1* at chr2:61.5 Mb a landmark gene) and 2p16.1 (*BCL11A* at chr2:60.45-60.55 Mb a marker) respectively (Fig. 14–7), the phenotypes due to deletion in each not greatly dissimilar, although Soblet et al. (2018) insist, in respect of *BCL11A*, on a specific effect upon orofacial praxis and language development due to haplo-insufficiency at this locus. Loviglio et al. (2017) observed physical

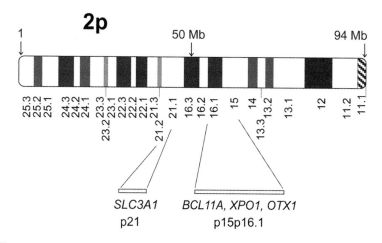

FIGURE 14–7

interaction, at the level of chromatin, between the *XPO1* locus at 2p15 and chromosome 16p11.2, and noted the similarities in the phenotypes of individuals with imbalances at these two loci. In the larger deletion, the phenotype is more severe, and may include structural brain abnormality on imaging. Abnormal genital development is a frequent concomitant, and Jorgez et al. (2014) propose that loss of the *OTX1* gene (chr2:63.0 Mb) may be the basis of this. De novo inheritance is the rule.

del 2p21 This extremely rare syndrome is unusual in being seen in only the homozygous state (Bartholdi et al. 2013), and thus displaying an autosomal recessive mode of inheritance. The loci implicated are *PPM1B*, *SLC3A1*, *PREPL*, and *CAMKMT*. *SLC3A1* is the basis of the cystinuria seen in the syndrome (a smaller deletion including just *SLC3A1* and *PREPL* leads to the hypotonia-cystinuria

syndrome). Seizures, intellectual disability, and a Prader-Willi-like facial dysmorphism are observed.

del 2q11.2 Sequences within the segment chr2:96.1-98.0 Mb are prone to recurrent rearrangement. Deletion leads to a neurobehavioral phenotype, with soft facial dysmorphism, and marked short stature. The condition can arise de novo, or be inherited from either parent (Riley et al. 2015). *LMAN2L* is a landmark locus (Fig. 14–8).

del 2q13 A recurrent deletion at chr2:110.6-112.3 Mb is associated with a syndrome of intellectual deficiency, autism, and dysmorphism, but it is equally associated with normality (Hladilkova et al. 2015; Riley et al. 2015). In some, major cardiac and craniofacial malformation is reported. The loci *BCL2L11*, *FBLN7*, and *TMEM87B* may be wherein lies the pathogenesis (Russell et al. 2014).

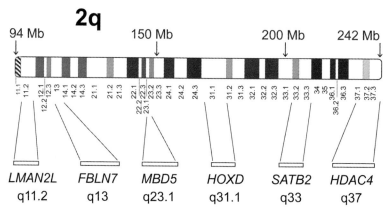

FIGURE 14–8

This deletion is typically inherited. The carrier parent may or may not show any sign; this may well reflect the influence of variation elsewhere in the genome, and the concept of the "second-hit" CNV is likely germane. This issue of incomplete penetrance is particularly problematic in counseling, and interpretation of a possible second-hit scenario may here become a question of practical relevance. With this, and indeed with other del/dups of incomplete penetrance, we will await the accumulation of data concerning penetrance in the absence of any other CNV, and compared with penetrance in the presence of a particular CNV (or sequence variant).

del 2q23.1 This syndrome is one of the more frequently seen of the microdeletions (Talkowski et al. 2011). Deletions range very considerably in size, from ~300 kb to 20 Mb, but all including *MBD5*. All cases have been de novo. There is a resemblance to Angelman and Rett syndromes, with features of severe mental retardation with absent speech, stereotypic repetitive behavior, microcephaly, ataxia, and a coarse facies. Severe epilepsy (infantile spasms) is recorded (Du et al. 2014). The crucial gene, *MBD5*, is located at chr2:148.0 Mb. This gene interacts with several autism-associated loci implicated in other deletion syndromes, including *RAI1* in del(17)(p11.2) Smith-Magenis syndrome, *TCF4* in del(18q) Pitt-Hopkins syndrome, *UBE3A* in del(15)(q11.2q13.1) Angelman syndrome, *EHMT1* in del(9)(q34.3) Kleefstra syndrome, and *MEF2C* in the del(5)(q14q21) syndrome; thus, the final common neurobehavioral phenotypic outcome in all these conditions is similar. Mullegama and Elsea (2016) speak of *MBD5*-associated neurodevelopmental disorder (MAND) whether due to deletion, duplication, or variation within the *MBD5* locus.

del 2q24q31 Deletions in the region chr2:164-177 Mb fit between, or slightly overlap, those of the foregoing and the following entries, and they are reviewed in Pescucci et al. (2007). A cluster of SCN (sodium channel) genes, including *SCN1A*, may be the basis of the epilepsy seen in this condition. Syndactyly of the hands and feet brings to mind the autosomal recessive disorder Filippi syndrome (Lazier et al. 2014), and this could be due to *HOXD* insufficiency (see next entry). De novo inheritance is the rule.

del 2q31.1 This is a syndrome which displays variable deletion, mostly within (occasionally beyond) chr2:171-178 Mb. Loss of the *HOXD* cluster at chr2:176.09-176.19, when this is within the deleted segment, is the presumed cause of the limb malformation, such as great toe duplication and clinodactyly (Dimitrov et al. 2011). Variable dysmorphism, in some presenting a distinctive facial gestalt, and neurocognitive capacity from essentially normal to substantially compromised, may correlate with the compass of the deletion. Parent-to-child transmission, and indeed grandparent-to-grandchild transmission, is recorded (Mitter et al. 2010; Tsai et al. 2009).

del 2q33.3q32.3 (del 2q33) A syndrome due to this deletion was proposed by Van Buggenhout et al. in 2005, and further reports have since appeared (Balasubramanian et al. 2011; Tomaszewska et al. 2013). There is considerable variation in the extent of the deletion, ranging from 35 kb to 10.4 Mb in size in the series of Balasubramanian et al., and indeed in some patients there is no common region of overlap. A behavioral phenotype of hyperactivity, and a "happy" affect, but with bouts of anxiety or aggression, are reported; intellectual deficiency can be severe. Dysmorphism may be subtle; a Marfanoid appearance is sometimes observed. *SATB2* may be an important gene, albeit that in a few, this locus is not deleted (Rosenfeld et al. 2009). De novo inheritance is the rule.

del 2q37.3q37.1: Albright-like Syndrome This well-known deletion should specifically be sought in patients with a morphological phenotype somewhat reminiscent of Albright hereditary osteodystrophy (short stature, short metacarpals), a quite distinctive facies, intellectual deficit with autistic behavior, and often obesity (Leroy et al. 2013). It is among the more frequent of the deletion syndromes. Deletions, which may vary quite considerably in size, typically from 2.6 to 9.9 Mb, lie within the cytogenomic range chr2:229.8-242.2 Mb. Parent-to-child transmission is very rare, but has been observed, in cases in whom the deletion is of smaller extent (Villavicencio-Lorini et al. 2013; Jean-Marçais et al. 2015). The latter authors describe a father and his three children with a small 0.49 Mb 2q37.3 deletion, and probably others in the family likewise affected. This case allowed an inference that deletion of the *TWIST2* and *HDAC4* genes may be necessary to produce the classic phenotypic features. Transmission from a mosaic parent is noted in Freitas et al. (2012).

Chromosome 3 Deletions

del 3p14p12 The extent of the deletion can vary considerably, the largest up to 27 Mb, practically the entire p12, p13, and p14 bands; no recurrent deletion is yet identified (Dimitrov et al. 2015). No single gene is implicated as central to the phenotype, but for certain loci, a plausible case can be made, such as *FOXP1* and *MITF* at 3p14.1, and *ROBO1* and *ROBO2* at 3p12.3 (Fig. 14–9). A broad, high forehead is a distinctive physical sign, while malformations of heart, eye, and urogenital tract are common. Death in infancy is recorded. Smaller deletions within this segment are noted in Schwaibold et al. (2013), 6.55 Mb and 4.76 Mb de novo deletions of 3p14.1p14.3, associated with a somewhat less marked but still important phenotype of severe intellectual deficiency, autistic features, and mild facial dysmorphism. No familial case of del 3p12p14 is known.

del 3p22.3, del 3p21.31 These two separate microdeletions have each been recorded in only single-digit numbers. Marangi et al. (2013) studied a family in which a 2.5 Mb del 3p22.3 (chr3:33.4-35.9 Mb) was carried by a mother and her three children, the genes *CLASP2* and *ARPP21* of plausible pheno-critical effect. Other CNVs carried by either parent may have had a second-hit exacerbating effect upon the phenotype of minor physical anomalies and intellectual disability (a concept that, of course, and as already noted, applies to many of the smaller microdeletions).

Eto et al. (2013) describe the three known cases of 3p21.31 deletion, characterized by a distinctive facies, developmental delay, and the neuromuscular correlates of white matter abnormality and elevation of the muscle enzyme, creatine kinase. The shortest region of overlap (chr3:49.1-50.2 Mb) included the possibly crucial *BSN* gene at chr3:49.6 Mb.

del 3p26.2, del 3p25.3p26.1, del 3p25p26 In contrast to the rarity of more proximal 3p deletion, deletions at distal 3p are well recognized and command considerable attention. These may comprise interstitial segments or may include the terminal region, and these differing degrees of distal 3p deletion are associated with phenotypes of differing severity (Shuib et al. 2009). Certain loci are proposed to be of central importance in determining the phenotypes. Within 3p25.3p26.1, a shared 124 kb overlap region includes the *SETD5* and *SRGAP3* loci (chr3:9.0-9.4 Mb), which are likely of central importance (Kellogg et al. 2013; Grozeva et al. 2014; Kuechler et al, 2015). Two genes of interest within distal 3p deletions are *ITPR1* (3p26.1, chr3:4.4-4.8 Mb) and *VHL* (3p25.3, chr3:10.1 Mb), and haploinsufficiency of which causes spinocerebellar ataxia type 15 and Von Hippel-Lindau disease, respectively. Thus, a del(3p) patient whose deletion included one or both of these genes, and surviving well into adulthood, might develop the corresponding ataxic and tumor-associated syndrome.

del 3p36.3p26.2 Terminal deletions of one or both of the distalmost two 3p bands, of up to about 10 Mb in extent, may lead to minor dysmorphism and developmental delay, but equally may be seen in normal persons. Moghadasi et al. (2014) describe a family in which all six tested individuals with a 2.9 Mb deletion (chr3:1-2,856,137 bp) other than the

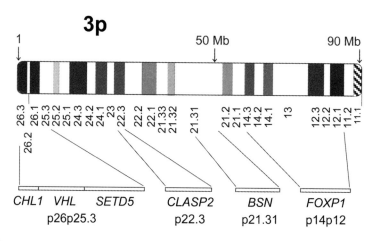

FIGURE 14–9

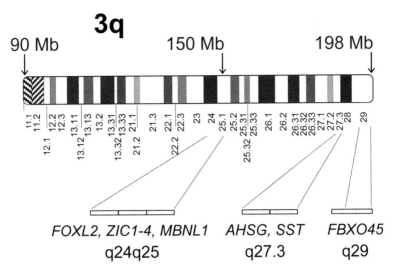

3q

FOXL2, ZIC1-4, MBNL1
q24q25

AHSG, SST
q27.3

FBXO45
q29

FIGURE 14–10

proband, and including his great grandmother, were essentially normal people. Very small terminal deletion, up to just 1 Mb, in 3p36.3, comprises its own syndrome, and may lie in the loss of just one gene, *CHL1*. Poor verbal development is the most notable trait. The condition is often familial, but again the transmitting parent may be of entirely normal phenotype (Tassano et al. 2014). A role for second-hit CNVs in the presenting symptomatology of del(3) (p26.2p36.3) probands remains well open.

del 3q24q25 According to the extent of deletion within this chromosomal region, the phenotype may include features of blepharophimosis-epicanthus inversus syndrome (BPES),[13] the Dandy-Walker cerebellar malformation, and the Wisconsin syndrome. Ferraris et al. (2013) define three critical regions within which the deletions of the observed cases have fallen. Deletions that remove *FOXL2* produce BPES; loss of *ZIC1* and *ZIC4* likely contributes to the cerebellar defect (but this component is of incomplete penetrance); and deletions extending into 3q25.2 may lead to Wisconsin syndrome (Fig. 14–10). Thus, a child described in Ferraris et al., who carried a large 3q22.1q25.1 deletion, 19.2 Mb in length, chr3:132.7-152.0 Mb, and which removed the *FOXL2*, *ZIC1*, and *ZIC4* genes, had both BPES and Dandy-Walker malformation as part of the overall complicated clinical

picture. The Wisconsin syndrome, characterized by a distinctive facial gestalt, may reside more distally in chr3:151.9-152.7 Mb, with the locus *MBNL1* at chr3:152.268-152.465 Mb plausibly the key factor (Bertini et al. 2017).

del 3q26.33q27.2 This rare syndrome is due to deletion, of variable (2.1-4.3 Mb) extent, which includes at least the segment chr3:183.3-185.4 Mb, within 3q27.1q27.2 (Mandrile et al. 2013). A distinctive facies, intellectual disability, and severe growth retardation characterize the clinical picture. Where studied, cases have been of de novo origin.

del 3q27.3 This syndrome gained definition through perusal of the DECIPHER database. Thevenon et al. (2014) collected recorded patients with variable deletions within an 8.2 Mb segment of 3q27.3q28 (chr3:184.6-192.8 Mb), in whom two regions of overlap were identified. A thin and narrow face with a hooked nose is very distinctive; the *SST* gene (contained within overlap region chr3:186.7-188.1 Mb) may be responsible for the neuropsychiatric picture ranging from autism to psychosis, and the *AHSG* gene (contained within overlap region chr3:186.0-186.7 Mb) for the rather Marfanoid skeletal phenotype. Most arise de novo, but parental transmission is known.

---

13 Isolated BPES may be due to a translocation having one breakpoint in this region, but distant from the actual gene—a laboratory diagnosis that might be missed unless a karyotype is preformed (Yang et al. 2014).

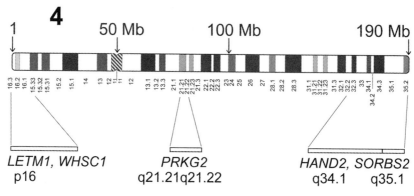

FIGURE 14-11

del 3q29 A recurrent 1.6 Mb deletion encompasses chr3:196.0-197.6 Mb (Città et al. 2013). Variable behavioral traits, mild-to-moderate mental retardation with microcephaly, and mild facial dysmorphism are core features of the phenotype. Some, in addition, have clefting and genitourinary malformation. The deletion predisposes very significantly to schizophrenia, indeed a 41-fold increased risk (Mulle 2015), and Torres et al. (2016) assess the potential roles of "neurodevelopmental genes" contained within the segment, *FBXO45* being an attractive candidate. Glassford et al. (2016) were able to recruit a cohort of 44 cases and documented neuropsychiatric traits including anxiety disorder, panic attacks, depression, and bipolar disorder, as well as schizophrenia. These numbers surely suffice to allow 3q29 syndromal status. Familial transmission is rare but recorded (Clayton-Smith et al. 2010), and both abnormal and reportedly normal parental neurocognitive aspects are observed.

Chromosome 4 Deletions

del 4p: Wolf-Hirschhorn Syndrome This well-known deletion syndrome identified in the prebanding era is one of the few that can, in its typical form, be confidently recognized clinically. The "Greek warrior helmet" craniofacial appearance is very characteristic. The natural history of WHS is discussed in Battaglia et al. (2015). The smallest deletions are confined to the distalmost band, 4p16.3, and are of less than 3.5 Mb size. Much the commonest observed is a terminal deletion of 5–18 Mb, which may extend into 4p15. (Larger, 22–25 Mb deletions, might be described as "WHS plus.") Deletions typically include two short contiguous "WHS critical regions," WHSCR1 (proximal) and -2 (distal), contained approximately within chr4:1.79-1.94 Mb,

in distal 4p16.3 (Fig. 14–11). The *WHSC1* gene at chr4:1.9 Mb is presumed to have a key role in determining the classic dysmorphology, and *LETM1* at chr4:1.8 Mb may influence nervous system functioning; but no one gene commands the phenotype, and this is a true contiguous gene syndrome, with a presumed contribution of several p16.3 genes, within chr4:0.4-1.9 Mb. While de novo occurrence is the typical observation, almost half may be revealed as having arisen as unbalanced translocations, some showing additional phenotypic features in consequence (Wieland et al. 2014; Battaglia et al. 2015).

A deletion just centromeric of the typical WHS extent, at 4p15.2-p15.32, leads to a quite different disorder, in some respects resembling Marfan syndrome (Basinko et al. 2008). A point of interest is that inheritance had been from a mosaic mother.

del 4q21 The first major series of patients with this deletion was reported in 2010 by Bonnet et al. A number of further cases have since appeared in the literature, concerning this syndrome of marked growth and developmental retardation, with poor or absent spoken language, along with a quite distinctive facial appearance. The brain defect of polymicrogyria is described (Dobyns et al. 2008). Most deletions are in the range 2.0–15 Mb; the smallest is 761 kb. The 1.4 Mb critical region lies in 4q21.21q21.22, chr4:81.1–82.5 Mb. Important genes therein are *PRKG2* and *RASGEF1B*, which likely underlie the cognitive phenotype (Hu et al. 2017); Zarrei et al. (2017) present also a case for the loci *HNRNPD* and *HNRNPDL*, at chr4:82.3 Mb. If the deletion extends into 4q22 and removes the *PKD2* gene, the very specific feature of polycystic kidney disease ensues (Sakazume et al. 2015).

All cases have been de novo; nevertheless, a parental insertional translocation is prudently to be excluded.

del Distal 4q, 4q32.3/q35.2qter Many cases are on record of distal 4q deletions ("4q deletion syndrome"), mostly terminal or at least subterminal, some interstitial; but this is a heterogeneous collection, as almost all are nonrecurrent rearrangements. Heart malformation is frequent, and the *HAND2* (in q34.1) and *SORBS2* (q35.1) genes are implicated. The very specific observation of ulnar ray defect may reside in 4q34.1 (Lurie 2016). In the review of Strehle et al. (2012), the distal segments in seven patients ranged from 4q32.2q35.2 to 4q35.2q35.2, and of sizes 464 kb to 24.0 Mb. It is not uncommon that a parental rearrangement, such as a balanced translocation, is identified.

Phenotypic severity is not necessarily proportional to segment length. Indeed, in a normal woman identified incidentally in the course of a miscarriage investigation, a 10 Mb deletion in 4q34.2q34.3, of minimum extent chr4:171.8-181.5 Mb, was seen; this represents apparent nonpenetrance (Bateman et al. 2010). A 4q35.1 deletion in the series of Strehle et al. (2012) was of only 464 kb (chr4:185.6-186.0 Mb), but the child was dysmorphic with heart and palatal malformation. The del(4)(q35.1q35.2) child in Vona et al. (2014) was able to attend a normal school, albeit that he had required much hospitalization for the management of cardiac anomalies, hearing loss, and cleft palate and a velopharyngeal insufficiency. The 6.9 Mb deletion was de novo, chr4:183.1-189.9 Mb. A marginally smaller deletion, chr4:183.7-189.5 Mb, was seen in a mother and her two daughters, who were in fact normal, in Yakut et al. (2015b). This observation again speaks

to a nonpenetrance of this segment, and it also illustrates that these distal deletions are capable of parental transmission.

Chromosome 5 Deletions

del 5p: Cri du Chat Syndrome Most of the deleted segments of this famous syndrome are terminal and vary considerably in length. The clinical severity corresponds substantially, but not always precisely or consistently, to deletion size. The *cri* in the newborn is characteristic, and may even allow the diagnosis to be suspected, sight unseen, as one enters the neonatal nursery. The cri region is pinpointed to a 700 kb region containing only two genes (*ADAMTS16, ICE1*) in p15.32 (Fig. 14–12), while certain other components of the phenotype can be attributed to certain other p15 segments (Nguyen et al. 2015; Zhang et al. 2016a). Van Buggenhout et al. (2000) document in quite some detail, with several photographs, the phenotypes in seven older individuals, teenagers and adults; and Nguyen et al. provide detail collected from a support group (the 5p Minus Family Database). Cognitive compromise is typically mild/moderate in more distal small (5p15.31pter) deletions; moderate to severe with deletions from 5pter to 5p14.1; and profound in those extending into 5p13.2p13.3 (Marignier et al. 2012). Extraordinarily, cases of normal intellect are, very rarely, discovered, such as a man (a physician) presenting only with infertility, who carried a de novo interstitial 15.5 Mb deletion at 5p13.3p14.3, chr5:18.4-33.9 Mb, this region being described as a "gene desert" (Papoulidis et al. 2013).

While most cases are sporadic, about 10% are due to a familial translocation, and this possibility should be checked for in each case; a rare cause is a

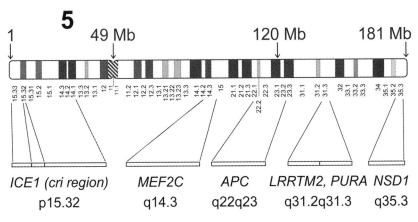

FIGURE 14–12

large parental inversion (Ohnuki et al. 2010). One case of recurrence of del(5)(p15.2), identified at prenatal diagnosis, attests to the reality of parental gonadal mosaicism (Hajianpour et al. 1991). Very seldom, in milder cases, parental transmission may be seen; here, a distal breakpoint at chr5:17.630 Mb is common. These transmitting parents typically display a compromised cognitive and behavioral phenotype; but remarkably, Zhang et al. (2016a) describe one del(5p) father who had a cat-like cry as a baby, learning difficulty at school, and who was yet able to graduate with a bachelor's degree in computer science. These rare cases allow inference about the *cri* region, as mentioned above.

del 5q14q21, del 5q14.3 This condition has some resemblance to Rett syndrome. Hotz et al. (2013) make the case that *MEF2C* at 5q14.3 is the pheno-critical gene in this deletion syndrome. The severe intellectual deficit is associated with the brain malformation, microcephaly with simplified gyral pattern. Deletions may be small enough that only *MEF2C* (at chr5:88.8 Mb) is removed, and these cases can be considered as 5q14.3 deletion syndrome; most deletions are of 1–10 Mb, within chr5:86-96 Mb, and could more widely be described as del(5)(q14q21).

del 5q22q23: Polyposis Plus Syndrome A minor degree of facial dysmorphism and mild to moderate mental retardation are nonspecific features seen in deletions in the region of 5q22q23; the unique feature is adenomatous polyposis of the bowel, and indeed it was such a deletion that led to discovery of the *APC* (adenomatous polyposis coli) gene (Hockey et al. 1989). Absence of one *APC* allele (at chr5:112.7-112.8 Mb) of itself allows polyps to develop, and any subsequent mutation/loss of the allele on the intact chromosome 5 then leads to loss of the tumor suppressor function of this gene (Hodgson et al. 1994).

Other similar examples exist of constitutional deletions that convey, in addition to congenital abnormality, a cancer predisposition (Lucci-Cordisco et al. 2005). As with the polyposis example, the typical scenario is that loss of one allele of a tumor suppressor gene on the deleted chromosome comprises the "first hit" in the process of tumorigenesis. The 13q14 deletion associated with retinoblastoma, noted below, is the classic example.

Jacoby et al. (1997) describe a deletion of 10q22.3q24.1 in a patient with multiple congenital malformations and juvenile polyposis, the latter presumably reflecting the loss of one copy of the *PTEN* gene. A 9q22.32q31.1 deletion has been associated with a "Gorlin syndrome plus" phenotype, and an increased risk for cancer is to be expected (del 9q22.32q31.1 entry below). Lucci-Cordisco et al. identified a de novo 2p16p21 deletion in a mildly dysmorphic woman with a moderate degree of mental retardation, who had presented with bowel cancer at age 37 years; her disease was on the basis of the constitutional loss of one *MSH2* mismatch-repair allele.

del 5q31.2q31.3 The clinical picture in this rare deletion syndrome is predominantly neurodevelopmental, with severe intellectual deficit, marked hypotonia, apneic episodes, and poor feeding. A particular observation is abnormal movements in the neonatal period resembling a seizure, but with no epileptic activity on the electroencephalogram (EEG). Brain MRI shows poor frontal lobe structure (Brown et al. 2013). Bonaglia et al. (2015) record the life history of the oldest known patient, who survived to age 26 years. *PURA*, at chr5:140 Mb, and *LRRTM2*, at 138.8 Mb, are proposed as key loci. Deletion sizes range from approximately 1 to 5 Mb. Two small deletions—which do not overlap—are the 360 kb deletion (chr5:139.949-140.309 Mb) of Bonaglia et al. above, and the 0.9 Mb deletion (chr5:138.387-139.323 Mb) in Kleffmann et al. (2012). We may need to consider that two "subsyndromes" exist: one defined by loss of *PURA*, another by loss of *LRRTM2*, and most del5q31.2q31.3 deletions combine the two. All cases have been de novo.

del 5q35.3: Sotos Syndrome A curious observation in the genetics of Sotos syndrome (cerebral gigantism) is a racial difference: About half of Japanese cases are due to a microdeletion at 5q35.3, but only 10% of a U.K. population (the remainders having an *NSD1* point mutation). Furthermore, deletion lengths varied quite considerably in U.K. cases, from 0.5 to 5.0 Mb; but in the Japanese, most had a recurrent 1.9 Mb deletion, chr5:176.1-178.0 Mb. A similar picture is seen in Korean patients (Sohn et al. 2013). These differences likely reflect an ethnic heterogeneity of "genomic architecture," and specifically, the nature of flanking low-copy repeats, which

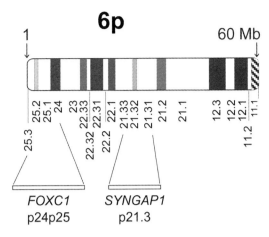

6p

1

60 Mb

25.2 25.1 24 23 22.33 22.31 22.1 21.33 21.32 21.31 21.2 21.1 12.3 12.2 12.1 11.1

25.3 22.32 22.2 11.2

FOXC1   SYNGAP1
p24p25   p21.3

FIGURE 14–13

may predispose to rearrangement (Tatton-Brown et al. 2005; Mochizuki et al. 2008). A large majority of deletions occur on the paternal chromosome. More extensive 5q35 deletions are recorded, which may include bands 5q35.1 and q35.2 (Rauch and Dörr 2007).

Chromosome 6 Deletions

del 6p21.3 The *SYNGAP1* locus at chr6:33.4-33.5 (Fig. 14–13) may be the key basis of the neurofunctional phenotype (intellectual deficiency, severe speech impairment, epilepsy) in deletions at 6p21.3 (Writzl and Knegt 2013). Deletions are reported ranging from 50 to 200 kb.

del 6p25p24 Terminal deletions at 6p25 may involve just that band, or extend into 6p24 or further. Qi et al. (2015) summarize the literature cases, and Figure 14–14 is taken from their work. The "commonly deleted region" includes the *FOXC1* gene. Brain imaging can show a cerebellar malformation, dilated vascular (Virchow-Robin) spaces, and variable leukoencephalopathy (Cellini et al. 2012; Delahaye et al. 2012). Eye defects, of the anterior segment,[14] are common (Cornelis et al. 2015). Prenatal diagnosis, following ultrasonographic demonstration of multiple anomalies, is recorded (Delahaye et al. 2012; Ergin et al. 2015). Vernon et al. (2013) report an adult, of normal intelligence (certainly an atypical observation),

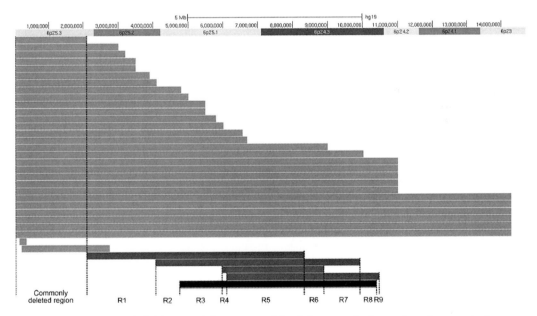

FIGURE 14–14 Recorded deletions of chromosome 6 distal short arm. Light gray bars show terminal deletions; dark gray and black bars (*lower*) show interstitial deletions. The interstitial deletions enable a division into nine subregions (R1–R9).

Source: From Qi et al., Haploinsufficiency and triploinsensitivity of the same 6p25.1p24.3 region in a family, *BMC Med Genom* 8: 38, 2015. Courtesy J. Yu, and with the permission of BioMed Central, as per the Creative Commons Attribution License.

---

14 The anterior segment: the front part of the eye, including the cornea, iris, ciliary body, and lens. Axenfeld-Rieger anomaly refers to a dysgenesis of the anterior segment components. Cataract and glaucoma are classic anterior segment diseases.

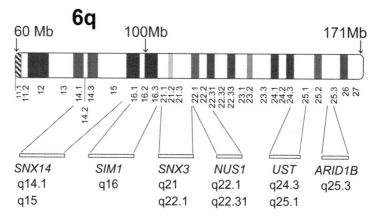

FIGURE 14–15

with a "CADASIL-like"[15] leukoencephalopathy, who showed a del 6p25.3p25.2 (chr6:0.2-2.7 Mb) karyotype, *FOXC1* included in the deleted segment. A notable familial case is described in Qi et al. (2015): A mother mosaic del(6p)/dup(6p)/normal for the somewhat more proximal segment 6p25.1p24.3 (chr6:4.74-10.38 Mb; black bar in Fig. 14–14) had a del(6p) daughter with mild speech delay and minor dysmorphism, and a dup(6p) son of normal development, and the softest of soft dysmorphic signs. The mother's chromosomal state likely arose from an unequal sister chromatid exchange in early embryogenesis.

del 6q14.1q15 This deletion can determine a clinical picture of dysmorphic features, congenital malformation, and neurobehavioral difficulty, but within these bounds, quite some variation is seen (Quintela et al. 2015). Body habitus has been described with the opposite observations of a resemblance to Marfan or Prader-Willi syndrome (Lowry et al. 2013). All are intellectually affected; Quintela et al. ponder upon a possible second-hit role of a concomitant Xp22.31 CNV in contributing to their patient's autism. A 5 Mb segment, chr6:83-88 Mb in 6q14.2q14.3 (Fig. 14–15), appears to comprise the pheno-critical component of the syndrome; it contains several plausible genes, of which *SNX14*, a "brain gene," is one. No familial case is known.

del 6q16 Two very closely linked[16] loci, *POU3F2* at 6q16.2 (chr6:98.8 Mb) and *SIM1* at 6q16.3 (chr6:100.3 Mb), determine two factors involved in an appetite pathway (the leptin → melanocortin → SIM1 → oxytocin pathway) (El Khattabi et al. 2015; Kasher et al. 2016). A deletion including just one, or just the other, or indeed both of these two genes, leads to a syndrome in which obesity associated with hyperphagia is a cardinal observation, along with cognitive compromise; the condition has been called Prader-Willi-like. Most cases are de novo, but very rare familial transmission of an ~1 Mb *POU3F2*-containing deletion is recorded. The breakpoints are almost all nonrecurrent.

del 6q21q22.1 This segment, at chr6:105.5-117.2 Mb, and the following, 6q22.1q22.31, are adjacent, and some deletions take in both. The phenotype includes that of the acrocardiofacial syndrome, previously thought to be an autosomal recessive condition (Hudson et al. 2014). Several loci lie within the deleted segment, and while, for example, *SNX3* may be an important contributor to one component (the ectrodactyly), the full picture presumably reflects haploinsufficiency for a number of contiguous genes.

del 6q22.1q22.31 Epilepsy and tremors are the notable clinical observations in this deletion; dysmorphology is borderline or essentially absent. Intellectual deficiency is moderate or severe. Deletion sizes range from 0.2 to 16 Mb, with chr6:117.6-117.9 Mb in 6q22.1 assessed as the likely

---

15 CADASIL = cerebral autosomal dominant arteriopathy with subcortical infarcts and leukoencephalopathy.

16 Genetically linked, that is. Apparently, the near-contiguity of these functionally very closely related loci is a coincidence of evolution (Kasher et al. 2016).

critical segment, and the loci *NUS1* and *SLC35F1* in particular implicated (Szafranski et al. 2015).

del 6q23.2q24.2 Only one case is on record, but this is worth noting, given the clinical picture: a 3-year-old girl del(6)(q23.2q24.2), whose development was "completely normal to advanced," and who had only been karyotyped as a newborn because of low birth weight (Kumar et al. 1999). While the facies was distinctive, she was said to resemble her family. One might imagine that this particular segment contains no critical brain loci.

del 6q24.3q25.1 Deletion at the distal long arm, 6q24.3q25.1, is well recognized, albeit that most cases are nonrecurrent (Salpietro et al. 2015). A very few cases extend into q24.2 or q25.2, or, as in Stagi et al. (2015), into both. Notable traits are a joint hypermobility, reminiscent of Ehlers-Danlos syndrome, and a mild degree of cerebellar hypoplasia; speculatively, the *UST* gene at chr6:149.0 Mb could underpin both. Deletion of *TAB2* at chr6:149.3 Mb dictates the high likelihood of a cardiological defect (Cheng et al. 2017).

del 6q25.3 The *ARID1B* gene (mutation in which causes Coffin-Siris syndrome) at chr6:157.0 Mb is the basis of this deletion syndrome (Sim et al. 2015; Ronzoni et al. 2016). Deletions are of variable extent, falling within the wide range of 6q24.3 to 6q27 (and thus some having overlap with the del(6)(q24.3q25.1) described above), but nevertheless there are some breakpoints in common. The clinical picture includes intellectual disability, poor speech acquisition, dysmorphism, dysgenesis of the corpus callosum, and hearing loss. Apart from one child with an inherited very small 403 kb deletion, not including *ARID1B* (Peter et al. 2017), all cases have been de novo.

Chromosome 7 Deletions

del 7p13: Greig Cephalosyndactyly Syndrome Plus This acrocephalopolysyndactyly syndrome, classically inherited as an autosomal dominant, is due to mutation at the *GLI3* locus at chr7:42.1 Mb (Fig. 14–16). Recorded deletions in this region are up to 12 Mb in extent. Loss of other loci is the basis of a combined Greig syndrome with neurodevelopmental defect, seizures, and other abnormalities. Loss specifically of the glucokinase gene at chr7:44.2 Mb leads to one form of maturity-onset diabetes of the young (MODY; Zung et al. 2011).

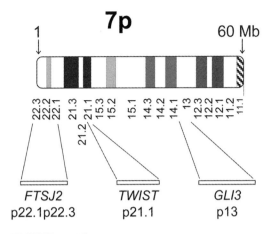

FIGURE 14–16

del 7p21.1: Saethre-Chotzen Syndrome Plus Most Saethre-Chotzen syndrome (another type of acrocephalosyndactyly) is due to point mutation in the *TWIST* gene at 7p21.1 (chr7:19.2 Mb). Cytogenetic forms include microdeletions within this chr7:15.3-27.0 Mb region, which may remove other genes and impose a broader phenotype (Busche et al. 2011; Cho et al. 2013a). A larger (13 Mb) deletion, 7p21.1p14.3, including the *HOXA13* gene, produced a more severe Saethre-Chotzen plus hand-foot-uterus syndrome phenotype in a child described in Fryssira et al. (2011). The skull defect in Saethre-Chotzen syndrome is premature fusion of cranial bones; a duplication ("triplo-excess") at this locus can produce the opposite effect, an underdevelopment of the cranial bones (see below, Fig. 14–51).

del 7p22.3p22.1 Deletions in distalmost 7p are rarely reported, and Richards et al. (2011) accumulated just nine cases (in five of which, the deletion extended through to 7p21 or 7p15). Their own, de novo, 0.3 Mb del 7p22.2p22.3 (chr7:1.99-2.32 Mb) case had a complex heart malformation, leading these authors to deduce that the genes within this segment underlaid the heart defect. But none of the loci within the segment stood out as candidates; for want of better understanding, the gene *FTSJ2* is chosen as a landmark in the diagram above. A radial ray defect in the case in Vergult et al. (2013a), a de novo more proximal deletion of 1.4 Mb at 7p22.1 (5.33–6.74 Mb), may have been due to *RAC1* haploinsufficiency; the child was also microcephalic.

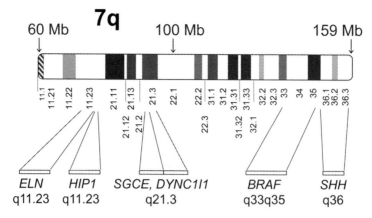

7q

60 Mb   100 Mb   159 Mb

ELN   HIP1   SGCE, DYNC1I1   BRAF   SHH
q11.23   q11.23   q21.3   q33q35   q36

FIGURE 14–17

del 7q11.23: Williams Syndrome Most (95%) Williams[17] syndrome (WS), also known as Williams-Beuren syndrome, is due to a 1.5 Mb deletion at chr7:73.3-74.8 Mb (Fig. 14–17), and it can arise equally in the gamete of either parent (Pober 2010). Sperm studies in control donors show similar frequencies of deletion and duplication for this segment (the WS critical region, WSCR), consistent with an NAHR mechanism (Molina et al. 2011). A parent who carries an inversion inv(7) (q11.23) including the WSCR (this polymorphism is present in 6% of the general population) has odds tilted in favor of meiotic generation of the deletion; inversion heterozygotes have a prior risk to have a child with WS of about 1 in 1,750, which is fourfold the overall population risk (1 in 7,500) (Hobart et al. 2010).

The characteristic neuropsychological phenotype is that of a mild intellectual disability, with overfriendliness to strangers, and a lacking in social judgment; an abnormally developed amygdala (a brain structure subserving social behavior and the recognition of emotional facial expressions) may be the basis of these traits (Martens 2013). Abnormal development of another specific brain structure, the right superior longitudinal fasciculus (a major white matter tract), may underlie the visuospatial deficit, of which one commonly given example is a hesitancy in stepping from one type of floor (e.g., carpet) to another (e.g., floorboards) (Hoeft et al. 2007). Earlier impressions that aspects of language might be intact have been refuted (Donnai

and Karmiloff-Smith 2000). The problem of which components of the deletion segment contribute to which components of the neurofunctional phenotype remains to be well elucidated (Broadbent et al. 2014). The deleted loci within the WSCR include the elastin gene *ELN*, which is responsible for the cardiovascular component (supravalvular aortic stenosis) of the phenotype. Growth indices (height, weight, head circumference) for deletion-proven WBS have been compiled (Martin et al. 2007). Affected monozygous twins generally have a rather similar phenotype (Castorina et al. 1997).

Recurrence of WS in a subsequent child is almost, but not entirely, unknown. Scherer et al. (2005) describe two instances of recurrence, one of which was associated with the paternal inversion polymorphism noted above. These authors suggested that family members of a WS proband found to be inv(7)(q11.23) heterozygotes consider prenatal testing, albeit that the risk figure is, objectively speaking, very low. In the other instance, maternal gonadal mosaicism was suggested, but not proven.

Rare instances of parent-to-child transmission are known, and Farwig et al. (2010) address the challenging question of counseling persons who themselves have WS.

del 7q11.23, Distal A deletion just distal to the WS segment, albeit within the same cytogenetic band, produces a very different clinical picture, of variable epilepsy, cognitive impairment, and neurobehavioral disorder (Ramocki et al. 2010). The key locus

---

17 The custom of removing the apostrophes from the names of authors associated with syndromes has led to the occasional misspelling of this condition as "William syndrome." Similarly, the terminal "s" of Edwards and of Sotos is sometimes erroneously dropped.

is *HIP1* (chr7:75.5-75.7 Mb), with possibly a contribution from *YWHAG* in some having a slightly larger deletion. Notably, transmission from a nonpenetrant parent is the rule; the overt symptomatology in probands may reflect the agency of a "second hit."

del 7q21.3 DLX6 and *DLX5* are limb development genes under the control of enhancer *DYNC1I1*; the *SGCE* gene codes for epsilon sarcoglycan. Loss of these neighboring two loci contained within chr7:94.58-97.03 Mb can lead to a split hand/foot malformation, and myoclonus-dystonia, respectively; deletion of adjacent loci contributes to a broader phenotype. Delgado and Velinov (2015) describe a family with an inherited 1 Mb chr7:95.1-96.2 Mb deletion, which removed *DYNC1I1* (*DLX6* and *-5* intact), and some centromeric loci (but not *SGCE*). A father and three sons had variable intellectual deficiency, and ectrodactyly in just two of the sons, this latter observation illustrating a presumed reduced penetrance with respect to *DYNC1I1* deletion.

Saugier-Veber et al. (2010) review 7q21.3 deletions associated with myoclonus dystonia "plus"; they identify a 0.5 Mb segment at chr7:93.23-93.72 Mb, a little centromeric of *SGCE*, that may well be the basis of the mental retardation that is seen in some cases. Their own case concerned father-to-son transmission of a 7q21.3 deletion, chr7:92,774,747-94,652,905 bp. The son, who had an IQ of 30, developed "shock-like" jerks of limbs and trunk (myoclonus) at age 12 years; the father was less affected. Psychosis may be a concomitant of *SGCE* haploinsufficiency (Dale et al. 2012).

del 7q33q35 Dilzell et al. (2015) review 12 cases of various q33q35 interstitial deletions, de novo except for an instance of familial insertion. Their own case involved a 9.9 Mb deletion at chr7:133-143 Mb. A gene in this region, at chr7:140.7-140.9 Mb, which will otherwise be familiar to the counselor, is *BRAF* (in the germline, activating missense mutations cause cardiofaciocutaneous syndrome; somatically, mutations occur in certain "cancer cascades"); whether it is contributory to the phenotype in the 7q33q35 deletion is an open question. The phenotype is of intellectual deficiency, dysmorphism, epilepsy, and susceptibility to infection.

del 7q36qter: Holoprosencephaly Plus Syndrome Terminal 7q deletions can involve as much as q33qter, but are more usually of q36qter (Lukusa et al. 2005). Holoprosencephaly is a developmental brain defect that can vary from devastatingly severe to rather mild, and there are several different genetic causes. The pheno-critical locus in this deletion is *SHH*, albeit that penetrance is incomplete (Linhares et al. 2014). De novo deletion is the rule, but inherited holoprosencephaly has been recorded in the setting of a familial 7q36 translocation (Hatziioannou et al. 1991). The cognitive phenotype is typically severe.

Chromosome 8 Deletions

del 8p23.1pter Distal deletions of 8p can be divided into those which are telomeric of the *GATA4* locus at chr8:11.7 Mb in p23.1, and those which include *GATA4* (Burnside et al. 2013) (Fig. 14–18). Considering the more distal cases, a landmark locus is *DLGAP2* in p23.3 at chr8:1.5 Mb, this gene having a role in synaptic integrity, and potentially influencing behavioral and cognitive traits. In some individuals with the distal deletion,

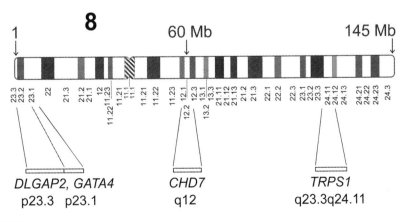

FIGURE 14–18

frustration tolerance is very low, but behavior seems to improve in later adolescence. Some have even been able to gain employment. Dysmorphism is mild. Almost all are of de novo generation; parent-to-child transmission is rare.

If *GATA4* (a cardiac transcription factor) is deleted, either in a more extensive terminal deletion or due to interstitial deletion, heart malformation is likely. Diaphragmatic hernia may be a characteristic component (Keitges et al. 2013). These cases are de novo (except for one remarkable instance of a mentally retarded but nondysmorphic mother with an interstitial deletion chr8:7.06-12.67 Mb, who had had cardiac surgery as a child, and whose fetus on ultrasound had an atrioventricular canal defect; she died when at 22 weeks gestation, probably of a ventricular arrhythmia; Guimiot et al. 2013).

An allied disorder is the inversion duplication/ deletion of 8p; this is a more severe condition, in which a duplication of a variable amount of 8p proximal to 8p22 is added to the imbalance of a del 8p23.1 deletion (García-Santiago et al. 2015). The foregoing 8p rearrangements each arise consistently in maternal meiosis—which thus allows the assumption of sporadic generation, and a very low recurrence risk—and had been facilitated by a common (26% population rate) maternal heterozygosity for an inversion polymorphism within p23.1, involving the segment chr8:7.6-12.3 Mb (Giglio et al. 2001).

del 8q12 Variable deletions in 8q12 thus far have all included 8q12.2, and extending into 8q12.1, 8q12.3, or both. Deletions involving 8q12.1, and which include the *CHD7* locus (chr8:60.8 Mb), curiously may not show a CHARGE phenotype (Palumbo et al. 2013). All cases have been de novo.

del 8q23.3q24.11: Langer-Giedion Syndrome The facies is distinctive, the bulbous nose a remarkable feature, and diagnosis can be made with some confidence on clinical grounds. The condition is due to a deletion that removes the gene for trichorhinophalangeal syndrome type I (*TRPS1*, at chr8:115.5 Mb), and a bone growth control gene (*EXT1*, which causes exostoses, at chr8:117.8-118.1 Mb), along with several other genes, to give the broader picture of Langer-Giedion syndrome (Maas et al. 2015). Deletions around this segment are of variable extent; some breakpoints are recurrent. Intellect is affected, to a degree, but may yet be within a normal range (Schinzel et al. 2013). These latter authors provide a useful narrative about four cases living into young or older adulthood (and comment about the paucity, in general, of long-term data in many of these syndromes of chromosome imbalance). The deletion may arise de novo on the chromosome 8 of either parent (Nardmann et al. 1997).

Chromosome 9 Deletions

del 9p13.3p13.1 This rare deletion, of chr9:33-39 Mb, shows a distinctive "square" facies and is associated with a learning difficulty. Tremor is a notable feature. No particular gene within the deleted segment presents itself as an attractive candidate (Crone and Thomas 2016). Inheritance is de novo.

del 9p24p22: 9p Deletion Syndrome, Alfi Syndrome A number of 9p deletion cases involving the p22p24 region are recorded, more than 100, and they present a characteristic phenotype. Many are confined to a region of about 5 Mb at 9p22.3, and a proposed critical region resides within this segment. Trigonocephaly is a classic craniofacial malformation, and this may relate to loss of *FREM1* at 9q22.3, chr9:14.8 Mb (Spazzapan et al. 2016) (Fig. 14–19).

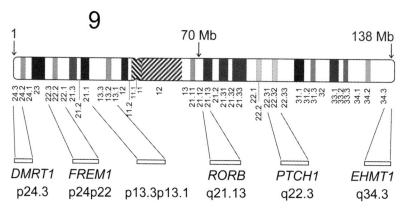

FIGURE 14–19

The brain is abnormal, and a curious imaging observation is a widening of the Sylvian fissure, the major cerebral sulcus. The deletion is equally likely to have happened on the paternal or maternal chromosome 9. Other deletions extend further in either direction, and some that may at first sight have seemed to be simple deletions turn out, on further analysis, to be due to other more complicated rearrangements (Swinkels et al. 2008; Onesimo et al. 2012). If the deletion extends through to 9pter, and thus removing 9p24.3, a gonadal phenotype may be seen, as noted in the next section.

del 9p24.3 These deletions occur distal to the 9p deletion syndrome critical region (see above), and typically within the segment chr9:pter-7.6 Mb. This condition is notable in having pointed the way to discovery of the *DMRT1* gene (chr9:0.84-0.97 Mb). This is the most conserved of any known sex-determining gene, and it is actually on the Z chromosome (the homogametic chromosome) of birds. Its expression is normally greater in the male than in the female embryo, and this dosage is the basis of its testis-inducing action. Loss of one *DMRT1* allele in the deleted segment brings the amount of product down below this threshold, and thus potentially leading to a disorder of sex differentiation, of varying form (hypospadias through to gonadal dysgenesis or male-to-female "sex reversal"), in the 46,**XY**,del(9)(p24.3) person. This observed variable expressivity, but also, in some, a nonpenetrance such that normal male development is seen, may reflect that other loci are intact or absent; that is, a second-hit scenario may apply (Quinonez et al. 2013). Concerning the 46,**XX**,del(9)(p24.3) female, Bartels et al. (2013) report primary ovarian dysfunction, proceeding to menopause in young adulthood, and suggest that this may be a reflection of the *DMRT1* haploinsufficiency. They advise that this diagnosis be considered in the investigation of premature ovarian failure (but surely it must be a rare cause). Loss of adjacent genes contributes to a wider phenotype, of mild dysmorphic features, and modest developmental delay, or at least a neurocognitive status that is less than the norm for that family.

del 9q21.13 This rare syndrome may have haploinsufficiency of *RORB* at chr9:74.4 Mb as its basis

(Boudry-Labis et al. 2013; Baglietto et al. 2014). Of academic interest is the case in Genesio et al. (2015a), in whom the deleted chromosome 9 had undergone chromothripsis:[18] Multicolor banding provided a beautiful visual demonstration of the internal restructuring of the chromosome. The IQ of their patient, a dysmorphic 16 year-old, was 46.

del 9q22.3 A notable feature of this deletion syndrome is the involvement of the *PTCH1* gene at chr9:95.4 Mb in 9q22.32, and thus the Gorlin basal cell nevus syndrome is a component of the phenotype (Muller et al. 2012). Deletions are mostly within the range chr9:95-97 Mb, but can extend further into adjacent bands. Other aspects include craniosynostosis with trigonocephaly, hydrocephalus, overgrowth, facial dysmorphism of no consistent character, and intellectual deficiency. De novo generation is the rule.

del 9q34.3: Kleefstra Syndrome This subtelomeric microdeletion syndrome of intellectual deficit typically of severe degree, difficult behavior, distinctive facies, and multiple malformation may be, after 1q36 and 22q13, the third most frequent of the subtelomeric deletion syndromes. Haploinsufficiency of (and also point mutation in) the gene *EHMT1*, at chr9:137.7 Mb, the penultimate gene on chromosome 9, determines the core phenotype, and varying degrees of the extent of deletion may impose further compromise (Willemsen et al. 2012). The protein encoded by this gene, Eu-HMTase1, has a role in maintaining the integrity of histones that comprise a key component of the architecture of the chromosome; this syndrome can thus be considered as a disorder of chromatin remodeling. Parental somatic-gonadal mosaicism with recurrence in offspring has been recognized, but the large majority represent a de novo occurrence.

Chromosome 10 Deletions
del 10p12.1p11.23 The first major report of this proximal p arm interstitial deletion is of recent appearance (Wentzel et al. 2011), and a review in 2014 is provided by Mroczkowski et al. All deletions have been of differing extents and lengths (0.5–10 Mb), but analysis of overlapping segments has allowed proposition of a probable 1.1 Mb critical region at p12.1 (chr10:27.7-28.8 Mb) (Fig. 14–20).

---

18 A word invented in the twenty-first century meaning "chromosome shattering" (mostly used in cancer cytogenetics). See also p. 226.

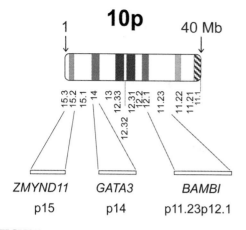

FIGURE 14-20

Within this, two subregions may determine the phenotypic components of cryptorchidism (the *MKX* locus at chr10:27.7 Mb the likely culprit) and craniofacial malformation (*BAMBI* at chr10:28.6 Mb the possible basis). The variable pattern of dysmorphism presumably reflects specific deleted regions. In one autopsy case, no malformation beyond those externally visible was identified (Sosoi et al. 2015). Developmental delay in survivors has been universal.

del 10p14: "HDR" Syndrome, Barakat Syndrome All three components of this syndrome—hypoparathyroidism, deafness, and renal dysplasia (HDR)—inhere in deletion (or point mutation) of *GATA3* at chr10:8.1 Mb. Haploinsufficiency of adjacent genes leads to a broader phenotype, with typically severe mental retardation; the deletion can extend proximally within p14 or further, and likewise distally within p14 or further, indeed as far as pter (Lindstrand et al. 2010). Centromerically extending deletions may remove a segment of approximate extent chr10:11.0-11.2 Mb within 10p14, which has been labeled the critical region for a DiGeorge-like syndrome, DGS2, although no specific genes have been implicated. But this distinction may not be entirely clear; a DGS-like phenotype is not consistently observed (Benetti et al. 2009; Melis et al. 2012). Sporadic occurrence is typical in 10p14 deletions (but see p. 164, familial HDR due to a segregating insertional translocation).

del 10p15: DeScipio Syndrome This quite new syndrome was delineated in detail in 2012 by DeScipio et al. Deletions largely fall into two categories. First, those confined to subtelomeric p15.3, the region chr10:pter-645 kb (which contains only two genes, *ZMYND11* and *DIP2C*). Deletion size is up to 64 kb; some are interstitial and as small as 154 kb. Second, those extending beyond, some into p15.2 and some (barely) into p15.1, and which may range 1.1–4.0 Mb in size. The important clinical aspect is typically a severe neurocognitive compromise, often with dystonic cerebral palsy, associated with cortical abnormality identifiable on brain imaging (Vargiami et al. 2014). Surprisingly, there is little difference clinically between those with the smaller and those with the larger deletions; this supports the view that the *ZMYND11* and *DIP2C* genes (chr10:134-690 kb) are the likely key pheno-critical factors (DeScipio et al. 2012; Cobben et al. 2014; Eggert et al. 2016). Almost all cases have been de novo, but two known or assumed transmitting mothers are on record (Eggert et al. 2016).

del 10q22.3q23.2 This rare condition is due to recurrent deletion at chr10:79.9-87.2 Mb, reflecting a role for flanking low-copy repeats. The clinical phenotype is fairly nonspecific, with facial dysmorphism and, in most, delayed language development (but in one case, as an infant, language development was judged to lie within normal limits; Petrova et al. 2014). The *BMPR1A* gene at 10q23.2, chr10:86.8 Mb (Fig. 14–21), is proposed to be pheno-critical. Juvenile polyposis syndrome might be predicted, along with features of Banayan-Zonana syndrome, if the deletion extends more distally into 10q23.2 and removes *PTEN*, although in fact such observation is rare (Jacoby et al. 1997; Singh et al. 2011). Most del q22.3q23.2 cases have arisen de novo, but two are recorded of maternal inheritance.

del 10q25.3q26.13 This deletion syndrome, if *EMX2* at chr10:117.5 Mb in 10q26.11 is involved, is associated very notably with a disorder of sex development, and the XY male may present with genital ambiguity. Piard et al. (2014) describe micropenis, dysgenetic testes, and a "Mullerian recessus" (a uterine rudiment) entering the urethra, in a nondysmorphic child with developmental delay including failure of acquisition of language. He had a deletion chr10:117.1-121.0 Mb. A very similar case is reported in Tosur et al. (2015), with a slightly larger deletion chr10:115.3-123.5 Mb, a child in whom facial dysmorphism was of distinctive character. In deletions extending into 10q26.13, *CTBP2* (chr10:125.0 Mb) is a candidate for the typically observed renal tract abnormality, and a 1 Mb

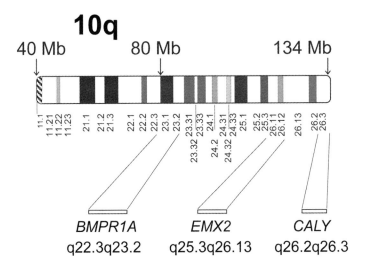

10q

40 Mb   80 Mb   134 Mb

BMPR1A   EMX2   CALY
q22.3q23.2   q25.3q26.13   q26.2q26.3

FIGURE 14–21

segment at chr10:122.7-123.7 Mb may determine a risk for malformation of the cranial bones (Piard et al. 2014; Vera-Carbonell et al. 2015; Faria et al. 2016). Loss of other genes contributes to a wider phenotype.

del 10q26.2q26.3 Terminal deletions in distal 10q may comprise loss within only bands 10q26.2q26.3; or, they may be of larger extent and include the segment 10q25.3q26.13 as described in the section above; or, they may involve more proximal segments, such as were identifiable on classic cytogenetics, and called the 10q– syndrome. Focusing on those deletions confined to the terminal bands 10q26.2q26.3, the clinical picture is one of moderate intellectual disability, growth retardation, and mild facial dysmorphism. The neurobehavioral phenotype is variable, with some exhibiting attention deficit and hyperactivity; the *CALY* gene at chr10:133.3 Mb (the seventh-last gene on the chromosome) may be implicated (Plaisancié et al. 2014). Lacaria et al. (2017) mention ataxia and hyperemia of hands and feet as notable observations. A familial case, a mother and her two daughters, is recorded in Plaisancié et al., while two siblings in Lacaria et al. came from a mother with an inv(10)(p15.3q26.2).

Chromosome 11 Deletions

del 11p11.2: Potocki-Shaffer Syndrome The clinical phenotype includes the notable features of multiple exostoses and craniofacial dysostosis with enlarged parietal foramina, along with mental retardation and micropenis in males. Most deletions are

above 2.1 Mb in extent. These genes are proposed as pheno-critical for these phenotypic aspects: *EXT2* (chr11:44.1 Mb) for the exostoses; the adjacent *ALX4* gene (chr11:44.2 Mb) for the skull bone defect; and *PHF21A* (chr11:46.0 Mb) contributory to the intellectual deficit and craniofacial picture (Labonne et al. 2015) (Fig. 14–22). A lesser deletion, leaving *PHF21A* intact, is recorded in a child with a normal intellect, indeed scoring well above the mean in several educational test assessments, albeit that the neurobehavioral phenotype was somewhat affected (McCool et al. 2017). Familial transmission is recorded in the setting of a parental balanced insertion in the original family (Shaffer et al. 1993). An exceptional case is described in Chuang et al. (2005) of a del(11)(p11.2) child whose phenotypically normal mother carried the same deletion, but with a supernumerary 11p11.2 neocentromeric marker chromosome, and thus having an overall balanced genotype. But de novo occurrence is much the rule.

del 11p13: WAGR Syndrome Haploinsufficiency of the *PAX6* morphogenesis gene at chr11:31.8 Mb causes aniridia (absence of the iris), with visual loss in consequence. Loss of one *WT1* allele (chr11:32.4 Mb) can comprise the first hit in the sequence of events to cause Wilms tumor, and it is also responsible for the abnormality of genital development. These two genes, among others, are removed in the 11p13 deletion, and the *tout ensemble* adds up to the WAGR (Wilms tumor, aniridia, genital defects, mental retardation) syndrome. Deletions are of

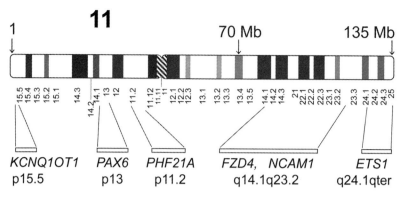

FIGURE 14–22

very variable extent; should the deletion include *BDNF* in 11p14.1, at chr11:27.5 Mb, cognitive functioning and adaptive behavior (adjusted for the visual handicap) are negatively impacted upon (Han et al. 2013). Isolated aniridia is often due to deletion restricted to just the *PAX6* locus, or in smaller 11p13 deletions which do not include *WT1* (Wawrocka et al. 2013). Less commonly, aniridia-causing 11p13 deletions spare *PAX6*, but affect a *PAX6* cis-regulatory element that resides in the adjacent *ELP4* gene. A familial case of del11p13 is recorded in Dolan et al. (2011), due to a father carrying an ins(11)(p13) in balanced state.

del 11p15.1 This segment is well-known as containing imprintable growth control loci which can be the basis, when perturbed, of Beckwith-Wiedemann syndrome (BWS), or, contrariwise, of Russell-Silver syndrome (RSS). Deletions removing the maternal allele, either de novo or inherited, cause BWS, whereas deletions of the paternal allele can lead to RSS (Begemann et al. 2012). We note here the remarkable case of a healthy father mosaic for a 60 kb deletion chr11:2.66-2.72 Mb, but in two pregnancies of his, severe fetal growth retardation occurred, with demise at 27 weeks (De Crescenzo et al. 2013). The deletion had removed the growth control factor *KCNQ1OT1* (p. 399).

del 11q14.1q23.3 This deletion, detectable even on "solid-stain" cytogenetics, removes almost half of 11q, pointing to a sparseness of critical survival genes within the region. Shiohama et al. (2016) describe a mildly dysmorphic and globally delayed, blind 6-year-old, with a 34 Mb deletion, chr11:82-116 Mb. She had presented with a neuroblastoma (the fifth such case), which may have reflected a "first-hit" hemizygosity for the neighboring *NCAM1*

or *CADM1* loci, at chr11:113 and 115 Mb, respectively. The visual defect is due to exudative vitreo-retinopathy; this is attributed to haploinsufficiency of *FZD4* at chr11:86.9 Mb.

del 11q24qter: Jacobsen Syndrome The clinical phenotype includes, along with an intellectual disability, congenital cardiac malformation, thrombocytopenia, and immunodeficiency (Dalm et al. 2015; Favier et al. 2015; Blazina et al. 2016). The diagnosis is defined according to the genes deleted: at minimum, *BSX*, *NRGN*, *ETS1*, *FLI1*, and *RICS*, contained within 6 Mb from chr11:123 to 129 Mb. Lesser deletions, which may be confined to a phenotype of intellectual disability, produce "partial Jacobsen syndrome." Specific genes have been linked to aspects of the clinical picture. Thus, *ETS1* dictates failure of development of both B and T lymphocytes, and hence predisposing to recurrent bacterial and viral infection; this gene is also the basis of the heart maldevelopment. *FLI-1* is likely the basis of the platelet deficiency. Loss of *RICS* may predispose to autism (Akshoomoff et al. 2015). The classic deletion condition is typically of sporadic occurrence, but it is of historic interest that in the original family, multigenerational inheritance was observed, due to an 11;22 translocation (Jacobsen et al. 1973).

Chromosome 12 Deletions

del 12p13.1 Very few cases are known (more surely will be), but a picture of mild dysmorphism and moderate mental retardation, with in particular poor speech acquisition, is forming (Dimassi et al. 2013). *GRIN2B* (Fig. 14–23) may well prove to be the important gene whose haploinsufficiency determines the observed functional neurology.

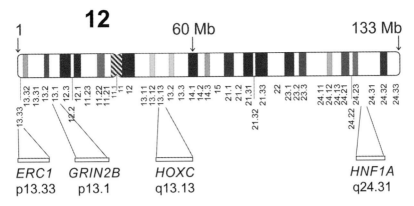

FIGURE 14–23

del 12p13.33 The notable observation in this subtelomeric microdeletion is of a speech apraxia: that is, an inability to "put words together," due both to compromise of voluntary intention of speech generation and to the neural control of the mechanical aspects of vocalization. Speech might be comprehensible only to the parents. The neurobehavioral phenotype includes a proneness to attention deficit and hyperactivity, but the IQ may be within a normal range. Otherwise, any dysmorphism is very mild, or arguably not present. *ERC1* is a good candidate as the key gene, at chr12:1.0-1.5 Mb. Deletions are of variable extent, ranging from 1.3 to 4.8 Mb, and are nonrecurrent. Parental inheritance is frequent, perhaps in one-half of cases, and, in retrospect, a history of poor language development in that parent's childhood can be elicited (Thevenon et al. 2013).

del 12q13.13 This is another very rare (thus far) deletion, in which an interesting clinical observation relates to hypermobility of some joints, and flexion contractures of others, along with a long, narrow thorax. There is intellectual disability. The *HOXC* gene cluster at chr12:54 Mb is a plausible phenocritical segment (Hancarova et al. 2013); the family of *HOX* genes have a fundamental part to play in setting out the anteroposterior body plan of the embryo.

del 12q24.31 Nonrecurrent deletions in 12q24.31 typically lead to global developmental delay and a characteristic dysmorphism (Palumbo et al. 2015a). This disorder is added to the list of conditions displaying café au lait macules. A 39-year-old man described in Verhoeven et al. (2015), with the deletion chr12:120.3-122.0 Mb, was notable in being able to have gainful employment (as a clerk), but his intellectual function, while formally within a normal range (IQ of 93; considerable inconsistency between domains), was well below that of his tertiary-educated parents. He had been diabetic since age 10 years, presumably due to haploinsufficiency for the *HNF1A* gene, at chr12:120.9 Mb, the basis of MODY type 3. *SETD1B* (at chr12:121.8 Mb) may be important in determining the intellectual phenotype.

Chromosome 13 Deletions

del 13q12.3q14.11 In contrast to the chromosome 13 imbalances discussed below, deletions confined to segments proximal to the *RB1*-containing band 13q14.2 are rare indeed (Fig. 14–24). Cirillo et al. (2012) propose a syndrome in some ways resembling ataxia-telangiectasia, with cerebellar and immunological symptomatology, along with facial dysmorphism and intellectual deficiency (IQ of 40), in their patient having the de novo deletion chr13:31.38-43.34 Mb.

13q– Syndrome The "13q– syndrome" was first described in detail in 1969 by Allderdice et al., and the association with retinoblastoma recorded, in the days of "solid-stain" cytogenetics. The no. 13 chromosomes were distinguished from the others of the D group on the basis that no. 13 was later replicating during the cell cycle, and using the (long-since discarded) methodology of treating cells in culture with tritiated thymidine (autoradiography). In 1993, Brown et al. reviewed the syndrome in light of the sophisticated cytogenetics of the day, and they proposed three main categories: Group 1 within q12.2q31, with a phenotype of minor abnormalities, mild or moderate mental retardation, and

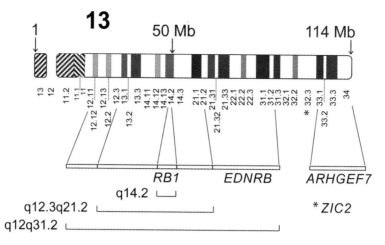

FIGURE 14–24

susceptibility to retinoblastoma; Group 2 within q12.2q32, with particular reference to band q32, in cases with major malformation and severe mental retardation; and Group 3, comprising those with deletion of the distal segment q33q34, with severe mental retardation, but typically without major malformation. The risk for retinoblastoma lay in the *RB1* gene in q14, at chr13:48.3-48.5 Mb, loss of which by deletion comprises a classic first-hit of carcinogenesis, as initially proposed by Knudson (1971).

A review in Ballarati et al. (2007) noted that the grouping as above did not always hold true. In 2011, Mitter et al. offered an updated and more molecular categorization for deletions which included *RB1*-containing 13q14: small deletions within q14 of less than 6 Mb; medium deletions within q12.3q21.2 and of size 6–20 Mb; and large deletions within q12q31.2, of greater than 20 Mb in extent (Fig. 14–25). The foregoing assessments inform the following entries. (For the record, possibly the largest constitutional deletion ever reported may be del(13)(q13.3qter), encompassing 75.7 Mb, in a fetus diagnosed at 16 weeks gestation with cerebellar hypoplasia; Ballarati et al. 2007.)

del 13q14.2q14.3 Small (less than 6 Mb, and as low as 0.15 Mb) deletions lead to a syndrome of mild or only borderline intellectual deficiency, with language acquisition in particular affected, and a mild, "soft" facial dysmorphism. As noted above, loss of one *RB1* gene predisposes to a very high risk for retinoblastoma, 50% or more. The considerable

majority of deletions arise de novo, but familial cases are recorded, such as a father and two sons with a 3.33 Mb deletion, and an aunt and nephew with a 1.17 Mb deletion, recounted in Mitter et al. (2011). Of these, the father had a retinal scar, likely a spontaneously regressed tumor; one son had a unilateral and the other a bilateral retinoblastoma; and the aunt and niece both had a unilateral tumor. A parental insertional translocation may be the basis of some familial cases (Punnett et al. 2003).

del 13q12.3q21.2 Deletions of 6–20 Mb extent within these chromosomal bands are, as in the entry foregoing (which this larger segment encompasses), at very high risk for retinoblastoma. Delayed motor and speech development are the rule, as is growth retardation. Physical features include a distinctive facies. Almost all cases are of de novo origin.

del 13q12q31.2 Larger deletions, above 20 Mb in size, generally produce a more marked phenotype, in comparison to the above entry, in terms of the neurodevelopmental compromise, and a more notable facial dysmorphism. Microcephaly is seen in some. Those deletions removing the *EDNRB* locus at q22.3 (chr13:77.8 Mb) are associated with variable signs of Waardenburg-Shah syndrome[19] (Tüysüz et al. 2009). Again, the high risk for retinoblastoma applies. Practically all are de novo.

del 13q32 Deletions which include this cytoband, and however extensive otherwise, typically present a severe neurodevelopmental picture

---

19 Waardenburg-Shah syndrome: deafness; hypopigmented skin, hair, and irides; and Hirschsprung disease.

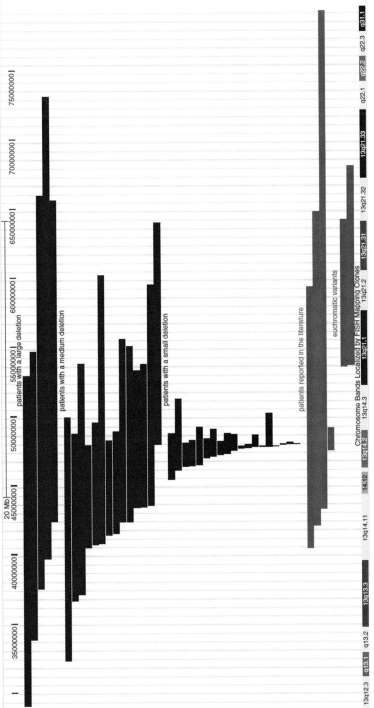

FIGURE 14-25 The range of molecularly defined 13q deletions including the *RB1* locus at chr13:48 Mb in band 13q14.2, from a cohort of retinoblastoma patients. These are divided into large (>20 Mb), medium (6–20 Mb), and small (<6 Mb) sizes. Note that deletions are not recurrent, suggesting nonhomologous end-joining as the generative mechanism. The cases in black are from a retinoblastoma clinic in Essen, Germany, and the remaining four in gray are from the literature. Of interest, two 13q21 euchromatic variants are also shown (and see p. 373).

Source: From Mitter et al., Genotype-phenotype correlations in patients with retinoblastoma and interstitial 13q deletions, *Eur J Hum Genet* 19: 947–958, 2011. Courtesy D. Mitter, and with the permission of Macmillan Publishers Ltd.

(Ballarati et al. 2007). A key gene in this respect may often be *ZIC2*, at chr13:99.9 Mb, in subband q32.3, although other as yet unidentified loci may also contribute (Myers et al. 2017).

del 13q33q34 These distal deletions can be interstitial or terminal. Microcephaly and mental retardation are typical in those encompassing both cytobands. Genital malformation is often seen in the male, and a considerable resemblance to the VACTERL (vertebral, anal, cardiac, tracheaesophageal, renal, limb association) syndrome has been observed (Walczak-Sztulpa et al. 2008; Dworschak et al. 2013). The *EFNB2* and *ARHGEF7* genes, at chr13:106.5 Mb and chr13:111.1 Mb, respectively, may be instrumental in determining aspects of the phenotype. Smaller deletions, restricted to 13q34, may present a different picture, such as the child in Yang et al. (2013), a mildly retarded boy (IQ of 71), with four-limb hexadactyly and heart disease (a single atrium), who had a 1 Mb terminal deletion, chr13:113.3-qter Mb; the terminal deletion of somewhat larger extent (chr13:103.1-qter) in the patient of Myers et al. (2017) was due to recombination from a maternal inversion 13. A more proximal and interstitial deletion within q34, of 4 Mb, is described in Witters et al. (2009), in a child whose IQ measured 72, and in whom was identified an agenesis of the corpus callosum.

Chromosome 14 Deletions

del 14q12: FOXG1 Syndrome Cytoband 14q12 contains the *FOXG1* locus at chr14:28.7 Mb (Fig. 14–26), and loss of this gene as part of a typically 0.4–4.0 Mb microdeletion leads to the "*FOXG1* syndrome" of marked postnatal microcephaly (head circumference with a standard deviation [SD] of –4 to –6), severe mental retardation, and absent language acquisition; a resemblance to Rett syndrome is noted (Ellaway et al. 2013). The facies is unremarkable. Bertossi et al. (2014) speak of a "dyskinetic encephalopathy of infancy," a movement disorder which may include jerks, athetosis, chorea, and dystonia. In 14q12 deletions not actually removing *FOXG1*, the clinical picture is very similar, and a dysregulation of the *FOXG1* pathway, due to loss of a nearby *cis*-acting regulatory element, may lead to the same end result of a *FOXG1* functional haplo-insufficiency (Allou et al. 2012; Ellaway et al. 2013; Perche et al. 2013).

del 14q13.1q21.1 This rare deletion has been associated with the brain malformation holoprosencephaly, which in its complete form is devastatingly severe, but a wide spectrum exists. Piccione et al. (2012) report a blind and severely intellectually disabled teenager, in whom the brain anatomic defect, at least as defined on imaging, was confined to the visual system (hypoplastic optic chiasma and one optic nerve, along with bilateral microphthalmia). It may be that loss of *NPAS3* (chr14:32.9-33.8 Mb), the locus in common in five reviewed cases (deletions of 5–9 Mb), causes severe functional neurological deficit, which may or may not be manifest in structural holoprosencephaly.

del 14q24q32 Deletions within q24q32 can vary in size from 10 Mb to 20 Mb, although the children reported in Nicita et al. (2015) and Stokman et al. (2016) revealed smaller 5.5 Mb and 4.5 Mb segments, respectively, at chr14:73.4-78.9 Mb and

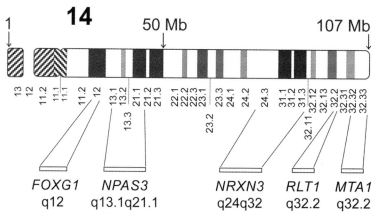

FIGURE 14–26

chr14:72.6-77.2 Mb. Thus, while given considerable genetic heterogeneity, a phenotype of intellectual deficit is typical, and brain scans can show structural defects. The facies is abnormal. The region in common between most reported cases lies in 1.6 Mb at chr14:77.3-78.9 Mb, within cytoband 14q24.3; a gene of interest therein, at chr14:78.4 Mb, is *NRXN3*, a "brain gene." The deletion in Stokman et al. does not quite extend this far; these authors postulate *IFT43*, at chr14:76.0 Mb, as a pheno-contributory gene. Inheritance is de novo.

del 14q32.2: Kagami-Ogata Syndrome, Temple Syndrome This deleted segment contains loci subject to imprinting, and thus the phenotype can resemble one of the UPD14 syndromes (p. 401). These loci may include *DLK1, DIO3*, and *RTL1* (expressed from the paternal chromosome) and *MEG3, RTL1antisense*, and *MEG8* (*MEG* = maternally expressed gene), all residing within chr14:100.7-100.9 Mb (Martinez et al. 2016).

If the deletion is on the *maternal* chromosome, the *MEGs* and *RTL1antisense* loci have nil expression, while *RLT1* in particular is overexpressed, and the Kagami-Ogata upd(14)pat-like syndrome results (Ogata and Kagami 2016). Pre- and postnatal overgrowth, developmental delay, and a distinctive facies are phenotypic features, and a notable clinical observation is that of a narrow chest, flaring inferiorly (Fig. 14–27). A milder phenotype may accompany smaller deletions; familial occurrence is recorded in this setting (van der Werf et al. 2016).

If the deletion is on the *paternal* chromosome, the upd(14)mat-like Temple syndrome results, in which hypotonia, growth failure, and precocious puberty are clinical observations (Rosenfeld et al. 2015). Broader phenotypes likely reflect the loss of other (nonimprinted) loci within the deleted segments. Deletions have been both nonrecurrent and recurrent, the latter reflecting nonallelic homologous recombination due to flanking TGG_n repeats (Béna et al. 2010). Most cases have been de novo, but Rosenfeld et al. report transmission of a chr14:100.83-100.98 Mb deletion from a phenotypically normal mother.

del 14q32.3 Deletions are mostly in the range 3–6 Mb and most include qter; the smallest recorded deletion, of 0.3 Mb, chr14:105.16-105.46 Mb, is interstitial (Engels et al. 2012; Holder et al. 2012). The pheno-critical factor may lie in the *MTA1* gene at chr14:105.4 Mb, which is deleted in common in

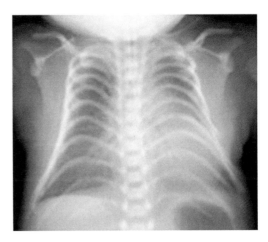

FIGURE 14–27   Chest X-ray of a child with Kagami-Ogata syndrome, in this case due to an epimutation in the 14q32.2 imprinted region. The thorax is narrow in its upper and mid parts, and flaring below. The ribs have an increased "coat-hanger" angle.

Source: From Ogata and Kagami, Kagami-Ogata syndrome: A clinically recognizable upd(14)pat and related disorder affecting the chromosome 14q32.2 imprinted region, *J Hum Genet* 61: 87–94, 2016. Courtesy T. Ogata, and with the permission of Nature Publishing Group.

all cases. The usual clinical picture is one of malformation in several organs, intellectual handicap, and facial dysmorphism. A single familial case is on record, the father-to-son transmission of the 0.3 Mb deletion just mentioned in Holder et al.

Chromosome 15 Deletions. We may be, as *Homo sapiens*, hostage to our evolution, at least in respect of proximal 15q deletions. "Recent" (somewhat less than 1 million years ago) reorganization of the 15q11.2q13.3 region has led to the embedding of segments that can now impose a particular vulnerability to nonallelic homologous recombination (Antonacci et al. 2014). The five major segments of our particular interest are referred to as breakpoints 1 through 5 (BP1-BP5) (Fig. 14–28). These segments contain sequences of the GOLGA8 family. For example, GOLGA8Q at chr15:30.55 Mb identifies BP4, while BP5 resides in its palindromic partner, GOLGA8N, at chr15:32.59 Mb. BP1-BP2 relate to Burnside-Butler syndrome; BP2-BP3 deletion is the basis of most Prader-Willi/Angelman deletion; and BP4-BP5 bookend the segment of the 15q13.3 deletion syndrome. Figure 14–29 outlines points of interest in 15q11.2q13 (and see also Fig. 14–60 below, and color insert). The 15q11.2q13.3 region contains

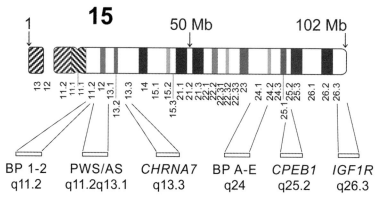

FIGURE 14–28

certain "brain genes," and autism is a frequent concomitant of imbalance (Hogart et al. 2010).

del 15q11.2: Burnside-Butler Syndrome This condition is also known as 15q11.2 BP1-BP2 microdeletion syndrome. The minimum deletion region is chr15:22.78-23.04 Mb, containing the loci *NIPA1, NIPA2,*[20] *CYFIP1,* and *TUBGCP5*. Albeit that the deletion can vary in size (from 0.25 to 1.5 Mb, most commonly 0.5 Mb), only these four loci are ever lost (De Wolf et al. 2013). Any of the four could plausibly be implicated in the neurobehavioral phenotype seen in the deletion state. Previously this segment had been considered not subject to imprinting, but differential methylation, based on parent of origin, has been detected at *TUBGCP5*, suggesting there may in fact be a parent-of-origin effect (Joshi et al. 2016). The background population carrier rate may be as high as 0.25% (1 person in 400), and about double that, 0.57%, in a cohort of those of neurobehavioral phenotype (Cafferkey et al. 2014).

The clinical picture is very largely (but not entirely) confined to a neurocognitive/behavioral/psychiatric phenotype (Cox and Butler 2015). Learning is affected, especially with respect to reading and writing. Attention deficit and hyperactivity are commonly seen, as also may be oppositional defiant disorder. It is one of the most common cytogenetic disorders to be found in children with autism. Schizophrenia is a risk. This chromosome imbalance is a classic example of the incompletely penetrant microdeletion/CNV. It is typically an inherited deletion (in 80%–85%), but often (50%) the parent is reportedly unaffected; the remaining

cases are of de novo origin (Vanlerberghe et al. 2015). A penetrance estimate of 10% might be slightly low, and it would likely vary according to the stringency of phenotypic assessment of carriers: In other words, if microsigns of neurobehavioral disorder in parents were sought, the penetrance could well be higher. On the other hand, Hashemi et al. (2015) counsel against overinterpretation of a pathogenic effect, and they urge further study.

del 15q11.2q13.1: Prader-Willi Syndrome, Angelman Syndrome See Chapter 18.

del 15q13.3 This deletion, between BP4 and BP5, usually involves chr15:30.6-32.1 Mb. Uncommonly, larger ~4 Mb deletions can encompass BP3-BP5, or smaller deletions can be "nested" within BP4 and BP5. The associated phenotype is essentially one of neuropsychiatric expression, and Lowther et al. (2015) determined these fractions, corrected for ascertainment: intellectual disability in 58%, epilepsy in 28%, poor speech development in 16%, autism spectrum disorder in 11%, schizophrenia in 10%, mood disorder in 10%, and attention deficit hyperactivity disorder in 7%. A similar inference comes from Torres et al. (2016), who determined high odds ratios for epilepsy, intellectual deficiency, autism, and schizophrenia. The average nonverbal IQ in the series of Ziats et al. (2016) was 60, and one-third of cases met criteria for a diagnosis of autism spectrum disorder. About 85% of cases are inherited, and in 62 transmitting parents studied by Lowther et al., half had been diagnosed with a neuropsychiatric condition, although none

---

20 The naming of these two *NIPA* genes is of interest, according to what they are *not*: "not imprinted in Prader-Willi or Angelman."

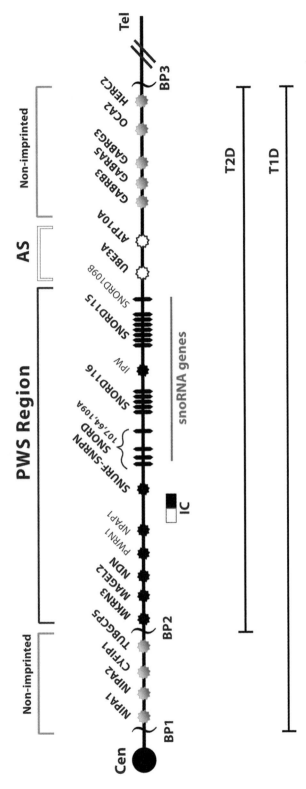

FIGURE 14–29 (Also shown as Fig. 18–7.) The regions and loci of interest within the segment 15q11.2q13 (see also Fig. 14–60). AS, Angelman syndrome; BP, (numbered) breakpoint; IC, imprinting center; PWS, Prader-Willi syndrome; T1D, type 1, T2D, type 2 deletion. Coding (black, white, gray) indicates, respectively, PWS-related, AS-related, and non-imprinted loci.

Source: From Driscoll et al., Prader-Willi syndrome, *GeneReviews* 2016 (updated, personal communication D. J. Driscoll, and with the permission of the University of Washington.

had schizophrenia; those with schizophrenia in their study had all been probands in their own right. Thus, we have a further example of a molecular chromosomal imbalance of incomplete penetrance and variable expressivity; however, the fact that Lowther et al. found no cases in 23,838 adult controls suggests that penetrance is, in fact, high. The crucial factor, in terms of the phenotype, is haploinsufficiency for the gene *CHRNA7*, which is located within the deleted segment, at chr15:32.03-32.17 Mb (Hoppman-Chaney et al. 2013). In the company of another genetic defect, the clinical severity is exacerbated, such as Ehmke et al. (2017) show in a child who had no speech, and in whom was seen both a de novo del 15q13.3 and a de novo mutation in the *ZBTB18* gene.

In what may be the first example of a genetically targeted pharmacological management in a deletion syndrome, Cubells et al. (2011) report a substantial improvement in aggressive behavior in an adult male with the use of a drug (galantamine) which acts as an agonist for the acetylcholine receptor due to *CHRNA7*. It is reasonable to imagine that this drug stimulation enabled maximal activity of the reduced quantum (due to *CHRNA7* haplo-insufficiency) of these receptors on brain neurons, and that the neurons thus stimulated allowed an improved function within the neural substrate that subserves control of behavior.

del 15q24 The breakpoints of this imbalance are for the most part founded upon a series of five low-copy repeats, breakpoints (BPs) A through E, which can promote nonallelic homologous recombination, a 3.1 Mb deletion at BP A-D (chr15:72.65-75.81 Mb) being the most frequently observed (Mefford et al. 2012). This genomic variation matches a variable phenotype. Speech development is severely affected in many, some being nonverbal, and some show attention deficit hyperactivity. The BP C-D region, chr15:75.3-75.8 Mb, wherein lies *SIN3A*, may be central to the pathogenesis (the SIN3A protein interacts with the Rett syndrome protein, MeCP2; Witteveen et al. 2016). Facial dysmorphism is mild or "soft," with a large forehead a common observation. No familial case is known.

del 15q25.2 Several of these deletions are recurrent, at chr15:82.5-84.1 Mb, and these are flanked by

GOLGA6 sequences; others extend in either direction. Of several plausible candidate genes within the segment in common, *CPEB1* at chr15:82.3 Mb is one that might have a role in the neurocognitive phenotype (Burgess et al. 2014). The hematological disorder Diamond-Blackfan anemia is a notable concomitant (Doelken et al. 2013). All cases have been de novo.

del 15q26.3 A particular phenotypic feature of this terminal deletion, which can be of variable extent, is growth retardation, with height and weight often 2–4 SD below the mean (Jezela-Stanek et al. 2012). This reflects loss of the *IGFR2* growth factor gene, at chr15:98.6-98.9 Mb (as also in the ring 15, p. 215). Intellectual handicap is typical; school attendance may be possible in some, but special tuition is required.

Chromosome 16 Deletions. Rearrangements in chromosome 16p are among the more often seen in the genetic clinic. As with proximal 15q, the proximal short arm of 16 is of evolutionary interest, being a site of particularly active rearrangement in primate speciation, and accumulating, in the time of *H. sapiens*, loci having putative roles in autism. This region has come to command a major role among CNVs associated with intellectual deficiency and, in particular, with psychosis. There is also a link with growth, as measured by body mass index, and head circumference. A considerable number of loci within the region, at least 65, makes it difficult to implicate with confidence specific culprit genes. There are five listed breakpoint (BP) regions within 16p11.2p12.2, numbering 1–5 from telomeric to centromeric (distal to proximal), enabling classification of different segmental imbalances (Newbury et al. 2013) (Fig. 14–30). There is considerable similarity in phenotypes across these different deletions, and the counselor should take care that it is the correct condition being addressed. Again, concomitant CNVs elsewhere in the genome may, as second (or first) hits, aggravate the clinical picture.

del 16p11.2: BP4-BP5 (Proximal del 16p11.2) This deletion is of sufficient frequency, and of such phenotype, that many counselors could expect to meet a family. BP4 and BP5 define an ~600 kb segment, within sequence coordinates chr16:29.5-30.2 Mb, and this is the most commonly encountered of the canonical imbalances within the BP1-BP5 region. *TBX6* is a useful landmark locus. Deletion presents a

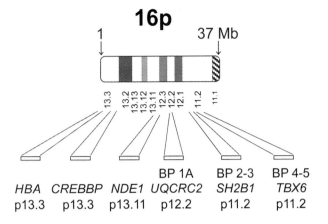

FIGURE 14–30

neuropsychological picture which may include intellectual impairment, epilepsy, poor language acquisition presenting as childhood apraxia of speech, clumsiness, and behavioral disturbance (Zufferey et al. 2012; Hanson et al. 2015; Fedorenko et al. 2016; Steinman et al. 2016; Torres et al. 2016). The clinical picture may quite closely resemble classic autism (and this is one of the most commonly seen CNVs in individuals with autism; D'Angelo et al. 2016), but there are some subtle differences; indeed, Duyzend and Eichler (2015) propose that the genotype-first approach may enable more precise diagnostic categorizations within the autism spectrum.

White matter tracts within the brain are abnormally formed (Owen et al. 2014). Paroxysmal kinesigenic dyskinesia (PKD), in which an abnormal body positioning is triggered by sudden movement, may be due to loss of the PRRT2 gene[21] at chr16:29.8 Mb. Macrocephaly is a frequent observation, albeit that the cerebral cortex is thin (this contrasts with the microduplication, with microcephaly). The increase overall in brain size relates to increases in certain brain regions, notably those with roles in the reward pathway, and presumably reflecting aberrant neurogenesis; a specific malformation is the Chiari cerebellar defect (Maillard et al. 2015; Steinman et al. 2016). An increased body mass index with marked obesity is common and may have, as its basis, disturbance of the reward pathway, such that

appetite is excessive. There may or may not be a mild degree of dysmorphism.

The deletion is more usually de novo, but can be inherited; the phenotype is more abnormal in the familial case (Duyzend and Eichler 2015). Rosenfeld et al. (2013) estimate a penetrance of 47% (95% confidence interval [CI], 32%–64%).[22] A concomitant second hit may exacerbate the phenotype (Bassuk et al. 2013, Newbury et al. 2013).

del 16p11.2: BP2-BP3 (Distal del 16p11.2) A short recurrent 220 kb deletion lies between BP2 and BP3, chr16:28.8-29.1 Mb. Haploinsufficiency of *SH2B1* (chr16:28.86 Mb) is presumed to be the basis of the severe early onset obesity that is typically observed (Barge-Schaapveld et al. 2011; D'Angelo et al. 2016). The phenotype is one of intellectual deficit, difficult behavior, mild facial dysmorphism, and, as mentioned, obesity. An association with schizophrenia is noted (Guha et al. 2013). Penetrance is high, 62% (Rosenfeld et al. 2013). It is often inherited.

del 16p12.2p11.2: BP1-BP5 Deletions of up to ~8 Mb from BP1 at chr16:21.8 to variably 28.8–30.2 Mb, BP2-BP5, are associated with intellectual disability, severely delayed speech development, and dysmorphic features. Recurrent ear infections may be due to loss of *OTOA* which overlaps

---

21 Mutation within the *PRRT2* gene causes familial isolated PKD (Termsarasab et al. 2014).

22 These estimates (and see Table 4–1) will be at the level of a clinically diagnosed neuropsychological/cognitive phenotype. Stefansson et al. (2014) address the question whether subtler personality traits might, on careful observation, be seen, that could yet be considered to lie within a normal population range, with respect to a number of CNVs. In the case of the 16p11.2 deletion, they note impairments in several cognitive domains tested in control carriers, and record the observation of a reduced verbal IQ. They prefer to speak of "variable expressivity" rather than "reduced penetrance," and there is some merit in this view.

BP1 (Hempel et al. 2009). Heart defects and short stature are occasional features. Rosenfeld et al. (2013) estimate a penetrance of 62% (95% CI, 27%–94%). Further heterogeneity of deletion within 16p11.2p12.2 is observed: Some larger deletions may extend from BP1 through to BP5, or yet beyond; some may encompass BP3-BP5 (Egger et al. 2014; Pebrel-Richard et al. 2014).

del 16p12.2:[23] *BP1A* Girirajan et al. (2010) identified a recurrent 520 kb deletion at chr16:21.93-22.45 Mb, which imposed a phenotype of neuropsychiatric disorder, and which was especially susceptible to the exacerbating effect of second-hit CNVs elsewhere in the genome: Second-hit CNVs were seen with a much higher frequency in cases (24%) than in controls (0.4%). If a risk for schizophrenia might otherwise have been the case, possession of this deletion, typically as a single-hit imbalance, increases the risk (Rees et al. 2014b). Minor craniofacial anomalies may coexist. Just three OMIM genes lie within the segment: *CDR2*, *EEF2K*, and *UQCRC2*, the latter implicated in autism (Kanduri et al. 2016). Parental transmission is usual: A carrier parent is likely to have had a learning difficulty and mental disorder, such as depression or bipolar disease, but less severely so than in his or her affected offspring. De novo cases are occasionally seen.

del 16p13.11 This deletion was discovered "genotype-first," in five patients from a large cohort screened by microarray analysis (Hannes et al. 2009). It is associated with mental retardation, microcephaly, and, in some patients, short stature, cleft lip, and other midline defects. Epilepsy has a particular association (Mullen et al. 2013). The typical deletion is 1.65 Mb in size, at approximately chr16:14.7-16.3 Mb, and contains at least 15 genes, of which *NTAN1* and *NDE1* (at chr16:15.0 and 15.6 Mb, respectively) were seen as good candidates to have a causative role (Sajan et al. 2013); *MYH11* is another landmark locus. Paciorkowski et al. (2013) describe a severe structural brain defect in sibs, in whom the deletion exposed a *NDE1* mutation on the other chromosome 16. Contrariwise,

Liu et al. (2012) found no abnormality, at the histological level, in brain tissue (removed at temporal lobe surgery for epilepsy) of two adults of normal learning capacity, they both having a deletion of chr16:15.38-16.22 Mb, within which smaller segment lies *NDE1*.

del 16p13.3: α-Thalassemia and Mental Retardation This is one of two α-thalassemia and mental retardation (ATR) syndromes (the other being an X-linked Mendelian condition). In the del(16p) ATR syndrome, there is monosomy for a segment at the very tip of the chromosome, which includes at least the α chain globin loci (at chr16:176 kb). Previously, the thalassemia would have been a key observation leading to the diagnosis; but as Gibbons (2012) comments, nowadays "the widespread use of array-based screening for genomic deletions is identifying cases with little regard for the phenotype." Deletions are of variable size. Smaller ones, from about 0.3 to 1 Mb, may present no evident cognitive compromise, but those in the range 1 to 2 Mb usually do. A larger deletion, extending proximally beyond 2 Mb, determines a broader phenotype, which may include tuberous sclerosis and polycystic kidney disease (due to the *TSC2* locus at chr16:2.0 Mb and *PKD1* at chr16:2.1 Mb), over and above the ATR syndrome. De novo occurrence is often so, but parental rearrangements are not infrequent and should always be sought.

del 16p13.3: Rubinstein-Taybi Syndrome The Rubinstein-Taybi syndrome[24] (RTS) has a distinctive phenotype, and the facies and the broad thumbs are very characteristic. Most cases are due to point mutation in the *CREBBP* gene (chr16:3.72 Mb), but approximately 10%–25% have a small (1–15 kb) deletion that removes part or all of *CREBBP* (Wójcik et al. 2010). There is no obvious clinical distinction between those RTS patients with or without the microdeletion, suggesting closely adjacent genes may not be dosage-sensitive (Rusconi et al. 2015). The range of observed severity presumably reflects a variable expressivity of the abnormal genotype, and the case of monozygous twins with RTS having rather different neurobehavioral phenotypes

---

23 This deletion is often referenced as del(16)(p12.1). However, because the segment as defined in Girirajan et al. (2010) lies entirely within 16p12.2, according to the UCSC browser, the coordinates having been converted to build hg38 (chr16:21,935,203-22,455,963), we are here making the call as del 16p12.2, as do Pizzo et al. (2017). Similarly, we prefer del 16p11.2 (not p12.1) for the BP2–BP3 deletion.

24 A similar condition due to mutation in the *EP300* gene, a paralog of *CREBBP*, has been called RTS type 2 (Hamilton et al. 2016).

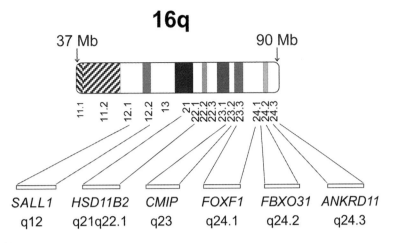

16q

37 Mb   90 Mb

11.1   11.2   12.1   12.2   13   21   22.1   22.2   22.3   23.1   23.2   23.3   24.1   24.2   24.3

SALL1   HSD11B2   CMIP   FOXF1   FBXO31   ANKRD11

q12   q21q22.1   q23   q24.1   q24.2   q24.3

FIGURE 14–31

supports this suggestion (Preis and Majewski 1995). The oldest putative case, from 500–900 AD, is that of a skeleton excavated at the Yokem site in Illinois (Wilbur 2000); some kind of record would be set were this case ever to yield to a paleocytomolecular genetic analysis!

del 16q12 This rare syndrome may be defined, in particular, by loss of the *SALL1* gene at chr16:51.1 Mb (Fig. 14–31), which leads to an attenuated form of Townes-Brock syndrome,[25] along with aspects such as moderate to severe developmental delay, presumably due to loss of other loci. Deletions are from 2.6 to 6.9 Mb in size (Morisada et al. 2014). A more extensive deletion at 16q12.1q12.2, including representative loci *ZNF423* and *FTO*, leads to a more severe syndrome (Shoukier et al. 2012).

del 16q21q22.1 Yamamoto et al. (2008) reported a series of 14 cases, including some of classical cytogenetic description; and Genesio et al. (2013) reviewed those six examples of a precise molecular definition. Pre- and postnatal growth retardation, microcephaly with psychomotor retardation, and facial dysmorphism are observed. The smallest deletion, of 0.27 Mb,

involved chr16:67.37–67.64 Mb; all deletions were encompassed within chr16:62.2-68.9 Mb. Loss of *HSD11B2* at chr16:67.4 Mb might be the basis of the growth retardation. Notably, a partially overlapping region just centromeric (chr16:59.90-65.67 Mb) can be deleted without any effect upon the phenotype; this is a "euchromatic variant," reflecting a very low gene density in this segment of 16q21 (Barber 2005; Coussement et al. 2011) (p. 373).

del 16q23 The smallest deletion is recorded in Van der Aa et al. (2012), at chr16:81.3-81.6 Mb, in a 5-year-old girl with autism, but no dysmorphism. A role for the gene *CMIP*, one of only two genes deleted, is suggested. The rearrangement was de novo. Jobling et al. (2013), in a larger deletion, report an association with nephrocalcinosis, along with psychomotor delay, unusual skull shape (trigonocephaly), and an abnormal vascular connection between the portal vein and the inferior vena cava, bypassing the liver (portocaval shunt).

del 16q24 Three separate or overlapping syndromes involve band 16q24. First, the *del 16q24.1* syndrome, as well as implying neurocognitive

---

25   Townes-Brock syndrome is due to dominant-negative *SALL1* mutation, and it presents a triad of imperforate anus, thumb malformation, and dysplastic ears with hearing loss. Kidney and heart disease are also associated. The attenuated form in the 16q12 deletion indicates that haploinsufficiency of *SALL1* (an act of omission) is a less deleterious genetic mechanism than is gain-of-function mutation (an act of commission). A similar interpretation applies to the 16q24.3 deletion discussed below, of Grønborg et al. (2015), in which haploinsufficiency of *TUBB3* leads to a less abnormal MRI brain picture than is seen in Mendelian mutation; and likewise with the 17q24.2q24.3 deletion (below) including the *KCNJ2* gene, mutation in which causes cardiac conduction abnormality, but this is attenuated or absent in the haploinsufficient state.

deficit, may also predict certain organ malformations, according to the regions of deletion: the severe and usually lethal lung disorder, alveolar capillary dysplasia; bilateral hydronephrosis, likely consequential upon urinary tract obstruction; and heart and gut defects (Stankiewicz et al. 2009). For the most part, deletions, of range 100 kb to 2 Mb, are confined to the segment chr16:85.1-87.9 Mb;[26] a few are larger. *FOXF1* (chr16:86.5 Mb) is a key pheno-critical candidate in many. One instance of parental transmission is recorded, of a 131 kb deletion that did not include *FOXF1*, from an essentially normal mother; this observation might reflect a paternal imprinting status of the region, but interpretation is complicated (Stankiewicz et al. 2009; Szafranski et al. 2014). All others have been de novo.

> This syndrome provides an example of a phenotype which can be due not to haploinsufficiency of a gene but, rather, to haploinsufficiency of a distant enhancer of a gene. Thus, Szafranski et al. (2016) show that deletion removing an upstream enhancer of *FOXF1* (a long non-protein coding RNA, *LINC01081*, at chr16:86.2 Mb), while the *FOXF1* gene itself, some 272 kb away, remains intact, can nevertheless lead to a functional nonexpression of the gene, and in consequence, the typical lung disease.

Second, *del 16q24.2* is associated with autism and intellectual disability, often of severe degree, and minor craniofacial dysmorphism (Handrigan et al. 2013). Deletions are mostly confined to the segment 16q24.2 (chr16:87.0-88.6 Mb), ranging from 27 kb to 2.7 Mb in size. One of the contained genes, *FBXO31* at chr16:87.3 Mb, is plausibly a key factor in the neurobehavioral phenotype; another gene implicated is *ANKRD11* at chr16:89.3 Mb, in those in whom the deletion spans into 16q24.3 (see below). Deletions extending into 16q24.1 (see above) may be associated with urinary tract disease, but this is also seen in some cases restricted to 16q24.2. Parental transmission is quite frequently observed, with the deletion size in these being less than 1 Mb; an instance of maternal mosaicism for the deletion is known.

Third, *deletion of 16q24.3* leads to a syndrome in which intellectual disability, minor facial anomalies, macrodontia, and short stature are typical observations (Kim et al. 2015). Deletions range up to about 2 Mb in size. Loss of *ANKRD11*, at chr16:89.3 Mb (and the gene responsible for KBG syndrome), is the central factor; loss of neighboring genes extends the phenotype (Novara et al. 2017). Familial transmission is recorded, including from a mosaic mother (Sacharow et al. 2012; Khalifa et al. 2013).

Chromosome 17 Deletions

del 17p11.2: Smith-Magenis Syndrome The Smith-Magenis syndrome (SMS) comprises a picture of dysmorphology, mental defect, and fractious behavior. Brain anatomy may be abnormal (Maya et al. 2014). Sleep disturbance is a characteristic feature (associated in most cases with a reversal of the normal circadian pattern of melatonin secretion); and a habit of self-mutilation, and a markedly diminished pain sensitivity, can manifest as "onychotillomania" (pulling out nails). To the practiced eye, the facies may be distinctive (Allanson et al. 1999). Most (>90%) patients have an ~3.8 Mb deletion at chr17:16.8-20.6 Mb, arising by NAHR between "SMS repeat sequences"; a larger deletion may be associated with a more complicated phenotype (Park et al. 2002; Vieira et al. 2012). The crucial locus within the deleted segment is *RAI1*, at chr17:17.7 Mb (Fig. 14–32), haploinsufficiency of which may compromise the activity of a number of downstream genes (cf. del 2q23.1 above), and each of these, thus compromised, then contributing to a component of the syndrome. Recurrence is very rare, but one case is recorded due to low-level (25% on blood) parental somatic, and inferentially gonadal, mosaicism (Campbell et al. 2014). A single instance of maternal transmission, in this case due to *RAI1* mutation, is reported in Acquaviva et al. (2017).

del 17p12: Hereditary Pressure-Sensitive Neuropathy A 1.4 Mb deletion at chr17:14.2-15.6 Mb is the typical basis of hereditary pressure-sensitive neuropathy (HPSN), which has the alternative names of hereditary neuropathy with liability

---

26 One report describes a child with poor language development, in whom a de novo 159 kb 16q24.1 deletion somewhat centromeric of the others noted here, included the locus *ATP2C2* (chr16:84.4 Mb), and this loss was likely the pheno-critical factor in this instance (Smith et al. 2015).

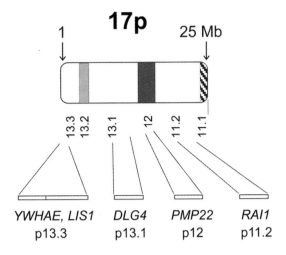

17p

1   25 Mb

13.3
13.2
13.1
12
11.2
11.1

YWHAE, LIS1   DLG4   PMP22   RAI1
p13.3   p13.1   p12   p11.2

FIGURE 14–32

to pressure palsies (HNPP) and tomaculous neuropathy (Chance 2006). It is the reciprocal deletion of the Charcot-Marie-Tooth neuropathy duplication (see below).[27,28] The deletion of a particular "nerve gene," the *PMP22*, or peripheral myelin protein 22 gene, at chr17:15.2 Mb, leads to abnormal myelination of the peripheral nerves, and this compromises their function. A typical presentation is the backpacker who complains of numbness (sensory nerves) and weakness (motor nerves) in the arms after a day's hiking, and these symptoms are due to the pressure of the shoulder straps on the nerves leading to the upper limb. Almost all HPSN is due to this type of deletion; imbalance of the few other genes within the 1.4 Mb segment seems not to be of any phenotypic effect (Zhang et al. 2010). The former mainstay of cytogenetic diagnosis was by FISH, using a probe that hybridized to the region; Figure 14–33 is still useful, in giving a direct pictorial demonstration of the deletion. The deletion can arise de novo or, as is more usual, can be transmitted from an affected parent, in which case the risk to transmit the disease is 50%.

Rare deletions encompassing both the above loci, *RAI1* and *PMP22*, lead to a clinical picture comprising both phenotypes. These deletions are nonrecurrent (Yuan et al. 2016).

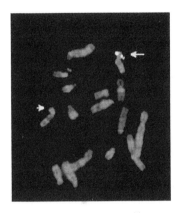

FIGURE 14–33   Hereditary pressure-sensitive neuropathy. The FISH probe to 17p12 has failed to hybridize to the proximal short arm of one of the no. 17 homologs (short arrow), while hybridizing normally to the other (longer arrow). This reflects the absence of the p12 segment on the deleted chromosome.

del 17p13.1 Deletions of 17p13.1 are of differing extents, mostly within the region chr17:5.5-8.4 Mb. Microcephaly with profound mental retardation is typical, and these children are nonverbal. A critical region at chr17:7.1-7.3 Mb contains proposed

27   17p12 rearrangements arising from maternal gametogenesis, which can be either deletions or duplications, are due to an *intra-chromosomal* mechanism, either an unequal sister chromatid exchange or, in the case of deletion, excision of an intrachromatid loop. If the rearrangement occurs in paternal gametogenesis (the more common scenario), it comprises a deletion or duplication and arises by unequal meiotic crossing-over between the two no. 17 chromosomes (cf. Fig. 14–1), an *interchromosomal* mechanism.

28   An extraordinary coincidence is for one no. 17 chromosome to carry a *PMP22* deletion, and the other a *PMP22* duplication, and thus a balanced genome, and the person free of either neuropathy (Hirt et al. 2015).

important loci including *ASGR1*, *ACADVL*, *DVL2*, *DLG4*, and *GABARAP*. Carvalho et al. (2014) propose an "oligogenic" model, whereby the microcephaly flows from a perturbed epistatic interaction between these four genes (rather than an independent effect of each locus; see also Figure 3–11, p. 51). A gene coding for a cell adhesion molecule having a role in the formation and functioning of synapses, *NLGN2*, at chr17:7.40-7.41 Mb, may well play a key role in those in whom the deletion extends to here (Parente et al. 2017). In all studied cases, inheritance has been de novo.

del 17p13.3: Miller-Dieker Syndrome This well-known syndrome of "lissencephaly plus" is not uncommonly diagnosed following prenatal ultrasonography (Chen et al. 2013a). Three specific loci in 17p13.3 are of note, from proximal to distal: *LIS1* (more recently known as *PAFAH1B1*) at chr17:2.6 Mb; *OVCA1* (also known as *DPH1*) at chr17:2.0 Mb (Yu et al. 2014); and *YWHAE* at chr17:1.3 Mb. A proneness to rearrangement in 17p13.3 reflects a local richness in *Alu* sequences (Gu et al. 2015), and deletions of variable extents, interstitial or terminal, may remove some or all of these loci. Loss of all three, and including others in the vicinity, leads to classic Miller-Dieker syndrome (Fig. 14–34). If *LIS1/PAFAH1B1* is intact but the other two are lost, a neurodevelopmental syndrome with dysmorphism results, of variable severity, in which brain imaging may or may not be abnormal (Enomoto et al. 2012). Most 17p13.3 deletions arise de novo, but a parental balanced rearrangement is occasionally recognized.

del 17q12 Dixit et al. (2012) reviewed the small number of reported cases of this syndrome, in which a key observation is that of renal cystic disease. Developmental delay is usually of mild degree, but autism is a possibility. Facial dysmorphism may be moderate, "soft," or essentially absent. Pancreatic, liver, and genital abnormality may be seen, and some have had diabetes (MODY type 5). A crucial gene is *HNF1B* at chr17:37.7 Mb (Fig. 14–35), which, as a Mendelian mutation, is responsible for the renal cysts and diabetes (RCAD) syndrome. Mother-to-child transmission is recorded.

del 17q21.31: Koolen-de Vries Syndrome This is a condition that could, in retrospect, be seen as a syndrome, but in which the collection of features did not impress sufficiently that recognition was likely to have been achieved ahead of the laboratory discovery ("genotype-first") of this recurrent deletion

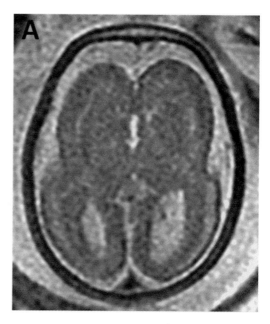

FIGURE 14–34   Lissencephaly ("smooth brain") in Miller-Dieker syndrome, prenatal diagnosis. Brain imaging (MRI) of a 31-week fetus with a de novo del 17p13.3, chr17:1-3,262,236×1. Frontal lobe in upper part of image, occiput in lower. The surface of the brain (the cortex) is smooth, lacking the normal furrowed appearance at this gestation. The occipital ventricles are mildly enlarged, reflecting a reduction in brain parenchyma.

Source: From Chen et al., Chromosome 17p13.3 deletion syndrome: aCGH characterization, prenatal findings and diagnosis, and literature review, Gene 532: 152–159, 2013. Courtesy C.-P. Chen, and with the permission of Elsevier.

(Tan et al. 2009). Poor speech development, epilepsy, and "hypersocial behavior" may be seen as having a resemblance to Angelman syndrome. *KANSL1* (chr17:46.1 Mb) is the relevant gene (point mutation can also produce the syndrome); a 990 kb inversion polymorphism spanning 17q21.31 is a necessary predisposing element (Zollino et al. 2015; Koolen et al. 2016).

Recurrence is very rare. One case is known of mother-to-child transmission (Rendeiro et al. 2016). Koolen et al. (2012) studied two instances of recurrence due to low-grade maternal mosaicism. One mother had the deletion chr17:45.6-46.1 Mb in 8% of buccal mucosal cells, and in the other mother there was an essentially similar deletion in 3% of peripheral lymphocytes. They calculated a general risk of recurrence of 1/9,446 (0.01%), which is about twice the baseline population risk of

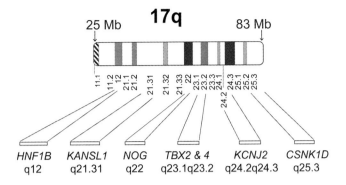

FIGURE 14–35

1/16,000. This overall calculation is based upon the separate risks according to the parental genotypes for the inversion polymorphism mentioned above; the interested reader is referred to p. 60 for a full exposition.

del 17q22 Deletion of the *NOG* locus (chr17:56.59 Mb) is a finding in common in a group of del 17q22 cases reviewed in Laurell et al. (2013), and this is presumably the basis of the bone and joint aspects of the syndrome, including symphalangism (fusion of joints of fingers and toes) and other digital defects, joint contractures developing through childhood, and conductive hearing loss. Intellectual disability associated with microcephaly, and a distinctive facial dysmorphism, are also noted. De novo inheritance is more usual, but parent-to-child transmission is recorded.

del 17q23.1q23.2 An inconsistency of phenotype mirrors the considerable range of deletions within this region (some of which flow into 17q22), as reviewed in Coppola et al. (2013b). In those in whom the deletion removes the adjacent transcription factor genes *TBX2* and *TBX4* at chr17:61.4 Mb, heart and limb defects are characteristic (Ballif et al. 2010). All cases have been de novo.

del 17q24.2q24.3 This rare deletion determines a distinctive facies, which is well illustrated in serial photographs of two unrelated cases in Lestner et al. (2012). The deletion removes the *KCNJ2* gene (chr17:70.1 Mb), albeit that an electrocardiographic defect is not seen, or is only subtly present (cf. mutation in this gene leads to the Andersen-Tawil syndrome of dysmorphology and cardiac conduction abnormality). *MAP2K6* (chr17:69.4 Mb), a gene on the well-known Ras-MAPK cascade, is a potential pheno-critical candidate; a role may also inhere in *KCNJ2*. These cases have been of de novo generation.

del 17q25.3 Various deletions, terminal and interstitial, are reviewed in Probst et al. (2015). Neurocognitive deficits were present in all cases, and cardiac malformation was almost universal. Brain MRI revealed abnormality in several. A plausible case could be made for the pathogenicity of number of genes in the deletion intervals, one such, with respect in particular to the heart defects, being *CSNK1D* (chr17:82.2 Mb). All cases in which parental testing was done were of de novo origin.

Chromosome 18 Deletions

del 18p: de Grouchy Syndrome The most frequent 18p deletion involves a whole-arm loss, the breakpoint at the centromere (thus "centromeric 18p– syndrome"), seen in almost one-half of del 18p cases (Sebold et al. 2015). *TGIF1* and *AFG3L2* (at chr18:3.4 Mb and 12.3 Mb, respectively) (Fig. 14–36) are two of several genes reviewed in Hasi-Zogaj et al. (2015) that may be contributory to the phenotype. Albeit that this is a homogeneous cytogenetic material, the clinical picture can vary quite considerably. Intellectual handicap may be relatively mild, with an IQ range around 50–100, an average of 70 (Hasi-Zogaj et al. 2015); Turleau (2008) gives a lower range of 25–75, although acknowledging some to be of normal or borderline mental development. Coping with everyday life is difficult. Autism is seen in a minority. Facial dysmorphism is "soft," shading into normality. Most cases occur de novo, but there are rare instance of parental (all maternal) transmission. Partial 18p deletion breakpoints are recorded along the whole length of the short arm, very few of which are

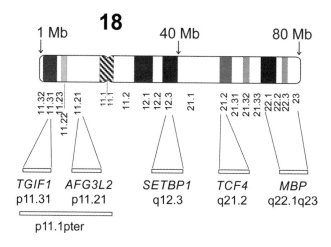

FIGURE 14-36

recurrent. In principle, the milder the phenotype, the less the degree of 18p loss. In any 18p deletion, parental rearrangement is prudently to be excluded.

del 18q Terminal deletions, of differing lengths, up to 30 Mb, are the more usually observed, but about one-fourth are interstitial. Cody et al. (2015) assess which genes may contribute to which aspect of the phenotype, and divide deletions into those proximal and those distal to the region chr18:49.8-50.9 Mb (within which no deletion has ever been observed). Two loci of note in the distal segment are *TCF4* at chr18:55.2-55.6 Mb and *MBP* at chr18:76.9 Mb. Mutation in the former is the basis of Pitt-Hopkins syndrome (next entry), and the latter directs white matter myelination. The *TCF4* locus, intact or deleted, serves as a further subdivision among the distal deletions; those with loss of *TCF4* have a Pitt-Hopkins phenotype superimposed. Concerning the proximal segment, one of the genes therein, *SETBP1*, at 18q12.3 (chr18:44.7 Mb), is associated with severely deficient expressive but intact receptive speech. The *CELF4* locus at chr18:37.2 Mb may influence development of an autistic presentation (Barone et al. 2017).

del 18q21: Pitt-Hopkins Syndrome Mutation in, or deletion of, the *TCF4* gene at chr18:55.22-55.58 Mb is the basis of Pitt-Hopkins syndrome. Whole gene deletion is seen in 30%, and these deletions may extend contiguously, while under 10% are—as is the child in Figure 14–37—due to partial gene deletion (Marangi and Zollino 2015). The condition includes developmental delay, and disordered respiratory control with episodes of hyperventilation

and apnea. Gonadal mosaicism is well recognized (Fig 14–37), and a small risk of recurrence is to be acknowledged (Kousoulidou et al. 2013).

del 18q22.1q23 While most 18q deletions are nonrecurrent, Cody et al. (2014) were able to assemble a group of patients in whom the deleted terminal segments (chr18:64-80 Mb) all had breakpoints at various sites within a 2 Mb segment between two

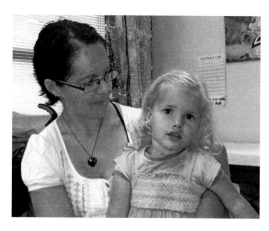

FIGURE 14–37   Mother and child with del(18)(q21), attending a genetic clinic. Mother, completely normal physically and intellectually, had, on microarray, a "slight negative shift" at 18q21, and on FISH, 4/18 cells showed deletion of *TCF4*. Blood was the only tissue analyzed. Daughter is nonmosaic for the deletion at chr18:55.36-55.95 Mb and has Pitt-Hopkins syndrome.

Source: Case of J. Watt, in Doudney et al. (2013). Reproduced with kind permission of the parents.

consecutive genes (*SERPINB8* and *CDH7*). These removed the same suite of 38 genes, among which *TMX3, NETO1, ZNF407, TSHZ1, NFATC,* and *MBP* are judged attractive as contributory to the clinical picture. These authors speak of this as the "distal 18q– reference group." Diminished cognitive capacity (of low-normal degree), growth retardation, and hearing loss were commonly observed traits. The deletion can, very rarely, be transmitted. For example, Margarit et al. (2012) describe a mother and her two daughters each with a 4.8 Mb deletion comprising essentially all of 18q23 (chr18:75.4-80.2 Mb). The mother was intellectually disabled; one daughter had an IQ below average but well within the normal range; the other was of borderline intellect.

Chromosome 19 Deletions

del 19p13.11 This rare deletion, in the region chr19:16.3-17.6 Mb, has the interest that imbalance of the *EPS15L1* gene at chr19:16.3-16.4 Mb (Fig. 14–38) may lead to distal limb defects such as syndactyly (Bens et al. 2011).

del 19p13.2 We may attempt a division, albeit not a clear-cut one, into two groups within this chromosome band. Deletions in a more distal group fall within chr19:10-12 Mb, with the *SMARCA4* locus (chr19:11.0 Mb) common to several; and a more proximal group, at chr19:12-14 Mb, in which *NFIX* (chr19:13.0 Mb) may be a pheno-critical locus (Shimojima et al. 2015; Welham et al. 2015). Some of the latter deletions may "flow over" into the adjacent bands 19p13.13 and 19p13.12, and several of these having loss of the *LPHN1* locus

(chr19:14.2 Mb) in common (Bonaglia et al. 2010). Welham et al. made a detailed analysis of the psychology and behavior of those with these deletions, acknowledging a heterogeneous material and assessing such domains as mood, interest, pleasure, and liability to challenging behavior (some prone to self-destructive acts). We have seen a man with a de novo del chr19:10,759,332-12,358,697, from a family otherwise of high achievers, who had been incarcerated for numerous crimes, including arson and indecent assault, and diagnosed with a (risperidone-responsive) psychosis.

Sibship recurrence is recorded: Two sisters had the same del 19p13.13 chr19:13.04-13.44, but the parents tested normal on (presumably) peripheral blood (Nimmakayalu et al. 2013). Naturally, one must have been a gonadal mosaic.

del 19p13.3 Again, we may need to consider two distinct categories, but in this instance, there is no overlap between them: deletion within a very distal segment, chr19:0.2-1.2 Mb; and within a more proximal, chr19:3-5 Mb segment. The distal segment deletion is reviewed in Peddibhotla et al. (2013), and in two families, transmission from a parent was recorded.

THEG is a common deleted locus. If the deletion includes the *STK11* gene at chr19:1.21-1.23 Mb, Peutz-Jegher syndrome will be added to the phenotype otherwise of learning difficulty, dysmorphism, and congenital anomalies (Kuroda et al. 2015).

The more *proximal* segment lies within chr19:3-5 Mb, and having a common deleted region of chr19:3.81-4.14 Mb. This region contains several loci, of which *DAPK3* is just one candidate for

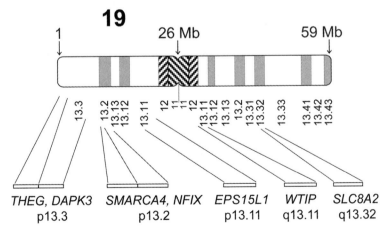

FIGURE 14–38

having a pheno-critical role. A phenotype of facial dysmorphism, multiple health problems, and intellectual deficiency is seen. All tested cases have been de novo.

del 19q13.11 Nonrecurrent deletions of varying lengths within this band (and in some extending into the adjacent bands) lead to a clinical picture including intellectual deficiency, hypospadias in the male, and the notable observation of an ectodermal dysplasia. Skin, hair, and nails are affected, and in some, there is an actual cutis aplasia of the scalp. Some children diagnosed as having Dubowitz syndrome, in which eczema and sparse hair are typical, may in fact have this microdeletion (Urquhart et al. 2015). A previously defined shortest region of overlap (SRO), chr19:34.62-34.95 Mb, has not held up universally, albeit that it is included in most deletions. Two contiguous loci on the immediate centromeric flank of this SRO, *UBA2* and *WTIP*, lying between chr19:34.43-34.51 Mb, may relate to the ectodermal aspects and the genital defect, respectively (Chowdhury et al. 2014; Melo et al. 2015). Deletion of *TSHZ3* (chr19:31.27-31.34 Mb) in 19q12, a gene having a role in development of cortical projection neurons (nerve cells that connect to others in the cerebral cortex), may account for the neuropsychological phenotype in those in whom the deletion extends this far (Caubit et al. 2016).

del 19q13.32 This syndrome has barely been defined, but there are some distinctive observations, and further reports will surely fill out the picture. A deletion of the "full region," chr19:46.77-47.68 Mb, leads to a phenotype of severe mental retardation, facial dysmorphism, and certain neuromuscular deficiencies, affecting innervation of the eye (with gaze palsy) and gut (with colonic atony and chronic constipation). These traits are not seen in lesser deletions telomeric of chr19:47.3 Mb, and in these a low-normal or mild intellectual deficit, and minor dysmorphism, are recorded (Castillo et al. 2014). Candidate pheno-critical genes include *NPAS1* at chr19:47.0 Mb and *SLC8A2* at chr19:47.4 Mb (Travan et al. 2017).

Chromosome 20 Deletions

del 20p11.2 Dayem-Quere et al. (2013) describe their own patient with a 4.2 Mb deletion, chr20:19.8-24.0 Mb, in which panhypopituitarism was a notable observation, and review the small number of other similar cases. Deletions may extend from p11.2 into adjacent bands, with p11.22 (chr20:20.0-22.3 Mb) (Fig. 14–39) the segment deleted in common. Facial dysmorphism, mental retardation, and autism are recorded in some. *FOXA2* (chr20:22.5 Mb) presents a plausible case as being instrumental in the genesis of the pituitary defect. In one instance, there had been mother-to-child inheritance, the (normal) mother mosaic for the deletion (Garcia-Heras et al. 2005); all others were de novo.

del 20p12.2: Alagille Syndrome The characteristic features of this syndrome are stenosis of the peripheral pulmonary arteries, and insufficient development of bile ducts within the liver (thus, "arteriohepatic dysplasia"), along with certain eye and skeletal defects, and a distinctive facies; intellect is typically normal. Genomic deletions are an

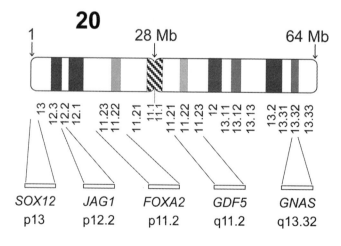

FIGURE 14–39

uncommon cause; most are in fact due to mutation in the *JAG1* gene at chr20:10.6 Mb. In the <5% of cases of Alagille syndrome with a deletion, those of smaller size, up to 4 Mb and contained within chr20:7.4-12.8 Mb, typically convey no further phenotypic burden beyond that imposed by *JAG1* haploinsufficiency (Sahoo et al. 2011). Parental transmission is recorded, at least from an affected father, and from a mosaic unaffected mother (Laufer-Cahana et al. 2002).

del 20p13 An et al. (2013) define the phenotype as comprising cognitive disability, autistic traits, and dysmorphic features but with no clearly discernible pattern. Landau-Kleffner syndrome is reported. Some achieve an IQ within a normal range. Most deletions are terminal, and most are nonrecurrent. Deletion size is typically from kilobase to 1–2 Mb in extent. The subtelomeric genes *NRSN2* and *SOX12* (chr20:325-354 kb) are proposed to be pheno-critical. Where tested, de novo inheritance has been universal.

del 20q11.21q11.23 This rare disorder typically presents, along with psychomotor retardation, the particular features of a visual defect due to retinal pigment epithelium atrophy, craniofacial dysmorphism, and certain skeletal anomalies (Posmyk et al. 2014). Deletion extents vary considerably, from about 2 to 8 Mb. Jedraszak et al. (2015c) identify a 1.6 Mb critical region at chr20:35.2-36.8 Mb. *GDF5*, *EPB41L1*, and *SAMHD1* within this segment are plausible pheno-contributory candidates. One of a pair of non-identical monozyous twins in Meredith et al. (2017) had the smallest recorded deletion, likely in constitutional mosaic state, with only *GDF5* deleted of the three genes just named; intriguingly, his phenotypically normal co-twin also showed mosaicism for the deletion, presumably as a consequence of chimerism confined to blood, reflecting that the two had shared a placenta. A mitotic origin of the deletion in one twin, after the splitting of the conceptus, is a probable basis of the abnormality.

del 20q13.33 Epilepsy, along with neurocognitive compromise, is a particular component of the phenotype due to this deletion. A 20q terminal deletion might remove only the last two genes on the chromosome (*MYT1* and *PCMTD2*,

at chr20:64.1-64.2 Mb), or, if of wider extent, genes of possible epileptic susceptibility (*KCNQ2* and *CHRNA4*, at chr20:63.3-63.4 Mb) could be included (Mefford et al. 2012). However, albeit that these latter two genes express a neuronal channel and neuronal receptor, respectively, Okumura et al. (2015) could not confirm that the epilepsy (typically benign neonatal seizures resolving in early infancy) was indeed related to loss of these loci. More proximally, deletion of *GNAS* (chr20:58.8 Mb) is associated, although not consistently, with pseudopseudohypoparathyroidism[29] (Balasubramanian et al. 2015; Garin et al. 2015).

Chromosome 21 Deletions

del 21q22, Braddock-Carey Syndrome Clinical observations include neurocognitive compromise typically of severe degree, agenesis of the corpus callosum, the Pierre Robin sequence, facial dysmorphism, heart malformation, and, in some, congenital thrombocytopenia (Braddock et al. 2016). This latter trait is due to loss of the *RUNX1* gene (chr21:34.8 Mb) (Fig. 14–40); in Braddock-Carey syndrome in which this gene is intact, platelet production is normal. *ITSN1* and *SON* are two of several other genes that might play a contributory role (Izumi et al. 2012; Fukai et al. 2014; Takenouchi et al. 2016). To our understanding, all cases of this syndrome have been of de novo generation.

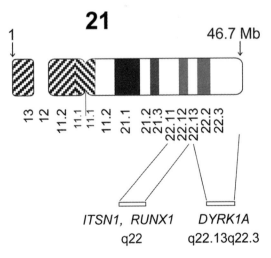

FIGURE 14–40

29 This clumsy term describes a phenotype resembling the nonresponse of target tissues to parathyroid hormone as in Albright hereditary osteodystrophy, but in fact not being due to a defect in the hormone receptor.

del 21q22.13q22.3 Valetto et al. (2012) review the few published cases of this deletion, in which the clinical picture is one of mental and growth retardation of marked degree, along with epilepsy, and various types of brain malformation on imaging. Facial dysmorphism is notable. Deletions are mostly in the range 0.5–10 Mb, within the segment chr21:34.7-46.7 Mb, immediately adjacent to the region of Braddock-Carey syndrome (as above). *DYRK1A*, at chr21:37.4 Mb, is a deleted locus in common, this gene having a role in development of the intellect (Bronicki et al. 2015). Deletions confined to the terminal band 21q22.3 are associated with hypoplastic left heart syndrome (Ciocca et al. 2015).

Chromosome 22 Deletions

del 22q11.21 Before their common cytogenetic basis was understood, the 22q11 deletion clinical presentations had a number of labels, including DiGeorge syndrome (DGS), velocardiofacial (VCF) syndrome, and Shprintzen syndrome.[30] DGS was the name typically applied to a child with heart defect, parathyroid abnormality, and immunodeficiency; in Shprintzen syndrome a cleft or deficient palate was the notable feature; while VCF syndrome emphasized the facial appearance, along with palatal ("velo") clefting and a heart defect. Kousseff syndrome and Cayler syndrome were names given to variants with a neural tube defect, and asymmetric crying facies plus cardiac outflow defect, respectively. A phenocopy of oculo-auriculo-vertebral spectrum is a rare observation (Digilio et al. 2009).

The intellect is affected. Difficulty in social interaction may relate mostly to the degree of intellectual disability (Campbell et al. 2015). A psychiatric/behavioral component is frequent, with susceptibility to psychosis and autism; if other features are absent, the chromosomal diagnosis may be delayed until adolescence or adulthood (Furuya et al. 2015; Fonseca-Pedrero et al. 2016). Those in whom the intellectual deficit is more marked have a greater tendency to develop a psychotic disorder (Vorstman et al. 2015). The evolution of the *tout ensemble* phenotype in the adult, with whom neuropsychiatric disease is the main cause for concern, presents its own challenges (Fung et al. 2015).

With a birth incidence of about 1 in 4,000, this is the most common human site of deletion, and

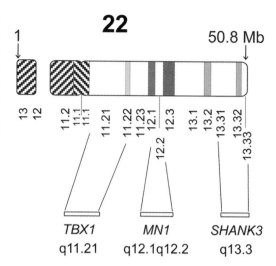

FIGURE 14–41

this vulnerability resides in the existence of low-copy repeats in the 22q11 region, LCR22 A through D. The most frequently observed (90%) deletion, of ~3 Mb, lies between LCR22A-D, while 8% span the ~1.5 Mb segment LCR22A-B: respectively, these involve chr22:18.6-21.4 Mb and chr22:18.6-20.3 Mb. Rare deletions occur at other sites (Burnside 2015). *TBX1* is the locus seen as key to the cardiac defects, and possibly also contributory to the psychopathy (Hiramoto et al. 2011); this gene lies between LCRs A and B, at chr22:19.7 Mb (Fig. 14–41). A number of other loci have been implicated in the psychiatric phenotype.

Incomplete penetrance for components of the syndrome, and variable expressivity for those that are present, is very much the rule. Monozygous twins are often discordant (Singh et al. 2002b). In the familial case, a parent can, for example, show mild features of the condition or have a predominantly Shprintzen facial and palatal phenotype, with a child showing a characteristic DGS cardiac and endocrine phenotype (Devriendt et al. 1997). Hart et al. (2016) rehearse issues in sensitively raising with parents the risk for psychosis. The condition is typically more severe in second-generation subjects, although ascertainment bias is a likely explanation (Cirillo et al. 2014). Variable expressivity with respect to facial appearance is compounded due to ethnic differences, and Kruszka et al. (2017)

---

30 In true acknowledgment of the first definition of the syndrome, in the Czechoslovakian literature in 1955, Sedláčková syndrome may be the most fitting name (Turnpenny and Pigott 2001).

propose that digital facial analysis technology is a more accurate "observer" than a clinician.

Most cases are de novo, but about 10% may be inherited. (Since the condition is not rare, occasional instances will happen of more than one case in a family, purely coincidentally; Saitta et al. 2004). Earlier estimates of a larger fraction of affected parents may have been biased due to studying more remarkable families (Swillen et al. 1998). Indeed, Smith and Robson (1999) report only 5% of parents to have had the deletion in an Australian series of 59 cases. In advising about recurrence risk, genetic counseling must take account of the possibilities of a parent being so mildly affected that the condition had not been recognized, and thus parental chromosomal analysis is appropriately offered. Vergés et al. (2014), in a study of fathers of children with the 22q11 deletion, found two of nine fathers with levels of del(22q11) sperm that were approximately threefold higher than those of controls. No increase in levels of dup(22q11) sperm was observed, leading the authors to propose a tendency to intrachromatid NAHR as a causative mechanism.[31] Gross et al. (2016) have conducted a pilot study of noninvasive prenatal testing by SNP analysis, which in principle could be offered to a whole pregnant population, or targeted to couples with a previously affected child or to increased-risk mothers (e.g., heart defect seen on ultrasound).

del 22q12.1q12.2 The clinical picture in this rare deletion includes the notable observations of cleft palate and susceptibility to schwannoma (Breckpot et al. 2016). The *MN1* gene at chr22:27.7 Mb may be the basis of the cleft palate, while the nervous system tumors are consequential upon loss of the *NF2* gene or its promoter (chr22:29.6 Mb). Other traits include intellectual deficiency, in some with severe language deficiency, and facial dysmorphism, of which micrognathia is one feature. Breakpoints are nonrecurrent. De novo inheritance is seen in all cases in which parental testing has been done.

del 22q13.3, Phelan-McDermid Syndrome A particular trait of this well-known condition is a failure to develop expressive language, and high pain tolerance is also notable; the physical phenotype comprises rather "soft" dysmorphism, if any. Autism spectrum in childhood, and psychosis in adulthood, may compound the neuropsychiatric picture. A characteristic electroencephalographic pattern is reported, which may or may not be associated with seizures (Figura et al. 2014). Most deletions are terminal (with telomere healing), while a few are interstitial; in scarcely any is the proximal breakpoint recurrent. Size varies from 122 kb to 9 Mb, such that cytogenetic nomenclature can range from del(22)(q13.31q13.33) to del(22)(q13.33) alone (Bonaglia et al. 2011). The key locus is *SHANK3* (chr22:50.6 Mb), the antepenultimate gene on the chromosome,[32] and whose role involves crucial interaction with a neuronal glutamate receptor (Vicidomini et al. 2017). Interplay with other genes within the deleted segment (e.g., *IB2*, adjacent to *SHANK3*, and the microRNA *hsa-mir-1249* at some distance from it, at chr22:45.2 Mb), as well as the presence of a variant in the remaining *SHANK3* allele, may influence the degree to which autism and global developmental delay evolve (Oberman et al. 2015). An intriguing suggestion is that intranasal insulin may improve the neurobehavioral picture (Zwanenburg et al. 2016).

Recurrence due to parental gonadal mosaicism for the deletion is very rare but not unknown (Tabolacci et al. 2005). A balanced parental translocation is slightly less rare and should always be checked for. However, almost all cases arise de novo. The deletion may be in the form of a ring chromosome (p. 217).

DUPLICATIONS

While there are certainly very many individual duplication cases on record, rather fewer duplication phenotypes have acquired eponymic status than with deletions, and we do provide a somewhat shorter catalog than the listing of deletion syndromes above. The dosage effect due to a duplication is referred to as triplo-excess, or triplo-sensitivity, in contrast to the haploinsufficiency of the deletion.

---

31 As noted earlier, rates of NAHR, as measured in sperm, vary up to sevenfold between different males, and possibly this may be the explanation for the variability seen in this study. An alternative explanation is that there are hitherto undetected differences in genomic architecture at 22q11.2, that influence the rate of NAHR at this locus.

32 Argument in the correspondence columns of the *American Journal of Medical Genetics* turns on the question of interstitial deletions which do not remove *SHANK3*, such as those reported in Disciglio et al. (2014). Do these represent a new syndrome, or merely variants of Phelan-McDermid syndrome (Mari et al. 2015; Phelan et al. 2015)? The view of she who gave her name to the syndrome might perhaps hold sway.

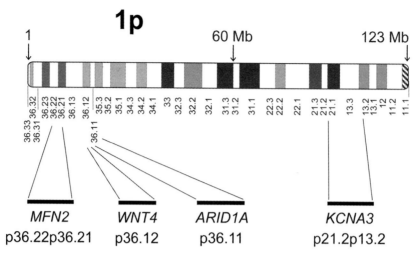

FIGURE 14–42

The expression partial trisomy is sometimes used, especially for larger classical duplications. Some duplications do have a countertype deletion; in the case of those with no recorded reciprocal deletion, it may be that haploinsufficiency is nonviable. The same comment applies, that only "pure" imbalances are listed here; those duplications with a concomitant imbalance on another chromosome are not considered. We make no distinction between the direct duplication (genomic sequence in the same direction) or indirect duplication (sequence in the reverse direction). A very few triplications (trp) are also included. We remind the reader again that the genome coordinates here, unless otherwise indicated, are given in the hg38 build (most having been converted from the hg18 or hg19 builds in the papers cited).

Chromosome 1 Duplications

dup 1p21.2p13.2 Piccione et al. (2010) describe their case of a de novo 10.4 Mb deletion in p21.1p13.2, chr1:102.0-112.4 Mb, in a mildly retarded teenager with "soft" dysmorphism. A potassium voltage-gated channel gene *KCNA3* at chr1:110.6 Mb (Fig. 14–42) is one of numerous possible candidates as contributory to the phenotype. These authors review a very heterogeneous collection of other rare/unique 1p duplications, including p11p13, p13.3p22.1, p21p31, p21.2p32,

p22.3p32.3, p34p31, p34.1p34.3, and p36.3pter, but these had not been subject to molecular characterization.

dup 1p36.11 A single de novo case of this 190 kb duplication, chr1:26.67-26.86 Mb, is of note in that the *ARID1A* gene, the basis of some Coffin-Siris syndrome, is included (Coutton et al. 2013). The child was severely developmentally delayed, with facial dysmorphism, and postaxial hexadactyly of all four limbs (in Coffin-Siris syndrome, the little finger is hypoplastic).

dup 1p36.12 This duplication is of interest in that it contains the *WNT4* gene at chr1:22.1 Mb, which acts upon *DAX1* at Xp21 to cause sex reversal in the 46,XY,dup(1)(p36) individual (Jordan et al. 2001). Duplication of *DAX1* of itself (p. 537) similarly causes sex reversal.

dup 1p36.22p36.21 The physical phenotype is that of "focal facial dermal hypoplasia type 3," also known as Setleis syndrome, characterized by atrophic facial lesions and otherwise facial dysmorphism, and aberrant hair growth. Deletions are nonrecurrent and of varying extents; the 1.3 Mb minimal overlapping region of the duplication (or, in some, triplication) is chr1:11.63-12.86 Mb.[33] No genes within this segment can particularly be implicated; *MFN2* at chr1:11.98 Mb is an arbitrarily

---

33 Thus, this duplication does not overlap the two critical regions involved in the common 1p36.33 deletion (Fig. 14-5). Curiously, isolated duplication of 1p36.33, as a reciprocal countertype to the common deletion, is scarcely ever reported (Heilstedt et al. 1999).

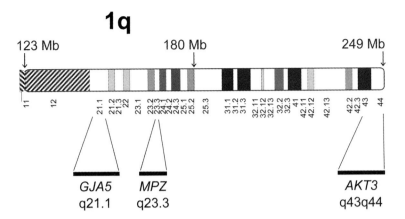

1q

123 Mb   180 Mb   249 Mb

GJA5   MPZ   AKT3
q21.1   q23.3   q43q44

FIGURE 14–43

chosen landmark gene (a gene otherwise of interest, mutation in which being the basis of one form of Charcot-Marie-Tooth neuropathy). Of the few cases thus far reported, developmental delay has been a feature in most, but an example is also on record of an intellectually normal man with Setleis syndrome, who had inherited the duplication from his phenotypically normal (and nonmosaic) carrier father (Lee et al. 2015a).

dup 1q12q22, dup 1q12q23 Sawyer et al. (2007) report a dysmorphic infant initially suspected of having Turner syndrome, with a 1q12q22 duplication extending to chr1:156.4 Mb (the proximal breakpoint, in the heterochromatin of 1q12, not precisely measurable) (Fig. 14–43). Development at 15 months was delayed. A similar case of a newborn testing dup(1)(q12q23) on classical karyotype (not tested molecularly) presented with diaphragmatic hernia and arthrogryposis multiplex (Otake et al. 2009). These duplications (both de novo) encompass the segment of dup 1q21.1, as below.

dup 1q12q31 A very large 50 Mb duplication, chr1:143-193 Mb (~40% of the length of the long arm), is reported in Sifakis et al. (2014), concerning a fetus of 23 weeks gestation with multiple malformations. They review a very heterogeneous prenatally diagnosed dup(1q) material; in almost all, termination had been chosen, while in the pregnancies going to livebirth, survival was mostly measured in minutes or days. The even larger

duplication described as 1q21qter, a length of fully 100 Mb, causes multiple severe, lethal malformation (Machlitt et al. 2005).

dup 1q21.1 The typical recurrent duplication at 1q21.1 has been reported as a 1.35 Mb chr1:147.0-148.4 Mb rearrangement, although Bernier et al. (2016) note that the important material is the 800 kb of unique sequence at chr1:147.1-147.9 Mb (the 1.35 Mb segment included a considerable amount of flanking segmental duplication, and presumably not contributory, of itself, to the phenotype). The phenotype of this duplication includes mental retardation, or at least borderline cognitive functioning, and autism. Bernier et al. measured verbal IQ scores, with a mean of 80.5 and a range 62–105; for nonverbal IQ scores, the respective figures were 86.0 and 57–123. These numbers compare with 108.3/77–128 (verbal) and 111.4/89–140 (nonverbal) in noncarrier parents and siblings, giving about a 25–28 IQ points shortfall for the dup heterozygotes.[34] As the deletion leads to microcephaly, so does the duplication cause macrocephaly; brain scanning may show reduced white matter volume. Dolcetti et al. (2013) document an increased risk for schizophrenia, noting the genes *BCL9, GJA8, PDZK1,* and *PRKAB2* as candidates in this respect. A range of heart defects are seen (tetralogy of Fallot having a particular association), likely relating to a triplo-excess of *GJA5* at chr1:147.7 Mb (Soemedi et al. 2012; Digilio et al. 2013). In the review of Bernier et al., of those patients whose parents were

---

34 This is a greater shortfall than in the del(1q21.1), an uncommon example of the dup exhibiting a more marked effect than in the del.

studied, all but one were familial cases. It is true to say that incomplete penetrance and variable expressivity complicate interpretation and counseling; an important factor here is likely the role of CNVs elsewhere in the genome (Qiao et al. 2017).

A larger, 5 Mb duplication 1q21.1q21.2 in Brisset et al. (2015) was in company with a 16p11.2 deletion, and the phenotype in the child more severe than a simple "sum of the parts": a multiplicative two-hit. The dup 1q21 had come from the father, and the del 16p11.2 from the mother; the father suffered from psychopathy and mild intellectual deficiency, and the mother from depression. A yet larger duplication, 1q21.1q44, is recorded in mosaic state in brain tissue from a nondysmorphic child suffering from intractable epilepsy, who had had surgical resection of a part of one frontal lobe (Conti et al. 2015). On imaging, and subsequently on histopathology, the cerebral cortex was dysplastic. Loss of *AKT3* (see dup 1q43q44, below) may have led to the brain defect. The duplication was not seen in blood or saliva; the abnormality likely arose at a postzygotic mitosis in neurectodermal tissue at an early stage of embryonic development, and was confined to this lineage. Triplication of 1q21.1 is described in Van Dijck et al. (2015).

dup 1q23.3 A familial dup chr1:161.2-161.4 Mb is described in Speevak and Farrell (2013), a presumed benign copy number variant including two genes, *MPZ* and *SDHC*, seen in three generations: a grandfather, father, and one child. But in a second child, the duplication was itself duplicated, to give a 1q23.3 "quadruplication." This infant presented with a severe form of Charcot-Marie-Tooth (CMT) neuropathy, due to the excess dosage of the *MPZ* gene (mutation in which is the usual basis of CMT type 1B). The quadruplication may represent a second NAHR event on this no. 1 chromosome in the family, the first having occurred one cannot say how many generations ago.

dup 1q32.1q44 These deletions are of substantial size and readily detectable on classical cytogenetics. Balasubramanian et al. (2009) estimate a size of 42 Mb. The clinical picture is one of a distinctive facial dysmorphism, due in particular to craniofacial bone maldevelopment, along with developmental delay.

dup 1q43q44 One de novo case is on record, a child with megalencephaly and developmental delay (Wang et al. 2013a). The interest here is the proposed role of the *AKT3* gene (chr1:243.7 Mb), which is a component of the important PI3K growth control pathway. (Deletion of this gene leads to microcephaly; Gai et al. 2015, and see del(1) (q44q45) above.)

Chromosome 2 Duplications

dup 2p16.1p15 In their 2015 review, Mimouni-Bloch et al. list only a single-digit number of reports, although it is notable that three were of very similar extent. The reported cases spanned the 2p segment from *BCL11A* (chr2:60.4 Mb) to *COMMD1* (chr2:62.1 Mb), a length of 1.7 Mb (Fig. 14–44); some extended beyond *BCL11A* into gene-less DNA. Little clinical information was available for these other cases (from the DECIPHER and ISCA

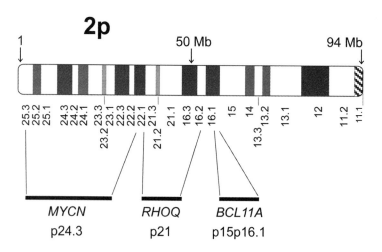

FIGURE 14–44

databases); the child in Mimouni-Bloch et al. had a mild developmental delay, attention deficit and oppositional behavior, and mild dysmorphism. *BCL11A*, which was duplicated in every case, bids fair as a pheno-critical candidate. All those in whom parental studies were noted were of de novo generation.

dup 2p22p16, 2p25p22 In an acerbic response to an earlier paper, Lurie (2014) notes that neural tube defect, diaphragmatic hernia, and susceptibility to neuroblastoma may all reside in components of a partial 2p trisomy. The neuroblastoma risk is due to duplication of the *MYCN* locus at chr2:15.9 Mb, in 2p24.3, while the susceptibility to neural tube defect may be conveyed by duplication of loci within the rather substantial segment 2p13p25.3. A 1.9 Mb duplication within 2p21, chr2:45-47 Mb, may account for the (hormone-resistant) growth retardation seen in children whose 2p imbalance includes this particular segment; *EPAS1* and *RHOQ* (at chr2:46.5 and 46.7 Mb) are plausible candidate genes for this aspect (Blassnig-Ezeh et al., 2013).

dup 2q11.2 Short stature is a particular observation, and for example, Russell-Silver syndrome might be suspected. Mild facial dysmorphism and developmental delay are typical. The duplication may arise de novo, or it may have been inherited from an affected or an (apparently) unaffected parent (Riley et al. 2015). Duplication sizes are in the range 1.38–1.47 Mb, encompassing chr2:95.88-97.61 Mb (Fig. 14–45), and are presumed to be generated due to NAHR. *LMAN2L* is a landmark locus.

dup 2q13 This duplication is the reciprocal of the 2q13 deletion. In four cases studied in Riley et al. (2015), developmental delay or intellectual disability was observed in all. Two (an uncle and a nephew) were from a three-generation kindred, and the connecting relative was described with a learning difficulty. The patriarch in generation I was apparently unaffected. The duplications were of sizes 1.62 and 1.71 Mb, spanning chr2:110.63-112.34 Mb. *FBLN7* is a landmark locus.

dup 2q23.1 Mullegama et al. (2014) review this syndrome and report a picture not unlike that of the countertype deletion, although not quite as severe, with respect to the core phenotype of intellectual deficiency, autistic features, and minor dysmorphisms; an "affable personality" is common. The duplicated segments, which are mostly nonrecurrent, vary very considerably in size; most are less than 10 Mb, and several are less than 1 Mb. All contain the pheno-critical gene *MBD5* at chr2:148.0 Mb. Most arise de novo, although Mullegama et al. do record rare cases of mother-to-child transmission; detailed information was not available for these transmitting parents, but on best advice, they were not considered to be affected. In other words, nonpenetrance is observed.

dup 2q32q33 Duplications in this chromosomal region are of varying lengths, and several overlap in the segment containing *SATB2, KCTD18*, and *ADAM23*, at chr2:199.4-206.4 Mb, as Usui et al. (2013) document in their review. Their own case, of a child with severe developmental delay, autism, ataxia, and mild facial dysmorphism, had the de novo duplication chr2:188.2-207.7 Mb. Some duplications extend into 2q31 and 2q24.3; if the imbalance includes the *DLX* loci at chr2:172.0 Mb, this may engender epilepsy (Lim et al. 2014).

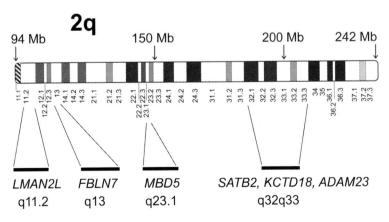

FIGURE 14–45

dup 2q37 The 2q37 duplicated state may be associated with an intellectual capacity within the normal range and little or no dysmorphism (Batstone et al. 2003), in obvious contradistinction to the deletion.

Chromosome 3 Duplications

dup 3p24.1p26.2 Pure duplication in this region has been seen in only two children in whom molecular analysis has been done (Bittel et al. 2008; Natera de Benito et al. 2014). The segments involved are large, one of 26 Mb (chr3:3.9-29.6 Mb), and the other contained within, at 3p25.3p26.2, chr3:4.3-13.0 Mb (Fig. 14–46). The *GHRL* gene at chr3:10.2 Mb is plausibly a basis of the observed obesity, quite strikingly reminiscent of a Prader-Willi phenotype. Both had a mild pervasive developmental disorder. At least the larger duplication was confirmed de novo; it is likely both were.

dup 3q22.2q29 Duplications within this segment are of considerable length, and can be >60 Mb; for example, in the child in Shanske et al. (2010), the duplication spanned chr3:134.8-195.9 Mb. This is large enough that the condition—named the "dup(3q) syndrome"—was detectable on classical cytogenetics as early as 1966 by Falek et al. The clinical phenotype is notable in a resemblance to Cornelia de Lange syndrome (and indeed this dup(3q) misled early efforts to locate the gene). Other duplications within the segment of interest are the 14.7 Mb dup(3)(q26.32q28) described in Pavone et al. (2016) and the de novo direct tandem 7.9 Mb dup(3)(q26.32q27.2) in Dworschak et al. (2017). These latter authors propose that the anorectal malformations observed in dup(3q) may relate to the genes *DVL3* and *EPHB3*, located respectively at chr3:184.1 and chr3:184.5 Mb, in

3q27.1. A pheno-contributory role for *TBL1XR1* is proposed in Riehmer et al. (2017), who studied a familial case in which a mother and two offspring were duplicated for a very small segment of 521 kb, at 3q26.32. A syndrome resembling the oculo-auriculo-vertebral spectrum is described in association with a small (<1 Mb) duplication at 3q29, of chr3:194.4-195.1 Mb (Guida et al. 2015).

dup 3q29 Adjacent to the foregoing on distal 3q is the reciprocal duplication of the 3q29 microdeletion syndrome (chr3:196.0-197.6 Mb). This has the notable feature that the majority of cases are familial, in contrast to the deletions, which almost always arise de novo (Ballif et al. 2008; Lisi et al. 2008). *DLG1* and *PAK2*, at ch3:197.0 and 197.7 Mb, may be key loci (Dworschak et al. 2017). Mild to moderate mental retardation and microcephaly are the most commonly observed traits in index cases. The normality or near-normality of a transmitting parent, which is sometimes observed (Aleixandre Blanquer et al. 2011), may reflect an incompletely penetrant genotype, and other genetic factors may influence expression.

Chromosome 4 Duplications

dup 4p16.3 Heterozygotes for this duplication can be of fairly unremarkable phenotype, and they may be able to function independently, albeit at undemanding level, in society. Macrocephaly and tall stature were observations in a three-generation family described in Schönewolf-Greulich et al. (2013), the imbalance of extent chr4:73 kb-30.7 Mb. These authors review similar cases, in whom the common region of duplication comprised chr4:1.57-1.86 Mb (Fig. 14–47). The *FGFR3* locus at chr4:1.79 Mb could have a role in the mild degree of overgrowth; other duplications have included the

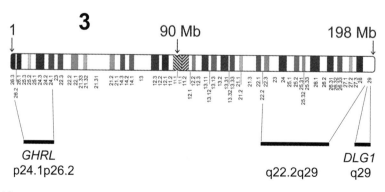

FIGURE 14–46

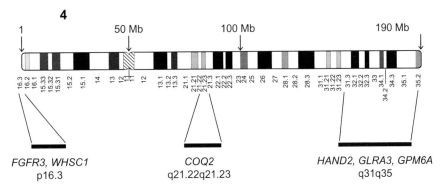

4

FGFR3, WHSC1
p16.3

COQ2
q21.22q21.23

HAND2, GLRA3, GPM6A
q31q35

FIGURE 14–47

Wolf-Hirschhorn region *WHSC1* at chr4:1.87-1.98 Mb (Carmany and Bawle 2011; Cyr et al. 2011). Schönewolf-Greulich et al. suggest that underdiagnosis of distal 4p duplications might reflect the mild degree of affection.

dup 4q21.22q21.23 The very specific disease associated with this duplication is myoclonic-astatic epilepsy, at least in one reported de novo case in Ottaviani et al. (2015). Their patient had the duplication chr4:83.1-83.8 Mb; one DECIPHER subject with dup chr4:82.1-85.0 Mb showed complete overlap of that segment, but epilepsy was not mentioned in this child. *COQ2* at chr4:83.2 Mb is a locus of interest, coding as it does for a mitochondrial factor.

Distal dup 4q A 4q duplication syndrome has been recognized for some time, and Thapa et al. (2014) review several cases from as early as the 1970s, in which the breakpoints ranged from q22 to q31.3[35] proximally, to q32.3 to qter distally. Two cases were familial, from mother to child (dup 4q31.1q32.3 and dup 4q31.3q33). Thapa et al. describe two patients with smaller duplicated segments, dup q32.1q35.2 and dup q32.2q34.3, whose segments of imbalance were precisely defined. They conclude that the region 4q33q34 may be critical in conveying the (fairly nonspecific) phenotype of dysmorphism and intellectual deficiency in distal 4q duplications. The genes *HAND2*, *GLRA3*, and *GPM6A*, resident between chr4:173.5-175.6 Mb, are proposed to have key roles; it is of interest that 4q34 contains quite a large "gene desert."

Chromosome 5 Duplications

dup 5p13 Novara et al. (2013) review this condition, which is associated with a phenotype of intellectual deficit that can be severe, along with EEG and brain MRI abnormality, and facial dysmorphism. The key locus, in 5p13.2, is *NIPBL* (which is well known otherwise as the basis, when deleted, of Cornelia de Lange syndrome), at chr5:36.8 Mb (Fig. 14–48). The duplicated segment ranges in size from 0.25 to 13.6 Mb. The only familial example on record relates to an insertional translocation of 5p13.2 into Xp, with a carrier mother of karyotype der(X)ins(X;5) (p. 164).

dup 5q14 The neurocognitive phenotype of this rare imbalance inheres in the *MEF2C* locus, at chr5:88.8 Mb. Duplications are of varying size; that in Cesaretti et al. (2016) comprised chr5:86.8-91.4 Mb. These authors documented, at the level of macroscopic fetal neuropathology, partial agenesis of the corpus callosum. All cases have been de novo.

dup 5q22.1q23.2 This large duplication, of variable extent, and obvious on classical cytogenetics, is associated with a clinical picture of variable intellectual disability, typically microcephaly, minor facial dysmorphism, and short stature. In the cases reported in Schmidt et al. (2013) of an affected mother and her two children, the (inverted tandem) duplication extended approximately from the *CAMK4* to the *ZNF608* loci, encompassing chr5:110.7-124.9 Mb, slightly more than 14 Mb in length.

dup 5q35.2q35.3 and Hunter-McAlpine Syndrome This dup (5)(q35.2q35.3) is the countertype

---

35 This is the breakpoint in the siblings with essentially dup(4)(q31.3) whose photograph appears in the frontispiece.

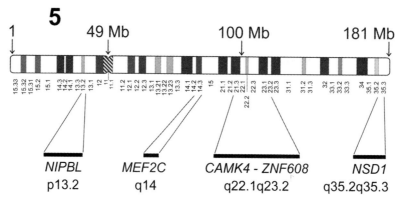

FIGURE 14–48

of the ~2 Mb deletion which is the basis of some cases of the Sotos overgrowth syndrome. Growth is in the opposite direction to Sotos syndrome, with mean length and head circumference being approximately –2.0 and –3.5 SD, respectively; bone age is delayed (Rosenfeld et al. 2012a; Novara et al. 2014). Radial ray defects are seen in some. *NSD1* (the "Sotos gene"; chr5:177.1 Mb) has the central role in pathogenesis; *FGFR4* (chr5:177.0 Mb) and, in larger duplications, *MSX2* (chr5:174.4 Mb) have also been implicated. Parental transmission has been recorded, albeit that the majority represent de novo cases. A duplication of somewhat greater distal extent, typically to 5qter, is referred to as Hunter-McAlpine syndrome (Jamsheer et al. 2013; Žilina et al. 2013).

Chromosome 6 Duplications

dup 6p Castiglione et al. (2013) review a heterogeneous 6p dup (partial trisomy) material, with many cases having a concomitant imbalance from another chromosome. Their own example of a father and two daughters with dup(6)(p23p25.3) (chr6:pter-13.8 Mb) is notable, in that all three were

judged to be of normal cognitive capacity; *FOXC1* (Fig. 14–49) was included in the duplicated segment. A more proximal imbalance is that reported in Savarese et al. (2013) comprising a 13.8 Mb segment at 6p21.31-p12.3 (chr6:35.4-49.3 Mb, including *RUNX2*), and transmitted from mildly retarded mother to her daughter; these two bear a most striking facial resemblance to each other. Contained within this segment is band 6p21.1, and Varvagiannis et al. (2013) focus on the dup(6) (p21.1) syndrome, noting that the most remarkable feature was a craniosynostosis, and proposing that an additional dose of *RUNX2* may be the basis of this.

dup 6q21q22 A very few cases of duplication involving the q21q22 segment are recorded, just one of which (chr6:111.2-115.7 Mb) was familial (Pazooki et al. 2007). The clinical picture is mostly rather nonspecific, with mild to moderate intellectual deficiency, growth deficiency, and facial dysmorphism, but the observation of an intention tremor in the mother and daughter in Pazooki

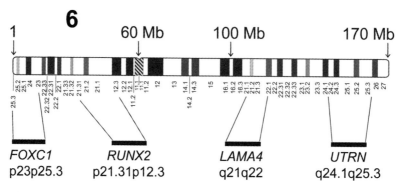

FIGURE 14–49

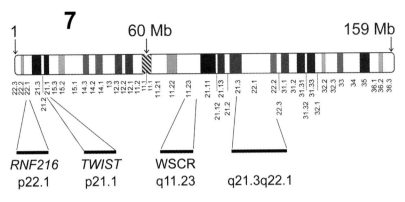

FIGURE 14-50

et al. is of interest. A landmark locus is *LAMA4* at chr6:112.1 Mb.

dup 6q24.2q25.3 A dozen cases of duplication in this region are on record, all de novo. The clinical picture has been referred to as the "dup 6q syndrome": severe mental retardation, microcephaly, facial dysmorphism, and, notably, joint contractures ("arthrogryposis"). Tabet et al. (2010), in their report of a child with a 13 Mb dup 6q24.2q25.3 (chr6:144.5-157.9 Mb), suggest that the utrophin (*UTRN*) gene at chr6:144.3-144.9 Mb may be the basis of the arthrogryposis. Utrophin has considerable similarity to dystrophin (the Duchenne gene), and it is plausible that disordered muscle function due to overexpression could result in reduced movements, and in consequence, joints "seizing up."

Chromosome 7 Duplications

dup 7p21.1 A duplication which includes the *TWIST* locus at chr7:19.1 Mb (Fig. 14–50) may lead to underdevelopment of the skull, with a large and confluent fontanelle (Stankiewicz et al. 2001c) (Fig. 14–51). As mentioned above, this is an example of the "type and countertype" of a del/dup: Haploinsufficiency of *TWIST* causes premature cranial bone fusion (craniosynostosis), while triplo-excess leads to underdevelopment.

dup 7p22.1 This syndrome is associated with intellectual disability and craniofacial dysmorphism. A triplo-excess of *RNF216* at chr7:5.6 Mb, a gene with a similar function to the *UBE3A* of Angelman syndrome, may be a particular factor in the evolution of the behavioral phenotype, which can include an autistic component (Goitia et al. 2015). The smallest duplication (386 kb) is that of

the child in Ronzoni et al. (2017); given the observation here of renal dysplasia, these authors propose a pheno-contributory role also for the *ACTB* gene at chr7:5.5 Mb, known otherwise to be associated with

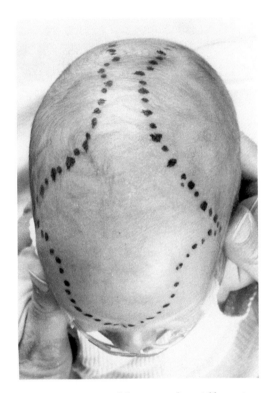

FIGURE 14-51 Widely separated cranial bones in a child with dup(7)(p14.2pter). The ink marker shows the palpable outline of the skull bones, and demarcates the extent of the widely patent fontanelle. This observation reflects duplication of the *TWIST* gene at 7p21.1, which is included within the imbalanced segment in this child; in contrast, deletion of *TWIST* is associated with premature cranial bone fusion.

kidney disease. De novo inheritance is recorded in all cases in which parental studies have been done.

dup 7q11.23 This duplication is the reciprocal recombination product to the Williams syndrome (WS) deletion, chr7:73.3-74.8 Mb. Familial cases are not uncommon, and in the series of Morris et al. (2015), about one-fourth of probands had an affected parent; Earhart et al. (2017) report an affected father of four affected children. Of de novo probands in this series, about one-fourth had an inversion of the q11.23 segment on their duplicated chromosome, and in all of these cases, one parent had the WSCR inversion polymorphism which is seen in 6% of the general population (Hobart et al. 2010). As with WS, this inversion polymorphism is presumed to foster the formation of an intrachromosomal loop, which in turn sets the stage for illegitimate recombination.

The phenotype is variable, with neurological function the major focus of concern. Macrocephaly and also brain anomalies on imaging are observed (Morris et al. 2015). An expressive language delay is in contrast to the loquacity of WS (Orellana et al. 2008; Torniero et al. 2008); this trait was more severely manifest in a child with a triplication of the WS segment (Beunders et al. 2010). Aortic dilatation is recognized (Parrott et al. 2015). A somewhat subtle observation of "straight, neat eyebrows" is noted (Dixit et al. 2013b).

dup 7q21.3q22.1 A small number of duplications of variable extents, in which band 7q21.3q22.1 is held in common, are on record, most coming from the era of classical cytogenetics (Alfonsi et al. 2012). The considerable heterogeneity of imbalance precludes making a firm karyotype-phenotype analysis. Some duplications are rather large, comprising as much as half or more of 7q; one of the smaller (but yet of 18.7 Mb) is described in Alfonsi et al., a child with a clinical picture not unlike Russell-Silver syndrome, having a de novo duplication of chr7:87.5-106.2 Mb.

Chromosome 8 Duplications

dup 8p23.1 Duplications within 8p23.1 (Fig. 14–52) present challenges in distinguishing between those that are pathogenic and those that are normal (or uncertain) variants (Barber et al. 2015). These authors advise upon a distinction between imbalances involving telomeric (chr8:8.3-9.5 Mb), centromeric (chr8:11.1-11.9 Mb), and "medial" (chr8:9.5-11.1 Mb) segments within this cytoband. These three regions lie within the bounds of olfactory receptor (REPD) and defensin (REPP) repeat sequences. When the entire 3.6 Mb segment is involved, this is referred to as the "8p23.1 duplication syndrome."

Two key pathogenic loci are *SOX7* at chr8:10.7 Mb (within the medial segment) and *GATA4* at chr8:11.7 Mb (in the centromeric segment). Duplication of *SOX7* determines a neurobehavioral phenotype, while *GATA4* may be responsible for congenital heart malformation. Duplication of the telomeric segment may be, of itself, without a phenotype; thus, this is seen as a normal variant, which can have been transmitted by an unaffected parent, and ascertainment is typically due to a fortuitous coincidental presentation. Smaller duplications within the medial and centromeric segments may also be nonpathogenic, and identified in a normal parent. The interested reader is referred to the detail in Barber et al. (2015).

Chromosome 9 Duplications

dup 9p24.3cen: Trisomy 9p Syndrome This is one of the more common partial trisomies, indeed said to be fourth in frequency after the three major full

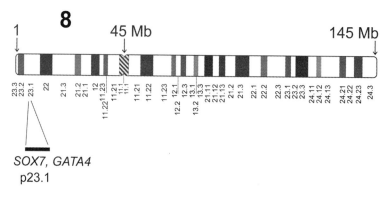

FIGURE 14–52

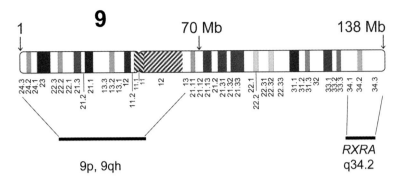

FIGURE 14–53

trisomies, and known since 1970 (Guilherme et al. 2014). In many, the duplication extends into the 9qh heterochromatic region, 9q11q12, and occasionally as far as q21.11 (Fig. 14–53). A paucity of dosage-sensitive loci within 9p, and a concentration of repeat sequences within the pericentromeric region, are the basis of its viability. Most cases in fact occur in the setting of a rearrangement with another chromosome (in these, the recurrence risk relates to the parental carrier status), but isolated examples are well recorded. The craniofacies is characteristic. Intellectual deficiency is typical, and Martínez-Jacobo et al. (2015) report in addition psychotic behavior; brain abnormality is often seen on imaging. However, one case with a partial 9p duplication of large size, 34 Mb (dup 9p13.3pter, chr9:0.6-34.5 Mb), had a normal IQ of 95 (Bouhjar et al. 2011), and Bouhjar et al. record a few other cases, with somewhat smaller 9p duplications, in whom intelligence was also within a normal range.

dup 9q34 Amarillo et al. (2015) review this condition, in which there is considerable heterogeneity of extent of the duplication. They propose that the heart malformation frequently seen in those in whom the duplicated segment includes 9q34.2 may be due to the *RXRA* locus at chr9:134.3 Mb. An intriguing story of a congenital vocal cord paralysis that resolved by age 21 months is described in Gadancheva et al. (2014), the child duplicated for chr9:129.9-135.9 Mb. Recurrence has been observed in the context of a parental balanced translocation (Mizuno et al. 2011).

Chromosome 10 Duplications

dup 10p Most 10p duplications are due to a parental rearrangement; a few cases arise de novo. The extents of duplication (Fig. 14–54) are variable, and likewise the associated phenotypes, as Mégarbané et al. (2001) discuss in considering their own case of dup(10)(p11.2p12.2).

dup 10q11.21q11.22 Manolakos et al. (2014) evaluate this condition, accumulating just eight cases; they speculate that the growth factor genes

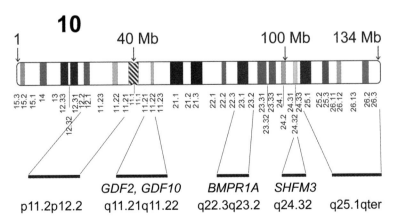

FIGURE 14–54

GDF2 and *GDF10* (chr10:47.3 Mb) may have an important role. Microcephaly with neurological deficit is typical. De novo inheritance is the rule.

dup 10q22.3q23.2 This is one of several microduplications that raises a dilemma when seen at prenatal diagnosis, due to its incomplete penetrance, and a paucity of recorded information. Kong et al. (2016) describe prenatally diagnosed cases, in the context of one parent being a carrier, and with a causal link between genotype and (variable) phenotype being uncertain. One case concerned a (presumably monozygous) twin pregnancy, both twins typing as dup chr10:77.83-87.32 Mb. While the index fetus was growth retarded and had ventriculomegaly, the "internal control" twin and the carrier mother were considered to be phenotypically normal. This illustrates the point that phenotypic abnormality is often the basis of ascertainment, and thus subject to bias. With this, and with so many other of the del/dups of uncertain significance, the collection of family data beyond the proband, and this being available internationally, is a desideratum of high degree. This recurrent duplication is the countertype of del(10)(q22.3q23.2) in which, by contrast, a phenotype is typically present.

dup 10q24.3: Split Hand Foot Malformation Syndrome Type 3 Duplications of small (kb size) extent in the 10q24.3 region are associated with this malformation syndrome; dysregulation of the *BTRC* and *SHFM3* genes at 10q24.32 (chr10:101.4 and 101.6 Mb, respectively) may be the key factor (Sowińska-Seidler et al. 2014). Neurocognitive functioning is typically intact, and familial transmission in an autosomal dominant pattern is common (Dai et al. 2013). Sibship recurrence due to maternal somatic-gonadal mosaicism is on record

(Dimitrov et al. 2010; Filho et al. 2011); we have seen 30% mosaicism in an unaffected father of a child with split hand foot malformation.

dup 10q25.1q25.3: Distal 10q Trisomy Syndrome Large duplications of distal 10q, involving most or all of 10q25, have been known for some time, the first reports appearing in the 1970s (Al-Sarraj et al. 2014). The clinical picture includes intellectual deficiency, microcephaly, facial dysmorphism (often with blepharophimosis), and distal limb defects. Most cases have been due to the malsegregation of a parental translocation, but some have reflected a de novo event, and the duplication being, in that case, "pure."

Chromosome 11 Duplications

dup 11p13 WT1 (chr11:32.4 Mb) and *PAX6* (chr11: 31.8 Mb) are well-known loci contained within this genomic segment (Fig. 14–55). Given the severity of the classic WAGR 11p13 deletion, the mild effect seen in some duplications of the similar segment is notable, as Dolan et al. (2011) emphasize in a dup chr11:30.0-35.1 Mb. Their patient had a slight delay in developing language, but by age 4 years was considered to be at an age-appropriate level; ophthalmology was normal, other than ptosis. (Ascertainment had been via his younger sibling with a typical WAGR syndrome, the father an insertion heterozygote.) However, a child with a small de novo duplication, chr11:31.68-31.84 Mb, involving only the *PAX6* "eye gene," had poor vision but no definite anatomic eye malformation; she was microcephalic, of short stature, and developmentally delayed (Aradhya et al. 2011). Defects of retina and iris were seen in the child in Aalfs et al. (1997), in whom the de novo duplication (chr11:22.3-33.6 Mb) also included *PAX6*. A different phenotypic effect was seen in the

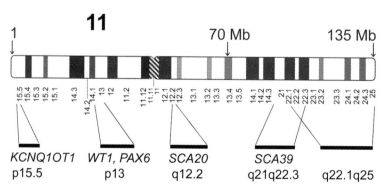

FIGURE 14–55

closely overlapping de novo dup chr11:31.5-35.6 Mb reported in Palumbo et al. (2014), a child presenting a picture resembling Russell-Silver syndrome. These apparent inconsistencies in karyotype-phenotype correlation are perplexing.

dup 11p15.5 Duplications at this locus can result in Beckwith-Wiedemann syndrome (BWS), Silver-Russell syndrome (SRS), or no phenotype, depending on the location of the duplication and the parental origin of the duplicated chromosome (Begemann et al. 2012; see also p. 413). The effect of genomic imbalance at this locus is rather complicated, reflecting changes in gene expression due both to altered copy number and to altered expression patterns.

Larger duplications that encompass both of the 11p15.5 imprinting control regions, ICR1 and ICR2, lead to SRS when maternally inherited, and BWS when paternally inherited. A familial three-generation duplication chr11:1,828,124-3,094,843 is one of the smallest on record to contain ICR1 and ICR2 (Vals et al. 2015): A grandfather with BWS had a daughter with the same diagnosis, and in turn, his granddaughter presented with the growth restriction of SRS. The pattern is different when the duplication is confined to just one of the ICRs. Duplications of the entire paternally-originating ICR1 (including *H19* and *IGF2*) cause BWS, whereas duplications of the maternal ICR1 are not associated with an aberrant phenotype. In contrast, duplications of the entire maternal ICR2 cause SRS, but they are phenotypically silent when paternally inherited. The correlation between genotype and phenotype is even more complex for smaller duplications. Maternal duplications that are restricted to just the *H19* portion of ICR1 cause an SRS phenotype, whereas paternal *H19* duplications are silent. Maternal duplications within ICR2 that are restricted to the *KCNQ1OT1* DMR, or to the *CDKN1C* enhancer region, cause a BWS phenotype.

dup 11q12.2, dup 11q21q22.3 These two duplications, of 0.3 and 7.5 Mb, respectively, have the interest that each is associated, and possibly causally, with a dominantly inherited adult-onset spincocerebellar ataxia: SCAs 20 and 39, respectively (Knight et al. 2008; Johnson et al. 2015). Which actual gene may be responsible for the ataxia is unknown. In SCA20, no other phenotypic effect is seen, presumably reflecting a triplo-insensitivity otherwise of the 10 genes within the chr11:61 Mb segment concerned. Some of the SCA39 family manifested mild intellectual disability, hearing impairment, and chest and foot deformity; these other aspects may inhere in overexpression of one or some of the 44 loci contained within chr11:96.1-103.6 Mb.

dup 11q22.1q25, Distal 11q Trisomy, Emanuel Syndrome A variety of duplications are observed, some encompassing the full length of 11q22.1qter—about half of the q arm—and some of more limited extent, such as dup(11)(q23.3q24.2) and dup chr11:110.2-119.2 Mb (Burnside et al. 2009; Chen et al. 2013d). Most are upon the basis of parental rearrangement, but de novo cases are known (Ben-Abdallah-Bouhjar et al. 2013). The Emanuel syndrome, essentially due to dup(11)(q23qter) from an inherited der(22)t(11;22)(q23;q11), is discussed on p. 87 and illustrated in Figure 5–10.

Chromosome 12 Duplications

dup 12p: Trisomy 12p Syndrome Duplication of the entire p arm (Fig. 14–56) was first reported in

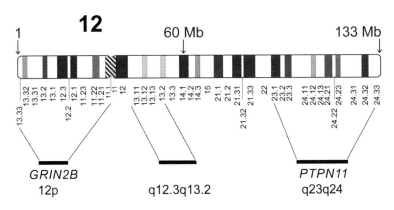

FIGURE 14–56

the 1970s, and it remains a rare condition. Partial duplications, more often terminal than interstitial, are similarly rare. The phenotype in the full 12p duplication is well recorded, including a distinctive craniofacial appearance and mental retardation (Poirsier et al. 2014). Inheritance is about equally de novo, or from malsegregation of a parental rearrangement. Only two instances are known of parental transmission, both involving small interstitial duplications: a father and son with an inv dup(12)(p12.3p11.2), and a mother and son with inv dup(12)(p12.3p13.1), respectively chr12:17.6-28.8 Mb and chr12:13.3-19.8 Mb. Albeit these duplicated segments were mostly non-overlapping, the phenotypes of a mild intellectual disability, and soft facial dysmorphism, were similar. Poirsier et al. make the case for GRIN2B at chr12:13.5 Mb as contributory to the neurocognitive phenotype in those persons with this gene duplicated. A remarkable story in Lim et al. (2013) describes twins with de novo mosaic full 12p trisomy; a somatic error likely occurred in very early embryogenesis, before the splitting which generated the twinning.

dup 12q12.3q13.2 Only four cases are on record in which these bands are included in the duplication, two being mosaic. The molecular description in the smallest (but still the repository for 40 genes) is chr12:52.5-53.7 Mb (Bertoli et al. 2013). Interestingly, the facial appearance in this case and that of the other nonmosaic child both resembled that of Wolf-Hirschhorn syndrome. All have been de novo.

dup 12q23q24 Bouman et al. (2013) review distal 12q duplications, of which the reported number is small, and most being unique. Their own case, a teenage boy with rudimentary speech, facial dysmorphism, and the inability to walk independently, represented the segment chr12:106.4-123.3 Mb. De novo cases and inheritance due to a parental rearrangement are both observed. Several genes that will be familiar to the counselor reside within 12q23q24, including *PTPN11, TCTN1, ATXN2*, and *TRPV4* (respectively genes for Noonan syndrome, Joubert syndrome, spinocerebellar ataxia type 2, and several pleiotropic phenotypes with *TRPV4*).

Chromosome 13 Duplications

dup 13q Partial trisomy 13, of large segments, is often viable, an unsurprising fact given observations in the full trisomy. With the availability of G-banding from the 1970s, a number of cases of partial trisomy 13 came to light, and the conclusions from that period quite considerably hold today (Rogers 1984). Duplications are grouped broadly into proximal and distal, with bands 13q14q22 as the dividing region (Fig. 14–57). Those of substantial size are invariably associated with psychomotor retardation. Certain features are peculiar to the segment: Thus, polydactyly is seen only in the distal duplication. Most cases are due to a parental rearrangement, while some are de novo, and of these, several involve the attachment of a 13q segment to another chromosome, as an "add."

Smaller duplications yield to FISH and molecular methodology. Thus, Bertini et al. (2010) describe a de novo proximal duplication of 13q11q13.2 (chr13:19.1-35.0 Mb), associated with severe mental retardation. Jobanputra et al. (2012) observed clinical normality in an infant with a de novo dup 13q32.2, chr13:99.8-100.4 Mb; these authors conclude that the *ZIC2* gene resident within this segment does not lead, in the dup state, to

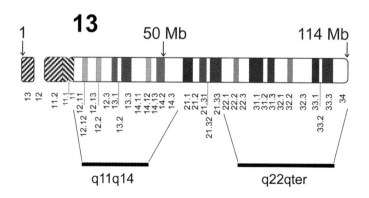

FIGURE 14–57

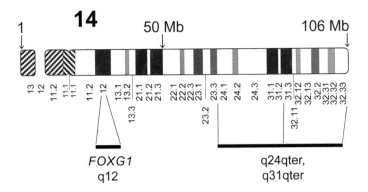

FIGURE 14-58

holoprosencephaly (which is does when deleted). Mascarenhas et al. (2008) report the prenatal diagnosis, in the case of severe fetal abnormalities seen on ultrasound, of a neocentromeric supernumerary marker chromosome, derived from a de novo inverted duplication of 13q31qter, and imposing a tetrasomy for this region.

Chromosome 14 Duplications

dup 14q12 Duplications within this band, or in some cases extending into the adjacent bands p11.2 and p13.1, are associated with epilepsy and mental retardation, along with a mild facial dysmorphism (Brunetti-Pierri et al. 2011). An additional copy of *FOXG1* at chr11:28.7 Mb (Fig. 14–58) is presumed a pheno-critical element (this gene is otherwise implicated in a Rett-like syndrome). De novo inheritance is the rule, but malsegregation from a parental translocation is on record.

dup Distal 14q Duplication of this large segment is seen with growth retardation, developmental delay, and facial dysmorphism. A parental inversion is always to be considered in the context of a terminal duplication of an acrocentric chromosome, as was the case in the children in Sgardioli et al. (2013) and Kurtulgan et al. (2015), with dup(14)(q31.3qter) and dup(14)(q24qter), respectively chr14:85.8-106.8 Mb and chr14:64.3-106.8 Mb.

Chromosome 15 Duplications

dup (or trp) 15q11.2q13.1 In this syndrome of intellectual impairment and autism but usually without dysmorphism, the imbalance exists either as a triplication due to a supernumerary chromosome (inv dup or isodicentric 15) or as an interstitial tandem duplication. Of the inv dup and idic, the typical triplicated segment, of ~6 Mb, lies between BP1 and BP3; while of the duplication, the classical segment consists of the ~5 Mb between BP2 and BP3 (Al Ageeli et al. 2014) (Fig. 14–59). At the molecular level, BP1-BP3 is chr15:22.6-28.5 Mb, and BP2-BP3 comprises chr15:23.4-28.5 Mb; both encompass the Prader-Willi/Anglelman region (Figs. 14–29 and 14–60).[36] It is with maternal transmission that the typical syndrome is seen; the phenotype may be normal on paternal inheritance (discussed below).

The intellectual impairment ranges from borderline to severe ("pervasive developmental disorder"), with autism often a prominent feature (Battaglia 2008; Hogart et al. 2009). Epilepsy is recognized, and gastrointestinal symptoms are common (Coppola et al. 2013a; Shaaya et al. 2015). The considerable majority of probands are of de novo generation, but transmission of the interstitial duplication from a parent (affected or unaffected), and indeed grandparent, is known (Bonuccelli et al. 2017). Rare duplications other than BP1-BP3 and BP2-BP3 are documented in Al Ageeli et al. (2014) and Isles et al. (2016).

Of particular interest is the susceptibility to schizophrenia due to the duplication. Almost exclusively, it is in those in whom the duplication is of maternal origin that this psychiatric disease is seen. The penetrance for schizophrenia in the maternally inherited dup(15)(q11.2q13.1) is 12%, compared to only 1%—essentially the

---

36 These imbalances are not to be confused with the nonpathogenic 15q11.2 euchromatic variant due to constitutional cytogenetic amplification, which does not involve the PWS/AS region (Barber 2005).

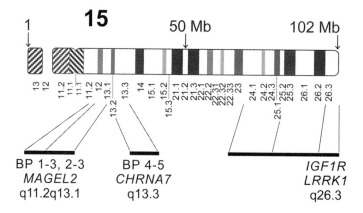

FIGURE 14-59

population figure—in paternal transmission (see color insert Fig. 14–60; Isles et al. 2016). The penetrance with respect to developmental disability, autism spectrum disorder, and multiple congenital anomaly also shows a bias, but less markedly so, toward maternal transmission: The respective parental penetrances with respect to these traits are 50% (mat) and 20% (pat). These differences presumably reflect the differing roles of imprinted genes with the segment. Note that these are the same imprinted genes[37] that are implicated, when deleted, in Prader-Willi and Angelman (and Schaaf-Yang) syndromes.

An isodicentric inv dup(15) which contains no euchromatin—the breakpoint presumed to be proximal to BP1—is classified as a nonpathogenic "small supernumerary marker chromosome" (sSMC) or, in the analysis of Webb (1994) from classical cytogenetics, a group 1 inv dup(15). Oracova et al. (2009) review this sSMC and report a familial example, a father and son, both normal men, the son having presented due to couple infertility. On sperm study (the son), one-quarter of cells were 24,+sSMC, and there was a slight increase (1.0% cf. 0.1% baseline) in cells disomic for chromosome 15. In vitro fertilization was unsuccessful, the cause obscure.

dup 15q13.3 This is one of the most frequently seen of the microduplications. The typical segment comprises ~2 Mb at chr15:30.38-32.39 Mb, involving BP4 and BP5 (Hassfurther et al. 2016). The pheno-critical locus contained therein is *CHRNA7* (chr15:32.03-32.16), coding for an acetylcholine receptor (Gillentine et al. 2017a). The clinical picture with the duplication is quite similar to that of the deletion, predominantly one of intellectual impairment, difficult behavior, autistic features, and subtle dysmorphism. (The dup/del similarity may reflect that, while excess *CHRNA7* components are produced in the duplication, chaperones cannot cope with the excess, and thus—as with the deletion—fewer than normal are actually assembled and trafficked to the cell membrane; Gillentine et al. 2017b.) Counseling is complicated by the incomplete penetrance and variable expressivity of this genomic disorder (Miller et al. 2009; van Bon et al. 2009).

dup Distal 15q Duplications can involve more than half the length of 15q. Zollino et al. (1999) propose a distinction between duplications of 15q21qter and 15q25qter. A clinical difference is that the former, larger imbalance is associated with microcephaly and unremarkable growth indices, whereas the smaller q25qter duplication is seen with macrocephaly and craniosynostosis, and tall stature; Tatton-Brown et al. (2009) refer to a "15q overgrowth syndrome." Intellectual handicap and facial dysmorphism are observed in both forms. A phenocritical locus with respect to the overgrowth may be the insulin-like growth factor receptor type 1, *IGF1R*, at chr15:98.6 Mb, albeit that Leffler et al. (2016; see next entry) make a case for *LRRK1* at chr15:100.9 Mb. These duplications are often the result of malsegregation of a parental translocation or inversion, but de novo examples exist (Chen et al. 2011a; Kim et al. 2011a).

---

37 A locus of particular pheno-contributory importance in these duplications/triplications may be *MAGEL2* at chr15:23.6 Mb.

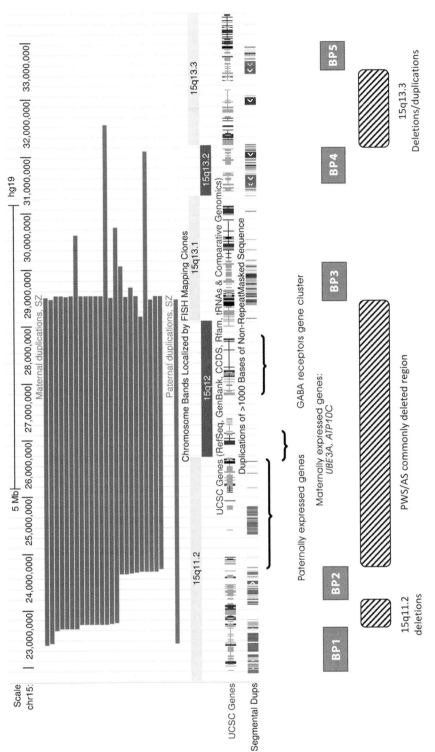

FIGURE 14–60 Susceptibility to del/dups rearrangement within the 15q11.2q13.3 region. The five important breakpoints, which define the extent of the several del/dups occurring in this region, are shown, BP1-BP5; these breakpoints coincide with the repeat sequences shown in the segmental duplications track. Above, in red (maternal) and blue (paternal) are the duplications[38] in a series of patients with schizophrenia; most are defined by BP1-BP3 and BP2-BP3. (Compare Fig. 14–29; See also the color insert.)

Source: From Isles et al, Parental origin of interstitial duplications at 15q11.2-q13.3 in schizophrenia and neurodevelopmental disorders, *PLoS Genet* 12: e1005993, 2016. Courtesy M.J. Owen and G. Kirov, and with the permission of the Public Library of Science, as per the Creative Commons public domain.

38 The degree to which sequences are homologous (and thus predisposing to illegitimate recombination) are color-coded in the segmental duplications track: light/dark gray 90%–98% homology; light/dark yellow 98%–99%; orange >99% (as seen in the color insert of this figure).

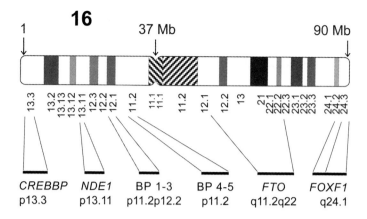

| 16 |
| 1 | 37 Mb | 90 Mb |

CREBBP | NDE1 | BP 1-3 | BP 4-5 | FTO | FOXF1
p13.3 | p13.11 | p11.2p12.2 | p11.2 | q11.2q22 | q24.1

FIGURE 14–61

dup 15q26.3 Duplication of this much smaller distal segment (which does not include *IGF1R*) is likewise associated with a syndrome of overgrowth as a particular feature. The intellectual compromise is of only mild degree, such that familial transmission is observed, in an autosomal dominant fashion (Leffler et al. 2016).

Chromosome 16 Duplications

dup Proximal 16p11.2, BP4-5 BP4 and BP5 encompass an ~600 kb segment within chr16:29.5-30.2 Mb (Fig. 14–61); *TBX6* at chr16:30.08-30.09 Mb is a useful landmark locus. This region provides another modern example of Lejeune's 1960s concept of type and countertype. The del (see above) leads to hyperphagia and obesity; the dup is associated with underweight (Jaquemont et al. 2011). In deletion carriers, upon a particular type of brain imaging (diffusion tensor imaging) that detects variation in the microstructure of white matter tracts, there are increases of "fractional anisotropy"[39] in the white matter, contrasted, in the duplication heterozygote, with decreases; and this reflects opposite influences upon the formation and integrity of white matter (Chang et al 2016). There is a 14-fold risk of psychosis and a 16-fold risk of schizophrenia (Giaroli et al. 2014). From a very large international study (*n* = 1,006), D'Angelo et al. (2016) show a full-scale IQ in probands of 26 points below that of noncarrier relatives, and in non-probands (whose ascertainment is therefore less biased), about 15 points below. Dysmorphism, if present, is mild. Parental transmission is frequent, and some relatives may be apparently unaffected. Rosenfeld

et al. (2013) estimate a penetrance of 27% (95% CI, 17%–41%), and thus a majority of heterozygotes would display a phenotype within the normal population range (but again the question arises that more thorough examination might reveal subtler differences, and in comparison with noncarrier relatives).

The discovery of a dup 16p11.2 might not necessarily explain a clinical presentation. Dastan et al. (2016) show this duplication in a child with facial dysmorphism and global developmental delay; his normal mother carried the same dup(16). To cast light on the mother–child difference, a whole exome study was done in the child, and this showed compound heterozygosity at *VPS13B*; thus, in retrospect, a diagnosis of Cohen syndrome could be appreciated. The dup(16) in the child was merely coincidental, of little or no discernible effect per se.

dup Distal 16p12.2p11.2, BP1-BP3 Breakpoint 1 is at chr16:21.8 Mb and BP3 at 29.1 Mb. Duplication of BP1-BP3 may lead to a syndrome including delayed motor development, mild to severe intellectual disability, autism, obsessive or stereotyped behavior, and a mildly dysmorphic facies (Barber et al. 2013; Okamoto et al. 2014). Rosenfeld et al. (2013) estimate a penetrance of 11% (95% CI, 6%–20%). Rare duplications may extend from BP1 through to BP5 at chr15:30.2 Mb (Tabet et al. 2012).

dup 16p13.11 Duplication for the same p13.11 deletion noted above may predispose to a range of neurodevelopmental disability, including intellectual deficiency, attention deficit disorder, autism,

---

39 Fractional anisotropy is used as a measure of fiber density, axonal diameter, and myelination.

and, less often, epilepsy (Ramalingam et al. 2011; Coe et al. 2014). Congenital anomalies and dysmorphism are seen in some. Segmental repeat sequences around chr16:15.0, 16.5 and 18.4 Mb define sites of rearrangement, leading to some heterogeneity of duplication extent. The most commonly observed imbalance, of ~1.3 Mb, lies between repeat sequence sites at chr16:15.0 and 16.5 Mb, with *NDE1*, at chr16:15.6 Mb, a sentinel gene. Larger, ~3 Mb duplications can extend to 18.4 Mb. The phenotype may be susceptible to the influence of a second-hit CNV elsewhere. Males are more susceptible, or, stated differently, females are more resistant, to the inimical effects of the imbalance (Tropeano et al. 2013). Both de novo and transmitted inheritance are observed, the transmitting parent, more often the mother, of either normal or (usually mildly) abnormal neurocognitive phenotype. Homozygosity for a chr16:15.0-18.7 Mb duplication (from a consanguineous union) has been reported, the neurocognitive phenotype, curiously enough, not particularly different from the heterozygous state (Houcinat et al. 2015).

dup 16p13.3 Duplications in this chromosomal region are the "countertypes" of the ATR-16 deletions above, including the key *CREBBP* locus (chr16:3.7 Mb), and are of similarly variable sizes. In the smallest kilobase-size duplications, *CREBBP* may be the only gene involved (Mattina et al. 2012). Intellectual disability with poor speech, mild periorbital dysmorphism, micrognathia, and proximally implanted thumbs are notable features (Demeer et al. 2013; Li et al. 2013). De novo inheritance is almost always the case, but nonpenetrance has been observed in two parents, who had "followed normal schooling, function normally in society, and do not present the typical face" (Thienpont et al. 2010). Inheritance from an affected parent is reported in Lee et al. (2016). Rare duplications not including *CREBBP* are known (Ciaccio et al. 2017).

dup 16q11.2q22 Lonardo et al. (2011) review "pure" proximal 16q duplications, concerning the segments q11q13, q21q22, and q23q24, to which they respectively refer as proximal, intermediate, and (rarely seen) distal. The small number of duplications on record are categorized as proximal, proximal-intermediate, intermediate, and intermediate-distal, and they are, for the most part, nonrecurrent. Both

de novo and, for some of the smaller imbalances, familial cases are observed. The heterogeneity of genotype hampers phenotypic correlation, although it is to be noted that obesity is seen in some (Odak et al. 2011). The *FTO* gene at 16q12.2, chr16:53.7-54.1 Mb, had been proposed as a susceptibility locus, but this was not supported by studies of the families in van den Berg et al. (2010) and in Davies et al. (2013). In the latter family, segregating a small 680 kb duplication, chr16:53.3-54.0 Mb, *RBL2* may have been pheno-contributory to the overweight.

dup 16q24.1 Two separate kilobase-length imbalance segments are recorded in 16q24.1, and in just one case, a duplication including both segments. Dharmadhikari et al. (2014) report three duplications of size 15–500 kb, all including the *FOXF1* locus (chr16:86.5 Mb), and all three familial. Phenotypes varied from normal psychomotor development to behavioral abnormality and autism, and bowel maldevelopment, in a three-generation pedigree. A 250 kb duplication at chr16:85.6-85.9 Mb is described in Quéméner-Redon et al. (2013), and with a severe phenotype, including epilepsy and spastic paraplegia; but the clinical picture was actually less marked in the single case in Dharmadhikari et al. spanning both segments (chr16:85.4-87.1 Mb). A microRNA, *MIR1910*, at chr16:85.7 Mb, is potentially a pheno-contributory factor. Quéméner-Redon et al. review other cases of 16q2 duplication, mostly from the classical era, and comprising large segments.

Chromosome 17 Duplications
dup 17p11.2: Potocki-Lupski Syndrome This condition was predicted to exist, as the reciprocal recombination product of the Smith-Magenis deletion (Potocki et al. 2000). The clinical picture is less severe than in Smith-Magenis syndrome, and it includes such rather nonspecific features as mental retardation, infantile hypotonia, and failure to thrive (Potocki et al. 2007; Lee et al. 2012). The key locus is *RAI1* (Fig. 14–62).

dup 17p12: Charcot-Marie-Tooth Neuropathy The most common form (40%) of Charcot-Marie-Tooth neuropathy, CMT1A, is due to the duplication of about 1.7 Mb in 17p12, which encompasses the *PMP22* (peripheral myelin protein 22) gene (Murphy et al. 2012).[40] It is the countertype of the

---

40 The duplicated segment of chromosome 17 is some 1.7 Mb in size, but it is "gene-sparse." The very few other genes contained therein appear to imply no phenotypic consequence, due to their being in imbalanced state.

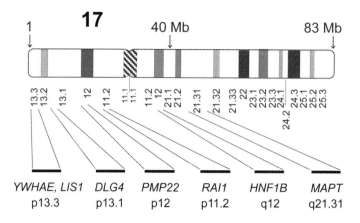

FIGURE 14–62

deletion which causes pressure-sensitive neuropathy. The duplication leads to the production of a 150% amount of the PMP22 protein, and this excess mars the capacity for proper functioning of the peripheral nerve. The sensory nerves are affected, but the major functional effect is on the motor nerves, and weakness is the important consequence. The nerves to the peroneal muscles (on the outside of the leg, with tendons passing around the ankle to the foot) are particularly vulnerable, and an alternative name for the condition is peroneal muscular atrophy. A rare circumstance is that of homozygosity for the duplication: effectively, a partial 17p tetrasomy, which leads to a more severe manifestation of the neurological phenotype (Pareyson et al. 2003).

A former laboratory diagnostic test was based upon FISH, which had the benefit of giving a direct visual demonstration of the duplication, with probe hybridizing twice to the duplicated chromosome, and seen as two adjacent fluorescent spots, with the third spot due to fluorescence from the other chromosome appearing elsewhere in the nucleus. The demonstration being so pretty, and as a nod to history, an example is shown in Figure 14–63.

Lebo (1998) proposes that prenatal diagnosis should be made available for CMT, notwithstanding that CMT can be a relatively mild handicap, and comments: "Given the slow rate of progress toward curing all forms of human genetic disease, patients with degenerative diseases who already have irreversible nerve pathology should not be offered undue hope for intervention by gene therapy." Couples will make their own decisions.

dup 17p11.2p12 Duplication encompassing both *RAI1* and *PMP22* produces a syndrome showing features of both Potocki-Lupski syndrome and Charcot-Marie-Tooth type 1A neuropathy (Yuan et al. 2015). Segmental lengths range from 3.2 to 19.7 Mb. These duplications are nonrecurrent, and all tested cases have been of de novo origin.

dup 17p13.1 A duplication of the same 17p13.1 region listed above as the deletion encompasses the same critical region chr17:7.1-7.3 Mb, within which lie proposed important loci including *DLG4*, *GABARAP*, *CTDNEP1*, and *GPS2*. Very few duplications are on record, and the segment extents differ

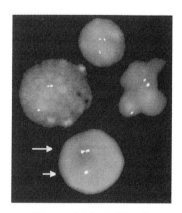

Charcot-Marie-Tooth
neuropathy type 1A

FIGURE 14–63   Charcot-Marie-Tooth neuropathy. FISH probe to 17p12 applied to an interphase cell, showing three signals. Two of the signals are closely adjacent, reflecting the duplicated segment. The remaining signal is from the normal homolog.

(sited between chr17:6.1 Mb through chr17:9.3 Mb), but all including the critical region (Coutton et al. 2012; Kuroda et al. 2014b; Mooneyham et al. 2014). Intellectual disability, of varying degree, is seen in common. All cases studied have been de novo.

dup 17p13.3 Duplication of the "Miller-Dieker region" produces a variable phenotype of intellectual deficiency and behavioral abnormality, in some diagnosed as autism, along with structural brain defects in a minority, especially of cerebellum and corpus callosum (Curry et al. 2013). Some have IQs in the normal range; curiously, mental capacity does not correlate well with dup size or location. Dysmorphism is subtle. No recurrent imbalances are seen; duplications range from kilobase size up to 4 Mb. Curry et al. group these into small telomeric duplications at chr17:0.8-1.6 Mb which include *YWHAE* at chr17:1.4 Mb; larger duplications encompassing most of 17p13.3; and small centromeric duplications of chr17:2.0-3.0 Mb, which include *LIS1* at chr17:2.6 Mb (Fig. 14–64). De novo and familial inheritance are seen with similar frequency. Affected parents are typically less affected than their (proband) child; somatic-gonadal and (presumed) confined gonadal mosaicism, with normal parents, are both recorded.

dup 17q12 A recurrent 1.4 Mb duplication, chr17:36.4-37.9 Mb, is associated with variable intellectual deficiency, difficult behavior, occasionally epilepsy, inconsistent minor facial dysmorphism, and certain mostly fairly minor malformations, but esophageal atresia as an uncommon major defect (Smigiel et al. 2014; Mitchell et al. 2015). *HNF1B* (ch17:37.7 Mb) is a useful landmark locus. Parental transmission is the rule, with the parent displaying, or not, some of the syndromic traits. Second-hit CNVs elsewhere in the genome may exacerbate the phenotype.

dup 17q21.31 The reciprocal duplication of the deletion for this segment had been considered to lead to a variable neurocognitive capacity, from moderate handicap to a normal IQ (Natacci et al. 2016). Anxiety with poor social interaction and autistic features were observed. However, Le Guennec et al. (2017) propose rather that the phenotype is one only of an early-onset dementia, and that the previous observations of intellectual disability were merely coincidental. The crucial gene is probably *MAPT* (chr17:45.9 Mb), duplication of which leads to an over-production of tau, this protein being the basis of the neurofibrillary tangles characteristic of Alzheimer's disease. Most cases have been de novo, but familial transmission is recorded. Thus, checking for this chromosome abnormality may come to be an appropriate test in cases of early-onset Alzheimer-like dementia; when the diagnosis is made in an index case, we expect that genetic counseling would follow the model as for other dominantly-inherited adult-onset neurodegenerative disease. Its unanticipated discovery at chromosome analysis would raise an ethical question (p. 13). This 17q21.31 rearrangement (deletion and duplication both) is associated with a particular inversion polymorphism in the parent that facilitates non-allelic homologous recombination between low-copy repeats flanking the region (p. 60).

Chromosome 18 Duplications

dup 18p, Trisomy 18p Jedraszak et al. (2015b) describe their patient with trisomy 18p (Fig. 14–65), only the 25th such to be reported, a man of mild intellectual deficiency, able to be employed, and with borderline facial dysmorphism. Three cases of maternal transmission are recorded; azoöspermia may be a basis of the non-observation of paternity. A recurrent (but very rare) rearrangement causing trisomy 18p is the curious supernumerary chromosome with a centromere derived from 13/21 material, but the euchromatin comprising only 18p (Plaja et al. 2013).

trp 18p, Tetrasomy 18p Sebold et al. (2010) review this syndrome, characterized by dysmorphism and numerous minor and some major malformations. Intellectual deficiency ranges from mild or borderline normal to severe and profound (O'Donnell et al. 2015). In all in whom parental studies were done in the large series of Sebold et al., the anomaly had been of de novo generation. However, recurrences are known, either from demonstrable somatic-gonadal mosaicism or from presumed gonadal mosaicism (Abeliovich et al. 1993; Boyle et al. 2001).

dup 18pterq12 Duplications comprising the whole p arm, plus the q arm to q12, are associated with a severe clinical picture, whereas a segment of lesser extent, a de novo dup(18)(p11.21q12.1), chr18:10.3-29.5 Mb, was identified in a child who had presented with an anorectal malformation, but successfully attending primary school (Schramm et al. 2011).

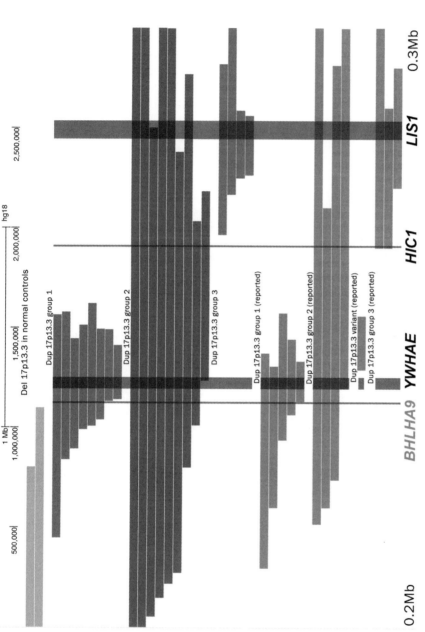

FIGURE 14–64   The range of 17p13.3 duplications from the study of Curry et al. (2013), considered in three groups, along the segment chr17:0.2–3.0 Mb. As the heterogeneity of segment size attests, nonrecurrence is the rule. Group 1 comprises smaller dups within chr17:0.8-1.6 Mb, and which include *YWHAE*. Group 2 comprises larger dups. Group 3 comprises smaller dups within chr17:2.0–3.0 Mb, with *LIS1* the key landmark locus. The thick vertical lines give positions of *YWHAE* and *LIS1*; thin vertical lines denote positions of (*left*) *BHLHA9* at chr17:1.2 Mb and (*right*) *HIC1* at chr17:2.0 Mb as "sentinel" loci. The upper groups are from the study of Curry et al.; the lower "reported" cases are from the literature otherwise. Two nonpathogenic 17p terminal deletions are shown at the top. Scale at top is in build hg18.

Source: From Curry et al., The duplication 17p13.3 phenotype: Analysis of 21 families delineates developmental, behavioral and brain abnormalities, and rare variant phenotypes, *Am J Med Genet* 161A: 1833–1852, 2013. Courtesy C. J. R. Curry and W. B. Dobyns, and with the permission of John Wiley & Sons.

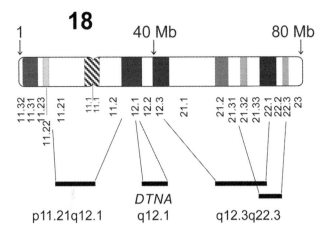

FIGURE 14–65

dup 18p11.32p11.31 This (genomically and genetically) small segment on distal 18p may be, when duplicated, associated with a mild degree of intellectual deficiency and difficult behavior, but without effect upon the physical phenotype. The picture is sufficiently mild that familial transmission is quite possible (Balasubramanian et al. 2016).

dup 18q12.1 Two de novo 4–6 Mb duplications including the *DTNA* locus (chr18:34.7 Mb) have been associated with autism, along with mild to moderate intellectual deficiency, seizures, and short stature (Wang et al. 2013b).

dup 18q Rare duplications within 18q12q22 have an association with intellectual deficiency and epilepsy. In one case with precise molecular distinction, a de novo duplication at chr18:43.9-69.8 Mb, dup(18)(q12.3q22.1), was documented in a man with a severe

intellectual disability, a lack of sphincter control, epilepsy, and minor dysmorphisms (del Gaudio et al. 2014). A partially overlapping more distal 12 Mb duplication involving 18q21.31q22.2 is of interest in that three affected children had been born to a (university graduate) mosaic mother, mos46,XX,dup(18)(q21q22)[90]/46,XX[10] (Ceccarini et al. 2007). An inherited 18q21q23 dup apparently slightly larger, of chr18:59.4-73.2 Mb, is in Henson et al. (2012); but in contrast to Ceccarini et al., the phenotypes in mother and daughter in this latter case could be seen as falling within a normal range.

Chromosome 19 Duplications
dup 19p Very few 19p duplications are recorded, and Ishikawa et al. (2013) provide a review. The imbalances are nonrecurrent and vary in size from 0.8 to 8.9 Mb, within 19q13.2 and 19q13.3 (Fig. 14–66); all have been de novo. Their own case

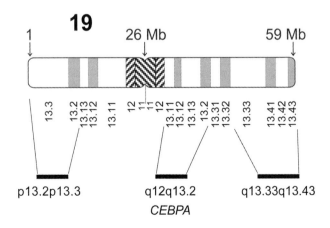

FIGURE 14–66

with a dup 19p13.3, chr19:0.3-6.1 Mb, presented with a severe psychomotor deficit and a distinctive facies.

dup 19q12q13.2 Variable microcephaly/macrocephaly, developmental delay, obesity, and an unusual facies characterize these proximal 19q duplications (Davidsson et al. 2010; Lugli et al. 2011). The obesity can be of severe degree, and *CEBPA* at chr19:33.3 Mb, whose gene product modulates the expression of leptin and influences the insulin receptor, is one of a number of candidate loci. The several involved segments are nonrecurrent and lie approximately between chr19:28-42 Mb; the overlapping region in common is chr19:33-40 Mb, within 19q13.11q13.2. All cases have been de novo.

dup 19q13.33q13.43 Distal 19q is (as is the chromosome as a whole) particularly gene-dense, and very few duplications from the molecular era are recorded. Carvalheira et al. (2014) reviewed terminal duplications, ranging in size from 0.4 to 10.6 Mb, some of which were familial due to a parental rearrangement. The largest such was their own case, which concerned a girl with minor dysmorphism, intellectual disability, and epilepsy, and whose de novo dup chr19:47.9-58.5 Mb was due to a translocation of the 19q segment onto 21p. Two other cases in DeScipio et al. (2008) also involved translocation to an acrocentric short arm, but in these cases coming from a maternally-transmitted translocation.

Chromosome 20 Duplications

dup 20p Bartolini et al. (2013) review trisomy for all, or almost all, of 20p, most cases coming from the premolecular literature. Their own patient had a de novo 17.98 Mb dup, at chr20:8.0-26.1 Mb, cytogenetically (20)(p12.3p11.21) (Fig. 14–67). The syndrome entails mental retardation with speech delay, finger abnormalities, and moderate facial dysmorphism. An isochromosome 20p, which endows a tetrasomy 20p (trp20p), leads to severe multiple malformation (Fryer et al. 2005).

dup 20p12.3 This single cytoband duplication, at chr20:7.5-8.3 Mb, is associated with the cardiac conduction anomaly, Wolff-Parkinson-White syndrome (WPWS). The child in Mills et al. (2013) presented as a newborn with heart failure due to tachyarrhythmia, but responded well to treatment. She was otherwise, at age 5 months, essentially unremarkable. Her father and uncle, both diagnosed with attention deficit, and the latter also with WPWS, carried the duplication. WPWS is seen also in the corresponding 20p deletion, supporting the contention of a causal link. *PLCB1* at chr20:8.3 Mb is a sentinel locus.

dup 20q11.2 Avila et al. (2013) delineate the syndrome due to dup(20)(q11.2), the region in common being chr20:31.6-38.7 Mb. The notable clinical feature is trigonocephaly with ridging of the metopic suture, along with psychomotor delay, poor speech acquisition, and short hands and feet. *ASXL1*, at chr20:32.2 Mb, is a plausible phenocontributory locus, and Avila et al. draw attention to a clinical similarity with Borhing-Opitz syndrome, which is due to mutation in this gene. All cases have been of de novo generation.

Distal 20q Duplication Blanc et al. (2008) review reports concerning duplication within 20q13.1qter,

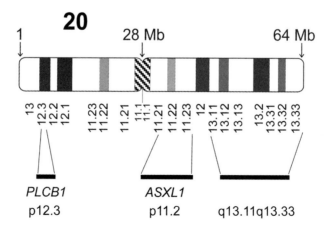

FIGURE 14–67

and it is true that very few examples exist of "pure" 20q duplication. Some comprise a large fraction of 20q and include 20qter; others, including the case in Blanc et al., concern an interstitial dup, theirs comprising a de novo dup (20)(q13.2q13.2). The clinical picture includes craniofacial dysmorphism and a wide range of neurodevelopmental delay, especially affecting language.

Chromosome 21 Duplications

dup 21q22.11q22.13 A particular point of interest concerns the Down syndrome critical region (DSCR) at 21q22.1 (Fig. 14–68). Broadly speaking, a duplication in which this segment is included leads to a DS picture; duplications elsewhere may convey only partial effects, or merely hints, of the overall DS phenotype (Korenberg et al. 1994; Ohira et al. 1996). The roles of certain genes, and the precise extent of the DSCR, are not fully determined. (It may have been a misnomer to have thus labeled the *DSCR1* gene, and its alternative name of *RCAN1* may be more suitable; the case for *DYRK1A* (chr21:37.4 Mb) as the major DS determinant is stronger: Eggermann et al. 2010b; Park and Chung 2013). The dementia of DS is due to duplication of the *APP* locus; a dup of 21q21.3 alone, containing *APP*, is of itself a determinant of early onset dementia (Meschino et al. 2016; see also p. 14).

dup 21cenq21.3 A duplication comprising about the proximal half of 21q, to chr21:30 Mb, may lead to developmental delay with poor speech acquisition, hypotonia, and joint hyperlaxity, these being fairly nonspecific DS features; but not with the DS facies (Korenberg et al. 1994; Capkova et al. 2014).

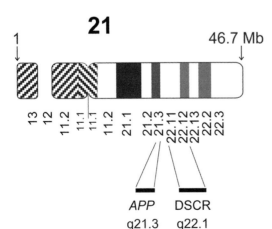

FIGURE 14–68

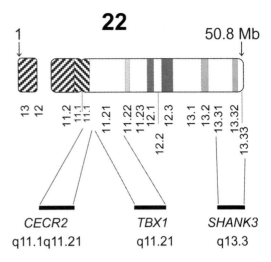

FIGURE 14–69

Chromosome 22 Duplications

dup, trp 22q11.1q11.21: Cat-Eye Syndrome, Schmid-Fraccaro Syndrome The cytogenetics of this imbalance varies, and it can be seen typically as a supernumerary inv dup(22)(q11.21) or der(22) (q11.1q11.21), but also as an intrachromosomal duplication or triplication. The eponymous eye sign is iris coloboma; developmental delay, ear tags, renal and anal anomaly, and occasionally the severe cardiovascular malformation, total anomalous pulmonary venous return, are variably associated. The segment involved is chr22:17.3-17.9 Mb, and *CECR2, SLC25A18,* and *ATP6V1E1* are proposed as pheno-contributory loci (Fig. 14–69). Both the intrachromosomal and supernumerary forms can be familial, and it would be obligatory to offer parental testing (Belangero et al. 2012; Knijnenburg et al. 2012; Jedraszak et al. 2015a). Mosaicism is common. One mother had 4.5% mosaicism in blood, while her two affected sons had levels of 85% and 70%; and reproductive study in one mosaic man, the father of three mosaic children, showed 50% of sperm to carry the inv dup(22) (Kvarnung et al. 2012; Jedraszak et al. 2015a). The genetic landscape of 22q11, with respect to this and the adjacent del/dup 22q11.21 (next entry), is reviewed in Tan et al. (2010).

dup 22q11.21 The countertype of the common del(22)(q11) is a duplication for the same ~3 Mb segment, chr22:18.7-21.6 Mb (Portnoï 2009). Theoretically, the dup(22)(q11) should be similarly common, but it is not—or to be precise, it is not as commonly recognized. The clinical picture is quite diverse, ranging from essential normality to multiple malformation, including defects as severe as the genitourinary defect, exstrophy-epispadias complex (Draaken et al. 2010). In perhaps a first for a chromosomal imbalance, dup heterozygotes may have, in at least one respect, *better* mental health than a general population: There may be a protective effect against schizophrenia (Rees et al. 2014a). This neurofunctional benefit does not, however, extend to intellectual capacity, and equally, susceptibility to autism is increased. Nevertheless, among parents of diagnosed children, some dup carriers, functioning normally, will be discovered. This very wide range of expressivity, and merging into nonpenetrance, makes for challenging counseling (Dupont et al. 2015); the coexistence of CNVs elsewhere in the genome may be the basis, in part at least, of this phenotypic variation (Fig. 14–70).

Recurrence from chromosomally normal parents has not, as yet, been reported, but a theoretical risk exists. Demaerel et al. (2016) report siblings of normal parents, one with dup 22q11, the other with del 22q11, both coming from the mother. Familial examples are known, including one case of a three-generation family, in which eight individuals had the dup(22), evincing a range of fairly minor malformation and neurobehavioral phenotypic effects (Yu et al. 2008).

dup 22q13 The countertype of Phelan-McDermid syndrome presents with developmental delay, very limited language acquisition, and mild dysmorphism (Okamoto et al. 2007). *SHANK3* in 22q13.33 (chr22:50.6 Mb) is the relevant locus. Both de novo and familial cases due to a parental translocation are known.

TRIPLICATION

A few examples of trp have been included in the dup listing above. With very few cases reported, an empiric recurrence risk cannot usefully be determined for the typical sporadic case. Parental gonadal mosaicism remains a possibility, as illustrated by the example in Eckel et al. (2006) of a phenotypically normal mother with a 46,XX,trp(12)(pter→p11.22::p11.22→p12.3::p12.3→qter)[6]/46,XX[44] karyotype, her son having the triplication in nonmosaic

form; see also the trp(22)(q11.1q11.21) entry above. Such examples oblige caution. Rare instances are reported of a nonpathogenic duplication in a parent leading to a pathogenic triplication in a child (López-Expósito et al. 2008).

SMALL SUPERNUMERARY MARKER CHROMOSOMES: 47,+MAR

A small (smaller than a chromosome 20) supernumerary chromosome, the identity of which could not readily (or at all) be determined on classical methodology, has been referred to as a "marker" (mar). The expression "mar" is becoming somewhat outdated, as molecular methodology now allows the supernumerary chromosome to be identified precisely, and, in recurring examples, a specific syndromal status may be assigned (Jafari-Ghahfarokhi et al. 2015). Most are derived from an acrocentric chromosome. A number have been listed above under the category "Duplications": the 11p11.2 neocentromeric sSMC; the inv dup or isodicentric 15 (pathogenic and nonpathogenic); the 18p sSMC whose centromere is of 13/21 material; and the inv dup(22)(q11.21) or der(22)(q11.21) sSMC of cat-eye syndrome. Some sporadic cases may derive from more than one chromosome (Manvelyan et al. 2015). Some small isochromosomes (next section) have been referred to as sSMCs.

If the parental blood karyotypes are normal, parental mosaicism is unlikely, but not completely excluded. The load in gametes may be less than seen on peripheral blood, at least in the case of the male (Cotter et al. 2000; Oracova et al. 2009). The dup(22)(q11.21) of cat-eye syndrome (above) is exceptional in that mosaicism, and which can be familial, is commonly observed.

ISOCHROMOSOMES (NONACROCENTRIC)

We deal in detail with isochromosomes in relation to their discovery at prenatal diagnosis in Chapter 21, and including the following derived from a nonacrocentric[41] chromosome: 47,+i(5p), 47,+i(8p), 47,+i(9p), 47,+i(10p), 47,+i(12p), 47,+i(18p), 47,+i(18q), and 46,i(20q). A couple having had a child with an isochromosome, for a chromosome

---

41 As for the acrocentric-derived isochromosome (Chapter 7), a postzygotic mechanism may be the rule, and thus of optimistic outlook for a subsequent pregnancy (Riegel et al. 2006).

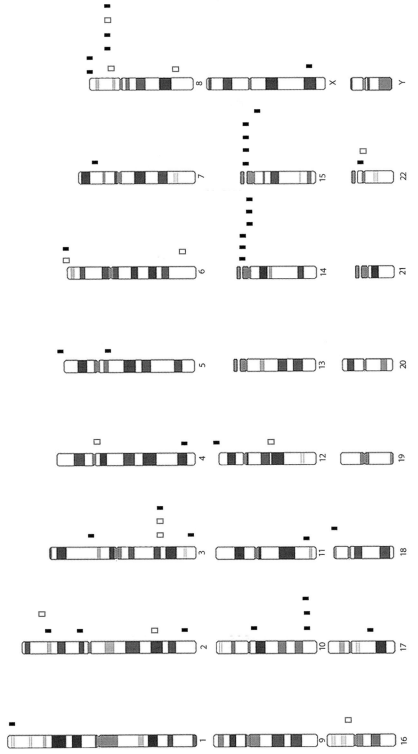

FIGURE 14–70   Locations of copy number variants coexisting with the dup 22q11.21 in 11 individuals out of a cohort of 17. Filled bar = duplication; open bar = deletion. These several accompanying CNVs may contribute to the variable expressivity seen in this duplication syndrome (a concept that may apply rather widely). Several cases have more than one CNV, with a maximum, in one case, of eight; the detail of which patients carried which CNVs is recorded in the original paper.

Source: From Dupont et al, Prenatal diagnosis of 24 cases of microduplication 22q11.2: An investigation of phenotype-genotype correlations, *Prenat Diagn* 35: 35–43, 2015. Courtesy C. Dupont, and with the permission of John Wiley & Sons.

other than an acrocentric, can generally be given encouraging advice, especially if the child is mosaic. The major mechanisms of generation are considered to operate either at meiosis II or postzygotically, and in either case no discernibly increased risk of recurrence would be implied, albeit that a premeiotic mechanism may apply in some (de Ravel et al. 2004; Rittinger et al 2015). Very rare exceptions exist: The history in Boyle et al. (2001) (above: trp 18p, tetrasomy 18p) is most remarkable—two half-sisters both with 47,XX,i(18p), their mother an inferred gonadal mosaic.

15

SEX CHROMOSOME ANEUPLOIDY AND STRUCTURAL REARRANGEMENT

THERE ARE FOUR MAJOR sex chromosome abnormalities due to *complete aneuploidy*. Otherwise unassisted, infertility is practically inevitable in XXY Klinefelter syndrome and 45,X Turner syndrome. The other two conditions, XXX and XYY, apparently have little effect on fertility; furthermore, they are not discernibly associated with any increased risk for chromosomally abnormal offspring. Mosaic forms need to be considered on their own merits, albeit that infertility is often the case with Klinefelter and Turner mosaicism, at least in those cases coming to clinical attention. As for recurrence, to parents who have had a child with one of these aneuploidies, typically, the risks are low.

Structural rearrangement of X or Y leads to a partial imbalance. This may involve a large amount of chromatin, such as in substantial deletions, a ring, or an isochromosome. Or, deletion or duplication may involve only a small segment (of kilobase, or a few megabases, in extent). Some of the latter may have little effect upon fertility, and reproductive risk assessment becomes of practical importance. The recurrence risks vary.

BIOLOGY

We need briefly to consider why X chromosome aneuploidy can be associated with so little phenotypic abnormality, compared with autosomal imbalance. The important factor is dosage compensation. Only one X in each cell needs to be fully active. Thus, potentially detrimental effects of an X chromosomal imbalance are mitigated (although not exactly canceled out) by *in*activating a supernumerary or abnormal X, or by *not* inactivating a sole remaining X, as the case may be.

The conceptus with an X chromosome complement in excess of the normal 46,XX or 46,XY accommodates to this imbalance by inactivating any additional X chromosome; or, as Migeon (2007) emphasizes, by maintaining, in each cell, just one X in the active state. This is nearly successful in the 47,XXX female and the 47,XXY male, in each of whom there is apparently normal in utero survival and a relatively mild postnatal phenotype. The fact that some loci are not subject to inactivation, and may therefore function in the X disomic (XXY), trisomic (XXX), or even quintasomic (49,XXXXX) states, is likely the predominant reason for the phenotypic abnormalities associated with these karyotypes.

In females with abnormal X chromosomes, the pattern of X-inactivation is usually nonrandom, particularly when the imbalance due to the abnormality is "large." In the 46,X,abn(X) karyotype, with one normal X and one abnormal X—an "abn(X)," as we write it here—the abnormal X is characteristically the inactive one. However, if the abnormality is a microdeletion or microduplication, the inactivation pattern can be random. In the case of the X-autosome balanced translocation heterozygote, the normal X is usually, although not invariably, inactive (Chapter 6).

Laboratory Test for X-Inactivation. Analyzing the pattern of X chromosome methylation with molecular methodology shows whether inactivation is random or nonrandom. A useful assay is methylation-specific polymerase chain reaction based on the androgen receptor gene, located at Xq13 (or any other gene with a convenient polymorphism). A highly skewed pattern, with one X mostly methylated and the other mostly not, is indicative of nonrandom inactivation (Kubota et al. 1999). While this test is performed routinely on a blood sample, there are grounds for believing that the assay result may, at least to some extent, fairly represent the state in other body tissues (Bittel et al. 2008). The former tests of Barr body and late-labeling BrdU analysis are of historic interest; both assays still provide a nice visual illustration of the concept of X-inactivation (Figs. 15–1 and 15–2).

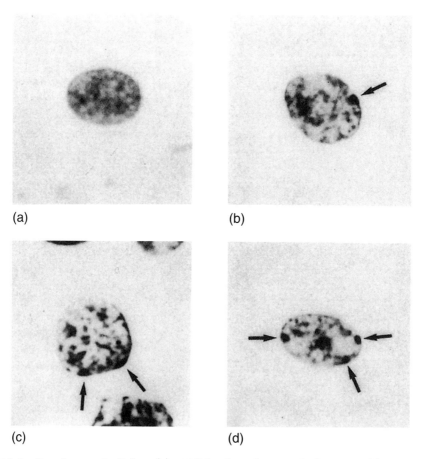

(a)

(b)

(c)

(d)

FIGURE 15–1 Buccal mucosal cells from (a) a 45,X female, with no Barr body present; (b) a 46,XX female showing the inactive X as a Barr body; (c) a 47,XXX female showing two Barr bodies; and (d) a 48,XXXX female with three Barr bodies.

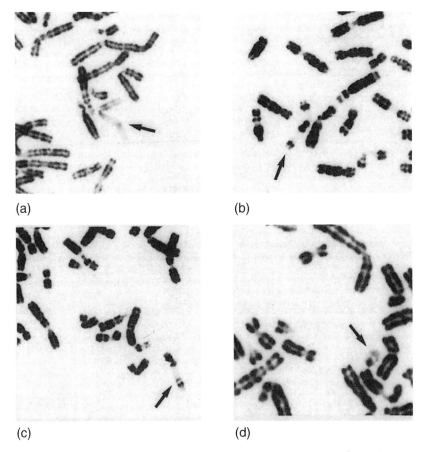

(a)　(b)　(c)　(d)

FIGURE 15–2　Partial metaphases showing X-inactivation: (*a*) a normal X chromosome, (*b*) an isochromosome of X long arm, (*c*) an X with a short arm deletion, and (*d*) a ring X. BrdU had been added for the last 6 hours of culturing. The inactive chromosomes, replicating at this late time in the cell cycle, incorporate BrdU extensively, and thus are palely stained. The active X stains darkly.

Y chromosome imbalance is similarly mild in its effects, but for a quite different reason, namely the very low gene carriage of this chromosome, and the very narrow scope of activity—male gonadal development—of most of these genes. As discussed elsewhere, the *SRY* gene on the Y short arm has the critical role of directing the gonad to form as a testis; other loci, most notably the *DAZ* family of genes within the AZFc region on the long arm, determine aspects of spermatogenesis (Krausz and Casamonti 2017).

Complete Aneuploidy

DETAILS OF MEIOTIC BEHAVIOR

Meiosis proceeds differently in persons with each of the various sex chromosome abnormalities, and each warrants separate consideration.

XXX

On theoretical grounds, one might have expected the three X chromosomes to display 2:1 segregation, with the production of equal numbers of X and XX ova. But this is not the case. No discernible increased risk for chromosomally abnormal offspring of these women has been demonstrated: In the extensive review of Otter et al. (2010), only one case had ever been reported of an XXX mother having had an XXX daughter. Apparently, only normal ova, with a single X, are regularly produced. It may be that the extra X is lost before meiosis occurs (Neri 1984), with meiosis then proceeding as in the normal XX female. Fertility may, however, be affected, due to premature ovarian failure (Tartaglia et al. 2010).

XXY AND XXY MOSAIC STATES

Barring medical intervention, infertility is almost inevitable in nonmosaic Klinefelter syndrome (KS), although some remarkable exceptions exist (Terzoli et al. 1992); undetected XY/XXY mosaicism could account for some of these cases. Bergère et al. (2002) showed both XY and XXY cell populations in testicular biopsies from three of four men who, on blood karyotyping and fluorescence in situ hybridization (FISH) analysis, were nonmosaic 47,XXY. These three men had small numbers of sperm identified in the biopsied tissue (one went on to have a child by in vitro fertilization [IVF]).

Van Saen et al. (2012b) list three subgroups of adult men with KS, according to findings on testicular biopsy: one group in which mature spermatozoa can be retrieved by testicular extraction, a group with no testicular spermatozoa but in which germ cells are present, and a third group with no germ cells at all. Several workers have karyotyped sperm from XXY men, and all find an excess, albeit not a large one, of 24,XX and 24,XY sperm. Possibly, these XY and XX sperm come from XXY spermatogonial stem cells, in which an asymmetric disjunction has occurred. Alternatively, the abnormal gonadal environment may of itself predispose to gonosomal nondisjunction in the XY tissue; and from that stance, autosomal segregation may also be vulnerable, as indeed sperm studies indicate: There is a higher rate of disomy 21 on sperm studies from Klinefelter men, 6.2% versus 0.4% in controls (Hennebicq et al. 2001; Bergère et al. 2002). As for XY/XXY mosaicism, Samplaski et al. (2014) showed better androgenization on a number of criteria in these men, including a higher rate of men having sperm in the ejaculate (half, compared to only 4% in nonmosaic XXY).

XYY

The clinical observation is that XYY men have no *discernible* increase in risk to have children with a sex chromosome aneuploidy (and XYY or XXY would have been the theoretical risk outcomes, from an XYY trivalent at meiosis). A true increased risk of a fraction of a percent could be distinguished only with great difficulty, when the background population risk is of a similar order of magnitude. On laboratory study, XYY spermatocytes proceeding through meiosis encounter checkpoints that may lead to elimination of most of the abnormal forms (Milazzo et al. 2006), but nevertheless, some men may have a small increased fraction of 24,YY and 24,XY spermatozoa in the ejaculate, and in some also, of autosomal disomies.

A distinction may be drawn between XYY men presenting with infertility and those whose fertility is intact, with the sperm aneuploidy rate somewhat higher in the former. Rodrigo et al. (2010) studied the cytogenetics of the preimplantation embryo, from five infertile XYY men having had IVF. The rates of chromosome abnormality were double that of a control group, with particular elevations in XY aneuploidy and triploidy. In one man with azoöspermia, having come to testicular biopsy, both Y chromosomes were present and in synapsis in all meiotic spermatocytes, and in association with—but not synapsing with—the X chromosome, and this configuration may possibly have been the cause of spermatogenic arrest (Wu et al. 2016a). Such a scenario may apply in the minority of XYY men presenting with infertility.

NONMOSAIC 45,X TURNER SYNDROME

The great majority of women with 45,X Turner syndrome (TS) are infertile and do not spontaneously menstruate or develop secondary sexual characteristics. The ovaries initially appear to be normal but typically begin to degenerate in midfetal life. Oöcytes undergo apoptosis and disappear at an accelerated rate and, in most cases, are gone by the age of 2 years: "The menopause occurs before the menarche" (Federman 1987; Modi et al. 2003). It may be that a 45,X oöcyte could not proceed through meiosis I, given that the sex chromosome has no homolog with which to pair. In one series of 18 45,X girls, none had ovarian follicles on biopsy in childhood or teenage (Borgström et al. 2009).

Completed pregnancy in women with an apparent 45,X karyotype is very rare. In a Danish study based on a national TS register, none of 200 45,X women achieved a natural pregnancy (one had twins by ovum donation) (Birkebaek et al. 2002). In a large French study, coming from seven endocrine units nationwide, 480 adult women with TS were recruited (Bernard et al. 2016). Of the 181 with monosomy X, only two had achieved pregnancy, although presumably not all had been attempting motherhood (Table 15–1; other chromosomal forms of TS also listed here). Sybert (2005) was able to record a total of 18 45,X women having had 42 pregnancies, and observed that the risks for spontaneous abortion, sex chromosome aneuploidy, and trisomy 21 were all elevated. Only 17 of the

Table 15–1. Data from 480 Adult Women with Turner Syndrome, According to Karyotype and Reproductive Outcomes

CHARACTERISTICS	PREGNANT TS PATIENTS (*n* = 27)	NONPREGNANT TS PATIENTS (*n* = 453)
Age at diagnosis*	20 (0–45)	10 (0–64)
45,X	2/27 (7%)	179/453 (40%)
45,X/46,XX	19/27 (70%)	111/453 (25%)
Mosaicism with Y	1/27 (4%)	20/453 (4%)
Mosaicism with ring X	2/27 (7%)	30/453 (7%)
Isochromosome X	1/27 (4%)	27/453 (6%)
Other	2/27 (7%)	86/453 (19%)
Spontaneous menarche	25/27 (93%)	70/453 (15%)
Age at first pregnancy (years)	27.5 (18–38)	n/a
Delay to conceive (months)	6 (0–84)	n/a

*Years, median and range.
n/a, not applicable; TS, Turner syndrome.
Source: From Bernard et al. (2016).

pregnancies proceeded to live birth, including two cases of 45,X and one of trisomy 21.

What is the explanation for fertility in these rare cases? An obvious point to consider is gonadal mosaicism, with a 46,XX cell line in the ovary. This has often been suggested, but rarely proven (Birkebaek et al. 2002). Jacobs et al. (1997) undertook a systematic search in 84 subjects with TS whose standard blood karyotype was 45,X, with molecular testing of blood and of a second tissue (buccal cells) and found only two cases of X/XX mosaicism. One very thorough study is that reported in Magee et al. (1998b), concerning a 45,X woman who had had seven pregnancies, five miscarrying, one producing a healthy male, and the last terminated following demonstration of fetal cystic hygroma and a 45,X karyotype on amniocentesis. Biopsies of skin, uterus, and ovary at subsequent gynecological surgery all gave a 45,X karyotype, but molecular testing showed two alleles in ovarian DNA, indicating the presence of occult 46,XX tissue. A similar investigation is reported in Sugawara et al. (2013) of a woman 45,X on standard blood karyotype, but other XX and XXX cell lines seen when 500 cells were analyzed by FISH, and skin and cumulus tissue studied (and even, inexplicably, 4/260 cumulus cells were XY). It is difficult to know, but fair to consider, whether such subtly occult mosaicism might be the explanation for the very rare instances of true natural fertility in (apparently) nonmosaic 45,X TS.

X/XX, X/XX/XXX, AND X/XXX MOSAICISM TURNER SYNDROME

The relative fractions of the various karyotypes—at least as may be judged on standard peripheral blood analysis—are listed in Table 15–2 and

Table 15–2. Relative Frequencies of Turner Syndrome Karyotypes

CLASSIC MONOSOMY	45,X	46%
X mosaicism	X/XX, X/XXX, X/XX/XXX	7%
Isochromosome Xq	45,X/46,X,i(Xq), 46,X,i(Xq)	18%
Ring	45,X/46,X,r(X)	16%
Deletion Xp	45,X/46,X,del(Xp), 46,X,del(Xp)	5%
Structural abnormality of Y		6%
Other		2%

Source: Jacobs et al. (1997).

illustrated in Figure 15–3. In the X/XX state, some gonadal function is likely to be retained if the 46,XX fraction reaches 10%, as evidenced by a spontaneous menarche (Castronovo et al. 2014). Among the TS categories, the X/XX karyotype is associated with the best chance for pregnancy, natural or IVF-assisted, but nevertheless the odds are poor (Doğer et al. 2015; Bernard et al. 2016). The survival of 45,X cells in the gonad may be enabled by support from surrounding 46,XX oögonia; such a 45,X cell might, in theory, be able to produce a nullisomic X egg, if its sole X is sequestered to the polar body at meiosis I. This could be the basis of the observation in Uehara et al.

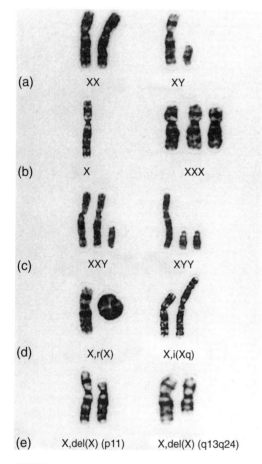

(a) XX   XY

(b) X   XXX

(c) XXY   XYY

(d) X,r(X)   X,i(Xq)

(e) X,del(X) (p11)   X,del(X) (q13q24)

FIGURE 15–3   Some sex chromosome complements: (a) normal female XX and normal male XY; (b) X and XXX females; (c) XXY and XYY males; (d and e) abnormal chromosomes from females with a ring X, an isochromosome of X long arm, an X short arm deletion, and an X long arm deletion.

(1999c) of a woman with 45,X/46,XX having had three monosomic X pregnancies, all showing fetal hydrops; she also had a normal son. Pubertal development may often be apparently normal in the 45,X/47,XXX case (Lim et al. 2017). The X/XXX patient in Bouchlariotou et al. (2011) had two normal children, and one (unkaryotyped) deceased severely growth retarded baby; while Sahinturk et al. (2015) report a woman with 45,X[8]/47,XXX[12] who had had five miscarriages and one healthy 46,XX daughter.

The variability of phenotype according to the degree of mosaicism is well illustrated in the report of Lespinasse et al. (1998), who studied monozygous (but not identical) triplets with 45,X/46,XX mosaicism. One child with typical TS had only 6% 45,X cells on blood karyotyping but 99% on fibroblast analysis. One sister with only mild features to suggest TS had 43% of fibroblasts with 45,X, and the third sister, of normal phenotype, had just 3%. Presumably, the mosaicism existed from a very early stage, and the three-way division of the 45,X/46,XX blastocyst, or (if marginally later) of the inner cell mass, happened to cut across an asymmetric disposition of normal/monosomic cells.

Low-Level 45,X/46,XX Mosaicism in Phenotypically Normal Women. This category is to be distinguished from that of TS due to 45,X/46,XX mosaicism discussed above, and it is supposed to be without reproductive consequence; advice from the European Cytogeneticists Association a propos is presented on p. 436. Loss of one X to give an occasional 45,X cell is a normal characteristic of aging in the 46,XX female (Ziętkiewicz et al. 2009). The phenomenon may reflect variation in a number of cell-cycle factors, similarly to, but less markedly than, the male equivalent, mosaic loss of the Y, as discussed below (Wright et al. 2017). Russell et al. (2007) reviewed data from a large number of women having had a peripheral blood cytogenetic analysis, and correlated the degree of X chromosome loss (XCL) with age, documenting a clear association. Up to age 30 years, 1% or less of cells showed XCL, but rising to an average 2%, 3%, and 5%, at median ages of 40, 50, and 65 years, respectively. The lost chromosome is more likely to have been the inactivated one (Machiela et al. 2016). To give a sense of where a threshold might lie between normality and the possibility of a significant effect, these workers considered the 99th centiles of the fractions of observed

XCL, for different cell counts. On a 30-cell count, for example, the 99th centiles were as follows: 6% at 30 years, 9% at 40 years, 13% at 50 years, and 17% at 60 years. Machiela et al. identified an absence of any XCL effect in relation to reproductive loss or infertility. Curiously, the opposite observation applies to women with X/XX mosaic TS: in them, the fraction of 46,XX cells actually increases with age (Denes et al. 2015).

45,X/46,XY AND 45,X/47,XYY MOSAICISM IN THE MALE

X/XY mosaicism is occasionally found in males presenting with hypogonadism and infertility with oligo/azoöspermia; in some, the Y chromosome has a deletion at Yq11 (Telvi et al. 1999; Cui et al. 2007). The maleness presumably reflects the fact that the gonad contained XY cells with a functioning *SRY* gene, that were able to induce effective testicular differentiation with consequent androgenizing capacity. Reddy and Sulcova (1998) did testicular biopsy on an X/XY man and demonstrated absence of spermatogenesis; about half of the Sertoli supporting cells showed a Y-signal on FISH. One X[10]/XY[90] man with moderate oligoasthenoteratozoöspermia showed a two- to threefold rate for XY disomy and 18 disomy in sperm (using 18 as a representative autosome) (Newberg et al. 1998). In contrast, a man with 45,X/47,XYY mosaicism reported in Dale et al. (2002) showed normal gonosomal complements in 99.9% of sperm. He had presented with infertility due to oligospermia; a normal 46,XY pregnancy

was achieved with intracytoplasmic sperm injection (ICSI). A meiotic mechanism in these men may favor the production of normal sperm (Ren et al. 2015).

Low-Level 45,X/46,XY Mosaicism in Phenotypically Normal Men. A curious fact is this: Mosaic loss of the Y (mLOY) is the most common chromosome abnormality in the postnatal population. Long considered merely to be an incidental observation more prevalent in older men, in more recent years it has been appreciated as having an association with increased morbidity and mortality (Forsberg 2017). The effect is more marked in smokers (Fig. 15–4). It may be that mLOY is an epiphenomenon, reflecting an underlying basis in variation in a number of cell cycle factors (Wright et al. 2017); an attractive candidate among these is *MAD1L1*, which halts the cell cycle until the chromatids are bi-oriented at the equator. This susceptibility could lead to vulnerability of the Y during mitosis in a rapidly-dividing tissue such as blood, the LOY line thereafter having unimpaired survival, as hematogenous tissue has little or no need of Y-based genes. More importantly, the putative cell-cycle susceptibility could predispose to certain diseases, including cancer and atheroma. The practical value to which this evolving understanding may be put is yet to become clear.

SEX CHROMOSOME POLYSOMY

The 48,XXXX female characteristically has diminished ovarian function, and fertility in pure XXXX

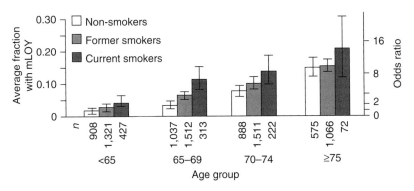

FIGURE 15–4   Mosaic loss of a Y chromosome (mLOY) on peripheral blood in older men, and according to smoking status (non, former, current). The *y* axis shows the proportions of men in whom X/XY is seen, from 2% of nonsmokers age under 65 years to 20% of smokers age 75 years or older. Numbers of subjects in each category are shown under x axis.

Source: From Zhou et al., Mosaic loss of chromosome Y is associated with common variation near TCL1A, *Nature Genet* 48: 563–568, 2016. Courtesy S. J. Chanock, and with the permission of Nature Publishing Group.

is on record in only one case (ascertained through a Down syndrome child) (Gardner et al. 1973b; Kara et al. 2014). Sterility is presumably invariable in XXXY and XXYY males, who have a further sex chromosome superadded upon the Klinefelter karyotype (Linden et al. 1995).

Recurrence to Parents Having Had a Child with a Sex Chromosome Aneuploidy

XXY (KLINEFELTER SYNDROME), XXX, AND XYY

These aneuploidies occur at roughly similar frequencies, approximately 1 per 1,000 of the appropriate sex. Approximately 75% of XXX and about 40% of XXY KS is due to a maternal meiotic error, and in three-fourths of each of these it is the first meiotic (MI) division that is involved, this MI group showing a maternal age effect.[1] It is noteworthy that almost half of KS results from a paternal MI error (MacDonald et al. 1994). Fathers of paternally originating KS may have marginally elevated levels of disomic XY sperm in comparison with fathers of maternally originating cases, possibly reflecting an inherent tendency among a small minority of these men to produce aneuploid sperm (Eskenazi et al. 2002). In what may have been the only known example of a recurrence, Woods et al. (1997) report two XXY brothers. The karyotype in both reflected a paternal meiosis I error. Manifestly, XYY of meiotic origin must be due to a paternal error, at MII. All three sex chromosomes aneuploidies can have a postzygotic mitotic generation, which may present as mosaicism.

45,X TURNER SYNDROME

In approximately three-fourths of TS, it is the paternal X chromosome that is absent (Hassold et al. 1990a; Uematsu et al. 2002). Mostly, the error is a meiotic one and resides in paternal gametogenesis, possibly reflecting an absence of pairing along most of the X-Y bivalent with a consequential vulnerability in the process of disjunction (Jacobs et al. 1997). Fathers of nonmosaic 45,Xᵐ Turner girls may have a marginally increased risk to produce

sperm nullisomic for a sex chromosome. Martínez-Pasarell et al. (1999) analyzed sperm from four fathers and eight controls, and there was a slight increase in nullisomic sperm (0.48%) and 24,XY sperm (0.22%) in the fathers, compared to the fractions in controls (0.32% and 0.11%, respectively). This might suggest that some fathers of nonmosaic 45,Xᵐ Turner girls have a slight proneness to produce sperm nullisomic for a sex chromosome; but if so, the near-absence of recurrences would point to a very minor influence.

An alternative explanation is that the loss occurred postzygotically, and the "45,X" child is actually a 45,X/46,XX mosaic, with a very low proportion of XX cells; but this is apparently an uncommon event (Jacobs et al. 1997). Wiktor and Van Dyke (2005) describe 22 patients with apparently nonmosaic 45,X in whom, upon further study, three had a minor XX cell line, and 19 were apparently pure 45,X; no XY cell lines were seen. To the contrary, Uematsu et al. (2002) suggest that most TS may actually be due to a structurally abnormal gonosome (X or Y) having been generated in paternal meiosis, with a 46,X,abn(X) conception resulting, and subsequent mitotic loss of the abn(X) leaving a 45,X karyotype. In a Brazilian cohort of 74 cases of TS, cryptic Y-chromosome material was detected in 2.7% (Bispo et al. 2014).

These theories notwithstanding, the observational data point to a very low recurrence risk. In the literature review of Kher et al. (1994), they could find only one instance of 45,X recurrence in sisters. From the Birth Defects Register of Victoria, Australia, over the period 1995–2008, of 245 prenatal diagnoses of 45,X, in none had the indication been of a previous chromosome abnormality (J. L. Halliday, personal communication 2010). In the case of a postzygotic origin, if it could be presumed to have been an event that occurred at random in a single mitosis in the early embryo, the risk of recurrence would be regarded as not being raised at all. Kher et al. did, however, report a unique family with occurrence of 45,X/46,XX in sisters.

RARE POLYSOMIES

Polysomies such as XXXX, XXYY, XYYY, XXXY, XXXXX, and XXXXY are very rare. Successive nondisjunctions in one parent, the other contributing a single sex chromosome, is the mechanism

---

1 For convenience, detailed age-related sex chromosome risk data are included in Chapter 13, Table 13–6, alongside equivalent autosomal risk data.

in most if not all (Hassold et al. 1990b; Deng et al. 1991). Apart from the extraordinary circumstance of (hypothetically) a familial tendency to mosaicism, these polysomies arise sporadically (Bergemann 1962; Kher et al. 1994). Rare reports of coincidence with some other aneuploidy in the family may more likely reflect chance than a causal link (Court Brown et al. 1969). In the particular case of pentasomy X, no maternal age effect is observed (Pirollo et al. 2015).

GENETIC COUNSELING

Persons with a Sex Chromosome Aneuploidy

XXX

XXX mothers have no discernibly increased risk of bearing chromosomally abnormal children. A theoretical increased risk for children with an X aneuploidy has not been demonstrated in practice. Despite reports of chromosomally abnormal children born to XXX women, it should be emphasized, as did Dewhurst and Neri in 1978 and 1984, respectively, that when biased ascertainment is taken into account, no excess of abnormal offspring has been reported. Near silence subsequently in the literature on this issue suggests at least a considerable rarity of X-aneuploid pregnancy outcomes; one such case, an XXX daughter of an XXX mother, is mentioned in passing in Haverty et al. (2004). A possibility of premature ovarian failure with 47,XXX can be brought to the attention of these women, which may assist in decisions about the timing of childbearing.

XXY

Hardly ever will these men father children, without recourse to testicular sperm extraction and IVF. This requires the surgical opening of the testis, with microdissection of seminiferous tubules under the operating microscope, and analysis, on site, by an embryologist, for the presence of sperm; the procedure is preferably undertaken on the day before programmed oöcyte retrieval from the female partner. The few single sperm obtained are injected into the egg (ICSI).[2] The success rate is variable, with sperm retrieved in approximately 40%–70%

of men, and about half of couples achieving pregnancy (Denschlag et al. 2004; Schiff et al. 2005; Van Saen et al. 2012b). The chances might be improved if anticipatory sampling for storage is done in adolescence or young adulthood (Plotton et al. 2015; Rohayem et al. 2015; Gies et al. 2016; Nahata et al. 2016). A possible benefit of testicular sampling and storage of spermatogonial stem cells, at around the onset of puberty (and necessarily supposing the diagnosis to have been made by that age), remains currently in the research realm (Van Saen et al. 2012a). Gamete donor from a brother or father is a means to have a child with shared genetic heritage.

The chromosomal outcome for the child conceived from an XXY man appears very promising, with only one case known of fetal XXY in more than 100 pregnancies (Lejeune et al. 2014). Thus, one may propose an approximate risk figure of 1% for a sex chromosomal abnormality in the child. However, at preimplantation genetic diagnosis (PGD), the rate of aneuploidy, both for the sex chromosomes and for autosomes 18 and 21 in particular, may be slightly higher in XXY patients; and this is consonant with the observed higher rate of disomy 21 on sperm study mentioned above. This being so, PGD could be offered to these couples as part of the IVF procedure (Staessen et al. 2003).

XYY

To our knowledge, there is no report of a discernibly increased risk for the XYY male to have chromosomally abnormal children. A slight increase in gonosomal imbalances in sperm (see above, and Rives et al. 2003) might nevertheless lead some to choose prenatal diagnosis. The risk might, in theory, be greater in those XYY men who need fertility treatment (as some do; Kim et al. 2013) and for whom PGD might therefore be offered as an "add-on" to the IVF process.

NONMOSAIC 45,X TURNER SYNDROME

Infertility is almost always the case. However, successful pregnancy outcomes from natural conception, albeit very few in number, are on record (Bernard et al. 2016). A 45,X woman who has spontaneous menses may possibly be fertile. Endocrine

---

2 It is an intriguing thought that, in those cases proceeding to fatherhood through intervention with assisted reproductive technology, the situation may be presented of the homogametic sex being the one to provide the greater quantum of gametes, albeit by a small margin: an extraordinary contrast from the typical vast imbalance due to the heterogametic male of the species.

and ultrasound studies may clarify whether ovulation is occurring, or likely to occur (Paoloni-Giacobino et al. 2000a). Any period of fertility is likely to be short-lived; thus, a woman with 45,X TS who wishes to have a child should not delay unduly in trying for a pregnancy. In some centers, timely sampling and storage of oöcytes in early adolescence, or ovarian cryopreservation in prepubertal girls, might offer a future possibility (Oktay et al. 2016).[3] An increased risk for miscarriage, X aneuploidy, and autosomal trisomy is to be noted (Sybert 2005). (As discussed above, occult mosaicism may in fact be the basis of retained ovarian function in apparent nonmosaic TS.) Gametes donated from a mother or a sister would offer, in principle, the opportunity to have a child with a shared genetic inheritance, albeit that ova are more difficult to store and reanimate than are sperm. This and other options (gestational surrogacy, adoption) are reviewed in Hovatta (2012), Grynberg et al. (2016), and Oktay et al. (2016).

MOSAIC 45,X TURNER SYNDROME

Women with 45,X mosaicism and a TS phenotype presumably carry the 45,X cell line in much of the soma and gonad. Categories include X/XX, X/XXX, and X/XX/XXX. Ovarian function is often intact, although premature failure is common (Blair et al. 2001; Sybert 2005; Lau et al. 2009); normal cells in the gonad may provide support for monosomic cells that otherwise would not have survived. A few may, as adolescents, have ovarian tissue suitable for biopsy and storage for possible future use, as mentioned above with respect to nonmosaic TS. There is apparently an increased risk for X monosomy in a child, and this is consonant with theoretical expectation; autosomal trisomy is also seen (Sybert 2005; Bernard et al. 2016). The risk for miscarriage is increased; it is of interest that the miscarriage rate is greater with natural conception than in pregnancy due to donation of (presumably normal) eggs (Homer et al. 2010; Bryman et al. 2011; Doğer et al. 2015; Bernard et al. 2016). In a large French study, most pregnancies that continued through to live birth produced phenotypically normal children: Of 30 newborns, 13 were normal boys, 15 normal girls, and two girls had

an X chromosome abnormality presumably related to the maternal karyotype (Bernard et al. 2016).

Ovum Donation, Mosaic and Nonmosaic Turner Syndrome. For the great majority of TS patients, mosaic and nonmosaic, who cannot make their own eggs, ovum donation with IVF may be one route to achieve childbearing (Hovatta 2012). Foudila et al. (1999) report their experience with 18 women with TS, and although the rates of embryo transfer were similar to those of other women with primary ovarian failure, the miscarriage rate was high (40%); possibly, this may have been due to uterine factors. Bodri et al. (2009) report a similarly discouraging experience. Fénichel and Letur (2008) insist on the advisability of transferring a single embryo only. Any genetic risk to the TS patient bearing children via ovum donation is due to that of the biological donor parents. A related donor (mother, sister) would have obvious attraction, and the improving methodology of ovum storage offers the possibility of maternal donation well ahead of the time of potential use (Schoolcraft et al. 2009). Gidoni et al. (2008) report a 33-year-old mother having "oöcyte vitrification" for the potential use of her daughter with isoXq Turner syndrome. These authors discuss the ethical issues involved and conclude that the procedure is reasonable and acceptable, with the mother's motives purely altruistic, and she "is simply providing an option for her daughter"; these ethical issues are similarly canvassed in Grynberg et al. (2016). Anticipating possible artificial fertility, the offer should be made of hormone treatment from the age of 10–12 years, in order to avoid uterine hypoplasia (Leclercq et al. 1992). Otherwise, obstetric management must take account of possible cardiovascular complication (Folsom and Fuqua 2015).

Low-Level 45,X/46,XX Mosaicism in Phenotypically Normal Women. This category is to be distinguished clearly from that of the preceding section on "Mosaic 45,X Turner Syndrome." The discovery of a low-level (a single-digit percentage) of 45,X cells in a woman presenting no phenotype traits of TS is not to be overinterpreted, nor is a reproductive risk to be exaggerated. Indeed, no such risk may apply (Horsman et al. 1987). We have observed a number of healthy

---

3 Although a pregnancy has yet to be achieved following ovarian cryopreservation in a woman with Turner syndrome, a successful pregnancy was reported in a 46,XX woman in whom ovarian tissue had been cryopreserved prior to menarche (Demeestere et al. 2015), demonstrating feasibility of the approach, at least in 46,XX women.

pregnant women identified by noninvasive prenatal testing as having low-level 45,X/46,XX mosaicism, the presence of 45,X cells in the mother leading to a "false positive" increased risk result for TS in the fetus. In those presenting with infertility, and having 45,X levels of 3%–10%, Kláskov á et al. (2015) observed no increase in aortic abnormality (a Turner concomitant). Otherwise, loss of an X chromosome is a normal concomitant of aging (see also "Biology" section).

X/XY MALE

Infertility is probable. If there is any sperm production, an IVF pregnancy might be possible. Given a possible increased risk for aneuploidy, gonosomal or autosomal (Newberg et al. 1998), PGD is to be considered in that setting. (Mosaic loss of the Y in older men is a different matter altogether; see "Biology" section).

SEX CHROMOSOME POLYSOMY

Many XXXX women are of low-normal or borderline intelligence, and the questions of fertility and genetic risk may well be raised by their carers. In fact, it appears that sterility is almost always the case. XXXY and XXYY men are undoubtedly sterile.

Parents Having Had a Child with a Sex Chromosome Aneuploidy

XXX, XXY, XYY, 45,X, AND OTHER SEX CHROMOSOME ANEUPLOIDY

There is no firm evidence that a recurrence risk above the age-specific figure exists, and indeed in respect of XXX and XXY, no recurrences, of either homotrisomy or heterotrisomy, were observed in the study of Warburton et al. (2004). Prenatal diagnosis in a future pregnancy would be discretionary.

Structural Rearrangement

As in the preceding chapter on autosomal rearrangements, we are here dealing with a *segment* of a chromosome existing in an imbalanced state, mostly with respect to the X, but the Y chromosome making a small appearance. Broadly, we may

consider two categories: large rearrangements that have been known from the early days of cytogenetics; and microrearrangements, originally detected on G-banding, and now including deletions and duplications seen only with molecular karyotyping. Typically so, the large rearrangements are associated with disorders of gonadal development, and variant forms of TS predominate among these. Here, X-inactivation enables an otherwise massive genetic imbalance to become functionally viable. The viability of large Y imbalances reflects the very small component of active genes on this chromosome. Contrariwise, microimbalances of the X chromosome in the female are not necessarily subject to "correction" by inactivation; and they may be damaging, but not lethal, in the male. Thus, the implications may be, in some respects, similar to the autosomal microimbalance. (Again, we mention that genomic coordinates noted with microrearrangements are according to the hg38 build, unless otherwise indicated.[4])

We list here selected deletions and duplications of the X and Y chromosomes. As for the X, for the most part we categorize, as commented above, according to (1) large "classic" rearrangements and (2) microdeletions and microduplications. Y abnormalities, although so few, follow suit.

LARGER X DELETIONS

del Xp Turner Variant. Substantial Xp terminal deletions, many of which had been seen on the solid-stain analysis of the early days of cytogenetics, typically lead to variant or incomplete, "formes frustes" of TS (Fig. 15–3). These deletions can remove up to most of, or even all of, the short arm. X-inactivation is markedly skewed toward the abnormal X (Zinn et al. 1997). Short stature is largely due to haploinsufficiency of the *SHOX* growth control gene at chrX:0.63 Mb in the pseudoautosomal region.

Ovarian function may be retained, in part at least, with the more distal Xp deletions, but is typically absent in proximal deletions (Zinn et al. 1997; Lachlan et al. 2006). In those women who achieve fertility—and numerous examples of transmission of a del(Xp) are on record (Periquito et al. 2016)—presumably a partial synapsis occurs at meiosis in

---

4 The cytoband boundaries as shown on the UCSC genome browser are very precise, to a nucleotide. Applying the nucleotide coordinates in a cited case sometimes comes up with a different band than had been reported. For the most part, we have chosen to accept the band as determined on the UCSC browser.

the 46,X,abn(X) oöcytes, with the intact segment of the abnormal X pairing with the homologous region of the normal X. A segregation ratio of 1:1 would be expected, with equal frequencies of gametes carrying either the normal X or the abnormal X, from that part of the gonad tissue containing the abn(X).

Not infrequently, mosaicism is recognized. Palka et al. (1994) describe an apparently nonmosaic 45,X woman who had an abnormal child with an interstitial Xp deletion, del(X)(p22.2p11.3). Upon restudy, the mother herself had one 46,X,del(X) out of 450 cells, allowing the presumption of a somatic-gonadal mosaicism. In a more direct demonstration of gonadal mosaicism, Varela et al. (1991) studied a woman with TS and normal menstruation, and who had had a 46,X,del(X)(p21) daughter. They showed 5/100 cells with 46,X,del(X)(p21) in one ovary, while all cells from the other ovary, fibroblasts, and lymphocytes were 45,X. Gonadal function can vary in a family, as Zinn et al. (1997) show for a familial del(X)(p21.2). The 45,X/46,X,del(X) mother had had three pregnancies, including one miscarriage, and had normal menses till age 39 years. Her two daughters were both 46,X,del(X). The elder was amenorrheic at age 15 years, while the younger had spontaneous menarche at age 14½ years, with regular cycles 1 year later. A very similar family is on record in Adachi et al. (2000).

An Xp deletion might coexist with an Xq duplication, the consequence of recombination within an inversion chromosome. Stoklasova et al. (2016) report a four-generation family—clearly fertility was retained—of women with the karyotype 46,X,rec(X)inv(p21.1q27.3). A great-great-grandparent may have been the heterozygote in whom the recombinant arose.

del Xp22.12pter. This deletion, and others of lesser extent, may be associated, in the female, with only the short stature component of TS, this segment including the *SHOX* gene. Cho et al. (2012) report a deletion Xp22.12pter (chrX:1 nt-19.9 Mb), which had been passed from a mother to her two daughters. The mother's height was just a little above the range seen in classic TS at 148.7 cm (−3.3 SD); her young daughters plotted somewhat higher, on −2.1 and −1.8 SD, respectively, at their ages of close to 9 and 12 years. The mother's pubertal development had been normal.

del Xq Turner Variant. Deletions may be of very substantial size, up to 74 Mb, or approximately three-fourths of the q arm length. Mercer et al. (2013) reviewed the clinical picture in a series of 10 del(Xq) cases, of whom eight were nonmosaic (two had a concomitant 45,X cell line). Of the nonmosaic cases, six had terminal deletions, with proximal breakpoints from Xq21.1 to Xq25 (chrX:81.9-129.7 Mb); where parental testing had been done, all were de novo. The clinical presentations had been due to primary amenorrhea, premature ovarian failure, infertility, and in one child, short stature. If puberty commences naturally, it remains the case that premature ovarian failure is likely; and it is practical advice that child-bearing, if wished, and of course other things being equal, should be embarked upon sooner rather than later. Assuming 1:1 segregation (a fair assumption), the deleted X would be transmitted in 50% of ova.

Ring Turner Variants. The imbalance in the classic 46,X,r(X) Turner syndrome is essentially due to distal Xp and Xq deletion, the deletions of variable extent. Rare reports of fertility exist. Blumenthal and Allanson (1997) record a woman with mosaic ring X TS, 45,X/46,X,r(X), who had been amenorrheic until being given hormone replacement therapy. She had three pregnancies: a healthy 46,XY son, a 12-week miscarriage, and a healthy daughter with the same 45,X/46,r(X) karyotype. The latter was presumably 46,X,r(X) at conception, with postzygotic loss of the r(X) in some tissue. Other such cases are known (Uehara et al. 1997; Sybert 2005). A rather different example is that in Matsuo et al. (2000), in which a mother and daughter were 45,X/46,X,r(X) (p22.3q28), the ratios of X:X,r(X) being 97:3 in the mother and 73:27 in the daughter. The ring comprised an almost complete X, but small distal Xp and Xq segments were deleted. The two X chromosomes were randomly inactivated, and in consequence, presumably, some "brain genes" would have been functionally nullisomic in those cells having the normal X-inactivated. Thus, mental function in the mother, and more so in the daughter, was compromised. A male with r(X) is almost unknown, but Ellison et al. (2002) describe transmission from a nonmosaic 46,X,r(X) mother to her nonmosaic 46,Y,r(X) son, mother and son both short statured. The breakpoints were very distal, within and beyond the Xp and Xq pseudoautosomal regions, respectively.

The *"tiny ring X syndrome,"* with the karyotype 45,X/46,X,r(X), is a quite different entity. There may be a functional X disomy, and it is typically, but not universally, seen with a severe phenotype of physical and mental defect, in some resembling Kabuki syndrome. The severity of the phenotype has been attributed to a functional X disomy, due to the ring lacking the *XIST* locus and thus not undergoing inactivation; this scenario may not necessarily apply, and the clinical picture may merely be that of Turner syndrome (Migeon et al. 2000; Turner et al. 2000; Rodríguez et al. 2008). Similarly, in the male with the tiny ring as a supernumerary chromosome, usually as 46,XY/47,XY,+r(X) mosaicism, the clinical picture is typically abnormal, and in some severely so (Baker et al. 2010). Chen et al. (2006d) report a notable exception, from the prenatal diagnosis at amniocentesis of 46,XY[17]/47,XY,+mar[6], the marker chromosome turning out to be a very small *XIST*-negative r(X). The infant boy, on whose blood the proportions of the two cell lines were similar to the amniocentesis findings, was normal physically and developmentally, on follow-up to 1 year of age. These various phenotypic differences, in male and female, may reflect the composition, proportion, distribution, and activation status of the abnormal chromosome.

LARGER X DUPLICATIONS

Isochromosome Xq Turner Variant. The imbalance in i(Xq) Turner syndrome is a monosomy of Xp and a trisomy of Xq. The condition is, apparently, invariably associated with an infertility.

Isochromosome Xq Klinefelter Variant. In this rare form of Klinefelter syndrome, 47,X,i(Xq),Y, there is a monosomy of Xp and trisomy of Xq (as with i(Xq) TS), along with a normal Y complement. Infertility is usual, but rare fertility, with recourse to IVF, is on record (Stabile et al. 2008; Sabbaghian et al. 2011).

dup Xq21q26. Large duplications of (and microduplications within) this segment are noted below. A functional disomy can influence the clinical picture, according to the pattern of X-chromosome inactivation (Armstrong et al. 2003).

LARGER Y REARRANGEMENTS

Y Isochromosome, Isodicentric Y. The inactivation of one of the two centromeres allows this chromosome to be mitotically functional. The distinction here is between Yp and Yq isochromosomes;

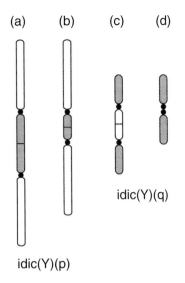

idic(Y)(p)

FIGURE 15–5   Formation of the isodicentric Y chromosome (Yp chromatin, gray; Yq chromatin, white). The idic(Y)(p) has mirror copies around a distal (*a*) or mid (*b*) Yp breakpoint, whereas the idic(Y)(q) has mirror copies around a Yq breakpoint (*c*) or practically at the centromere, Yq11.1 (*d*). Thus, heterogeneity of chromosome length relates to a heterogeneity of breakpoint site.

or, since typically there are two copies of the centromere, they are usually called Yp and Yq isodicentric chromosomes—thus, i(Y)(p) and i(Y)(q), or idic(Y)(p) and idic(Y)(q). Or, more fully, for example, idic(Y)(pter→q11.22::q11.22→pter); note the identical, palindromic sequences on either side of the :: breakpoint. Note also that the Yp or Yq designation refers to the site of breakpoint, and that the idic(Y)(p) has two complete Yq copies, while vice versa, the idic(Y)(q) has two complete copies of Yp.[5] There is considerable heterogeneity of size, according to the site of breakpoint (Fig. 15–5). An idic(Y)(p) with a breakpoint at distal Yp, with mirror copies of the remainder of the Y, would comprise almost a double copy of the whole chromosome (Fig. 15–5a). An idic(Y)(q11.223) would convey a double copy of Yp, and a double copy of the proximal long arm (Fig. 15–5c). A breakpoint at Yq11.1 would give an idic(Y)(q), with a double copy of only the short arm, and absence of long arm material (Fig. 15–5d). Generation is de novo, typically in (obviously)

5 This can sometimes lead to muddling of nomenclature. Beaulieu Bergeron et al. (2011) note that "when referring to an idic with unspecified breakpoints, some authors use idicY(p) or idicY(Yp) when two copies of the short arm are present, and idicY(q) or idic(Yq) when two copies of the long arm are present, therefore creating some confusion among readers." ISCN (2016) does not adjudicate.

paternal gametogenesis, and reflecting a vulnerability due to the apposition of similar Y sequences; uncommon cases may be due to a postzygotic event.

Mosaicism very frequently accompanies as a postzygotic event, with 45,X and a second abn(Y) the usual additional cell lineages. The clinical presentations range from a majority with male infertility (e.g., the idic(Y)(p11.3) in Fig. 15–6), male with mild cognitive impairment, through ovotesticular disorder of sex development (DSD) or mixed gonadal dysgenesis with genital ambiguity, to TS; the gonadal phenotype is presumably directed in keeping with the regional presence or absence of SRY. In a series of 14 cases in Kalantari et al. (2014), all with idic(Y)(q11.22), 13 were men with azoöspermia (note that this chromosome would lack the b and c AZF spermatogenic factors). Most had a concomitant 45,X cell line. Immature germ cells in the ejaculate were, overall, of fairly similar fractions of haploid 23,X and 23,idic(Y) karyotypes, indicating that the first stage of meiosis, division of the primary spermatocyte, had been entered. The only woman had a Turner-like clinical picture, and about half of cells, on blood, were 45,X; in comparison, in the series of Beaulieu Bergeron et al. (2011), four women all had gonadal dysgenesis. Ambiguous genitalia with ovotesticular DSD/mixed gonadal dysgenesis was the presenting sign in three children in Mekkawy et al. (2012) and in the infant in

Becker and Akhavan (2016). The Y isochromosomes were idic(Y)(p11.32) in two and idic(Y)(q11.222) in two; all were mosaic for at least 45,X, and two with an additional idic(Y)(p11.32)×2 line.

Ring Y. The usual case is of 46,X,r(Y)/45,X mosaicism, although it is likely that the 45,X line had arisen secondarily, following postzygotic loss of the ring. Double and interlocked rings are occasionally seen, as late mitotic events. Retention of the SRY locus at chrY:2.78 Mb determines a male phenotype, and provided that cells within gonadal tissue retain the r(Y); nevertheless, testicular gametic function is compromised. Loss of loci in the AZF regions in Yq11.23, if the ring breakpoint in Yq is proximal to these loci, adds further insult to gametogenic potential. Short stature is common, and loss of SHOX (chrY:0.63 Mb) in the pseudoautosomal region is the presumed basis of this. If the gonad is 45,X, a Turner-like phenotype is seen; or, if the gonad comprises both 45,X and 46,X,r(Y) lineages, a mixed gonadal dysgenesis, possibly with a genital ambiguity, may be the consequence (Milenkovic et al. 2011). A Turner-like habitus, albeit in a male, may in any event arise, if the ring is very small and lacks any Yq material (Tzancheva et al. 1999).

In the ring Y man, azoöspermia is usual, and less than 1% of cases have been inherited from a ring Y father (Arnedo et al. 2005). In the rare event of spermatogenesis proceeding, almost always fertility could only ever be achieved through IVF. In theory, and since only the 46,X,r(Y) gametocytes are "meiotically competent" (Blanco et al. 2003), sperm would be equally 23,X and 23,r(Y). Thus, normal 46,XX daughters and (probably mosaic) ring(Y) sons would be the predicted outcomes, although a 45,X cell line arising in the latter could potentially lead to a disorder of sex development. PGD would have an obvious place (Spinner et al. 2008).

X;Y Translocation. See Chapter 6.

Inversion Y. This normal variant is mentioned in Chapter 9.

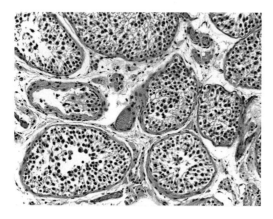

FIGURE 15–6 Testicular histology in an infertile man with 45,X[9]/46,X,mar[3]/46,X,idic(Y)(p11.3) [33]. There is a maturation arrest at the level of the primary spermatocyte, reflected in the azoöspermia of this man. The idic(Y) had the format as in Figure 15–5a.

Source: From Lehmann et al., Isodicentric Yq mosaicism presenting as infertility and maturation arrest without altered SRY and AZF regions, *J Assist Reprod Genet* 29: 939–942, 2012. Courtesy M. A. Fischer, and with the permission of Springer.

GENETIC COUNSELING

Larger Rearrangements

TURNER SYNDROME VARIANTS

Lachlan et al. (2006) reviewed their own experience and the published literature, and they noted fertility with respect to these terminal Xp deletions: p11.4, p21, p21.1, p22.1, p22.12, and p22. Presumably, the risk to transmit the del(Xp) is 50:50. The implications for offspring differ according to the gender of the child. The limit of viability for the hemizygous deletion male is defined by the cases studied in Melichar et al. (2007), with the maximum survivable loss being ~10 Mb. The phenotype is very abnormal and includes severe psychomotor retardation, Léri-Weill syndrome, chondrodysplasia punctata, ichthyosis, Kallmann syndrome, and ocular albinism. Periquito et al. (2016) describe a woman with 45,X/46,Xdel(Xp) Turner syndrome, who had been advised that she would be infertile but who went on to have two (nonmosaic) 46,X,del(X) (p11.4) daughters and a 46,XY son.

Fertility in women with a terminal Xq deletion is rare but reported. As with the del(Xp), the risk of transmission is presumed to be 50:50, but the outcome is dependent upon the gender of the child. A male pregnancy with a degree of nullisomy Xq is presumed to be nonviable.

Fertility with a ring X is known. An r(X) mother can have chromosomally normal children or an r(X) daughter. As for the isochromosome X, we know of no example of an i(Xq) TS woman reproducing. A unique case concerns a mother mosaic for an X chromosome with a small interstitial insertion at Xq26: 45,X/46,X,add(X)(q26); she had two daughters with essentially the 47,XXX syndrome (one of the three X chromosomes being the addXq26) (Ramachandram et al. 2013).

KLINEFELTER SYNDROME VARIANTS

Infertility is the rule. In one example, normal daughters were born to a man with the karyotype 47,X,i(Xq),Y, following IVF with ICSI (Stabile et al. 2008).

MICRODELETIONS AND MICRODUPLICATIONS

Chromosome X deletions

del Xp11.3p11.23 The striking phenotype in the male is a progressive visual loss from boyhood, due to retinal cone-rod dystrophy, and reflecting loss of the *RP2* gene at chrX:46.8 Mb (Delphin et al. 2012) (Fig. 15-7). If the deletion is confined to chrX:46.4-46.9 Mb, no other abnormality is seen, and specifically, intellect is normal. A more extensive deletion removing two microRNA loci, *mir221* and

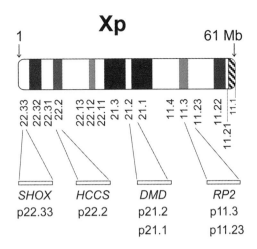

FIGURE 15-7

mir222 at chrX:45.7 Mb, causes intellectual disability. The female heterozygote is typically unaffected.

However, in a more extensive deletion, extending into Xp11.4, the carrier female may display, at least to some extent, the components of a contiguous gene deletion. We have seen a young woman with retinitis pigmentosa, chronic granulomatous disease, and ornithine transcarbamylase (OTC) deficiency, having an Xp deletion which removed these neighboring loci. She suffered recurrent upper respiratory tract infections and had a history of surgery for mastoid osteomyelitis and lung abscess; her peripheral vision was poor; and she unconsciously self-managed the OTC deficiency by avoiding high-protein foods. X-inactivation was random. She came to prenatal diagnosis and elected to terminate a male pregnancy with the deletion, the predicted phenotype being severe (Coman et al. 2010b).

del Xp21 Cytogeneticists can claim some credit for the initial location of the gene for Duchenne muscular dystrophy at Xp21.1p21.2, chrX:33.1-33.2 Mb (Lindenbaum et al. 1979), and at least for that historical reason, we include a mention of deletion in this region. As noted above, loss of neighboring loci within chrX:30.3-33.2 Mb in the hemizygous male leads to a contiguous gene syndrome, sometimes referred to simply as the "Xp21 deletion syndrome." The condition is often familial; while the carrier mother is typically unaffected, rare cases of clinically affected girls with a de novo deletion are reported (Heide et al. 2015).

del Xp22.2 Some deletions in the 46,X,del(Xp) female which include this segment, either as an interstitial or as a terminal deletion, lead to the syndrome of microphthalmia and linear skin defects (MLS). The key gene is *HCCS*, at chrX:11.1 Mb, this gene directing a component of the mitochondrial respiratory chain.[6] The intriguing question is this: Why is MLS seen in only some deletions of Xp22.2? Unfavorable X-inactivation is the reasonable explanation, and in theory, inactivation of the normal X could lead to a functional nullizygosity of *HCCS*. Thus, in tissue derived from neural crest destined to contribute to skin and eye, mitochondrial failure could lead to cell death, and hence the MLS phenotype. Favorable inactivation, skewed toward the del(Xp), could see the normal X hold sway (Morleo and Franco 2008). If there is mosaicism with a 45,X cell line, this may be protective, by virtue of retained activity of *HCCS* when the gene is present on a single, active X. Wimplinger et al. (2007) suggest this to be the basis of a mildly affected mosaic 45,X/46,X,del(X)(p22.2) mother with MLS having a more severely affected nonmosaic 46,X,del(X)(p22.2) daughter.

Another example of mother-daughter difference is seen in Margari et al. (2014), in this case with a large (and apparently nonmosaic) Xp22.2pter deletion. The mother was of short stature, and she had had one eye removed in infancy; the daughter was blind due to bilateral eye involvement, short, dysmorphic, had lost language ability, and developed signs of autism. Both showed, at least on blood, preferential inactivation of the del(Xp), of ratios 10:90 in daughter and 15:85 in mother. The smallest deletion, of ~200 kb, removing only *HCCS* and part of one other gene (*ARHGAP6*), is described in Vergult et al. (2013b) and concerned a mother and daughter, both of normal intellect, each with only one eye affected, and skin lesions only in the mother; X-inactivation was completely skewed in both.

It is presumed that an Xp22.2 deletion in a male conceptus would lead to inevitable early abortion. Thus, the risk to the female carrier to have a living affected child is one-third, the segregation ratio of 1:1:1 applying to normal female:affected female:normal male.

del Xq21.1q21.33 One case in the del(Xq) series of Mercer et al. (2013) had a deletion encompassing chrX:80.9-98.2 Mb. She had presented due to the prenatal diagnosis of the deletion in a male. She herself was essentially normal. *PCDH11X* at chrX:91.8 is a landmark locus (Fig. 15–8).

del Xq22.1q22.3 Deletions of ~3 Mb in Xq22.1q22.3 are seen only in the heterozygous female, and the non-observation of males points to a lethality of the nullizygous state. Intellectual deficit can be severe; one patient is described as "aphasic and incontinent." Sleep disturbance is typical. Facial dysmorphism is of "soft" degree. Yamamoto et al. (2014) propose three potential pheno-critical regions—A, B, and C—within chrX:102.1-104.5 Mb. Loci of interest are the *BEX* (brain-expressed X-linked) genes at chrX:102-103 Mb, in their region B. A smaller (nullisomic) deletion of 1.4 Mb, removing regions A and B, of de novo generation, is reported in the only known male case, a profoundly neurologically affected child, in Shirai et al. (2017).

Deletions are nonrecurrent. Most have been de novo, but maternal transmission is recorded. Interpretation is not straightforward, and the influence of X-inactivation is uncertain, as proposed in the family in Grillo et al. (2010). These authors report a mother with a smaller (1.1 Mb) deletion within band Xp22.1, involving the region A of Yamamoto et al. (2014), who was rather mildly affected, but her daughter was severely retarded. This may have reflected the effects of favorable skewing of X-inactivation in the mother, and an influence of the paternal genetic contribution on the daughter's phenotype.

del Xq22.3q23 A contiguous gene syndrome within this segment encompasses, in the hemizygous male, Alport syndrome, intellectual disability, facial dysmorphism, and a curious red cell anomaly, elliptocytosis (Gazou et al. 2013). The basis of the Alport syndrome of renal failure and deafness in this syndrome is well understood, namely the *COL4A5* gene at chrX:108.4 Mb. Deletions are nonrecurrent, and if *COL4A5* is not included, naturally Alport syndrome is not seen; the intellectually deficiency may reside in loss of the *ACSL4* gene (chrX:109.6 Mb). Familial cases are well known. Mothers can have the

---

6 A small minority of MLS is due to other X-borne loci, *COX7B* at Xq21.1 and *NDUFB11* at Xp11.3, which, like *HCCS*, code for components of mitochondrial function (Indrieri et al. 2012; Van Rahden et al. 2015). Thus far, *COX7B* and *NDUFB11* cases have been due to point mutation or intragenic deletion, not X chromosomal microdeletion.

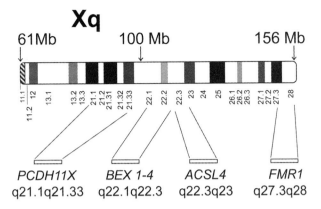

Xq

| 61Mb | 100 Mb | 156 Mb |

PCDH11X BEX 1-4 ACSL4 FMR1
q21.1q21.33 q22.1q22.3 q22.3q23 q27.3q28

FIGURE 15-8

slightest sign of renal impairment; it may well be that skewed X-inactivation is protective (Rodriguez et al. 2010).

del Xq27.3q28 This rare deletion removes loci for the fragile X syndrome and Hunter syndrome (a mucopolysaccharidosis): *FMR1* at chrX:147.9 Mb and *IDS* at chrX:149.4 Mb, respectively. X-inactivation in the female heterozygote is variable. If inactivation is skewed to the deleted X, physical signs of Hunter syndrome and fragile X syndrome are not seen, as Marshall et al. (2013) describe in their patient, a 4-year-old girl with global developmental delay, having the de novo deletion chrX:145.1-155.6 Mb.

Chromosome Y Deletions. The most common Y deletion is seen in the isodicentric chromosome, as a del/dup. The deletion in the idic(Y)(q) may involve a distal part of Yq, in company with duplication of proximal Yq and all of Yp, and vice versa in the idic(Y)(p), with a partial distal del(Yp) and dup(Yq), as discussed above and in Chapter 19.

del Yp11.2 The pseudoautosomal region 1 (PAR1) on the Y extends from Ypter to about chrY:2.70 Mb in band Yp11.2 (Fig. 15–9). Deletions that are confined to within PAR1, and which contain the *SHOXY* counterpart of *SHOX* at chrY:0.6 Mb, are rare, and indeed we know of no example of a "pure" Yp11.2 deletion including *SHOX* (this locus at the telomeric bound of band Yp11.2, essentially adjacent to Yp13.1). Should one be identified, short stature would be predicted. This was the observation in a boy with a de novo t(Y;22), who was otherwise quite normal, and in whom the effective imbalance was of a deletion from Ypter to at least *SHOX*, but

not as far as the sex-determining factor *SRY* (which is just beyond the PAR1 bound, at chrY:2.78 Mb) (Borie et al. 2004). Deletions more proximally within Yp11.2, and which include the *AMELY* gene (chrY:6.8 Mb), are nonpathogenic copy number variants (Jobling et al. 2007).

del Yq11.21q11.23 This de novo deletion was identified in a man with pervasive developmental disorder (IQ below the first centile), short stature, and some dysmorphisms (Tyson et al. 2009). The deletion is within Yq euchromatin, at chrY:11.6-25.5 Mb. Six cases in Salo et al. (1995), with de novo Yq deletions of varying (but less precise) extents, presented with cognitive compromise of varying degree, and minor dysmorphism. Genital defect is common. These authors mention a reservation

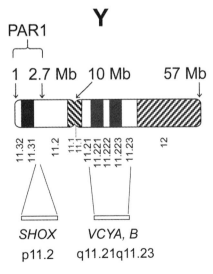

Y

PAR1

| 1 | 2.7 Mb | 10 Mb | 57 Mb |

SHOX VCYA, B
p11.2 q11.21q11.23

FIGURE 15-9

that intellectual impairment could possibly reflect ascertainment bias, and acknowledging that normal intellect has been reported in a man with a complete Yq deletion. Nevertheless, as Tyson et al. note, two genes in Yq11.21q11.23, VCY and VCY1B (chrY:13.9 and 14.0 Mb, respectively), may have a role in brain development, and this deletion would leave only the VCX X-homologous loci on Xp22.31 functional. The case for a causal relationship is plausible but unproven. Transmission is not recorded.

Chromosome X Duplications

dup Xp11.23p11.22 (Region 1) A recurrent duplication at Xp11.22p11.23 involves the segment chrX:48.4-52.6 Mb (Giorda et al. 2009; Evers et al. 2015; Nizon et al. 2015; Grams et al. 2016). The pheno-critical component may lie at chrX:50.3-50.7 Mb, wherein reside the genes *SHROOM4* and *DGKK* (Fig. 15–10). Males show a phenotype essentially the same as with the female. This may reflect that disomy of the chrX:48.4-52.6 Mb segment expresses the same in the male as in the female (in whom, curiously, the abnormal X is preferentially active, as mentioned below); of course, the male's single X is active. Intellectual deficiency ranges from mild to severe degree, with language in particular impaired; in one case, the IQ, at 86, was within a normal range. Autistic behavior and epilepsy (or at least an abnormal electroencephalographic pattern) are recorded. Brain scan can show minor anomalies or, in one case, actual cortical atrophy. Early puberty is observed. Facial dysmorphism is of mild or subtle degree.

All inherited cases of this duplication have come from a carrier mother. In these, the inheritance pattern could be described, in essence, as X-linked dominant. Most cases, however, have been de novo, and in these, the abnormal X has consistently been of paternal derivation. In female de novo cases, X-inactivation, where measured, has been nonrandom, and markedly skewed toward the *normal* X—a most remarkable observation (Di-Battista et al. 2016). Thus, the *abnormal* X is preferentially activated, and loci within the duplicated segment may express a functional, and therefore potentially damaging, disomy.

dup Xp11.23p11.22 (Region 2) Variable duplications within chrX:52.9-54.2 Mb, but overlapping the segment chrX:53.13-53.68, and having in common the inclusion of *HUWE1*, have been grouped by Grams et al. (2016) into a "Region 2" dup Xp11.22p11.23 class, albeit that most may actually be confined to the p11.22 band. Some recurrent breakpoints are observed, sited at points of long terminal repeats. The clinical picture includes intellectual deficiency, with a particular focus on poor speech acquisition. Mild facial dysmorphism and very minor digital anomalies are noted. In contrast to the Region 1 duplication, epilepsy is not a feature. Familial transmission, consistently from the mother, is recorded. In one notable family, in which the duplication encompassed both Region 1 and Region 2, inheritance from grandmother to mother to male child was observed.

dup Xp11.22 A small duplication within Region 2 above, but not including *HUWE1*, is reported in Moey et al. (2016). Three different but very similar duplications are described, each including *TSPYL2*, *KDM5C*, and *IQSEC2*, encompassed within chrX:53.08-53.23 Mb. All were maternally

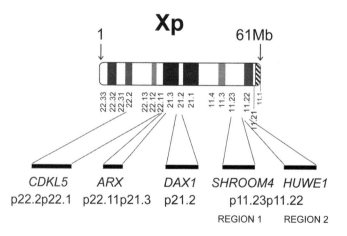

FIGURE 15–10

inherited. One child had two affected male cousins, these boys being the sons of three carrier sisters; one of the maternal grandparents was likely a mosaic hemizygote or heterozygote. The observed phenotype in the affected male is one of intellectual deficiency and attention deficit/hyperactivity.

dup Xp11.23p11.4 In a single de novo case, Monnot et al. (2008) report a young girl with a severe language deficit and minor dysmorphism, in whom X-inactivation was random. Thus, she had a functional partial Xp disomy for the p11.23p11.4 segment.

dup Xp21 A locus of important effect in this duplicated state is *DAX1* (also known as *NR0B1*) at Xp21.2, chrX:30.3 Mb, which may lead to sex reversal in the 46,dup(X),Y genetic male. Barbaro et al. (2012) review cases in which small (<1 Mb) duplications, encompassed within chrX:2.99-3.08 Mb, are associated with gonadal dysgenesis of differing forms in the affected phenotypic females. The 46,X,dup(X)(p21) female carrier is normal (seven carriers in the six-generation kindred in Barbaro et al.), and X-inactivation is random.

Cognitive capacity with these small duplications in Xp21 is unimpaired; but this is not so with larger imbalances, in which there is intellectual deficiency of variable degree. Speculatively, an additional copy of *IL1RAPL1* may be contributory. In some of these larger duplications, male gender may develop substantially normally; mild facial dysmorphism is also seen, as illustrated in the 12 Mb dup(X)(p21.3p11.4),Y case in Wu et al. (2013). This duplication extended from chrX:29.4-41.7 Mb; the phenotypically normal carrier mother showed preferential inactivation of the abnormal X chromosome. De novo cases are also recorded. (An additional complete copy of the Duchenne gene *DMD* at Xp21.1 seems to be without obvious effect.)

dup Xp22.11p21.3 Popovici et al. (2014) discuss the difficulty in determining pathogenicity in a duplication carried by some intellectually disabled persons, but then also identified as a de novo event in a child of superior IQ (who had presented due to a supravalvular aortic stenosis); and likewise seen in the unaffected maternal grandfather of a severely disabled child with the very similar duplication. These duplications within chrX:24.5-25.3 Mb included the *ARX* locus (chrX:25.0 Mb), this gene the basis of the ATR-X mental retardation syndrome. Popovici et al. debate whether *ARX* duplication has no phenotypic effect per se, or possibly that this imbalance may sometimes be vulnerable to the malign influence of regulatory factors. This uncertainty hampers counseling.

dup Xp22.2p22.1 Sismani et al. (2011) describe a family in which a mother heterozygous for a 9 Mb duplication chrX:9.8-19.0 Mb, dup Xp22.2p22.13, had four mentally retarded sons, there of whom died in childhood. She herself and her carrier daughter were of short stature but normal intelligence. These authors compare two similar duplications within the region Xp22.11 to Xp22.2, each with different breakpoints, but encompassing in common seven known X-linked mental retardation loci. One of these, *CDKL5*, at chrX:18.4 Mb in Xp22.13, is shown as a landmark locus in the ideogram above.

dup Xq12q13.3 Three families (one a five-generational pedigree) are on record segregating very similar duplications, with the segment chrX:67.5-74.7 Mb in common (Apacik et al. 1996; Kaya et al. 2012; Prontera et al. 2012). The affected males are microcephalic with marked intellectual deficiency, and in Apacik et al., with a slightly more extensive duplication, multiple malformations were associated with death in early infancy. Female carriers are phenotypically normal, but with completely skewed inactivation of the dup(X); the inheritance pattern is essentially that of an X-linked recessive disorder. A locus of particular interest within this segment is *XIST*, the X-inactivation center (Fig. 15–11).

Large Duplication Within Xq21q26 A number of dup(Xq) cases have been reported, of varying lengths, within this large (~60 Mb) Xq segment. Some are extensive and readily detectable on classical cytogenetics, while others (see below) warrant the appellation of microduplication. Both genders are seen; the clinical picture in the female, more so in the larger duplication, is often mitigated by skewed X-inactivation. One of the largest in a *female* is a de novo dup(X)(q21.1q25) initially diagnosed prenatally due to intrauterine growth retardation, in a girl whose circumstance at age 2 years remained one of a substantial physical and neurodevelopmental handicap (Tachdjian et al. 2004). These authors list reports of a variety of relatively large Xq duplications in affected females. Cheng et al. (2005) review

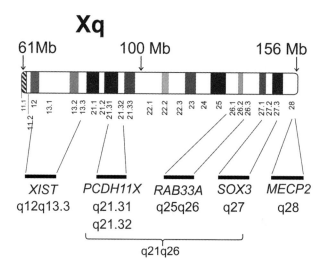

FIGURE 15–11

a number of reports of *male* cases of large duplication and present their own patient with 46,Y,dup(X)(q21.32q35), a profoundly retarded 2-year-old boy. Mostly, these are inherited from a heterozygous mother; grandpaternal meiosis may be the usual origin of the duplication.

dup Xq21 Gabbett et al. (2008) describe a boy with poor motor and language development, who became a "food seeker" as an infant, and who is described as presenting a Prader-Willi phenocopy, in whom a dup(X)(q21.1q21.31) was identified. His mother, who had had "learning difficulties" at school, proved (on blood analysis) to be a mosaic carrier of the duplication, with a random pattern of X-inactivation. Chromosomally adjacent to this case (but not overlapping), Basit et al. (2016) report a family in which five mild to moderately intellectually disabled brothers were the offspring of a consanguineous couple, but in fact a 3.95 Mb dup(X)(q21.31q21.32) at chrX:89.1-93.1 Mb proved to be the causative factor. Some displayed a facial dysmorphism; one was epileptic. Hyperphagia with obesity, dry skin, and self-mutilation were further observations. The phenotypically normal carrier mother and one sister showed markedly skewed X inactivation with respect to the abnormal X. Of the three genes within the duplicated segment, *PCDH11X* bids fair to be a pheno-critical locus; the other two are *TGIF2LX* and *PABPC5*.

Yet, some microduplications in this region are not to be over-interpreted: they may in fact be harmless, that is to say, a benign copy number variant. Maurin et al. (2017) make this point in their report of a 3.6 Mb microduplication at Xq21.33, discovered incidentally at prenatal diagnosis, and inherited, through the mother, from a normal grandfather. The fact of this being a gene-sparse region—only two loci resident therein, *DIAPH2* and *RPA4*, at chrX:96.6-97.6 Mb—is the likely basis of the non-pathogenicity, with these genes tolerating duplication. This principle applies more widely: a large CNV is not necessarily pathogenic.

dup Xq25 Di Benedetto et al. (2014) define a minimal segment of this proposed syndrome, encompassing the loci *XIAP* and *STAG2*, lying within the short segment chrX:123.8-124.1 Mb. Intellectual deficiency is of mild to moderate degree. Both affected and unaffected female carriers are observed.

dup Xq25q26.2 Møller et al. (2014) studied eight families in which a dup(X)(q25q26.2) was segregating. The 46,Y,dup(X) males manifested growth retardation and microcephaly with facial dysmorphism, digital anomalies, and abnormal genitalia. The heterozygous mothers were less affected, and mostly of normal intelligence; X-inactivation patterns in them were inconsistent. The duplications were nonrecurrent and fell within chrX:128.6-134.8 Mb. Some duplications did not overlap, allowing these authors to propose three pheno-critical segments: chrX:130.13-130.17 Mb containing the genes *AIFM1* and *RAB33A*, predisposing to intellectual disability; chrX:130.49-130.90 Mb leading to microcephaly, ptosis, and digital anomalies; and a broader segment, chrX:130.1-134.2 Mb, the basis of the syndromic facial dysmorphism, small hands and feet, and genital abnormality. They further identified a "polymorphic" segment at chrX:131.5-132.4 Mb, duplication of which was without phenotypic effect.

dup Xq26q27 A number of duplications within this region have been recognized, with the observations in common of growth retardation due to pituitary hypoplasia (Stagi et al. 2014). The pheno-critical gene is *SOX3* at chrX:140.5 Mb. Inheritance can be either de novo or due to maternal transmission. Skewed X-inactivation does not necessarily protect the female, as Stankiewicz et al. (2005) illustrate in their study of a short-statured mother and daughter. The dup(X)(q27) is also associated with XX sex reversal, and for example Vetro et al. (2015) describe a de novo 46,X,dup(X)(q27.1q27.3), chrX:140.4-146.0 Mb, with random X-inactivation, in a mildly developmentally delayed phenotypic male. *SOX3* is again implicated (and see Chapter 19).

dup Xq28, Lubs Syndrome The crucial locus in this syndrome of severe neurodevelopmental defect is *MECP2*, the Rett syndrome gene (at chrX:154.0 Mb) (Lim et al. 2017); duplication of the close-by *L1CAM*, *FLNA*, and *IKBKG* genes may also, in some, be pheno-contributory. In the large series of El Chehadeh et al. (2017), most duplications lay within the region chrX:153.6-154.6 Mb; a few may extend well into Xq27.3. Brain malformation is observed on imaging. The condition can be inherited from a carrier mother (who may herself be mildly affected) or of de novo generation. Rare female patients are affected, often, but not necessarily, less markedly than in the male; this may reflect the influence of random or unfavorable X-inactivation (Fieremans et al. 2014; Scott Schwoerer et al. 2014).

A most remarkable case is described in Magini et al. (2015), concerning a four-generation pedigree in which the original diagnosis had been of an X-linked syndrome of ataxia with psychomotor retardation, myoclonic encephalopathy, macular degeneration, and recurrent bronchopulmonary infections. The root cause was in fact a duplicated and deleted X, rea(X)(qter→Xq28::Xp22.33→qter), which carried a distal Xq dup at chrX:152,364,518-155,611,794, and a 1.2 Mb deletion at distal Xp.

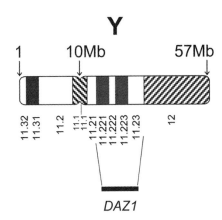

FIGURE 15–12

Two of the mothers, of normal neurological fusion, had a Madelung wrist deformity, a reflection of loss, on their rea(X), of the *SHOX* locus.

Chromosome Y Duplications. Y chromosome duplications, which largely refer to the isodicentric Y with a del/dup combination, are noted above. A single family is recorded with an inter-arm insertional Yq duplication of band Yq11.2 into the distal p arm, 46,X,insdup(Y)(pter→p11.32::q12→q11.1::p11.32→qter), presumed transmitted from a normal father to two normal sons; a locus therein is *DAZ1* (Fig. 15–12). The wife of one had presented with two miscarriages, which may or may not have been related (Engelen et al. 2003).

GENETIC COUNSELING

Many of the gonosomal structural rearrangements are associated with infertility, or at least subfertility. Some present a phenotype of relatively mild abnormality. Whether prenatal diagnosis is chosen, in those who are able to achieve pregnancy, may depend on the parents' perception of the seriousness of the potential abnormal outcome. Inference from prenatal X-inactivation analysis, in abn(X) cases, may be fraught with uncertainty.

SEX CHROMOSOME DELETIONS AND DUPLICATIONS

Del(X), dup(X). If the female del(X) or dup(X) carrier is fertile, the risk to transmit the abnormal chromosome will presumably reflect equal segregation, 1:1. If passed from a 46,X,del(X) mother to a *daughter*, the daughter's phenotype may be the same as that of the mother (which may well be quite normal). But a firm statement cannot be made. If the rule of selective Lyonization holds, the abn(X) is consistently the inactivated one, and normality might, in theory, be expected; while if the rule fails, random inactivation could, in theory, lead to an attenuated functional partial disomy, with phenotypic abnormality.

If a del(X) is passed from a 46,X,del(X) mother to a 46,Y,del(X) *male* conceptus, the hemizygous male fetus will be nullisomic for loci within the compass of the deletion. Viability may be possible, but the absence of loci will lead to a "contiguous gene syndrome." A classic example is the variable combination of Duchenne muscular dystrophy, adrenal hypoplasia, glycerol kinase deficiency, and mental retardation, due to deletion within Xp21, chrX:30.3-33.2 Mb. Larger microdeletions will often be lethal in utero, due to nullisomy for the segment concerned.

Fertility is usually an academic question in the male hemizygote for a del(X) or dup(X) (but the reader will well understand that, were his Y chromosome to be passed on, the child would, other things being equal, be normal).

Del(Y), dup(Y), r(Y). Fertility is achievable, with medical assistance, in some rea(Y) hemizygotes. In these cases, a 50:50 segregation with respect to the X and the rea(Y) chromosomes is to be assumed. A son inheriting the rea(Y) would very likely recapitulate his father's reproductive phenotype. In the specific case of the idic(Y), infertility affects the male and female. IVF may enable fertility in those few males with extractable sperm, but with a high risk to offspring, in principle 50%, and with postzygotic karyotypic evolution unpredictable, as per the phenotypic range outlined elsewhere (Chapter 19).

16

CHROMOSOME INSTABILITY SYNDROMES

A DEFECT OF DNA repair is the factor underlying the chromosome instability syndromes, also known as chromosome breakage syndromes (Brewer et al. 1997; Michelson and Weinert 2000; Taylor 2001). The "instability" refers to the predisposition of the chromosomes to undergo rearrangement, or to display other abnormal cytogenetic behavior. Their inclusion in this book is warranted in that special cytogenetic techniques may be useful in clinical diagnosis and prenatal diagnosis, albeit that direct molecular analysis is having an increasing role, as more is learned of the mutational basis of these syndromes.

The classic chromosome instability syndromes are Fanconi pancytopenia syndrome, Bloom syndrome, and ataxia-telangiectasia. The main cytogenetic features are listed in Table 16–1. They are Mendelian conditions, and in each the mode of inheritance is autosomal recessive. There is genetic heterogeneity in Fanconi syndrome, with cells homozygous for one mutation able to correct

in vitro cells homozygous for another mutation ("complementation"). We briefly note three other rare mutagen-hypersensitivity syndromes: the Nijmegen breakage syndrome; the immunodeficiency, centromeric instability, facial anomalies (ICF) syndrome; and Seckel syndrome. Proneness to cancer is a common concomitant of several of the breakage syndromes (Duker 2002). Some of these genes have in common their interaction with the breast cancer susceptibility gene *BRCA1*, their protein products forming a "BRCA1-associated genome surveillance complex" (Futaki and Liu 2001).

Rare or even unique families with various clinical presentations have been associated with chromosomal instability, and some representatives are mentioned in this chapter. Chromosome instability has been reported as an occasional observation in quite a number of known conditions. This list includes, among others, the Cockayne/ cerebro-oculo-facial-skeletal syndrome spectrum,

Table 16–1. The Three Classic Chromosome Instability Syndromes

SYNDROME	CYTOGENETIC FEATURES
Fanconi pancytopenia	Increased spontaneous and inducible chromosome breakage
Ataxia-telangiectasia	Increase in chromosome breaks; presence of clones with translocations having specific breakpoints in 7, 14, and X
Bloom syndrome	Increased spontaneous and inducible sister chromatid exchange; increased spontaneous chromatid breakage with production of symmetrical quadriradials

xeroderma pigmentosum, Rothmund-Thomson syndrome, Werner syndrome, Dubowitz syndrome, and Riyadh chromosome breakage syndrome. But in several the associations are not clear, the relevance for genetic counseling is uncertain (other than in supporting a diagnosis), and we do not consider them here. Likewise, chromosome instability is a feature of many cancers, and it may indeed be a crucial factor in the process of carcinogenesis; but this is a somatically acquired attribute and not of relevance in the present context.

A different cytogenetic observation is that of premature sister chromatid separation. This is a feature of Roberts syndrome, Cornelia de Lange syndrome, variegated aneuploidy syndrome, Warsaw breakage syndrome, and the chronic atrial and intestinal dysrhythmia syndrome, and we make brief mention of these conditions. The genes underlying these disorders code for cohesins, which contribute to the control of sister chromatid segregation at cell division, and thus are dubbed "cohesinopathies." Cohesins are one component of the "structural maintenance of chromosomes" (SMC) complexes, the other two being condensin and the SMC5-SMC6 complex (Uhlmann 2016). SMC complexes are a major component of the chromosomes of all living things; they control chromosome condensation and sister chromosome cohesion, as well as playing a role in DNA repair.

CLINICAL GENETICS AND CYTOGENETICS

The three classic chromosomal breakage syndromes, as well as Roberts syndrome, Nijmegen breakage syndrome, and the ICF syndrome, are of autosomal recessive inheritance, and the recurrence risk, for parents who have had one affected child, is 1 in 4. In those rare instances in which parenthood for the affected person is achievable, the risk to the child will in most cases be very low. Cornelia de Lange syndrome is almost always due to a de novo mutation.

Fanconi Pancytopenia Syndrome

This uncommon disorder of protean manifestation (also known simply as Fanconi anemia [FA]) is the least rare of the breakage syndromes (Tischkowitz and Hodgson 2003; Kennedy and D'Andrea 2005). Originally described as a disorder of short stature, characteristic facies, and certain malformations along with progressive bone marrow failure, the picture has now widened. In one-third of FA there are no major congenital malformations, although many of these will have minor anomalies, skin pigmentary abnormalities, microphthalmia, and growth indices below the 5th centile (Kee and D'Andrea 2012). Myelodysplastic syndrome and acute myeloid leukemia are common complications, and solid tumors may present at an unusually young age. Some patients whose clinical condition resembles the VACTERL[1] association may, in fact, have FA, and tests for chromosome breakage can enable the distinction to be made (Faivre et al. 2005).

Chromosomes show a range of abnormalities, including an increase in chromosome breakage, both spontaneously and upon exposure to DNA cross-linking agents (Fig. 16–1). There is little or no hypersensitivity to radiation damage. The increase in chromosome breakage after exposure of cells to a cross-linking agent such as diepoxybutane (DEB) provides, when it is observed, a reliable diagnostic test (Esmer et al. 2004; Castella et al. 2011).

As Joenje et al. (1998) note, most cytogenetic laboratories will see a case of true FA only very infrequently, and it may be difficult to maintain technical expertise in the practice

---

1 Vertebral, anal, cardiac, tracheo-esophageal, renal, limb.

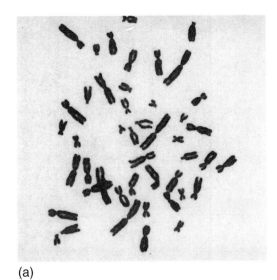

(a)

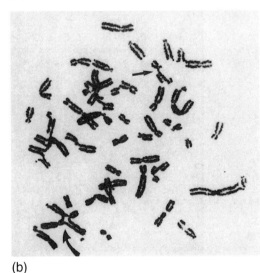

(b)

FIGURE 16-1 Metaphase from (a) a control and (b) a patient with Fanconi anemia after exposure to diepoxybutane. Note the high level of chromatid breakage in the patient metaphase. One chromatid break is indicated (straight arrow), and a quadriradial figure is shown (curved arrow).

of clastogen-challenge test protocols. Thus, a negative result might not absolutely exclude the diagnosis. Another reason for a misleading negative result is in vivo "correction" of the functional defect in blood-forming tissue by intragenic homologous recombination, with

proliferation of the corrected stem cell population. Joenje et al. refer to patients with typical FA who converted from a positive test result on blood sampling to apparent false negative over a period of years.[2] Skin fibroblasts maintain the clastogen-sensitive phenotype, and diagnosis following fibroblast study should be reliable.

There is genetic heterogeneity in FA, with at least 15 loci identified, mostly listed sequentially as *FANCA, FANCB*, and so on, to *FANCP*. With the exception of the X-linked *FANCB*, all are autosomal recessive. The gene products from these different loci contribute to the control of cellular DNA repair (Kee and D'Andrea 2012). One of the less common of these genes is the breast cancer susceptibility gene *FANCD1*, better known to the counselor as *BRCA2*; biallelic mutation leads to a particularly severe form of FA, with a very high cancer risk (Alter et al. 2007).

Prenatal diagnosis by mutation detection will be possible in those cases with a known mutation. Preimplantation diagnosis has been successfully applied, not only to select an unaffected embryo but also to select one with the same HLA typing, in order to enable blood stem cell donation to a pre-existing affected sibling, an approach not without controversy (Verlinsky et al. 2001b). Otherwise, DEB-induced chromosome breakage in amniotic fluid or chorionic villus cells should provide a satisfactory approach (Auerbach et al. 1986). We have seen a case in which, at routine fetal ultrasonography, upper limb defects were identified, and the couple chose to terminate the pregnancy; subsequent analysis of fetal tissue showed the characteristic cytogenetics of FA. This same cytogenetic testing was offered in subsequent pregnancies. Merrill et al. (2005) report somewhat similar experiences, although they were able to offer targeted testing for a specific mutation enriched in the Jewish population, following ultrasound suspicions of FA.

Bloom Syndrome

Bloom syndrome (BS) is a rare disorder that has its highest prevalence in Ashkenazi Jews, but also seen in many other ethnic groups. It is characterized clinically by proportionate short stature, a characteristic facies, sun-sensitive skin rash, immunodeficiency, and

---

2 This reversion to a normal cell line may work as a natural "self-treatment," whereby the normal marrow clone arising could have a proliferative advantage and ameliorate the disease state (Gross et al. 2002).

a marked susceptibility to cancer (German 1993). Infertility seems to be invariable in the male; females have difficulty conceiving, but a few have given birth (Martin et al. 1994). The Bloom gene, *BLM*, was originally mapped to 15q25qter by the elegant approach of determining the region of isodisomy in a child with BS and concomitant Prader-Willi syndrome due to uniparental disomy 15 (Woodage et al. 1994). *BLM* codes for a recQ DNA helicase that monitors DNA integrity during the S phase of the cell cycle (German and Ellis 2011). (Other members of this gene family are the basis of Rothmund-Thomson syndrome and Werner syndrome.)

The diagnostic cytogenetic finding in BS is a markedly increased level of spontaneous sister chromatid exchange (SCE). The normal is 6–10 exchanges per cell; in BS, it is more than 50 per cell (Fig. 16–2), although some normal cells may be present in BS patients.[3] The other cytogenetic abnormality is an increased incidence of spontaneous chromatid aberrations, giving the classic symmetrical quadriradial configuration. Intriguingly, this effect can manifest in the haploid state, with the heterozygous male producing an excess of sperm with chromosome breaks and rearrangements (Martin et al. 1994).

Prenatal diagnosis may be based upon observation of increased SCEs in chorionic villus cells (Howell and Davies 1994). Specific mutation analysis would be applicable if the family mutations were known; a Bloom mutation register is maintained (German et al. 2007). For the affected woman's reproductive outlook (in those few surviving to adulthood), the standard Mendelian advice, with consideration of the likelihood of the spouse being heterozygous, applies (Chisholm et al. 2001). As noted earlier, the male is infertile.

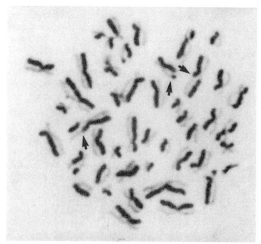

(a)

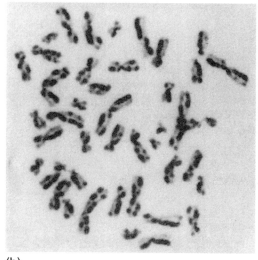

(b)

FIGURE 16–2   Metaphase from (*a*) a control and (*b*) a patient with Bloom syndrome, showing very high sister chromatid exchange (SCE) in the latter. Three points of SCE are indicated (arrows) on the control metaphase.

> We have identified a *Bloom syndrome variant* in two children, the offspring of consanguineous parents, who presented with slow growth and multiple café au lait macules, and whose cells exhibited a "Bloomoid" phenotype of markedly elevated levels of SCE (Hudson et al. 2016). The siblings were homozygously deleted for the gene *RMI2*, which encodes for one of the four proteins that make up the *BLM* complex.

Ataxia-Telangiectasia

Ataxia-telangiectasia (AT) is the archetype of a group in which the basic pathogenetic process is a failure in one of the monitoring and repair systems that keep watch for DNA damage. The group includes AT itself

---

3 Interestingly, and analogous to the FA "self-treatment" noted above, the normal cells may be due to a "correcting" genetic event occurring in a bone marrow cell, and which then leads to a heterozygous cell line having a normal in vitro phenotype. The correcting event may be either a somatic recombination between the two sites of *BLM* mutation in the homologs in the BS individual with compound heterozygosity, or a back mutation in a homozygote (Ellis et al. 2001).

and Nijmegen breakage syndrome (below), and both exhibit chromosome instability. The genes for AT and Nijmegen breakage syndrome encode proteins that are part of a complex that senses abnormal DNA structures and monitors post-replication DNA repair (Michelson and Weinert 2000).

The clinical presentation of AT is as a brain/immune/cancer syndrome. It is characterized by cerebellar ataxia and oculomotor apraxia (difficulty in performing voluntary eye movements), oculocutaneous telangiectasia, immunodeficiency, and increased cancer predisposition. The cytogenetic hallmarks of AT include frequent nonrandom rearrangements of chromosomes 7, 14, and occasionally X, in T-lymphocytes; nonspecific chromosome breakage in fibroblasts; and normal chromosomes in bone marrow. The breakpoints in the lymphocyte rearrangements are at 7p14, 7q35, 14q12, and 14q32, involving the T-cell receptor and immunoglobulin heavy chain genes. Clones with rearrangements may be harbingers of a T-cell malignancy, and these clones evolve as the disease progresses. Breakage is exacerbated, in vitro, by exposure of cells to ionizing radiation and to radiomimetic chemicals such as bleomycin (Kojis et al. 1991).

Most *ATM* mutations are null, but missense and splicing mutations that allow a limited amount of functional product to be produced may lead to milder clinical and cytogenetic phenotypes. Some of these "milder" mutations may, on the other hand, promote an increased cancer risk, including breast cancer in the female heterozygote (Chenevix-Trench et al. 2002).

Prenatal diagnosis of classic AT could be approached cytogenetically on amniocyte analysis, but direct mutation analysis of the *ATM* gene on chorionic villus tissue is preferred due to its greater accuracy (Gatti and Perlman 2016). Preimplantation genetic diagnosis may be successful (Hellani et al. 2002).

Nijmegen Breakage Syndrome

This is another brain/immune/cancer syndrome, and it is rare indeed. The clinical picture includes microcephaly with brain dysgenesis, immune deficiency, and risk for lymphoreticular malignancy. It shares with AT certain cytogenetic features (preferential involvement of chromosomes 7 and 14 in rearrangements) and radiation hypersensitivity (Antoccia et al. 2006). The causative gene, called *NBS1*, interacts with the *ATM* gene, noted above. A founder mutation, 657del5, is common among the Slavic

population, and most patients are 657del5 homozygotes (Seemanová et al. 2006). Prenatal diagnosis is preferably achieved by specific mutational analysis.

Roberts Syndrome

Roberts syndrome (RS) is a syndrome of craniofacial abnormalities and limb defects that are often severe, and the archetype of the "cohesinopathies." Cohesinopathies are genetic instability syndromes that are associated with defects in the regulators and structural components of the cohesion complex, which is responsible for maintaining sister chromatid cohesion during mitosis, from synthesis to separation. In RS, the phenotype is so very distinctive that it is unsurprising that case reports date back some centuries, the first appearing in 1672 (a "Portrait d'un enfant monstre"), well before Roberts' description from 1919 (Bates 2003; Kompanje 2009). Intellect is normal.

Most affected individuals (~80%) exhibit a chromosomal phenomenon known as premature chromatid separation (PCS), sometimes described as "tram-tracking" or "railroad track appearance," and also referred to as "heterochromatin repulsion," as the sister chromatids bulge away from each other. The gene is *ESCO2* (Vega et al. 2010), and its product enables proper disposition of the chromatids. In its absence, there is an abnormality of sister chromatid apposition around the centromeres, particularly noticeable for those chromosomes with large blocks of heterochromatin (Fig. 16–3). It is best seen in plain-stained or C-banded chromosomes; G-banding obscures the phenomenon (Van Den Berg and Francke 1993). In this particular instance, classical cytogenetics is the more powerful diagnostic tool, and it may enable recognition of an atypical case; microarray would miss the abnormality (Gerkes et al. 2010).

Prenatal diagnosis based upon the presence or absence of PCS at chorionic villus sampling or amniocentesis, and abnormality or normality of limbs on first-trimester fetal ultrasonography, should be valid in at least the majority. It would be prudent to follow up an interpretation of normality at second-trimester ultrasonography. Molecular testing can be applied when the specific mutation is known (Schulz et al. 2008).

Cornelia de Lange Syndrome

The clinical phenotype of Cornelia de Lange Syndrome (CdLS) is, in the classic case, very

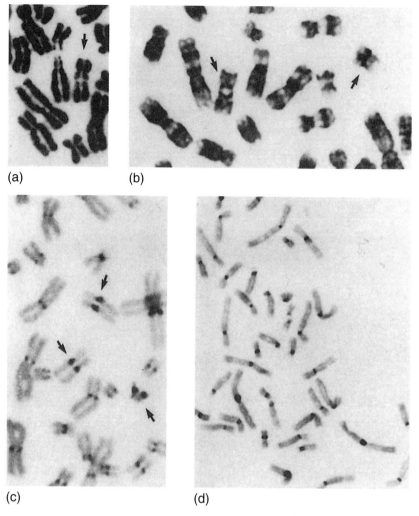

(a)   (b)

(c)   (d)

FIGURE 16–3   Unusual appearance of the chromosomes in Roberts syndrome: puffing at the centromeres (*a* and *b*); a C-banded preparation showing separation of the heterochromatic segments (*c*) is compared with a C-banded preparation from a control showing the normal centromere appearance (*d*).

Source: From Mann et al., Roberts syndrome: Clinical and cytogenetic aspects, *J Med Genet* 19: 116–119, 1982, with the permission of the British Medical Association.

distinctive. To date, five causative genes are known: *NIPBL* (the most frequently seen); *SMC1A* and *RAD21* cause autosomal dominant CdLS, typically due to de novo mutations; and mutations in *SMC3* and *HDAC8* are the basis of X-linked CdLS (Boyle et al. 2015). The cytogenetic phenotype is PCS, and thus CdLS is another cohesinopathy. Be that as it may, testing for PCS is not useful in the diagnosis of CdLS, with one study showing it to be no more frequent in CdLS patients than in controls (Castronovo et al. 2009).

VERY RARE SYNDROMES

ICF (Immunodeficiency, Centromeric Instability, Facial Anomalies) Syndrome. The ICF syndrome is characterized by immunodeficiency, an unusual facies, and growth and developmental retardation; and a most remarkable tendency of chromosomes 1, 9, and 16 to form "windmill" multiradials by interchange within heterochromatic regions (Fig. 16–4). This instability of the pericentromeric heterochromatin reflects hypomethylation of satellites II and III, which are important components

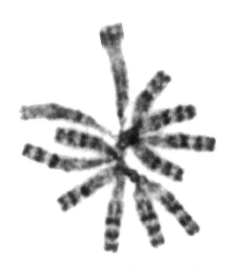

FIGURE 16–4   A "windmill" or "starburst" multiradial chromosome 1 in the ICF syndrome.

Source: From Sawyer et al., Chromosome instability in ICF syndrome: Formation of micronuclei from multibranched chromosomes 1 demonstrated by fluorescence in situ hybridization, *Am J Med Genet* 56: 203–209, 1995. Courtesy J. R. Sawyer, and with the permission of Wiley-Liss.

of its structure. Hagleitner et al. (2008) document the variability of the phenotypic range. The phenotype, physical and cytogenetic, can be considered to be secondary to a failure of methylation. Most cases are due to autosomal recessive mutations in either DNA methyltransferase 3B (*DNMT3B*, ICF1) or *ZBTB24* (ICF2) (van den Boogaard et al. 2017).

Mosaic Variegated Aneuploidy. The core phenotype of this recessively inherited syndrome comprises microcephaly with functional neurological abnormality, growth retardation, and susceptibility to childhood malignancy, with most of the lymphocytes and about half of skin fibroblasts showing premature chromatid separation. Many cells are aneuploid, with trisomies, double trisomies, and monosomies, with almost every chromosome represented (Bohers et al. 2008; García-Castillo et al. 2008). In mosaic variegated aneuploidy (MVA) type 1, the underlying defect in the cell cycle involves one of the checkpoint proteins (BUB1B) that control progression through the mitotic process, maintaining an alert for chromosome malsegregation. The *BUB1B* heterozygote may display the tendency in a proportion of lymphocytes, and some mitotic cells may present the striking observation of a 92-chromosome count. MVA type 2 is caused by mutations in *CEP57*, coding for a centrosomal

protein that stabilizes microtubules (Snape et al. 2011). Prenatal diagnosis has been reported, based on conventional cytogenetics, the abnormalities being very obvious (Plaja et al. 2003; Chen et al. 2004c).

Seckel Syndrome and Primary Autosomal Recessive Microcephalies. This spectrum of disorders presents with microcephaly of prenatal onset, an absence of visceral malformations, and variable cognitive impairment and short stature. Mutations in at least 16 different genes are responsible. Although these disorders are well suited to diagnosis by multigene sequencing panels, chromosome analysis may also have a role. Premature chromosome condensation, initially described by Neitzel et al. (2002) as a novel syndrome in siblings with microcephaly and cognitive impairment, is now known to be caused by mutations in *MPCH1*. In a group of five patients with Seckel syndrome of unknown genotype, Bobabilla-Morales et al. (2003) demonstrated excessive chromosomal breakage with mitomycin C, although not an excess of SCEs. Casper et al. (2004) discovered, in patients with SCKL1 (due to the *ATR* gene, which interacts with *ATM*), increased breakage rate at known fragile sites.

Warsaw Breakage Syndrome. A severely growth-retarded and microcephalic teenager showed both chromosomal breakage and premature chromatid separation, and his case represents a further cohesinopathy, named Warsaw breakage syndrome for the city of his residence (van der Lelij et al. 2010). The causative gene is *DDX11*, having some sequence similarity to the gene for Fanconi anemia type J, and coding for a helicase. Inheritance is autosomal recessive, although there is a hint the heterozygote may have an increased cancer risk. Additional families are reported in Capo-Chichi et al. (2013), Bailey et al. (2015), and Eppley et al. (2017).

Chronic Atrial and Intestinal Dysrhythmia Syndrome. This rare autosomal recessive disorder has the cytogenetic phenotype of "railroad track" heterochromatin repulsion at the centromere (Chetaille et al. 2014). The clinical presentation is with cardiac arrhythmia and intestinal pseudo-obstruction, in the first four decades of life, in the absence of birth defects or signs of other cohesinopathy.

Syndromes Reported in Only One or Two Families (A Few Examples)

- Ishikawa et al. (2000) reported a single family with a dominantly inherited chromosome instability syndrome. The major clinical observations are mild to moderate mental retardation, depression, and a spastic ataxia, with striking abnormalities of cerebral white matter and the basal ganglia, and an atrophic spinal cord. All three affected individuals having a cytogenetic analysis showed a low frequency of a t(7;14), with a common 14q11.2 breakpoint in each, and a hypersensitivity to radiation and radiomimetic drugs.

- A unique Austrian family appears to present a sex-limited chromosome breakage syndrome with ovarian failure (Duba et al. 1997). The index case had presented with primary hypogonadism, and karyotyping showed a high proportion of cells with breaks, acentric fragments, triradial rearrangements, and dicentric chromosomes. Two healthy brothers had essentially the same chromosome findings. The cytogenetic picture most closely resembled that of Fanconi anemia, and the three siblings also demonstrated an elevation in α-fetoprotein, which is a feature of AT. Lespinasse et al. (2005) report a similar case, but in this instance, a sister and a brother were both infertile, and the α-fetoprotein was normal.

- Bakhshi et al. (2006) describe a 17-year-old boy with growth retardation and dysmorphic facies, with mitomycin-sensitive chromosomal breakage, who developed a B-cell lymphoma; they proposed this as a new syndrome, distinct from FA.

- We have described two families in which biallelic mutations in SPRTN caused a novel chromosome instability syndrome, with progeroid features and early onset hepatocellular cancer (Lessel et al. 2014). Nonclonal structural chromosome abnormalities, comprising spontaneous breaks, rearrangements, deletions, and marker chromosomes, were present in peripheral blood, comparable with "variegated translocation mosaicism," a phenomenon previously described in cells of the Werner premature-aging syndrome.

- van der Crabben et al. (2016) identified a new chromosome breakage disorder associated with defective T and B cell function, and leading to fatal lung disease, in four children from two unrelated families. Peripheral blood cells showed multiple de novo chromosome rearrangements and variable numbers of de novo supernumerary marker chromosomes. This is another disorder of the SMC complex (see above), due to biallelic missense mutations in the NSMCE3 gene, which encodes a subunit of the SMC5/6 complex essential for DNA damage response and chromosome segregation.

- The Bloom-like syndrome described by ourselves is noted above.

PART THREE

CHROMOSOME VARIANTS

17

NORMAL CHROMOSOMAL VARIATION

One definition of human genetics is "the study of inherited human variation." Variation can be normal: traits such as height, blood pressure, and intelligence. Abnormal variation may be clearcut: dwarfism, hypertension, and intellectual deficiency. But the distinction may blur at the edges: short stature, borderline blood pressure, and low-normal IQ. There is somewhat of a parallel in the study of chromosomes. Some variation is quite normal, and well understood as such. And of course an observation such as a large deletion is abnormal. But some chromosomal variation does not admit of straightforward interpretation.

The word "variant" has gained considerable currency in the genetic lexicon of this century (Bruno et al. 2012). Molecular laboratories may issue reports concerning a Mendelian gene, referring to a "pathogenic variant," in preference to the formerly favored expression, "mutation." The word variant does allow, in principle, for a nuanced interpretation, and conventionally the gamut runs a sliding scale from pathogenic, through likely pathogenic, of uncertain significance, likely benign, to benign/nonpathogenic. A similar construction is now applied to chromosomal variants of small size, detectable only upon molecular karyotyping. The matter is further complicated by variation within a variant: It may be harmless in one setting and pathogenic in another. The expressions "microdeletion/microduplication" may more usefully be reserved for cases in which the abnormality is taken unequivocally to be pathogenic.

We may consider variation within two major categories, essentially reflecting analysis due to either classical or molecular methodology: heteromorphisms ancient and modern, so to say. First, there is variation in size, staining qualities, and certain other attributes, from the microscopic analysis of chromosomes. Second, we have the copy number variants (CNVs) revealed in molecular karyotyping. As for the genetics, in either category the likelihood of transmission of a variant from parent to child is simple Mendelian, 50/50 (transmission naturally being gender-specific for X-linked variants). More so with CNVs, de novo generation is not uncommon. The particular difficulty lies in the occasional penetrance of some (usually) nonpathogenic CNVs.

CLASSICAL CYTOGENETICS

Microscopists from the era of classical cytogenetics became very familiar with the appearances of chromosomes and learned readily to distinguish normal structural variation. The counselor of the twenty-first century may yet need to refer to historic literature and should have at least some familiarity with these classical concepts. Homologs could differ in the respects discussed next.

BANDING PATTERN: HETEROCHROMATIN

Heterochromatin is made up of highly repetitive DNA that has been distinguishable from euchromatin for the larger part of a century (Heitz 1928).[1] Heterochromatic variants are best seen on C-banding, which specifically stains the extensive tracts of heterochromatin adjacent to the centromeres of each chromosome (hence, the C), substantially comprising alpha-satellite DNA consisting of hundreds of thousands of copies of a 171 base pair repeat. Certain chromosomes show quite marked differences in their C-band pattern, particularly chromosomes 1, 9, 16, and the Y, and the large blocks of heterochromatin thus stained are labeled 1qh, 9qh, 16qh, and Yqh.[2] They are of no phenotypic effect.[3]

ACROCENTRIC SHORT ARMS

The short arms of the acrocentric chromosomes (13, 14, 15, 21, and 22) can vary quite considerably in their lengths. Indeed, some p arms are apparently completely absent, and others are several times the typical length. This reflects variation in the three components of the short arm: the centromeric heterochromatin, the satellite stalk, and the satellite material, identified as bands p11, p12, and p13, respectively. Band p12 contains multiple copies

of genes coding for ribosomal RNA; because the nucleolus of the cell is formed by an aggregation of rRNA, this region is also called the nucleolar organizing region (NOR). Acrocentric short arm variation appears to be without any phenotypic effect.

BANDING PATTERN: EUCHROMATIN

Most of a chromosome consists of euchromatin, which contains the active genetic material, resident in greater amount in G-light bands (pale-staining on Giemsa banding) than in G-dark bands. The light microscope cannot reliably enable detection of alterations of less than 3–5 Mb, and most deletions and duplications of more than this size can be presumed to have phenotypic consequences. Exceptions to this rule include, first, euchromatic variants that involve common copy-number variable regions that become visible when copy number is high enough, or when the size of the copy-number variable tract is large enough. Second, there are chromosomal segments whose deletion or duplication has no phenotypic consequence.

EUCHROMATIC VARIANTS

Euchromatic variants (EVs) due to copy-number variable tracts (Table 17–1) can be considered, in a sense, as extreme forms of CNVs, either because their copy number is at the high end or higher than the normal range or because their size is greater than 3 Mb (at which point they are excluded from the Database of Genomic Variants; see below). Thus, EVs and the molecular CNVs (below) essentially form a continuum, with no fundamental genetic distinction. For example, Tyson et al. (2014) analyzed the *REXO1L1* gene and pseudogene cluster which resides within a 12 kb tandem repeat in band 8q21.2, and of which the diploid copy number ranges from approximately 100 to 200. This repeat may account for almost half of band 8q21.2 and, at the upper end of this range, additional G-light material is discernible (Fig. 17–1). Albeit that D'Apice et al. (2015) proposed that deletion of this segment (but with several copies yet remaining) could be

---

1 The seminal contributions of Emil Heitz to the science of cytogenetics are reviewed in Passarge (1979).

2 Variation in the size of Yqh in an extended Canadian kindred could inferentially be traced back over three centuries, allowing Genest (1973, 1981) to claim that it was "the oldest known chromosome aberration."

3 This has been the prevailing, if not universal view, for quite some time. Reproduction may, however, be a vulnerable sphere; and Tempest and Simpson (2017) review the reported associations with infertility and unfavourable reproductive outcomes.

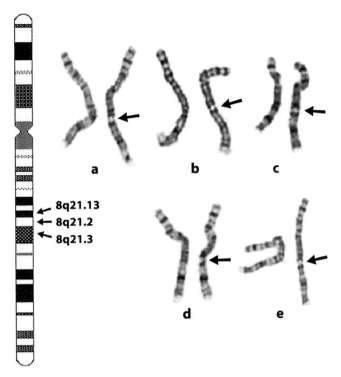

FIGURE 17–1   The likely benign euchromatic variant at 8q21.3, which reflects copy number variation of the *REXO1L1* gene and pseudogene cluster. This observation could be viewed, in a sense, as an intermediary between classical and molecular cytogenetic variation.

Source: From Tyson et al., Expansion of a 12-kb VNTR containing the *REXO1L1* gene cluster underlies the microscopically visible euchromatic variant of 8q21.2, *Eur J Hum Genet* 22: 458–463. 2014. Courtesy J. C. K. Barber and C. Tyson, and with the permission of Nature Publishing Group.

Table 17–1. Euchromatic Variants due to Copy-Number Variable Tracts

EUCHROMATIC VARIANT (EV)	REPEAT/SEGMENT SIZE	CONTROL COPY NUMBER	EV COPY NUMBER
dup 8p23.2	2.5 Mb	2	3
amp 8p23.1	>260 kb	2-9	8–12
amp 8q21.2	12 kb	97–277	265–270
amp 9p12	~1 Mb	1–3	7–12
del/dup 9p11.2p13.1	~5 Mb	4	3–5
dup/trp/ins 9q12	~5 Mb	4	5–6
del/dup/trp/amp 9q13q21.1	~5 Mb	4	3–8
amp 15q11.2	~1 Mb	*IGVH* 1–3; *NF1* 1–4	*IGVH* 4–9; *NF1* 5–10
amp 16p11.2	692–945 kb	3–8	8–10

Abbreviations: amp, amplification; dup, duplication; EV, euchromatic variant; ins, insertion; IGVH, immunoglobulin variable heavy chain; NF1, neurofibromatosis 1; trp, triplication.

Source: From Tyson et al. (2014).

the basis of a new microdeletion syndrome, Barber et al. (2016) argue that, more likely, it may typically be a benign EV. The same interpretation of innocuousness likely applies to the other EVs listed in Table 17–1.

Some of these EVs may have been confused, on classical karyotyping, with pathogenic imbalances. On microarray analysis, however, the distinction should be clear; and in fact many microarrays exclude the repetitive regions that EVs involve.

IMBALANCES OF CHROMOSOMAL SEGMENTS WITH NO APPARENT PHENOTYPIC EFFECT

In a review in 2005, Barber found only 23 examples of families with directly transmitted autosomal segmental imbalance in which two or more carriers were unaffected, and a few have since been published (Table 17–2). These cases were often ascertained for incidental reasons, such as prenatal diagnosis for maternal age. The gene content is often lower than

Table 17–2. Euchromatic Duplications and Deletions (and One Quadruplication) Detectable by Microscope Cytogenetics, and Without Phenotypic Effect, as Inferred from the Observation of Transmission from Phenotypically Normal Parent to Normal Child

CHROMOSOME	DEL	DUP	QDP
1		p21-p31	
		q31.1-q32	
2	p12-p12 (x2)		
	q13-q14.1		
3	p25.3-pter (×2)	q28-q29	
4	q34.1-q34.3	p16.1-p16.1	q12q13.1
5	p14.1-p14.3 (×2)		
6	q22.31-q23.1		
7		p22.3-pter (×2)	
8	p23.1/2-pter	p22-p22	
	q24.13-q24.22	p23.1-p23.3	
9	p21.2-p22.1	p12-p21.3	
10	q11.2-q21.2	p11.1-q11.22	
		p13-p14	
11	p12-p12		
	q14.3-q22.1		
12		q21.31-q22	
13	q14.3-q21.33	q13-q14.3	
	q21-q21	q14-q21	
	q21.1-q21.31		
	q21.1-q21.33		
16	q13q22 (×4)		
18	p11.31-pter	p11.2-pter	
		q11.2-q12.2	
22	q11.21-pter		

Notes: The estimated sizes of the deletions and duplications range from 4.2 to 16.0 Mb (del) and from 3.4 to 31.3 Mb (dup). The numbers of studied families, where more than one, are shown in parentheses.

Source: From Barber (2005), and the Chromosome Anomaly Collection website at http://www.ngrl.org.uk/wessex/collection (updated information is posted in the "What's New" section). Additional material due to Chen et al. (2011b), Coussement et al. (2011), Kowalczyk et al. (2013), and Liehr et al (2009b).

the genome average, and the lack of phenotype is attributed to the absence of dosage-sensitive genes, or to dosage compensation by related genes. Similar imbalances with no phenotypic consequence are recorded in more than one family for the gene-poor G-dark bands 2p12, 5p14, 13q21, and 16q21. Most of the families listed in Table 17–2 remain as isolated examples and may yet turn out to reflect segmental incomplete penetrance. This may apply, for example, to the distal 3p cases, as other families with similar deletions are more often phenotypically affected. This question of penetrance, in these few cases of cytogenetically visible imbalances, is somewhat of a harbinger of the immense challenge that came to be presented by the flood of CNVs of twenty-first century molecular analysis, as we discuss at length below.

Inversions. We mention normal variant inversions seen in certain chromosomes (1, 2, 3, 5, 9, 10, 16, and Y) in Chapter 9.

Fragile Sites. Under certain stressed culturing conditions, some, indeed most, chromosomes show apparent rupture in one or, less commonly, both chromatids (Sutherland and Hecht 1985; Sutherland and Baker 2000; Arlt et al. 2003; Sutherland 2003). This is almost always without phenotypic implication. The spectacular exception is the fragile site FRAXA at Xq27, and indeed this laboratory observation lent its name to the well-known fragile X syndrome, originally referred to as a "marker" X (Lubs 1969). The fragile site observed by the microscopist reflected the trinucleotide expansion within the *FMR1* gene. Three other sites in the same region are FRAXB, FRAXD, and FRAXE, of which only the latter is pathogenic. Otherwise, only two fragile sites may be of clinical import. FRA11B, at 11q23.3, is possibly the basis of some (not all) Jacobsen syndrome 11q deletions (Michaelis et al. 1998; and see p. 288). A single case of a man with 46,XY,fra(16)(q22.1), the fragile site classed FRA16B/C, in whom 1% of sperm and two out of 10 PGD embryos showed chromosome 16 imbalance, is to be noted (Martorell et al. 2014). We mention the fragile site FRA10A at 10q23, which

may or may not be relevant at prenatal diagnosis, on p. 495.

COPY NUMBER VARIANTS

The molecular lens, when it began to be applied from the late twentieth century, came up with a somewhat surprising observation: Short genomic segments could exist in deleted or duplicated state, invisible on routine classical cytogenetics, among individuals in the general, normal population. They are certainly common, indeed universal: each of us has, on average, 1,000 CNVs of >450 bp, compared to a reference genome (Conrad et al. 2010). The word "variant" can allow, as noted above, for agnosticism in terms of pathogenicity; adjectives and adjectival qualifiers can be added, accordingly as the interpretation unfolds, and a descriptive classification conferred (Figure 17–2):

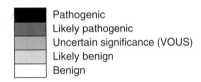

FIGURE 17–2   CNV Gradations.

What is the actual basis of the variation? A short segment of chromatin—a "copy"—would normally exist on a chromosome in single state, and thus with one copy on each autosome (and one on each or one X chromosome, according to gender). Variation lies in the presence of these copies in absent or double (sometimes triple or quadruple or higher) states on a chromosome, and hence the expression *copy number* variant. The copy size can vary from less than 1 kb to approximately 1 Mb.[4] Some segments are in "gene deserts"; others contain known genes. If there is an observation that no untoward effect exists in the presence of a single, triple, or higher multiple amount of these genes, this then allows the inference that these genes are not dosage-sensitive.

The difficulty lies in determining that a CNV is, indeed, a normal variant and of no phenotypic import (Hehir-Kwa et al. 2013). The harmlessness

---

4 The lower limit of size may be taken as 1 kb (a clinical viewpoint), or to as low as 50 bp (as seen by a molecular scientist) (Martin and Warburton 2015; Zarrei et al. 2015). Elements below 50 kb are known as insertions or deletions, or "indels." An upper limit of 1 Mb is proposed, although many cases in the literature involving segments of up to a few megabases have been called CNVs. The DGV database uses an arbitrary, somewhat higher cut-off of 3 Mb; this could be seen as a pragmatic border between the euchromatic segmental variants described above and the CNVs as discussed here.

of many CNVs is attested by their segregation within a family, in which only the proband (through whom the CNV was ascertained) may have been of abnormal phenotype. In these, the CNV can usually be taken as benign/nonpathogenic, and its discovery merely coincidental. The finding of a de novo change may more reasonably be considered as likely causative; but the gene content of this genomic segment should be considered in the context of the patient's phenotype, and not losing sight of the fact that de novo CNVs are not uncommon in healthy individuals. Interpretation may need to account for ethnicity: The frequencies of some CNVs vary depending on the background of the individuals tested. Had it been possible to make a clear distinction between all "CNVs" consistently harmless, and all those consistently pathogenic, the discussions in this chapter and in the chapters on autosomal and sex chromosomal microdeletions and microduplications (Chapters 14 and 15) could have been quite self-contained. But that is not the case—at least as at the present writing.

The five-part classification is not necessarily as clear-cut as the grayscale above might imply. With what confidence can a CNV be called indeed pathogenic, or benign? The bar is high: Only those "practically certain" to be so, can be called so. How likely is "likely"? In the similar setting of Mendelian variants, an expert group[5] views 90% as a suitable cut-off (Richards et al. 2015). That leaves another 80% or so in the "variant of uncertain significance" (VOUS) territory. Every counselor can expect to encounter, and to deal with, VOUSs.

The genic content of a CNV would seem, intuitively, to be a key—possibly the key—factor determining pathogenicity, or not. This "common-sense" viewpoint is given formal support in Rice and McLysaght (2017), who determined that a pathogenic CNV is more likely to contain a gene or genes that are dosage-sensitive, that have a role in embryonic development, or that are evolutionarily conserved. "Ohnologs" (footnote p. 264) are especially represented in pathogenic CNVs. Applying this understanding may, in due course, be helpful in allowing a more precise interpretation of which CNVs are of clinical significance.

We mentioned in Chapter 14 the concept of a deletion "unmasking heterozygosity"

of a recessive allele coincidentally on the other chromosome. The similar scenario may obtain with an otherwise benign deletion CNV, if a locus therein happens to code for a Mendelian recessive disease. Thus, Liu, Li, et al. (2016) diagnosed autosomal recessive spastic ataxia of Charlevoix and Saguenay (ARSACS) in a patient with a SACS mutation at 13q12.12 on one chromosome, and a 1.33 Mb CNV deletion encompassing the SACS locus on the other. We have seen a very similar case, in a woman with ataxia and a Charcot-Marie-Tooth-like neuropathy inheriting a (normally non-pathogenic) paternal 0.2 Mb CNV deletion which removed SACS, and an accompanying maternal SACS mutation on the other homolog, and thus enabling a diagnosis of ARSACS.

DATABASES

The counselor dealing with a family in which a CNV has been shown, has formidable resources to which to appeal. Collaborative efforts from around the world bring together data, and repositories are assembled to which enquiry may be made. An important resource is DECIPHER, the Database of Chromosomal Imbalance and Phenotype in Humans Using Ensembl Resources. This database lists known or possibly pathogenic variants and also VOUSs. The Internet link is http://decipher.sanger.ac.uk. A panel displays CNVs that either match with or overlap with a segment of interest. Duplications are shown in blue, and deletions are shown in red. The distinction between pathogenic variants and VOUSs is indicated by the differing color intensity (the darker, the more likely to be pathogenic). The user will note that many cases show DDD as the data source: This is the database Deciphering Developmental Disorders, and it is accessible at http://www.ddduk.org.

A complementary resource is ClinGen, a "National Institutes of Health-funded resource dedicated to building an authoritative central resource that defines the clinical relevance of genes and variants for use in precision medicine and research." Each listed variant has a thumbnail sketch of the

---

5 American College of Medical Genetics and Genomics and the Association for Molecular Pathology.

clinical history alongside; the link is http://www.clinicalgenome.org.[6]

A more encyclopedic collection, including the smallest normal variants, is that due to DGVa—the *Database of Genomic Variants* (version *a*)—which is curated at The Center for Applied Genomics at the Hospital for Sick Children, Toronto, Ontario, Canada. The Center records "genomic alterations that involve segments of DNA that are larger than 50 bp. . . . The content of the database is only representing structural variation identified in *healthy control samples.*" The data derive from upwards of 14,000 individuals, carrying more than 77,000 deletions and 660 duplications (MacDonald et al. 2014; Zarrei et al. 2015). The database is accessed directly at http://dgv.tcag.ca/dgv/app/home. Continuing refining of the data leads to increasing accuracy and confidence, and a special track within the DGVa lists "gold standard structural variants" (GSSVs). The UCSC (*University of California, Santa Cruz*) genome browser site at http://genome.ucsc.edu is another useful resource. The site simultaneously displays information from DECIPHER, the Copy Number Variation Morbidity Map of Developmental Delay, OMIM, RefSeq genes, and GeneReviews.

The data from the laboratory need to be clearly conveyed to those for whom the report is intended, which will very often be the genetic counselor. A pictorial display, with accompanying written detail, is a style of document with which the twenty-first century counselor is becoming well familiar, such as that produced by the Genoglyphix database (see Fig. 17–6 below).

Copy Number Variants and the Brain. The most complex organ, the brain, is the most susceptible to CNV imbalance, and typically presenting as cognitive/behavioral dysfunction; indeed, in most CNV imbalances, there is no observable physical phenotypic abnormality. In a large study of children with intellectual deficiency/developmental delay, an excess of those with a CNV compared to controls emerged significantly at a CNV size of 400 kb, and became more evident at 1.5 Mb (Cooper et al. 2011). At least some of these CNVs, therefore,

would have been pathogenic. Again unsurprisingly, larger (>1.5 Mb) CNVs were overrepresented in de novo cases; presumably this reflects a reduced reproductive fitness of those with larger, and pathogenic, CNVs. Similar conclusions are reached in Coe et al. (2014). McCormack et al. (2016) recorded frequencies of benign versus pathogenic CNVs in an abnormal population (Fig. 17–3). A subtler study was performed in Estonia (Männik et al. 2015); in this study, the CNV status of a large population was shown to correlate with educational attainment (Table 17–3). These subjects had been selected due to attendance at a general medical practice, and could be considered as quite close to a true random population sampling. Of the CNVs analyzed in these subjects, only smaller (0.25–1 Mb) duplications appeared to be consistently benign. A detailed review of CNVs associated with a neurodevelopmental disorder is presented in Torres et al. (2016): These authors list, in particular, CNVs at 1q21.1, 3q29, 15q11.2, 15q13.3, 16p11.2, 16p13.1, and 22q11.

Autism spectrum disorder (ASD) is a clinical diagnosis for which molecular karyotyping is the first genetic investigation.[7] The counselor may deal rather frequently with the challenge of interpreting a finding of a CNV, or of CNVs, and which may be de novo or inherited. In a segment for which a causal link is well established, such as the del(16)(p11.2) (p. 296), the expression microdeletion/duplication may be more apposite, and counseling may be (relatively) straightforward. For less well-understood segments, and especially when in combination, our understanding is a work in progress. Certain regions, with spectacular contributions of chromosomes 15, 16, and 22, harbor ASD-related CNVs (Fig. 17–4).

Developmental coordination disorder, also called dyspraxia or the "clumsy child syndrome," is not uncommonly diagnosed in school-age children, and quite often in coexistence with attention deficit disorder (Gibbs et al. 2007). In a relatively small Canadian cohort of such children, the burden of CNV deletions or duplications in the 0.5–1.0 Mb range was significantly increased, and CNVs more often spanned brain-expressed genes, compared with a control population (Mosca et al. 2016).

6 This database also provides a list of loci according to their dosage sensitivity, at https://www.ncbi.nlm.nih.gov/projects/dbvar/clingen (Hunter et al. 2016).

7 It is necessary to distinguish "idiopathic autism" from neurogenetic syndromes which may include, in some, autistic-like features (e.g., Rett syndrome, fragile X syndrome, tuberous sclerosis). Harris (2016) offers a useful commentary; he refers to CNVs in idiopathic ASD as "common variation, individually of small effect, [which] may have substantial impact *en masse.*"

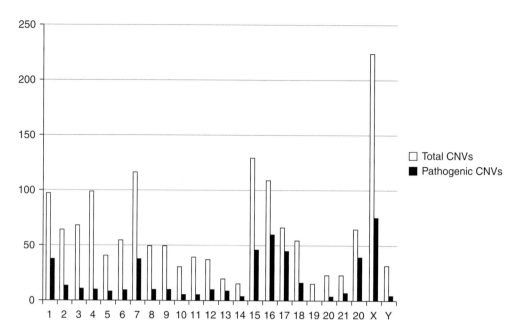

FIGURE 17–3   Frequencies of pathogenic CNVs, compared to total CNV frequencies, in an abnormal population. These data derive from a series of 5,369 postnatal (single or multiple congenital abnormalities, neurodevelopmental delay with or without neuropsychiatric disorders) and prenatal (two or more abnormalities detected on ultrasound) samples.

Source: From McCormack et al., Microarray testing in clinical diagnosis: An analysis of 5,300 New Zealand patients, *Mol Cytogenet* 9: 29, 2016. Courtesy D. R. Love and A. M. George, and with the permission of BioMed Central, per the Creative Commons Attribution License.

Table 17-3. Educational Attainment in Three Estonian Cohorts, with Respect to Copy Number Variant Carriage

GROUP	TOTALS	EDUCATIONAL ATTAINMENT*	NOT REACHING SECONDARY EDUCATION	
			NO.	%
Estonian population	7,877	4.08	2,000	25
DECIPHER-listed CNV carriers	56	3.64	28	50
Deletion carrier by CNV size				
>1 Mb	37	3.51	17	46
500 kb–1 Mb	47	3.93**	16	34.0
250–500 kb	164	3.84	50	30.5
Duplication carrier by CNV size				
>1 Mb	115	3.69	45	39.1
500 kb–1 Mb	149	4.10	43	28.9
250–500 kb	319	4.14	78	24.5

Notes: In the general population, the average attainment score is 4.08. In those with DECIPHER-listed CNVs, it is less, at 3.64. The averages in those with other deletion CNVs is also less, ranging from 3.51 to 3.93. Likewise, the score is less in the larger duplication category (>1 Mb), but in those with smaller (0.25–1 Mb) duplications, it is essentially the same as that for the general population. These average figures match those of the fractions of those not reaching secondary education.

*The mean educational attainment score is derived from these levels, based on the Estonian education curriculum: less than primary, 1; primary, 2; basic, 3; secondary, 4; professional or college, 5; university or academic, 6; and scientific degree, 7.

**This fraction, although slightly less than that of the general population, does not reach statistical significance.

Source: From Männik et al. (2015).

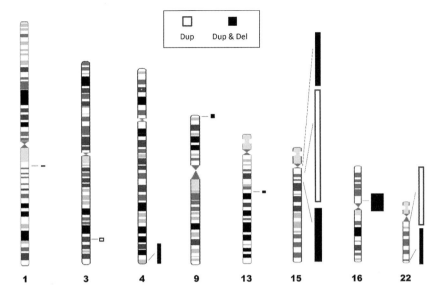

FIGURE 17–4   Chromosomal locations of the top-ranked 11 autism spectrum susceptibility CNV loci. Copy number gains (duplications) are open bars; copy number losses and gains (both duplications and deletions) are filled bars. The length and width of bars are proportional to the CNVs' genomic size and burden score, respectively; note the disproportionate roles of chromosomes 15 and 22 in particular, and also of chromosomes 4 and 16.

Source: From Menashe et al., Prioritization of copy number variation loci associated with autism from AutDB—An integrative multi-study genetic database, *PLoS One* 8; 8: e66707, 2013. Courtesy I. Menashe, and with the permission of the Public Library of Science, according to the Creative Commons Attribution License.

The X chromosome is rich in CNVs. Isrie et al. (2012) studied a cohort of 2,222 males with intellectual disability and found 3% to have an X-borne CNV. Some could quite confidently be termed as pathogenic; in others, the interpretation was unclear. These authors developed a decision tree, whereby a CNV could be "called." Those interpreted as pathogenic ranged in size[8] from 0.5 kb to 4.4 Mb; those regarded as VOUSs were of a rather similar range, 1 kb to 4.3 Mb, but the distribution skewed toward smaller sizes. An inference is, therefore, that many of the smaller ones would have been nonpathogenic CNVs. Family studies can cast light, as we exemplify in the family with a trp(X)(q27.1) mentioned below. CNVs comprising a duplication of a specific segment within Xp22.33 which includes, but may extend beyond, the *SHOX* locus convey a low-penetrance risk for autism (3.6%) or other neurodevelopmental disorder (8.6%) (Tropeano et al. 2016).

PENTRANCE AND EXPRESSIVITY

The concepts of variable penetrance and expressivity,[9] more traditionally invoked in Mendelian genetics, impose a real concern with respect to the CNV (Grayton et al. 2012). A CNV may be, in one genomic environment (e.g., in a parent), of no clinical effect, but it may be pathogenic in a child, if a different CNV—a "second hit"—comes from the other parent. Subtle examples come from studies in autism (Coe et al. 2014). Or, a microduplication or microdeletion of recognized incomplete penetrance may become penetrant in the company of a CNV (Fig. 17–5). The concept of "digenic inheritance" may, in some, understate the genetic complexity: Oligogenic, or even polygenic, mechanisms may be the basis of some CNV combinations determining a boundary beyond which phenotypic abnormality appears. Or, to use the common terminology, a two-hit or more-hit scenario may apply. The other issue to add into this mix is the matter of defining a boundary of abnormality—which can be a

---

8 One outlier of size 11 Mb, a triplication at Xq27 encompassing 48 loci, including *FMR1*, and visible on karyotyping, might be seen as a microtriplication rather than a CNV.

9 Penetrance refers to the proportion of individuals with an imbalance that shows any trait resulting from that imbalance, whereas expressivity refers to the variability in phenotype of those who carry the imbalanced region.

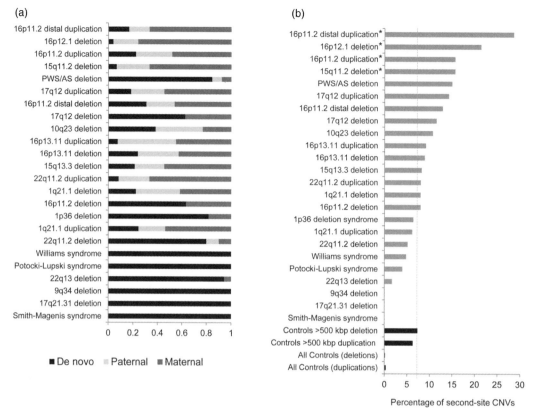

FIGURE 17–5 A display of microduplications and microdeletions (*a*), alongside concomitant second-hit CNVs (*b*) that may influence phenotype, typically for the worse. Microduplications and microdeletions are ranked, from top down, according to the frequency with which second-hit CNVs are observed. Those at the top of the list can sometimes be (apparently) nonpenetrant, and thus the second-hit CNV may be necessary to lead to overt pathogenicity (in the top four, asterisked in *b*, the enrichment of CNVs is statistically significant). Those further down the list have second-hit CNVs at no greater frequency than in the control population, and are "stand-alone" pathogenic. The fractions of microduplications and microdeletions due to parental or de novo origin are indicated in panel *a*, according to the shading of the bars. Compare Figure 14–70, which shows second-hit CNVs in the dup(22)(q11.12) syndrome.

Source: From Girirajan et al., Phenotypic heterogeneity of genomic disorders and rare copy-number variants, *N Engl J Med* 367: 1321–1331, 2012. Courtesy S. Girirajan, and with the permission of the Massachusetts Medical Society.

subtle question in the case of intellectual and behavioral traits. The Estonian study noted above leads to an inference that earlier assumptions, that some heterozygotes for "syndromic CNVs" could be unaffected, may be incorrect, albeit that the degree of affection is quite mild (Lupski 2015; Männik et al. 2015).

IN PRACTICE

The following is a very common situation the counselor faces: An imbalance is detected on

molecular karyotyping, and the segment concerned contains CNVs and possibly known genes. An example is a 268 kb triplication at Xq27.1, trp chrX:138,414,910-138,683,873,[10] that we have seen in a child with epilepsy and intellectual deficiency. The extent of the segment is displayed in Figure 17–6, according to the Genoglyphix database. Two known genes are included, Factor IX (*F9*) and *MCF2*; the latter is incompletely present and thus unlikely to be of pathogenic significance.

---

10 These coordinates according to hg19, as this is the build Genoglyphix, ClinGen, and DECIHPER were using at this writing.

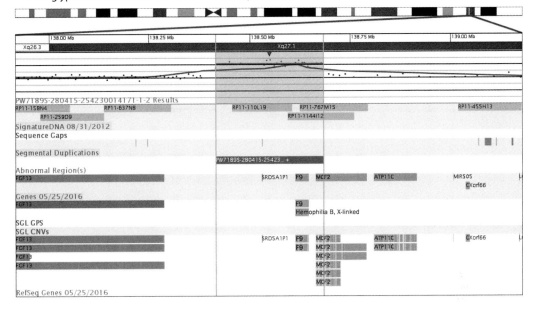

Abnormality Details

Genome Build	UCSC 2009 hg19 assembly
Copy Number	Two Copy Gain
Chromosome Band	Xq27.1
Genomic Coordinates	chrX:138414910-138683873
Estimated Minimum Size	268.96 kb
Estimated Maximum Size	318.51 kb
Number of Probes	27
Avg Value	1.075
StartGap	35.56 kb Cen
EndGap	13.99 kb Tel

FIGURE 17–6   An example of a CNV display using the Genoglyphix database, based on the trpX:139,332,751-139,601,714 bp described in the text (here seen according to the hg19 numbering, chrX:138,414,910-138,683,873). The Factor IX gene (*F9*) is completely contained within the segment; the *MCF2* gene is partially included. (Case of J. Watt.)

If this sequence is interrogated in DECIPHER, a list is displayed of several segments of larger and smaller size, which overlap with the sequence of interest. The closest in this example is a case of dup X:138,556,249-138,764,448, and this segment can be called up and displayed in the row "This patient: copy number variants" (Fig. 17–7). This case is annotated (click on the "Affected patient" bar) as "Paternally inherited, constitutive in father." No comment is made under Pathogenicity, and the curators have left this interpretation open (perhaps awaiting further cases; and this one of ours has since been submitted).

But the assessment is not inconsistent with the CNV being, at least in terms of brain function, benign.

A summary of the genes resident within a region and a commentary on haplo/triplo-sufficiency status where applicable, and with links to synoptic data about each locus, are accessible through ClinGen (https://www.clinicalgenome.org). The display according to the trp(X) under discussion is shown in Figure 17–8 (on hg19).

By going to the DGVa link[11] mentioned above and entering the coordinates of the trp(X) (q27.1), the CNVs contained therein are displayed

---

11 Or, if a segment is identified in the University of California Santa Cruz (UCSC) browser, and the track "DGV Struct Var" under the Variation category is chosen, the region will be displayed, and segments of deletion (red) and duplication (blue) within the vicinity indicated. Clicking on to a CNV within the segment of interest will link to the DGV database.

(a)

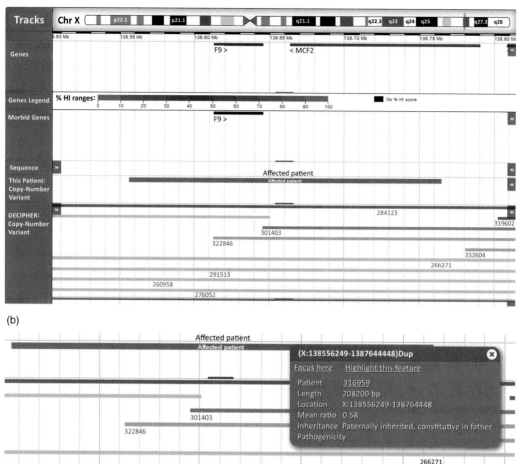

(b)

FIGURE 17-7 (*a*) An example of an interrogation using the DECIPHER database, based on the trpX:139,332,751-139,601,714 bp described in the text (here seen according to the hg19 numbering, chrX:138,414,910-138,683,873). Entering these coordinates, and then scrolling through a list of cases that DECIPHER presents with some degree of overlap, the closest variant is dup X:138,556,249-138,764,448. Choosing this case, it is then shown as the prominent bar "Affected patient" in the track "This Patient: Copy Number Variants" (*upper*). (*b*) Clicking on this bar (*lower*) gives a dialog box with detailed information, although in this case a call was unable to be made on pathogenicity. In the track below, other annotated CNVs from the DECIPHER database are depicted.

(Fig. 17-9). The largest is a 15,273 bp deletion, and smaller dels and dups are listed. But these, by definition in DGVa, are normal variants and can therefore be dismissed as pheno-contributory. Only two genes are noted, and one of these, MCF2, is disrupted by the distal breakpoint and thus, as mentioned above, unlikely of concern (and no Mendelian disease is due to this gene). The remaining gene, coding for clotting Factor IX, could in principle be associated with a disorder of coagulation.

The important next step is a family study, if feasible. In the example just given, it transpired that the brother and mother both had the same trp(X) *and* were both normal intellectually. But interestingly, they had both suffered thrombotic episodes, with elevated levels of Factor IX. The conclusion to be drawn is that the neurological compromise[12] in

---

12 Brain imaging was normal, and there was no evidence that cerebral vascular thromboses could have been the basis of her abnormality.

Location search results

Gene Symbol	Haploinsufficiency score	Triplosensitivity score	Curation Status	Region Location	Relationship to Submitted Location	ISCA ID
SNURFL	N/A	N/A	Awaiting Review	chrx:138,444,099-138,444,641	Contained	ISCA-2512
SRD5A1P1	N/A	N/A	Awaiting Review	chrx:138,528,978-138,531,132	Contained	ISCA-20697
F9	3	0	Complete	chrx:138,612,895-138,645,617	Contained	ISCA-25959
MCF2	N/A	N/A	Awaiting Review	chrx:138,663,930-138,790,381	Overlap	ISCA-20739

FIGURE 17-8 The display according to the ClinGen database, of the trpX:139,332,751-139,601,714 (on hg19) described in the text. The links at the right (ICSA ID) take the reader to synoptic data about each locus.

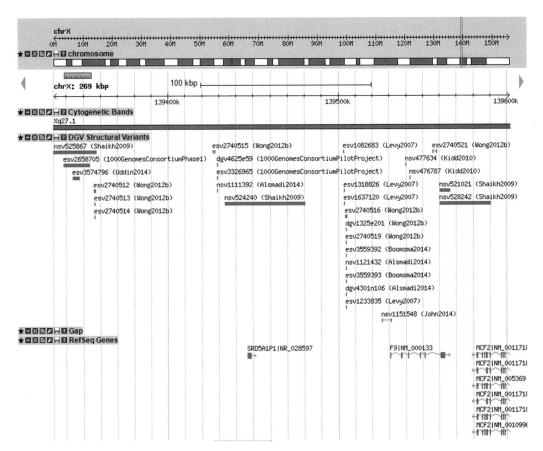

FIGURE 17-9 An example of an interrogation using the Database of Genomic Variants (DGVa) based on the trpX:139,332,751-139,601,714 bp described in the text. The website is accessed at http://dgv.tcag.ca/gb2/gbrowse/dgv2_hg38. Nucleotide numbers are entered according to the appropriate "build" chosen (here, hg38). Duplicated CNV segments (blue on screen; here, dark gray) and deleted CNV segments (red; here, light gray) are presented. These are mostly labeled *nsv* and *esv* (*sv*, structural variant, archived and accessioned by dbVAR and DGVa, respectively). The largest duplication is nsv524240 (*upper center*), whereas esv2658705 (*upper left*) is the largest deletion. Clicking on each entry links to detail about the variant, including the lengths (here, 46,585 and 15,273 bp, respectively). The default display also shows actual genes (here, *F9* and *MCF2*) within the chosen segment, by exons (blocks) and introns (wavy lines).

the presenting child is likely coincidental. A genetic diagnosis yet awaits, if indeed there is one. (The reader may well have similar stories to tell.)

A Rare Complexity

The Multiple De Novo CNV Phenotype Whereas de novo CNVs are generated at a mutation rate considerably higher than that seen in Mendelian genetics, the number of independent de novo CNVs observed in this rare "CNV mutator" phenotype is on an altogether different scale and reflects a different mechanism (Liu et al. 2017). The original cases, through whom the syndrome had been delineated, were defined by the possession of four or more independent de novo CNVs of >100 kb, and they had been ascertained at a frequency of 1 in 12,000 among children with "various developmental disorders" referred for clinical microarray testing. These CNVs are typically duplications, and they may number in the low single digits to just double digits; an example is shown in Table 17–4.

Further investigation of the de novo CNVs in these individuals suggests that they arise in the perizygotic time interval, due to a transient fault in the DNA replicative repair process. According to one proposed construction, a de novo mutation arising in the gamete leads to the production of a mutant mRNA that compromises the repair of DNA replicative error,

thereby leading to the "CNV mutator" phenotype. In the male, the homolog harboring the mutation in a meiotic spermatocyte is preferentially segregated into a daughter nontransmitted sperm, leaving the actual fertilizing sperm to have the normal homolog, but yet retaining some of the abnormal mRNA. The chromosomes of this sperm are vulnerable to this mRNA, but the effect is short-lived, and by the time the zygote comes into existence, no mRNA is left; thus, the de novo CNVs are all of paternal origin. In the female, albeit that the homolog with the mutation is, in similar fashion, directed out of harm's way into the polar body, mRNA is nevertheless retained in the cytoplasm of the oöcyte, and its influence carries over into the zygote and the first one or two mitoses. Thus, the de novo CNVs are of both maternal and paternal origin (e.g., the case in Table 17–4). Thereafter, these CNVs are transmitted stably in the soma.

GENETIC COUNSELING

Classic Cytogenetic Variant

A person carrying a classical chromosome variant has, practically by definition, no increased risk for having abnormal offspring, pregnancy loss, or any other reproductive problem. Some view it as at best pointless and at worst counterproductive even to mention to the individual that a variant chromosome has been found; others feel obliged to pass on the observation. If it is discussed, it must be made clear that it is a normal finding—perhaps interesting but of no practical importance. For the heterochromatic size variants (C-band and NOR) and euchromatic variants, the point can simply be made that some chromosomes come in short, medium, and long forms, and where a chromosome happens to fit in this continuum is without significance. For segmental imbalances ascertained in apparently unaffected individuals, careful clinical assessment should be made, if practicable, of carriers from the same family; incomplete penetrance and variable expressivity should be borne in mind in assessing innocuousness, or not, of the variant. Fragile sites are, almost always, normal findings. The primacy, in the twenty-first century, of molecular karyotyping in fact means that discovery of variants such as these will be rather infrequent events.

There is considerable potential for iatrogenic anxiety, whereas in reality the biology of the supposed

Table 17–4. Nine De Novo Copy Number Variants Observed in a Child with the Multiple De Novo Copy Number Variant Phenotype

SITE	SIZE	NATURE	PARENTAL ORIGIN
1p34p35	1.7 Mb	Dup	Maternal
3p14p21	4.2 Mb	Dup	Maternal
8q24	4.5 Mb	Dup	Maternal
10q24q25	4.7 Mb	Dup	Maternal
16p11	322 kb	IDD	Paternal
16q23	4.2 Mb	IDD	Maternal
16q24	312 kb	Dup	Maternal
19q13	4.3 Mb	Dup	Maternal
Xp11	214 kb	Dup	Maternal

Dup, duplication; IDD, insertional double duplication.
Source: From Liu et al. (2017).

anomaly has no pathogenic implication. The counselor may thoroughly understand the presumed harmlessness of a variant chromosome, but the person in whose family it has been discovered may react "nonscientifically." To put a stark setting, the worst possible response might be for a couple to choose to terminate a pregnancy because of an overinterpreted variant chromosome, as has actually happened with the 16p11.2 euchromatic variant (López Pajares et al. 2006). *Primum non nocere*: First do no harm.

Copy Number Variants

The distinction between harmful and harmless variants is a much subtler exercise in the case of CNVs. As we outlined above, interrogating databases such as DECIPHER and DGVa may be a first court of appeal. If a parent, or other family member, has the same variant, and is of normal phenotype, the CNV may be adjudged a "likely benign" variant; or, other data, and especially pedigree data, in the public domain, may be sufficiently powerful to indicate indeed a nonpathogenic CNV. A qualitative assessment of the genic content, as mentioned above, and as understanding progresses, may well be valuable. A

de novo CNV may need to be considered as "likely pathogenic" unless there is solid evidence otherwise; a data resource is the website http://denovo-db.gs.washington.edu (Turner et al. 2017).

A detailed format for the practical assessment of a CNV is outlined in Di Gregorio et al. (2017), who assessed a little over 1,000 individuals with developmental delay/intellectual disability (Fig. 17–10). These variants were classified into CNVs of size greater than 3 Mb (which we might equally call microdeletion/duplications); del/dups associated with known syndromes; CNVs spanning known Mendelian disease genes; likely pathogenic CNVs, and noting the genes contained within them; and VOUSs/likely benign. These authors referred to the databases of a number of publicly-available sources, including material from large autism repositories, in order to judge the possible pathogenicity of abnormal copy number of the loci contained within CNVs. In some, a diagnosis was clear enough at the outset, with a number of known syndromes seen. In others, it required a detailed weighing of the nature of the loci, and appealing to information from the several sources. The reader wishing further demonstration of the rationale in CNV assessment is referred to this paper.

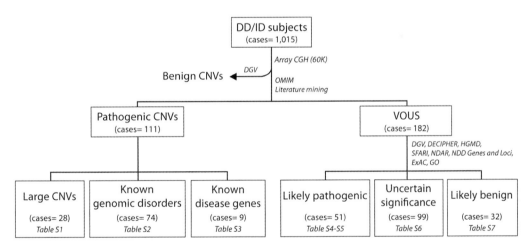

FIGURE 17–10   A schema for the analysis of copy number variants. The data from a series of 1,015 cases of developmental delay/intellectual disability were assessed, and in 10%, a pathogenic CNV was identified. The criteria by which the CNVs were judged are set out in fine detail in the Tables S1-S7 in the original paper. Sources referred to: DGV, DECIPHER as noted above; OMIM, Online Mendelian Inheritance in Man; HGMD, Human Gene Mutation Database; SFARI, Simons Foundation Autism Research Initiative; NDAR, National Database for Autism Research; NDD, neurodevelopmental disorders; ExAC, Exome Aggregation Consortium; GO, Gene Ontology Consortium.

Source: From Di Gregorio et al., Copy number variants analysis in a cohort of isolated and syndromic developmental delay/intellectual disability reveals novel genomic disorders, position effects and candidate disease genes, *Clin Genet* 92: 415–422, 2017. Courtesy A. Brusco and G.B. Ferrero, and with the permission of John Wiley & Sons.

The question of nonpenetrance, or at least reduced expressivity, of a CNV is a challenging one. Attempting to dissect out "micro-phenotypes" in a parent may prove rather fraught. Adding to this is the problem of "second hit" CNVs, and the degree to which they may modify or exacerbate a phenotype. In the meantime, in advising about the risk to a future child, the counselor will need to consult current sources and to seek expert advice. A problem of long familiarity in genetic counseling, that of dealing with uncertainty, certainly applies here (Wilkins et al. 2016). Conveying the information about a CNV to counselees is an exercise to which genetic counselors are becoming more accustomed, which is not to say that they find it straightforward. Finally, a question of well-considered clinical judgment, and of which the answer might differ between families: Having discovered a CNV that would qualify as a VOUS, would it, or might it not, be helpful to pursue a family study?

Concerning the CNV-mutator phenotype, if the theory of a fresh mutation at a meiotic stage (see above) is correct, then occurrence would be sporadic, and no increased risk would apply to a subsequent pregnancy.

PART FOUR

DISORDERS ASSOCIATED WITH ABERRANT GENOMIC IMPRINTING

18

UNIPARENTAL DISOMY
AND DISORDERS
OF IMPRINTING

UNIPARENTAL DISOMY IS A FASCINATING and important pathogenetic mechanism, albeit that it is the basis of only a small number of well-defined clinical conditions. At the outset, we may list the following nine well-described uniparental disomy (UPD)[1] syndromes, representing chromosomes 6, 7, 11, 14, 15, and 20, approximately in order of frequency:

Beckwith-Wiedemann syndrome
Prader-Willi syndrome
Angelman syndrome
Silver-Russell syndrome
Kagami syndrome
Temple syndrome
Transient neonatal diabetes

Maternal UPD 20
Pseudohypoparathyroidism type 1B

Some of these can be due to genetic causes other than uniparental disomy, and for convenience we include a discussion of the other causes in this chapter. In a category by itself, UPD can be the cause of homozygosity for an autosomal recessive gene. Nevertheless, the fact remains that most UPDs appear to be without any phenotypic consequence, and a number of syndromes that had originally seemed fair candidates turned out not to be due to UPD (Kotzot 2002).

A distinction is to be made between UPD where both chromosomes are identical (uniparental *iso*disomy, UPID) and where they are

---

1 As a general rule, abbreviations for "uniparental disomy" are in uppercase (UPD, UPHD, UPID) when making broad reference to the concept of uniparental disomy/heterodisomy/isodisomy, and in lowercase (upd, uphd, upid), according to the rules of cytogenetic nomenclature, when attention is more focused upon a specific case.

(a)

Parents

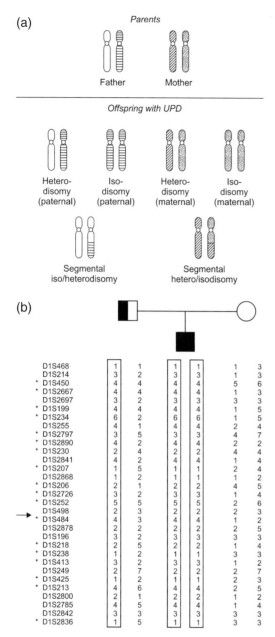

Father Mother

Offspring with UPD

Hetero-disomy (paternal) Iso-disomy (paternal) Hetero-disomy (maternal) Iso-disomy (maternal)

Segmental iso/heterodisomy Segmental hetero/isodisomy

(b)

Marker	Father		Child		Mother	
D1S468	1	1	1	1	1	3
D1S214	3	2	3	3	1	3
* D1S450	4	4	4	4	5	6
* D1S2667	4	4	4	4	1	3
D1S2697	3	2	3	3	3	3
* D1S199	4	4	4	4	1	5
* D1S234	6	2	6	6	1	5
D1S255	4	1	4	4	2	4
* D1S2797	3	5	3	3	4	7
* D1S2890	4	2	4	4	2	2
* D1S230	2	4	2	2	4	4
D1S2841	4	2	4	4	1	4
* D1S207	1	5	1	1	2	4
D1S2868	1	2	1	1	1	2
* D1S206	2	1	2	2	4	5
* D1S2726	3	2	3	3	1	4
* D1S252	5	5	5	5	2	6
D1S498	2	3	2	2	2	3
→ * D1S484	4	3	4	4	1	2
D1S2878	2	2	2	2	2	5
D1S196	3	2	3	3	3	3
* D1S218	2	5	2	2	1	4
* D1S238	1	2	1	1	3	3
* D1S413	3	2	3	3	1	2
D1S249	2	7	2	2	2	7
* D1S425	1	2	1	1	2	3
* D1S213	4	6	4	4	2	5
D1S2800	2	1	2	2	1	2
D1S2785	4	5	4	4	1	4
D1S2842	3	3	3	3	3	3
* D1S2836	1	5	1	1	3	3

FIGURE 18–1 (*a*) The distinction between uniparental heterodisomy and uniparental isodisomy. The four parental homologs are shown in different patterns. In the child with *hetero* disomy, the two homologs are different. In *iso* disomy, they are identical. Meiotic crossing-over can lead to segmental iso/heterodisomy, and the pattern can reveal whether the initial nondisjunction had been at meiosis I or II (see text). (*b*) The molecular picture of a child with paternal uniparental isodisomy 1. The markers run from D1S468 at the top of chromosome 1 down to

different (uniparental *hetero*disomy, UPHD) (Fig. 18–1a). UPD is normally demonstrable only at the molecular level: Typically, although not invariably, the UPD pair of chromosomes are cytogenetically normal, and the (classical) karyotype appears normal, 46,XX or 46,XY. The pattern of polymorphic DNA markers shows that both chromosomes have the same haplotype as just one of the chromosomes from one of the parents (isodisomy); or, the two chromosomes have the same haplotypes as the chromosome pair from one of the parents (heterodisomy). For example, the chromosome 1 haplotypes from parents and child set out in Figure 18–1b show that the child has two identical copies of one of the father's chromosomes: thus, paternal uniparental isodisomy. This UPD had been discovered fortuitously, when the child was investigated for a clinical diagnosis of congenital insensitivity to pain, an autosomal recessive disorder (Miura et al. 2000). He proved to be homozygous for a mutation in the appropriate gene (*TRKA*, located at 1q21q22, chr1:156.86-156.88 Mb), and his father carried the mutation, but his mother did not. This scenario—a child with a recessive disorder for which only one parent is heterozygous—is commonly the circumstance behind the discovery of UPIDs that would otherwise have been without clinical effect, and it is sometimes referred to as the "unmasking" of a recessive gene. The other typical route to recognition of harmless UPDs is through the incidental discovery of long continuous/contiguous stretches of homozygosity

D1S2836 at the bottom. Both the child's chromosome 1 haplotypes are the same, and the same as one of his father's no. 1 chromosomes. He has no chromosome 1 from his mother. (The arrow points to the position of the *TRKA* locus. Homozygosity for an abnormal *TRKA* allele was the cause of his having the recessive condition congenital insensitivity to pain, which had led to his ascertainment.)

Source: From Miura et al., Complete paternal uniparental isodisomy for chromosome 1 revealed by mutation analyses of the TRKA (NTRK1) gene encoding a receptor tyrosine kinase for nerve growth factor in a patient with congenital insensitivity to pain with anhidrosis, *Hum Genet* 107: 205–209, 2000. Courtesy Y. Indo, and with the permission of Springer-Verlag.

on single nucleotide polymorphism (SNP) microarray.

The state of iso- or heterodisomy can allow an inference as to the site of the initial chromosomal error. Isodisomy for an entire chromosome typically reflects a meiosis II nondisjunction (in the absence of recombination) or a mitotic error (including monosomy rescue). In contrast, heterodisomy for an entire chromosome is due to nondisjunction at meiosis I. More commonly, recombination at meiosis I results in the coexistence of partial heterodisomy and partial isodisomy for the same chromosome pair. For example, a crossover at meiosis I in, for example, the distal long arm, followed by meiosis I nondisjunction, could lead to a disomic gamete isodisomic for distal long arm, and heterodisomic for proximal long arm (Fig. 18–1a, lower right). If the nondisjunction were at meiosis II, the isodisomy and heterodisomy would be the other way around, involving the proximal and distal segments, respectively (Fig. 18–1a, lower left). Recognizing some forms of UPD can be achieved on SNP array, and we discuss this below.

Epigenetics and Imprinting

In epigenetic variation, a core consideration is that a phenotype may differ according to whether a DNA sequence is active, or inactive, but with the DNA sequence itself remaining unchanged. Our focus is on the activity, or nonactivity, of a gene (or chromosomal segment), according to the parental origin of the chromosome upon which the gene (or segment) is located. Thus, a chromosomal segment can receive an "epigenetic mark"—or is "imprinted"—as it is transmitted from parent to child, depending upon whether it is the mother or the father who had contributed that chromosomal segment, and this determines whether this segment will be genetically active or not active ("silent"). This is spoken of as a "parent-of-origin" effect. The major physical basis of this epigenetic effect is due to methylation of the DNA (i.e., a methyl group attached to cytosine bases), modification of the histone scaffolding of chromatin, and to the actions of noncoding RNAs, which severally or separately can then prevent the expression pattern of the relevant gene(s). There are certain chromosome segments (in sum, only a small fraction of the whole genome) that are subject to imprinting. Slightly counterintuitively, imprinting refers to *non*activity: An imprinted chromosome segment is silenced, while the nonimprinted chromosome segment is the *active* one.

In the normal setting, with biparental inheritance, imprintable segments (or loci) function monoallelically. That is, it is only the segment of maternal origin, or only the segment of paternal origin, as the case may be, which is genetically active.[2] But if both segments originate from one parent, there will be either double the amount (biallelic) of expression or no (nulliallelic) expression, according to the gender of the contributing parent. (Some imprinting is tissue specific, in which case, the aberrant expression is confined to that tissue.) It is this functional imbalance that is the root cause of the phenotypic effect in the UPD syndromes. If a chromosome is not subject to imprinting, UPD does not of itself cause abnormality, other things being equal. The only other factor due to UPD, and specifically UPID, which can lead to defect, is homozygosity for a recessive mutation ("isozygosity"), as noted above.

Although the list of classic UPD syndromes, as in the introduction above, is not long, imprinting as a process is by no means confined to the "big six": chromosomes 6, 7, 11, 14, 15, and 20. Joshi et al. (2016) analyzed samples from 57 individuals with UPDs for many (not quite all) chromosomes, searching for segments within these chromosomes showing a parent-of-origin methylation bias. These segments allowed a recognition of 77 "differentially methylated regions" (DMRs) (Fig. 18–2). However, it remained an open question as to a possible pathogenic or harmless effect of these DMRs, with some of the cohort being phenotypically normal.

---

2 Apart from imprinting, two other epigenetic mechanisms can lead to expression of only one allele of a gene: X-inactivation; and random monoallelic expression (RME). RME is the mosaic, mitotically stable, inactivation of one allele of an autosomal gene, and it may occur for approximately 2% of all genes (Gendrel et al. 2016). Unlike imprinting, RME involves expression, in a random and clonal fashion, from either the paternal or the maternal allele. Although the role of RME is poorly understood, it may contribute, at the level of transcription, to some of the phenotypes associated with chromosome imbalance, particularly those associated with haploinsufficiency.

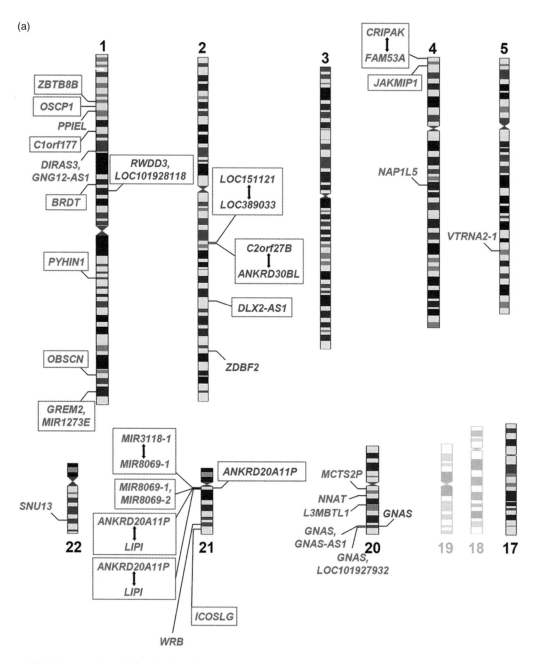

FIGURE 18–2   (*a* and *b*) A display of autosomal segments subject to an imprinting effect, from a cohort of 57 cases of UPD. Differentially methylated regions (DMRs) are designated according either to a locus within or very close by that region or by a segment flanked by two loci, with the ↕ arrow between. Loci to the left of each chromosome are maternally imprinted; those to the right, paternally. Novel DMRs are boxed. Grayed chromosomes (10, 11, 18, 19) were not represented in the cohort, and thus otherwise known DMRs on these chromosomes are not shown here. *Source:* From Joshi et al., DNA methylation profiling of uniparental disomy subjects provides a map of parental epigenetic bias in the human genome, *Am J Hum Genet* 99: 555–566, 2016. Courtesy A. J. Sharp and G. Kirov, and with the permission of Elsevier.

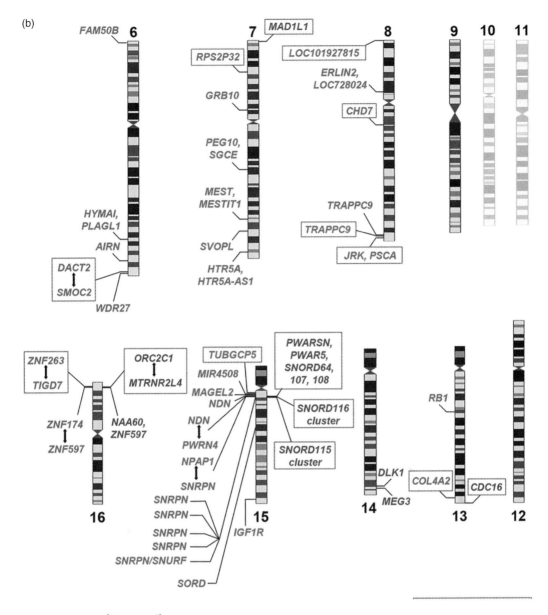

FIGURE 18–2 (Continued)

Uniparental Disomy for a Complete Chromosome

In UPD for a complete and intact chromosome, both members of a homologous pair come from the one parent. Four routes to lead to this state are the following (and see Figs. 18–3 and 18–4):

- Gametic complementation
- Trisomic rescue
- Monosomic rescue
- Mitotic error

Gametic complementation is mentioned first, as the simplest and classic example, but in truth it must hardly ever be that UPD is the consequence of a meiotic error happening coincidentally in both parents (Park et al. 1998; Shaffer et al. 1998).

Trisomy "rescue" or "correction"[3] is the mechanism behind most UPD. The cause of the trisomy

---

3 It might be more accurate to speak of a "failed rescue," or better a "foiled rescue," since the end result is an unfortunate one. Or, "mistaken correction."

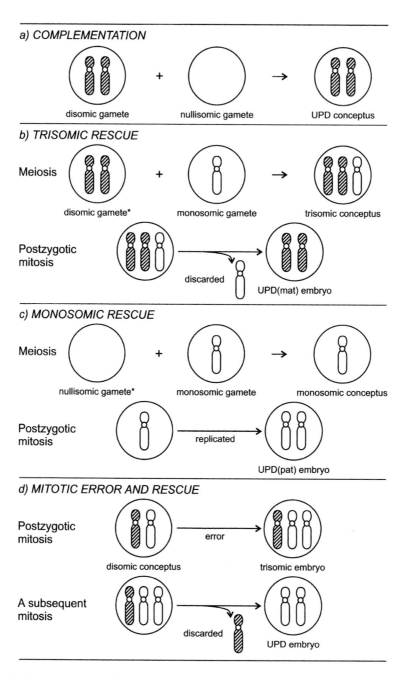

FIGURE 18–3   Mechanisms whereby complete UPD may be generated. (*a*) Gametic complementation, with one parent producing a disomic gamete, and the other a nullisomic gamete. (*b*) Meiotic nondisjunction in one parent to produce a disomic gamete, with a trisomic conceptus following fertilization, and subsequent mitotic loss of the homolog from the other parent. This is uniparental heterodisomy, from the parent in whom the nondisjunction had taken place. (*c*) Meiotic nondisjunction in one parent to produce a nullisomic gamete, with monosomic conceptus following fertilization, and subsequent mitotic reduplication of the homolog from the other parent. This is uniparental isodisomy, from the parent who had contributed the normal gamete. The reduplication may produce a free homolog or an isochromosome. (*d*) Two sequential mitotic errors.

*Since most meiotic nondisjunction occurs in maternal gametogenesis, these asterisked gametes can be imagined to be oöcytes, with UPD(mat) and UPD(pat) resulting accordingly.

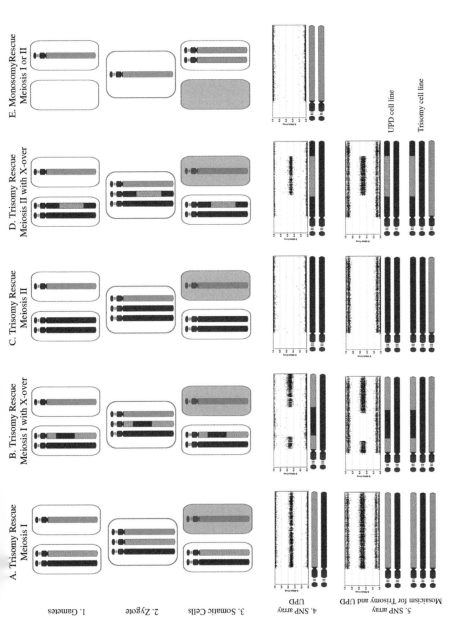

FIGURE 18–4   The several routes by which UPD may arise, and the observations on SNP array that may inform interpretation. (*A* and *B*) Meiosis 1 nondisjunction with postzygotic trisomy rescue: UPD with centromeric heterodisomy ± distal isodisomy. (*C* and *D*) Meiosis 2 nondisjunction with postzygotic rescue: UPD with centromeric isodisomy ± distal heterodisomy. (*E*) Postzygotic monosomy rescue: complete isodisomy.[4] (*See color insert.*)

Source: From Kearney et al., Diagnostic implications of excessive homozygosity detected by SNP-based microarrays: Consanguinity, uniparental disomy, and recessive single-gene mutations, *Clin Lab Med* 31: 595–613, 2011. Courtesy H. M. Kearney and L. K. Conlin, and with the permission of Elsevier.

4 Note that in the absence of recombination, meiosis 1 nondisjunction will not cause excessive homozygosity, and SNP array will be normal.

is a typical meiotic nondisjunction that happened in one of the two conceiving gametes. The rescue process takes place in a cell of the trisomic conceptus at a very early postzygotic stage (possibly even in the zygote), with one of the trisomic chromosomes being discarded, perhaps due to anaphase lag.[5] This enables a cell line within the conceptus to be restored to disomy, but if it is the "wrong" chromosome that is eliminated— that is, purely by chance, the discarded chromosome happens to be the one that came from the normal gamete—the remaining two are from the same parent, and UPD results. In this scenario, the two chromosomes will comprise one of each of the homologs of that parent: thus, uniparental heterodisomy. This would be expected to happen, by chance, in one-third of such rescues, biparental inheritance being maintained in the other two-thirds (close to these ratios was observed in a large study of UPD 16; Yong et al. 2002). The 46-chromosome cell with UPD that results from this process may be the progenitor of the cells which produce the inner cell mass, which in turn gives rise to the embryo. Any remaining trisomic cells may go on to form the placenta, leading to confined placental mosaicism; or, they may also contribute to the inner cell mass, leading to trisomy/disomy mosaicism of the embryo. Thus, the phenotypes in some UPD states are complicated by the additional effects of compromised placental function due to trisomy, and/or of fetal trisomy mosaicism.

Monosomic rescue also comes into play following a nondisjunctional event. If a nullisomic gamete is generated at meiosis, then the conceptus will be monosomic (assuming a normal gamete from the other parent). Mitotic correction then takes place, and this is achieved by replication of the single, normal, homolog received from the other parent. In this case, the UPD will be an isodisomy.

The fourth possibility is a *mitotic error* in an initially normal conception, leading to either trisomy or monosomy. In the case of a trisomy, this is followed soon thereafter by loss, in this cell line, of the nonreplicated trisomic chromosome. In the case of a mitotic nondisjunction resulting in monosomy, the remaining homolog is then duplicated. In both cases, the UPD is isodisomic.

Note that each of these four scenarios requires there to be two separate abnormal events, occurring either contemporaneously (the first scenario)

or sequentially (the latter three). These errors can be meiotic (the first), meiotic followed by mitotic (second and third), or both mitotic (the fourth). In whichever case, the original abnormality will practically always have been a sporadic event, with no discernible increased risk of recurrence due to having had one affected child; and indeed, to our awareness, as yet not one instance is known of a recurrence of UPD in the setting of normal parental karyotypes.

Which of these various states applies in a particular case can be discovered on SNP array. The telling observation is of long stretches of homozygosity (typically >13.5 Mb) on a single chromosome (Papenhausen et al. 2011); and the pattern of homozygosity gives insight into the etiology of the UPD (see color insert Fig. 18-4).

One risk factor is known, and this is increasing maternal age. The link here is that meiotic nondisjunction, the root cause of most UPD, is more prevalent in women of older childbearing age. The meiotic errors noted earlier as leading to trisomic rescue and monosomic rescue are typically of maternal origin. Ginsburg et al. (2000) have shown that maternal age is higher in the subset of patients with Prader-Willi, Angelman, and Russell-Silver syndromes due to UPD, compared to those due to other causes. A causative factor for the meiotic error leading to UPD 15 may be (as also in the classic disorder with a maternal age association, namely Down syndrome) a reduced level of recombination (Robinson et al. 1998). It is worth noting that paternal UPD also has a maternal age effect, which seeming contradictory statement can be appreciated upon considering the mechanism of monosomic rescue after mostly maternal nondisjunction, this being the usual initiating cause of UPDpat.

Rare mechanisms to generate complete UPD include the following:

• Correction of interchange trisomy
• Correction of interchange monosomy
• Isochromosome formation
• Correction of imbalance due to small marker chromosome

If one parent carries a reciprocal translocation, asymmetric segregation of the chromosomes may lead to an interchange trisomy (p. 90) at conception, in which the translocation chromosomes,

---

5 Studies of human preimplantation embryos (see Chapter 22) have revealed that the two requisite events for trisomy rescue, trisomic conception and postzygotic chromosome loss, are, individually, common occurrences, and so the phenomenon of trisomic rescue is not seen as improbable.

plus one of the normal homologs, are transmitted. Postzygotic correction by the loss of one homolog restores disomy, but if it is the other parent's chromosome that is lost, UPD is the consequence. Or, if a nullisomic gamete meets a normal gamete (interchange monosomy), the normal gamete may replicate the homolog in question, to restore disomy (just as in monosomy rescue, mentioned above).

Liehr (2014) records 84 examples of UPD associated with a Robertsonian translocation, involving UPDs for chromosomes 13, 14, 15, 21, and 22. Uniparental disomy is observed less frequently in the setting of a reciprocal translocation, with only 10 known examples, the involved chromosomes being 7, 15, 16, and 20. In the case of parent with a Robertsonian translocation, the most common mechanism leading to UPD is a trisomy rescue after nondisjunction. A monosomic acrocentric chromosome, after nondisjunction from a Robertsonian translocation parent and fertilization with a normal gamete, could replicate as an isochromosome in a monosomy rescue (Berend et al. 2000; McGowan et al. 2002). Complementary isochromosomes

(p. 225), of which scarcely a double-digit number have ever been described, can even allow the circumstance of "contraposed UPD": That is, there may be UPD of the p arm from one parent and UPD of the q arm from the other. Finally, in the setting of a supernumerary small marker chromosome (SMC), there may be a coexisting UPD for the same chromosome from which the SMC was derived (James et al. 1995; Liehr 2014).

Segmental Uniparental Disomy

Segmental UPD may be acquired as the consequence of a postzygotic somatic recombination, between the maternal and paternal homolog (Fig. 18–5), and in that case it will necessarily be an isodisomy (Kotzot 2008a). An assessment of "long contiguous stretches of homozygosity" may prove a useful means to demonstrate the state (Papenhausen et al. 2011). The UPD segment lies distally, the rest of the chromosome pair having a normal biparental disomy. The classical karyotype is normal. An alternative sequence is the following: meiotic nondisjunction

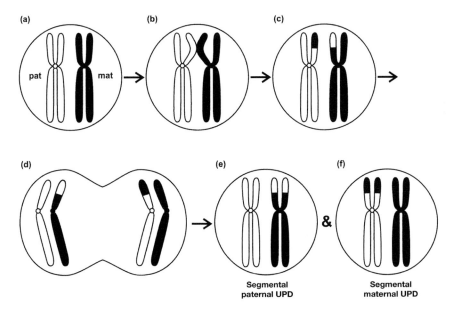

FIGURE 18–5   A mechanism whereby segmental uniparental (iso)disomy may be generated. In one cell of the early conceptus, the paternal and maternal homologs of a chromosome pair (a) undergo somatic recombination between the short arms (b and c). Segregation at mitosis (d) produces daughter cells with segmental UPD: In one (e), the short arm distal segments of both chromosomes are now of paternal origin, and in the other (f), they are both of maternal origin. These cells can then be the source of segmentally UPD tissue in a part of the conceptus.[6]

---

6 The same mechanism may apply in the setting of somatic mosaicism for a Mendelian condition, as Happle and König (1999) discuss in the case of a boy with a variegated manifestation of the rare skin condition epidermolytic hyperkeratosis of Brocq.

producing a disomic gamete, a trisomic conception, a mitotic crossing-over between a maternal and a paternal chromatid, and finally loss of one of the chromosomes that had come with the disomic gamete. A different mechanism is the repair of a double-strand DNA break via break-induced replication.

Segmental UPD can have an effect if the particular chromosomal segment incorporates loci subject to imprinting. If the recombination occurs in a cell after the formation of the inner cell mass (which gives rise to the embryo), the segmental UPD will involve only some cells; in other words, there is *mosaic segmental UPD*. Beckwith-Wiedemann syndrome, Russell-Silver syndrome, UPDs for chromosome 14, and transient neonatal diabetes mellitus are conditions in which segmental UPD may apply. If the segment harbors a recessive allele, "unmasking" of a recessive disorder can be the consequence (see above). If the segmental UPD arises at a later stage of somatic development (thus, mosaic segmental UPD), conversion to homozygosity might affect only a localized tissue, such as, for example, Amyere et al. (2013) show with mosaic segmental upd(1p) in the development of cutaneous glomovenous malformations, in carriers of a *GLMN* mutation, the locus being at 1p22.1. This is very rarely recognized.[7]

A partial trisomy might have different abnormal phenotypic effects according to the parental origin of the duplicated segment, if that segment is subject to imprinting. Trisomy for distal 14q provides an example. A similar picture of dysmorphology and psychomotor deficit is seen in either paternally or maternally originating 14q trisomy. But low birth weight, sometimes less than 2000 grams for a full-term baby, is a specific observation when the duplicated 14q segment comes from the mother (Georgiades et al. 1998). A classic example is the dup15q11.2q13.1 (p. 323): Inherited from the father, there is frequently no phenotypic consequence, but when the duplication is transmitted maternally, the child is at high risk of autism.

ABERRANT IMPRINTING IN A BIPARENTAL SETTING

Differential methylation at a particular imprinted locus can be due to (1) loss of imprinting, leading to expression from both alleles, or (2) gain of imprinting, leading to loss of expression. Aberrant imprinting can be further classified according to whether the maternal or paternal allele is affected. When imprinting is lost, a chromosomal segment that is normally imprinted (thus, inactive) may lose its imprint and become active. This is "relaxation" (or inappropriate erasure) of the imprint effect, and it may be termed an "epimutation"; to re-emphasize the point, the DNA sequence remains unchanged. Consider Beckwith-Wiedemann syndrome (BWS). In some BWS with normal biparental inheritance of chromosome 11, the *IGF-2* (insulin-like growth factor 2) and *KCNQ1OT1* loci on distal 11p show biallelic expression; normally, only the paternal alleles should be functional. This overexpression of genes contributes to the overgrowth that is characteristic of the syndrome (as discussed in more detail below). An iatrogenic cause of aberrant imprinting may relate to pregnancy following assisted reproductive technology; aspects of the process of artificial ovulation stimulation, or of the embryo's environment in vitro, may disturb DNA methylation (Kagami et al. 2007; Amor and Halliday 2008; Katari et al. 2009; Uyar and Seli 2014).

Uniparental Disomy Phenotypes

Uniparental disomy is rare. Extrapolating from the frequency of UPD 15, Robinson (2000) estimated that UPD for any chromosome is present in about 1 in 3,500 births; more recently, King et al. (2014) arrived at a similar estimate, 1 in 2,800, by analyzing exome data from nearly 17,000 samples. Uniparental disomy has been observed for every chromosome except 19 (Liehr 2014). For most chromosomes, as already mentioned, there is no apparent phenotypic consequence. For others, there may be, and we list below some of the syndromes of UPD. The reader seeking more detail is referred to Kotzot (2008a), Yamazawa et al. (2010), and Liehr (2014). In the case of UPD arising from incomplete trisomic rescue, additional factors of trisomy of the placenta, and/or a residual low-level trisomy of the fetus, may also contribute to the eventual phenotype. De Pater et al. (1997) note that a fetal trisomic cell line may not be detected unless the possibility of mosaicism

---

7 UPD can be a factor in some adult-acquired cancers. For example, the well-known V617F mutation in the *JAK2* gene at 9p24.1, occurring in bone marrow as a somatic event, may be the initiating cause of myelofibrosis, polycythemia rubra vera, or essential thrombocytosis. As clonal hematopoiesis advances, UPD can convert a lineage to 9p isozyosity, producing a greater V617F 'allele burden', and presumably, in consequence, accelerated disease (Hinds et al. 2016).

is painstakingly pursued, and Benn (1998) uses the expression "occult mosaicism" to denote an unprovable suspicion. Because mosaicism can never be completely excluded, and neither can homozygosity for an unknown recessive mutation, one should generally incline in the direction of accepting that there is an absence of any UPD effect, when instances are known both of normal and of abnormal phenotypes, or when the observed abnormalities are inconsistent (Kotzot 1999). The abnormal phenotypes will more likely be due to non-UPD mechanisms.

Certain clinical groups might be considered as candidates to harbor cases of UPD. Intrauterine growth retardation (IUGR) is one obvious category. Eggermann et al. (2001) studied 21 patients with pre- and postnatal growth retardation, choosing chromosomes 2, 7, 9, 14, 16, and 20 for analysis, and identified one with upd(14)mat and one with upd(20)mat. Another major category is developmental disability and congenital malformation. Combining data from three large surveys (Conlin et al. 2010; Bruno et al. 2011; King et al. 2014), more than 8,000 cases in total, in which testing employed whole genome genotyping with SNP arrays and exome sequencing, UPD was identified in 1 in 325 (10 times the population UPD frequency). Specific UPDs included, not unexpectedly, chromosomes 6, 7, 11, 14, and 15. UPDs of other chromosomes may have been pathogenic due to unmasking of a recessive gene mutation, or occult mosaicism; some may have been incidental findings. Concerning a possible contribution to spontaneous abortion, Levy et al. (2014) identified a similarly increased frequency of UPD in miscarriage samples of 1 in 265, but a clear causal link could not be assumed.

We have already noted the UPD (UPID) effect of reduction to homozygosity of a recessive mutation, and the consequential unmasking of the respective Mendelian condition. The list of disorders due to this mechanism continues to grow, and even includes rare examples of two recessive diseases in the one individual, when the loci happened to be on the same UPD segment/chromosome (Engel and Antonarakis 2002; Yamazawa et al. 2010; Zeesman et al. 2015).

We now list, by individual chromosome, the UPD syndromes, or associations with normality, that are on record.[8] We frequently comment that there is no known phenotype due to the UPD per se, and that unmasking of a recessive disorder, as

mentioned above, is often the only consequential effect (and often the route to the diagnosis of UPD). Likewise, we make frequent mention that an undetected residual trisomy might contribute to a phenotype, when the UPD mechanism has been trisomy correction. Nevertheless, while recognizing that the classic UPD phenotypes are limited to six chromosomes, imprinted loci are predicted to be present on all chromosomes (Choufani et al. 2011; cf. Fig. 18–2), and it thus remains possible that more subtle and/or later-onset phenotypes, such as effects on behavior and intelligence, a risk for cancer, and other complex disease predisposition, may have (as yet) escaped notice. The case is not closed.

Chromosome 1. Maternal UPD of chromosome 1 may have of itself no effect (provided no recessive mutations are unmasked, as exemplified in Miura et al. 2000, and illustrated in Fig. 18-1b). Field et al. (1998) made the serendipitous discovery of UPD 1 in a normal diabetic adult in the course of a genetic study of diabetes, as did Miyoshi et al. (2001) in their investigation of two normal persons with anomalous Rh blood grouping results: upd(1) mat in the former, mosaicism for paternal isodisomy 1 in the latter. Unmasking of recessive genes, rather than an effect of imprinting, may have been the basis of phenotypic abnormality in a unique case of upd(1)pat described in Chen et al. (1999b). A woman of normal intelligence had a myopathy, short stature, sterility, and deafness. In this case, there was a paternal isodisomy, with the chromosome 1 elements present in the form of two isochromosomes, i(1)(p10) and i(1)(q10). Using SNP arrays and whole exome sequencing, Roberts et al. (2012) identified maternal UPID for all of chromosome 1 in an infant with severe combined immune deficiency and isozygosity for a maternally inherited *CD45* mutation. Of additional interest in this case, seven other homozygous variants were detected that were predicted to be pathogenic, but the child apparently without symptoms. Chromosome 1p harbors the maternally imprinted tumor suppressor gene *DIRAS3* (Niemczyk et al. 2013), suggesting (no more than that) a possible elevated tumor risk in those with maternal UPD 1.

Chromosome 2. About 20 cases of UPD 2 have been reported (Carmichael et al. 2013), with a range of phenotypes which, importantly, include apparent normality for both maternal UPD 2 and paternal UPD 2 (Bernasconi et al. 1996; Keller et al. 2009). In five patients with UPD2mat, the recurrent observations included intrauterine and postnatal growth retardation (four of five cases), atypical bronchopulmonary dysplasia/hypoplasia (three cases), and hypospadias (two cases) (Shaffer et al. 1997; Wolstenholme et al. 2001b). Isozygosity for a recessive mutation, in this case the *ABCA12* gene located at 2q34 that is the basis of severe harlequin ichthyosis, was the result of trisomic rescue in a case reported by Castiglia et al. (2009), an interpretation underpinned by the observation of nonmosaic trisomy 2 at chorionic villus sampling. In an example of the use, and challenges, of exome sequencing, Carmichael et al. describe a girl with UPD 2 and a complex phenotype comprising skeletal and renal dysplasia, immune deficiencies, growth failure, retinal degeneration, and ovarian insufficiency. Exome sequencing identified homozygosity for 18 potentially pathogenic variants, yet none was proven to be causal.

Chromosome 3. Paternal UPD 3 was identified as an incidental finding in a healthy patient who was genotyped as part of a linkage study (Xiao et al. 2006). Maternal UPD 3 has been reported as unmasking the recessive phenotypes of GM1 gangliosidosis (King et al. 2014), Fanconi-Bickel syndrome (Hoffman et al. 2007), and dystrophic epidermolysis bullosa (Fassihi et al. 2006); but in none of these cases was there any evidence of an additional phenotype that might be specific to maternal UPD 3.

Chromosome 4. UPD4mat, isodisomic or heterodisomic, may be another of the UPDs without a phenotype per se: In all the reports to date, the clinical presentations are explicable on the basis of the unmasking of recessive alleles (Spena et al. 2004; Cottrell et al. 2012; Ding et al. 2012). Cottrell et al. report a case of (autosomal recessive) limb girdle muscular dystrophy type 2E, for which the suggested sequence of events was as follows: mother heterozygous for recessive mutation; advanced maternal age; aberrant recombination between chromosome 4 homologs at maternal meiosis; meiotic nondisjunction; trisomy 4 conception; trisomy rescue; maternal UPD 4; isozygosity of the causative gene. Paternal isodisomy for all of chromosome 4 led to a mild form of maple syrup urine disease

in an otherwise well 21-year old, due to homozygosity for a paternally inherited mutation in the *PPM1K* gene (Oyarzabal et al. 2013). Middleton et al. (2006) report a patient with major depression who was genotyped as part of a research study and who had upid(4)mat as a presumed incidental finding. Upid(4)mat may also have been an incidental finding in the child with mild intellectual disability in Palumbo et al. (2015b), although possibly the upid(4)mat unmasked a recessive gene for intellectual disability.

Chromosome 5. UPD 5 is rare, but there is no evidence of an effect of the UPD per se. Maternal UPD 5 in a patient with the skin disease Netherton syndrome (Lin et al. 2007) and paternal isodisomy for chromosome 5 in a child with spinal muscular atrophy (Brzustowicz et al. 1994) were presumably simply the cause of the reduction to homozyosity of the respective recessive genes.

Chromosome 6. The defining feature of transient neonatal diabetes mellitus (TNDM) is hyperglycemia requiring treatment with insulin, with a gradual resolution to normal glucose metabolism in the first few months of life, although with a risk subsequently for non-insulin-dependent diabetes in adult life. About two-thirds of patients with TNDM have aberrations at the TNDM region at 6q24, causing overexpression of two imprinted genes, *PLAGL1* and *HYMAI* (Docherty et al. 2013). The three reported mechanisms, occurring in approximately equal proportions, are UPD6pat, maternal hypomethylation of the differentially methylated region (DMR) at 6q24, and paternally inherited duplication of 6q24, this latter accounting for all familial cases (one example due to a familial insertion involving this segment is in Temple et al. 1996). Docherty et al. noted an apparent increase in the incidence of congenital abnormalities in the TNDM patients with UPD compared to the other two categories. But upd(6)pat can be without apparent effect, as witness an otherwise normal girl with thalassemia whose family was being studied to find a donor for marrow transplantation, and who turned out to have paternal UPID 6 (Bittencourt et al. 1997).

Hypomethylation of multiple imprinted loci is a related disorder that presents with TNDM accompanied by variable manifestations of other imprinting disorders such as intrauterine growth retardation, macroglossia, heart defects, and developmental delay. The underlying mechanism is not UPD but, rather, autosomal recessive mutations in *ZFP57* that result in hypomethylation of maternally methylated loci (Boonen et al. 2013). A separate and apparently sporadic entity is the multi-locus hypomethylation that is observed in a minority of patients with BWS and Silver-Russell syndrome, and which can affect both maternally and paternally methylated loci (Azzi et al. 2009).

No consistent phenotype has been associated with upd(6)mat, although intrauterine growth retardation has been noted in about half of reported cases (Sasaki et al. 2011). Parker et al. (2006) describe a child with congenital adrenal hyperplasia (the 21-hydroxylase gene being on chromosome 6) and Klinefelter syndrome, 48,XXY,+mar(6), with maternal isodisomy for both chromosomes 6 and X. "Correction" of fetal trisomy 6 was the probable basis of the upd(6)mat identified by Cockwell et al. (2006) in a case of fetal death in utero.

Chromosome 7. Silver-Russell syndrome (SRS) has as its major feature intrauterine and postnatal growth retardation, often with a concomitant limb asymmetry. Genetic causes include maternal UPD 7 (~10%), and 11p15 epimutation and structural 11p aberrations (see *Chromosome 11* below); SRS due to UPD7mat presents with more speech and language difficulty, but less incidence of congenital abnormality (Wakeling et al. 2010). The specific loci responsible for UPD 7 imprinting have not been identified, but one or more genes in the *MEST* imprinted region at 7q32.2 may play a role (Eggermann et al. 2010a; Carrera et al. 2016). There is a maternal age association: Very few SRS children born to mothers under age 35 years have UPD 7, but approximately half of those born to mothers age 35 years or older are due to upd(7)mat (Ginsburg et al. 2000); most are consequential upon 'trisomy rescue' from an initial maternal meiotic nondisjunction (Chantot-Bastaraud et al. 2017). Two cases are recorded of SRS in the setting of a maternal reciprocal translocation involving chromosome 7 (Dupont et al. 2002; Behnecke et al. 2012): In both instances, the conception was probably an interchange trisomy, with subsequent loss of the paternal chromosome 7 producing the balanced state, but with a maternal UPHD 7.

As for paternal UPID7, Liehr et al (2014) collated five cases that were identified following a diagnosis of cystic fibrosis (CF). We have seen a similar example, which was in fact the only instance of a child being born with CF from more than 10,000 women who had screened negative for CF carrier status (Archibald et al. 2014). The other reported case was a woman of normal linear growth, and a normal intellect, and it was only because she had a recessive condition with its locus on chromosome 7 (congenital chloride diarrhea) that she had been investigated (Höglund et al. 1994). Apart from unmasking of recessive genes, there does not appear to be a phenotype associated with paternal UPD 7.

Chromosome 8. UPID 8 (pat) is apparently without any phenotypic effect, and one may suppose that this reflects a lack of imprinted genes on this chromosome. Benlian et al. (1996) had made the fortuitous discovery in an otherwise normal child with lipoprotein lipase deficiency, a recessive condition for which the locus maps to 8p22. Similarly, Karanjawala et al. (2000) discovered maternal isodisomy 8 by chance in a man participating in a research study.

Chromosome 9. Maternal UPD 9 appears to be without effect (Björck et al. 1999; Engel and Antonarakis 2002). Homozygosity due to upid(9) at these loci has been reported in children with the corresponding recessive disease: *SURF-1* with Leigh syndrome, and *FOXE* with syndromic congenital hypothyroidism (Tiranti et al. 1999; Castanet et al. 2010).

Chromosome 10. Maternal UPD 10 appears to be without effect of itself, and it is only pathogenic when a recessive disease is unmasked, the latter including familial lymphophagocytic histiocytosis and mitochondrial DNA depletion syndrome (Jones et al. 1995; Al-Jasmi et al. 2008; Nogueira et al. 2013). In a case of uphd(10)mat with concomitant trisomy 10 mosaicism, it was presumably the trisomy rather than the UPD that caused a severe phenotype (Hahnemann et al. 2005).

Chromosome 11. There are growth regulation loci in 11p15 that are expressed monoallelically, according to the parent of origin of the allele. These include the paternally expressed genes *IGF2* and *KCNQ1OT1*, and the maternally expressed genes *H19* and *CDKN1C*. *IGF2* and *H19* are located within one of two "differentially methylated regions"[9] (DMR1), such that *IGF2* is only expressed from the paternal allele, and *H19* only from the maternal allele. Similarly, *KCNQ1OT1* (paternal expression) and *CDKN1C* (maternal expression) are under the control of the second region, DMR2 (Manipalviratn et al. 2009; Weksberg et al. 2010). Perturbation of these regions and genes can lead to two syndromes of opposite growth disorder: BWS, of which overgrowth and hemi*hyper*plasia are characteristic, and SRS, in which growth retardation and hemi*hypo*plasia are key features.

Beckwith-Wiedemann Syndrome Mosaic segmental upd(11p)pat is the basis of approximately 20% of sporadically occurring BWS. That BWS patients with paternal UPD always show mosaicism[10] indicates a mitotic origin and suggests that nonmosaic paternal UPD 11 is an embryonic lethal. In BWS, the striking clinical picture is that of overgrowth of tissues and organs. Thus, in upd(11p)pat, *IGF2* and *KCNQ1OT1* are expressed biallelically, and *H19* and *CDKN1C* are silenced ("nulliallelic"). This imbalance is the basis of the excessive growth, and the associated increased risk of tumors (Ibrahim et al. 2014). Hemihyperplasia is a clinical indicator of this category, and those tissues with the greater fraction of upd(11p) cells may show a correspondingly greater degree of overgrowth. Itoh et al. (2000) describe a child with BWS having a normal adrenal gland on the right and a very enlarged one on the left: 30% of cells in the right gland had upd(11)pat, compared with 88% on the left. Epigenetic mechanisms exist due to other than UPD, noted in the section below on "Genetic Counseling" and as outlined in Figure 18–6 and Table 18–1. BWS due to 11p15 epimutation, affecting in particular the DMR2, has a particular association with in vitro fertilization (IVF) (Amor and Halliday 2008; Lim et al. 2009; Manipalviratn et al. 2009).

Paternal UPD 11 for larger extents of chromosome 11, and maximally the whole chromosome, may lead to typical or to more severe forms of BWS, or to a phenotype with severe intrauterine growth retardation, the differences likely reflecting tissue distribution of the UPD lineage (Grati et al. 2007).

Silver-Russell Syndrome SRS due to 11p anomaly can be considered the countertype to BWS, both clinically and at the molecular level (Schönherr et al. 2007). In SRS due to upd(11p)mat, or to 11p "epimutation" (hypomethylation of DMR1), the maternally active gene *H19* functions biallelically, whereas *IGF2* is underexpressed (Horike et al. 2009). Isolated hemihypoplasia, with shorter limbs on one side, has been recorded with an epimutation (Zeschnigk et al. 2008). Upd(11p)mat appears to be a particularly rare cause of SRS, having been reported on only five occasions (Bullman et al. 2008; Netchine et al. 2007; Luk et al. 2016). SRS can also be due to upd(7)mat, as noted above; the two genetic forms have different underlying causes of the growth retardation (Binder et al. 2008).

Wilms Tumor In a study of 437 (nonsyndromic) Wilms tumor patients, Scott et al. (2008a) showed, in 13 of them, 11p15 abnormalities of the same sort that may be seen in BWS: upd(11p), epimutations, a microinsertion, and a microdeletion, in DMR1. A sibling of the child with a maternally inherited DMR1 microdeletion had a clinical diagnosis of BWS, illustrating that the identical genetic factor, although presumably with differing levels and distribution of postzygotically arising mosaicism, can underlie the two disorders.[11]

Chromosome 12. Maternal isodisomy for chromosome 12 resulted in the transmission of type 3 von Willebrand disease (Boisseau et al. 2011), and vitamin D-resistant rickets (Tamura et al. 2015), whereas paternal isodisomy 12 was the cause of isolated sulfite oxidase deficiency (Cho et al. 2013b). In none of these three instances was there evidence of an additional phenotype attributable to the UPD.

Chromosome 13. Neither maternal nor paternal UPD 13, iso- or heterodisomy, appears to have any effect upon the phenotype (Berend et al. 1999; Soler et al. 2000). A unique example of familial UPD 13, paternal and maternal, emphasizes this point: A normal mother with presumed 45,XX,i(13q)pat had a normal child with 45,XY,i(13q)mat (Slater

---

9 There is a multiplicity of nomenclature of these regions. DMR1 and DMR2 may be referred to as Imprinting Control Regions 1 and 2, ICR1 and ICR2. DMR1 is also known as H19 DMR, and the telomeric cluster; and DMR2 is also known as KvDMR1, KCNQ1OT1 DMR, LIT1 DMR, and the centromeric cluster.

10 Using diagnostic SNP array, we have detected mosaic segmental upd(11p)pat in individuals with no clinical features of BWS. We presume that in these cases the mosaic upd(11p) is restricted to tissues that do not contribute to the BWS phenotype.

11 In BWS with isolated DMR2 loss of methylation (the most common form; see Table 18–1), Wilms tumor is not seen, and this knowledge can inform clinical management.

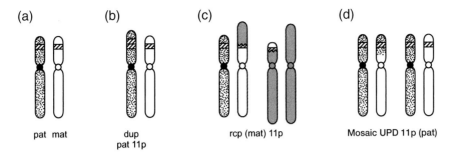

FIGURE 18–6 The no. 11 chromosomes in different chromosomal bases of Beckwith-Wiedemann syndrome (BWS). The maternal homolog is shown open, the paternal homolog is speckled, and the BWS critical region at 11p15 is shown cross-hatched. (*a*) The normal state of biparental inheritance of intact no. 15 chromosomes. (*b*) Paternal duplication of distal 11p. (*c*) Maternal reciprocal translocation disrupting the BWS critical region, with the other chromosome shown in gray. (*d*) Mosaic segmental paternal UPD of 11p, showing the chromosome 11 pairs of the two cell lines. The pair on the left shows paternal UPD for distal 11p (the speckled segments).

Table 18–1. Different Causes of Beckwith-Wiedemann (BWS) and Silver-Russell (SRS) Syndromes (see also Fig. 18–6)

	FRACTIONS (%)	
GENETIC FORM	BWS	SRS
Gain/loss of methylation at DMR1	5 (gain)	35–50 (loss)
Loss of methylation at DMR2	50	
Uniparental disomy	20 (upd11pat)	5–10 (upd7mat)
Large duplication (DMR1 + 2)	<1 (paternal)	1–2 (maternal)
Smaller CNV	1–3	<1
Inversion, translocation	<1	<1
CDKN1C mutation	10	
Unknown	10	40

Notes: Fractions (rounded) indicate relative frequencies; these data may be influenced by the clinical index of suspicion. False-negative results for methylation testing and UPD testing may occur due to mosaicism.

DMR1 and -2, differentially methylated regions 1 and 2. DMR1 gain of methylation causes overexpression of *IGF2* and nonexpression of *H19*. DMR2 loss of methylation causes overexpression of *KCNQ1OT1* and nonexpression of *CDKN1C* (and see text).

In a minority of cases with imprinting changes at DMR1 and/or DMR2, the imprinting change has been shown to be due to a copy number variant at 11p15 (Baskin et al. 2014).

Sources: Algar et al. (2007), Manipalviratn et al. (2009), Eggermann et al. (2010a), Wakeling et al. (2010), Zollino et al. (2010a), and Ibrahim et al. (2014).

et al. 1995). She may have been the result of monosomic rescue, and her son due to trisomic rescue! Maternal isodisomy for chromosome 13 has been seen in autosomal recessive *GJB2*-associated deafness (Alvarez et al. 2003).

Chromosome 14. Chromosome 14 contains an imprinted locus at 14q32, and UPD 14 produces different syndromes according to the paternal or maternal basis of the disomy (Sutton and Shaffer 2000; Engel and Antonarakis 2002). Either may be seen in the setting of a normal karyotype, or with a Robertsonian translocation (or "acrocentric isochromosome"). A balanced 45,der(13;14) Robertsonian translocation may reflect correction of an initially 46,der(13;14),+14 conception, while the 45,der(14;14) case might in fact result from a 45,−14 conception which then corrected by reduplication of the single chromosome 14 to give an i(14q) with isodisomy. Isodisomy may be present in the setting of a normal karyotype, and it may thus be less rare than is appreciated (Chu et al. 2004).

Kagami-Ogata Syndrome Paternal UPD 14 is the more severe of the UPD 14s, with obstetric complication (polyhydramnios and premature labor), a particular pattern of malformation, growth retardation, and major functional neurological compromise (Sutton et al. 2003; Stevenson et al. 2004; Ogata et al. 2016). Survival is poor. The bell-shaped thorax (Fig. 14–27), reminiscent of Jeune syndrome, is a particular clinical pointer, and it has been observed at 23-week ultrasonography; this anatomy may improve during childhood in those who survive (Chu et al. 2004; Kagami et al. 2005; Curtis et al. 2006).

Temple Syndrome Maternal UPD 14, or more specifically maternal UPD at the 14q32 imprinted locus, causes Temple syndrome, which can also result from an epimutation (hypomethylation at key loci within 14q32) or from paternal deletions at 14q32 (Ioannides et al. 2014). The syndrome is characterized by pre- and postnatal growth retardation, small hands and feet, early puberty, subtle dysmorphism, mildly reduced intellectual ability, and, in approximately half of patients, obesity. Mitter et al. (2006) pointed out the overlap with the Prader-Willi phenotype, and we now have a biological basis for this similarity: Loss of expression of paternally expressed genes at the Prader-Willi syndrome locus at 15q11q13 leads to upregulation of maternally expressed genes at 14q32 (Stelzer et al. 2014).

Chromosome 15. Prader-Willi syndrome (PWS) and Angelman syndrome (AS) are the two UPD 15 syndromes. It may be an oversimplification, but equally a useful perspective, to think of these as each being caused by absent activity of a particular single genetic segment—the PWS region and the AS region, respectively—within 15q11q13. The chromosomal region of interest is illustrated in Fig. 18–7 (and replicated in Fig. 14–60).

Prader-Willi syndrome is a contiguous gene syndrome, with the phenotype being due to loss of transcription of several genes and RNA transcripts on the *paternal* chromosome 15. Among these, deficiency of a particular cluster of small nucleolar RNA genes (snoRNAs) called SNORD 116 (previously HBII-85) is responsible for the key features of PWS (Sahoo et al. 2008; de Smith et al. 2009). Different components of the PWS phenotype are therefore mediated via perturbed functioning of different genetic targets of these snoRNAs. Another RNA transcript from the paternal chromosome 15, IPW, has been shown to downregulate transcription of maternally expressed genes at the 14q32 imprinted region, providing an explanation for the similarity in phenotypes between PWS and maternal UPD 14, as just mentioned above.[12]

Angelman syndrome is due to absent activity of a single gene, *UBE3A*, on the *maternal* chromosome

15. SNORD 116 and *UBE3A* lie in close proximity on 15q11q13, and both are under the influence of an imprinting control center (IC): From centromeric to telomeric on the chromosome, the order is IC, SNORD 116, and the *UBE3A* gene (Fig. 18–7).

The absence of gene activity in PWS and AS is due either to the loss, or to the nonfunctioning, of this PWS/AS region on one chromosome 15 homolog. *Loss* is most commonly due to a simple interstitial deletion ("classical deletion"). Low-copy repeats on either side of the region can come together and set the stage for nonallelic homologous recombination, leading to deletion of the PWS/AS region. Whether the phenotype comes to be PWS or AS depends upon which parent contributed the deleted chromosome. *Nonfunctioning* of (structurally normal) genes within 15q11q13 is due to the imprint status. This is most commonly the consequence of UPD 15, with the phenotype determined according to the parent of origin of the disomic pair of chromosomes. A rare cause is failure of, or damage to, the chromosome 15 IC. Study of these IC-damaged cases has cast much light on the processes of molecular pathogenesis in PWS and AS, and so the length of their commentaries that follow is quite out of proportion to their frequencies. In the case of AS, *mutation* in the *UBE3A* gene is a further category of mechanism.

The 15q11q13 Imprinting Center Normal persons have one paternally imprinted chromosome 15 and one maternally imprinted chromosome 15. The imprinting state of a chromosome 15 is set and reset as it is transmitted down the generations, according to the sex of the transmitting parent. This resetting—an "epigenetic modification"—is dictated during gametogenesis from the *cis*-acting IC, with the methylation of genes comprising, in large part at least, the crux of the process. The IC is bipartite, with a centromeric element, the AS-IC, and 35 kb distant a telomeric element, the PWS-IC, this latter including exon 1 of *SNRPN*. Interaction between these two elements directs the process. In *maternal* gametogenesis, the AS-IC has responsibility for initiating a paternal→maternal switch on the chromosome 15 that the mother herself had received from her father. The chromosome 15 she got from her mother retains a maternal imprint. With an active

---

12 Also of interest is the single exon gene *MAGEL2*, which is expressed from the paternal allele. Truncating mutations in paternal allele of *MAGEL2* cause Schaff-Yang syndrome, which shares with PWS the features of neonatal hypotonia and intellectual disability, but also has joint contractures as a prominent feature. Intriguingly, cognitive impairment in Schaff-Yang syndrome is frequently more severe than in PWS or in patients with whole gene deletions of *MAGEL2* (Fountain et al. 2017).

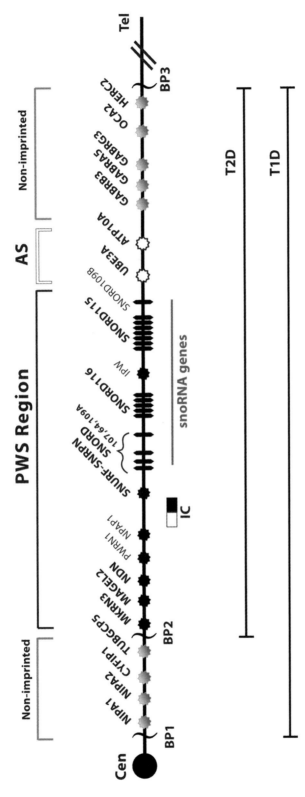

FIGURE 18–7 (Replicate of Fig. 14-29) The regions and loci of interest within the segment 15q11.2q13.3. AS, Angelman syndrome; BP, (numbered) breakpoint; PWS, Prader-Willi syndrome; T1D, type 1, T2D, type 2 deletion. Black, white, and gray shading indicates, respectively, PWS-related, AS-related, and non-imprinted loci. IC, imprinting center: The black IC segment is the PWS-IC, influencing the black-coded loci in the PWS region; the white IC segment is the AS-IC, influencing the white-coded loci in the AS region.

Source: From Driscoll et al., Prader-Willi syndrome, GeneReviews 2016 (updated, personal communication, D.J. Driscoll, 2016). Courtesy D.J. Driscoll, and with the permission of the University of Washington.

AS-IC, the *UBE3A* gene, lying approximately 1 Mb distant, is free to function in the embryo to which this ovum gives rise. Vice versa, *paternal* gametogenesis serves to effect a maternal→paternal switch, or to retain a paternal status, on the chromosome 15 that the sperm contributes to the embryo. In consequence, a number of genes under its aegis are able to function, in part at least, by being demethylated. The *UBE3A* gene's activity is prevented. These epigenetic modifications operate only in *cis*, and so the maternal and paternal chromosomes continue to function autonomously, with their different repertoires of expression, during the life of the individual.

A scheme for the various molecular defects of PWS and AS is presented in Figure 18–8. Table 18–2 sets out the test results for the different types of PWS and AS.

Classical Deletion This is the most frequent basis of the two syndromes, accounting for approximately 70% of both PWS and AS (Horsthemke and Buiting 2006). The deletion removes 5.9 Mb (class I) or 5.0 Mb (class II) within 15q11q13, encompassing the PWS and the AS genetic elements, and including the IC (types 1 and 2 deletions in Fig. 18–7). There is one common distal breakpoint (BP3), and two variable proximal deletion breakpoint regions (BP1, BP2), due to duplicons at these sites. Nonallelic homologous recombination between the distal and whichever proximal duplicon then causes the deletions (Ji et al. 2000). The behavioral phenotype is a little worse with the class I BP1-BP3 deletion than the class II BP2-BP3 deletion (Bittel et al. 2006). Larger deletions are infrequent, and they are associated with a more severe phenotype (Sahoo et al. 2007).

If the deletion occurs on a *paternally* originating chromosome, it will cause the PWS phenotype to develop;[13] and vice versa, a *maternal* deletion produces AS. In a sense, there is an "unmasking of the silent elements" on the other chromosome. As well as the crucial PWS and AS genetic elements, a number of other loci may be deleted, and so the expression "contiguous gene syndrome" is not inappropriate, albeit having a somewhat different sense from its usage elsewhere in this book. One of the least important of these other loci is the *P* gene that contributes to normal pigmentation, and so children with PWS and AS due to classical deletion typically have fairer complexions than do their siblings.[14] Mosaicism may lead to a milder phenotype (Golden et al. 1999; Tekin et al. 2000). In very rare cases of PWS with concomitant 47,XXY Klinefelter syndrome, the coincidence of the two conditions is merely by chance (Nowaczyk et al. 2004).

Prader-Willi and Angelman Syndromes due to Deletion, Associated with Uncommon Rearrangement Loss of the PW/AS region can be due to transmission of an unbalanced translocation or an inversion involving chromosome 15. The male carrier of a balanced reciprocal translocation in which one breakpoint is in the region of 15q13 can transmit an unbalanced complement to produce a deletion PWS child (Hultén et al. 1991; Smeets et al. 1992), and the female carrier can have a child with deletion AS (Stalker and Williams 1998). There may be an additional effect from the concomitant imbalance involving the other chromosome of a translocation, such as the case in Torisu et al. (2004), a child who displayed features both of AS and the 1p36 deletion syndrome, due to a tertiary monosomy for these two segments, the mother being a balanced translocation carrier. A handful of PWS cases have been due to a Y;15 translocation with breakpoints in Yp and at 15q12q13, deleting the PWS region, having the karyotype 45,X,der(Y),t(Y;15) (Vickers et al. 1994). A grandmother heterozygous for an inverted insertion of chromosome 15 had a PWS grandchild through her carrier son and an AS grandchild through her carrier daughter (Collinson et al. 2004). Loss of the PW/AS region can be due to a de novo rearrangement, such as Dang et al. (2016) exemplify in a PWS child with a translocation t(15;19)(q12;p13.3).

Uniparental Disomy and Prader-Willi Syndrome About one-third of PWS is due to UPD (Horsthemke and Buiting 2006). The cytogenetic study typically shows a normal 46,XX or 46,XY karyotype. Both chromosomes 15 come from the *mother*, and so neither of the PWS critical regions is expressed. This functional lack causes the PWS phenotype. In most (80% or more), the UPD had its origin in a maternal meiosis I error. A maternal age effect is clear: Five times as many PWS children born to mothers younger than age 35 years have a deletion as have UPD, but the reverse applies

---

13 An aide-mémoire: Prader-Willi due to Paternal deletion.

14 An additional copy of this gene leads to hyperpigmentation (Akahoshi et al. 2001). This is a good example of a simple dosage effect: One copy of the *P* gene = pale skin, two copies = normal pigmentation, three copies = hyperpigmentation.

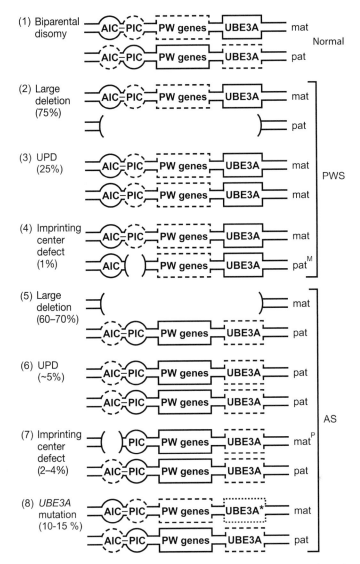

FIGURE 18–8 An outline of the different genetic forms of Prader-Willi syndrome (PWS) and Angelman syndrome (AS). The PWS/AS critical region of chromosome 15 is depicted. A bipartite imprinting center with AS and PWS components (AIC and PIC) controls, in *cis*, the activity of a set of PWS genes and the *UBE3A* gene. A switched-on IC and an actively functioning gene are shown in unbroken line; a switched-off IC and an unactivated gene are shown in dashed outline. A mutated *UBE3A* gene is shown starred and with a dotted outline. (1) Normally, the *UBE3A* gene is transcribed only from the maternal chromosome (mat), and the PWS genes only from the paternal chromosome (pat), with each chromosome thus functioning appropriately for its parent of origin. In PWS there is nonfunctioning of the PWS genes because: (2) the PWS genes have been removed by a typical large deletion from the paternal chromosome; (3) both chromosomes are of maternal origin; (4) a microdeletion of, or mutation in, the PIC has fixed a maternal imprint status on the paternal chromosome. In AS there is nonfunctioning of the *UBE3A* gene because: (5) the *UBE3A* gene has been removed by a typical large deletion from the maternal chromosome; (6) both chromosomes are of paternal origin; (7) a microdeletion of, or mutation in, the AIC has fixed a paternal imprint status on the maternal chromosome; (8) there is a mutation in the *UBE3A* gene on the maternal chromosome. A further category (9) is not shown, comprising the 10%–15% in which no genetic defect can be shown. Approximate percentages of each PWS/AS category are indicated; in another ~10% of AS, no genetic defect can be identified. pat^M, a maternally functioning chromosome of paternal origin; mat^P, a paternally functioning chromosome of maternal origin.

Table 18–2. Assessment of Genetic Category of Prader-Willi and Angelman Syndromes According to Results of Molecular Testing

		DELETION ON MICROARRAY	LOH ON SNP MICROARRAY	METHYLATION PATTERN OF NO. 15S	PARENTAL ORIGINS OF NO. 15S	*UBE3A* GENE
Prader-Willi syndrome	Classical deletion	+	+	Mat	Bi	
	upd(15)mat	N	±	Mat	Mat	
	Imprinting center microdeletion	N	N	Mat	Bi	
	Other imprinting center defect	N	N	Mat	Bi	
Angelman syndrome	Classical deletion	+	+	Pat	Bi	Deleted
	upd(15)pat	N	±	Pat	Pat	"Intact"
	Imprinting defect	N	N	Pat	Bi	"Intact"
	UBE3A mutation	N	N	Bi	Bi	Mutated
	Epigenetic error	N	N	Bi	Bi	"Intact"

Notes: LOH, loss of heterozygosity. A normal chromosome microarray result is indicated by N, an abnormal result by +. An inconsistent result is shown as ± (LOH will be seen in all UPD due to meiosis II error or UPD of postzygotic origin, but will only be seen in UPD due to meiosis I error when there has also been recombination). Bi, biparental; Mat, maternal; Pat, paternal. "Intact" means that the DNA sequence of the gene is normal, but its function is epigenetically compromised.

to those born to mothers age 35 years or older, in whom there is a fivefold excess of those showing UPD (Ginsburg et al. 2000). The phenotype is very similar to classical deletion PWS, although the facies may be less "typical" with the UPD form of PWS, learning and behavior problems are less prominent, and some of the minor manifestations are less likely to occur; in consequence, diagnosis may be delayed in comparison to deletion PWS (Cassidy et al. 1997; Gunay-Aygun et al. 1997). The UPD form of PWS is particularly associated with a psychiatric phenotype, typically presenting in young adulthood and characterized by a fluctuating psychosis and bipolar mood disorder (Verhoeven et al. 2003). A more severe form of UPD PWS is associated with a concomitant trisomy 15 mosaicism (Olander et al. 2000). In rare instances, UPD may be mosaic, arising from rescue of a post-fertilization error and resulting in an incomplete PWS phenotype (Morandi et al. 2015).

Uniparental Disomy and Angelman Syndrome Approximately 7% of AS is due to UPD. As

with PWS due to UPD, the karyotype is normal 46,XX or 46,XY. Both chromosomes 15 are from the *father*, and neither chromosome expresses the AS critical region. Most cases involve a postzygotic origin of the extra paternal chromosome, resulting in isodisomy for the entire chromosome that is readily recognizable as such on SNP microarray. This probably follows the "correction" of monosomy 15 due to a nullisomic ovum (as outlined above) and, as with PWS, is likely a maternal age effect. Very few AS children born to mothers younger than age 35 years have UPD, but those born to mothers age 35 years or older have about equal numbers due to deletion and UPD (Ginsburg et al. 2000). A few are due to a paternal second meiotic error (Robinson et al. 2000). In parallel with the observations in UPD PWS noted above, the phenotype in AS due to UPD is not quite as severe as in the deletion form, with these children showing a lesser frequency of seizures, and some having a few words (Fridman et al. 2000). But it remains true that the handicap is severe.

Prader-Willi and Angelman Syndromes due to Uniparental Disomy, Associated with Chromosome 15 Rearrangement Uniparental disomy can result from a variety of rearrangements involving chromosome 15. The male carrier of a reciprocal translocation involving chromosome 15 could transmit a disomic 15 spermatocyte from 3:1 nondisjunction, with the maternal chromosome 15 then being lost, and have a child with UPD AS; and vice versa, the female carrier could have a PWS child (Calounova et al. 2006; Heidemann et al. 2010). Similarly, a familial nonhomologous Robertsonian translocation in which one of the component chromosomes is a no. 15 giving a trisomic 15 conception, and with postzygotic loss of the chromosome 15 from the other parent, would lead to upd(15) with either PWS or AS, according to the sex of the carrier parent (Fig. 7–6) (Tsai et al. 2004). The same thing could happen if the translocation were de novo. A maternally originating de novo homologous der(15;15) (which may actually be a 15q isochromosome), with no chromosome 15 contributed from the father, would cause PWS (Robinson et al. 1994); and vice versa, AS would result from a paternal isochromosome 15q (Tonk et al. 1996). Smith et al. (1994) describe AS from asymmetric segregation of a paternal 8;15 translocation (Fig. 12–4). The heterozygous father passed on his der(8) and his normal chromosome 15 (thus, paternal UPD), and there was absence of a maternal chromosome 15. Some PWS children with a 47,+idic(15) karyotype may actually have UPD of the two intact chromosomes 15, and the small idic(15) is a phenotypically irrelevant relic of the original process of abnormal chromosomal behavior (Robinson et al. 1993).

Imprinting Center Defects A very small group of PWS and AS patients, approximately 1% and 3%, respectively, have normal biparental inheritance and no classical deletion, but a uniparental pattern of methylation and gene expression (Horsthemke and Buiting 2006). Most of these cases reflect *abnormal function* of the IC, while a minority, around 10%–20%, have an actual IC *microdeletion*. The latter category can be strongly suspected when there is a positive family history, while in the former, sporadic occurrence has been universally observed. Whether PWS or AS is seen depends upon which component of the IC is deleted or nonfunctional.

Functional Imprinting Center Defect Buiting et al. (2003) analyzed 44 PWS and 76 AS patients with a failure of IC functioning, an IC deletion or point mutation having been excluded; these aberrant epigenetic states are referred to as epimutations.[15] All cases were sporadic. Some shared with an unaffected sibling the 15q11q13 haplotype on their paternal (PWS) or maternal (AS) chromosome, supporting the presumption of a de novo defect. With PWS, the basis of the epimutation may be a failure to erase the maternal imprint, as an act of omission. Thus, for example, the father of such a PWS child passes on his maternal chromosome 15 with its maternal imprint still in place, and the child inherits two maternally imprinted no. 15 chromosomes. In AS, the typical scenario may be the imposition of an anomalous imprint status. This can be thought of as an act of commission: The mother inappropriately applies a paternal imprint to the chromosome 15, or fails to reset her paternal chromosome 15 that she passes to the child; or (since some maternal epimutations are mosaic) the error may occur postzygotically. If the error is incomplete, a milder AS phenotype may be seen (Brockmann et al. 2002).

AS due to an imprinting defect, with loss of methylation of the maternal allele, may have an association with subfertility and artificial reproductive technology (Manipalviratn et al. 2009). If the association is indeed causal, the biological basis may be in the subfertility per se, or due to the superovulation treatment as part of IVF protocol, which leads to a failure to acquire normal *UBE3A* activation status in the ovum.

Microdeletion of Imprinting Center Microdeletions of the IC, generally of kilobase size, remove one or other of its major component parts, either the PWS-IC or the AS-IC. The inability to reset an appropriate imprint status leads to the "fixation of an ancestral epigenotype" (Saitoh et al. 1997). Only a handful of cases have been identified worldwide (Hassan and Butler 2016; Horsthemke and Buiting 2006). Their particular importance to the counselor lies in the high recurrence risk, if a parent is heterozygous: The mode of inheritance is essentially sex-influenced (the *parent's* sex, that is) autosomal dominant, with a 50% risk for the heterozygous father (for PWS) or the heterozygous mother (for AS), according to which component part of the IC is deleted. De novo mutations are also reported.

---

15 The word *mutation* is normally taken to indicate that there is a change in the DNA sequence (from the Latin *mutare*, to change). By definition, no such change has occurred in an epimutation. But there has been a change in the functioning of the DNA.

In *Prader-Willi syndrome due to IC microdeletion*, the father would have received the deletion on his mother's chromosome 15. He is normal, since an erased paternal imprint on his maternal chromosome is, naturally, correct. The deletion could have originated in his mother, or antecedent to her, provided transmission had been exclusively matrilineal. But when he passes this chromosome 15 with its fixed maternal epigenotype to a child of his, with the maternal→paternal imprint switch unable to function, the child has, effectively, a functional maternal UPD 15. Such a family is illustrated in Ming et al. (2000). Of 10 children, all of them normal and with normal karyotypes on standard cytogenetics, four inherited an IC microdeletion, presumably from their deceased mother (their father was proven not to have the deletion). Two of these children were male, and each went on to have, in the next generation, a child with PWS: an example of "grandmatrilineal inheritance."

In *Angelman syndrome due to IC microdeletion*, the scenario is essentially the obverse of the above. A microdeletion on the maternal chromosome 15 removes the AS-IC. The defect may have arisen de novo from the maternal grandfather of the AS child, or alternatively, there could have been patrilineal transmission of the mutation, harmlessly, for any number of previous generations. Transmission from the grandfather to the mother would be without phenotypic consequence, since a paternally originating chromosome 15 would in any event have its AS-IC inactivated. But in oögenesis in the mother, the normal paternal→maternal switch on the abnormal chromosome cannot be effected (thus, "fixation" of the ancestral paternal epigenotype). If the child receives this chromosome 15 from the mother, both homologs carry a paternal imprint. In consequence, the child has AS. Two such Japanese families, independently ascertained and reported, had exactly the same 1.487 Mb deletion and may well have represented distant branches from the same, presumably male, ancestor (Sato et al. 2007).

Angelman Syndrome due to UBE3A Gene Mutation Classical point mutation, affecting the *UBE3A* (ubiquitin protein ligase 3A) gene, is an important contributor to AS etiology (Abaied et al. 2010). This gene is expressed from both parental chromosomes in some tissues, but, in the brain, from only the maternal chromosome. The (normal) paternal allele does not function in embryonic brain, or at least in particular parts of the brain. Thus, if the maternal gene is mutated, there is no UBE3A expression, and in consequence brain

development is compromised (Rougeulle and Lalande 1998). In a mouse knockout model, *Ube3a* expression was compromised in certain cells of the hippocampus, a crucial structure in learning and memory, and of the cerebellum, which may have a role in learning as well as its classic role in coordination (Albrecht et al. 1997). The human situation is quite likely to be similar. (Mouse knockout models for PWS are lethal.)

Approximately 70% of inherited "non-deletion non-UPD non-IC" AS is due to *UBE3A* mutation of maternal origin. The severity of phenotype in the mutation form falls between the deletion and UPD cases (Abaied et al. 2010). Multigenerational transmission may be seen, with the revealing observation that AS children are born only to carrier daughters of carrier males (Fig. 18–9). The mutation transmitted by the father has no effect in his child since this chromosome 15 region would in any event carry a paternal imprint and be silenced. Intragenic deletions within the *UBE3A* gene are a rare basis of AS, with only seven such cases reported (Aguilera et al. 2017).

Angelman Syndrome with No Deletion, No Uniparental Disomy, No Imprinting Mutation, and No UBE3A Mutation In some 15%–20% of AS, no genetic defect can be found (Hitchins et al. 2004; Horsthemke and Buiting 2006). There is a normal karyotype, with no deletion demonstrable on fluorescence in situ hybridization (FISH), normal methylation analysis (at least on the sampled tissues), biparental inheritance, and an apparently intact *UBE3A* gene. There may be an epigenetic influence whereby a normal *UBE3A* gene on the maternal chromosome fails to activate normally during embryogenesis. Or there may be some other AS genetic basis, as yet unknown.

Chromosome 16. This is one of the more commonly seen UPDs, and it is almost always due to correction of trisomy 16 of maternal meiotic origin. Thus, it is typically a *maternal* UPHD or UPHID. It has been difficult to separate out the effects of the UPD, and of a placental insufficiency due to confined placental mosaicism for trisomy 16, this typically being the route by which the UPD comes to be recognized, following chorionic villus sampling; and in addition, a possible residual occult fetal trisomy mosaicism always remains as a potential confounder. Opinions differ. Yong et al. (2003) showed in a large series of mosaic trisomy 16 discovered at prenatal diagnosis that the degree of fetal growth restriction, and probably the malformation rate,

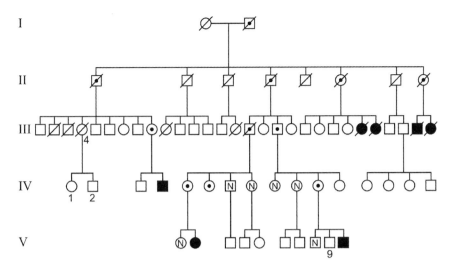

FIGURE 18–9   A family with inherited Angelman syndrome, due to a *UBE3A* mutation, reported in Moncla et al. (1999). Filled symbol, Angelman syndrome; bull's-eye symbol, mutation carrier, demonstrated or inferred; N, demonstrated noncarrier. Note that all the affected children are born to carrier *mothers*, but that these mothers are related to each other through the *male* line. Some normal children have been proven to be noncarriers with molecular testing (N in symbol), but the reader can also determine that any unaffected child of a potential carrier mother, such as IV:1 and 2, the children of III:4, or V:9, the sibling of an affected child, cannot be carriers. An inherited imprinting center mutation could present a similar pedigree.

was greater in those with upd(16)mat than in those with biparental inheritance, thus suggesting a role of the UPD per se. Imprinting of the *FOXF1* locus at 16q24.1 has been proposed as a mechanism underpinning some phenotypic features of upd(16)mat (Szafranski et al. 2016). In contrast, Scheuvens et al. (2017) suggest that upd(16)mat is, of itself, without phenotype and may serve merely as a biomarker for an underlying trisomy 16 mosaicism. As for *paternal* UPD 16, it seems probable that it has no clinical consequences (Engel and Antonarakis 2002).

The usual rare risk from isozygosity for a recessive gene applies, as exemplified in Wattanasirichaigoon et al. (2008), who note a child with hydrops fetalis due to hemoglobin Bart's, consequential upon upd(16)mat. Hamvas et al. (2009) reported three infants with paternal isodisomy 16 resulting in surfactant deficiency due to *ABCA3* mutation, but none of whom exhibited a nonpulmonary phenotype.

Chromosome 17.   Three cases of complete upd(17)mat have been described. One 46,XY child was normal, ascertainment having been via the discovery of trisomy 17 mosaicism at amniocentesis (Genuardi et al. 1999). Lebre et al. (2009) identified the UPD in an infant with cystinosis, a recessively inherited multiorgan storage disease, the

locus of which is on chromosome 17p, and this segment being in isodisomic state in the child; and upid(17)pat was the basis of a case of junctional epidermolysis bullosa, the relevant locus, *ITGB4*, being on this chromosome (Natsuga et al. 2010). A recessive etiology was suspected in a girl with developmental delay, microcephaly, and seizures, in whom mat upd(17) was identified by exome sequencing, although no definite causative mutation was found (King et al. 2014).

Chromosome 18.   Given the frequency of trisomy 18 at conception, it is rather surprising that there have been no reports of UPD for the entire chromosome 18, either with or without phenotype. Kariminejad et al. (2011) presented a fascinating example of segmental maternal UPD of 18p and segmental paternal UPD of 18q in a girl whose consanguineous parents both carried a pericentric inversion inv(18)(p11.31q21.33). The healthy child received two recombinant chromosomes 18, from the mother a derivative chromosome 18 with dup(18p)/del(18q), and from the father a derivative chromosome 18 with dup(18q)/del(18p).

Chromosome 19.   This is the only chromosome for which neither maternal nor paternal UPD has been reported. Of potential relevance, the paternally expressed imprinted gene *PEG3*, located at 19q13, has been implicated in embryogenesis, behavior, and carcinogenesis (Jiang et al. 2010).

Chromosome 20. Eggermann et al. (2001) reviewed three reported cases of upd(20), one paternal and two maternal, with a major malformation phenotype in the former, and growth retardation the common observation in the latter two. But it took until 2016 for *maternal* UPD 20 to be confirmed as a bona fide imprinting syndrome, following the diagnosis of eight new cases, due in large part to improved ascertainment via SNP microarray (Mulchandani et al. 2016). Features present in all cases are intrauterine growth restriction, short stature, and prominent feeding difficulties with failure to thrive, frequently needing tube feeding. Development is typically normal, and there is no consistent dysmorphism. The predominant mechanism is trisomy rescue after maternal meiosis II nondisjunction.

Pseudohypoparathyroidism type 1b (PHP1b) is caused by imprinting defects in *GNAS*, which, in certain tissues, such as renal proximal tubules, is predominantly expressed from the maternal allele. Hence, symptoms of PHP1b would be expected to accompany *paternal* UPD 20, and indeed some patients with sporadic PHP1b have upd(20)pat, either involving the whole chromosome or, more commonly, as a segmental mitotic error (Fernández-Rebollo et al. 2010; Bastepe et al. 2011). Dixit et al. (2013a) reviewed six reported cases of PHP1b due to upd(20)pat and suggested that large birth weight, obesity, and macrocephaly may be additional features of the upd(20)pat phenotype.

Chromosome 21. UPD 21, maternal or paternal, appears to be without effect (Engel and Antonarakis 2002).

Chromosome 22. Maternal UPD 22 has generally not been causally associated with any defect (Kotzot 1999; Engel and Antonarakis 2002). Intrauterine growth retardation, if present, may more likely reflect the influence of a trisomic 22 placenta, or low-level "occult" mosaicism of the fetus (Balmer et al. 1999; Bryan et al. 2002). A der(22;22)(q10;10q) has been reported in association with both maternal and paternal UPD 22, typically having presented with recurrent miscarriage in otherwise healthy individuals (Liehr et al.

2014), although Ouldim et al. (2008) report the unexpected transmission of a der(22;22)(q10;10q) from a father to (normal) son (and see p. 152). An instance of homozygosity for a *PLA2G6* mutation, leading to neurodegeneration with brain iron accumulation, in monozygous twins from an IVF conception, was due to paternal UPD 22 (Tello et al. 2017).

Chromosome X. Neither upd(X)mat nor upd(X)pat appears to have any consequence in the 46,XX person, with the usual exception of homozygosity for a recessive mutation (Quan et al. 1997). However, there may be a subtly different neuropsychological phenotype according to the parent of origin in monosomy X (self-evidently a uniparental condition). In a British study, 80 girls with Turner syndrome underwent behavioral evaluation, 55 of whom were 45,X^M and 25 were 45,X^P. The 45,X^P girls were more socially adept and more articulate than the 45,X^M girls. Speculatively, this may represent the effect of an imprintable X-borne "locus for social cognition" that is functional on the X chromosome transmitted from a father, and nonfunctional on the X from a mother (Skuse et al. 1997). Autism, which is a male-susceptible condition, is associated with 45,X^M in the case of autistic girls with Turner syndrome (Donnelly et al. 2000). In terms of response to growth hormone, it makes no difference whether the child is 45,X^M or 45,X^P (Tsezou et al. 1999).

Upd(X)pat offers the intriguing scenario of father-to-son transmission of an X-linked gene. A 24,XY gamete from a hemizygous father could produce a 47,XXY zygote, which could subsequently lose the maternally contributed X; or the ovum could be nullisomic X, with sex chromosomal complementation producing 46,XY. Either mechanism could explain the observations in a family with the X-linked form of ectodermal dysplasia, as presented in Ferrier et al. (2009).

Uniparental Disomy for the Entire Chromosomal Complement

Nonmosaic paternal uniparental disomy (UPDpat) for the full diploid complement—all 46 chromosomes are of paternal origin—produces the placental disorder of complete hydatidiform mole. When, in addition to a double set of paternally derived chromosomes, there is also a haploid maternal set (triploidy, with a total chromosome count of 69), a partial hydatidiform mole results. Hydatidiform mole is discussed in more detail in Chapter 19.

UPDmat of an oöcyte, following failure of a premeiotic or of a meiotic cell division, leads to benign cystic ovarian teratoma, an unusual tumor of the ovary in which several embryonic tissues may be represented (Miura et al. 1999).

Mosaicism for Complete Uniparental Disomy. Abnormal cytogenetic events around the time of fertilization—such as two sperm entering an ovum to produce a zygote with three pronuclei, or an ovum undergoing a mitosis, and then cell lines of different (but diploid) genetic constitution being produced—can be the basis of a mosaicism for UPD. This can be UPDmat/biparental or UPDpat/biparental mosaicism, and it may be confined to the placenta, or also involve the fetus.

Complete UPD*pat*/normal mosaicism in the placenta (androgenetic/biparental mosaicism) leads to the histological phenotype of mesenchymal dysplasia (p. 442). If the UPDpat line also involves the fetus, a complex clinical picture may be observed, comprising features of different paternal UPD syndromes, such as BWS, AS, and transient neonatal diabetes. Malignant and nonmalignant cystic lesions, and a cystic placenta, are frequently present (Inbar-Feigenberg et al. 2013); and there is the additional possibility of unmasking an autosomal recessive disease carried by the father (Ohtsuka et al. 2015). The *tout ensemble* of observation presumably reflects the cellular distribution of the UPD tissue. Darcy et al. (2015) reported a 6-month-old girl who was mosaic for a complete UPD*pat* cell line and a Down syndrome cell line, her phenotype comprising features of both conditions. Complete UPD*mat*/normal mosaicism affecting the fetus is rarely observed, and can lead to a SRS-like phenotype with associated cognitive impairment (Strain et al. 1995; Horike et al. 2009).

Two unique cases cast light on how aberrant chromosomal behavior in the perizygotic period can lead to UPD-related pathology. A 46,XX/46,XY male child described in Strain et al. (1995) with growth asymmetry had complete maternal isodisomy in the 46,XX cell line and biparental inheritance in the 46,XY line. It may be that an ovum had completed a mitosis on its own, and then one of its daughter cells received the sperm (for the 46,XY line) while the other underwent endoreduplication (for the 46,XX,upd(mat) line): thus, biparental/gynogenetic mosaicism. A diploid sperm may have been the basis of the case in Hsu et al. (2008), in which the pregnancy from an apparently normal IVF embryo ended in intrauterine fetal death, with a portion of the placenta of molar appearance, at 14 weeks. Three separate genetic constitutions could be determined. The molar tissue was androgenetic 46,XX,uphd(pat); the fetus and placenta, both 46,XX, shared the same maternal genome but had different paternal genomes. Any explanation for this circumstance is necessarily complex.

GENETIC COUNSELING

Uniparental Disomy for Individual Chromosomes

No instance of recurrence of full UPD for a particular chromosome, with a 46,XX or 46,XY karyotype, is known, and we assume there to be no discernibly increased recurrence risk. The association with increasing childbearing age is to be noted, but in reality the increase in risk for older mothers would be very small.

Segmental Uniparental Disomy

Segmental UPD arising postzygotically, and which is karyotypically 46,XX or 46,XY, we presume to imply no increased risk for a future pregnancy. UPD due to rearrangement would have a risk according to the nature of the specific rearrangement.

Five Imprinting Syndromes with More Than One Genetic Basis

TRANSIENT NEONATAL DIABETES MELLITUS

Risks to family members depend on the underlying mechanism, as outlined below. Reduced penetrance has been reported for TNDM (Valerio et al. 2004).

Uniparental Disomy 6. About one-third of cases are due to paternal uniparental disomy of chromosome 6, a sporadic event with no known risk of recurrence.

Paternal Duplication of 6q24. Duplication of 6q24 can be either de novo or inherited. For de novo deletions, there is presumably a very low risk of recurrence, acknowledging a possibility of gonadal mosaicism. If the father has the 6q24 duplication, then the risk to offspring is 50%. For a female proband with a paternally inherited 6q24 duplication, her children would have a 50% chance of inheriting the duplication, but would not be at risk of developing TNDM.

Maternal Hypomethylation of the 6q24 Region. Isolated hypomethylation at the 6q24 DMR is typically a sporadic event with a low risk of recurrence. For TNDM caused by autosomal recessive mutations in *ZFP57* (hypomethylation at multiple imprinted loci), the risk to sibs is 25%.

BECKWITH-WIEDEMANN SYNDROME

The considerable majority (~85%) of BWS occurs sporadically, including the two more common categories of UPD 11 and epigenetic error. UPD 11 is diagnosed readily by SNP microarray (Keren et al. 2013), but detection of epimutation requires more specialized testing. The other categories that may have an important recurrence risk are recognized by an abnormal cytogenetic report and/or by a positive family history. A detailed treatment is given in Weksberg et al. (2010).

Uniparental Disomy 11. Approximately one-fifth of sporadic cases are due to mosaic segmental paternal UPD of 11p. This category of BWS can be suspected clinically if there is hemihyperplasia. No increased recurrence risk applies in the setting of segmental UPD and a normal karyotype.

Epigenetic Error. In sporadic BWS with biparental disomy, the underlying cause is an epigenetic error ("epimutation") affecting the ovum or early conceptus. This is the basis of a little over half of all cases. There is biparental inheritance with aberrant methylation on the maternal chromosome of either DMR1 (gain of methylation, ~5% of cases) or DMR2 (loss of methylation, ~50% of cases), the latter combination particularly associated with IVF. No cases of recurrence in this setting are known, and this fits the understanding of a typical postzygotic generation of the epimutation (Scott et al. 2008b) (but note recurrences in the section on "Silver-Russell Syndrome", epimutations of 11p15). Theoretically, there might be a very small increased risk, if the same susceptibility factors (subfertility, IVF) were operating.

The application of methylation-sensitive MLPA, a test which detects both methylation abnormalities and genomic alterations at 11p15 (Baskin et al. 2014), shows that in a small fraction of cases of BWS diagnosed with an epigenetic error, there is actually an underlying 11p15 copy number variant (CNV; a maternal deletion or a paternal duplication). Detection of these CNVs, which may be de novo or inherited, will alter recurrence risk counseling. Molecular testing for chromosome 11p15-associated imprinting disorders is complicated by molecular heterogeneity and the complexity of this region; the reader seeking detailed advice is referred to Eggermann et al. (2016).

11p Rearrangement. Chromosome rearrangements are rare causes of BWS. A *balanced* reciprocal translocation or an inversion with one breakpoint in distal 11p, if of maternal transmission, may lead to BWS (Li et al. 1998). An *unbalanced* distal 11p15 duplication, if of paternal origin, leads to double expression of *IGF2* in the 11p15 region, and this brings about the growth pattern of BWS (and if of maternal origin, a Silver-Russell growth retardation phenotype results). Functional trisomy of nonimprinted 11p segments, or other imbalance due to a translocation, may contribute to the clinical picture (Han et al. 2006; Russo et al. 2006; South et al. 2008b; Bliek et al. 2009). An extraordinary familial case, in Jurkiewicz et al. (2017), is due to triplication of the 11p15.5 imprinting region: a father with SRS, and his daughter with BWS. The recurrence risks for these various circumstances will depend upon the nature of the rearrangement and the parental karyotypes.

Mendelian Mutation. Autosomal dominant BWS accounts for about 10% of cases, the major locus being *CDKN1C*. Typically, only the offspring of female heterozygotes are affected. Careful review of the pedigree in the maternal line is necessary to identify mildly affected individuals, and bearing in mind the amelioration of phenotype with time (Elliott et al. 1994; Hunter and Allanson 1994), and that mutations in *CDKN1C* are associated with a high risk of abdominal wall defects and a very low risk of abdominal tumors (Mussa et al. 2016). One might consider the very rare case of deletion of the differentially methylated region DMR1 also to be in the category of Mendelian mutation; a child receiving this deletion from a mother has BWS, due to consequential biallelic *IGF2* expression (Sparago et al. 2004). A rare recessive basis of a maternal susceptibility to have a BWS child resides in the *NLRP2* gene, with failure to impose a proper imprint upon ova (Meyer et al. 2009).

SILVER-RUSSELL SYNDROME

About half of SRS can be traced to an anomaly of chromosome 7 (UPD) or chromosome 11p15 (epimutation), the latter mirroring the mechanism in BWS, as outlined above. Both these genetic forms typically imply a low risk of recurrence (Eggermann et al. 2010a).

Chromosome 7. Upd(7)mat is seen in up to 10% of cases, and the clinical phenotype is particularly associated with speech and language difficulty (Wakeling et al. 2010). Sporadic occurrence has been the universal observation.

Chromosome 11. Epimutations of 11p15, with hypomethylation of the *IGF2/H19* differentially methylated region (DMR1), comprise the largest

single category: According to the stringency of clinical criteria, these account for up to half of all SRS. This category may be associated with conception by IVF (Wakeling et al. 2010). Sporadic occurrence is very much the rule, albeit that very rare recurrences are on record, due to parental heterozygosity or parental gonadal mosaicism (Bartholdi et al. 2009). Structural rearrangement of 11p15, such as microduplication involving the differentially methylated region DMR2, is a rare cause (Eggermann et al. 2009). A familial translocation, such as the t(11;15) (p15.5;p12) described in Eggermann et al. (2010c), in which one segment comprises distal 11p, could lead to either SRS, if maternally transmitted, or BWS, if from the father.

PRADER-WILLI SYNDROME

A summary of the different genetic forms of PWS, and the associated risks of recurrence, is set out in Tables 18–2 and 18–3.

Classical Deletion 15q11q13. The empiric observation of zero recurrences out of some thousands of "trials" underscores the very considerable unlikelihood of significant paternal gonadal mosaicism for the deletion observed in the PWS child. This is the basis of the substantial optimism

Table 18–3. Approximate Relative Frequencies and Recurrence Risks, to Parents Having Had an Affected Child, for the Different Categories of Prader-Willi and Angelman Syndromes

	CATEGORY	RELATIVE FREQUENCY (%)	RECURRENCE RISK
Prader-Willi Syndrome	Classical deletion	70	Extremely low*
	upd(15)mat	25	Extremely low*
	Imprinting center deletion	<0.5	50%
	Imprinting center epimutation	2	Extremely low*
	15q translocation/inversion	Rare	According to rearrangement
Angelman Syndrome	Classical deletion	70	Extremely low**
	upd(15)pat	7	Extremely low*
	Imprinting center deletion	0.5	50%
	Imprinting center epimutation	2.5	Extremely low*
	UBE3A mutation	10–15	50%
	15q translocation/inversion	Rare	According to rearrangement
	Unknown	10	Presumed very low

*No case yet recorded.
**Only two cases in the world recorded (Kokkonen and Leisti 2000; Sánchez et al. 2014).

that can be offered to parents in terms of any further pregnancies. A figure of approximately 0.1% may be a fair one to offer for the risk of recurrence. Nevertheless, the theoretical possibility of paternal gonadal mosaicism, or of a paternal predisposition to undergo chromosome 15 deletion in spermatogenesis (Molina et al. 2011), obliges acknowledgment that the risk is not absolutely zero. If prenatal diagnosis is pursued, chorion villus sampling (CVS) can be offered using microarray for deletions, or the *SNRPN* methylation test (Buiting et al. 1998).

Uniparental Disomy 15, Karyotype 46,XX or 46,XY. We know of no recorded instance of recurrence of upd(15)mat PWS in a chromosomally normal couple, and we would otherwise assume, on theoretical grounds, any increased risk in a future pregnancy to be practically negligible, the modest maternal age effect notwithstanding.

Functional Defect ("Epimutation") of Prader-Willi Syndrome Imprinting Center. These extremely rare cases of IC defects will require individual expert advice. They can be suspected if a child has typical PWS clinically, but there is neither classical deletion nor UPD demonstrable. All cases of functional IC deficiency have so far been sporadic (but very few are known).

Prader-Willi Syndrome Imprinting Center Microdeletion. The recognition of these cases will require referral to a specialist laboratory. A positive family history, if observed, would oblige the assumption of this category, unless or until otherwise proven. Assuming the father carries the genetic defect, the recurrence risk is high, namely 50%. *SNRPN* methylation testing on CVS can identify an affected pregnancy. The father's brothers would have a 50% likelihood to be heterozygous (making the assumption that their mother would have carried the mutation), and in that case, these brothers would also have a 50% risk to have a PWS child. Equally, his sisters could be carriers, but their children would all be unaffected, and it would only be *their* sons who might, in the next generation, have the risk for a PWS child. The siblings of the affected child would themselves have no different genetic risk than the general population. The reader should work through the reasoning behind these various risk assessments, even though most counselors will never encounter this actual circumstance in the clinic.

Uncommon Cytogenetically Detectable Rearrangement. The nature of the rearrangement, and the parental karyotypes, will determine the recurrence risk in each type.

PWS Phenocopies. A duplication of the segment Xq21.1q21.31 may lead to a clinical picture very reminiscent of PWS in the older child, while deletions distal to Xq25 are associated with a phenotype more resembling infantile PWS (Gabbett et al. 2008). A small fraction of males with fragile X syndrome present a PWS-like phenotype. A focused Xq analysis, and a fragile X study, may thus be warranted in patients in whom a diagnosis of PWS is suspected on clinical grounds, but in whom chromosome 15 tests are normal. Deletion at 6q16.2, and the 1p36 deletion, may also be associated with a PWS-like clinical picture (D'Angelo et al. 2006; Varela et al. 2006; Bonaglia et al. 2008), and some features of PWS are seen in maternal UPD 14.

ANGELMAN SYNDROME

A summary of the different genetic forms of AS, and the associated risks of recurrence, is set out in Tables 18–2 and 18–3. More detail is given in the reviews of Stalker and Williams (1998), Clayton-Smith and Laan (2003), Van Buggenhout and Fryns (2009), and Buiting et al. (2015).

The clinical diagnosis of AS is sometimes easy (parents have recognized the condition in their child having seen a television program), but at other times, more challenging. Of course, if accurate genetic advice is to be given, an accurate clinical diagnosis is crucial. The possibility of Rett syndrome may need to be considered (Scheffer et al. 1990). The counselor must obtain a detailed family history. A genetic defect could have been transmitted through males for some generations, and only causing AS when it had been passed from a daughter of such a male. Figure 18–9 shows a family in which some quite distant relatives, including second cousins once removed and first cousins twice removed, had AS due to an inherited *UBE3A* mutation.

Classical Deletion 15q11q13. Similarly to PWS, approximately 70% of AS is due to a de novo interstitial deletion. Recurrence in siblings of a typically sized deletion is extraordinarily rare, and in the two known cases reflected presumed gonadal (Kokkonen and Leisti 2000) or somatic-gonadal (Sánchez et al. 2014) maternal mosaicism. Thus, as for classical deletion PWS, we presume a very low—but clearly not quite zero—recurrence risk. There are two recorded examples of deletion AS in cousins, which manifestly represented coincidental de novo events in these families, in that different ancestral chromosomes were involved (Connerton-Moyer et al. 1997). The comments on prenatal diagnosis in PWS (see above) apply similarly here.

Uniparental Disomy 15, Karyotype 46,XX or 46,XY, Parents' Chromosomes Normal. AS due to paternal UPD 15 is uncommon; as discussed above, the initial error may actually reflect a maternal age effect. Interestingly, the AS phenotype may be somewhat milder in UPD 15, and in some children it was only after an electroencephalogram showed typical findings that the diagnosis was suspected (Bottani et al. 1994). But this does not mean that some upd(15)pat AS children may not be severely affected (Prasad and Wagstaff 1997). No recurrence is on record (Chan et al. 1993), and we assume on theoretical grounds that no usefully measurable increased risk would exist.

Angelman Syndrome Imprinting Center Microdeletion. Assuming the mother carries the genetic defect, there is a high recurrence risk, namely 50%. *SNRPN* methylation testing on CVS can identify an affected pregnancy. The possibility of maternal gonadal mosaicism for an IC mutation complicates the picture (Stalker et al. 1998). The siblings of the carrier mother could also be carriers (assuming their father to be heterozygous). However, it would only be the sisters who would have the risk for an AS child.

Functional Defect ("Epimutation") of Angelman Syndrome Imprinting Center. The previous comments on PWS apply similarly here. All cases of AS due to a functional IC defect have so far been sporadic, but it would be prudent to offer prenatal diagnosis in a subsequent pregnancy (*SNRPN* methylation testing). Although the numbers are very small (but epimutation AS is rare), there are grounds for supposing there might be a link with infertility/IVF (Manipalviratn et al. 2009). Had there been such a reproductive history, this fact would need to be weighed.

UBE3A Mutation. If the mother carries the mutation, the risk for recurrence is 50%. Maternal mosaicism has been recognized (Malzac et al. 1998; Hosoki et al. 2005), and so nondemonstration (on blood) of the mutation in the mother does not necessarily exclude a genetic risk. Indeed, it may be that such mosaicism is not uncommon (Stalker et al. 1998). It may be appropriate to track the mutation through the patrilineal family, in order to be able to offer genetic counseling to female cousins who might be carriers. The reader should study the illustrative pedigree in Figure 18–9.

No Genetic Defect Demonstrable. In a small fraction of AS, approximately 10%, no cytogenetic or molecular defect, nor *UBE3A* mutation, is demonstrable. Some of these cases could conceivably reflect a mutation that has not been able to be detected. The family history, if positive, may compel the assumption of a mutation, and thus imply a high recurrence risk. A negative family history might support the inference of a low risk, but it would not allow a definite assumption. If a normal sibling carried the same 15q11q13 haplotype, on molecular study, a low-risk scenario would be probable. Expert advice should be sought.

Uncommon Cytogenetically Detectable Rearrangement. The nature of the rearrangement, and the parental karyotypes, will determine the recurrence risk in each type. The rare circumstance of UPD associated with a parental Robertsonian translocation is noted on p. 155.

Angelman Syndrome Phenocopies. A number of other conditions resemble AS (Tan et al. 2014). There is clinical overlap with Rett syndrome, Pitt-Hopkins syndrome, Mowat-Wilson syndrome, *MBD5* deletion (2q23.1), 22q13.3 deletion, and *MECP2* duplication, the latter three being readily detected by chromosome microarray.

A SIMPLIFICATION FOR ANGLEMAN SYNDROME

Some parents will not find it easy to come to grips with these various possible causes for their child's condition even if, in the end, they need only consider the category that applies to themselves. It may be helpful to discuss AS, and the risks of recurrence, in the following terms.[16] Let us say that AS is

---

16 See also the *European Journal of Human Genetics* Clinical Utility Card (Buiting et al. 2015).

due, simply, to a lack of the UBE3A protein, a very important protein that is necessary for the brain to grow normally. The gene for *UBE3A* works only on the chromosome 15 from the mother, while the gene on the father's chromosome is dormant. There is a switch on the mother's chromosome that makes this gene work.

- If the bit of the maternal chromosome that contains this gene is missing (deletion), or if the mother's chromosome is replaced by another one from the father (UPD), no UBE3A protein can be made. These two types happen as one-off events.
- If the switch fails on the mother's chromosome, then the gene remains dormant, and no protein is made (imprinting center fault). This type can happen one-off, as though the switch "gets stuck," for reasons that we do not well understand. Or, there may be a genetic fault in the actual switch, and in this case the defect could be passed to a subsequent child.
- If the *UBE3A* gene itself is faulty on the mother's chromosome (mutation), no protein is made, or only an abnormal protein that cannot function. The genetic risk depends on whether the faulty gene started with the child (no increased risk) or if the mother is a carrier (high risk). Note that the mother can be a carrier and still be perfectly normal, since the faulty gene would be the one she got from her father, and so in any event it would be switched off.
- Sometimes the *UBE3A* gene fails to work, even though the maternal chromosome is normal and has a normal switch. We do not know why this happens (there has been a suggestion that one cause *may* be if there had been difficulty achieving the pregnancy, either naturally or with IVF). This type is a one-off event.

A common question parents have is whether their normal children might, in the next generation, have an AS child. Or the aunts and uncles of an AS child might want advice about risks to their future children or to their grandchildren. The answers are as follows:

- The normal siblings of an AS child have no increased risk, for any genetic category, with the possible exception of a familial translocation. Even if the AS child has (or had) a potentially heritable type of *UBE3A* genetic defect, the fact that the sibs themselves are normal self-evidently declares that they cannot have received it. If they had got the abnormal gene, they would have AS; since they do not have AS, they cannot have the gene. The sex of the siblings is immaterial.
- Aunts and uncles have an increased risk for children or grandchildren of theirs only if a heritable type of AS is involved (imprinting center defect, *UBE3A* mutation). In that case, an uncle could be a carrier, but his children would not be at risk, since the *UBE3A* gene would be dormant anyway. Daughters of his, however, could have an AS child. A carrier aunt would have a high risk (50%) to have an AS child. But her grandchildren, through her normal sons and daughters, would have no increased risk. Her normal children would have declared themselves, by their very normality, not to have inherited the genetic defect.

UNIPARENTAL DISOMY FOR THE ENTIRE CHROMOSOMAL COMPLEMENT

UPD for the entire *paternal* chromosome set (hydatidiform mole) is associated with an increased recurrence risk; this is discussed in detail in Chapter 19. There is no discernibly increased risk for the recurrence of UPD for the entire *maternal* chromosome set (ovarian teratoma).

DIAGNOSTIC TESTING FOR UNIPARENTAL DISOMY

The Canadian College of Medical Genetics has published guidelines for when diagnostic testing for UPD should be offered (Dawson et al 2011), summarized in Table 18–4. Much UPD (between 50% and 100%, depending on origin of UPD) is detectable on SNP microarray, although a normal SNP array cannot exclude UPD originating in meiosis I.

In relation to prenatal diagnosis, two scenarios warrant specific mention. First, a small risk of UPD applies for non-Robertsonian translocations if one or both chromosomes carry imprinted genes, specifically when there is a risk of 3:1 nondisjunction, and where trisomy or monosomy rescue or gamete complementation could occur. Reports of this (very rare) occurrence are listed in Table 18–5.

Second, if a parent is a carrier of a Robertsonian translocation involving chromosome 14 or 15, a risk of UPD, in the setting of a normal prenatal karyotype, appears to be extremely small. Although Dawson et al. (2011) recommend that UPD studies be performed, we note that this recommendation is based on a single

Table 18–4. Circumstances in which Diagnostic Testing for UPD should be Offered

PRENATAL TESTING (CVS OR AMNIOCENTESIS)	POSTNATAL TESTING
1. A balanced Robertsonian translocation or iso-chromosome (inherited or de novo) involving chromosome 14 or 15	1. Patients with congenital abnormalities and developmental delay who have: • A Robertsonian translocation involving chromosome 13 or 14 • A supernumerary marker chromosome derived from chromosome 14 or 15
2. A normal karyotype when a parent is a carrier of a Robertsonian translocation involving chromosome 14 or 15	2. Newborns with neonatal diabetes mellitus
3. A de novo supernumerary marker chromosome with no apparent euchromatic material	3. Patients with clinical features of mat or pat UPD 14
4. Level II or level III mosaicism for trisomy or monosomy of chromosomes 6, 7, 11, 14, or 15	4. Patients who are homozygous for an autosomal recessive disease when only one parent is a carrier
5. Ultrasound features of pat UPD 14	5. As part of the diagnostic workup for SRS, BWS, PWS, and AS, depending on the result of other investigations

AS, Angelman syndrome; BWS, Beckwith-Wiedemann syndrome; mat, maternal; pat, paternal; PWS, Prader-Willi syndrome; SRS, Silver-Russell syndrome.

Source: The Canadian College of Medical Genetics, Dawson et al. (2011).

report of a child with complete paternal isodisomy of chromosome 14 and a normal karyotype, whose mother had a rob(13;14) (Potok et al. 2009).

Diagnostic Implications of Excessive Homozygosity Detected by SNP-Based Microarrays

SNP-based microarrays, in addition to detecting CNVs, also allow the recognition of homozygosity. An excessive degree of homozygosity is most often observed with one or more uninterrupted regions of homozygous SNP alleles, having a copy number state of 2. Such a region is frequently referred to as a "long-contiguous stretch of homozygosity"

(LCSH). A LCSH in excess of ~5 Mb is considered to be of potential clinical significance, albeit that excessive homozygosity of itself is not diagnostic of any particular condition, and may be benign (Kearney et al. 2011).

When LCSH is present on two or more chromosomes, this is assumed to represent regions identical by descent (IBD), implying consanguinity, and the concomitant association, therefore, with autosomal recessive disease. The total proportion of LCSH across the genome can be used as a crude measure of degree of parental relationship, as summarized in Table 18–6. A LCSH fraction of above one-eighth (12.5%) should arouse suspicion of incest, but it does not provide information about the specific

Table 18–5. Imprinting Syndromes due to Malsegregation of a Parental Translocation

TRANSLOCATION	PHENOTYPE	REFERENCE
t(8;15)(p23.3;q11)pat	AS	Smith et al. (1994)
t(7;16)(q21;q24)mat	SRS	Dupont et al (2002)
t(8;15)(q24.1;q21.2)mat	PWS	Calounova et al. (2006)
t(2;15)(p11;q11.2)mat	PWS	Heidemann et al (2010)
t(7;13)(q11.2;q14)mat	SRS	Behnecke et al. (2012)

AS, Angelman syndrome; PWS, Prader-Willi syndrome; SRS, Silver-Russell syndrome.

Table 18–6. Correlation Between Degree of Parental Relationship and Percentage of Long Contiguous Stretches of Homozygosity (LCSH)

DEGREE OF RELATIONSHIP	EXAMPLE	PREDICTED LCSH IN CHILD (%)
First	Parent/child Full siblings	25
Second	Uncle/niece Aunt/nephew Grandparent/ grandchild	12.5
Third	First cousins	6
Fourth	First cousins once removed	3
Fifth	Second cousins	1.5

parental relationship. A LCSH of >12.5% may also reflect, in parents who are first cousins, additional consanguinity in preceding generations.

The percentage of LCSH correlates with the risk of autosomal recessive disease, and the coordinates of the specific regions of LCSH can be used to focus the search for candidate autosomal recessive genes. A specific bioinformatics tool that combines clinical data with LCSH data is available for this purpose (Wierenga et al. 2013).

LCSH restricted to a single chromosome could be due to either isodisomy or IBD. If LCSH extends along the whole chromosome, this can be assumed to represent isodisomy for that chromosome. When LCSH involves only part of the chromosome, distinguishing IBD from UPD is more complex. Papenhausen et al. (2011) showed that in proven cases of UPD, LCSH always exceeded 13.5 Mb, suggesting that a single chromosomal LCSH of >13.5 Mb should trigger additional investigation for UPD. In practice, a more conservative threshold of 10 Mb may be used, particularly in the context of an imprinted chromosome. Once the presence of UPD is confirmed, the pattern of isodisomy and heterodisomy can be used to infer the origin of the UPD (Fig. 18–10).

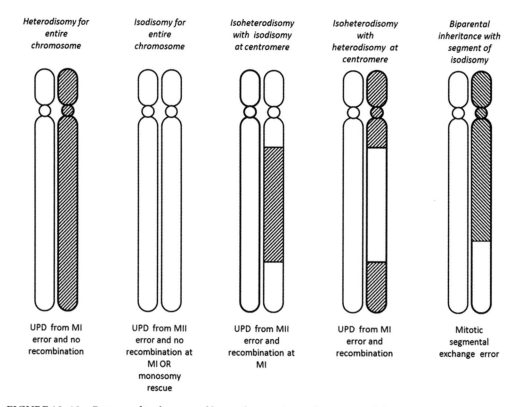

FIGURE 18–10 Patterns of isodisomy and heterodisomy observed in UPD and their associations with the mechanisms of UPD.

PART FIVE

REPRODUCTIVE CYTOGENETICS

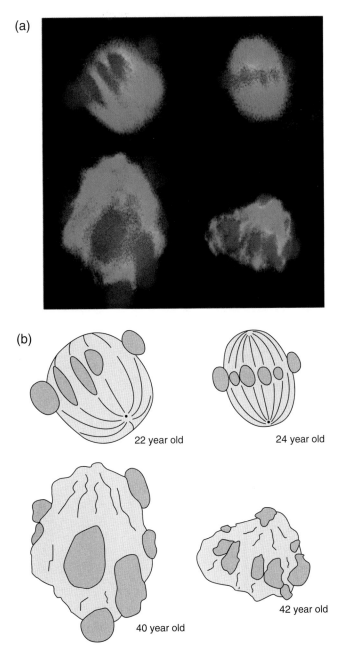

FIGURE 3–7   (*a*) Meiosis II oöcytes from younger and older women, illustrating what may be the physical basis of the maternal age effect. The microtubules of the spindle stain green, and the chromosomes stain orange. (*b*) The tracing identifies these components, and the smooth or wavy lines suggest, respectively, an intact or a degenerating spindle apparatus (the ages of the women indicated). The chromosomes are well organized at the metaphase plate at the equator of the cells in the younger women (the 22-year-old's oöcyte, on the upper left, is viewed on a tilt). In contrast, the 40-year-old's oöcyte shows the chromosomes in disarray. The 42-year-old woman's oöcyte has one chromosome, at the top, dislocated from the metaphase plate, and the disposition of the other chromosomes at the equator is not as regular as in the younger women.

Source: From Battaglia et al., Influence of maternal age on meiotic spindle assembly in oöcytes from naturally cycling women, *Hum Reprod* 11: 2217–2222, 1996. Courtesy D. E. Battaglia, and with the permission of Oxford University Press and *Human Reproduction*.

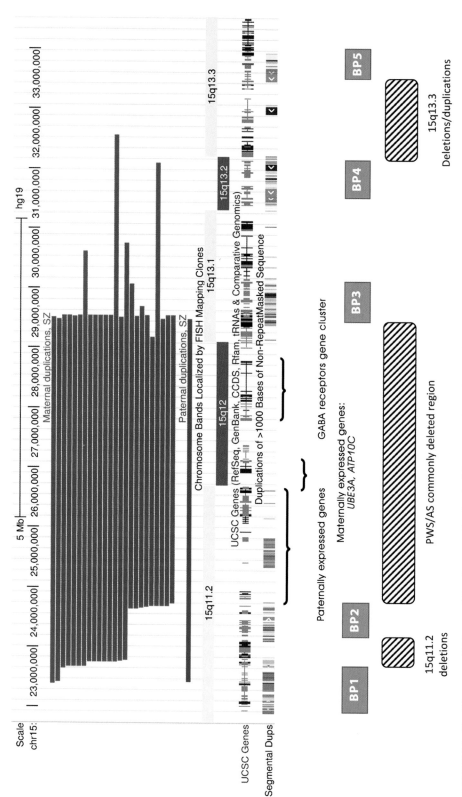

FIGURE 14–60   The susceptibility to schizophrenia in the dup(15)(q11.2q13.1) syndrome. The five important breakpoints, which define the extents of the several del/dups occurring in this region, are shown, BP1-BP5; these breakpoints coincide with the repeat sequences shown in the segmental duplications track. Above, in red (maternal) and blue (paternal) are the duplications in a series of patients with schizophrenia; most are defined by BP1-BP3 and BP2-BP3. (Compare Fig. 14–29)

Source: From Isles et al., Parental origin of interstitial duplications at 15q11.2-q13.3 in schizophrenia and neurodevelopmental disorders, *PLoS Genet* 12: e1005993, 2016. Courtesy M.J. Owen and G. Kirov, and with the permission of the Public Library of Science, as per the Creative Commons public domain.

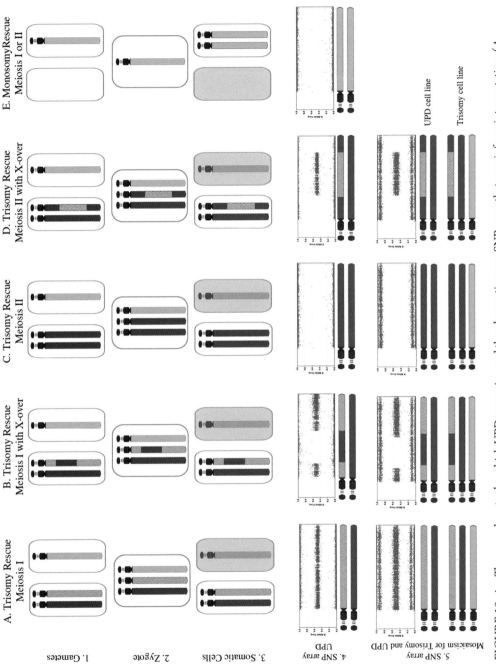

FIGURE 18–4   The several routes by which UPD may arise, and the observations on SNP array that may inform interpretation. (*A* and *B*) Meiosis 1 nondisjunction with postzygotic trisomy rescue: UPD with centromeric heterodisomy ± distal isodisomy. (*C* and *D*) Meiosis 2 nondisjunction with postzygotic rescue: UPD with centromeric isodisomy ± distal heterodisomy. (*E*) Postzygotic monosomy rescue: complete isodisomy.

Source: From Kearney et al, Diagnostic implications of excessive homozygosity detected by SNP-based microarrays: Consanguinity, uniparental disomy, and recessive single-gene mutations, *Clin Lab Med* 31: 595–613, 2011. Courtesy H. M. Kearney and L. K. Conlin, and with the permission of Elsevier.

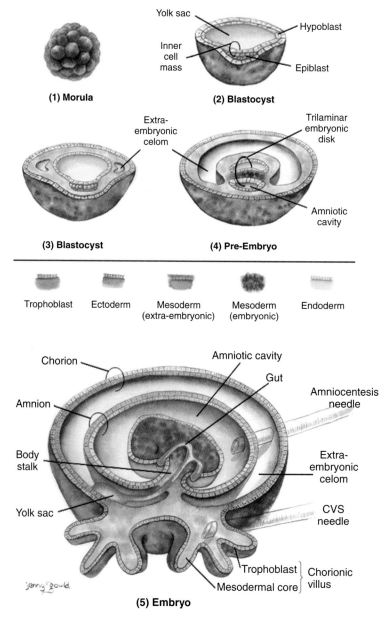

(1) Morula

Yolk sac

Hypoblast

Inner cell mass

Epiblast

(2) Blastocyst

Extra-embryonic celom

Trilaminar embryonic disk

Amniotic cavity

(3) Blastocyst   **(4) Pre-Embryo**

Trophoblast   Ectoderm   Mesoderm (extra-embryonic)   Mesoderm (embryonic)   Endoderm

Chorion

Amniotic cavity

Gut

Amniocentesis needle

Amnion

Body stalk

Extra-embryonic celom

Yolk sac

CVS needle

jenny gould

Trophoblast ⎫
Mesodermal core ⎭ Chorionic villus

(5) Embryo

FIGURE 21–1   Developmental origins of tissues sampled at prenatal diagnosis (simplified; color-coding of tissues shown on the color insert). (1) Morula, 3–4 days postconception, a sphere with trophoblast cells at its surface. (2) Cross-section of blastocyst at beginning of second week, showing outer rim of trophoblast, the inner cell mass comprising epiblast (orange) and hypoblast (yellow), and the yolk sac cavity lined by an inner rim of cells of hypoblastic origin. (3) Blastocyst toward end of second week. The hypoblastic cells of the yolk sac have given rise to extra-embryonic mesoderm. Lacunae are beginning to appear in this mesoderm, and these will coalesce to form the extra-embryonic celom. (4) "Pre-embryo." The amniotic cavity and the yolk sac bound the dorsal and ventral surfaces of the embryonic disk. The extra-embryonic celom has now cavitated the extra-embryonic mesoderm. Note that the embryonic mesoderm (middle layer of the trilaminar embryonic disk) arises from the epiblast, and thus it has a different lineage from the extra-embryonic mesoderm. (5) Composite embryo/early fetus. (Rotation has reversed the relative positions of the yolk sac and amniotic cavity.) The three embryonic tissue types (ectoderm, mesoderm, endoderm) all had origin from the epiblast, as did the amniotic epithelium. Epithelial cells from the embryo's ectodermal surface are shed into the amniotic cavity, as also are amniotic epithelial cells (both these tissues shown orange). Cells from endodermal derivatives (respiratory and urinary tracts, which originate from the gut, shown in yellow) pass into the amniotic cavity. Chorionic villi comprise mesenchymal core (of extra-embryonic mesodermal origin), gloved by trophoblast. Extra-embryonic and embryonic mesoderms are continuous at the body stalk, albeit that some embryonic mesodermal cells may then migrate into the amniotic mesoderm (Robinson et al. 2002).

19

REPRODUCTIVE FAILURE

HUMAN CONCEPTION and pregnancy is both a vulnerable and a robust process. Vulnerable, in that a large proportion of all conceptions are chromosomally abnormal, with the great majority of such pregnancies aborting. Robust, in that more than 99% of the time, a term pregnancy results in a chromosomally normal baby; unbalanced chromosomal abnormalities are seen in less than 1% of newborns (Table 1–3). But the economic cost of chromosomally abnormal conceptions is not horrendous; it is measured largely in terms of miscarriage, seen or unseen. The occasional chromosomally abnormal child is, relatively speaking, an exceptional outcome—the tip of an iceberg (Fig. 19–1).

Most of this chromosomal vulnerability lies in the process of producing eggs and sperm. Meiosis hangs, literally and figuratively, upon "tender filaments,"[1] and often the meiotic chromosomes are incorrectly distributed to the daughter cells (Hassold and Hunt 2001). Indeed, 46,XX and 46,XY humans are more prone to produce aneuploid germ cells than any other species studied (McFadden and Friedman 1997).[2] The small group who are exceptionally likely to produce abnormal gametes are carriers of balanced chromosome rearrangements, and much of this book is devoted to that fact.

Advances in reproductive technology now enable many otherwise infertile couples to have children. Translocation carriers may have recourse to preimplantation genetic diagnosis (PGD) as a means to improve their chances of achieving a successful pregnancy. In the case of men with poor

---

1 "I that have examined the parts of man, and know upon what tender filaments that fabric hangs"—Thos. Browne MD, Religio Medici, 1642.

2 Dorothy Warburton suggested that this error rate conveyed an evolutionary advantage in former times: Miscarriage due to aneuploidy led to a wider spacing of offspring, allowing a woman to devote scarce resources to a more manageable number of children, more of whom would survive to contribute their genes to the following generation. What was beneficial in a prehistoric society has been quite the opposite for many women, now hostage to their biology, in the present century (a concept not without several other examples).

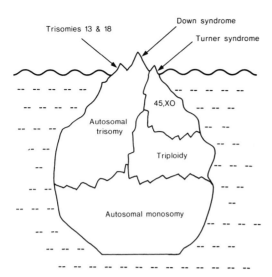

FIGURE 19–1   The iceberg of chromosomal pregnancy loss.

sperm production, intracytoplasmic sperm injection (ICSI) at in vitro fertilization (IVF) is a means to get a single sperm into an egg. Success with IVF is not necessarily easy to achieve, neither is it a certain outcome, and counselors dealing with infertile couples need a particular awareness of the psychological and practical difficulties they may face (Boivin et al. 2001). A "failed embryo transfer" following IVF may be considered as a form of pregnancy loss not unlike that of the natural miscarriage of a wanted pregnancy.

BIOLOGY

Gametic Cytogenetics

Many more sperm are made than eggs, by orders of magnitude, and logically one might have expected a higher standard of meiotic fidelity in the scarcer gamete (Hunt and Hassold 2002). But in fact it is the other way round, and so it is the egg that commands most of our attention, in terms of the practical relevance of gametic chromosomal pathology.

OÖCYTES AND POLAR BODIES

IVF is widely applied in the management of infertility, and one consequential benefit of this has been the access afforded to study of the oöcyte and its minor partner, the polar body. Many eggs sampled prove to be surplus to the requirements of

the couple, and they are often willingly donated for research. Overall, a fifth to a quarter of oöcytes were cytogenetically abnormal in the study of Pellestor et al. (2006); a remarkably higher fraction, almost a half, is deduced from analyzing polar bodies as surrogates for the egg (Kuliev et al. 2011). Most of the abnormalities are accounted for by hyperhaploidy with a 24-chromosome count (an additional double-chromatid or single-chromatid chromosome), hypohaploidy with a 22-chromosome count (a missing homolog), or a 23-chromosome count that could be described as "22½" (one homolog represented by only a single-chromatid chromosome), and diploidy with 46 chromosomes. It is the smaller chromosomes that are the more vulnerable to error (Cupisti et al. 2003).

These data are necessarily influenced by the source of the material: The ova mostly come from women being treated for infertility, who are typically of an older childbearing age. What does nevertheless seem apparent is that somewhere between one-fifth and one-half of eggs—the fraction very much age-dependent—from at least this population of women, are chromosomally abnormal. The maternal age link is well illustrated in the work of Battaglia et al. (1996), showing how the structural integrity of the oöcyte's meiotic apparatus declines as a woman gets older (see color Fig. 3–7); a detailed discussion of the underlying biology is given in Webster and Schuh (2017). One particular type of abnormal egg, the giant binucleate oöcyte, is typically diploid (Balakier et al. 2002; Rosenbusch et al. 2002).

SPERM

The gamete whose chromosomes are most readily accessible to analysis is the sperm, and with fluorescence in situ hybridization (FISH), very large numbers can be analyzed. On conservative criteria, approximately 2½% of sperm are aneuploid. Diploidy and sex chromosome disomy are the most commonly observed imbalance, at approximately 0.2% each (Donate et al. 2016); the average disomy rate for each of the autosomes ranges around the 0.1% to 0.2% mark (Shi and Martin 2000b). No ethnic differences have come to light, at any rate comparing Caucasians and Chinese (Shi and Martin 2000a). There is no clear correlation with paternal age, except possibly with respect to XY disomy.

Fathers of Aneuploid Children. There are very few data on 46,XY men who have actually fathered children with chromosomal abnormalities. Hixon et al. (1998) studied 10 fathers of paternal-error Down syndrome children (the error at meiosis I in three, meiosis II in six, postzygotic in one) and found no differences: These fathers had a mean of 0.15% disomic 21 sperm versus 0.17% in the controls. Similarly, Blanco et al. (1998) studied a group of 15 fathers of children with trisomy 21, and, overall, the fraction of disomic 21 sperm was little different from a control group: 0.31% versus 0.37%.[3] However, of the total of 25 fathers from the two studies, three stood out with twice the level of sperm disomy 21; and two of these also showed an increase in sperm disomic for chromosomes 13 and 22 (Soares et al. 2001a). As for monosomy X Turner syndrome, three-fourths of which may be the consequence of nullisomy X in the sperm, four fathers of Turner syndrome daughters reported in Martínez-Pasarell et al. (1999) and in Soares et al. (2001b) had increased levels of sperm with a sex chromosome aneuploidy, and also with disomies 13, 21, and 22. From the foregoing, it is tempting to suppose that a minority of normally fertile men may be predisposed to meiotic errors at spermatogenesis, whether generalized or restricted to one chromosome; but the data are as yet too insubstantial to make a firm statement.

Cytogenetics of the Preimplantation, Embryonic, and Early Fetal Period

An aneuploid gamete (nullisomic or disomic) will lead to an aneuploid conceptus (monosomic or trisomic). A diploid gamete, combining with a normal gamete, will give rise to a triploid conceptus. With many oöcytes aneuploid, and a few sperm, and simplistically supposing equal fertilizing/fertilizable capacity, the expectation is for a very considerable fraction of conceptions to be chromosomally unbalanced. On top of this, dispermy (two sperm fertilizing the one ovum) can cause triploidy. An abnormal postzygotic cell division can give rise to mosaicism, and this may be quite a common

happening. These several possibilities all add up to a substantial potential for chromosome abnormality in the very early conceptus, in the first days (even hours) of existence.

THE CLEAVAGE EMBRYO ("PRE-EMBRYO") (DAYS 1–3)

The development of the technology of PGD in association with IVF has offered a much clearer view of the frequency of chromosomal abnormalities in the zygote and in the first few days postconception.[4] Admittedly, couples presenting for PGD will not, in the main, be a true representation of all couples. One category of patient will, however, be close to "chromosomally typical": otherwise normally fertile women who are heterozygotes for a Mendelian condition, presenting for diagnosis of embryonic sex or for specific mutation testing. These embryos offer the best insight to the true background rate of chromosomal abnormality, with respect to the maternal age groups involved. Pellicer et al. (1999), assessing some or all of chromosomes 13, 16, 18, 21, 22, X, and Y, studied 10 Mendelian heterozygous women of mean age 34 years, range 30–36 years. These women had a total of 12 abnormal embryos out of 62 tested (19%), but a considerably higher figure (46%) was observed in a group of older mothers presenting for the same reason (see also Table 19–2 below).

The "atypical" group of patients presenting to the IVF clinic are of course a population of clinical interest, and thus the observations gained from study of them, however unrepresentative they might possibly be of the general population, are very germane to the agenda of the counselor. Earlier studies using FISH suggested that a substantial fraction of unused IVF embryos are karyotypically abnormal, the ranges observed from 30% to 65% (Wilton 2002). These findings have been essentially confirmed by molecular techniques that can examine all 24 chromosomes: Demko et al. (2016) studied more than 22,000 day-3 embryos tested using single nucleotide polymorphism (SNP) microarray and found that the proportion of aneuploid embryos remained

---

3 These considerable differences in control rates presumably reflect laboratory criteria, a point drawn out in Donate et al. (2016).

4 Strictly speaking, in utero life is divided into three periods: pre-embryonic (the first 2 weeks), up to formation of the primitive streak; embryonic (to the end of the 8th week) when the body forms and organs are constructed; and fetal (from 8 weeks to term), characterized by growth and changes in proportion rather than the appearance of new features. Often the word *fetal* is used loosely to refer to the entire period, and in IVF parlance (and in the present discussion) the word *embryo* is routinely applied in reference to the conceptus in the early cleavage stage during the first few days. "Conceptus," in theory, applies to any stage, but it generally refers to early pregnancy. The conceptus at the one-cell stage—the fertilized egg—is the zygote.

fairly constant at 65% between maternal ages 27 and 35 years, but increased markedly at older ages (and see Fig. 22–4).

Mosaicism of the very early embryo has been one of the more startling discoveries to emerge from the PGD laboratory (although again there is the caveat that it would be unsafe to draw too many conclusions from these laboratory observations, concerning the likelihood that mosaicism might happen in chromosomally normal zygotes, conceived naturally). Many IVF embryos are aneuploid or diploid/haploid mosaics, and even in normal-appearing embryos, the fraction, analyzing a limited number of chromosomes, ranges from 17% to 43% (Wilton 2002). This mosaicism presumably reflects the fact that the first few postzygotic divisions are particularly susceptible to errors in chromosomal distribution.[5] The main mechanism may be chromosome loss due to anaphase lag, but chromosome gain is also frequent; mitotic nondisjunction (different cells with the corresponding monosomy and trisomy) occurs in a small minority (Daphnis et al. 2008). When the mosaicism is extensive, exhibiting several different karyotypes, these embryos may be referred to as being chromosomally "chaotic." Voullaire et al. (2000b) showed, using comparative genomic hybridization (CGH) methodology to check on every chromosome, that a majority of surplus embryos from IVF patients were mosaic. A CGH study by Blennow et al. (2001), on embryos from translocation carriers which had been diagnosed as aneuploid on PGD, demonstrated, in some, that every cell could be different: the absolute maximum mosaicism.

THE MORULA AND BLASTOCYST (DAYS 4–5)

The short period during which the cleavage embryo advances through the morula stage and into the blastocyst may be an important hurdle during which the development of many chromosomally abnormal pre-embryos arrest, in particular those with extensive mosaicism (Bielanska et al. 2002a). Fragouli et al. (2008) studied 136 embryos donated for research, of good quality, and which they considered would not differ too greatly from the in vivo situation (although acknowledging that the embryos came from couples undergoing treatment for infertility, and with an average maternal age of 36 years). They cultured these embryos through to the blastocyst stage and analyzed them using CGH. Overall, 39% of these blastocysts were aneuploid, with 35 trisomies and 46 monosomies identified. Entirely as expected, the rate was very considerably higher in older (37 years or older) than in younger women, 48% versus 16%. The simplest state was a blastocyst with a single aneuploidy, with slightly more monosomies than trisomies; and the most complicated imbalance was monosomy for six chromosomes and trisomy for five. Only chromosomes 3, 4, 5, and 9 were not represented among the aneuploidies.

The number of monosomic blastocysts was an interesting observation: It had previously been considered that the monosomic conceptus could very rarely advance beyond the morula (day 4). The aneuploidy rate was close to the rate expected from the combination of sperm and egg rates, but less than that seen in cleavage-stage embryos, leading Fragouli et al. (2008) to conclude that the abnormalities in the blastocysts were of meiotic origin. The observation of equivalent fractions of trisomy and monosomy (and see Fig. 19–3 below) is consistent with the interpretation that meiotic nondisjunction produces equal numbers of disomic and nullisomic gametes, which have equal chances of fertilizing; and if so, that trisomies and monosomies have similar survivability through to the early blastocyst (but almost all autosomal monosomies presumably soon thereafter succumbing).

The more powerful approach of quantitative polymerase chain reaction (qPCR) or SNP array, using an established 24-chromosome assay, and applied to a very large number of cases, is the strength of the study due to Franasiak et al. (2014). These researchers analyzed more than 15,000 embryos of parents presenting at IVF/PGD for trophectoderm biopsy for a variety of reasons, and could thus derive rather precise estimates of aneuploidies according to maternal age. A small increase above baseline was seen in the youngest mothers, the least rate was in the 25- to 34-year-old age group, and progressively increasing steeply from age 35

---

5 The very earliest cause of failure of the embryo may apply at the very earliest mitoses, from as early as mitosis number 2. These initial mitoses require integrity of the *TLE6* and *PADI6* genes; mutation in these genes leads to embryonic arrest at this stage (Maddirevula et al. 2017).

years to the mid-forties (Fig. 19–2). Similar results were obtained by Demko et al. (2016), who studied more than 15,000 day-5 embryos using SNP microarray and showed that the aneuploidy rate remained at approximately 45% between ages 27 and 35 years but increased sharply thereafter. The range of aneuploidies is illustrated in Rodriguez-Purata et al. (2015), taken from a series of just over 1,000 embryos subject to trophectoderm biopsy at day 5/6, for preimplantation genetic screening. At this early stage, the frequencies of trisomy and monosomy per chromosome are rather similar, albeit that the rates between different chromosomes differ greatly, as the graphs in Figure 19–3 show.

"Chaotically mosaic" cleavage-stage embryos, aneuploid in many or all of their cells due to mitotic errors, will almost all fail at the embryo-morula hurdle (Bielanska et al. 2002a). In contrast, consider mosaicism that arises over the time frame of days 4–5, but which is not chaotic, and with the coexistence of a normal euploid lineage, this being the state which is detected in approximately 5% of human embryos. Such diploid-aneuploid mosaic embryos may undergo progressive normalization that can then, in due course, go on to produce a euploid fetus and a normal child (Fragouli et al. 2008; Greco et al. 2015). The abnormal cells fall by the wayside.

THE "EMBRYO PROPER" (WEEKS 3–6)

The embryo proper, in the sense that the body plan is beginning to be laid out, takes form in the third week, and is barely 1½ mm long; by the end of the sixth week postconception (8 weeks by dates), it will be 1½ cm. This is a time frame that is not easily studied. First, this appears to be a period during which the threshold for natural abortion is relatively high, and many abnormal embryos seem able to maintain existence (however imperfect that existence might be). Second, the practicalities of collecting intact embryos from very early spontaneous miscarriage, they being scarcely discernible among the products of conception otherwise (chorionic villi the main component), present obvious drawbacks.

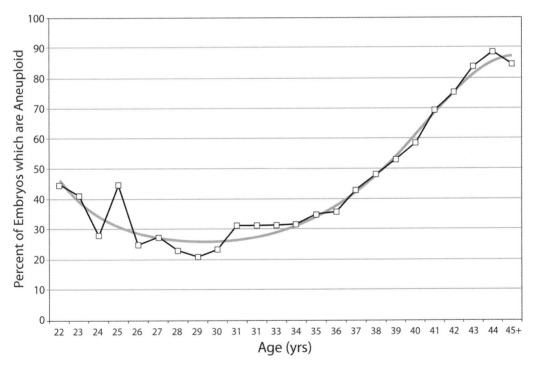

FIGURE 19–2   The rates of aneuploidy in blastocysts subjected to trophectoderm biopsy, according to maternal age. Regression curve (gray) is derived from the actual data points. The slight reduction at age 45+ years may reflect small numbers in this age group.

Source: From Franasiak et al., The nature of aneuploidy with increasing age of the female partner: A review of 15,169 consecutive trophectoderm biopsies evaluated with comprehensive chromosomal screening, Fertil Steril 101: 656–663.e1, 2014. Courtesy J. M. Franasiak, and with the permission of Elsevier.

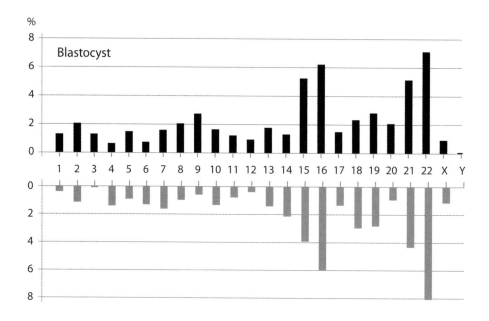

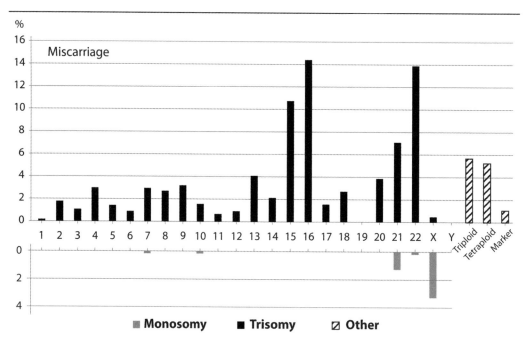

■ Monosomy ■ Trisomy ☑ Other

FIGURE 19–3 (*Top*) The range of aneuploidies observed in day 5–6 blastocysts subjected to trophectoderm biopsy and microarray, and their frequencies as a percentage of all aneuploidies. Note that trisomy and monosomy for each chromosome rather closely mirror their relative frequencies. (*Bottom*) A comparison with observations on products on conception at miscarriage (on classical karyotyping). The spread of trisomies is fairly similar, whereas the autosomal monosomies have all but disappeared, attesting to the differential early pregnancy survival of the two aneuploidy classes.

Source: From Rodriguez-Purata et al., Embryo selection versus natural selection: How do outcomes of comprehensive chromosome screening of blastocysts compare with the analysis of products of conception from early pregnancy loss (dilation and curettage) among an assisted reproductive technology population? *Fertil Steril* 104: 1460–1466.e1-12, 2015. Courtesy J. Rodriguez-Purata, and with the permission of Elsevier.

Nevertheless, Philipp et al. (2003) were able to study by endoscopy the anatomy of embryos in women prior to uterine evacuation for "missed abortion"; in some, growth had arrested, thus enabling a window upon an earlier developmental stage than a standard calculation of gestation-by-dates might have indicated. Some embryos (illustrated in their paper) showed no recognizable external structures (e.g., trisomy 16), while in some an outline embryonic form could be recognized (e.g., trisomies 4 and 7).

A French group has been able to look at an even earlier stage (and in which growth arrest might not yet have happened), in examining expelled products following very early elective abortion using the drug mifepristone (RU486), following which procedure there is little, if any, disruption of the embryonic anatomy (Golzio et al. 2006). One severely malformed embryo (Fig. 19–4), at 25 days postconception age, had failed to develop such crucial organs as the forebrain, the mesonephros (the kidney anlage), or the liver; and the pharyngeal arch system, a fundamental structural framework for the upper body, was absent. (Neither had limb buds developed, but this is normal at this stage.) The heart was grossly distorted. The chromosomal diagnosis was trisomy 8 (nonmosaic) due to a parental meiotic nondisjunction.

The practice of non-invasive cell-free DNA prenatal screening, now becoming widespread, has given clearer insight into the chromosomal picture of early pregnancy, at the time at which the blood sample would have been drawn (usually at the 10 week mark, or shortly thereafter). Pertile et al. (2017) analyzed findings due to just under 90,000 samples from on-going pregnancies, mostly from late first trimester, with a minority from second: thus, representing in particular the transition into the early fetal developmental stage. Some would have presented due to advanced maternal age, but ascertainment in the majority was, in all likelihood, essentially unbiased. Of these, 306 (0.34%) had a "rare autosomal trisomy", that is, a trisomy of other than 13, 18, 21, or sex chromosomal; and while the spread of abnormality was somewhat comparable to that seen at miscarriage (Fig. 19–6), with trisomies 15, 16, and 22 prominent, the largest single contributor was actually trisomy 7. Unsurprisingly, many of these pregnancies went on to miscarriage or intrauterine fetal death; some normal outcomes reflected placental mosaicism.

Cytogenetics of Very Early Pregnancy Loss

NONIMPLANTATION AND "OCCULT ABORTION"

Although the natural in vivo circumstance might differ from the observations in vitro, nevertheless it is a fair assumption that a substantial fraction of human conceptions have a lethal genetic burden and will not implant. It becomes a semantic question whether the existence of a nonimplanting morula or blastocyst could be described as a pregnancy, and whether its loss could be considered an abortion. Transient implantation may be associated with little or no perturbation of the menstrual cycle, although the woman may fleetingly feel pregnant as a hormonal response is briefly elicited. This is "occult abortion" (Miller et al. 1980). Monosomy, or extensive mosaicism, may be lethal around the time of blastocyst development, at least on in vitro observation, but some will enter into the blastocyst stage, as discussed above. Some trisomies impose an early developmental arrest. Trisomy 1 may exist in a small fraction of day-3 embryos in an IVF population, and yet it is almost unknown in an established pregnancy (just four recorded cases, presenting as empty sac[6]; Vičić et al. 2008). The frequency and range of trisomies seen in blastocysts is otherwise fairly similar to that seen at the stage of late first-trimester miscarriage (albeit that autosomal monosomies have by now practically all disappeared; cf. Fig. 19–3), and this is the next major period during which selective pressure is exerted.

Recurrent Implantation Failure at In Vitro Fertilization. More than one cause may apply, and a distinction is to be made between maternal ("uterine receptivity") and embryo characteristics. A subgroup of couples undergoing IVF may produce apparently normal embryos, but suffer repeated implantation failure or recurrent pregnancy loss (RIF, RPL) following transfer of embryos to the uterus. Voullaire et al. (2007) compared the frequency of aneuploidy at PGD in embryos from woman with RIF and found a higher rate of complex chromosome abnormality, which they defined as aneuploidy of three or more chromosomes, compared with those who had not. This effect was not related to maternal age. Thus, it may be that, in at

---

6 This expression refers to a conceptus in which a gestational sac and possibly a yolk sac exist, but no recognizable embryonic parts, or at most a "nubbin" of tissue. *Blighted ovum* and *anembryonic miscarriage* are other expressions meaning the same thing.

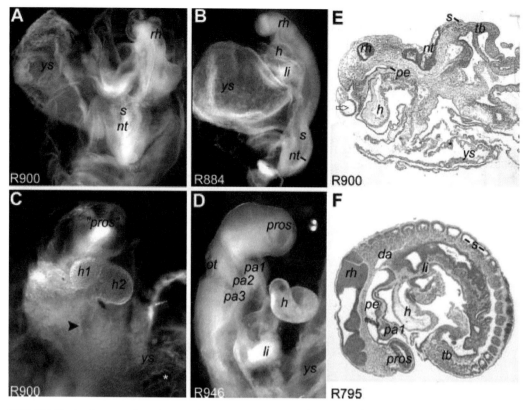

FIGURE 19–4   A very early embryo with nonmosaic trisomy 8 (A, C, and E), due to meiotic I nondisjunction. A normal embryo (B, D, and F) is shown for comparison; each is approximately 3 weeks post conception, and 3 mm in length. The trisomic embryo is devastatingly malformed. On sagittal section, normal brain structure (the prosencephalon [pros] and rhombencephalon [rh] nicely shown) and regular somite (s) development are clear to see in the normal embryo (F), compared with the gross deformity in the trisomic embryo (E). On ventral view of the trisomic embryo (C), the heart (h1, h2) is bifid, and no liver bud (li in the normal) has formed between it and the anterior intestinal portal (arrowhead). da, dorsal aorta; nt, neural tube; ot, otic vesicle; pa#, pharyngeal arch #; pe, pharyngeal endoderm; tb, tail bud; ys, yolk sac.

Source: From Golzio et al., Cytogenetic and histological features of a human embryo with homogeneous chromosome 8 trisomy, *Prenat Diagn* 26: 1201–1205, 2006. Courtesy H. C. Etchevers, and with the permission of Wiley-Blackwell.

least some of these women, there is an underlying susceptibly for embryos of theirs to undergo chromosomal error during the first two rounds of mitosis.

Taking a step back, the gametes from RIF couples may be analyzed. Vialard et al. (2008) analyzed the first polar body of the oöcyte and determined an average aneuploidy rate of 35% (range, 0%–86%). There may be a male factor: These workers also observed sperm aneuploidy rates of 2.1% in the male partner of RIF couples, compared with 0.6% from a comparison group of couples undergoing IVF, where a female factor had been identified as the cause of the infertility. Of 25 couples who had had both sperm and polar body studies, one-third demonstrated no increased chromosomal risk, but

in 60%, there was an increased aneuploidy rate in either polar body or sperm, whereas in 8%, the gametes of both of the RIF partners displayed a chromosomal susceptibility. These observations suggest that in two-thirds of RIF couples, recurring meiotic error may be the cause.

Cytogenetics of Spontaneous Abortion and Later Pregnancy Loss

CLINICAL MISCARRIAGE

At the late first-trimester miscarriage, at which stage tissue from "products of conception" is more readily obtainable, we have a clearer idea of how many

Table 19–1. Abnormal SNP Microarray Results from a Series of 7,396 Miscarriage Samples

ABNORMALITY	FREQUENCY OF ABNORMALITY (%)*
Single trisomy	63.3
Triploidy	11.8
Monosomy X	11.2
Multiple trisomy	3.2
Deletions/duplications	3.2
Hypertriploidy or hypotriploidy	2.2
Unbalanced translocations	1.3
Whole genome uniparental isodisomy (complete mole)	1
Monosomy X + trisomy	0.8
Sex chromosome abnormality	0.7
Monosomy (autosome)	0.6
Uniparental isodisomy	0.45
Multiple regions of homozygosity	0.15

*Among the 3,975 abnormal cases.
Source: From Sahoo et al. (2017).

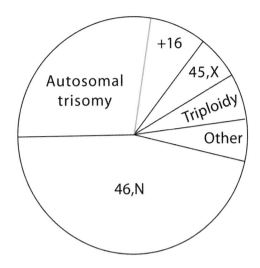

FIGURE 19–5   Chromosomal findings in products of conception from spontaneous abortions analyzed by microarray.

Source: After Sahoo et al. (2017).

conceptuses are chromosomally abnormal and what the abnormalities are. Of all recognized pregnancies (recognized in the traditional way, that is), approximately 10%–15% end in clinical miscarriage—"spontaneous abortion"—mostly toward the end of the first trimester.[7] If the products of conception are successfully cultured and karyotyped, in most studies somewhat over a half of abortuses are shown to have a chromosome abnormality (a figure that has increased with increasing expertise and experience, and the application of modern methodologies[8]; Rajcan-Separovic et al. 2010; Sahoo et al. (2017). Sahoo et al. studied 8,188 miscarriage samples, from which an SNP microarray result was obtained in 7,396 (Table 19–1). A clinically significant chromosome abnormality was seen in 54% of samples, and in almost all (94%), this was considered the cause of the miscarriage. If the embryonic anatomy

is taken into account, in the case of an empty sac, the fraction with a chromosomal abnormality is approximately 60%; this compares with close to 70% in cases in which embryonic/fetal parts are identifiable on ultrasound (Lathi et al. 2007) and over 80% in those in which multiple external defects are observed through an endoscope prior to operative evacuation (Philipp et al. 2003). The rates of abnormality are similar between natural and in vitro conception (Wu et al. 2016b). The type and frequency of abnormalities are presented in Table 19–1.

Trisomies account for about two-thirds of all cytogenetic abnormalities identified at spontaneous abortion (Fig. 19–5). The most commonly seen abnormal karyotypes are trisomy 16, monosomy X, and triploidy. As many as 1% of all human conceptions may have trisomy 16 (Benn 1998); and monosomy X and triploidy account for approximately 11% and 12% of all abnormalities, respectively (Sahoo et al. 2017). The full range of trisomies, and their relative frequencies,

---

7 The distinction between an embryo and a fetus (and see footnote 2) in this setting is not necessarily straightforward. Embryonic development may have arrested, and spontaneous abortion will be inevitable, but the pregnancy may continue for one or a few weeks ("missed abortion"), and using apparent gestational age would give a misleading impression. In this case, it is more useful to consider the developmental stage of the embryo in judging the effects of a particular aneuploidy (Philipp et al. 2003). For example, the triploid embryo (not fetus) shown in Figure 19–4 was retained in the uterus until 18 weeks, but development had arrested at the 7–8 week mark.

8 Molecular methodologies (MLPA and array-CGH) are powerful, but they may miss most triploidies. The use of SNP arrays and genotyping can, in principle, detect these abnormal ploidy states. Tetraploidy is not detected by CGH or SNP arrays.

are depicted in Fig. 19–6. Double trisomy (trisomy for two chromosomes) is infrequent, this being an observation in 2.2% in one large series (Diego-Alvarez et al. 2006); triple trisomy is extraordinarily rare (Reddy 1999; Sebire et al. 2016[9]). After aneuploidies and triploidies, structural rearrangements constitute most of the remainder ("other" in Fig. 19–5). The distribution of abnormality does not differ between pregnancies conceived naturally, at standard IVF, or at IVF by ICSI (Wu et al. 2016b).

The origin of the abnormality is, in most, an error at maternal meiosis I, and this includes most of the major trisomies: trisomies 13, 14, 16, 21, and 22, with trisomy 18 a possible exception. Robinson et al. (1999) analyzed the originating status of certain of the less studied karyotypes: trisomies for chromosomes 2, 4–10, 12, 15, 17, and 20. Around three-fourths showed three alleles for the trisomic chromosome, thus confirming a meiotic origin. Most of the remainder are presumed to have been due to

somatic errors; some might have been mosaic, but not detected as such. Trisomy 8 is unusual, in that all cases were due to a meiotic error, which stands in contrast to somatic errors being almost entirely the basis of the mosaic trisomy 8 syndrome that is diagnosed postnatally. Uniparental disomy appears not to be a causative factor in miscarriage (Shaffer et al. 1998; Smith et al. 1998; Robinson et al. 1999).

Phenotypes of the Embryo/Fetus. An embryo or fetus may or may not be identifiable in the products of conception collected at the time of spontaneous abortion due to chromosomal abnormality. Severe growth disorganization can be graded according to whether there is complete absence of any detectable embryonic parts, a tiny nubbin of tissue without recognizable embryonic landmarks, or an embryo in which cephalic and caudal poles can be distinguished (Philipp et al. 2003). The triploid embryo in Figure 19–7 is very deformed but with recognizable face, trunk, and limbs; it is not as

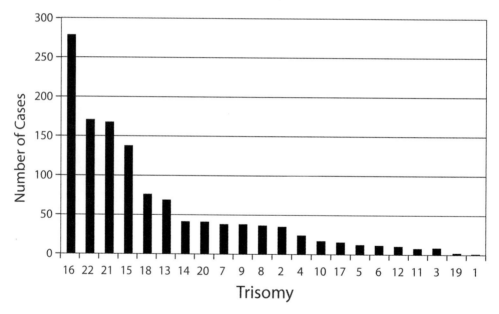

FIGURE 19–6   The relative frequencies of trisomies observed in products of conception, descending from the most often seen (trisomy 16) to the least (trisomy 1). These data are from the 1,872 abnormal results of a series of 5,457 consecutive samples of products of conception, on G-banding analysis. The findings are very similar to those of Rodriguez-Purata et al. shown in Figure 19–3.

Source: From Wang et al., Abnormalities in spontaneous abortions detected by G-banding and chromosomal microarray analysis (CMA) at a national reference laboratory, *Mol Cytogenet* 7:33, 2014a. Courtesy B. T. Wang, and with the permission of Springer Nature, according to the Creative Commons Attribution License.

9 These authors report a case in which trisomy 3, 7, and 8, along with upd16pat, were associated with a form of hydatidiform mole.

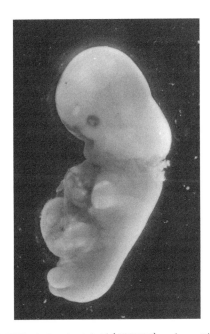

FIGURE 19-7   A triploid (69,XXY) embryo. The face has no landmarks other than eyes and a single opening. The anterior trunk is open, with the heart and liver visible. Spontaneous abortion occurred at 18 weeks gestation, but the length is that of 6–7 weeks gestation. The disrupted tissue at the neck was the site of biopsy for the cytogenetic analysis.

severely distorted as the trisomy 8 embryo in Figure 19-4. Seller et al. (2004) describe the only known case of (presumed) nonmosaic trisomy 2, a very severely deformed fetus that survived to 12 weeks gestation. Warburton et al. (1991) provide a graphic catalog of embryonic/fetal phenotypes from their material of approximately 1,300 karyotypically abnormal spontaneous abortuses collected over a 12-year period in New York state, and we have mentioned above the illustrations of aneuploid embryos in Philipp et al. (2003). What actually leads to expulsion of the conceptus from the uterus may be the declining vascular and endocrine function of the placental tissue, with decidual necrosis finally causing uterine irritation and contraction (Rushton 1981). The underlying process of decline, or at least a contributory factor, may be accelerated apoptosis: Qumsiyeh et al. (2000) observed a higher apoptotic index in villi of the abortus with an abnormal versus a normal karyotype.

Twinning. If an abnormal twin dies, the normal twin may ensure continuation of the pregnancy, and only a parchment-like vestige (*fetus papyraceus*) remains, preserved in the uterus along with the normal twin. A "vanishing twin" has plausibly been proposed in the study of a pregnancy in which two cell lines were identified at chorion villus sampling, 46,XX and 47,XY,+9. Amniocentesis gave a 46,XX result, and a normal girl was subsequently born. Analysis of a fibrotic area of the placenta gave the same two karyotypes, 46,XX and 47,XY,+9 (Falik-Borenstein et al. 1994). The likely explanation is that a 47,XY,+9 co-conceptus died, and the fibrotic placental tissue was the only remnant.

An extremely rare observation is the trisomy that would otherwise lead inevitably to early miscarriage, but in which a monozygous euploid co-twin allows some ongoing in utero survival. These cases may result from a very early postzygotic event that generates a trisomic cell line (or which generates a normal cell line from a trisomic conceptus), and the trisomic co-twin, among other grossly devastating defects, fails to form a heart ("acardius"). The normal euploid co-twin provides the blood circulation to the abnormal fetus ("twin reverse arterial perfusion"). This scenario has been reported with trisomies 2 and 11 (Blaicher et al. 2000; Mihci et al. 2009), and we have seen one case due to trisomy 3 (McGillivray et al. 2004).

FETAL DEATH IN UTERO, PERINATAL DEATH

Concerning mid-trimester loss, which, coming between miscarriage and stillbirth, may be referred to as fetal death in utero (FDIU) or in utero fetal demise (IUFD), chromosome abnormality may be present in about a half, although at this stage it is the "viable" rather than the invariably lethal aneuploidies that come to light (Howarth et al. 2002). For stillbirths, occurring after 20 weeks of gestation, 6%–13% are attributed to karyotypic abnormalities, in particular trisomy 18, trisomy 21, and monosomy X (Korteweg et al. 2008). The rate of chromosome abnormalities varies from 5% in morphologically normal fetuses to 35%–40% when anatomical abnormalities are present (Korteweg et al. 2008). Array methodology is more likely than karyotype analysis to provide a genetic diagnosis, primarily because of its success with nonviable tissue, and also because it enables the detection of subtler

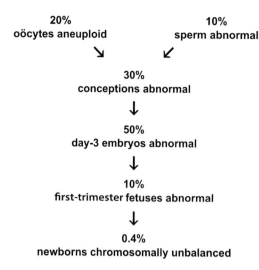

20%
oöcytes aneuploid

10%
sperm abnormal

↘   ↙

30%
conceptions abnormal

↓

50%
day-3 embryos abnormal

↓

10%
first-trimester fetuses abnormal

↓

0.4%
newborns chromosomally unbalanced

FIGURE 19–8   The frequency of chromosome abnormalities at gametogenesis and during pregnancy, demonstrating the effectiveness of selection against aneuploid states. The figures given for gametes through to embryos are very approximate, and considerable individual variation is probable. The oöcyte percentage varies very considerably according to maternal age. The day-3 embryo percentage, drawn from in vitro fertilization data, may exaggerate the true picture in vivo. The figures for fetal and newborn abnormality are quite accurate.

imbalances. In a series of 465 stillbirths successfully analyzed by microarray, Reddy et al. (2012) detected aneuploidy in 6.9% and a pathogenic copy number variant in 2.6%, for an overall yield of 9.5%. Similarly, a fraction of pregnancies going through to term, or at any rate to the third trimester, but with the baby stillborn or dying in the early neonatal period (perinatal death), are due to chromosomal abnormality, whether this be full or partial aneuploidy; a common representative of this group is trisomy 18. Again, array-CGH may increase the detection of chromosome abnormality or allow diagnosis when classic chromosomal analysis has been unsuccessful (Raca et al. 2009). Among liveborn babies, only 1 in 250 has an unbalanced chromosome abnormality on standard karyotyping (see Table 1–1). Thus, there has been a very effective selection against those conceptions that were abnormal (Fig. 19–8).

RECURRENT PREGNANCY LOSS

Two or more failed pregnancies is the criterion for "recurrence."[10] Do some couples, themselves karyotypically normal, miscarry due to a predisposition to produce aneuploid conceptions (Ulm 1999)? On the other hand, could recurrent aneuploid miscarriage, in the setting of a high background rate of aneuploidy in humans, simply reflect random biology, with increasing maternal age the only clear predisposing factor? A common event is common, and not uncommonly it may happen more than once.

This was a subtle question to dissect. While earlier studies (Hassold et al. 1993; Robinson et al. 2001) did not detect a susceptibility, evidence for a predisposition to recurring aneuploid conception subsequently emerged. In Rubio et al. (2003), the endpoint of observation was FISH analysis of the embryo at PGD, from a patient population having previously experienced multiple miscarriage, and stratified by maternal age. As Table 19–2 shows, more aneuploidy was seen in embryos of younger women, but not older, having suffered previous miscarriage. Bianco et al. (2006) showed an increase in the likelihood for an aneuploidy to be found at prenatal diagnosis in women who had had previous miscarriage, and this risk increased with the number of miscarriages. Similarly, in Marquard et al. (2010), older women (>35 years) who had had three or more miscarriages had an increased risk for a further loss, and trisomy much the most probable cause. A small effect indicating a predisposition to aneuploidy recurrence was discernible in Warburton et al.'s (2004) review of a very large body of prenatal diagnostic data, and more stringently supported in Grande et al. (2016). A tentative conclusion from the foregoing is that a fraction of recurrent abortion may be explained by a predisposition to recurrent aneuploidy, and that this effect is more of an issue in younger women.

It may seem counterintuitive, but for some couples who have suffered multiple miscarriages, it may be that an aneuploid abortion indicates a better chance for a normal live birth in a subsequent pregnancy than when a miscarriage is euploid (Ogasawara et al. 2000; Carp et al. 2001). Aneuploidy of the abortus may be *less* often observed in couples who have had a large

---

10 Definition from the American Society for Reproductive Medicine (2008): "Recurrent pregnancy loss is a disease distinct from infertility, defined by two or more failed pregnancies. When the cause is unknown, each pregnancy loss merits careful review to determine whether specific evaluation may be appropriate. After three or more losses, a thorough evaluation is warranted."

Table 19–2. Frequencies of Aneuploidies for Certain Chromosomes in a Cohort of Women Having Had Recurrent Miscarriage (559 Embryos Analyzed), Compared with a Presumed Normally Fertile Cohort (215 Embryos)

ANEUPLOID CHROMOSOME OF EMBRYO	RECURRENT MISCARRIAGE		COMPARISON GROUP	
	‹37 YEARS	≥37 YEARS	‹37 YEARS	≥37 YEARS
13	20%	19	7	21
16	24	29	7	16
18	10	12	5	15
21	23	27	9	30
22	18	25	5	14
X, Y	11	12	7	15

Notes: The two major classes of aneuploidy were autosomal monosomy and autosomal trisomy. Figures are percentages. Within each clinical category, distinction is made between women younger than age 37 years and those age 37 years or older. The rates of aneuploidy for chromosomes 16 and 22 show the most notable differences between the two cohorts, approximately two- to threefold, across both age groups. For the other autosomes (13, 18, 21), the marked differences are confined to the women <37 years. The comparison cohort comprised women having preimplantation genetic diagnosis for X-linked Mendelian conditions.

Source: From Rubio et al. (2003).

number of miscarriages, sometimes into double figures, than among those who have had fewer. The probable reason, in such cases, is that a chromosomally normal miscarriage reflected an underlying maternal factor that would apply to all pregnancies, whereas aneuploidy at least offers the hope that better fortune might attend the next ovulation.

Couples with Rearrangements. For the small group of people who are heterozygous for a chromosomal rearrangement, pregnancy loss may of course occur with a much higher frequency, and this briefly stated fact is the basis of much of what is written in this book. In about 5% of all couples suffering two or more fetal losses, one of the partners carries a balanced chromosomal rearrangement, which represents an approximate eightfold increase compared with the general population (Fryns and Van Buggenhout 1998; Celep et al. 2006; Zhang et al. 2011; Sudhir et al. 2016). These chromosomal rearrangements are typically of sufficient size to be readily detectable at standard karyotyping; and typically of sufficient size that imbalanced combinations will lead, very frequently, to inevitable miscarriage. A large study from China by Zhang et al. (2015), specifically examining the male partner, identified a number who were heterozygous for a reciprocal or Robertsonian translocation (Table 19–3).

Table 19–3. Translocations Observed in Men Whose Partners Had Had Recurrent Miscarriage, Among a Series of 3,319 Men Presenting to an Andrology Service

TRANSLOCATION	NO. OF MISCARRIAGES PER WOMAN
46,XY t(1;10)(p31.2;q26)	4
46,XY t(3;7)(p23;q21.2)	3
46,XY t(4;14)(q25;q24)	3
46,XY t(4;21)(q21;q12)	3
46,XY t(4;5)(q21;p15)	3
46,XY t(4;9)(q35;p13)	2
46,XY t(6;7)(q15;p15)	4
46,XY t(6;8)(p21;q24)	4
46,XY t(6;9)(q26;p13)	3
46,XY t(7;8)(q32;q22)	3
46,XY t(7;10)(q32;q21)	2
46,XY t(9;15)(p14;q22)	2
46,XY t(10;21)(p11;q22)	2
46,XY,t(10;22)(q25;q13)	3
46,XY,t(18;20)(p11;q11)	2
45,XY,rob(13;14)	2
45,XY,rob(13;14)	3
45,XY,rob(15;21)	2

Source: From Zhang et al. (2015).

An actual example of a chromosomally unbalanced pregnancy leading to spontaneous abortion in the first trimester is shown in Fig. 5–9; this was the third miscarriage out of three pregnancies for the couple, the wife being a t(13;16) carrier. Cryptic translocations can also be associated with a risk for miscarriage (Diego-Alvarez et al. 2007). The risk for miscarriage will depend upon the particular characteristics of the rearrangement. As a global figure, for couples, one of whom carries a reciprocal translocation, there is an increased odds of three- to fourfold, compared to chromosomally normal couples who have had repeated pregnancy loss, to have a subsequent further miscarriage (Ozawa et al. 2008). In contrast, the risk for a viable unbalanced form is very low in this group (Barber et al. 2010).

As well as translocations and other autosomal rearrangements, sex chromosome abnormalities may be identified in couples presenting with recurring pregnancy loss. Table 19–4 sets out the karyotypes seen in a Portuguese clinic population (Kiss et al. 2009). Although this was a small series, the spread and prevalence of chromosome abnormalities is quite similar to the findings at infertility investigation (cf. Table 19–5).

Table 19–4. Chromosome Abnormalities in a Series of 108 Couples Having Had Recurrent Pregnancy Loss

KARYOTYPE	NO.
Sex Chromosomal	
45,X/46,XX	2
47,XXX/46,XX	1
47,XXY/46,XY	1
47,XYY/46,XY	1
Autosomal	
Simple rcp	3*
rob	2*
inv (pericentric)	1

*One woman carried two rearrangements, a reciprocal translocation, and a Robertsonian translocation.
Source: From Kiss et al. (2009).

Table 19–5. Chromosome Abnormalities in a Series of Candidate Couples for Intracytoplasmic Sperm Injection (ICSI), Comprising 2,196 Men and 1,012 Women (Some Female Partners Not Studied, Since It Had Been Assumed the Infertility Was in the Male)

KARYOTYPE	NO. (FEMALE)	NO. (MALE)
*Sex Chromosomal**		
45,X/46,XY**	–	8
47,XXY	–	49
47,XXY/46,XY, etc.***	–	8
47,XYY****	–	8
Structural Y abn.	–	9
X or Y rcp with autosome	–	5
Autosomal		
Simple rcp	7	18
Mosaic rcp	–	2
Complex rcp	–	2
rob	7	18
inv (pericentric)	7	3
Structural abn., unbalanced	–	4
Total abnormal	21 (2.1%)	134 (6.1%)
None of the above	991	2,062
Totals	1,012	2,196

Note: Most, but not necessarily all, of these abnormalities will have been related causally to the infertility.
*Excluding a variety of low-level X chromosome mosaicisms in 28 women, of doubtful significance.
**Including one 45,X/46,XX/46,XY low-level mosaic.
***Including one 47,XXY/48,XXXY/46,XY mosaic and one low-level 47,XXX/47,XXY/46,XY mosaic.
****Including one 47,XYY/46,XY low-level mosaic.
Source: From a France-wide study 1995–1998 (Gekas et al. 2001).

Cytogenetics of Infertility

Infertility is defined as the inability to achieve conception.[11] Certainly, it is common, affecting approximately 15% of couples. It is worth emphasizing that infertility is to be seen in the context of the couple, not necessarily of the individuals separately. An

---

11 Definition from the American Society for Reproductive Medicine (2008): "Infertility is a disease, defined by the failure to achieve pregnancy after 12 months or more of regular unprotected intercourse. Earlier evaluation and treatment may be justified based on medical history and physical findings, and is warranted after 6 months for women over age 35 years." Using this definition, infertility is clearly a heterogeneous condition. Some of these couples will be permanently infertile, some will be "subfertile," and still others may simply be "unlucky."

oligospermic man may be fertile with a "superfertile" female partner, but not with a woman of average fertility, for example. Many causes of infertility exist, involving the male (Skakkebæk et al. 1994) and the female (Healy et al. 1994) partner, and a fraction of these are presumed to be genetically determined (Layman 2002; Feng et al. 2016; Huang et al. 2017; Mayer et al. 2017; He et al. 2017), and with demonstrable chromosomal causes seen in a minority. Sex chromosomal defects include XXY and XXY/XY in the male, typically presenting with azoöspermia and occasionally severe oligospermia in the nonmosaic state; and Turner syndrome and its variants in the female. The common Yq microdeletion is dealt with below. The "XX male" and XY female are rare (Chapter 23). Autosomal rearrangements as cause of infertility are noted in several chapters. The reciprocal translocation (especially when an acrocentric is involved) and the inversion may be associated, though infrequently, with severe hypospermatogenesis and moderate to severe oligospermia (Chapters 5 and 9). Robertsonian translocations are occasionally associated with infertility in the male or, less often, the female (Chapter 7). Translocation between a sex chromosome and an autosome is a rarely identified cause of infertility (Chapter 6). Complex rearrangements (Chapter 10) and rings (Chapter 11) typically present an insurmountable obstacle to cell division in the spermatocyte, resulting in azoöspermia; oögenesis is more robust.

The frequency of karyotypic abnormality in couples with infertility depends considerably upon the criteria of ascertainment, and quite wide ranges of figures have been produced. Couples presenting to ICSI programs might be supposed typically to manifest a male factor infertility; but van der Ven et al. (1998) were surprised to discover that female partners had about as many chromosomal abnormalities (X aneuploidy, reciprocal and Robertsonian translocations, inversions) as did the males, in a series of 305 couples presenting for ICSI; the experience of Meschede et al. (1998a) was not dissimilar. In an Italian series of 2,710 infertile couples, more men were identified with a chromosome abnormality in those who had had ICSI, compared with those having standard IVF, and the least seen in those men in whom simple intrauterine insemination (IUI) was considered appropriate; no such differential applied to the women (Riccaboni et al. 2008).

A large French study (Gekas et al. 2001) brought together all the ICSI programs in France over a 3-year period and included some 3,208 individuals,

2,196 men and 1,012 women, who had come forward as candidate couples for ICSI. Gynecologic causes of infertility had been excluded. Each individual had at least 20 metaphases examined. Sex chromosome mosaicism at a level of <10% was categorized as "minor." In the men, 6% showed a chromosomal abnormality, and in the women (excluding insignificant minor sex chromosome mosaicism), 2%, even though a basis of the infertility had been determined in the male partner. We return to the comment above about infertility being a couple condition. The abnormalities included numerical and structural sex chromosome abnormalities, reciprocal and Robertsonian translocations, inversions, and other structural abnormality (Table 19–5). The French group compared their own data with those of 10 other similar series, deriving consensus figures of approximately 5%–6% and 4%–5% for male and female karyotypic abnormality, respectively. The figure is rather higher (16%) in men presenting with azoöspermia. Considering just autosomal translocations, and in relation to the nature of the infertility, Stern et al. (1999) noted the rate of balanced rcp and rob carriers to be 3% in 219 couples (both partners tested) who had failed more than 10 embryo transfers, and 9% in 130 couples who had three or more consecutive first-trimester abortions. (In one notable couple from the latter group, both were translocation carriers.)

INFERTILITY: CHROMOSOMAL FACTORS IN THE FEMALE

Fertility in the 46,XX female begins to fall in the mid-thirties, as the ovarian reserve dwindles. The average maximum number of 300,000 ovarian follicles is reached in midfetal life, at 18–22 weeks gestation, falling to 180,000 by age 13 years, 65,000 by 25 years, 16,000 by 35 years, and with less than 1,000 remaining at the age of menopause (Wallace and Kelsey 2010). A diminishing ovarian reserve, as indicated by a low level of anti-Müllerian hormone, may point to an increasing risk for aneuploidy (Gat et al. 2017). An important age-related factor may be a decline in the functional competence of the meiotic spindle, compromising chromosomal distribution and leading to the generation of aneuploid gametes (color Fig. 3–7).

Various sex chromosomal abnormal states, mostly mosaic and containing a 45,X cell line, account for— or are at least associated with—a number of cases of female infertility; autosomal abnormalities are less frequent. Some illustrative karyotypes are listed in Table 19–5. In some, the infertility is primary (there has never been a period of fertility), and in others it is secondary (following a previous fertile period). In a Malaysian study, Ten et al. (1990) karyotyped 117 women with primary amenorrhea, who had previously been investigated for other causes, and one-third had a sex chromosome abnormality. They were classified as follows: X aneuploidies (8%), X structural abnormalities (7%), presence of a Y (14%), and presence of a gonosomal marker chromosome (2%). Six women were mosaic, all having a 45,X cell line. Secondary infertility may be due to premature ovarian failure, and Devi and Benn (1999) studied 30 women with unexplained secondary amenorrhea under the age of 40 years. Four (13%) had chromosomal abnormalities: an Xq isochromosome, Turner syndrome mosaicism (45,X/46,XX), an X-Y translocation, and an X-autosome translocation.[12]

The conundrum of how to interpret low-level X aneuploidy—for example, just one or two 47,XXX or 45,X cells—is addressed in a newsletter from the European Cytogeneticists Association (Madan and Lundberg 2015).[13] The salient points listed in this article are worth repeating:

• The frequency of low-level X aneuploidy is correlated with age and gender but not with reproductive history.
• There is no significant difference in the number of aneuploid cells between these two groups: women with recurrent abortions (1.64%) and age-matched controls (1.78%).
• Approximately 16% of women of reproductive age show X-aneuploidy in 2%–10% of blood cells.
• The finding of low-level X aneuploidy in peripheral blood of a mother is not a predictor of fetal aneuploidy.
• Low-level X aneuploidy is found in blood but not in skin or bone marrow.

Autosomal structural anomalies are an uncommon association with infertility due to premature ovarian insufficiency, accounting for only 2% of cases, and with only 25 cases on record, including 10 reciprocal and 10 Robertsonian translocations, in the review of Vichinsartvichai (2016). The association may reflect a nonspecific disturbance of meiosis, interruption of an autosomal locus, or simply coincidence. Recurrent implantation failure following embryo transfer at IVF treatment is a form of infertility, albeit that conceptions have occurred. The rate of nonmosaic autosomal translocation carriers in one series of 65 women who had had ≥15 failed transfers was 8%, two being sisters with the same translocation (Raziel et al. 2002). (Compare with the 3% translocation figure based upon rather larger numbers, and testing both of the couple, in Stern et al. 1999, noted above.) Failure of the meiotic apparatus, with no formation of the first polar body, may be a rare cause of female infertility, and possibly due to an autosomal recessive gene (Neal et al. 2002; Schmiady and Neitzel 2002). Genetic factors other than classic chromosomal are reviewed in Qin et al. (2015).

A Rare Complexity. A most remarkable coincidence leading to infertility in a young woman is described in Kuechler et al. (2010). Her father was heterozygous for a mutation in the *FSHR* (follicle-stimulating hormone receptor) gene, which is located at 2p16.3; and her mother carried an apparently balanced translocation, t(2;8)(p16.3;p23.1), but which in fact had a microdeletion at the 2p16.3 breakpoint, demonstrable on microarray. This microdeletion removed two exons of the *FSHR* gene. The daughter inherited this translocation, plus the paternal mutation, and in consequence, the former "unmasked" the latter, no normal FSHR was produced, and folliculogenesis was arrested.

INFERTILITY: CHROMOSOMAL FACTORS IN THE MALE

Fertility is not necessarily synonymous with normospermia and, as mentioned above, a man with oligospermia[14] may be fertile with a woman of

---

12 X-autosome rearrangements associated with ovarian failure may reflect a consequence of breakpoints in one of the Xq21 critical regions (CR1), which bring autosomal "ovarian genes" under the influence of X-heterochromatin at Xq21. In other words, it may be a position effect, whereby autosomal genes for ovarian function are downregulated due to epigenetic modification, rather than disruption of X-borne loci at the X breakpoint (Rizzolio et al. 2006; Moysés-Oliveira et al. 2015a).

13 See also Mosaic loss of the X, p. 342.

14 Oligospermia is defined as a sperm count of <20 million per milliliter. Oligoasthenoteratozoöspermia includes the observations of poor motility (*astheno*) and an increased fraction of abnormal forms (*terato*). Severe oligospermia is a count of <2 million per milliliter, moderate oligospermia is 2–5 million per milliliter, and mild is 5–20 million per milliliter. Azoöspermia is absence of sperm. A distinction is to be made between obstructive and nonobstructive azoöspermia; in the latter, the primary fault is a severe defect of spermatogenesis.

"superfertility" (Krausz and McElreavey 2001). Nevertheless, much couple infertility is associated with diminished sperm production in the male, and a fraction of this is associated with an abnormal karyotype (Table 19–5). In men presenting with azoöspermia or oligospermia, numerical and structural gonosomal abnormalities (mostly XXY and Y rearrangements) and structural autosomal abnormalities (mostly reciprocal and Robertsonian translocations) are identified in 3%–13% (De Braekeleer and Dao 1991; Meschede et al. 1998a; Stuppia et al. 1998; van der Ven et al. 1998; Causio et al. 1999; Dohle et al. 2002; Elghezal et al. 2006). Rare observations include complex rearrangements (Chapter 10) and the small isodicentric 15 and other small marker chromosomes (Eggermann et al. 2002; Ma et al. 2003; Wang et al. 2009b). A slight effect (not statistically significant) was seen in male partners of recurrent miscarriage couples, in the study of Neusser et al (2015), in whom sperm studies showed an increase in disomy 16.

X Chromosome Abnormalities. The XXY state is the most frequently observed classical karyotype; some of these may be, and more especially in men with extreme oligospermia rather than azoöspermia, very low-level XY/XXY mosaic (Elghezal et al. 2006). Otherwise, mosaicism with a 45,X cell line, 45,X/46,XY, is often associated with infertility (Newberg et al. 1998), as also may be 45,X/47,XYY (Dale et al. 2002), and true XX/XY mosaicism, or chimerism[15] (Sugawara et al. 2005). In some instances, if there is a residual spermatogenesis, artificial reproductive technology might enable fatherhood. The X-autosome translocation is dealt with in Chapter 6; the "XX male" is discussed on p. 537.

Y Isochromosomes. The Y isochromosomes, the karyotypes 46,X,i(Y)(q) and 46,X,i(Y)(p)[16] (Fig. 15–5), may be seen in nonmosaic and 45,X/46,X,i(Y) mosaic forms. While abnormal genital phenotypes may be associated with this karyotype (see p. 349), here we are discussing the otherwise normal male presenting with infertility. This is seen in either type: the iYq, in which Yq-located AZF spermatogenesis loci are lost, and the iYp, in which there is a double amount of Yq (Fig. 15–5)

(Codina-Pascual et al. 2004). The typical basis of this may be "Sertoli-only syndrome," in which the testis lacks germ cells (Lin et al. 2005). While testicular extraction may sometimes enable sperm retrieval in this syndrome, we know of no cases of success in men with a Y isochromosome. We have seen a man, tertiary-educated, with nonmosaic 46,X,i(Yp), in whom attempted testicular aspiration of sperm was unsuccessful (had IVF with ICSI been possible, PGD to select for an XX embryo would have been considered).

Yq Microdeletions. The most frequent chromosomal cause of male infertility resides in a Y chromosome microdeletion, with particular reference to the AZF (azoöspermia factor) regions in Yq11, wherein certain spermatogenesis factors have their loci (Fig. 6–1) (Foresta et al. 2001). The fraction varies according to patient selection, and when other causes of oligospermia/azoöspermia have been excluded, the proportion due to AZF deletion reaches 10%–20%. While the initial discovery had been made by cytogeneticists (Tiepolo and Zuffardi 1976), these Y-deletions are mostly not detectable cytogenetically, and are routinely analyzed using molecular methodology. There are three main AZF regions—a, b, and c—and deletions in one or more region can impair spermatogenesis or lead to its complete failure. The most commonly seen deletion involves the AZFc region, in Yq11.23, the causative mechanism being an inappropriate apposition of duplicons (Kuroda-Kawaguchi et al. 2001). AZFc contains the *DAZ*—deleted in azoöspermia—multigene family, the products of these duplicated loci being important (but not necessarily crucial) spermatogenesis factors. As a rule, AZFa or AZFb deletions are more severe in their effects than AZFc. Different causes for disordered spermatogenesis may coexist in an individual, and Jaruzelska et al. (2001) point to the need for cytogenetic studies, bringing to attention cases in which 45,X/46,XY mosaicism may have had an additive effect along with an AZFc deletion. Deletions due to a ring Y are noted on p. 350.

A male child conceived from a father with a constitutional Yq microdeletion would very likely have similar infertility (although, as noted below,

---

15 A man with 46,XY[79]//46,XX[22] chimerism in Higgins et al. (2014) had presented due to couple infertility, albeit that his reproductive indices were normal; the only abnormal sign in himself was hypomelanosis of Ito.

16 Some inconsistency in nomenclature, according to Yp or Yq breakpoint, is noted in footnote 5 on p. 349.

some men with a Yq deletion may retain fertility). Komori et al. (2001) formally demonstrated that a man with a del(Yq) on blood karyotyping could transmit the deletion, in showing the deletion actually to be present in sperm, as did de Vries et al. (2001) in all of seven infertile men with deletion of the *DAZ* gene cluster. The observation of the same deletion in the sons of men who had conceived via ICSI confirms the reality of vertical transmission (Cram et al. 2000; Mau Kai et al. 2008). The reduction in fertility may be relative, at least for AZFc deletions, and at a younger age, and perhaps with a partner of "excellent" fertility, a man with a deletion may father children with no obvious difficulty (Krausz and McElreavey 2001). Chang et al. (1999) report the example of an azoöspermic 63-year-old man with a *DAZ* deletion, but who had been fertile in his younger days, having had five children from when he was 25–38 years of age. His four sons all had the deletion, and the three of them tested (ages 24–37 years) were oligospermic or azoöspermic.

Translocation Carriers. In the setting of a balanced rearrangement, gametogenesis in the male heterozygote is vulnerable to the stumbling block imposed by a chromosomal abnormality, and infertility occasionally results. An important element in this male vulnerability may be the integrity at meiosis of the X-Y bivalent, synapsing and recombining at the pseudoautosomal regions at the tips of Xp and Yp—the "sex vesicle." Unpaired or aberrantly associating autosomal segments, particularly of the acrocentric chromosomes, might disturb this integrity, leading to disruption of spermatogenesis (Guichaoua et al. 1990; Oliver-Bonet et al. 2005; Vialard et al. 2006). Another element may be impaired synapsis of homologous segments in the normal and the rearranged chromosomes, which of itself prevents further progress in gametogenesis, and spermatogenesis may be more sensitive to this obstacle than is oögenesis (Hale 1994; Oliver-Bonet et al. 2005). Pinho et al. (2005) undertook testicular studies on a man with a de novo 46,X,t(Y;1)(q12;q12), demonstrating reduced Xp/Yp pairing, and showing that spermatogenesis had arrested at meiosis I, and that the germ cells had undergone apoptosis. If spermatogenesis is retained, a compromised testicular environment due to the presence of a translocation may nevertheless, of itself, predispose to the production of diploid sperm (Egozcue et al. 2000). A representative collection of translocations seen in infertile men is listed in Table 19–6.

Table 19–6. Translocations Observed Among Infertile Patients in a Series of 3,319 Men Presenting to an Andrology Service

46,XY,t(1;2)(q21;p23)	46,Y,t(X;2)(p22;p11)
46,XY,t(1;2)(q21;q37)	46,X,t(Y;4)(p11;p14)
46,XY,t(1;3;6)(p32;q29;q14)	46,X,t(Y;14)(q11;p11)
46,XY,t(1;4)(p36;q31)	45,X,t(Y;13)(p10;q10)
46,XY,t(1;9)(p32;p24)	45,X,t(Y;15)(p10;q11)
46,XY,t(1;12)(q42;q13)	45,XY,rob(13;14)
46,XY,t(1;13)(p22;q14)	45,XY,rob(13;21)
46,XY,t(1;18)(p32;q23)	45,XY,rob(14;15)
46,XY,t(1;20)(p13;p11.2)	45,XY,rob(14;21)
46,XY,t(7;15)(p15;q15)	45,XY,rob (14;21)
46,XY,t(10;13)(q10;q10)	45,XY,dic(17;22)(p13;q13)
46,XY,t(11;22)(q25;q13)	46,XY,dic(13;19)(p11;q12)

Source: From Zhang et al. (2015).

Notwithstanding the above, it remains true that fertility is usually unimpaired, or scarcely impaired, in male translocation heterozygotes. In their study of just over 10,000 sperm donors, all of proven fertility, the frequency of men carrying reciprocal and Robertsonian translocations, and also pericentric inversions, did not differ with statistical significance from the general population (Ravel et al. 2006a). The semen indices of these men were within normal ranges. This epidemiology indicates that while it is true that a few heterozygotes may have impaired fertility, their numbers are too small to sway the figures of a large carrier population into statistical significance.

Sperm Phenotypic Defects Associated with Chromosome Abnormality. Not only may the contained genetic material of the spermatozoön be faulty from the translocation heterozygote, but also the "container." Baccetti et al. (2003) studied by electron microscopy the sperm of an infertile man with a de novo t(10;15)(q26;q12) and showed essentially all sperm to be structurally abnormal. A syndrome of infertility associated with "*large-headed sperm*" is described in Benzacken et al. (2001). Polyploidy may be the explanation here. Benzacken et al. studied infertile brothers with oligoasthenoteratozoöspermia, half of all sperm having the large-head phenotype. FISH analysis (X, Y, 18) in one brother showed all sperm cells to be diploid or polyploid (3*n*, 4*n*, and >4*n*). The basic fault may lie in a failure of the cell to cleave at the two meiotic stages and, with brothers affected, a genetic cause may reasonably be presumed. Similar cases were reported by Devillard et al. (2002), Lewis-Jones et al. (2003), and Perrin et al. (2008). In the Lewis-Jones study, three men had complete teratozoöspermia (all sperm with abnormal forms, such as double heads, large heads, and multiple tails), and the frequency of chromosomal abnormality was very high, up to 100%. Another type of sperm defect is the "*tail stump syndrome*," in which the flagellum, the motor apparatus, forms abnormally. Ravel et al. (2006b) report this defect in infertile brothers, both of whom carried a balanced t(5;12). It may be that a "flagellum gene" at one of the breakpoints was compromised.

Normal Karyotype. Among infertile men whose karyotype is normal, and whose sperm count is abnormally low, there is an increase in the sperm aneuploidy/diploidy rate, with the sex chromosomes being the most prone to exhibit disomy (Shi and Martin 2001). This effect is more apparent in those men with severe oligospermia, and in those aged 40 years or older (Asada et al. 2000). Vegetti et al. (2000) assessed the influence of sperm count and motility, and showed that both these indices correlate with the frequency of sperm disomy, testing chromosomes 13, 18, 21, X, and Y. The observations at testicular biopsy in men with severe oligoasthenozoöspermia support this interpretation, with univalents or oligochiasmatic and achiasmatic bivalents frequently being seen (Egozcue et al. 2000). Men with severe sperm indices may have a slight increase in sex chromosome abnormalities in peripheral blood (as a representative somatic tissue), when a very large number (1,000) of cells are studied; and this may suggest a more generalized vulnerability of cell division, both meiotic and mitotic (De Palma et al. 2005). As for men with actual azoöspermia, in whom sperm can be obtained only by testicular or epididymal biopsy or aspiration, the data on fairly small numbers also show elevated disomy rates for some autosomes and the X and Y chromosomes (Martin et al. 2000; Burrello et al. 2002; Palermo et al. 2002; Gianaroli et al. 2005, Vozdova et al. 2012).

CONSIDERATIONS RELATING TO IN VITRO FERTILIZATION

It was reasonable to have imagined that IVF-conceived babies might be more likely to suffer a chromosomal abnormality, given the artificial circumstances of their conception, and in particular being aware of the increased rate of abnormality in the sperm of oligospermic men (Pang et al. 1999; Griffin et al. 2003; Silber et al. 2003). But the observation is of little, if any, such risk. One of the largest and most stringent studies addressing this question comes from Australia, in which 6,946 IVF babies born in the period 1991–2004 were compared with 20,838 controls (Halliday et al. 2010). The rate of chromosome abnormality in the IVF babies was 0.99%, compared with 0.97% in the non-IVF babies. Among chromosome abnormalities evident at birth (thus excluding some mosaics and sex chromosome imbalances), the respective rates were 0.69% and 0.80%. (Interestingly, the only category of malformation for which a statistically significant increase was discerned for IVF was in respect of "defects of blastogenesis," comprising a group of typically severe abnormalities which arise in the first 4 weeks postconception.)

Other studies have examined the issue of ICSI versus standard IVF, and there is a suggestion that a difference in chromosomal risk, albeit small, might exist. Possibly, the risks for (*a*) sex chromosomal aneuploidy and (*b*) de novo structural rearrangement may be increased in the children of severely oligospermic men (who will of course have needed ICSI to achieve conception). In a large French study (Bonduelle et al. 2002), documenting an 11-year experience comprising 1,586 ICSI pregnancies in which prenatal diagnosis had been done, de novo structural aberrations and sex chromosome anomalies were seen in 1.6% (cf. 0.5% in the general population). These comprised 10 sex chromosome aneuploidies (XXY, XXX, XYY, and X mosaicisms) and seven structural rearrangements (mostly *apparently* balanced translocations), along with eight cases of autosomal aneuploidy (mostly trisomies 18 and 21). All the gonosomal cases involved the father being severely oligospermic, and this male factor, rather than the ICSI procedure of itself, may have been the basis for the increase; the abnormality rate (gonosomal and autosomal) in children of men with sperm counts >20 million per milliliter was only 0.24%. We may conclude that an additional risk of chromosomal abnormality for children conceived from ICSI is marginal and may apply only in the case of men with very low sperm counts.

Karyotyping of the oligospermic man is prudently to be done before proceeding to ICSI (Bonduelle et al. 2002; Griffin et al. 2003). Bofinger et al. (1999) provided ICSI to a couple, the husband having severe oligospermia, and the wife being of older childbearing age. At amniocentesis, on the grounds of the mother's age, a 45,X/46,X,r(Y) chromosome constitution was discovered, and belatedly, the same karyotype was found in the father. The experience of Veld et al. (1997) is equally telling, concerning two men who both, having suffered reproductive misfortune following ICSI, turned out to have a Robertsonian translocation.

Epigenetic Effects. Fertilization occurring in vitro is occurring in an artificial environment. It may be that the delicate interplay whereby the epigenetic reprogramming of chromosomes is applied, according to parent of origin, is vulnerable in this artificial setting (De Rycke et al. 2002); and the question arises that children born from IVF could be at increased risk for an imprinting disorder (Amor and Halliday 2008). This is indeed the case with respect to Beckwith-Wiedemann syndrome due to epigenetic error, perhaps more so in the case of ICSI having been employed, and the risk is fivefold that of the general population (Vermeiden and Bernardus 2013). There is likely also a significant association between the incidence of Russell-Silver syndrome and IVF/ICSI, but the number of published cases is small. The case for Angelman syndrome is rather more tenuous: Vermeiden and Bernardus noted that between 2002 and 2012 there were just seven cases of Angelman syndrome with methylation errors born to couples with fertility problems; four were born after ICSI treatment and three after hormonal treatment, or in families with a history of fertility problems. Nevertheless, the fact of these cases all being the category of epigenetic error, and given the rarity of this type, must raise a valid concern. Equally, the statistical weight of the thousands of unaffected IVF children is not to be discounted, and this points to a low absolute level of risk.

Genetics and Pathogenesis of Hydatidiform Mole

Hydatidiform mole is an abnormal pregnancy that can be considered, in a sense, as a male chromosomal disorder (Petignat et al. 2003; Slim and Mehio 2007). Typically, there is either a completely paternal karyotypic origin (two haploid paternal sets, $2n = 46$) or an additional male haploid set (two paternal and one maternal haploid sets, $3n = 69$). The presence of two paternal chromosomal complements is referred to as "diandry." The chorionic villi undergo a degenerative change, forming fluid-filled sacs (hence *hydatidiform*; *mole* means mass). The characteristic appearance has long been recognized (Fig. 19–9). The phenotype is marked ("complete mole") when the genetic origin is completely paternal, and attenuated ("partial mole") in the presence of a maternal haploid contribution. Most cases are sporadic, but a specific genetic cause in rare recurrent cases may be maternal homozygosity for a predisposing gene.

COMPLETE MOLE

In the complete mole, there is placental tissue—swollen chorionic villi—but typically no embryo identified. The usual karyotype is 46,XX, looking, at first sight, like a normal female karyotype. This is due, in most, to a doubling (endoreduplication) of the chromosomal complement of a single 23,X sperm, while a minority are dispermic. In either case, there is no maternal chromosomal contribution. With the mole's nuclear genome being of entirely paternal origin, there is a total uniparental paternal disomy ("uniparental diploidy"). Moles due to doubling of a sperm chromosomal complement are entirely homozygous; in other words, they have a complete uniparental isodisomy. Complete

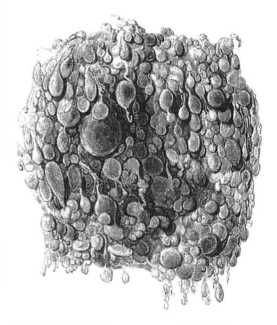

FIGURE 19–9 The appearance of hydatidiform mole, quite probably the first recorded depiction (Baillie 1799).

mole occurs more often at the beginning and end of reproductive life in the female: It is more common in the early teenager and in women in their forties (Bagshawe and Lawler 1982). Some diandric triploid molar pregnancies, when presenting earlier in pregnancy (before 8 weeks), may present a complete molar phenotype rather than the partial mole usually observed (Zaragoza et al. 2000).[17] A small minority of moles have a biparental diploid genotype, one causative factor of which may be maternal homozygosity or heterozygosity for mutation in the *NLRP7* gene, or rarely, homozygosity for *KHDC3L* (Qian et al. 2011; Slim et al. 2011; Nguyen et al. 2018). The *NLRP7* gene has a role in the acquisition of genomic imprinting as the ovum is produced, and it may also contribute to the ovum's safeguarding against polyspermy.

The original explanation was that this endoreduplication of the sperm's chromosomal complement represented an attempted correction following fertilization of an "effectively empty egg"—that is, an egg lacking a viable maternal pronucleus. This construction was challenged, and Golubovsky (2003) doubted the existence of the empty egg. He proposed instead a schema whereby diploidization (a sort of "triploid rescue") in very early mitoses follows a dispermic triploid conception and generates $2n$ cell lines. If it is the maternal complement which is discarded in each cell (perhaps just two cells, following the first mitosis), the genotype is androgenetic: A mole follows.

The complete mole typically presents either at early ultrasonography with a "snowstorm" pattern of the placenta on ultrasonography, reflecting the swollen villi, or at first or second trimester vaginal bleeding. There is a widespread and marked hyperplasia of the trophoblast. Where diagnosis is made early, and curettage performed, some nonchorionic elements (yolk sac, capillaries, amnion) may be identifiable, and very occasionally, embryonic parts (Zaragoza et al. 1997; Petignat et al. 2003). Immunostaining for the p57 KIP2 protein (the *p57 KIP2* gene being paternally imprinted) is a useful marker to discriminate between complete (staining-absent) and partial (staining-present) mole (Sebire and Lindsay 2006). The incidence of complete mole is about 1 in 1,500 diagnosed pregnancies, although regional/ethnic variations exist (Slim and Mehio 2007). In Japan, the incidence has apparently been falling, from about 1 in 400 in the 1970s to 1 in 650 by the late 1990s (Matsui et al. 2003).

There is a small but significant risk of recurrence following one mole, the risk increasing if a woman has had more than one. Recurrences can be of either kind of mole, complete or partial. In a subset of patients, recurrent complete mole is unusual in being diploid and biparental, and as noted above, the *NLRP7* gene has been implicated.

PARTIAL MOLE

An additional paternal haploid chromosome set is the basis of most cases of partial mole. This is triploidy, 69,XXX or 69,XXY (rarely 69,XYY), which may typically be the result of a normal ovum fertilized either with two sperm (dispermy) or with a diploid sperm, although other more complex scenarios are proposed (Zaragoza et al. 2000; Rosenbusch 2008).[18]

Partial moles typically present as threatened, incomplete, or missed abortion, during the late first or early second trimester, the mean at 12 weeks. There is hydatidiform change of some villi, and the placenta is abnormally large. It is underdiagnosed, and it may occur in as many as 1 in 700 pregnancies (a figure Jeffers et al. [1993] derive from a review of all 2,251 spontaneous abortions occurring in the catchment population of a Dublin hospital over a 3-year period during which there were 19,457 recorded pregnancies). Fetal development, in the very few cases proceeding far enough for this to be assessed, is characterized by a relatively normal growth pattern (McFadden et al. 1993). There appears to be little difference clinically between fetal development in 69,XXX and 69,XXY; the rare 69,XYY form has an earlier lethality (McWeeney et al. 2009). If the triploidy is confined to the placenta, and the fetal karyotype is normal, the pregnancy may proceed

---

17 A rare—or rarely recognized—scenario is that of confined placental mosaicism for molar and normal tissue, the infant being normal (Deveault et al. 2009). Photographs of the placenta in one such case give an obvious visual illustration of the mosaicism (Makrydimas et al. 2002). A possible mechanism is that the sperm underwent an inappropriate mitotic division to give two male pronuclei in the zygote, one of which fused with the female pronucleus (to give the cell leading to the normal child), and the other underwent endoreduplication (to produce a cell that gave the molar component). Or this may simply be the end result of chaotic mosaicism in the first few mitoses, with the two surviving cell lines happening one to be normal, and the other androgenetic.

18 Very uncommonly, partial mole has a normal diploid karyotype, with biparental inheritance. One very rare association is with large autosomal trisomy, such as trisomy for almost all of chromosome 4 (Fritz et al. 2000).

through to the late second or early third trimester, but the outlook for the infant is often dire (Sarno et al. 1993; Kawasaki et al. 2016).

Recurrences are on record, and a possible explanation is a genetically determined weakness in the zona pellucida of the ovum, which should act (the "zona reaction") to prevent more than one sperm penetrating. The double paternal contribution (diandry) is referred to as type I triploidy. Some cases of recurrence might reflect the effect of maternal homozygosity or heterozygosity for the *NLRP7* and *KHDC3L* genes, as discussed above. The fact that repeating moles can, in some cases, be of either type, partial or complete, is consistent with the proposition above due to Golubovsky (2003), that (perhaps maternally predisposed) early mitotic diploidization might be a mechanism to lead to either type.

Placental Mesenchymal Dysplasia. A possible clinical confounder, in that it rather resembles partial mole, but with apparently normal (or nearly so) fetal morphogenesis, is placental mesenchymal dysplasia (Ang et al. 2009; Faye-Petersen and Kapur 2013). This is a form of mosaicism. The placenta is, in part, normal, and this part has a biparental (and diploid) genotype. The dysplastic part is also diploid, but of paternal uniparental origin. Fetal growth may be affected; a number have been associated with Beckwith-Wiedemann syndrome (Wilson et al. 2008; Jalil et al. 2009). The pathogenetic process, at least in the majority, occurs in the zygote, as the first mitosis gets underway, and lies in a failure of replication of the maternal chromosomal complement, while the paternal complement replicates normally. One paternal complement then joins with the maternal complement to form a biparental cell; the other paternal complement undergoes endoreduplication and produces a uniparental (androgenetic) cell. These two cells then give rise to mosaicism with two lineages, the biparental lineage substantially going on to form the fetus, and the androgenetic lineage responsible for the dysplastic component of the placenta. Intrauterine or neonatal death is a frequent outcome.

GENETIC COUNSELING

Recurrent Miscarriage

People who have had one or perhaps two miscarriages generally do not come to a genetic clinic, and neither, as a rule, do they have cytogenetic analysis of the products of conception, or an analysis of their own karyotypes. Their physician or obstetrician may have advised them that this loss will very likely be part of the 15% or so of all pregnancies that miscarry, and the chance of a successful pregnancy in the future would be good. But having had three miscarriages requires investigation (although others propose testing at an earlier stage; see next paragraph). To use the jargon, such couples have had multiple abortions, recurrent miscarriage, or recurrent pregnancy loss (or to put it in Latin, *abortus habitualis*). The usual gynecological investigations, and a chromosome analysis of the couple, should be done at this point. If a chromosomal rearrangement is identified, this will probably be the underlying cause, but the possibility of a fortuitous discovery is not to be discounted. The precise nature of the rearrangement (consult the appropriate chapter), the reproductive history of any others in the family who have it, and the presence or absence of gynecological pathology allow one to make of judgment of its role in the etiology of the abortions. In the case of recurrent abortion due to a parent being a translocation carrier, Munné et al. (2000b) report that PGD can very substantially reduce the incidence of abortion, and "translocation couples" may wish to consider this option.

The majority of couples will have a normal karyotype, 46,XX and 46,XY. In most centers, cytogenetic analysis of abortus material (an expensive and time-consuming procedure) is not routinely done, and so chromosomal normality or abnormality cannot usually be demonstrated. Some have argued that this policy should shift, and Stephenson et al. (2002) speak of "this unfortunate omission" compromising the management of couples presenting with recurrent miscarriage. For women in their late thirties, who have already had miscarriages, trisomy is the major underlying cause; analysis of products of conception can be useful in offering advice to these women, in that the actual cause can now be known, when trisomy is discovered (Marquard et al. 2010). Since the discovery of an aneuploidy can avoid the necessity for further investigation, Stephenson et al. argue that routine karyotyping would actually be cost-effective and have the further benefit of helping couples understand, and thus come to terms with, their reproductive failure, as Sánchez et al. (1999) have also suggested. Wou et al. (2016a) propose that a quantitative fluorescence polymerase chain reaction (QF-PCR) assay containing markers on chromosomes 13, 18, 21, X, and Y applied to uncultured abortus tissue would enable a relatively inexpensive screen, followed by array-CGH analysis performed on the normal QF-PCR specimens. As for molecular methodology, the question of copy number variants (CNVs) arises, and Sahoo et al. (2017) identified a variant of uncertain significance in 2% of a large series of miscarriages. These CNVs were considered as incidental discoveries, but they were noted on the patient record as being possibly helpful in subsequent counseling for future pregnancies.

A miscarriage due to aneuploidy actually implies a lower risk for miscarriage of a subsequent pregnancy than if the abortus is euploid. However, a previous aneuploid miscarriage may elevate somewhat the risk for subsequent aneuploidy at prenatal diagnosis. IVF with PGD could benefit some women who have had several miscarriages, which might reduce the risk of another miscarriage. Recurrent implantation failure (which could be seen, in a sense, as a very early form of miscarriage) is often due to chromosomal aneuploidy; in that case, PGD may be useful (Vialard et al. 2008).

Sperm chromosome study is not often done, but Kohn et al. (2016) discuss the counseling issues that arise when seeing couples with recurrent miscarriage, when this may have been related to identified sperm aneuploidies in the male partner.

FETAL DEATH IN UTERO

Pregnancy loss in mid-trimester is less frequent than in the first trimester, and some may thus see a lower threshold for karyotyping the products of conception. In this case, Howarth et al. (2002) propose offering chorionic villus sampling or amniocentesis, rather than attempting culture of fetal tissue post delivery, in order to improve the chances of getting a definite chromosomal result. Compared to karyotype analysis, microarray analysis provides about a 40% increase in the detection of pathogenic abnormalities following stillbirth (Reddy et al. 2012).

WOMEN OF OLDER CHILDBEARING AGE

Maternal age is an important factor in recurrent miscarriage. The meiotic apparatus of the oöcyte deteriorates with age; returning to Figure 3–7, the reader can marvel at the disposition of the chromosomes in the eggs of the older women and appreciate how perfectly plausible it is that egg after egg could be aneuploid. The evidence from IVF points to a sharply increasing likelihood for aneuploid conception in women of older childbearing age. One cannot distinguish, just on the basis of history, which older couples are destined to experience reproductive misfortune. The counselor needs to recognize that many in this situation will go on to have successful pregnancies, but retaining quite some reservation that the risk may be "significant," and perhaps "substantial," for women who are getting into their late thirties or forties. For some, with concern that their reproductive years may be limited, IVF with PGD may seem an attractive option, but advice will need to be tempered by the evolving understanding of pregnancy outcomes from PGD for aneuploidy screening in this setting.

Infertility

Infertility is common, and, in Western countries at least, approximately 15% of couples wishing to have a child are affected (Foresta et al. 2002). Intrinsic fertility cannot be restored in men with persistent azoöspermia associated with seminiferous tubule failure, and neither in women who have had ovarian failure. The counselor will need to understand how disappointing and indeed devastating this may be to some couples (sometimes one of them more than the other) and to be prepared to deal with this. Those for whom assisted reproductive technology may offer hope need to be well aware that this is not necessarily an easy path, and neither can success be guaranteed.

Among the catalog of investigative tests that are available, a karyotype is well up on the list. A grouping of experts from the Italian professional community addressed the question of what tests should be done and when (Foresta et al. 2002). They propose that karyotyping should routinely be done in men with azoöspermia and oligospermia; and in the United Kingdom, karyotyping of men presenting for ICSI is "commonplace" (Griffin et al. 2003). Yq microdeletions should be checked for in men with nonobstructive azoöspermia and severe oligospermia, but this is unlikely to be the cause in lesser degrees of oligospermia (>5–10 million/ml) (Foresta et al. 2002; Quilter et al. 2003). Sperm karyotyping is not routinely practiced as a basis for informing genetic counseling.

Karyotyping should be routine in women presenting with primary ovarian dysfunction or recurrent miscarriage. Fragile X premutation analysis should be proposed in women with premature ovarian failure (Streuli et al. 2009); a consideration here is the requirement for informed consent, given the other genetic implications of making this diagnosis. Papanikolaou et al. (2005) pose the question, Is chromosome analysis mandatory in the initial investigation of normovulatory women seeking infertility treatment?—and answer in the negative. In other words, and having reviewed more than 1,000 infertile women with normal ovulatory cycles, the number and type of chromosome abnormalities detected differed scarcely from a normal neonatal population. A greater return came from karyotyping in women with secondary infertility.[19]

INFERTILITY WITH PARENTAL CHROMOSOMES ABNORMAL

If a chromosomal defect is discovered in one or other of the couple, this at least provides an explanation for the infertility and (according to the exact nature of the defect) may prevent the disappointment of undergoing pointless further investigation. In some, artificial reproductive technology may enable a normal/balanced gamete to be identified and retrieved, and used at IVF. Where this is impossible, artificial insemination or IVF using donor gametes offers an entrée to parenthood, and it may enable one of the couple to be a genetic parent.

Women. In women with a sex chromosomal abnormality having oöcyte donation, endocrinological management may be necessary to "prime" the reproductive tract (Devroey et al. 1988). But if the internal anatomy is intact, success may well follow, as is rather notably illustrated by the patient reported in Chen et al. (2003b), who had a Turner syndrome variant due to an isodicentric X, and who produced triplets following donation. In some cases, the woman's own mother, with whom of course she shares half her genes, has been the donor; sisters may also be willing. Artificially stimulated ovulation has been attempted in one case of a chromosomal state associated with secondary amenorrhea. Causio et al. (2000) describe a 29-year-old woman with a 46,X,t(X;16) karyotype, who had undergone premature ovarian failure, and in whom ovulation was then achieved by treatment with gonadotropin-releasing hormone and follicle-stimulating hormone (GnRH and FSH). But no pregnancy resulted.

Men. In men with complete spermatogenic arrest, gamete donation may be considered, and a brother or father might be willing. In those in whom the chromosome defect leads to oligospermia, rather than complete failure of spermatogenesis, IVF with ICSI is a possible means to achieve pregnancy, and PGD will often be appropriate. Otherwise, given the small increased risk for gonosomal aneuploidy following ICSI, a subsequent conventional prenatal diagnosis may appropriately be offered. *Translocations* and other rearrangements need to be assessed on their merits. A small (but growing) number of cases of fatherhood in men with *Klinefelter syndrome* have resulted from ICSI (p. 345). *Rare sex chromosome* abnormalities are judged individually. For example, a sperm study in the case of a man with sex chromosomal mosaicism (45,X/47,XYY), which gave normal findings, was instrumental in a decision not to have preimplantation diagnosis following an ICSI conception (Dale et al. 2002).

In the case of a *Yq microdeletion*, couples choosing the option of IVF with ICSI should know that a male child would be predicted to have, very probably, the same type of infertility (Foresta et al. 2001). Some might consider having PGD to ensure having a daughter; although Kim et al. (1998) comment that "interestingly, after genetic counseling, the decision to proceed with ICSI for the overwhelming majority of couples remains unchanged." Nap et al. (1999) assessed 28 such couples, and they interviewed the 10 counselors who had seen them, in six clinics in the Netherlands and in Belgium. A considerable majority of couples (79%) chose to continue with plans for ICSI, with only a few choosing donor insemination (7%) or opting out altogether (14%).

INFERTILITY WITH PARENTAL CHROMOSOMES NORMAL

Where the male has oligospermia, and if IVF with ICSI is to be attempted, there are the grounds (discussed earlier) for presuming a very slightly increased risk for de novo structural aberration or gonosomal aneuploidy. It may be prudent to offer prenatal diagnosis for an ICSI-produced pregnancy. However, given the immense investment couples will have made to achieve the pregnancy, there may be reservation about proceeding to an invasive prenatal diagnostic procedure, even being aware of a

---

19 Secondary infertility refers to a couple having previously had a successful pregnancy, but who are currently unable to conceive.

possibly increased genetic risk. In a German population, Meschede et al. (1998b) reported that only 17% of a cohort of 107 women having undergone ICSI chose subsequent amniocentesis, the great majority preferring noninvasive ultrasonography or serum screening. This preference was more marked in those who had had genetic counseling prior to entering the ICSI program. In contrast, an Italian clinic recounted a very opposite figure, with 86% choosing invasive prenatal diagnosis (and 100% choosing ultrasound screening); these workers could see "no logical explanation for the great difference" (Monni et al. 1999). Noninvasive prenatal testing of cell-free DNA in maternal blood is an attractive alternative to an invasive procedure in this setting.

The known or suspected risks for an imprinting disorder (Beckwith-Wiedemann syndrome, Russell-Silver syndrome, and Angelman syndrome, as discussed above) in IVF-conceived children raise a question that it may be prudent to advise couples of these concerns, according to the accumulating understanding of these risks, and the availability and reliability of prenatal testing for methylation defects at imprinted loci. Counselors working in the IVF clinic will want to maintain a watching brief.

IN VITRO FERTILIZATION CONSIDERATIONS

Chromosomally Abnormal Children Following Pregnancy by Donor Insemination. If a pregnancy achieved through gamete donation turns out to be chromosomally abnormal, should that donor continue to be used? Kuller et al. (2001) surveyed a number of reproductive endocrinologists and obstetrical geneticists to determine the current practice, with particular reference to trisomy 21 and monosomy X. It was clear that no consistent policy was followed. For chromosomal abnormalities generally regarded as being sporadic (or where any predisposition might reside in the recipient rather than the donor), it would seem unnecessary to remove that donor from the panel.

In Vitro Fertilization and Multiple Pregnancy. Twinning and higher multiple pregnancies are common in IVF, for the obvious reason that more than one embryo may be transferred following IVF, this being a standard policy in some centers, in order to improve the chances for a successful implantation. The more conservative number of transfers is two, so that if both embryos do implant, no more than twins will result (unless a single embryo might go on to produce monozygous twins). Some clinics transfer more, sometimes for the simple economic reason that if couples can only afford one IVF cycle and transfer, using three (or even more) embryos increases the chance of pregnancy. The disadvantage is, of course, that if most or all of the embryos implant, a high multiple pregnancy results. Whatever might be the risk for aneuploidy,[20] that risk will apply to each embryo individually, thus increasing the overall risk that one at least might be chromosomally abnormal. If both abnormal and normal fetuses are present, and diagnosed at subsequent amniocentesis, selective feticide of the chromosomally abnormal fetus may be chosen, or for a lethal aneuploidy (trisomy 13, trisomy 18) the parents may opt to continue the pregnancy in the expectation that the abnormal fetus will die (Sebire et al. 1997). One of the claims made for PGD is that single embryo transfers—which many IVF clinics view as a desideratum—can be done with a better expectation of success, and a twin pregnancy avoided.

Hydatidiform Mole

The risk of recurrence in a subsequent pregnancy is approximately 1% (Garrett et al. 2008), and recurrence can be either of the same (complete or partial) or of the other type. Ultrasonographic surveillance is advisable in a future pregnancy. Having had a second mole, the risk for a third is considerably higher, on the order of 20% (Berkowitz et al. 1994).

A few of the single cases, but possibly most of the multiple recurrences, may be due to maternal homozygosity for mutation in the *NLRP7* or *KHDC3L* gene. These repeating cases typically show biparental inheritance, in contradistinction to the androgenetic basis of the majority of moles. Fisher et al. (2000) suggest that parental origin is worth establishing in those couples who might have been considering IVF with ICSI (to ensure entry of a single sperm), or PGD for ploidy diagnosis, as a means to diminish the risk in a subsequent pregnancy, since such approaches would be futile if the mole(s) had

---

20 If donor eggs are used, it is the age of the donating woman that counts in determining the age-related aneuploidy risk.

been biparental. In these cases, ovum donation offers the best chance for parenthood, although spontaneous normal pregnancy, while very rare, is not unknown (Akoury et al. 2015).

A major aspect of management is that the mole may undergo neoplastic transformation (gestational trophoblastic disease). With *complete mole*, the risk for the development of invasive mole is approximately 15%, and for the more dangerous choriocarcinoma, it is 3%. The risks are much less with *partial mole*, the respective figures being 0.5% and 0.1% (Seckl et al. 2000). These facts need to be borne in mind by those women choosing to attempt a further pregnancy.

We are unaware of any reports of recurrence of placental mesenchymal dysplasia.

20

PRENATAL TESTING PROCEDURES

THE MEANS to diagnose the fetal karyotype provides medical cytogenetics with one of its major areas of application. The discovery of an abnormality allows the option of termination of the pregnancy or, later in gestation, a more suitable obstetric management. The main indications for prenatal cytogenetic diagnosis are the following: (1) the pregnant woman being of older childbearing age, (2) parental heterozygosity for a chromosome rearrangement, (3) the birth of a previous child with a chromosome defect, (4) increased risk on maternal screening test, and (5) fetal anomaly detected on ultrasonography.

PRENATAL LABORATORY DIAGNOSTIC PROCEDURES

Prenatal diagnosis (PND) of chromosome disorders was first widely performed from the early 1970s, by the culturing of amniotic fluid cells obtained from amniocentesis at approximately 16 weeks of pregnancy, and analyzed according to classical methodology. A number of other approaches to PND have

since been developed, ranging from preimplantation genetic diagnosis (following in vitro fertilization), through chorion villus sampling (CVS), to the testing of cell-free DNA in maternal plasma.

Naturally, parents-to-be are anxious to have results as early as possible. A desire for an early result needs to be balanced against a number of considerations, which can include complexity of the procedure, both clinically and in the laboratory; procedural complication; reliability of results; cost; and the prior risk for a fetal abnormality. Four particular analytical procedures have enabled a faster return of results for common aneuploidies, compared with classical cytogenetics, namely FISH, QF-PCR, MLPA, and microarray analysis (and see also Chapter 2).

FLUORESCENCE IN SITU HYBRIDIZATION

Fluorescence in situ hybridization (FISH) using multiple colored probes and targeting the chromosomes most prone to survivable aneuploidy (13, 18, 21, X, and Y) bypasses the need for culture, whether the cells are from amniotic fluid or CVS, and the result can be given within the space of one working day (Morris et al. 1999). By way of example, in one small series with particular reference to the third trimester, Aviram-Goldring et al. (1999) showed an aneuploidy in 23% of pregnancies with intrauterine growth retardation and structural abnormalities: five with trisomy 21 and two with trisomy 18. Feldman et al. (2000) similarly applied amniotic fluid cell FISH to high-risk pregnancies (that is, with ultrasonographic abnormalities). They detected 14 cases of trisomy 21, 10 of trisomy 18, three of trisomy 13, four of monosomy X, and one triploid, in 4,193 samples over the period 1996–1998, for a total abnormality rate of 11%.

The question arises of false-negative results. Weremowicz et al. (2001) reviewed their experience over 1992–2000, during which time they applied FISH (using probes for 13, 18, 21, X, and Y) to approximately 8% of the 11,000 amniocentesis samples coming into their laboratory for routine karyotyping, this 8% including cases with an increased risk (abnormalities on ultrasound, serum screen result). In the whole material, of 89 potentially detectable abnormalities, 75 (84%) were found. The missed cases included eight with an inconclusive result, one with no result, and—more important—five false negatives. Of these latter five, the true karyotypes were trisomy 18 (two cases) and trisomy 21 (three cases). Technical problems related to poor hybridization efficiency (e.g., low copy number of the DNA repeats being probed) and maternal blood contamination of the fluid sample were plausible explanations.

As have others, Weremowicz et al. (2001) note the usefulness of the FISH approach in being able to provide a rapid answer, particularly when there are grounds for suspecting an abnormality, or if the pregnancy is more advanced; but they also emphasize the need for careful counseling so that patients are aware of the limitations. With respect to trisomy 21, Witters et al. (2002) had an encouraging record: In a similar study comprising 5,049 amniotic fluid samples, in which interphase FISH was applied in parallel with conventional karyotyping, all 70 cases of trisomy 21 were detected, and no

false-positive result arose. One false positive is on record, however, probably due to technical aspects of probe hybridization (George et al. 2003). On the question of mosaicism, Van Opstal et al. (2001) note that FISH on uncultured cells may provide a more accurate picture than on cultured cells, the latter possibly being subject to selective pressure in vitro and the abnormal cells more prone to fail in culture. On the other hand, the class of amniocyte that grows preferentially in culture (namely amniotic mesoderm) might, according to the reinterpretation of Robinson et al. (2002), more closely reflect the true embryonic state.

Focused FISH can be applied in specific circumstances. The ultrasound discovery of a cardiac outflow tract abnormality would, for example, point to the need for 22q11 analysis. A rapid diagnosis is particularly to be desired in the setting of parental heterozygosity for a chromosome rearrangement in which there may be a high risk for abnormality, and FISH can provide this. Thus, Cotter and Musci (2001) used subtelomeric probes for 5pter, 5qter, and 14qter to enable rapid diagnosis for a pregnant woman with the karyotype 46,XX,t(5;14)(p14.2;p13), she having had a previous child with cri du chat syndrome. Similarly, Pettenati et al. (2002) applied this approach in the circumstance of parental heterozygosity for a number of reciprocal and Robertsonian translocations.

FISH tests only that segment of the chromosome to which the probe binds. Inferentially, the complete chromosome is present; but this is not necessarily so. With chromosome 18, it is the centromere which the FISH probe recognizes. We have seen a case in which amniocentesis was done on the basis of a maternal age of 40 years, albeit that the risks based on serum screening were lowered for age (trisomy 21, 1 in 164; trisomy 18, 1 in 8,030). FISH showed three chromosome 18 signals. Fetal growth and morphology on ultrasonography were normal. The couple considered whether they might request termination, but wanted to await the result of karyotyping. This showed a supernumerary minute marker—barely a speck—which appeared to comprise only chromosome 18 centromere: The karyotype was 47,XX,+mar.ish der(18)(D18Z1+) dn[13]/46,XX[4] (case of M. D. Pertile). The pregnancy continued. The child subsequently born was 3 years old at most recent contact, and while she manifested a familial shortness, her cognitive and personality development were entirely normal (S. Fawcett, personal communication, 2010).

QUANTITATIVE FLUORESCENCE POLYMERASE CHAIN REACTION

Quantitative fluorescence polymerase chain reaction (QF-PCR) relies on the use of molecular markers that display a high level of heterozygosity, such that the presence of three alleles—that is, a trisomy—can reliably be detected. Similarly to FISH, when compared to karyotyping, QF-PCR has the advantages of lower cost, shorter turnaround of results, and lower technical complexity. The major disadvantage is that QF-PCR will only identify common aneuploidies: Most deletions and duplications, along with balanced rearrangements, will not be detected. Cirigliano et al. (2009) assessed the relative performances of QF-PCR (for chromosomes 13, 18, 21, X, and Y) and karyotyping in a series of 43,000 amniocentesis samples tested over a 9-year period. The QF-PCR assay detected 95% of all clinically relevant chromosome abnormalities, and there were no false-positive results. In a smaller study, de la Paz-Gallardo et al. (2015) suggested that if karyotyping were restricted to samples where there was an ultrasound abnormality, and QF-PCR were used for lower risk samples, laboratory costs could be halved, with minimal reduction in the detection of clinically significant abnormalities. Nevertheless, viewed against noninvasive prenatal testing (see below), the advantages of QF-PCR become less compelling.

MULTIPLEX LIGATION-DEPENDENT PROBE ANALYSIS

Multiplex ligation-dependent probe analysis (MLPA) is a PCR-based assay that can combine probes to many chromosomal loci, and which again has the advantage of a short turnaround time (Schouten et al. 2002; Shaffer and Bui 2007). In a comparison with standard chromosome analysis of 4,585 amniocentesis specimens, MLPA had 100% sensitivity and specificity for identifying common aneuploidies, but it failed to pick up 26 other abnormalities that were detected by karyotyping, including 12 with potential clinical significance (Boormans et al. 2010). A targeted application enables the diagnosis of microdeletion syndromes that would otherwise escape detection (Konialis et al. 2011).

MICROARRAY

Chromosome microarrays have been used in prenatal diagnosis since the mid-2000s (Le Caignec et al. 2005; Rickman et al. 2006), but their use only became widespread after the publication in 2012 of two large prospective studies that demonstrated their superior diagnostic yield compared to conventional karyotyping (Shaffer et al. 2012; Wapner et al. 2012). Microarray analysis can be applied to CVS and amniocentesis samples, with or without prior culture. Results can be delivered within several days, although in practice it may take longer due to the efficiency benefits for laboratories afforded by "batching" samples. The additional diagnostic yield is greatest (~10%) in fetuses with multiple ultrasound abnormalities, but benefit is also apparent, at a level of approximately 1%, in lower-risk women, such as those of advanced maternal age. A possible drawback is that microarrays can show copy number variants (CNVs; Chapter 17), which may introduce an uncertainty into the diagnostic interpretation. In approximately 1% of tests, a variant of uncertain significance (VOUS) is found (Hillman et al. 2013); or, a CNV may be detected that is of reduced penetrance or that is associated with a range of phenotypes not able to be assessed in the prenatal setting.

PRENATAL DIAGNOSTIC CLINICAL PROCEDURES

BLASTOMERE DIAGNOSIS AT IN VITRO FERTILIZATION

This technique of "very early prenatal diagnosis" is reviewed in Chapter 22.

CHORIONIC VILLUS SAMPLING

Chorionic villus sampling (CVS) is typically a first-trimester procedure, the usual time being at 10–11 weeks gestation. The normal approach is transabdominal (transvaginal CVS was formerly used). The operator inserts a needle through the lower abdominal wall, under ultrasound guidance, to penetrate to the placental tissue; with gentle negative pressure on the syringe, a small amount of chorionic villus tissue is aspirated. (The expression "placental biopsy" could also be applied, although in practice this term is used when the testing is done in later pregnancy; see below). The earlier period of diagnosis permitted by CVS, compared with amniocentesis, may be seen as more useful in the setting of a higher genetic risk. If a genetic abnormality is identified, and abortion is chosen, this can be, prior to 14 weeks, a more private matter, and the termination procedure is an operative intervention (curettage or suction evacuation of the uterus) (Verp et al. 1988). There is potential in CVS for diagnostic difficulty due to the occasional detection of confined placental mosaicism (which may, for some chromosomes, carry a risk also for uniparental disomy). Nonmosaic results for the common aneuploidies are, however, highly reliable (Smith et al. 1999). In experienced hands, there is a high degree of safety (Brun et al. 2003): A meta-analysis concluded that the risk of procedure-related miscarriage in women who had undergone CVS was only 0.22% (approximately 1 in 500 procedures) (Akolekar et al. 2015).

Direct, Short-Term, and Long-Term Chorionic Villus Sampling. Chorionic villi can be analyzed directly (same day), after short-term culture (next day or two), or after long-term (a week or so) culture. For microarray analysis, uncultured cells are typically used as the source of DNA, but "backup" cultures are established that are available if the microarray fails or if a microarray finding requires additional confirmation. For karyotype analysis, most laboratories offer only long-term CVS, in which the mesenchymal core of the villus is the source of the analyzed cells. Trophoblast is the source of the cell population studied at direct and short-term CVS culture; these cells are no longer extant after the first few days in culture (and see color insert Fig. 21–1).

> In the early 1990s, there were disconcerting reports of an increased incidence of transverse limb deficiencies and tongue and jaw defects—"oromandibular-limb hypogenesis"—following early CVS (before 10 weeks, and especially up to 8 weeks). The association appeared likely to be causal, and one line of circumstantial evidence was that the rate of anomalies fell with increasing gestational stage from 9 to 11 weeks (Firth 1997). Various mechanisms were proposed: oligohydramnios, bradycardia, hypovolemia, thromboembolism, vasoconstriction, antibody-mediated reaction, and increased apoptosis following disruption of end arteries (Luijsterburg et al. 1997). Given these observations, it became normal practice for CVS not to be done earlier than 10 weeks.

AMNIOCENTESIS

Transabdominal amniocentesis, at about 15–17 weeks gestation, with culture of cells for chromosome analysis, has been the standard cytogenetic prenatal

diagnostic procedure since the 1970s. It has a high degree of safety to both mother and fetus: Maternal complications, or fetal injury due to direct trauma, are practically unknown. The risk for maternal Rhesus immunization (Rh-negative mother, Rh-positive fetus) can be circumvented by administering an antibody injection. In their meta-analysis, Akolekar et al. (2015) concluded that the risk of procedure-related miscarriage in women who had undergone amniocentesis was 0.11% (approximately 1 in 1,000 procedures). The cytogenetic results are very reliable. The biological sources of error are, first, that maternal rather than fetal cells, or a mixture of both, are sampled. In practical terms, this rarely causes a problem. Second, fetal mosaicism may go undetected, since only a limited number of cells can feasibly be examined. Very few examples of this error are recorded.

Amniotic fluid culture has a high success rate. Persutte and Lenke (1995) suggested that if amniotic cells fail to grow, for no obvious reason, there may be a substantial risk for fetal aneuploidy (13% of 32 cases in their preliminary study). This assessment was supported in a large systematic study from London (Reid et al. 1996), in which 42 failures (1%) among 4,134 amniocenteses were followed up. Complete information could be obtained on all but one of these 42 cases. Karyotyping was ultimately done in most (78%) of these failed cases, and of these, 19% revealed an abnormality (compared with a 4% abnormality rate in the whole material). The clear lesson from these studies is that women having had a failed amniocentesis culture should be offered careful review and retesting. Prior cell culture is not necessary for microarray analysis, but as with CVS, "backup" cultures may be established for use only if the microarray fails, or if an abnormal microarray result requires confirmation or additional analysis.

The obvious disadvantage of amniocentesis is that the results are not to hand until about 16–18 weeks. If the reason for the amniocentesis had been an abnormality on second-trimester ultrasound, the procedure may not be done until 18–20 weeks, aggravating this difficulty. The outlook for the long-term health of the child does not differ between CVS and amniocentesis (Schaap et al. 2002).

NONINVASIVE PRENATAL TESTING USING CELL-FREE DNA FROM MATERNAL BLOOD

Noninvasive prenatal testing (NIPT) for fetal aneuploidy detection, using cell-free DNA from maternal blood, has been implemented in the clinical setting since 2012. Although in reality NIPT is a screening test (some write NIPS) rather than a diagnostic test, in practical terms it is such a good test that we are considering it separately from other screening modalities.

Cell-free DNA (cfDNA) testing takes advantage of the fact that everyone has free DNA (i.e., not within the nucleus of cells) circulating in the bloodstream, and in pregnant women, a proportion of that DNA is derived from the fetus. Or more specifically, it is derived from the placenta, and in fact from apoptosing cells of the cytotrophoblast. This is the "fetal fraction" of the maternal sample, which typically comprises approximately 10% of the whole. cfDNA can be analyzed by massively parallel sequencing, using either whole genome analysis or by methods that target specific chromosomes, and can also be quantified by microarray (Stockowski et al. 2015). Although it is possible to distinguish fetal DNA from maternal DNA by analyzing single nucleotide polymorphisms (SNPs) within the cfDNA sample, most methodologies simply measure the total amount of DNA (i.e., maternal and fetal contribution) derived from each chromosome and compare each chromosome with other chromosomes within the sample.

For example, in a euploid pregnancy with fetal fraction of 10%, for each chromosome, the total amount of DNA is 90% maternal and 10% fetal. In the setting of a Down syndrome pregnancy, the fetal contribution from chromosome 21 increases by 50%, to 15%. The total DNA derived from chromosome 21, as measured in maternal blood, and compared to other chromosome in the sample, increases to 105% (90% maternal plus 15% fetal). The fact that such a small difference can be measured accurately is testament to the power of massively parallel sequencers as a molecular counting tool.

NIPT can also be used for the detection of aneuploidy in twin pregnancies, but the test failure rate is higher, and the detection rate may be lower than in singletons (Bevilacqua et al. 2015).

NIPT for the Common Trisomies. NIPT using cfDNA for trisomies 21, 13, and 18 has very high sensitivity and specificity (Table 20–1). A related, and possibly more relevant, measure of test accuracy

Table 20–1. Sensitivity and Specificity of NIPT for Common Aneuploidies

ANEUPLOIDY	SENSITIVITY	SPECIFICITY
Trisomy 21	0.994	0.999
Trisomy 18	0.977	0.999
Trisomy 13	0.906	1.000
Monsomy X	0.929	0.999

Source: The meta-analysis of Mackie et al. (2017).

is the positive predictive value (PPV), which equates to the proportion of women with an abnormal result who actually do have an aneuploid fetus. The PPV incorporates the pretest likelihood that the aneuploidy is present, and therefore increases with maternal age. Even when an NIPT test has very high sensitivity and specificity, in a young woman with low pretest risk of having an aneuploid fetus, the PPV for a rare aneuploidy such as trisomy 13 will be low. Estimates of PPV for common aneuploidies detected by NIPT, at different maternal ages, are presented in Table 20–2, and they serve as a useful reminder that high-risk NIPT results should always be followed up with an invasive test. Any decision to terminate a pregnancy should not be based upon positive NIPT results alone.

While early trials focused on women from high-risk groups, more recent studies have demonstrated the clinical utility of NIPT in low-risk and average-risk women. Although the use of NIPT in low-risk women is associated with a lower PPV than

Table 20–2. Positive Predictive Values of NIPT Results at Different Maternal Ages

	PPV (%) AT MATERNAL AGES			
ANEUPLOIDY	25 YEARS	30 YEARS	35 YEARS	40 YEARS
Trisomy 13	7	10	21	50
Trisomy 18	15	21	39	69
Trisomy 21	51	61	79	93

PPV, positive predictive value.
Source: The online calculator at http://secure.itswebs. com/nsgc/niptcalculator/index.html, and using test sensitivity and specificity from Gil et al. (2015).

is the case for higher-risk women, leading to more false-positive results, NIPT still outperforms conventional screening by a very considerable margin (Gregg et al. 2016).

NIPT for Other Trisomies. It is technically straightforward to expand NIPT to autosomes other than 13, 18, and 21, and in fact NIPT methods that use whole genome sequencing already collect the necessary sequencing data. But the clinical utility of this information is not clear. Whole chromosome aneuploidy, other than the three common aneuploidies, typically results in fetal loss, and detection of these abnormalities may lead to parental anxiety and unnecessary diagnostic procedures. That is not to say that the detection of these aneuploidies is without any clinical benefit. In rare instances, discovery of certain aneuploidies might have direct implication for the pregnancy, one example being the detection of trisomy 15 in cfDNA leading to the diagnosis of Prader-Willi syndrome due to uniparental disomy of chromosome 15 (Bayinder et al. 2015). Nevertheless, as of 2016, the American College of Medical Genetics and Genomics has recommended against screening for autosomal aneuploidies other than 13, 18, and 21 (Gregg et al. 2016).

NIPT for Sex Chromosome Aneuploidies. NIPT for sex chromosome aneuploidies has a detection rate of >90% and a PPV of approximately 50%, similarly to the other common aneuploidies (Gregg et al. 2016). But caution is required when applying NIPT. Sex chromosome aneuploidies are more common than autosomal, in one series being detected in 1 in 272 amniocentesis samples (Forabosco et al. 2009). Therefore, inclusion of sex chromosome aneuploidies in an NIPT test will result in an additional 1% of samples yielding a false-positive result, increasing considerably the overall number of invasive tests required. The phenotypes in the sex chromosome abnormalities are typically less severe than autosomal aneuploidies, and in some cases may not be clinically apparent (as discussed in the following chapter). Careful pretest counseling should accompany NIPT for sex chromosome abnormalities, and some pregnant women may choose to restrict testing to autosomal trisomies.

NIPT for Microdeletions, Microduplications, and Copy Number Variants. NIPT can be extended to detect microdeletions such as those of 1p36, 15q11q13, and 22q11.2. These microdeletions are associated with severe phenotypes, and on that basis, they are appropriate for prenatal screening. NIPT can detect microdel/dups with high sensitivity and low false-positive rate; but a concern is that as greater proportions of the genome are analyzed, false-positive results will accumulate, leading to unnecessary invasive tests (Gregg et al. 2016). Improved sequencing and analytical techniques may assuage this concern. Lefkowitz et al. (2016) retrospectively analyzed 1,166 NIPT samples, including 42 known to harbor CNVs: All but one of the 42 CNVs were detected, and there was only one false-positive result, attesting to the feasibility of whole genome CNV analysis using cfDNA.

False-Positive and False-Negative NIPT Results. Cell-free fetal DNA is, as noted above, placental in origin, and so NIPT by cfDNA shares the major pitfall of CVS, namely being susceptible to confined placental mosaicism (CPM; see Chapter 21). False-positive results due to CPM cannot be overcome by technical improvements (Brady et al. 2016). NIPT results are, in principle, concordant with the CVS finding, and thus amniocentesis may be necessary to confirm that the aneuploidy is (if this is the case) confined to the placenta. In the event that NIPT shows trisomy for an imprintable chromosome, testing for uniparental disomy should be considered, if amniocentesis is chosen.

Early and undetected co-twin demise, or *"vanished twin,"* may lead to a false-positive test result (Brady et al. 2016). Chromosome abnormalities are common in vanished twins, and the involuting placenta of an aneuploid vanished twin may continue to release aneuploid DNA into the maternal bloodstream for weeks after demise. Using an SNP-based technology to identify fetal haplotypes, Curnow et al. (2015) were able to identify haplotypes from a vanished twin in 0.18% of pregnancies tested, with fetal demise having occurred between 2 and 8 weeks prior to maternal blood sampling.

CNVs or mosaic aneuploidy in the mother may affect test interpretation. Unidentified maternal sex chromosome mosaicism (45,X/46,XX or 47,XXX/46,XX) is an important cause of false-positive NIPT results for sex chromosome abnormalities (Wang et al. 2014b). We have also found Y chromosome material in maternal DNA, which has led to a high-risk result for sex chromosome aneuploidy in the fetus. Less commonly, mosaicism in the mother for other chromosomes, or chromosome segments, can lead to false-positive NIPT results (Brady et al. 2016). If NIPT is extended to CNVs, the possibility of unidentified CNVs being present in the mother and detected by NIPT will need to be considered, both in pretest counseling and in interpretation of results.

A particularly devastating cause of aneuploidy detectable in cfDNA is *maternal malignancy.* Bianchi et al. (2015) identified 10 cases of occult malignancy from a series of 125,426 NIPT samples. Maternal malignancies were typically associated with a "tumor-like" aneuploidy profile, comprising copy number gains and losses across multiple chromosomes, a pattern that is unlikely to be mistaken for fetal aneuploidy.

Follow-Up Procedures Following Abnormal NIPT Results. Invasive testing is recommended to confirm a high-risk cfDNA finding, with CVS the preferred modality, in order to allow for a more timely return of results. In a minority of cases, the CVS result will be mosaic; and this will necessitate a second procedure, amniocentesis, in order to distinguish CPM from true fetal mosaicism. If mosaicism is likely, there is an argument for bypassing CVS and using amniocentesis as the first-line invasive test.

Grati et al. (2015) addressed this question by estimating the frequency with which a CVS, performed after a high-risk cfDNA result, would require a follow-up amniocentesis due to suspected placental mosaicism. The authors did not actually undertake cfDNA testing but, rather, modeled data based on results from more than 50,000 CVS karyotypes obtained from cytotrophoblast (direct preparation), mesenchyme (long-term culture), and followed by confirmatory amniocentesis. Central to this modeling was the assumption that the fetal fraction of cfDNA originates mainly from the cytotrophoblast layer of the chorionic villus; and so, as noted above, the cfDNA test result should be concordant with direct, rather than long-term, cultures. The findings, along with the likelihood of mosaic CVS results being confirmed by amniocentesis, are shown in Table 20–3. Based on these data, CVS is the recommended procedure following a high-risk cfDNA result for trisomy 21 or trisomy 18, but with the caveat of a 2%–4% risk of an inconclusive result, which would require a follow-up amniocentesis. For trisomy 13 and monosomy X, the benefit of an early diagnosis by CVS is to be balanced against the likelihood of an inconclusive result, with an amniocentesis then needed.

Table 20–3. Likelihood of Mosaicism at CVS Following High-Risk cfDNA Results for Common Aneuploidies, and Likelihood of Mosaicism at CVS Being Confirmed by Amniocentesis

ANEUPLOIDY	LIKELIHOOD THAT A HIGH-RISK cfDNA RESULT WILL BE FOLLOWED BY DETECTION OF MOSAICISM AT CVS	LIKELIHOOD THAT A MOSAIC CVS RESULT WILL BE CONFIRMED BY AMNIOCENTESIS
Trisomy 21	2%	44%
Trisomy 18	4%	14%
Trisomy 13	22%	4%
Monosomy X	59%	26%

CVS, chorion villus sampling.
Source: Grati et al. (2015).

EXPERIMENTAL, LESS USED, OR FORMER TECHNOLOGIES

POLAR BODY DIAGNOSIS AT IN VITRO FERTILIZATION

This technique of "very early prenatal diagnosis," indeed preconceptual diagnosis, is reviewed in Chapter 22.

BLASTOCOEL FLUID ANALYSIS

Fluid aspirated from the blastocyst, at the time of in vitro fertilization, contains DNA of embryonic origin and is analyzable by microarray. But an important degree of discordance between this analysis and the results from the inner cell mass led Tobler et al. (2015) to conclude that "using blastocoel fluid DNA for preimplantation genetic testing is not yet advised." On a similar bent, two groups have demonstrated that embryo-derived cfDNA is present in the culture media of blastocyst-stage embryos (Shamonki et al. 2016; Xu et al. 2016) and also that following whole genome amplification, this could, in principle, be used to perform "noninvasive" preimplantation genetic screening without the need for embryo biopsy.

EARLY AMNIOCENTESIS

In the late 1980s, early (10–13 weeks) amniocentesis was proposed as an alternative to CVS. In a carefully controlled comparison, Nicolaides et al. (1994) found a 2%–3% additional fetal loss rate in early amniocentesis and, possibly, a higher incidence of talipes among subsequently born children. Daniel et al. (1998), comparing 10–14 week procedures with 15 weeks and upward, observed that the early amniocentesis samples were not quite as satisfactory, multiple needle insertions were more often required, and the pregnancy loss rate was greater. On the whole, the differences were not great, other than the loss rate of 2.2% in the early group compared with 0.6% in the mid-trimester group. Similar figures were reported in Collins et al. (1998). In the Canadian Early and Midtrimester Amniocentesis Trial, the findings for 11wk 0d through to 13wk 6d were somewhat more disconcerting, with more complications, and a higher culture failure rate (Delisle and Wilson 1999). The procedure is rarely undertaken now.

FETAL BLOOD SAMPLING

Fetal blood is aspirated by direct puncture of a blood vessel, usually in the umbilical cord (cordocentesis). Before FISH analysis of uncultured cells (see above) came to be more widely used, cordocentesis was useful when speed of diagnosis was of the essence, in the setting of the detection of a fetal anomaly at ~18-week ultrasonography. The procedure once had a role in assisting resolution of mosaicism in amniotic fluid culture (Shalev et al. 1994), but this was largely replaced by the use of FISH.

PLACENTAL BIOPSY

In principle, this is the same as first-trimester CVS. The placenta is sampled by a transabdominal approach, and this is a straightforward procedure. The main application had been when a rapid result was needed, although newer methodologies have largely bypassed that imperative. An insufficient amount of amniotic fluid remains an indication.

FETAL CELL ISOLATION FROM MATERNAL BLOOD

In 1969, Walknowska et al. identified cells with a male karyotype during the cytogenetic analysis of lymphocyte cultures from pregnant women, and they recognized the potential to use these cells for prenatal diagnosis. The two important cell types that are released from the fetal tissue into the maternal circulation are the nucleated red blood cell and the trophoblast (Dhallan et al. 2007; Maron and Bianchi 2007). Fetal cells circulating in maternal blood are an obvious target for noninvasive prenatal diagnosis, yet with a concentration of only one fetal cell in each 2–3 ml of maternal blood (Kolvraa et al. 2016), their isolation is a considerable challenge. For this reason, cell-based NIPT approaches have fallen somewhat out of favor, particularly with the successful implementation of NIPT approaches that use cfDNA. Nonetheless, researchers continue to explore the potential of fetal cell-based techniques. Two groups have successfully isolated fetal trophoblasts by the technique of immunostaining with antibodies directed against these cells. Whole genome amplification was then performed on single cells, and the DNA was used successfully for analysis by microarray and next-generation sequencing (Breman et al. 2016; Kolvraa et al. 2016).

CELOCENTESIS

The extra-embryonic celom, which exists only during the first trimester, is a source for (nondividing) cells originating from extra-embryonic mesoderm. Given its anatomical continuity with the cytotrophoblast (see color insert Fig. 21–1), Makrydimas et al. (2006) comment that it could be thought of as "a liquid extension of the placenta." The procedure has the attraction of an earlier timing (6–9 weeks) than CVS and NIPT, but so far its use has been limited by uncertainty about the safety of the technique, the low amount of DNA recovered, and by high levels of maternal cell contamination (Giambona et al. 2016). But possibly new molecular techniques, that allow the isolation and genetic analysis of single cells, may prompt a new interest in celocentesis, particularly if concerns about safety could be allayed.

CYSTIC HYGROMA AND PLEURAL EFFUSION

Cystic hygroma has a strong association with fetal aneuploidy, especially monosomy X. A concomitant oligohydramnios may make amniocentesis difficult. Fluid from cystic hygroma and pleural effusion contains lymphocytes, and these cells can be analyzed, using cytogenetic or molecular techniques, within the time frame of a few days. In one small series, three out of four cystic hygroma analyses showed aneuploidy (trisomy 21, monosomy X) (Costa et al. 1995).

CERVICAL LAVAGE OR CYTOBRUSH

Trophoblast cells may migrate from the confines of the uterine cavity and enter the endocervical canal, and they can be collected for molecular analysis by endocervical irrigation and aspiration (lavage), or by insertion of a "cytobrush" (Bischoff and Simpson 2006). The attraction, in principle, is of diagnosis as early as 5 weeks, and a (relatively) noninvasive procedure. Cells of maternal origin outnumber fetal cells at a ratio of 2000:1 (Imudia et al. 2009), but fetal cells can be isolated by incubating with specifically binding antibodies attached to magnetic particles. Fetal cells are then separated with a magnet and subjected to molecular analysis (Fritz et al. 2015).

PROTEOMIC FINGERPRINTING

Proteomic fingerprinting of amniotic fluid assesses the expression profile of proteins coded from specific chromosomes, or otherwise expressed in the context of a specific aneuploidy, and this could be considered as a functional assay for trisomy (Mange et al. 2008; Koster et al. 2010).

"Primum non nocere"

"First, do no harm" is a cornerstone of medical practice. Yet, almost inevitably, having a prenatal diagnostic procedure causes anxiety. Rothman (1988), in her book *The Tentative Pregnancy*, is particularly critical of what she viewed as a medicalized distortion of the normal process of being pregnant. Hodge (1989) describes her personal experience of *Waiting for the Amniocentesis*, and we reproduce her letter in full:

> I drafted the following letter to the editor one week before I expected to hear the results of my amniocentesis:
> "I am 40 years old and 19 weeks pregnant with what will presumably be my third child. I am on the basic science faculty of a medical school. When I teach medical students about amniocentesis, I occasionally mention the difficulty for the woman of having to wait

until well into the second trimester to receive her results.

"I am in that situation myself now, awaiting my results. And before experiencing it, I was unprepared for two phenomena. One was just how difficult the wait is. Pregnancy is always a time of waiting, but now time has slowed down to an extent I did not anticipate. The other, more disturbing phenomenon is how the waiting has affected my attitude toward the pregnancy. At many levels I deny that I really am pregnant 'until after we get the results.' I ignore the flutterings and kicks I feel; I talk of 'if' rather than 'when' the baby comes; I am reluctant to admit to others that I am pregnant. I dream frequently and grimly about second-trimester abortions. In some sense I am holding back on 'bonding' with this child-to-be. This represents an unanticipated negative side effect of diagnostic amniocentesis. And all this, even though my risk of carrying a chromosomal abnormality is less than 2 percent.

"I presume I am not alone in these reactions, yet I have not seen this problem mentioned in the literature, nor did my physician or genetic counselor discuss it with me. I am writing now to bring it to the attention of clinicians with pregnant patients undergoing diagnostic amniocentesis. I suggest to both clinicians and their patients that, when weighing the relative risk and benefits of prenatal diagnosis performed later (amniocentesis) as compared with earlier (chorionic villus biopsy), they not underestimate the negative effects of a 4½ month wait before the woman knows if she is 'really' pregnant."

The next day, before I had mailed this letter, I received the results, and unfortunately they were the dreaded ones: trisomy 21. I have since then had the grim second-trimester abortion. From my current perspective of grief and shock, I encourage clinicians to help their patients avoid the denial described in my letter. My husband and I spared ourselves no pain by holding back emotionally. It has become a cultural expectation that one will keep one's pregnancy a secret until one has had the "all clear" from the amnio. One reason, "If we get a bad result, we won't have to tell anyone." But I now believe that reasoning is wrong. After our bad result, my husband

and I did tell everyone. Sympathy and support from our friends, family, and colleagues have helped us to survive the ordeal of aborting a wanted pregnancy. By keeping the loss a secret, we would have cut ourselves off from such support when the feared outcome did happen.

Not every couple will react this way, some preferring to keep their personal affairs private, but many will. The counselor needs to acknowledge these criticisms and to rise to the challenge of providing a sympathetic and skillful service to clients/patients, according to their varying responses to deciding to have, to undergoing, and to waiting for the results of prenatal diagnosis, and then supporting those who do get an abnormal result. These issues are addressed in detail in *Prenatal Diagnosis: The Human Side* (Abramsky and Chapple 2004).

A considerable fraction of pregnant women are, in any event, opposed to invasive prenatal testing. In a study of pregnant women (age 37 years or older) who had not undergone prenatal diagnosis in Victoria, Australia, 33% had actively declined, with the two main reasons being concern about the safety of the test and a conviction that they would not in any event have a termination (Halliday et al. 2001). Hill et al. (2016) studied preferences for prenatal tests for Down syndrome among pregnant women from nine countries and found that women placed greatest emphasis on test safety and risk of miscarriage when choosing a prenatal test. In contrast, for health professionals, test accuracy was the most important factor in determining choice of prenatal test.

A practical question is pain: The thought of insertion of a needle, or of a catheter, sufficiently deeply to sample a pregnancy, would naturally be cause for some apprehension. Csaba et al. (2006) surveyed a number of women undergoing prenatal diagnosis in New York, asking them to quantify their anxiety ahead of the procedure (transabdominal CVS, transcervical CVS, or amniocentesis) and their perception of pain immediately afterward. In each procedure, the pain was typically seen as "mild," and three-fourths of the women thought it was the same or less painful than they had been expecting. Those who were more anxious—mostly the younger and nulliparous—felt the pain more keenly, and thus special reassurance should be given to these women.

SCREENING FOR FETAL TRISOMY

In broad terms, "screening" describes testing a whole population, or a whole segment of population, for a condition that in fact only a (typically small) fraction will have. This criterion applies to pregnancy screening for Down syndrome (DS) or other trisomy: All, or at least many, pregnant women in a population may be tested, but only a very few will turn out actually to have an affected pregnancy. A requirement of a screened condition is that the condition be well understood, and that an intervention be available. More precisely, screening in this context should meet three criteria: It should identify women who are at increased risk, prior to their having a definitive diagnostic test; it should be offered systematically to pregnant women, who are considered to be at only baseline population risk; and it should be viewed as beneficial to those who receive it, in terms of either choosing termination or being prepared for the birth of a child with DS (Weisz and Rodeck 2006).

Until the recent implementation of NIPT, the screening tools used were the taking of a maternal blood sample and the performing of an ultrasonogram, and these methods remain in widespread use. The methodology involves the analysis of data (maternal age, serum measurements, ultrasound findings), according to a sophisticated computed algorithm, in order to calculate a risk that the fetus is affected by DS. If the calculated risk is greater than that of a certain threshold risk figure (usually taken as 1 in 250), the pregnancy is regarded as being at "increased risk," and definitive testing is then offered. Since other aneuploidies can also influence the measured indices, the test procedure in practice becomes broader than just a trisomy 21 screen.

FIRST-TRIMESTER AND SECOND-TRIMESTER BIOCHEMICAL SCREENING

Certain biochemical markers in the mother's serum may have altered concentrations, whether increased or decreased, if she is carrying a trisomic pregnancy; presumably, these differences reflect perturbation in the trisomic fetoplacental unit. An assessment is made of the degree to which each level differs from expectation, and these data are factored into an algorithm that takes into account the prior risk due to maternal age (Spencer 2007). Sophisticated computer packages are employed to calculate an overall risk figure.

The two first-trimester analytes most commonly measured are the β component of human chorionic gonadotropin (β-hCG) and pregnancy-associated plasma protein-A (PAPP-A),[1] the former typically high and the latter low in a DS pregnancy. Interestingly, PAPP-A levels are also influenced by mode of conception, being lower in pregnancies that are conceived using in vitro fertilization, and leading to a higher rate of false-positive results in first-trimester screening for DS in these pregnancies (Amor et al. 2009). In the second trimester, the analytes measured in many jurisdictions comprise α-fetoprotein (AFP), estriol, β-hCG, and inhibin-A (four analytes: hence, the "quadruple test"[2]). In trisomy 21, the AFP is low, hCG high, uE3 low, and inhibin-A high.

With the increased uptake of noninvasive prenatal testing for DS, the question has arisen whether biochemical screening has a role in pregnancies that are also being screened by NIPT. Two arguments have been made in favor of retaining biochemical screening. The first is that although biochemical screening is aimed primarily at the detection of DS, in fact a range of other chromosome abnormalities may be seen, many of which would not be picked up on NIPT. The risk of a rare chromosome abnormality has been estimated to be 4% when PAPP-A levels are very low (<0.2 multiple of median [MoM]), and 7% when free β-hCG levels are very low (<0.2 MoM) (Petersen et al. 2014). Although it has also been argued, on the other hand, that the specific screening algorithms had not been set up for the purpose of finding rare chromosome abnormalities; and that using this screening to cast a wider net might have only a marginal benefit in terms of detection of other abnormalities, but would yet imply a significant increase in the false-positive rate (Yaron et al. 2016). The second argument in favor of retaining biochemical screening is that abnormal serum biochemistry, and particularly low levels of PAPP-A and free β-hCG, has been associated with third-trimester pregnancy complications such as pre-eclampsia, intrauterine growth restriction, and preterm birth (Krantz et al. 2004). Although on this latter point, Yaron et al. note that despite the recognized association, the sensitivity and predictive value of abnormal serum biochemistry for pregnancy complications fall short of what is required for clinically useful screening tests, and optimal management of women with these results has not been determined.

FIRST-TRIMESTER ULTRASONOGRAPHIC SCREENING

Ultrasonographic scanning is applied during the window of 11–14 weeks inclusive. This particular parameter is assessed: the degree to which the skin at the neck is separated from the underlying tissue by fluid. Since this fluid does not reflect the sound wave on the scan, it is referred to as "nuchal translucency"; "nuchal thickening" is another expression. Bekker et al. (2006) propose that the underlying cause is anomalous development of the lymphatic system in the region of the neck, and it appears that this development is susceptible to a chromosomal imbalance. An increased nuchal translucency is associated with DS, and combined with maternal age, the detection rate is 69%–75%, for a false-positive rate of 5%–8% (Rink and Norton 2016). An increase in nuchal translucency is not specific to DS, being also observed in trisomy 13, trisomy 18, monosomy X, and triploidy. Souka et al. (2005) have assessed risks in the setting of the specific finding of an increased nuchal translucency, related to the degree of separation (Table 20–4). Other ultrasonographic markers of DS are absence of the fetal nasal bone, tricuspid regurgitation, and abnormal blood flow in the ductus venosus (Rao and Platt 2016).

A practical question is this: If, following the observation of an increased nuchal translucency a CVS or amniocentesis is done, and the chromosomes are normal, is there a residual risk for some other type of fetal abnormality? If the translucency resolves, and if no defects (with particular focus on the fetal heart) are seen at 14–16 weeks gestation, the prognosis is good, with a better than 95% chance of a baby with no major abnormalities. If a cardiac defect is seen, which is observed in 1 in 16 fetuses with a nuchal translucency ≥3.5 mm, there

---

1 PAPP-A is produced by the syncytiocytotrophoblast, the development of which is impaired in a trisomic pregnancy. The syncytiocytotrophoblast is anatomically close to the maternal uterine vascular circulation, and also to the celomic cavity; the same applies to ADAM12, another first- and second-trimester marker (Wang et al. 2010b). Thus, these analytes have value as maternal serum markers (and also in celomic fluid analysis); but due to the barrier imposed by the amniotic membrane, they cannot be applied to amniotic fluid analysis (Makrydimas et al. 2006).

2 The "double test" uses AFP and estriol; the "triple test" is AFP, estriol, and β-hCG.

Table 20–4. Likelihood of a Microscopically Visible Chromosome Abnormality, and of Other Outcomes, in the Setting of Increased Nuchal Translucency

NUCHAL TRANSLUCENCY	CHROMOSOME ABNORMALITY (%)	MISCARRIAGE, FETAL DEATH (%)	MAJOR FETAL ABNORMALITIES (%)	ALIVE AND WELL (%)
<95th centile	0.2	1.3	1.6	97
95–99th centile	3.7	1.3	2.5	93
3.5–4.4 mm	21	2.7	10	70
4.5–5.4 mm	33	3.4	19	50
5.5–6.4 mm	51	10	24	30
>6.5 mm	65	19	46	15

Note: The row "<95th centile" describes the baseline population risks.
Source: From Souka et al. (2005).

remains a residual risk for some other type of fetal abnormality (Makrydimas et al. 2003). Noonan syndrome or other "RASopathy" require consideration, being present in approximately 15% of fetuses with a large nuchal translucency and normal karyotype (Croonen et al. 2013). On the question of neurodevelopment, Hellmuth et al. (2017) followed up more than 220,000 euploid children who had been screened in the first trimester, and they found a sixfold increased risk of mental retardation in children with a nuchal translucency above the 99th centile, although the absolute risk remained low (<1%).

FIRST-TRIMESTER COMBINED ULTRASONOGRAPHY AND BIOCHEMICAL SCREENING

A better detection is achieved through a combination of first-trimester nuchal translucency assessment and the measurement of maternal serum-free β-hCG and PAPP-A. If the blood test is done first, these results can be held pending the ultrasound, and the combined figure can be available soon after the scan is done. Detection rates are typically 80%–90%, for a false-positive rate of 5% or less (Spencer 2007). The validity of this approach in more precisely targeting an increased risk population is attested in the experience from Denmark, where a national program was put in place in 2004. The number of diagnostic procedures (amniocentesis or CVS) declined from 7,524 in 2000 to 3,510 in 2006; and yet, during the same period, the number of newborns with DS fell from approximately 50 to 30 per year (Ekelund et al. 2008).

While the prime focus of screening is on trisomy 21, a side benefit is the detection of other, and typically more severe, chromosomal disorders. Trisomy 13 and trisomy 18 both show reduced levels of β-hCG and PAPP-A at first-trimester screening, more so in trisomy 18, along with increased nuchal translucency or frank cystic hygroma. Few other trisomic pregnancies proceed through to the time of screening. Unsurprisingly, those that do so display abnormalities at screening. For example, in trisomy 22 at first-trimester screening, the β-hCG is very elevated, PAPP-A somewhat reduced, and fetal growth restriction is typical (Sifakis et al. 2008). In nonmosaic trisomy 9, the biochemistry is similar to that of trisomy 18 (Priola et al. 2007), and the same may apply in the mosaic case. In a triploid pregnancy, the biochemical indices at first-trimester screening are also quite abnormal, and very differently so according to the category of triploidy, digynic or diandric (p. 239). In the digynic form, β-hCG and PAPP-A are both much reduced, whereas in the diandric type, β-hCG is greatly elevated and PAPP-A marginally reduced. Likewise, ultrasonography is distinctly different, with severe growth restriction in the digynic type, and nearer normal growth but with an enlarged and partially molar placenta in diandric triploidy (Kagan et al. 2008).

SECOND-TRIMESTER ULTRASONOGRAPHY

A fetal anatomic survey in the second trimester may lead to the diagnosis of DS through the detection of a major structural abnormality such as a congenital heart defect or duodenal atresia. In addition, a number of "soft signs" on second-trimester ultrasonographic fetal assessment point to an increased likelihood for DS. An advantage is that this procedure is often done routinely, as part of normal obstetric management, and thus a de facto DS screen is added on, essentially at no additional cost. However, the observations do not lend themselves to a ready analysis in terms of adjusting the level of risk; furthermore, the frequency of these "soft signs" in normal fetuses leads to a high false-positive rate. A more rigorous approach is to adjust the patient's risk assessment using positive and negative likelihood ratios[3] which are available for each "soft sign" (Table 20–5).

Twin Pregnancies. In the case of biochemical screening, two fetoplacental units are expected to lead to the production of twice as much of the particular biochemical substance, which is then conveyed into the maternal bloodstream. Muller et al. (2003) examined the second-trimester analyte levels, and Spencer et al. (2008) the first-trimester analyte levels, in cohorts of twin pregnancies; and the MoM values were essentially double those of singleton pregnancies. The valid MoMs for risk evaluation can thus be derived by dividing the observed result by approximately 2. Intriguingly, monochorionic (and presumably monozygous) twins at first trimester have a somewhat lower PAPP-A mean (1.6 MoM) than do the dichorionic (2.1 MoM) (Madsen et al. 2011); if chorionicity is distinguishable at ultrasonography, adjustment can be made by applying the appropriate PAPP-A divisor. A theoretical complicating factor, in the case of one (dizygous) twin being trisomic 21, is that the normal co-twin might "dilute out" the abnormal serum biochemistry, and thus invalidate the test result. However, in a large French study addressing a second-trimester population, such an effect, if present, was marginal (and not significant statistically), and screening in this setting was considered to be effective (Garchet-Beaudron et al. 2008).

Concerning the ultrasonography, nuchal translucency screening allows each twin to be assessed individually, and the detection rate for aneuploidy is similar to singleton pregnancies (Cleary-Goldman et al. 2005). For monochorionic twins, a single risk estimate can be calculated for the pregnancy using the average of the two nuchal translucency measurements, whereas for dichorionic twins, a specific risk is calculated for each twin. When first-trimester serum markers and nuchal translucency results are combined, a detection rate of 90% can be achieved for a false-positive rate of 5.9% (Madsen et al. 2011).

Garchet-Beaudron et al. (2008) point out other issues relating to twin pregnancies. Logically, the age-related risk for DS might be expected to double

Table 20–5. Positive and Negative Likelihood Ratios of Sonographic Markers for Trisomy 21

MARKER	POSITIVE LR	NEGATIVE LR	LR ISOLATED MARKER*
Intracardiac echogenic focus	5.8	0.80	0.95
Cerebral ventriculomegaly	27.5	0.94	3.81
Increased nuchal fold thickness	23.3	0.80	3.79
Echogenic bowel	11.4	0.90	1.65
Mild hydronephrosis	7.6	0.92	1.08
Short femur	4.8	0.74	0.78
Short humerus	3.7	0.80	0.61
Aberrant right subclavian artery	21.5	0.71	3.94
Absent/hypoplastic nasal bone	23.3	0.46	6.58

*Calculated by multiplying positive LR for given marker by negative LR for all other markers.

LR, likelihood ratio.

Source: Adapted from Agathokleous et al. (2013).

---

3 The Likelihood Ratio (LR) is the likelihood that a given test result would be expected in a patient with the target disorder (e.g. Down syndrome) compared to the likelihood that that same result would be expected in a patient without the target disorder.

in a dizygous twin pregnancy. But such logic appears not to apply: Actual observation does not record such an increase. The technical procedures in the event of an increased-risk result are more demanding: double amniocentesis, with each sac sampled separately; and, if one twin is trisomic and selective termination is sought, the normal twin is placed at risk. Screening in twin pregnancies requires special expertise. In the case of a "vanishing twin" at the first trimester, as manifest by a second, empty sac, it may be prudent to confine the screening analysis to the nuchal translucency alone (Spencer et al. 2010).

INTERPRETATION OF SCREENING RESULTS

What do these various figures—detection rate, false positive rate, positive predictive value—mean? A little epidemiology is in order. Imagine a group of 10,000 pregnant women, of all ages. Assuming a birth prevalence for DS of 1.2 per 1,000, we can take it that 12 women would otherwise give birth to a baby with DS. If the particular screening approach has a detection rate of, for example, 85%, 10/12 of these DS pregnancies would be recognized as being at increased risk, and they could be identified at prenatal diagnosis. The remaining 15% who are carrying a DS fetus (2/12) would fail to be recognized. If the false-positive rate is, for example, 4%, 400 women would have an increased-risk report from screening, but they would go on to receive a normal result from the following amniocentesis or CVS. Putting these figures in the conventional format, we have (Table 20–6):

Table 20–6. Sensitivity, Positive Predictive Value, and Negative Predictive Value of DS Screening

TEST INTERPRETATION	FETUS WITH DS	FETUS NOT WITH DS	TOTAL
Test shows "increased risk"	10	400	410
Test shows "low risk"	2	9,588	9,590
Total	12	9,988	10,000

The *detection rate* (sensitivity) of the test is 10/12 (85%). Thus, 15% of women with a trisomic 21 fetus will be missed by the test. The *positive predictive value* of the test is only 10/410 (2.4%). Thus, 97.6% of women returning an "increased-risk" result will not have a baby with DS.[4] The *negative predictive value* is 9,588/9,590 (99.98%); in other words, a "low-risk" result means a 99.9% chance for an unaffected baby.

The false-positive rate is an important parameter: As noted earlier, this represents the fraction of women who will then go on to have an invasive definitive test, and which will return a normal chromosomal result. Clearly, the smaller this figure, the better. The trade-off is this: The smaller the false-positive rate, the less the detection rate. To judge the effectiveness and acceptability of the screening, we can declare a false-positive rate that is desirable, and this would then determine what the detection rate will be; or, we can choose a preferred detection rate, and accept the false-positive rate that this would incur. A typically desired false-positive rate is 5%; based upon this, the detection rate is noted as DR_5. Desired detection rates of 85%, or 90%, would come at a cost of false-positive rates noted as FPR_{85} and FPR_{90} (Weisz and Rodeck 2006).

THE UNDERSTANDING OF WOMEN WHO HAVE SCREENING

The interpretation of a DS screening test result to the patient is fraught with potential for confusion. The major pitfall is that an "increased-risk" test result may sometimes be understood by the woman and her medical advisor to mean that the pregnancy is likely to be affected. As we showed earlier, *the great majority of women who screen "positive" will go on to have a normal baby.* Counselors doing this work need a clear awareness of these issues so that they can enable their patients to understand, intuitively or explicitly, the concept and relevance of a low positive predictive value. The counselor is referred to Macintosh's (1994) essay "Perception of Risk" for a very readable and practical commentary upon these issues, and to Marteau and Dormandy (2001) for an overview of the complexity of the issues. The ideal is that those having a screening test for DS should have a basic awareness of the condition, and of the

---

4 Thus emphasizing the point that the expression to use is merely "increased risk," not "high risk."

rationale of the screening procedure, and that their beliefs and perceptions and attitudes should be reasonably consonant with the aims and practice of the program.

The ideal has not necessarily been met. Jaques et al. (2004), in a paper provocatively titled "Do Women Know That Prenatal Testing Detects Fetuses with Down Syndrome?" surveyed responses from pregnant women 37 years old or older in Victoria, Australia, in 1998–1999; and the answer to their question was, disconcertingly, that "Down syndrome" was not mentioned as a reason for undergoing pregnancy testing in almost 40% of respondents. Not every woman will respond "rationally" to an increased-risk interpretation, according to the view of rationality as seen by the providers of the screening program. Those who enter into a screening program without being properly aware of the implications may find themselves "in an untenable situation—anxious about a positive result, but unwilling to incur the risks of diagnostic testing" (Kuppermann et al. 2006). Depressive symptoms, and thus a reduced capacity to make clear decisions, may be exacerbated in those with a predisposition, and Hippman et al. (2009) see a role for the counselor in recognizing this. More recent reports have been rather more encouraging, suggesting that, latterly, those delivering the screening are becoming more skilled in advising their patients (Okun et al. 2008; Jaques et al. 2010).

For those who are better informed, understanding is by no means a neutral matter, and Rapp (1999) refers to the role of women as "moral pioneers," in coming to terms with the ethical issues that readily available screening may, in these modern times, present. Susanne et al. (2006) assessed responses in women who had had what turned out to be a false-positive screening result, following them prospectively through the pregnancy and after the baby was born. Several declared that they had "withheld" their pregnancy, and only returned to reacceptance after the normal chromosomal result from amniocentesis had been conveyed; nevertheless, most would have the same testing in a future pregnancy. Counselors need to be well attuned to these several complexities; and if a woman's family physician can share in the decision-making process, this is typically well received (Légaré et al. 2011).

Concerning the facts about DS itself in the context of pregnancy screening, leaflets are the simplest means of conveying information, and many clinics/jurisdictions produce their own material, the quality of which may vary (Murray et al. 2001); a number of online resources are also available. It is a fine matter to judge what should be the level and tone of the information. Bryant et al. (2001) reviewed the leaflets produced in a number of clinics in the United Kingdom and considered that the viewpoints expressed were, in the main, weighted unduly negatively toward DS. It is true that information ought to be couched in such terms that it will be useful, in the fullest sense of that word, to the wide range of people for whom it is intended (and see p. 15). Equally, the comment can be made that attempting to neutralize negative aspects of DS may send a mixed message, since being given the option of abortion in order to avoid having a DS child rather plainly implies that having such a child may not be a desirable outcome. The view that is offered should be clear, accurate, and even-handed.[5]

SECULAR TRENDS IN PRENATAL SCREENING AND DIAGNOSIS OF ANEUPLOIDY

The live birth prevalence of Down syndrome is influenced by two phenomena that, during the past 40 years, have occurred concurrently: changes in maternal age distribution (Chapter 13) and advances in prenatal screening technologies and policies. An example of the projected impact of prenatal diagnosis and elective termination of pregnancy on the birth prevalence of DS is presented in Figure 20–1. In general, these two factors might be expected to have opposite effects, with an increase in DS pregnancies resulting from women delaying childbearing to an older age, counterbalanced by an increase in prenatal diagnosis and termination of DS pregnancies. And indeed, to some extent, and in some countries, these two factors have largely cancelled each other out, with data from Britain (Morris and Alberman 2009) showing little change in the overall prevalence of DS births since the introduction of screening. In contrast, however, Australian data (Collins et al. 2008) showed an overall decrease in the birth prevalence of DS; while data from the United States (de Graaf et al. 2015) and the

---

5 These matters are dealt with in considerable detail in a document from the National Health Service of the United Kingdom, "Psychological Aspects of Genetic Screening of Pregnant Women and Newborns: A Systematic Review" (Green et al. 2004).

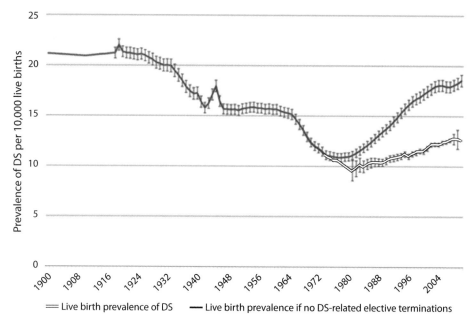

FIGURE 20–1   Estimated annual live birth prevalence of DS, if there had been no DS-related elective terminations, in the United States, 1900–2010 (filled line), and actual live birth prevalence, 1969–2010 (open line; the lower line from the bifurcation at 1969). Prenatal diagnosis began to be available from about 1969; the average maternal age also began to increase from this time. Error bars indicate 95% confidence intervals.

Source: From de Graaf et al. (2015).

Netherlands (de Graaf et al. 2011) showed a small increase over the period of study. (These data precede the introduction of NIPT for DS.) Another possible point to factor in to the overall picture may be a changing attitude toward pregnancy termination for an aneuploidy (Jacobs et al. 2016).

The increasing precision of screening has led to a reduction in the number of invasive procedures being done. Hui et al. (2016a) analyzed data for the years 1976–2013 from Victoria, Australia, and noted that while the total number of invasive tests climbed steadily from 1976 to 2000, it then declined, such that in 2013, fewer procedures were being done than at any time in the previous 25 years. At the same time, the number of prenatal diagnoses of DS was the highest recorded. This improved targeting reflected changes in the indications for invasive prenatal testing over the same period (Figure 20–2), and the number of invasive procedures performed per diagnosis of a major chromosome abnormality declined from 100 to six. Renshaw et al. (2013) have reported similar improvements in the United Kingdom, with the number of invasive procedures per syndrome diagnosis reducing from 46 to five between 1991 and 2010.

This trend is continuing since the introduction of NIPT, and in most centers, the number of invasive procedures has decreased by 50%–90% (Warsof et al. 2015). Figure 20–3 shows the picture in Australia. With fewer invasive tests being done, the question has been raised of how to maintain training and competency of obstetric sonologists, against this falling procedural load (Hui et al. 2016b).

FETAL ULTRASONOGRAPHIC ANOMALIES

We have discussed above ultrasonography in the specific setting of targeted screening. Otherwise, a mid-trimester ultrasound examination is, of course, a routine part of standard obstetric management. The discovery of a fetal malformation, in the course of a routine ultrasound, is a common indication for a fetal chromosome study. In Victoria, Australia, for example, approximately 20% of prenatal chromosome tests in 2013 were done on the grounds of ultrasound findings of a fetal malformation or of a marker of aneuploidy (Hui et al. 2016a). Certain major ultrasonographic defects are fairly specific: For example, holoprosencephaly predicts

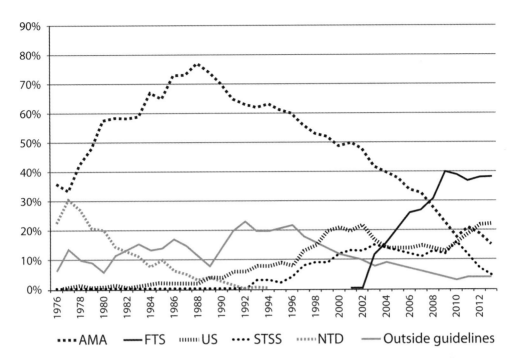

FIGURE 20–2   Indications for invasive prenatal diagnosis in Victoria, Australia, since 1976 as a percentage of total tests. AMA, advance maternal age; FTS, first-trimester screening; NTD, history of neural tube defect; STSS, second-trimester serum screening; US, ultrasound-detected fetal abnormality.

Source: From Hui et al. (2016a).

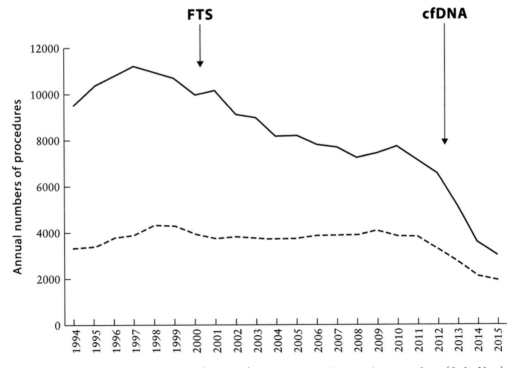

FIGURE 20–3   Uptake of amniocentesis (solid line) and chorionic villus sampling procedures (dashed line) in Australia 1994–2015, according to the introduction of first-trimester screening (FTS) and of maternal serum cell-free DNA (cfDNA) screening.

Source: From Hui et al. (2016a). Data extracted from Australian Medical Benefits Scheme billing records.

the likelihood of trisomy 13, fetal hydrops/cystic hygroma predicts monosomy X or trisomy 21, and an endocardial cushion defect or duodenal atresia predicts trisomy 21. Conotruncal defects are associated with the 22q11.2 deletion, and aortic narrowing suggests the 7q11.23 deletion of Williams syndrome (Krzeminska et al. 2009). Asymmetrical growth (head circumference vs. crown-rump length) may point to triploidy (Salomon et al. 2005). The acardiac fetus is often due to an otherwise unsurvivable autosomal trisomy, possibly tempered by mosaicism with a normal cell line, but their existence being maintained by a (karyotypically normal) monozygous co-twin (the "pump twin"). Certain renal defects have a frequent association with fetal aneuploidy, as do cardiac malformations generally (Amor et al. 2003; Wimalasundera and Gardiner 2004; Carbone et al. 2011). Up to one-third of heart defects are associated with fetal aneuploidy, although in most there will be additional anomalies; in the case of an isolated cardiac defect, microarray will detect a chromosome abnormality in 10% (Sukenik-Halevy et al. 2016). Cysts of the choroid plexus (tissue within the cerebral ventricles) are a "soft marker" for trisomy 18, but not trisomy 21 (Walkinshaw 2000); they are otherwise harmless (DiPietro et al. 2011).

On the specific question of rare autosomal abnormalities detected by conventional karyotyping (rare trisomies, deletions, duplications, supernumerary markers, various other structural rearrangements), a large European series based upon reports from malformation registers in several jurisdictions linked ultrasound findings to cytogenetic results (Baena et al. 2003). Nearly half of all rare autosomal abnormalities showed fetal anomalies on ultrasonography, with heart and brain defects and growth retardation more often seen with deletions, and cystic hygroma, hydrops, and nuchal translucency more typically associated with trisomies and duplications. These rare abnormalities comprised 7% of all chromosomally abnormal prenatal diagnoses.

In which cases should a chromosome analysis be conducted, following the discovery of structural anomalies by ultrasound examination? Staebler et al. (2005) examined the karyotypes (on classical cytogenetics) in 428 fetuses with ultrasound detected anomalies over a 10-year period. The karyotype was abnormal in 9% of cases with an isolated malformation, and in 19% of cases with multiple malformations. The following isolated defects were typically associated with a normal karyotype: hydronephrosis with high obstruction, unilateral multicystic dysplastic kidney, gastroschisis, intestinal dilatation, cystic adenomatoid malformation, pulmonary sequestration, vertebral anomaly, and tumor. Thus, one of these as a single malformation is not necessarily an indication, whereas, clearly enough, the presence of multiple malformations would warrant chromosome study. Daniel et al. (2003a) reviewed 1,800 cases in which an anomaly (an actual malformation or a minor marker of aneuploidy) had been detected at ultrasonography, and assembled a table of risks of aneuploidy according to the findings (Table 20–7).

Table 20–7. The Likelihood of Discovering a Microscopically Visible Chromosome Abnormality at Prenatal Diagnosis, According to the Pattern of Defects Identified at Fetal Ultrasonography, for All Maternal Ages

DEFECTS	LIKELIHOOD OF AN ANEUPLOIDY (%)
CNS/cranial shape plus cardiac*	53
Key malformation,** singly or in combination	37
CNS ± other***	21
Increased nuchal translucency, first trimester, ± other abnormality	25
Increased nuchal translucency, second trimester, ± other abnormality	13
Cardiac ± other abnormality	9
Pyelectasis/two vessel cord/echogenic bowel/ short femur	6
Other (singly or in combination)	3

Notes: Some percentages are considerably higher or lower for older and younger maternal ages, respectively. These data were obtained prospectively.

*Excluding anencephaly/spina bifida.

**Cystic hygroma/hydrops/exomphalos/severe IUGR/duodenal atresia/talipes.

***Excluding anencephaly/spina bifida/cardiac, including choroid plexus cysts.

CNS, central nervous system; IUGR: intrauterine growth retardation.

Source: From Daniel et al. (2003a).

The abnormal karyotypes included trisomies 13, 18, 21, triploidy, 45,X and mosaics, various autosomal and gonosomal duplications and deletions, rare trisomies, and de novo apparently balanced rearrangements.

The more precise tool of chromosome microarray provides a considerable additional yield above that which is detected by conventional karyotyping. Wapner et al. (2012), in a large prospective, blinded cohort study, showed that 6% of pregnancies with abnormal ultrasound findings and a normal (classical) karyotype had a clinically relevant CNV.[6] The superiority of microarray was confirmed by subsequent meta-analysis, which demonstrated that, in the setting of fetal anomalies, an additional 7% of abnormalities, compared with conventional karyotyping, were revealed (Hillman et al. 2013). Based on these findings, the American College of Obstetricians and Gynecologists (2013) recommended that microarray analysis be performed in patients with a fetus with one or more major structural abnormalities identified on ultrasound examination, and who are undergoing invasive prenatal diagnosis.

In karyotypically normal fetuses, certain ultrasound abnormalities are associated with a higher frequency of CNVs. Donnelly et al. (2014) performed a secondary analysis of the data from Wapner et al. (2012), using as a comparison group women who were having prenatal diagnosis for advanced maternal age, and in whom the frequency of CNVs with known or suspected pathogenicity was 1.7%. The yield of microarray was highest in fetuses with multiple ultrasound anomalies, 13% of which had a CNV with known or suspected pathogenicity. When the ultrasound abnormality was confined to one system, the yield of microarray was 5.6%, but varied according to the system involved, being higher in fetuses with renal anomalies (15%), cardiac anomalies (11%), and facial anomalies (10%) but lower when the abnormality affected the thorax (4.6%), central nervous system (3.2%), or skeleton (2.8%).

Twins. In the event of a twin pregnancy having been shown on ultrasonography, the question arises of an appropriate prenatal diagnostic procedure, if this is considered appropriate. A point to make here is that although monozygous (MZ) twins would be expected to have the same karyotype, and almost always do, this does not invariably apply. The ability to interpret monozygosity is not perfect; and those MZ twins in which the split occurred soon after conception, prior to the differentiation of the extrafetal tissues, may have the same ultrasound morphology of membranes (amnion and chorion) as would a dizygous pair. Thus, the advice is that dual amniocenteses, rather than CVS, may be the procedure of choice; and more especially so in the setting of discordance for an anatomical anomaly (Lewi et al. 2006).

---

6   As we discuss in Chapter 17, the expressions microdeletion/microduplication may also be appropriate, when a CNV is known to be pathogenic.

21

CHROMOSOME ABNORMALITIES DETECTED AT PRENATAL DIAGNOSIS

THE MAIN FOCUS of chromosomal prenatal diagnosis had been upon trisomy 21, usually in the context of older childbearing age, or of an increased-risk screening test. Trisomy 21 does remain, for most women and couples, the prime concern—the condition that most people are aware of— but with the sophistication of twenty-first century technology, the great majority of chromosomal imbalances are, in principle, diagnosable. Noninvasive prenatal testing—no more than a blood test for the woman—widens access and increases uptake very considerably. Routine fetal ultrasonography can detect quite subtle malformation, and genetic testing will often follow such a discovery. The counselor can expect to deal with a broad spectrum of chromosomal abnormality, presenting in the prenatal clinic.

DECISION-MAKING FOLLOWING PRENATAL DIAGNOSIS OF A CHROMOSOMAL ABNORMALITY

To some extent, the possibility of "other abnormalities besides Down syndrome" should have been raised at pretest counseling. But when a chromosomal abnormality is actually discovered, it is of course necessary to discuss in detail with the couple the implications of this particular abnormality, and to help them decide on a suitable course of action.

Outlines of the clinical consequences of these abnormalities follow, to serve as a basis for the decisions that these women and couples need to make. In transmitting the information, the counselor is obliged to be clear and accurate about the particular abnormality and to take care that the couple's autonomy in the decision-making process is not compromised. A decision for or against termination is the immediate one to be made. Some years ago, but their view remains valid, Engel et al. (1981) listed these factors influencing the parents' decision: their philosophy of life; their religious views; their socioeconomic status; and whether this was a first or wanted pregnancy or a later, unplanned pregnancy. More recently, Jacobs et al. (2016) assessed responses to the prenatal diagnosis of an aneuploidy in a Scottish population, observing a fall-off in the numbers choosing termination during the period 2000–2011. They suggested that this may have reflected "societal changes in accepting greater diversity" but acknowledged that "this interpretation is of course purely speculative."

Unsurprisingly, the severity of the condition influences decision-making. Drugan et al. (1990) found that 93% of parents having a prenatal diagnosis with a "poor prognosis" (autosomal trisomy, unbalanced translocation, 45,X with major anomalies on ultrasonographic examination) chose pregnancy termination, whereas only 27% of parents given a "questionable prognosis" (sex chromosome aneuploidy, 45,X with normal ultrasonography, de novo apparently balanced translocation or inversion) took this course. Shaffer et al. (2006) undertook a large retrospective review (1983–2003), analyzing parental decisions in 816 prenatal diagnoses of a major aneuploidy, at a San Francisco clinic. Termination was chosen in 86% of autosomal trisomy and in 60% with a sex chromosome aneuploidy. Of the latter, the rates of termination increased progressively from XXX (40%) to XYY (57%), 45,X (65%), and XXY (70%), in parallel with a perceived severity of phenotype. The rates did not differ significantly during the 21-year period, to the slight surprise of these authors. Drugan et al. make the interesting observation that ultrasound visualization of fetal defects "in a society dominated by the television screen" can be useful in helping parents better grasp the implications of the diagnosis; although seeing an image of the actual fetus can also sharpen the ethical dilemma inherent in confronting the possibility of termination of a pregnancy (Williams et al. 2005). In the specific case of Prader-Willi syndrome, among a group of 85 Israeli parents of a PWS child, whose views were sought at structured interview, all would allow prenatal diagnosis, but a minority (19%) were against termination (Even-Zohar Gross et al. 2017).

TRISOMY 21

Skotko et al. (2009) emphasize the need for the person conveying the news of a Down syndrome (DS) result to be well informed, whether that be a counselor, obstetrician, or other health professional (and of course this qualification is scarcely confined to a diagnosis of DS). Ideally, the news should be given in person; but where that is not feasible, a phone call should be at a prearranged time. Parents who decide to continue a trisomy 21 pregnancy, versus those who have chosen termination, would presumably come from different points of view. Skotko et al. note that contact with a DS support group might be useful for some couples in deciding the fate of a DS pregnancy, although they do observe that few

studies have assessed the views of those who have terminated a trisomic pregnancy, from whom the other face of the decision could be given a hearing.

A study of health professionals in Finland showed some inconsistency in comparing the points of view of midwives and public health nurses with the options available to their patients; and the acknowledgment was made that this difference could be viewed as a healthy sign, in recognizing that plurality of opinion is the way of the world (Jallinoja et al. 1999). Thus, most (79%) of these midwives and nurses agreed that all pregnant women should be offered a screening test, although only 44% personally accepted the concept of genetic abortion. An acceptance of abortion correlated with education and with a professional experience with DS patients. In the United States, Britt et al. (2000) studied 142 women who had had a prenatal diagnosis of trisomy 21, seen in Detroit over the period 1989–1998. Those who had already had children, and where the diagnosis of trisomy 21 was made earlier in the pregnancy, were more likely to choose termination. In the Netherlands, Korenromp et al. (2007) found that among women who had chosen termination following prenatal diagnosis of DS, "child-related" motivations (Table 21–1) were the most prevalent,

Table 21–1. The Five Most Acknowledged "Child-Related" Motivations of 71 Women Choosing Termination of a Trisomic 21 Pregnancy, from a Study Based in Eight Dutch Hospitals

MOTIVATION STATEMENT	PERCENTAGE OF WOMEN IN AGREEMENT WITH STATEMENT
I believed the child would never be able to function independently.	92
I considered the abnormality too severe.	90
I considered the burden for the child itself too heavy.	83
I worried about the care of the child after my/our death.	82
I considered the uncertainty about the consequences of the abnormality too high.	78

Source: From Korenromp et al. (2007).

but concerns about burden to the family were also important.

SEX CHROMOSOME ABNORMALITY

The grayest area is sex chromosome aneuploidy, and views have been changing somewhat over recent decades, at least in the West, generally in the direction of a more conservative response to the news of a chromosomal abnormality (Christian et al. 2000; Linden et al. 2002; Boyd et al. 2011). In Denmark in 1986, Nielsen et al. reported that approximately 80% of prenatal diagnoses of sex chromosome aneuploidy at that time were followed by the choice of abortion. In an English/Finnish study from the same period, termination (in ~60% overall) was more likely to be chosen in the case of the XXY and 45,X karyotypes, by younger parents with fewer previous children, and in all cases in which an ultrasonographic defect was identified (Holmes-Siedle et al. 1987). From a large survey of centers in five European countries, covering the years 1986 to 1997, the rate of choice of termination with respect to XXY was 44% (Marteau et al. 2002). In a German study over a similar period, termination was chosen by a much smaller fraction, only 13%, among parents who had been given a prenatal diagnosis of 47,XXX, 47,XXY, or 47,XYY (in contrast, just 2% of parents at the same clinic decided to continue a pregnancy with trisomy 21) (Meschede et al. 1998c). This may in part have reflected the practice of this clinic to emphasize the point that "the mean global IQ of around 90 falls well within the normal range and is compatible with a productive and socially well-adjusted life." In more recent years, a similar reduction in the choice of termination has been seen in France (Brun et al. 2004). A quite different experience comes from China, however (Liao and Li 2008; Liao et al. 2013). Almost all pregnancies with a fetal diagnosis of sex chromosome abnormality are terminated. In considerable part, this may have reflected the influence of the "one-child policy" of the time, with couples wanting the best outlook for their one and only child.

In the specific case of 45,X and variants, from 19 registries in 10 countries across Europe from 1996 to 1998, 79% of parents chose termination if morphological abnormality, and in particular cystic hygroma, had been seen on ultrasonography, versus 42% in which the diagnosis had not been led into by an ultrasonographic defect (Baena et al. 2004).

Parental attributes may be important in influencing the eventual outcome of these children. In the experience of the Denver group, for example, the parents choosing prenatal diagnosis were often of higher socioeconomic status, and the children of those who had made conscious decisions to continue the pregnancy, following the discovery of a sex chromosome abnormality, had generally done better than those identified in population newborn surveys (Linden and Bender 2002).

The way in which information is given has an important impact, and counselors need to be well aware of the weight that parents, in some emotional turmoil at the news they have just received, may put upon the news given them. Consider the example of 47,XXY Klinefelter syndrome. In the European survey mentioned above, Marteau et al. (2002) assessed responses to the prenatal diagnosis of XXY when counseling had been given by obstetricians, pediatricians, midwives, health visitors, or genetics specialists. Women counseled solely by genetics specialists were more than twice as likely (relative risk = 2.4) to continue the pregnancy versus those counseled either by other professionals or by other professionals along with a geneticist. It seems probable that these differences may reflect the style of counseling. Marteau et al. (1994) make the following distinctions in counseling types: nondirective counseling ("try to be as neutral as possible, covering both positive and negative aspects"), directive counseling for termination ("encourage termination" or "try to be as neutral as possible but overall convey more negative than positive aspects of the condition"), or directive counseling against termination ("encourage parents to carry to term" or "try to be as neutral as possible but overall convey more positive than negative aspects of the condition"). In a review of published reports, Jeon et al. (2012) noted the importance of these factors in influencing a decision: the specific type of sex chromosome abnormality, the gestational week at diagnosis, the parents' age, the providers' genetic expertise, and the number of children already had, or their desire for (more) children. They noted that among those parents choosing to continue a pregnancy, their socioeconomic status and ethnicity were particularly relevant. On the other hand, those parents choosing termination were characterized by a fear or anxiety of having a child with a sex chromosome abnormality, and also by having received directive counseling.

The desirability for a consistent approach, with access to accurate information, is to be emphasized, as is—of course—the requirement to enable women's choices to be well informed in the broadest sense, and for the counseling to be nondirective (Abramsky et al. 2001; Marteau and Dormandy 2001; Linden et al. 2002). Beyond the clinic, there are support groups, public information resources, and communicating with other parents, as means to become further informed about the implications of a sex chromosome abnormality (in the short period of time during which a decision must be made), and Linden et al. note the pros and cons of taking these paths; as noted earlier with respect to trisomy 21, the views of those who had previously chosen to terminate a pregnancy are less readily accessible. The prime responsibility for putting couples in the best position to make an appropriate decision lies with the counselor.

As for subsequently informing the children from the pregnancies that are continued, Sutton et al. (2006) emphasize the importance of telling them of their sex chromosomal diagnosis (specifically, Turner syndrome), and its implications, in a timely and sensitive manner, and of not "keeping secrets."

"MICROARRAY-LEVEL" REARRANGEMENT

Microarray analysis applied to prenatal samples is capable of detecting imbalance practically at the level of the operator's choice, according to which particular commercial or in-house microarray platform is used (Rickman et al. 2006; Shaffer and Bui 2007; Shaffer et al. 2008; Coppinger et al. 2009; Van den Veyver et al. 2009). The analysis can be performed on small amounts of material, and results may be obtained within several days. Microarrays can increase the prenatal diagnostic pick-up, following discovery of an ultrasound defect, by 7% (Hillman et al. 2013). The other side of this two-edged sword is the fact that some microimbalances are not pathogenic, and may simply reflect "copy number variation." Indeed, one commentator wrote, somewhat provocatively, that prenatal array testing is likely "to produce a flood of information that is overwhelming, anxiety-producing, inconclusive, and misleading" (Shuster 2007); and Werner-Lin et al. (2016a) provide some testament, in documenting frustration and anxiety of couples receiving uncertain results, that this prediction may not have been entirely inaccurate.

One response to this is to target the array: Ask the right question, if we want a useful answer. That is, we can interrogate only those chromosomal segments for which precedent exists as being causative of an abnormal phenotype, assessing in particular the known microduplication/microdeletion syndromes, along with subtelomeric and pericentromeric regions (South and Lamb 2009). Or, a little more broadly, to target, in addition, gene-dense regions, on the assumption that these might more plausibly be, when duplicated or deleted, pathogenic. (It is true that the considerable majority of pathogenic CNVs would not have been seen on classical cytogenetics. Replicating the general principle from classical cytogenetics that haplo-insufficiency is typically more deleterious than triplo-excess, CNVs judged to be pathogenic at prenatal diagnosis are more likely to be deletions, and those considered as variants of uncertain significance (VOUSs) are more often duplications.) Using these targeted approaches, results of unclear clinical significance are less often encountered, although the downside is that some unequivocally pathogenic copy number variants (CNVs) will be missed. Counselors need to be quite *au fait* with the interpretations and to maintain close liaison with expert scientists in the field (the science); they must also be aware of the particular subtleties that counseling in this circumstance will demand (the art) (Werner-Lin et al. 2016b). The uncertainty of a prenatal result, for those continuing the pregnancy, can flow over into the child's life: "They Can't Find Anything Wrong with Him, Yet," as Werner-Lin et al. (2017) title their paper apropos.

Be the foregoing as it may, we can nevertheless expect that experience of, and familiarity with, the concept of copy number variants, will improve; and it is surely inevitable, in the context of prenatal diagnosis, that consumer pressure to test 'everything possible' will see a wider application of testing for the generality of CNVs. In a survey of women presenting to prenatal clinics in Melbourne over 2014-15, who were in any event scheduled to have a CVS or amniocentesis (in most, due to an increased-risk screen), 60% chose 'extended' testing, while 40% were content with 'targeted' testing (Halliday et al. 2018). The 'extended' analysis included pathogenic CNVs, as well as those of incomplete penetrance, and VOUSs; the 'targeted' analysis looked only at abnormalities of known pathogenicity and 100% penetrance.

There are other ways in which the use of microarray is changing the face of prenatal chromosome analysis. The two notable categories are the identification of de novo balanced chromosome rearrangements, and very small marker chromosomes. Although typically benign, these abnormalities have historically necessitated detailed counseling and cytogenetic follow-up, and they have been a cause of anxiety for patients. The fact that these abnormalities may be invisible on microarray is a feature of the methodology that is, perhaps, almost an advantage in the prenatal setting. The capacity for next-generation sequencing (NGS) methodologies—"post-microarray" testing, one could almost say—to clarify the nature of apparently balanced rearrangements, is mentioned on p. 266.

MOSAICISM: CONFINED, CONSTITUTIONAL, AND PSEUDO

Mosaicism is the bane of cytogenetic prenatal diagnosis. Most times, it turns out to have been a false alarm, and the mosaicism in villus tissue or amniocytes does not reflect a true constitutional mosaicism of the embryo. This is a problem for the laboratory to resolve, inasmuch as they are able. We may list these two major categories: confined placental mosaicism, and true constitutional fetal mosaicism. A third category, pseudomosaicism, refers to an abnormality that arose during tissue culture in vitro ("cultural artifact"), but with the embryonic and extra-embryonic tissues being chromosomally normal.

A chromosomally abnormal cell line may exist only in the extra-embryonic tissues of the placenta (chorion, amnion), and the embryo is 46,N. This is confined placental mosaicism (CPM). CPM is encountered at CVS rather than at amniocentesis. It is uncommon that an observation of apparent CPM at CVS reflects a true constitutional mosaicism of the fetus. Grati (2014) offers an exhaustive treatment of the question of mosaicism at CVS, based upon an experience of more than 50,000 procedures, in which mosaicism was seen in 2.2%; of these, just 13% (0.3% of the total) proved to have a true fetal mosaicism (and see Table 21–2); she provides further authoritative review, with reference to the issues raised by noninvasive prenatal testing, in Grati (2016). Comparable fractions are seen on prenatal diagnosis by microarray: 1.8% of CVS, and 0.5% on amniocentesis, in the analysis of Carey et al. (2014a). Stetten et al. (2004) reviewed a series of 4,000 CVS studies done over the period 1998–2003, in which 29 cases (0.7% of the total) of CPM were defined. Testing of the newborns revealed two

as having (low-level) true mosaicism. A long-term follow-up study (Amor et al. 2006) is noted below.

Considerable discussion follows, but at the outset, we emphasize that true mosaicism of the fetus is infrequently observed, and that *the majority of mosaicism identified at prenatal diagnosis, more especially at CVS, does not presage an abnormal baby*. It is important to keep this perspective in talking with parents (according to the particular attributes of the mosaicism, as we go on to discuss) and to avoid causing any more anxiety than that which, inevitably, an "abnormal" result brings.

Applied Embryology

Interpreting mosaicism obliges an understanding of the earliest events of development of the conceptus, as we now outline (Bianchi et al. 1993; Robinson et al. 2002). The zygote undergoes successive mitoses to produce a ball of cells (morula) (Fig. 21–1,1, and see color insert). The morula then cavitates to produce an inner cyst, and it becomes the blastocyst (Fig. 21–1, 2); this is happening at the beginning of the second week postconception. The outermost layer of the blastocyst is composed of trophoblast, and this tissue becomes the outer investment of the chorionic villi. The inner cell mass protrudes into the blastocystic cavity, and this will give origin to the embryo. It comprises two different cellular layers, the epiblast and the hypoblast. In a 64-cell blastocyst, most cells are trophoblasts, the inner cell mass comprises about 16 cells, within which only about four (epiblast) cells will give rise to the embryo itself.

The hypoblast forms the spherical primary yolk sac (whose roof is, transiently, the ventral surface of the embryo). The primary yolk sac gives rise to the extra-embryonic mesoderm, sandwiched between itself and the outer cytotrophoblast, thus producing a three-layered sphere. The mesodermal cells now invade the blastocystic cavity (Fig. 21–1,3), and this mesodermal mass is in turn cavitated to produce the extra-embryonic celom, such that there are outer and inner layers of extra-embryonic mesoderm. The outer layer, underlying the trophoblast, gives rise to the mesenchymal core of the chorionic villus, and the inner layer becomes the outer (mesodermal) surface of the amniotic membrane. The amniotic cavity enlarges at the expense of the extra-embryonic celom (Figs. 21–1, 5 and 21–2) and eventually obliterates it (by the end of the first

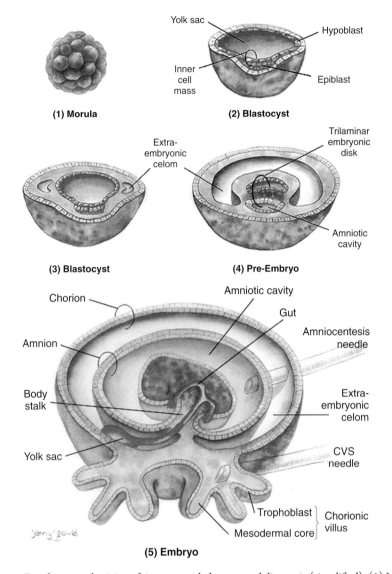

Yolk sac

Hypoblast

Inner cell mass

Epiblast

(1) Morula

(2) Blastocyst

Extra-embryonic celom

Trilaminar embryonic disk

Amniotic cavity

(3) Blastocyst

(4) Pre-Embryo

Chorion

Amniotic cavity

Gut

Amniocentesis needle

Amnion

Body stalk

Extra-embryonic celom

Yolk sac

CVS needle

Trophoblast

Chorionic villus

Mesodermal core

(5) Embryo

FIGURE 21–1   Developmental origins of tissues sampled at prenatal diagnosis (simplified). (1) Morula, 3–4 days postconception, a sphere with trophoblast cells at its surface. (2) Cross-section of blastocyst at beginning of second week, showing outer rim of trophoblast, the inner cell mass comprising epiblast (orange*) and hypoblast (yellow*), and the yolk sac cavity lined by an inner rim of cells of hypoblastic origin. (3) Blastocyst toward end of second week. The hypoblastic cells of the yolk sac have given rise to extra-embryonic mesoderm. Lacunae are beginning to appear in this mesoderm, and these will coalesce to form the extra-embryonic celom. (4) "Pre-embryo." The amniotic cavity and the yolk sac bound the dorsal and ventral surfaces of the embryonic disk. The extra-embryonic celom has now cavitated the extra-embryonic mesoderm. Note that the embryonic mesoderm (middle layer of the trilaminar embryonic disk) arises from the epiblast, and thus it has a different lineage from the extra-embryonic mesoderm. (5) Composite embryo/early fetus. (Rotation has reversed the relative positions of the yolk sac and amniotic cavity.) The three embryonic tissue types (ectoderm, mesoderm, endoderm) all had origin from the epiblast, as did the amniotic epithelium. Epithelial cells from the embryo's ectodermal surface are shed into the amniotic cavity, as also are amniotic epithelial cells (both these tissues shown orange). Cells from endodermal derivatives (respiratory and urinary tracts, which originate from the gut, shown in yellow) pass into the amniotic cavity. Chorionic villi comprise mesenchymal core (of extra-embryonic mesodermal origin), gloved by trophoblast. Extra-embryonic and embryonic mesoderms are continuous at the body stalk, albeit that some embryonic mesodermal cells may then migrate into the amniotic mesoderm (Robinson et al. 2002). *See color insert.

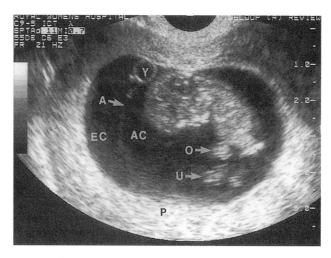

FIGURE 21–2   Ultrasound picture of embryo at 10–11 weeks gestational age, very close to actual size (note centimeter markers at right). Note amnion (A), amniotic cavity (AC), extra-embryonic celom (EC), umbilical cord (U), "physiological omphalocele" (O), yolk sac (Y), and placenta (P). The relative positions of embryo and other structures are similar to the depiction in the drawing in Figure 21–1, part 5.

Source: Courtesy H. P. Robinson.

trimester), with the mesodermal layer of the amnion fusing with the mesodermal layer of the chorion.

The epiblast gives rise to the amniotic cavity, the floor of which is the "dorsal" (ectodermal) surface of the embryo, and its roof is the amnion, these being continuous at their margins. Thus, the embryonic integument and the inner surface of the amniotic membrane—which are the source of the embryonic and amniotic epithelial cells present in amniotic fluid—have the same lineage. At the beginning of the third week, the primitive streak arises from the epiblast, and this in turn gives origin to both endoderm and intra-embryonic mesoderm. Endoderm gives origin, among other tissues, to urinary tract and lung epithelia, desquamated cells from which contribute to the cellular population of amniotic fluid. Albeit that the extra- and intra-embryonic mesoderms have different origins, there may be migration of some intra-embryonic mesodermal cells into the (extra-embryonic) amniotic mesoderm. Cells from the latter add a minor fraction to the population of amniocytes, but have a proliferative advantage, and may come to comprise most of the cells present following in vitro culture.

Amniocentesis is, therefore, a procedure that samples cells having origin from the epiblast of the inner cell mass, and these cells rather closely reflect the true constitution of the embryo. *Chorionic villus sampling*, on the other hand, samples more distantly related cells: trophoblast cells (direct and short-term culture), which were the first lineage to differentiate from totipotent cells of the morula, and villus core cells (long-term culture), which reflect the more recently separated lineage of the extra-embryonic mesoderm. The differing origins of tissues sampled by different means are set out in Fig. 21–3. *Noninvasive prenatal testing (NIPT)* samples cell-free DNA that originated from apoptotic trophoblast cells, and therefore is more closely related to CVS than to amniocentesis (indeed, it has been called a "liquid early CVS").

Mechanisms of Mosaicism

Mosaicism may involve aneuploidy for an intact chromosome or for an abnormal chromosome, along with a normal cell line. Two broad formats may apply, whereby the mosaicism arose: first, a mitotic error in an initially normal conceptus which gives rise to an abnormal cell line; or, second, an initially abnormal conceptus, typically due to a meiotic error, with a subsequent mitotic event generating a normal cell line (Fig. 3–8). The distribution of the normal and the abnormal cell lines in the fetus and the placenta depends upon the time and the place of the abnormal mitotic event. If, for example, a trisomic conceptus is "rescued" by the generation of a normal cell line, at a very early stage, in a cell that is going to give rise to the inner cell mass and to some of the extrafetal tissues, then the embryo may be

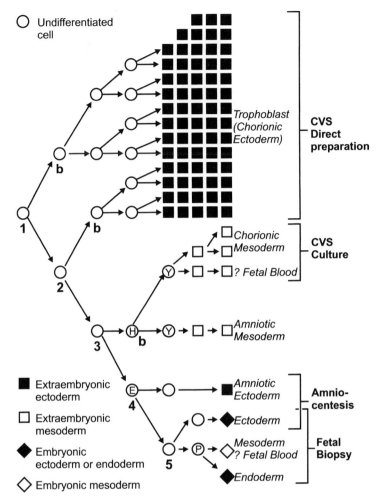

FIGURE 21–3 Diagram of cell lineages arising from differentiation in the very early conceptus. The fertilized egg (1) produces a trophoblast precursor (1b) and a totipotent stem cell (2), which in turn forms another trophoblast precursor (2b) and a stem cell (3) that produces the inner cell mass. The inner cell mass divides into stem cells for hypoblast (3b) and epiblast (4). The epiblast cell(s) (5) produces embryonic ectoderm and primitive streak, and the latter is the source of embryonic mesoderm and endoderm. The cell lineages sampled at various prenatal diagnostic procedures are indicated at right. E, epiblast; H, hypoblast; P, primitive streak; Y, yolk sac.[1]

Source: From Bianchi et al., Origin of extra-embryonic mesoderm in experimental animals: Relevance to chorionic mosaicism in humans, *Am J Med Genet* 46: 542–550, 1993. Courtesy D. W. Bianchi, and with the permission of Wiley-Liss.

46,N, and the placenta will show mosaic trisomy. If rescue occurred at a later stage, the placenta might be entirely trisomic, with a mosaic trisomy of the fetus. These and other possible combinations are depicted in Figure 21–4. The eventual phenotype will be influenced by the tissue distribution of the cell lineages that contain the trisomic chromosome, and the normal:trisomic proportions in various tissues. The important distinction between confined placental mosaicism and true fetal mosaicism, as identified at CVS and follow-up amniocentesis, is outlined in Tables 21–2 and 21–3.

---

1 This construction is to be compared with that of Kennerknecht et al. (1993b), in which three postzygotic mitoses occur, producing eight totipotent cells, before the cells begin to take on their tissue identities. Robinson et al. (2002) propose a further variation, with some cells of the embryonic mesoderm migrating into the (otherwise extra-embryonic) mesodermal layer of the amnion.

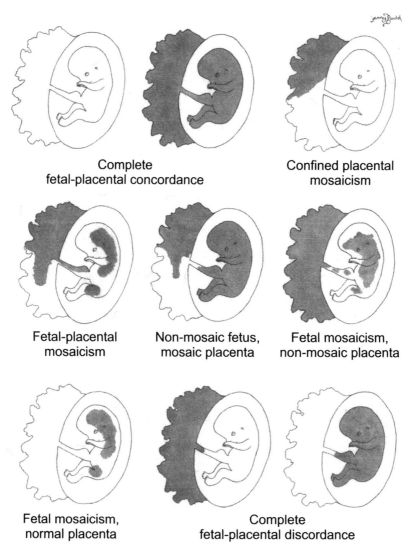

Complete
fetal-placental concordance

Confined placental
mosaicism

Fetal-placental
mosaicism

Non-mosaic fetus,
mosaic placenta

Fetal mosaicism,
non-mosaic placenta

Fetal mosaicism,
normal placenta

Complete
fetal-placental discordance

FIGURE 21–4   Types of mosaicism of the fetal-placental unit. Fetus depicted enclosed in its sac at right, with the chorionic villi comprising the placenta to left. Gray areas indicate an aneuploid cell line; white areas indicate karyotypic normality. In reality, the distributions of the two cell lines are unlikely to be as clear-cut as is shown here. In the examples showing placental mosaicism, the path taken by the sampling needle will determine whether the abnormality is detected or missed at chorionic villus sampling. The cartoon of the fetus, sac, and placenta is close to the form and about two-thirds of the size that actually exists at 10 weeks 0 days (gestational age as measured clinically, dated from the last menstrual period), when crown-rump length is approximately 30 mm.

The potential for widely differing tissue distributions of the different cell lines may confound interpretation at prenatal diagnosis. Consider the case of Jewell et al. (1992). A dup(12) chromosome was present in 87% of amnion cells, 60% of fetal blood, but only 2% of chorionic villi and in 0% of chorionic membrane. Kingston et al. (1993) provided a similar remarkable (and disconcerting) example. Amniotic fluid cells had 3% with an supernumerary marker chromosome; a sample of fetal blood showed all cells 46,N; and several tissues taken post termination had various fractions of mosaicism, including brain with 88% of cells aneuploid. Stankiewicz et al. (2001c) report an infant with the nonmosaic karyotype 46,X,der(Y)t(Y;7)(p11.32;p15.3) causing a 7p trisomy syndrome, following the CVS diagnosis of very low-grade mosaicism 46,X,der(Y)t(Y;7)[1]/46,XY[49], and yet with nonmosaic 46,X,der(Y)t(Y;7) at amniocentesis. These observations point to an early postzygotic origin of the translocation in an initially 46,XY conceptus, apparently affecting the entire inner cell mass, but only a very small minority of trophoblasts. These three cases, admittedly exceptional, are instructive in emphasizing that the proportions of abnormal cells in one tissue cannot necessarily be taken as indicative of proportions elsewhere.

Laboratory Assessment of Mosaicism

The resolution of mosaicism in the cytogenetics laboratory and in its clinical interpretation can differ for CVS and amniocentesis, and we will consider them separately. In terms of the laboratory result, we can apply to both CVS and amniocentesis the concept of different levels of in vitro mosaicism, originally developed for amniocentesis by Worton and Stern (1984), and refined by Hsu et al. (1992) and Hsu and Benn (1999), as follows:

Level I: A single abnormal cell is seen. With near certainty this is cultural artifact, and it is thus pseudomosaicism. The laboratory would not usually report the single cell observation, if the analysis of additional cells failed to confirm the abnormality.[2]

Level II: Two or more cells with the same chromosomal abnormality in a dispersed culture from a single flask, or in a single abnormal colony from an in situ culture (i.e., possibly or probably just a single clone). Some would also include the observation of two or more colonies from the same in situ culture. The abnormality is not observed in multiple colonies from other independent cultures. This form of mosaicism is almost always pseudomosaicism. It would not usually be reported to the physician if additional workup failed to confirm the trisomy, but it may be reported if additional studies were inadequate, if fetal anomalies had been identified, or in the case of certain chromosome abnormalities which are well recognized as existing in the mosaic

state (e.g., trisomy 16). A course of action to resolve the issue cytogenetically, in the case of amniocentesis, is given in Table 21–4.

Level III: Two or more cells with the same chromosome abnormality, distributed over two or more independent cultures. Level III is likely to reflect a true mosaicism, and the cytogeneticist will report this finding immediately. (Some allow level III to include more than one colony in only a single flask, although this could be an "overinterpreted level II" if two colonies in the one flask had arisen from a single cell whose progeny migrated and established separated clones.)

The distinction may not be quite as clear as this in practice, but this is a useful working definition. The mathematics of sampling comes into the picture: How many cells need to be looked at in order to establish what level of confidence that the possibility of mosaicism of what extent can safely be disregarded? Tables have been derived to assist in answering this question (Hook 1977; Sikkema-Raddatz et al. 1997a). Inevitably, low-level mosaicism will, on rare occasions, be missed. Given the reality that only a limited number of cells can be karyotyped on the classical approach, the statistics will sometimes conspire against the cytogeneticist, and only normal cells will be examined. This has to be accepted: The test is not perfect. For example, de Pater et al. (2003) describe their experience in reporting a normal result from amniocentesis, but in due course the child proving to be a r(12) mosaic, with a high level of 50% on blood. Critically reviewing their procedures, and indeed being able to see the ring chromosome when archived material from the amniocentesis was restudied, they nevertheless drew the conclusion that their original analysis has been appropriately performed. A similar example, with respect to a CVS case, is noted below, in the section on 47,+i(5p). In CVS, the exposure to error may relate to the part of the placenta the sampling needle happens to traverse.

NEWER METHODOLOGIES AND MOSAICISM

Microarray. Ballif et al. (2006) tested the system, using experimental dilutions of a 46,XY sample

---

2 An exception may be mosaicism for an isochromosome, as a handful of reports have demonstrated true mosaicism in the context of a single abnormal cell at prenatal diagnosis (see below).

with a 47,XY,+21 sample, in order to mimic trisomy 21 mosaicism; and they demonstrated that mosaicism of 20% or greater could confidently be identified. Similarly, Cross et al. (2007) set up mock samples from normal and trisomy 8 fibroblasts, and, by analyzing the extracted DNA with a 50K single nucleotide polymorphism (SNP) array, they established that down to a 20% level, mosaicism was readily recognized, but fading out at approximately 10%. In terms of actual experience, it is of interest that the threshold of detection, in practice, may be as low as 9% (Carey et al. 2014a). Filges et al. (2011) detected three cases of differing forms of mosaicism among 80 high-risk pregnancies tested by array comparative genomic hybridization (array-CGH), and show, unsurprisingly, that the same dilemmas can arise with confined placental mosaicism as seen in conventional karyotyping.

Quantitative Fluorescent Polymerase Chain Reaction. Mosaicism may be detected with reasonable efficiency on qualitative fluorescent polymerase chain reaction (QF-PCR). In one large retrospective study, Donaghue et al. (2005) reviewed 8,983 amniocentesis and CVS samples, from which 18 cases with mosaicism were identified. More (12) were detected by QF-PCR than by karyotyping (8), although neither approach picked up all. By their reckoning, a tissue load of 15% or more abnormal cells would allow detection of mosaicism by QF-PCR.

Noninvasive Prenatal Testing. Although NIPT is frequently referred to as the testing of cell-free fetal DNA, the primary source is of apoptotic placental cells of the cytotrophoblast, and so it is more accurate to speak of cell-free placental DNA. Thus, the question of mosaicism as with CVS applies similarly to NIPT, and it is an important cause of a false-positive result; the counsellor will find Figure 1 in Grati (2016) a helpful illustration. This is particularly relevant when considering the choice of an invasive procedure for the confirmation of a high-risk NIPT result. Given that NIPT is typically performed at 10–11 weeks gestation, a check CVS can be offered without delay, but in the awareness that the same false-positive (i.e., due to CPM) result

might be forthcoming.[3] Mardy and Wapner (2016) propose the following protocol: Offer CVS initially, and analyze using both fluorescence in situ hybridization (FISH) and long-term culture. If both FISH and CVS show a nonmosaic result, then the result is reported to the patient; but if mosaicism is observed in either, amniocentesis is recommended.

PREDICTION OF PHENOTYPE IN AN INDIVIDUAL MOSAIC CASE

Elegant theorizing notwithstanding, the pragmatic observations from published cases in the literature provide the mainstay of the advice that the counselor may offer the parents in an individual case. (Large series are better than single case reports, which are better than anecdote.) Are mosaicisms for some particular chromosomes, or types of aberration, of more concern than others? What is a low enough level of mosaicism, if any such exists, to have a degree of confidence that the child will be physically and mentally normal? We set out below summaries of the recorded examples from the literature, none of which necessarily provide a firm answer, but which may serve as the basis for discussion and counseling. The numbers in some are very small.

Another difficulty with these observational data is that, for the most part, the window of assessment of the child's phenotype was confined to the neonatal period. Of course, many children who are eventually diagnosed with significant handicap may have been well grown and morphologically normal at birth, with normal functional neurology (inasmuch as this may be assessed in a baby). On the other hand, it is possible to overdiagnose problems in babyhood, as a child who subsequently develops normally may prove (Warburton 1991; Joyce et al. 2001). An important concern in mosaicism is that a cell line inaccessible to analysis—specifically, in the brain—might contain the abnormal chromosome, notwithstanding a normal karyotype in the postnatal tissues which are normally examined, namely blood and possibly skin or buccal mucosa. If so, cognitive functioning could be compromised. Those few reports that include follow-up data for some years into childhood (Baty et al. 2001; Amor et al. 2006) are therefore most valuable. Nevertheless, no

---

3 This point can have a real clinical relevance, as Srebniak et al. (2014) describe in a diagnosis of 45,X at NIPT. A confirmatory uncultured CVS showed 45,X/46,X,idic(Y) mosaicism, and termination of the pregnancy was initially chosen. But a check amniocentesis showed nonmosaic 46,X,idic(Y), and a decision was then taken to continue the pregnancy, accepting that the male child would likely be infertile. In retrospect, it was concluded that the 45,X line was confined to chorionic villus.

Table 21–2. Different Types of Mosaicism Identified After Chorionic Villous Sampling*

TYPE	NATURE	TROPHOBLAST	MESENCHYME (DIRECT CVS)	AMNIOCYTES (CULTURE CVS)	RELATIVE FREQUENCY
I	CPM	Abnormal	Normal	Normal	34.8% (308/886)
II	CPM	Normal	Abnormal	Normal	42.3% (375/886)
III	CPM	Abnormal	Abnormal	Normal	10.2% (90/886)
IV	TFM	Abnormal	Normal	Abnormal	1.6% (14/886)
V	TFM	Normal	Abnormal	Abnormal	5.8% (51/886)
VI	TFM	Abnormal	Abnormal	Abnormal	5.4% (48/886)

*Based upon a series of 52,673 CVS procedures, in which 1,136 (2.2%) showed mosaicism, and of which 886 had follow-up amniocentesis.

CPM, confined placental mosaicism; CVS, chorionic villous sampling; TFM, true fetal mosaicism.

Source: From Grati (2014).

certainty can be offered, recognizing that every case of mosaicism will be unique, in terms of the extent and qualitative tissue distribution of the abnormal lineage.

CHORIONIC VILLUS CULTURE AND MOSAICISM, INCLUDING CONFINED PLACENTAL MOSAICISIM

CVS mosaicism is detected in 1-2% of procedures at the 10- to 11-week mark. Mosaicism from an early mitotic error in a single cell can give rise to *confined* mosaicism (confined to placenta, or to fetus) or to *generalized* mosaicism (present in both fetus and placenta), according to the destined lineage of that cell; the broad range of possibilities is shown in Figure 21–4. Depending upon the timing and site of the event producing the mosaic state, the karyotypes observed at CVS will vary. The extreme form is complete discordance, with a nonmosaic 46,N karyotype in fetus and nonmosaic aneuploidy in CVS, or vice versa.[4]

Clearly, an important distinction to make, inasmuch as it is possible to do so, is between a mosaicism confined to the placenta (CPM), and causing little or no compromise of its function, and the presence of an aneuploid cell line extending into the fetus, plus or minus an important effect upon the ability of the placenta to support fetal development. Follow-up amniocentesis is certainly advisable: A normal result, which is very often what eventuates, will substantially provide reassurance that the aneuploidy did not involve fetal tissue. In the large series of Grati (2014), as mentioned above, the great majority of mosaicism turned out to be CPM, with only a small fraction proving potentially to be true fetal mosaicism on follow-up amniocentesis (Table 21–2). As shown in Table 21–2, Grati uses the subclassification of CPM as follows: type I, aneuploidy confined to cytotrophoblast (recognized only at direct/short-term analysis); type II, aneuploidy confined to villous stroma; and type III, an aneuploid cell line in both cytotrophoblast and stroma. A proviso is given in Daniel et al. (2004), who assess that on the order of 10% of CVS mosaicism for certain "rare chromosomes"[5] interpreted as CPM may in fact reflect a cryptic fetal mosaicism, that would not be detected at follow-up amniocentesis, and which might or might not have important phenotypic consequence.

ORIGIN OF TRISOMY IN CONFINED PLACENTAL MOSAICISM

Robinson et al. (1997) studied 101 cases in which CPM had been identified at CVS, seeking to establish correlates of the origin of the trisomy. Some

---

4 CPM is the main, but not the only, cause of discrepancy between the CVS and fetal/child karyotypes. One very rare explanation is that there was a resorbed co-twin with a different karyotype, with the sampling instrument having traversed its placental remnant (Tharapel et al. 1989).

5 In this study, chromosomes 5, 8, 9, 10, 11, 12, 14, 15, and 16.

CPM trisomies are usually of mitotic (somatic) origin, the zygote having been 46,N. Others typically arise meiotically, and the zygote was trisomic *ab initio*. They determined that the meiotic or mitotic origins of the trisomy are substantially chromosome-specific. For example, trisomy 8 CPM is characteristically the consequence of a mitotic event, while in contrast, almost all cases of CPM for trisomy 16 have arisen at maternal meiosis I. From a meiotic origin, "correction" may generate a 46,N karyotype in the fetus, but there is a risk for this to be associated with uniparental disomy. Thus, of the trisomy 16 CPM cases, about half displayed UPD(16) in the fetus. A meiotic origin of the CPM typically implies a more guarded prognosis than if the error had arisen somatically. Trisomy 2 at CVS (see below) is an example of a mosaicism that conveys quite different implications according the meiotic or mitotic mechanism of its generation.

LEVEL III MOSAICISM IN CVS

Level III mosaicism in CVS raises an immediate concern. Management at this point (which will usually be around 12–13 weeks) is aimed at demonstrating, as much as possible, fetal normality; or, if it so transpires, confirming a true fetal mosaicism. Amniocentesis with rapid FISH analysis of a large number of cells, along with detailed ultrasonographic assessment of fetal morphology, is usually the next plan of action; or a microarray analysis might be performed on the uncultured or cultured amniocytes. In fact, the majority of cases will return normal results after this additional workup, since the mosaicism is likely confined to the placenta.

A large body of data on level III mosaicism for autosomal trisomy was gathered by the European Collaborative Research Group on Mosaicism in CVS (EUCROMIC) (Hahnemann and Vejerslev 1997), comprising information on just over 92,000 CVS procedures, from 79 laboratories, during 1986–1994. Mosaicism (or nonmosaic fetoplacental discrepancy) was seen in 650 (1.5%) cases. Of these, 192 were followed up in detail, with karyotyping of fetal fibroblasts, fetal blood, amniocytes, or neonatal tissues. Most, 84% of the 192, represented CPM. The abnormal cell line was present in either trophoblast (type I CPM; in 50%), villus mesenchyme (type II CPM; in 30%), or both (type III CPM; in 20%). Comparable numbers are due to a single Italian laboratory, based upon a total of 60,347 samples, of which 2.2% showed mosaicism (Malvestiti et al. 2015). Of the 1,001 of these going on to amniocentesis, in only 131 (13%; 0.2% of the whole) was a true fetal mosaicism actually demonstrated. A greater risk (18.6%) applied when the abnormality had been detected on villus culture. The likelihood of confirmation at amniocentesis varies considerably according to the specific chromosome abnormality, being greatest when the chromosome concerned was a sex chromosome, marker, or one of those involved in the common trisomies (Table 21–3). Malvestiti et al. emphasize the value and validity of follow-up amniocentesis.

Table 21–3. Likelihood of Confirmation of a Mosaic Chorionic Villous Sampling Result at Follow-Up Amniocentesis, According to Type of Chromosome Aberration

ABBERATION	PHILLIPS ET AL. (1996)	HAHNEMANN AND VEJERSLEV (1997)	MALVESTITI ET AL. (2015)	COMBINED LIKELIHOOD OF CONFIRMATION
47,+mar	8/30		22/65	30/95 (31.6%)
Sex chromosome aneuploidies	17/109		51/153	68/262 (26.0%)
Common trisomies (13, 18, 21)	15/79	15/66	29/151	59/296 (20.0%)
Rearrangements	3/35		18/178	21/213 (9.9%)
Polyploidy	1/28		2/63	3/91 (3.3%)
Other autosomal trisomies	6/188	5/126	9/391	20/705 (2.8%)

Notes. These data include cases in which the abnormal cell line was detected only in trophoblast (type I CPM). A greater risk is expected when the abnormality has been detected on villus culture.

CPM, confined placental mosaicism.

Sources: Data of Phillips et al. (1996), Hahnemann and Vejerslev (1997), and Malvestiti et al. (2015).

RANDOMNESS OF SAMPLING

The vagaries of sampling may influence the interpretation, as the following examples show. We followed to term a woman in whom first-trimester CVS had shown trisomy 7 mosaicism with 47,XY,+7 in three out of eight clones; and yet three out of four placental samples (one from each quadrant), and peripheral blood from the (normal) baby, karyotyped 46,XY. Just one placental sample, which was not histologically distinguishable from the others, was 47,+7 (Watt et al. 1991). Presumably, the CVS sampling catheter had traversed this unrepresentative region of the placenta, and most of the sample that was eventually analyzed came from here. Similarly, in a case of i(5p) diagnosis at CVS, following the birth of the (normal) baby, we identified a region of placental mosaicism (Clement Wilson et al. 2002). De Pater et al. (1997) did a CVS in a pregnancy of 37 weeks gestation in which severe growth retardation and a heart defect had been identified, and this showed nonmosaic trisomy 22. However, from a simultaneous amniocentesis, only two out of 10 clones were 47,XX,+22, the other eight being normal; and a cord blood from the (abnormal) baby gave a nonmosaic 46,XX karyotype. Skin fibroblasts demonstrated mosaicism, 47,XX,+22[7]/46,XX[25]. Of 14 placental biopsies studied by interphase FISH, only one showed trisomy 22 cells, and at a low (~20%) percentage. Again, it may be that a small focus of trisomic tissue happened to be in the path of the CVS sampling needle, and the sample was aspirated while the needle was at this very spot. (This case is an example of "fetal-placental mosaicism," as illustrated in Fig. 21–4.)

DIFFERENT TRISOMIES

Certain CVS trisomies are more or less likely to reflect the same trisomy in the fetus, and the pattern and distribution of the cell lines are also indicative. Trisomy 21 mosaicism on CVS is the most likely to represent a true fetal trisomy 21, whether in the nonmosaic or mosaic state. A risk applies also with trisomies 8, 9, 12, 13, 15, 18, and 20. On the other hand, CPM or fetoplacental discrepancy for trisomies 2, 3, 5, 7, 10, 11, 14, 16, 17, and 22 was never, in the EUCROMIC series, confirmed at fetal or postnatal studies. In some trisomies, a true fetal mosaicism may exist, but at such a low level that there might be no discernible effect upon the phenotype. Klein et al. (1994) reported such a case, a child born of a pregnancy in which trisomy 8 was observed in 81% of CVS cultured cells, 0% of amniotic fluid cells, and in 60% of a placental biopsy at delivery: The child had 4% and 1% mosaicism in blood at 2 and 7 months of age, and 0% on a skin fibroblast study, and was normal in appearance, growth, and developmental progress at age 30 months. Of course, any fetal morphologic defect shown on ultrasonography would indicate the very substantial probability of a major degree of true fetal mosaicism, and in that case the choice of termination is appropriately offered.

PROGNOSIS

The child subsequently born provides the direct evidence of a harm, or not, due to CPM. Amor et al. (2006) undertook a detailed postnatal follow-up, from ages 4 to 11 years, of 36 children from a "CPM pregnancy" and compared their outcomes according to a number of criteria, with a control group of 195 children having had a normal chromosome result from prenatal diagnosis. The mosaicisms included trisomies 2, 7, 8, 12, 13, 17, 18, 20, X aneuploidies, markers, and one translocation. The children from the CPM pregnancies did just as well in terms of general health, development, behavior, and intrauterine growth, as did the control group. Only in respect of postnatal growth was there a small difference in favor of the control group, their mean percentiles for height and weight being 64.0 and 66.4, and with the CPM children, 51.6 and 56.8 (this might have been an effect of subtly compromised placental function, but equally may have been random). These authors did note a statistically significant increase—which does not necessarily equate to biological significance—in CPM children being perceived by their mothers as "more active," and they were suitably cautious about this observation.

There have been a very few examples of presumed CPM suspected at prenatal diagnosis, a normal follow-up amniocentesis, but with the birth subsequently of a child with the same mosaicism (Stetten et al. 2004). In these, the mosaicism was, in retrospect, clearly *not* confined to the placenta, but was in fact a true fetal-placental mosaicism (Fig. 21–4). Notwithstanding these rare examples, a normal amniocentesis is almost always followed by the birth of a chromosomally normally baby.

UNIPARENTAL DISOMY AND CONFINED PLACENTAL MOSAICISM

A specific concern, when CPM for a trisomy is diagnosed, relates to uniparental disomy (UPD) (Kotzot 2008b). This is an issue in those trisomies involving an imprintable chromosome (namely 6, 7, 11, 14, 15, 16, and 20). The embryo may "correct" by postzygotic loss of the additional chromosome, while the placenta remains partly or wholly trisomic. The incidence of UPD in the setting of a mosaic CVS result is approximately 2% (Malvestiti et al. 2015). In the particular case of trisomy 15 on CVS followed by 46,N at amniocentesis, the Prader-Willi/Angelman methylation test can be applied. UPDs of the other chromosomes seem mostly to be without phenotypic effect per se, excepting the unlikely possibility of isozygosity for a recessive gene. Where the UPD concerned is associated, or possibly associated, with a major clinical phenotype (and see Chapter 18), prenatal testing for these UPDs (upd6pat, upd7mat, upd11p, upd14mat and pat, upd15mat and pat, upd16mat, and upd20mat) is justified.[6] Irrespective of imprinting, there remains also the question of a small residual trisomic cell line in the fetus, potentially contributing to an abnormal phenotype.

EFFECT UPON PLACENTAL FUNCTION

If a cytogenetically abnormal cell line is confined to the placenta, does this have any implication for placental function? A global statement cannot be made: Some trisomies may matter, and others not, and the fraction of placenta carrying trisomic tissue is likely an important variable. But for several trisomies at least, a placenta that is in part trisomic apparently retains a sufficient, or nearly sufficient, level of function, and mostly the (46,N) fetus is satisfactorily supported. Lestou et al. (2000) analyzed a series of 100 placentas from pregnancies producing a "viable and nonmalformed" infant, using the methodology of CGH with confirmatory FISH, and found one with CPM in only trophoblast (trisomy 13), two with CPM in the stroma (trisomies 2 and 12), and two with mosaicism in both compartments (trisomies 4 and 18); thus, in these cases, the CPMs were apparently harmless. However, Robinson et al.

(2010) observed placental autosomal trisomy (trisomies 2, 7, and 13) in 10% of pregnancies complicated by IUGR (and in some of these there was also the maternal complication of preeclampsia), but in none of 84 placentae from uncomplicated pregnancies. The more commonly observed CPMs at prenatal diagnosis involve chromosomes 2, 3, 7, and 8 (which mostly arise mitotically), and chromosomes 16 and 22 (mostly of meiotic origin, and typically affecting both trophoblast and villus core placental constituent parts); and it is mostly CPM of meiotic origin that is associated with a risk for pregnancy complication (Kalousek 2000). A quite different question is mosaicism with "placental mesenchymal dysplasia," in which there is a normal and a uniparental cell line (p. 442).

FALSE-NEGATIVE RESULTS FROM CHORIONIC VILLUS SAMPLING

False-negative results are very rare, and more so since many laboratories no longer use direct or short-term CVS culture. False negatives are presumed to have arisen due to an early postzygotic event, such that a normal cell line is generated in the extra-embryonic tissue from a basically abnormal conceptus; or, an abnormal cell line can arise from a normal conception, and this cell line then contributing to formation of the embryo (this latter scenario documented especially in the acrocentric isochromosome; Riegel et al. 2006). The largest formal series to address this question is due to van den Berg et al. (2006). These workers reviewed nearly 2,500 prenatal diagnoses from their own service, and comprehensively assessed the literature. In their own material, they had no false negatives. From the literature, most false negatives have been seen in the setting of a normal short-term culture, and then either an abnormal long-term result[7] or, if no further testing done, an abnormal pregnancy outcome. This highlights a relative instability of the cytotrophoblast karyotype, with a tendency, as the most usual scenario in this context, to lose the additional chromosome from an initially trisomic conception. From long-term CVS culture, true false negatives numbered only in single figures, and several of these were likely due to maternal-cell contamination. Thus, practically all of

---

6 If a SNP microarray has been used for karyotyping, evidence for UPD can be sought from the SNP profile; but it is important to note that some instances of UPD (specifically, meiosis I error where there has not been recombination) are not associated with stretches of homozygosity on SNP array.

7 Or an abnormal result from a simultaneous amniocentesis, typically done in the context of abnormal fetal ultrasonography.

the time, a normal long-term CVS result means that the baby will be chromosomally normal.

Fluorescence in situ hybridization, applied to direct uncultured CVS, may be chosen to enable a more timely diagnosis (a faster "turnaround time," in the laboratory jargon), and particularly in the circumstance of an ultrasound anomaly having been seen. This can target the common aneuploidies, which account for approximately 65% of all chromosome abnormalities. In one large series (Feldman et al. 2000), 115 direct CVS were analyzed by interphase FISH, from pregnancies in which 100 had a minor fetal anomaly by ultrasound, and 15 had a major anomaly. All of the FISH results were confirmed by routine cytogenetics, with no false positives or false negatives compared to the results after culturing. Although the authors did not separate the chromosome abnormalities found in CVS versus amniotic fluid, overall, they found aneuploidies by FISH in 10.6% of samples, with another 3.8% of cases having chromosome abnormalities by analysis of cultured cells that had shown a normal FISH result. Thus, the common aneuploidies are highly likely to be identified by uncultured, interphase FISH, but when the result is normal, routine karyotyping or microarray is still necessary to detect other abnormalities.

AMNIOTIC FLUID CELL CULTURE AND MOSAICISM

A mitotic error in the epiblast may produce mosaicism of both embryonic and amniotic tissue. A mitotic error in extra-embryonic epithelium causes mosaicism confined to the amniotic membrane. An in vitro cell division defect causes pseudomosaicism. Separating confined placental mosaicism and pseudomosaicism from true mosaicism is critical but not necessarily straightforward. The distinction is, in the first instance, based upon the number of abnormal cells seen, and whether one or more than one presumptive abnormal clone exists, according to the three levels I–III set out above. Level I mosaicism is seen in 2.5%–7% of amniocenteses, level II in 0.7%–1.1%, and level III in approximately 2 per 1,000 amniotic fluids (Wilson et al. 1989).

Once the laboratory studies are completed, the cytogeneticist will provide an opinion about the level of mosaicism, taking into account technical aspects of the cultures. There is generally no point, and indeed it could be counterproductive, to report level I mosaicism. The only exception would be a

single cell of a clinically relevant trisomy, and if the laboratory could not perform sufficient analysis, because of limited sample, to exclude substantial mosaicism. Some level II mosaicism and all level III mosaicism do, however, require to be conveyed to the patient, carefully and clearly interpreted.

LEVEL II MOSAICISM AT AMNIOCENTESIS

Level II mosaicism reflects a true fetal chromosomal abnormality in only 1% or less of cases (Worton and Stern 1984; Ledbetter et al. 1992; Fryburg et al. 1993; Liou et al. 1993). The nature of the "mosaic chromosome" is important. If it is one that has been recorded, in life, in the nonmosaic trisomic state, or in the mosaic state, the level of concern is higher. This includes, for example, mosaic trisomies 8, 9, 13, 14, 15, 18, and 21 and mosaic isochromosomes 5p, 9p, 12p, and 18p. Albeit that true mosaicism for many of the other trisomies has been observed in the malformed fetus in a pregnancy advancing well into the third trimester or in an abnormal liveborn child, these cases are so rare that a level II amniotic fluid mosaicism is still more likely due to artifact than a true significant fetal mosaicism. High-resolution ultrasonography provides helpful information in this context.

If further cytogenetic investigation is judged desirable—and it often is—repeat amniocentesis for interphase FISH analysis is the procedure of choice, with probe choice according to the chromosome in question. A large number of cells can be analyzed, and quickly. Fetal blood sampling, formerly the mainstay, is rarely used nowadays. (It is to be noted that not all mosaicism is necessarily present in blood, and for example fetal blood sampling only infrequently, if ever, detected a mosaic cell line in trisomy 5, 12, or 20, or i(12p); Berghella et al. 1998; Chiesa et al. 1998.)

Strictly speaking, no amount of investigation could ever completely exclude the possibility of a true mosaicism of the fetus, albeit the distribution of the abnormal cell line may be rather limited and quite possibly of unimportant phenotypic consequence. We have seen, for example, a case of level III 47,XX,+13/46,XX mosaicism at CVS, followed by the demonstration of very low-level mosaicism at amniocentesis (1/28 colonies trisomic) and fetal blood sampling (1/400 cells trisomic). At birth, a cord blood sample from the baby showed 47,XX,+13 in 1 out of

150 cells; 2/32 cells were trisomic in amnion and 1/30 and 3/30 in two placental villus biopsies (Delatycki et al. 1998). It only needed the colony from one amniocyte not to have been analyzable, or one lymphocyte to have been passed over at each blood sampling, for the true state in the baby to have gone unrecognized. The child was reviewed at age 13 years: She was an above-average student and unremarkable on clinical examination; on analysis of 400 cells (blood and buccal cell), none showed trisomy 13 (M. B. Delatycki, personal communication, 2009). Rare similar examples exist to disquiet the counselor (Terzoli et al. 1990; Vockley et al. 1991), but a sense of perspective is to be kept: For each autosome, only the tiniest number of level II mosaicisms (zero for most chromosomes) have

turned out to reflect, in fact, a recognized true mosaicism of the fetus.

LEVEL III MOSAICISM AT AMNIOCENTESIS

Hsu and Benn re-evaluated the issues in 1999, and they have set forth useful guidelines. These are presented in detail in Table 21–4. While every autosome has now had a mention as a mosaic trisomy at prenatal or postnatal diagnosis, some are very rare, and others are of questionable significance. Some reported associations may not necessarily have been causal. Hsu and Benn propose the stringent requirement that, before embarking upon an extensive workup, there be in the literature, for the particular chromosome, "two, or more, well-documented

Table 21–4. Guidelines for Workup for the Elucidation of Possible Amniocyte Pseudomosaicism/Mosaicism

FLASK METHOD	IN SITU METHOD
A. Indications for Extensive Workup	
(1) Autosomal trisomy involving a chromosome 21, 18, 13; or 2, 5, 8, 9, 21, 18, 13; or 2, 5, 8, 9, 12, 14, 15, 16, 20, 22 (SC, MC)	(1) Autosomal trisomy involving a chromosome 12, 14, 15, 16, 20, 22 (SC_o, MC_o)
(2) Unbalanced structural rearrangement (MC)	(2) Unbalanced structural rearrangement (MC_o)
(3) Marker chromosome (MC)	(3) Marker chromosome (MC_o)
B. Indications for Moderate Workup	
(4) Extra sex chromosome (SC, MC)	(4) Extra sex chromosome (SC_o, MC_o)
(5) Autosomal trisomy involving a chromosome 1, 3, 4, 6, 7, 10, 11, 17, 19 (SC, MC)	(5) Autosomal trisomy involving a chromosome 1, 3, 4, 6, 7, 10, 11, 17, 19 (SC_o, MC_o)
(6) 45,X (MC)	(6) 45,X (SC_o, MC_o)
(7) Monosomy (other than 45,X) (MC)	(7) Monosomy (other than 45,X) (SC_o, MC_o)
(8) Marker chromosome (SC)	(8) Marker chromosome (SC_o)
(9) Balanced structural rea (MC)	(9) Balanced structural rea (MC_o)
C. Standard, No Additional Workup	
(10) 45,X (SC)	(10) Unbalanced structural rea (SC_o)
(11) Unbalanced structural rea (SC)	(11) Balanced structural rea (SC_o)
(12) Balanced structural rea (SC)	(12) Break at centromere with loss of one arm (SC_o)
(13) Break at centromere with loss of one arm (SC)	(13) All single-cell abnormalities

Notes: Criteria for extensive (A), moderate (B), and standard (C) workup: A. Forty cells (20 cells from each of two flasks, excluding those cells analyzed from the culture with the initial observation of abnormality), or 24 colonies (excluding those colonies analyzed from the vessel with the initial observation). B. Twenty cells (from the flask without the initial observation), or 12 colonies (from vessels without the initial observation). C. Twenty cells (10 from each of two independent cultures), or 15 colonies (from at least two independent vessels).

MC, multiple cells (single flask); MC_o, multiple colonies (single dish); Rea, rearrangement; SC, single cell (single flask); SC_o single colony (single dish).

Source: From Hsu and Benn (1999).

independent reports of confirmed amniocyte mosaicism with abnormal pregnancy outcomes." The most extensive data treating the question are published in two reports from a collaboration of a number of American and Canadian laboratories: Hsu et al. (1997) with respect to the rare trisomies, and Wallerstein et al. (2000) on trisomies 13, 18, 20, and 21. We make much use of this material in the commentaries later, and every prenatal diagnosis laboratory will want to have a copy of these papers readily at hand. Ultrasonography provides useful adjunctive evidence, but apparent normality cannot be taken as a guarantee. Studies for uniparental disomy may need to be considered in the case of mosaicism for chromosomes known to be subject to imprinting. Further modifications to these guidelines can be anticipated, as new data come to hand.

One should always attempt to confirm a diagnosis of mosaicism, either on multiple fetal samples following pregnancy termination or on blood and placenta in an infant. A post-termination study that did not confirm the abnormality could cause parents great distress, and it needs deciding with them beforehand whether they wish to have the results. An unconfirmed abnormality could be misleading in a twin pregnancy in which the diagnostic sample had come from a vanishing abnormal twin, but the post-termination tissue had come from the normal co-twin (Griffiths et al. 1996). Fejgin et al. (1997) refer to the "hopeful possibility" of mosaicism as a comfort to parents, with the post-termination tissue having sampled only the normal cell line. It is true that even multiple tissue sampling cannot be taken as having ruled out mosaicism, and a diagnosis of "apparent phenotypic normality" in a fetus still leaves open that a functional brain defect could have come to pass.

TWIN PREGNANCY, DISCORDANT KARYOTYPES

Discordant karyotypes may be observed in the setting of either dizygous (DZ) or monozygous (MZ) twinning. Selective termination of the abnormal twin is an option, albeit one that cannot ensure that the normal twin will be unharmed; because twins may share circulations, the process of termination of the affected twin may lead to exsanguination of the normal one (Lewi et al. 2006). In MZ twins in which "trisomic rescue" has been the basis of one twin being karyotypically normal, a risk for UPD applies, and this would be a concern in the case of a "UPD-vulnerable" chromosome.

SPECIFIC ABNORMALITIES

In this section, we outline the risks for phenotypic abnormality of specific chromosomal abnormalities detected at prenatal diagnosis. Since the available data often derive from terminated pregnancies in which only major anomalies are recognized, many of these risk figures may be underestimates. For example, a trisomy 21 fetus may appear normal, to the inexpert eye, on external observation, but we naturally assume mental defect would have resulted; and the same may apply to several other chromosomal imbalances. New knowledge will continue to accumulate, and what appears here is printed on paper, not in stone.

The small number of aneuploidies that may exist in the true nonmosaic state are noted first. In the mosaic list, almost every chromosome is represented, although in the CVS section we do include also a few instances of nonmosaicism.

Autosomal Trisomy, Nonmosaic

Trisomies 13 and 18 (and extremely rarely 8, 9, 14, and 22) are practically the only nonmosaic autosomal trisomies besides +21 that are detected at amniocentesis. Others occur, but virtually all miscarry before the usual time of amniocentesis.[8] CVS, on the other hand, is done at a gestational stage when a number of trisomies destined to abort have not yet done so.

TRISOMIES 13 AND 18

There is a high likelihood of spontaneous abortion after amniocentesis, and it is somewhat higher if detection is at CVS. Earlier figures due to Hook (1983) are 43% for trisomy 13 and 68% for trisomy 18. More recent data from Won et al. (2005) indicated a rate of fetal death in utero following

---

8 Exceptionally, a nonmosaic aneuploidy might co-exist with a normal fetus, in the case of an apparent complete fetal-placental discordance (Fig. 21–4), as Maeda et al. (2015) show in an amniocentesis with 47,+20, and the child 46,XY (but the term placenta proving to be mosaic).

Table 21–5. Probabilities of Survival to 1 Week, 1 Month, and 1 Year, for Liveborn Infants with Trisomies 13, 18, and 21

	1 WEEK	1 MONTH	1 YEAR
Trisomy 13	0.42	0.20	0.03
Trisomy 18	0.52	0.30	0.03
Trisomy 21		0.98	0.95

Source: From Vendola et al. (2010).

amniocentesis-proven trisomy 18 of 32%, while Yamanaka et al. (2006) arrived at a figure of 27%; from a somewhat different viewpoint, Cavadino and Morris (2017) showed a 30% survival rate to term of prenatally diagnosed trisomy 18. Data for survival of a liveborn child are due to Vendola et al. (2010) and are set out in Table 21–5. Further data from Lakovschek et al. (2011), following prenatal diagnosis and a continued pregnancy, give live birth rates of 33% for trisomy 13 and 13% for trisomy 18, with deaths within days. But the outlook for a liveborn child is so bleak, with inevitable profound mental deficiency, barely a vestige of social response in those few who survive beyond early infancy, and typically a requirement for full nursing care, that termination is sought by the majority of couples.

Those who decide to maintain the pregnancy should know of the high perinatal and early infant mortality, the high likelihood of congenital malformation, and the rarity (but not impossibility) of survival beyond infancy (Bruns 2015a). The capacity for communication may be limited to "body movement," vocalization, and facial expression (Liang et al. 2015). Many would regard life-sustaining emergency surgery to the newborn as inappropriate (Bos et al. 1992), but nevertheless, some do have heart surgery (Maeda et al. 2011), and some parents may demand "aggressive" treatment (Takahashi et al. 2017). Carey (2012) emphasizes the need to bring the parents fully into the making of any decisions, and Chung et al. (2017) offer an alternative view, describing a family's positive and rewarding experience of looking after their infant with trisomy 13, with the help of pediatric palliative care staff; a view to be acknowledged, in the spirit of recognizing the plurality of opinion that is seen in the world.

An exceptional case exists in Chen et al. (2004e), in which nonmosaic translocation (or isochromosome) trisomy 13 was identified at CVS, but with only minor ultrasonographic findings; and mosaicism shown in subsequent amniocentesis (77%) and fetal blood sampling (14%). The child in due course had a major (but correctable) heart defect, some minor anomalies, and growth and development were judged normal at 8 months of age. Postnatal karyotyping of the placenta (46,XX,der(13;13)/46,XX/45,XX,-13), and post-surgical karyotyping of tissues from the child (46,XX), suggested that the initial chromosome constitution had been trisomy 13, but then with correction in a lineage which substantially contributed to the embryo.

TRISOMY 21

We expect most readers will have an expert appreciation of the predicted DS phenotype, but we do recommend Hunter's (2010) review as a full and balanced account. Marteau et al. (1994) appraised the views of obstetricians, geneticists, and genetic nurses to the prenatal diagnosis of DS, and recorded some remarkable differences. The respective proportions who would counsel nondirectively (see definitions above) were 32%, 57%, and 94%, and the respective proportions counseling directively in favor of termination were 62%, 40%, and 7%. Approximately 6% of obstetricians would counsel directively in favor of continuing the pregnancy, but practically no geneticists or genetic nurses would do so.

Having received a positive 47,+21 result, what personal factors influence the parental decision? A 7½ year study, over 1989–1997, reports the views of 145 women in Michigan (Kramer et al. 1998). Most (87%) elected to terminate the pregnancy.

The decision did not differ according to parity, race, religion, nor, perhaps surprisingly, with the presence or absence of ultrasonographic abnormality. Older mothers, those who had already had children, and those whose prenatal procedure was done at an earlier gestation were more likely to choose termination. A point to be aware of is that, with modern management, the survival of DS individuals approaches that of the general population (95% surviving at 1 year, according to recent data from Texas; Vendola et al. 2010, and see Table 21–5), but comorbidities become prevalent with age, raising questions of practicalities of care as the parents themselves age (Glasson et al. 2002). On the other hand, if fetal ultrasonography shows a heart malformation and/or growth retardation, there is a risk of prenatal demise or postnatal death (Wessels et al. 2003). In the study of Won et al. (2005), the rate of fetal death in utero after an amniocentesis diagnosis of trisomy 21, in 392 women who decided to continue the pregnancy, was 10%.

OTHER AUTOSOMAL TRISOMY (IN PARTICULAR 9, 10, 20, 22)

Never (almost) do other nonmosaic true fetal trisomies survive through to a stage of extrauterine viability. Schinzel (2001) catalogs no more than about two dozen each of trisomy 9 and trisomy 22, and barely one or two of possible trisomies 7, 8, and 14, with survival through to the third trimester. Miscarriage is nigh on inevitable, usually within the 8- to 14-week gestation range. An example is *trisomy 10*, of which very rare examples as nonmosaics at prenatal diagnosis are known, but survival to term is seen only in mosaic forms, and these infants are very abnormal (Hahnemann et al. 2005). If natural abortion has not already occurred by the time the chromosomal result is received, and if there is supportive evidence otherwise, such as ultrasonographic defect, for there being a true fetal involvement, termination is appropriately offered. Schwendemann et al. (2009) reviewed the sonographic findings of fetuses with nonmosaic *trisomy 9*; heart defects and central nervous system malformations were the most frequent anomalies seen. Concerning nonmosaic *trisomy 20*, Stein et al. (2008) record five cases at

prenatal diagnosis, the indication in each being the discovery of an anatomical abnormality on ultrasound, with early deaths in all except their own case, a child who in fact turned out to be mosaic on analysis of postnatal tissues; Morales et al. (2010) and Maeda et al. (2015) publish similar cases. Of all the other nonmosaic trisomies, it is only with *trisomy 22* that there might be, very rarely, the possibility of a term pregnancy, and in some, limited postnatal survival (Tinkle et al. 2003; Mokate et al. 2006; Barseghyan et al. 2009).

Autosomal Trisomy, Mosaic

DETECTION OF MOSAICISM AT CHORIONIC VILLUS CULTURE[9]

The substantial majority of mosaic trisomies for a single autosome are followed by a normal result at amniocentesis and at karyotyping of the child (or of the aborted fetus). In the EUCROMIC study, there were 192 gestations with mosaic or nonmosaic fetoplacental discrepancy for an autosomal trisomy, and in 84% CPM was confirmed. For mosaic trisomy 8, 9, 12, 15, and 20, only a single case of each was subsequently identified with aneuploidy in the fetus/child, compared with two each for chromosomes 13 and 18, and as many as seven for trisomy 21 (Hahnemann and Vejerslev 1997). With respect to mosaicism for multiple (>1) autosomal trisomies, the presence or absence of a normal cell line is the key point: A fetal involvement is practically never seen if there is a normal cell line, and practically always seen if there is no normal cell line (M. D. Pertile, personal communication, 2002).

The general rule that Robinson et al. (1997) advance is this: CVS mosaicism due to a preconceptual (meiotic) error conveys a significant risk for fetal trisomy/UPD, whereas a postconceptual (somatic) error is usually innocuous. Mosaic trisomies 15, 16, and 22 are mostly in the former category, for example, whereas trisomies 3 and 7 are typically of mitotic origin, and mosaic trisomy 2 can be either.

The possibility remains for a residual effect due to (*1*) undetected (and presumably low-level) mosaic trisomy of the fetus, (*2*) uniparental disomy of the fetus, and (*3*) placental dysfunction as a

---

9 As noted above, a few instances of apparent nonmosaic trisomy at CVS are also included here, on the assumption that—in the circumstance of a semblance of normal fetal development—a true fetal nonmosaic trisomy for that chromosome would in fact be improbable. We assume in these cases, rather, that this would be either "fetal mosaicism, nonmosaic placenta" or "fetal-placental mosaicism" with the sampling needle missing the karyotypically normal tissue, each of these scenarios being demonstrated in Fig. 21–4.

consequence of a regional placental trisomy. The risks for these scenarios differ for different chromosomes, and we provide specific commentaries following.

Mosaic Trisomy 1 at Chorionic Villus Sampling. One case was recorded by Malvestiti et al. (2015), and it was not confirmed at amniocentesis.

Mosaic Trisomy 2 at Chorionic Villus Sampling. Two broad groups of trisomy 2 mosaicism are recognized (Robinson et al. 1997; Albrecht et al. 2001; Wolstenholme et al. 2001b). In the first, a majority (~90% of the total) are characterized by a small fraction of trisomic cells, and usually seen only in cultured mesenchymal cells. The pregnancy outcome is typically normal; in the series of Sago et al. (1997), 11/11 pregnancies had a normal outcome; and of the 77 cases reported by Malvestiti et al. (2015), none was confirmed at amniocentesis. It may be that these cases reflect a postzygotic generation of the trisomic lineage in a restricted region of chorionic tissue in an otherwise normal conceptus, and this small trisomic region has no discernible effect upon placental function. The second, minority group is presumed due to trisomy "correction" in a 47,+2 conceptus, from either a maternal or a paternal error. The level of trisomic cells in the CVS is typically high, up to 100%, with the involvement of both trophoblast and the mesenchymal core. The placenta being substantially trisomic apparently compromises its function, and intrauterine growth retardation (IUGR) is a frequent observation, with a poor outcome (Roberts et al. 2003). One case is known of the very severe defect of "body stalk syndrome" associated with mosaic trisomy 2 at CVS (Smrcek et al. 2003). An atypical case in Chen et al. (2016c) showed 100% trisomy in cultured CVS, 14% in uncultured tissue (on array-CGH), 1 cell in 1/26 colonies on amniocentesis, 0/25 cells on fetal blood sampling, and in 13/134 urinary cells (on FISH) at age 2 weeks; the child was normal.

Mosaic Trisomy 3 at Chorionic Villus Sampling. In the EUCROMIC study, of 10 cases with trisomy 3 at either short- or long-term culture, none proved to have fetal involvement, apart from one child with a normal karyotype at amniocentesis, and a very low 1/100 trisomy 3 count on blood as a newborn (Hahnemann and Vejerslev 1997). Similarly, none of the 27 cases reported

by Malvestiti et al. (2015) had fetal involvement. Zaslav et al. (2004) identified a case of trisomy 3, in which the initial amniocentesis showed 47,XX,+3[8]/46,XX[27], and a repeat procedure 47,XX,+3[1]/46,XX[18]. Fetal blood was normal in 100 cells. The baby was apparently normal at birth, except for IUGR. FISH of placenta demonstrated the trisomy 3; thus, it would likely have been found by CVS, had this procedure been performed.

Mosaic Trisomy 4 at Chorionic Villus Sampling. This is very rare; there were none in the EUCROMIC study. Four instances of trisomy 4 at CVS are recorded in Malvestiti et al. (2015), of which one was confirmed by amniocentesis. That pregnancy was terminated, and the fetus had abnormalities of the heart, colon, and spleen. Two cases are noted in Kuchinka et al. (2001). In one case, subsequent amniocentesis gave a 46,XX karyotype, but fetal demise occurred at 30 weeks, associated with considerable growth retardation (although no externally observable malformations). Upd(4)mat was demonstrated. It remains open whether the unfortunate outcome was the consequence of the UPD or due to placental trisomy. The second case did not proceed to amniocentesis; biparental disomy 4 was demonstrated in the child. Follow-up at 1 year raised some reservation: Although development was judged to be normal, growth indices were low, including a head circumference at about the third centile (in other words, borderline microcephaly). To complicate the story, mother and child carried a balanced t(10;15). The case in Marion et al. (1990), and followed up several years later (Brady et al. 2005), was actually an amniocentesis diagnosis, but since postnatal studies showed trisomy 4 mosaicism in the placenta, it is not unreasonable to consider this is a potential CVS example. The child, at age 14 years, had a low-normal intellect and some physical body asymmetries (of hand, ear, and breast). Blood was 46,XX; skin biopsy confirmed constitutional +4 mosaicism. In another case, Gentile et al. (2005) identified mosaic trisomy 4 by amniocentesis (22% of cells). The pregnancy presented at 22 weeks gestation with micrognathia, abnormal brain development, and spinal and cardiac defects. At termination, trisomy 4 mosaicism was confirmed in placental and fetal skin cultured cells; the cord blood karyotype was normal. Molecular analysis excluded uniparental disomy of chromosome 4, but showed that the trisomy 4 was of maternal meiotic origin.

An extraordinary example of mosaic trisomy 4 at CVS with double mosaicism for trisomies 4 and 6 at amniocentesis, 47,XY+4/47,XY,+6/46,XY, is described in Wieczorek et al. (2003). The double trisomy mosaicism was confirmed on skin (but not blood) karyotyping in the child, whose phenotype, while certainly abnormal, was less so than might have been anticipated.

Mosaic Trisomy 5 at Chorionic Villus Sampling. Only three cases are recorded in the EUCROMIC study; in none was a fetal trisomy subsequently shown (Hahnemann and Vejerslev 1997). Another three cases are listed in Malvestiti et al (2015), again without fetal involvement.

Mosaic Trisomy 6 at Chorionic Villus Sampling. Very few examples are known. Malvestiti et al. (2015) record three cases, none confirmed on amniocentesis. A detailed case report is given in Miller et al. (2001). A young mother had a 12-week CVS because of ultrasonographic anomalies (crown-rump length at 11-week size, nuchal translucency), with 60% of cells in short-term culture and 22% of long-term cells showing 47,XX,+6. Amniocentesis was declined. An abnormal heart rate at 25 weeks led to emergency delivery, and a growth-retarded infant with numerous anomalies was born. Her blood karyotype was normal, but trisomy 6 cells were found in placenta and umbilical cord samples. Growth indices remained below the third centile. On follow-up at age 2¾ years, neurodevelopmental progress was "near normal." Skin taken at the time of surgery showed 3% (hand) and 20% (inguinal area) mosaicism.

Mosaic Trisomy 7 at Chorionic Villus Sampling. This is typically a mitotically arising mosaicism. Kalousek et al. (1996) looked at 14 cases of trisomy 7 CVS mosaicism and fetoplacental discordance, the fraction of trisomy ranging from 7% to 88% in 11, and with three showing 100%. Twelve infants were judged normal, and in the eight of these tested, all proved to have biparental inheritance. Two infants were of low birth weight, and the one of these tested was the only of the series with UPD and a meiotic origin; the cultured CVS in this case was 100% trisomic. In a case we studied, mentioned also above, three postnatal placental samples karyotyped normal, and one with trisomy 7; the baby was normal (Watt et al. 1991). In the EUCROMIC study, of 32 cases with trisomy at either or both short- and long-term culture (including three with nonmosaic trisomy), none proved to have fetal involvement (Hahnemann and Vejerslev 1997). The conclusion is that the great majority of trisomy 7 mosaicism detected at CVS arises mitotically, does not imply a risk for UPD, is confined to the placenta, does not obviously compromise intrauterine growth, and is associated with the birth of a normal baby.

Mosaic Trisomy 8 at Chorionic Villus Sampling. A well-recognized postnatal phenotype (Warkany syndrome) accompanies trisomy 8 mosaicism, which may also include an increased risk for cancer (Seghezzi et al. 1996; Altiner et al. 2016). Fetal defects are recorded on pathology examination (Jay et al. 1999). Typically, the mosaicism is the consequence of a postzygotic nondisjunction in an initially 46,N conceptus (Danesino et al. 1998). Van Haelst et al. (2001) reviewed their experience over the period 1986–2000, based on 33,870 prenatal tests, among which were six cases of trisomy 8 mosaicism diagnosed at CVS. These six CVS cases, as it transpired, each reflected a confined placental mosaicism, and from the five pregnancies continuing a normal baby was born. A seventh case had been reported as 46,XY normal on short-term CVS culture, but the abnormal baby had mosaic trisomy 8; thus, a false-negative diagnosis. This circumstance calls to mind the scenario proposed by Wolstenholme (1996): True fetal mosaicism is typically associated with low levels of trisomy 8 in trophoblast cells (short-term CVS culture), high levels in extra-embryonic mesoderm (long-term CVS culture), and low levels in amniocytes and fetal blood cells. Malvestiti et al. (2015) record 30 cases of mosaic trisomy 8 at CVS. Two of these (7%) were confirmed at amniocentesis, revealing true mosaicism; trisomy 8 cells were present in CVS mesenchyme, but not in trophoblast.

Mosaic Trisomy 9 at Chorionic Villus Sampling. Malvestiti et al. (2015) record 18 cases of mosaic trisomy 9 at CVS, none of which were confirmed at amniocentesis. In contrast, Saura et al. (1995) presented seven cases of trisomy 9, five of which gave a nonmosaic result, with the outcomes being abnormal in most. In the EUCROMIC study, of nine cases with trisomy 9 at either or both short- and long-term culture (including three with nonmosaic trisomy in one or both cultures), one proved to have fetal involvement (Hahnemann and Vejerslev 1997). This single case had nonmosaic trisomy at both short- and long-term culture. Slater et al. (2000) report a case of trisomy 9 nonmosaic at CVS, but with level II mosaicism found at amniocentesis, with only two cells 47,XX,+9. At fetal blood sampling, all 85 cells analyzed were 46,XX. Molecular studies revealed upd(9)mat. A blood sample from the newborn infant had the karyotype 47,XX,+9[4]/46,XX[50]; upon further review of the fetal blood, 3 of 102 cells were trisomy 9. Minor anomalies were noted in the child, who had been followed up to age 1 year. It is probable that this phenotype reflected a minor degree of residual trisomy in the child's soma.

Mosaic Trisomy 10 at Chorionic Villus Sampling. Malvestiti et al. (2015) list 10 cases of trisomy 10 at CVS, none of which were confirmed at amniocentesis. Jones et al. (1995) presented one case in which direct culture showed trisomy 10 mosaicism, while long-term culture and amniocentesis were 46,XY, but with upd(10)mat. The child subsequently born was apparently normal.

Mosaic Trisomy 11 at Chorionic Villus Sampling. In all five cases documented in Malvestiti et al. (2015), trisomy 11 cells were confined to the trophoblast, and none was confirmed at amniocentesis.

Mosaic Trisomy 12 at Chorionic Villus Sampling. Malvestiti et al. (2015) report 12 cases, one of which was confirmed at amniocentesis. Hahnemann and Vejerslev (1997) and Sikkema-Raddatz et al. (1999) describe three cases, two of which involved a true fetal mosaicism. Of these latter, one fetus appeared grossly normal post termination, and one infant was abnormal.

Mosaic Trisomy 13 at Chorionic Villus Sampling. A high level of trisomy 13 cells may well reflect significant mosaicism of the fetus. Ultrasonography and amniocentesis may clarify the picture. Mosaic trisomy 13 may present a very abnormal postnatal phenotype (Delatycki and Gardner 1997). A difficulty arises in the case of very low-level (a percent or so) mosaicism, in which case it is possible the child could be normal (Delatycki et al. 1998). In the EUCROMIC study, of 15 cases with trisomy 13 at either or both short- and long-term culture (including four with nonmosaic trisomy in one culture), two (14%) proved to have fetal involvement (Hahnemann and Vejerslev 1997). Malvestiti et al. (2015) record 42 cases of trisomy 13 at CVS, of which only one was confirmed at amniocentesis.

Mosaic Trisomy 14 at Chorionic Villus Sampling. Malvestiti et al. (2015) note 14 cases, none of which were confirmed at amniocentesis. Three examples of 47,+14/46,N were recorded in the EUCROMIC study, none showing fetal trisomy (Hahnemann and Vejerslev 1997). The case in Ralph et al. (1999) proceeded to follow-up amniocentesis, which also showed the mosaicism, and in addition maternal uniparental isodisomy 14. Fetal death in utero supervened; no morphological abnormality was identified. Other prenatal cases (or retrospectively diagnosed, on postnatal placental biopsy) with the syndrome of maternal UPD 14, following "correction" of trisomy, are known (Morichon-Delvallez et al. 1994; Towner et al. 2001; Engel and Antonarakis 2002). Growth restriction, and possibly dysmorphism and minor anomalies, may be associated.

Mosaic Trisomy 15 at Chorionic Villus Sampling. Malvestiti et al. (2015) report 26 cases, 16 of which were confined to the cytotrophoblast, and none of which were confirmed at amniocentesis. In two EUCROMIC studies, cases of trisomy 15 CPM were examined, in which direct and long-term cultures had been done (EUCROMIC 1999; Hahnemann and Vejerslev 1997). Few of these cases demonstrated true fetal mosaicism. Most often, the trisomy 15, mosaic or nonmosaic, was found in trophoblast and villus mesenchyme, and rarely in the fetus. The authors theorize that chromosome 15 (and 16) participates more often in trisomy rescue. This would increase the potential risk for UPD 15, and more often than not, the trisomy 15 would be meiotic in origin. The recommendation is that amniocentesis be offered to all patients with a CVS diagnosis of mosaic or full trisomy 15, prudently to check for the possibilities of UPD, and true fetal mosaicism. Redaelli et al. (2005) propose that the CPM might of itself lead to a phenotype, from their study of a case of severe IUGR and trisomy 15 CPM. At birth, mosaic trisomy 15 (84%) was shown by FISH on placental biopsy (which one could regard as equivalent to a CVS). The child had multiple malformations, including heart, gut, and genital, and an abnormal thymus. Postnatal chromosome analyses of blood and skin fibroblasts were normal, as had been an amniocentesis; upd15 was excluded. The child died at 6 months of age.

Mosaic Trisomy 16 at Chorionic Villus Sampling. Almost all CPM for trisomy 16 (which may present as mosaic or nonmosaic trisomy 16 on CVS) is due to a maternal meiosis I nondisjunction. The important follow-up investigation is an amniocentesis. If this gives a normal karyotype, CPM is very probable. IUGR with a low birth weight is common, but catch-up growth is typically observed. Malformation may be present, but usually these are minor or surgically reparable birth defects. Normal intellectual capacity is well recorded (Langlois et al. 2006; Neiswanger et al. 2006). However, a more severe phenotype may result, and ultrasonography may indicate this likelihood, the complications including major malformation, and fetal death in utero. The degree of severity may relate to the presence or absence of fetal trisomy (which may not be revealed until postnatal tissue sampling), or, in the case of CPM, to the existence of uniparental or biparental disomy of the fetus, although this latter point is controversial (Eggermann et al. 2004; Scheuvens et al. 2017). In the series of Malvestiti et al. (2015), 20 cases of trisomy 16 at CVS were recorded, two of which (10%) were confirmed at amniocentesis. If the mosaicism is seen at amniocentesis, the prognosis is less favorable (see below); and yet we have seen a normal postnatal outcome, on 2½-year follow-up, in this setting (Coman et al. 2010a).

Mosaic Trisomy 18 at Chorionic Villus Sampling. In the EUCROMIC study, of 29 cases with trisomy 18 at either or both short- and long-term culture (including eight with nonmosaic trisomy in one or both cultures), four (14%) proved to have fetal involvement (Hahnemann and Vejerslev 1997). In the study of Malvestiti et al. (2015), there were 53 CVS results showing mosaic trisomy 18, of which nine (17%) were confirmed at amniocentesis. Harrison et al. (1993) studied placental karyotypes from pregnancies in which trisomy 18 had been diagnosed, whether at pre- or postnatal diagnosis, and mosaicism was detected in seven of 12, involving the trophoblast. This supports the view that mosaic trisomy 18 at CVS may on occasion reflect a full trisomy of the fetus (and also leads to the conclusion that fetal survival may, in the context of this particular trisomy, be enhanced if there is a diploid placental fraction).

Mosaic Trisomy 19 at Chorionic Villus Sampling. Malvestiti et al. (2015) report two cases, one confined to cytotrophoblast and one to mesenchyme; neither was confirmed at amniocentesis.

Mosaic Trisomy 20 at Chorionic Villus Sampling. Mosaic trisomy 20 is one of the most common mosaicisms detected at amniocentesis (see below), but observation at CVS is less frequent. Malvestiti et al. (2015) list 29 cases, of which three (10.3%) were confirmed at amniocentesis. In the EUCROMIC study, of 12 cases with trisomy 20 at either short-term or at both short- and long-term culture (including four with nonmosaic trisomy in short-term culture), one (8%) proved to have fetal involvement (Hahnemann and Vejerslev 1997). Six cases were reported by Robinson et al. (2005), two of which had compromised outcomes: developmental delay in one, and growth retardation and stillbirth in the other; follow-up amniocentesis had shown trisomy at levels of 11% and 59%, respectively. Steinberg Warren et al. (2001) described a child, followed to age 8¾ years, normal other than hypomelanosis of Ito, from a pregnancy with a nonmosaic trisomy 20 diagnosed at CVS; culture from a subsequent amniocentesis failed. As the pigmentary skin sign in the child indicated, he was in fact mosaic, and proven so to be on skin culture; and this mosaicism would probably have been revealed had the amniocentesis been successful. We may presume the likely circumstance as depicted in "Fetal mosaicism, non-mosaic placenta" in Figure 21–4.

Mosaic Trisomy 21 at Chorionic Villus Sampling. Chromosome 21 naturally commands special attention. In the EUCROMIC study, of 22 cases with trisomy 21 at either or both short- and long-term culture (including eight with nonmosaic trisomy in one culture), in nine (40%) there transpired to be a fetal involvement (Hahnemann and Vejerslev 1997). In the study of Malvestiti et al. (2015), 19 (34%) out of 56 mosaic CVS results were confirmed at amniocentesis. Beverstock et al. (1998) report a "near false-negative" finding of mosaic trisomy 21, in which trisomic cells were observed in long-term CVS culture, and then, at follow-up amniocentesis, in only one culture. True mosaic trisomy was proven at fetal blood sampling, and at tissue culture post abortion.

Mosaic Trisomy 22 at Chorionic Villus Sampling. Malvestiti et al. (2015) report 11 cases of mosaic trisomy in cytotrophoblast and/or mesenchyme, none of which were confirmed at amniocentesis. When trisomy 22 is confirmed at amniocentesis, fetal defect is typically associated, but the degree may vary considerably. Wolstenholme et al. (2001a) described their own case of nonmosaic trisomy 22 diagnosed at direct and cultured CVS, with 47,XX,+22/46,XX mosaicism subsequently shown at amniocentesis (3/60 cells +22) and fetal skin biopsy (6/170 cells +22). Fairly subtle fetal dysmorphism was noted post termination, and multiple tissue samplings showed mostly low but consistent trisomy mosaicism: 1% trisomic cells in skin, muscle, blood, and kidney; 3% in lung; 5% in liver; and 21% in spinal cord. It is probable that neurological compromise would have eventuated, quite likely of severe degree, had a child been born. Wolstenholme et al. reviewed 11 other cases of mosaic and nonmosaic trisomy 22, the mosaicisms mostly being of high percentages at CVS, and (in the six cases proceeding to amniocentesis) low percentages at amniocentesis. Of nine cases in which post-termination samplings were done, six showed mosaicism in at least some tissues (see also the case of De Pater et al. 1997, mentioned above in the section on "Level III Mosaicism"). In the three cases with 0% trisomy at fetal sampling, all had manifested severe IUGR. This may have been the consequence of functional insufficiency of the trisomic 22 placenta; there is also the point that occult fetal trisomy can never be excluded. Bryan et al. (2002) studied a child born of a pregnancy with a nonmosaic 47,XY,+22 karyotype having been shown at CVS. There was IUGR, but the child apparently showed postnatal catch-up. He typed 46,XY on peripheral blood (with biparental disomy) and was phenotypically normal, except for hypospadias.

DETECTION OF MOSAICISM AT AMNIOTIC FLUID CELL CULTURE

Considering the three major trisomies, Hsu et al. (1992) have determined that mosaicism for chromosomes 13, 18, and 21 very frequently predicts fetal abnormality, in half or more of cases. As for rare trisomies, Hsu et al. (1997) undertook a wide survey, based on the experiences of a number of American and Canadian laboratories and drawing on previous reports in the literature; the reader wishing full detail will need to refer to the original document. Some mosaic trisomies are associated with a high risk for phenotypic abnormality in the fetus or term infant, with figures of >60% for mosaic trisomies 2, 16, and 22, whereas trisomies 7, 8, and 17 are toward the lower end of the scale (<20%). Ultrasonography has a role in the assessment: Most cases in which the mosaicism involves the fetus to a substantial degree will display morphologic/growth abnormality. Nevertheless, normal ultrasonography cannot allow firm reassurance. Some mosaic states might cause structural defects too subtle to be discerned at fetal imaging, and yet be associated in the child with considerable, possibly severe, functional neurological compromise. In chromosomes known to be subject to parent-of-origin imprinting, uniparental disomy needs also to be factored in to the assessment. Comments on individual trisomies follow (for the most part, we are here considering only abnormalities seen on amniocentesis as the first invasive prenatal procedure, and not follow-up amniocenteses done to clarify an abnormal CVS result).

These are rare observations, and in the survey of Forabosco et al. (2009), the most frequent mosaic autosomal trisomies recognized at amniocentesis were, in descending order: trisomies 21 (1 in 4,000 amniocenteses), 20 (1 in 5,000), 13 and 18 (1 in 22,000), 9 (1 in 30,000), and, each at 1 in 90,000, trisomies 2, 6, 7, 8, 15, and 17.

Mosaic Trisomy 2 at Amniocentesis. In Hsu et al.'s (1997) survey, trisomy 2 conveyed the highest risk of any of the "rare trisomic" autosomes for an abnormal outcome, namely 90%, with a variable pattern of major defects. It is probable that mosaic trisomy 2 detected at amniocentesis would be in the same group as the high-level mosaic CVS case (see above). Tuğ et al. (2016) report a case with severe fetal malformation initially identified on serum screening and ultrasonography, with amniocyte fractions 47,XX,+2[12]/46,XX[73]. A trisomic line in the fetus/child may take some diligence to find. Sago et al. (1997) reported a case in which there was level III mosaicism with trisomy 2 cells present in 27% of amniocytes (and biparental disomy). The child was severely abnormal, and while blood and skin karyotyped as 46,XY, 4% of liver cells were 47,+2. Similarly, Chen et al. (2013c) report a fetus with cardiac defect, polydactyly, and dysmorphism, and who had mosaic trisomy 2 at amniocentesis. Trisomy 2 cells had arisen due to maternal meiosis I error and comprised 100% of the placenta, 50% of the amniotic membrane, and 10% of the fetal liver, but fetal lung, skin, and blood showed a normal karyotype.

Mosaic Trisomy 3 at Amniocentesis. Only two cases were identified in Hsu et al.'s (1997) review, in one of which the child had multiple malformations, with the mosaicism confirmed on skin fibroblast culture. The child in the other case was normal. Marked intrauterine, and subsequently postnatal, growth restriction was the prominent feature in the cases in Zaslav et al. (2004) and Sheath et al. (2010); in both, development in early infancy was judged to be normal.

Mosaic Trisomy 4 at Amniocentesis. A very few cases have been reported, with normal and abnormal outcomes both, approximately proportional to the fraction of trisomic cells (Marion et al. 1990; Zaslav et al. 2000; Chen et al. 2004a; Gentile et al. 2005). A single-digit percentage of +4 cells has been associated with normality, on follow-up to 1 year of age. Likewise, normal ultrasonography is a positive pointer.

Mosaic Trisomy 5 at Amniocentesis. Hsu et al. (1997) recorded five cases. In one, a high level of trisomic cells (80%) was associated nevertheless with a phenotypically and karyotypically normal infant. In two, the child was abnormal, both showing the mosaicism on postnatal study. Brown et al. (2009) identified 50% mosaicism in a pregnancy in which an ultrasonographic heart abnormality had been seen, and subsequently terminated at 21 weeks. A dysmorphic facial appearance was noted, and the cardiac defect confirmed, at fetal pathology. The trisomy was confirmed in fetal tissues (excepting blood), although at a lesser level of mosaicism than that of the amniocyte culture. In their review, Chen et al. (2016a) add two further cases; of the total of eight, five had a normal outcome, and in three there was congenital malformation. A further case in Reittinger et al. (2017) may have reflected a 'correction' of trisomy, as the severely malformed infant eventually born had, on peripheral blood analysis, uniparental disomy 5 (and no trisomy).

Mosaic Trisomy 6 at Amniocentesis. Hsu et al. (1997) recorded three cases, each with the same low-level (6%) trisomy in amniocytes, and each with a normal outcome. Reports are on record of the diagnosis following recognition of fetal defects

at ultrasonography, the defects ranging from minor to severe (Wallerstein et al. 2002; Wegner et al. 2004; Destree et al. 2005). One case of fetal death in utero at 23 weeks was associated with 48% trisomy cells on fetal skin analysis (Cockwell et al. 2006). Chen et al. (2006b) report a case with low-level (3%–10%) mosaicism, with normal fetal blood karyotype, biparental inheritance, in which the parents chose termination, and the trisomy was absent on cultured fetal tissue. They suggest low-level trisomy 6 mosaicism may be a benign finding.

Mosaic Trisomy 7 at Amniocentesis. Hsu et al. (1997) recorded eight cases, with fractions of trisomic cells ranging from 5% to 48%. Only one resulted in the birth of a phenotypically abnormal child, but low-level 47,XY,+7/46,XY mosaicism was confirmed in two phenotypically normal children on foreskin analysis. Warburton (2002) emphasizes that this relatively low-risk assessment is the appropriate one to offer, and she notes also that UPD 7, while unlikely, may be worth testing for. A low-level mosaic case, taken to termination with pathology study and multiple fetal karyotyping, with entirely normal findings, led these authors (Chen et al. 2005a) to agree with the view that optimistic advice may usually be appropriate.

Other cases with abnormal outcome (and in which ascertainment was necessarily biased) include the following. Mosaicism was verified postnatally on skin fibroblast analysis in the child reported in Kivirikko et al. (2002), in whom fetal blood sampling and mid-trimester ultrasonography had been normal; there was facial asymmetry and mild dysmorphism along with rather impressive hypomelanosis of Ito, while mental development was "considered to be within normal limits," although no detailed assessment had been done. The fraction of trisomic colonies in the 47,XX,+7/46,XX case of Bilimoria and Rothenberg (2003) was rather high, at 41%, and in addition uniparental heterodisomy was shown in the 46,XX line; the pregnancy had come to attention because of an increased-risk maternal serum screen. On a neonatal blood sample, all cells were 46,XX, while on the contrary, all placental cells analyzed were trisomic. The child was small for dates and had some minor anomalies. These authors mention an anecdote of a trisomy 7 mosaic woman "graduating from college and getting married." Petit et al. (2012) describe a case of IUGR leading to amniocentesis, which was interpreted at the time as normal. The child proved to be retarded in growth and development, and displayed hypomelanosis of Ito. Blood analysis showed 46,XY with maternal UPD 7. The skin fibroblast karyotype, however, was 47,XY,+7/46,XY; and restudy of stored amniocytes from long-term culture showed mosaic trisomy 7. These authors provide a useful review.

Mosaic Trisomy 8 at Amniocentesis. Counseling is difficult, and advice must be cautious. An observation of trisomy 8 in amniocytes predicts a distinct probability, but by no means a certainty, of the clinical syndrome, namely Warkany syndrome. It is not possible to put a good figure on the level of risk. Vice versa, a true fetal mosaicism may not necessarily be detected at amniocentesis (Wolstenholme 1996). A finding of apparently normal morphology at fetal examination following termination in some 47,+8/46,N pregnancies might be misleading, since the physical component of the clinical syndrome is relatively minor (Hsu et al. 1997). In the series of van Haelst et al. (2001), the two cases of trisomy 8 mosaicism detected at amniocentesis both turned out to be pseudomosaicism.

Mosaic Trisomy 9 at Amniocentesis. The risk is high (Saura et al. 1995; Chen et al. 2003a). Hsu et al. (1997) recorded data on 25 cases, with pregnancy termination being done in 21. Abnormality was identified in most of the 21, and mosaicism was confirmed in the seven having skin fibroblast studies. In the four pregnancies continuing, one abnormal child was born, with 47,+9/46,N mosaicism on blood karyotyping, the other three pregnancies resulting in apparently normal newborns. An overall figure of 56% applies for the risk that the fetus is abnormal. This high percentage figure is not surprising, and indeed it may well be an underestimate of the risk for functional abnormality in the child (intellect not being assessable in the newborn), considering the well-recorded phenotype of mosaic trisomy 9 in older individuals. A review of the outcomes in surviving individuals is given in Bruns and Campbell (2015b).

Mosaic Trisomy 10 at Amniocentesis. In one case listed in Daniel et al. (2004), a 47,XX,+10[27]/46,XX[83] karyotype was associated with severe fetal defects, this observation being the basis of the referral for prenatal diagnosis. They were able to ascertain that the cause was a postzygotic duplication of the maternal homolog.

Mosaic Trisomy 11 at Amniocentesis. Of the four reported examples, all have had a normal outcome. One child came from a pregnancy with a 26% fraction of trisomic cells, with 46,N findings on postnatal tissues, and followed through to 1 year of age. Basel-Vanagaite et al. (2006) raise the question that this mosaicism may typically be a benign finding.

Mosaic Trisomy 12 at Amniocentesis. This is one of the more frequently described mosaicisms, and often implies a high risk. Hsu et al. (1997) accumulated 23 cases, comprising 12 continuing pregnancies and 11 terminations. In most of those proceeding to fetal or neonatal fibroblast karyotyping, the mosaicism was subsequently confirmed, albeit that most of the fetuses appeared to be normal. It is possible, however, that some subtle physical features, and possibly unsubtle neurological deficit, might have eventuated had these "normal" fetuses been born. The clinical range in the few recorded liveborn patients with true trisomy 12 mosaicism is very variable, from lethality in the newborn period through to an otherwise normal man with Kartagener syndrome being investigated for infertility (DeLozier-Blanchet et al. 2000). Of the 12 continuing pregnancies in Hsu et al., the outcomes were abnormal in five and grossly normal newborns in seven. Three of these normal infants followed for 5 months to 5 years were all judged to be continuing along normally, and Staals et al. (2003) add another 3-year-old to this list. The proportion of trisomic cells at amniocentesis apparently is not a very helpful guide in prognosis. In one case in Daniel et al. (2004), associated with fetal defect at 18-week termination, the trisomy had resulted from a postzygotic duplication of one homolog.

Mosaic Trisomy 13 at Amniocentesis. The risk for abnormality is very high. A collaboration of 23 American and Canadian laboratories provided data on the outcomes of 25 prenatal diagnoses of 47,+13/46 mosaicism (Wallerstein et al. 2000). Care was taken to exclude cases in which ascertainment had been biased by abnormal ultrasonography. In 21, the pregnancies were terminated. Various abnormalities were identified in 10 of these; the range of percentages of abnormal amniocytes was very wide, 6%–94%, average 58%. No defect was detectable in the remaining 11 aborted fetuses, although the assessment was limited to simple inspection. Four pregnancies proceeded to apparently normal live birth;

the percentages of abnormal amniocytes in these were lower, ranging from 5% to 13%. We mentioned above the very low-level mosiaicsm at a post-CVS follow-up amniocentesis in Delatycki et al. (1998), with a normal outcome.

Mosaic Trisomy 14 at Amniocentesis. Chen et al. (2013e) summarized 10 cases from the literature. In three of the 10 cases, the trisomy 14 resulted from an isochromosome 14. Four of the 10 pregnancies continued to term, from which three infants appeared normal, and one had multiple abnormalities resulting in neonatal death. Five pregnancies were terminated, in which four had multiple abnormalities, and one had micrognathia only. One pregnancy ended in intrauterine fetal death at 18 weeks gestation, in the absence of anatomical abnormality. A risk exists for UPD 14, over and above any defect due to the mosaic trisomy per se, and this should be checked.

Mosaic Trisomy 15 at Amniocentesis. Trisomy 15 is usually the consequence of a maternal meiosis I nondisjunction. Amniotic fluid mosaicism may well reflect a true mosaicism of the fetus. In Hsu et al. (1997), six of the 11 cases recorded had an abnormal outcome, the risk being greater when the trisomy level was higher (>40%). Zaslav et al. (1998) review seven cases of low-level mosaic trisomy 15 detected at prenatal diagnosis, in each the amniocentesis having been done for advanced maternal age. All seven chose to terminate, and a variety of defects were documented in most but not all. In their own case, the trisomic cell line in the initial amniocyte analysis was at a low level: 47,XX,+15[2]/46,XX[37]. Fetal tissues were also at low levels (lung 2%–5%, heart 8%–15%, skin 6%–10%, on metaphase and interphase analysis, respectively), but the placenta showed 100% trisomy on metaphase analysis, and 95% using FISH on interphase cells. These authors also document from the literature four cases of abnormal liveborns with trisomy 15 mosaicism. There is the additional question of upd(15)mat, the considerable phenotypic consequence of which—that is, Prader-Willi syndrome—may be superadded upon that of a trisomy 15 mosaicism.

Mosaic Trisomy 16 at Amniocentesis. Neiswanger et al. (2006) conducted an exhaustive literature review of trisomy 16 mosaicism diagnosed prenatally, including 36 cases from amniocentesis; and they reported their own findings in three cases in which no prior CVS had been undertaken. Of these three, all had abnormal outcomes: IUGR but with normal cognitive development as judged at 14 months; IUGR and major malformations including cardiac dextroposition; and IUGR with hypoplastic left heart, leading to neonatal death. In their literature review, the figures for complication were as follows: infant death, 33%; prematurity, 64%; IUGR, 69%; physical anomalies, 75%; and just one assessed as a normal outcome, 3% (these figures being considerably worse than for CVS diagnosis). They note that level II mosaicism, in this context, may well reflect a true fetal mosaicism. The presence of UPD appeared not to influence the rates of prematurity or infant death; and albeit that Scheuvens et al. (2017) have proposed that upd(16)mat is not, of itself, pathogenic, and that any associated phenotypic abnormality is actually the consequence of a cryptic trisomy 16 mosaicism, nevertheless, UPD was more frequent in those pregnancies in Neiswanger et al. with IUGR, or in the infants with anomalies. Yong et al. (2003) tested for UPD in a series of infants from mosaic trisomy 16 pregnancies, and the fraction with upd(16)mat, at 40%, was close enough to the one-third expectation from random loss of one chromosome; and these infants were more severely affected than those with biparental inheritance of 16. Mosaic trisomy 16 has a particular association with very low levels of pregnancy-associated plasma protein-A (PAPP-A) on first-trimester serum screening, and this carries a risk for the mother of preeclampsia (Yong et al. 2006; Spencer et al. 2014).

Thus, the earlier opinion of Hsu et al. (1998) is supported: "Mosaic trisomy 16 detected through amniocentesis is not a benign finding, but associated with a high risk of abnormal outcome, most commonly intrauterine growth retardation, congenital heart defect, developmental delay, and minor anomalies." Rieubland et al. (2009) diagnosed two cases postnatally, noting a considerable phenotypic difference between the two, one normally grown and developing at age 11 months, but with a severe hypospadias; the other with IUGR, body asymmetry, numerous physical anomalies, and dying at 7 months: yet further illustrating the challenge in offering advice at prenatal detection. Notwithstanding, we have seen an eventual normal outcome, the child assessed at 2½ years of age, albeit that delivery by cesarean section at 36 weeks had been necessitated due to fetal distress with IUGR. Trisomy 16 had been detected at high level on CVS and at amniocentesis, and low-level (8%) postnatally on buccal mucosal cells (Coman et al. 2010a).

Mosaic Trisomy 17 at Amniocentesis. DeVries et al. (2013) summarized 28 cases from the literature, a proportion at least of which had arisen mitotically. The most common outcome (19 of the 28, 68%) was the birth of a healthy infant, without evidence of trisomy 17 in blood and/or fibroblasts. In nine cases the trisomy was confirmed on fibroblasts, six after birth, and three following termination of pregnancy. In seven of the nine cases of true mosaicism, trisomy was not detected in blood, suggesting selection against trisomic cells in this tissue, and possibly explaining why so few postnatal cases are reported. In cases of true fetal mosaicism, the clinical phenotype includes cerebellar hypoplasia, ventricular septal defect, scoliosis, growth and intellectual retardation, and body asymmetry (Baltensperger et al. 2016). The longest follow-up is reported in Witters and Fryns (2008), a child at age 36 months, who was significantly delayed, with a developmental age of 26 months. And yet a number of normal outcomes are on record, as Abrams et al. (2005) document in their own case, with the child reportedly normal as a 2-year-old, and as they note similarly in a handful of other cases from the literature. They advise that an optimistic view is warranted, if the ultrasonography is normal. This view is supported in Chen et al. (2016d), whose patient had a prenatal diagnosis of 47,XX,+17[4]/46,XX[17], confirmed on repeat study with interphase FISH (5/105 cells); a normal child was in due course born, 46,XX on cord blood.[10]

Mosaic Trisomy 18 at Amniocentesis. The risk is very high. In the collaboration of Wallerstein et al. (2000), 31 prenatal diagnoses of trisomy 18 mosaicism were available for review. In just over half of these, the abortuses (induced termination or natural abortion) were abnormal. In 11, no defects were discerned at fetal examination. Just three pregnancies came to live birth, and these babies were apparently normal. The percentages of trisomic amniocytes in these three cases ranged from 2% to 20% (mean 9%), compared with 2%–95% (mean 37%) in those with abnormal outcome. A very rare abnormality is 45,X/47,XX,+18 mosaicism, in which

the phenotype can vary from fairly mild to severe (Schluth-Bolard et al. 2009; Tyler et al. 2009).

Mosaic Trisomy 19 at Amniocentesis. A single case is recorded in Hsu et al. (1997), and in which there was a normal outcome at live birth.

Mosaic Trisomy 20 at Amniocentesis. This is one of the most commonly observed mosaic aneuploidies. Trisomy 20 may exist in three forms: as confined placental mosaicism, as placental-fetal mosaicism with an apparently normal phenotype in the child that is subsequently born, or as a fetal mosaicism with phenotypic consequence (Hsu et al. 1991). There may be no dysmorphic features, or only some "soft" signs, or rarely an unambiguous facial dysmorphism; a characteristic, if subtle syndrome is proposed (Willis et al. 2008). In certain fetal regions in which the trisomy may exist, in particular kidney and gut, the imbalance apparently has no discernible untoward effect, and in fact aneuploid cells may be cultured from urinary sediment. (Recognizing that amniotic fluid has a substantial contribution from fetal urine production, presumably some of the "amniotic fluid cells" from which the diagnosis of trisomy 20 had been made may have actually had origin from the fetal urinary tract.)

In the collaboration of Wallerstein et al. (2000) comprising 152 diagnoses, 10 (7%) were recorded with an abnormal outcome (six liveborns, four abortuses). There was correlation with the level of mosaicism: Abnormality was observed in 20% of infants where there had been >50% trisomic cells at amniocentesis, and in 5% of those with <50%. Baty et al. (2001) reviewed 17 cases in which follow-up of the children extended beyond 1 year, of whom 12 (71%) had developed normally. The remaining five had various degrees of speech and motor delay. A more optimistic interpretation comes from James et al. (2002), who tracked down all cases diagnosed at amniocentesis in New Zealand from 1991 to 2001, numbering 13, with follow-up well into childhood for nine of these (the longest to age 10 years). The range of the trisomic fraction of amniocytes was 8%–50%. All were essentially normal, except for one child who had minor anomalies at birth, resolving by 6 months of age, and deformation due to breech delivery may have been the cause, although weight

---

10 The observation of 5/90 cells trisomic 17 on uncultured urinary cells from the child may well have reflected an occult constitutional mosaicism, but not necessarily so, since a low level of trisomic cells can be a normal finding in this tissue.

was below the third centile; and in the only case in which termination was chosen, rather subtle (indeed borderline) external fetal anomalies were noted, and cultured tissue showed low-level (skin 2%, kidney 7%) trisomy mosaicism. Baty et al. (2001) followed up two cases with higher fractions of trisomic cells at amniocentesis, 83% and 57% in one, and of 90% in the other, and the children, at ages 9 and 8 years, respectively, were of normal intelligence and of essentially normal morphological appearance. Each did, however, display quite prominent hypomelanosis of Ito, presumably reflecting a fairly widespread distribution of a trisomic 20 lineage, at least in skin.

Nevertheless, reservation must remain. Reish et al. (1998) offer the sobering example of a 15-month-old child with considerably delayed gross and fine motor skills and poor language acquisition, who had 54% trisomic cells from a skin biopsy (a normal karyotype on peripheral blood). In the pregnancy, amniocentesis had shown a 45% mosaicism, fetal ultrasonography was normal, and the parents had been "cautiously counseled." Likewise, Wallerstein et al. (2005) report a child who had seemed normal at birth, and 46,XX on blood, but who went on to manifest a "pervasive developmental disorder." Trisomy 20 had been present in only 4/63 colonies at amniocentesis; trisomy was further documented in urinary sediment at age 4 years. They comment that "optimism regarding developmental outcome should be tempered with some caution."

Bianca et al. (2008) summarize the issues and advise along these lines: A second CVS or amniocentesis would add little value; fetal blood sampling is not useful, and neither is UPD analysis; the level of mosaicism does not predict outcome (this agrees with the views of some and contradicts others, as noted above); and some reassurance may be gained from normal ultrasonography.

Mosaic Trisomy 21 at Amniocentesis. The risk for DS is very high. The collaborative study of Wallerstein et al. (2000) accumulated 96 cases for review. Half had an observably abnormal outcome, with confirmatory cytogenetic study performed in a minority. Most of these were fetuses post termination with various abnormalities; six were liveborns, five of these having a clinical diagnosis of DS, and one an isolated heart defect. An apparently normal appearance (assessment limited to inspection in 39, autopsy in two) was recorded in 41 aborted fetuses. Among these, 20 were submitted to further

cytogenetic analysis (repeat amniocentesis, fetal tissue, fetal blood, placenta), with eight showing 8%–90% trisomic cells, and 12 with 0%. Seven liveborns were normal, two being followed up beyond the newborn period; none had confirmatory karyotyping. The mean amniotic fluid proportion of trisomic cells was 17%, range 6%–31%, in these normal children. This compares with a mean of 35% in those with a demonstrably abnormal outcome. But even in the group with the lowest level of amniotic fluid trisomy, 3%–10%, half had an abnormal outcome. From the whole material, a risk for phenotypic abnormality of 50% should be seen as a minimum estimate, since subtler defects at fetal or neonatal assessment would have escaped notice, and a potential compromise of intellectual function was of course not assessable. However, the report in Chen et al. (2016e) illustrates that a confirmed true mosaicism in the child, if of low level (2/38 in this case, on postnatal cord blood), can be associated with phenotypic normality, at least as judged at age 7 months; two amniocenteses had returned trisomy 21 fractions of 5/53 and 6/26.

Mosaic Trisomy 22 at Amniocentesis. Hsu et al. (1997) determined a very high risk for abnormality for 47,+22/46, with seven out of 11 outcomes being abnormal. Berghella et al. (1998) described a normal fetal blood result following trisomy 22 mosaicism diagnosis at amniocentesis, but fetal skin biopsy showed 47,+22/46, and structural abnormalities were subsequently identified in the aborted fetus. Four cases are noted in the review of Wolstenholme et al. (2001a), these all having followed an initial detection at CVS. Three out of the four showed some degree of normal/trisomy mosaicism at fetal samplings post termination. Leclercq et al. (2010) record a normal phenotypic outcome in a single case, followed up to age 4 years, albeit that the child showed the mosaicism on skin, in 6% of cells. Three other cases were abnormal at autopsy study (two following fetal death in utero, and one a medical termination).

Mosaic Partial Trisomy at Amniocentesis. It is not feasible to list here recorded cases, and each must be judged on its merits. One specific example is worth noting, in that it may represent simply cultural artifact associated with a fragile site. This is mosaicism for a del(10)(q23). Zaslav et al. (2002) document a case of 46,XY,del(10)(q23)[9]/46,XY[45] detected at amniocentesis. The phenotypically normal child had the del(10q) in only 3/100 blood cells, this culture having been stressed by growth in a low-folate medium. We are aware of a handful of essentially similar case, all involving 10q23, and none resulting in a documented abnormal child. The biology here is uncertain, as amniotic fluid is normally cultured under conditions that suppress fragile site expression. Indeed, it is not clear that the known fragile site FRA10A at 10q23 is actually involved.

Polyploidy

TRIPLOIDY

Close to 100% of the time, triploidy aborts spontaneously, but in some cases not until the pregnancy is well advanced. In the prenatal diagnosis series of Lakovschek et al. (2011), in which no intervention was taken, no triploid infant was born alive. This being so, the offer of termination is appropriate when triploidy is diagnosed; the ultrasonographic observations are typically quite obvious (Zalel et al. 2016). Cassidy et al. (1977) described the emotional turmoil suffered by the family when a triploid infant, predicted to die immediately, survived for the extraordinary period of 5 months. Sarno et al. (1993) reported a unique case of complete placental/fetal discordance with triploidy on CVS, and a normal diploid karyotype on amniocentesis and fetal blood sampling, with the birth of a normal baby; such a possibility warrants consideration where triploidy on CVS accompanies an ultrasonographically normal fetus. Nonmosaic triploidy typically shows ultrasonographic anomalies, and according to the diandric (partial mole) or digynic (asymmetric IUGR) nature of the imbalance (p. 239).

True triploidy mosaicism is very rare (p. 241). Wegner et al. (2009) report a prenatal diagnosis, the pregnancy ending in fetal death in utero at 25 weeks, with the remarkable mixed-gender karyotype of 46,XX/69,XXY. Numerous abnormalities were revealed at anatomical pathological examination. They were able to demonstrate that the initial conception had been dispermic (one X- and one Y-bearing sperm), and that the 69,XXY lineage had arisen by the delayed incorporation of the Y-bearing male pronucleus into a cell with a 46,XX nucleus; they preferred the expression "mixoploidy" to describe this scenario.

A very rare case is "hypotriploidy" with 68 chromosomes. One case of 68,XX hypotriploidy was diagnosed prenatally, following an ultrasound picture which was similar to that of classic digynic triploidy (Pasquini et al. 2010).

TETRAPLOIDY

Tetraploidy seen at prenatal diagnosis, in the context of normal ultrasonography, is usually an in vitro cultural artifact, or possibly a vestige from the blastocystic stage of normally occurring trophoblastic tetraploidy (Krieg et al. 2009). Balkan et al. (2012) tell a salutary story, concerning a pregnancy with an increased-risk screen, mild fetal pyelectasis and hyperechogenic bowel on ultrasound, and the amniocentesis showing nonmosaic 92,XXYY; but cordocentesis then demonstrating 46,XY, and a normal child subsequently born. True tetraploidy is very rare, and Teyssier et al. (1997) recorded only 10 cases, two of which had been discovered at amniocentesis; further cases are listed in Stefanova et al. (2010), who describe their own case of a newborn who died at age 30 hours. Ultrasonographic demonstration of growth retardation and enlarged cerebral ventricles may be typical but rather nonspecific signs.

While tetraploid/diploid mosaicism is almost always a cultural artifact, Edwards et al. (1994), having observed true normal/tetraploid mosaicism in two severely retarded individuals, nevertheless caution that a tetraploid cell line is not absolutely certain to be an innocuous finding. The 2½ year old child in Stefanova et al. (2010) with mosaic tetraploidy was quite abnormal. In a prenatal case, Meiner et al. (1998) showed 92,XXYY/46,XY mosaicism on fetal blood sampling following the diagnosis of nonmosaic 92,XXYY at amniocentesis, in the setting of growth retardation discovered at ultrasonography, and confirmed at subsequent fetal pathology study.

Structural Rearrangement

Structural rearrangements are seen in about 1 in 1,000 cytogenetic prenatal diagnoses (Warburton 1991). It is typically a matter of urgency to do parental chromosome studies, in order to distinguish between a familial or a de novo rearrangement in the fetus. If one parent is discovered to have the same apparently balanced autosomal rearrangement identified at prenatal diagnosis, and in the context of normal ultrasonographic anatomy, there is no firm evidence for an increased risk of fetal abnormality, and many would counsel to the effect of no discernibly increased risk. Sex chromosome rearrangements require separate attention.

DE NOVO "APPARENTLY BALANCED" STRUCTURAL REARRANGEMENT

A major difficulty is posed by the de novo rearrangement that, at the level of classical cytogenetic analysis, is "apparently balanced," and when the interpretation at ultrasonography is normal. But even with the highest resolution banding, a submicroscopic abnormality (deletion or duplication, or gene disruption) may still be present. Fortunately, this uncertainty is now encountered less frequently, with the increasing use of microarray as a first-line genetic test: De novo rearrangements with no associated copy number gain or loss will not be detected, and they will be reported as normal. When the first-line test is classical cytogenetic analysis, microarray analysis should be offered as a second-tier test, as small deletions or duplications at the breakpoint may be identified; however, a true disruption of a gene, with no net gain or loss of DNA, would not be detected (De Gregori et al. 2007; Baptista et al. 2008). As for NGS, the extraordinary sophistication that this methodology can bring to bear is illustrated in Ordulu et al. (2016). As a harbinger of possibly where the future will lie, these authors showed how NGS could enable a minute dissection of loci at the breakpoints, or of loci potentially subject to a position effect, and allow an interpretation of a possible consequential functional influence. Nevertheless, we should emphasize the pragmatic observation that most pregnancies with prenatal diagnosis of a de novo inversion or simple reciprocal translocation go on to produce a normal baby. Presumably, these normal cases reflect breakpoints in DNA that does not code for a gene or for a control element (or if a gene is disrupted, its haplo-state is sufficient), and in which there is no concomitant microdeletion.

Of course, abnormal ultrasonography dictates a different perspective. Thus, for example, when Price et al. (2005) identified growth and anatomical abnormalities suggestive of Cornelia de Lange syndrome (CdLS), the subsequent finding of a presumed de novo translocation (father not available for testing) 46,XX,t(3;5)(q21;p13) enabled a clear interpretation, the CdLS gene being located at 5p13, and presumably disrupted by the rearrangement.

On postnatal observation, one can be wise after the event. If a child with a particular phenotype has a rearrangement involving a breakpoint known to be in the region of a Mendelian locus, or of other recorded rearrangements producing the similar phenotype, the conclusion could reasonably be drawn that the cytogenetic abnormality was the cause of that abnormal phenotype. For example, a child with a de novo inv(7)(p22q21.3) having a particular split hand/foot malformation would invite the inference of a causal link, given the similarity of the limb defect with other 7q21.3q22 rearrangements (Cobben et al. 1995). Sophisticated tools of the molecular cytogeneticist may reveal a hidden defect, such as an apparently balanced de novo 14q paracentric inversion in which Jiang et al. (2008) could actually show very small deletions at both breakpoints; these authors list the genes within the deleted segments, and they speculate about their possible contributions to the abnormal phenotype of the child in whom it was identified. In a normal person, on the other hand, an apparently balanced rearrangement we may take to be truly balanced. Caution should be exercised in the interpretation of apparently balanced translocations in which microarray testing detects an imbalance, and Gajecka et al. (2008a) provide several examples of gains and losses at the breakpoints in apparently balanced translocations in phenotypically normal individuals.

Empiric Risk Estimation. Warburton (1991) conducted a review of major laboratories in the United States and Canada over a 10-year period and collected data based on more than a third of a million procedures. We make frequent reference to this work. A de novo translocation was identified in about 1 in 2,000 amniocenteses, a Robertsonian translocation in about 1 in 9,000, and an inversion in 1 in 10,000. She emphasized that the outcome data are imperfect, given the lack of long-term follow-up and the questionable accuracy of phenotypic assessment in terminated pregnancies. Having made that point, she did say "there was no case in which a live birth originally reported as normal was later classified as abnormal after longer follow-up. In fact, the opposite tended to occur: Several cases described as having neonatal problems were later described as completely normal."

Small studies with follow-up into childhood have been undertaken (Gyejye et al. 2001), and these suggest that the figures presently offered are in the vicinity of the truth, but a clearer answer will require quite large numbers of children to be assessed. We undertook detailed follow-up, to mean age 6 years, in 16 children with prenatally detected de novo balanced chromosome rearrangements (Sinnerbrink et al. 2013). One congenital anomaly (congenital hip dysplasia) was reported; but compared to population norms, no significant differences were observed with respect to health care needs, intelligence, or mental health.

Given the long experience with prenatal diagnosis now accumulated, it is perhaps surprising that the data are as deficient as they are; or yet, if one considers the reality of what is involved in the logistics of long-term follow-up, perhaps not. A large collaborative exercise involving 29 Italian prenatal laboratories, covering the period 1983–2006, brought together the findings on a total of somewhat more than a quarter of a million diagnoses (amniocentesis, CVS, and fetal blood) (Giardino et al. 2009). From these, 246 de novo balanced rearrangements were identified: 177 reciprocal translocations, 45 Robertsonian translocations, 17 inversions, and seven complex chromosome rearrangements. But follow-up data, in the 80% of cases in which the pregnancy was continued, were insufficient to derive risk figures for clinical outcomes, due to logistic and legal considerations, albeit that the authors comment that "none of the newborns have been reported to display visible malformations." We hope others who might be in a position to access similar data will not be too discouraged; one can offer a note of reassurance for the researcher (and for members of ethics committees) that most parents, in the slightly different setting of having had the news of an ultrasound abnormality in pregnancy, are willing to respond to requests for information about how well their children subsequently did (Ramsay et al. 2009; and as we discuss on p. 19). Equally, it may be that microarray analysis will enable a clearer view, once our understanding of CNVs has settled (Martin et al. 2015); the fine focus due to microarray might bypass the need for a risk estimate by directly recognizing a balanced, or an unbalanced, genome.

The "Carrier Fetus" Who Will Become a Carrier Adult. We have discussed in the introductory chapter the issue of the genetic testing of children. In the case of prenatal diagnosis in which a de novo apparently balanced state is discovered, of course the child has already been tested, and "untesting" is not a practical matter. Consider the example of the mosaic test result mentioned below, the whole-arm translocation 46,XY,t(1;5)(p10;q10)/46,XY. Naturally, parents may want to know what reproductive implications this may have for their as-yet-unborn child. In this example, the genetic risk for the child will be, as the reader can readily determine, essentially that of a likely propensity to miscarriage, should the translocation cell line involve the gonad. It is the counselor's responsibility to communicate this sort of information in outline form to the parents, along with the advice that the child could, in the fullness of time, attend the clinic on his or her own behalf. The information must be clearly conveyed. It could be seen as a failure of the counselor's duty of care if, in the next generation, an affected child were born, the parents being unaware of the genetic risk (Burn et al. 1983; and p. 11).

We review hereunder the different categories of de novo apparently balanced autosomal structural rearrangements, in the context of their identification at prenatal diagnosis. Sex chromosomal rearrangements are considered separately.

DE NOVO BALANCED RECIPROCAL TRANSLOCATION

The starting point is an acknowledgment that precedents are recorded for a de novo translocation having disrupted or compromised a locus, and therefore that the discovery of such a rearrangement at prenatal diagnosis could potentially herald an abnormal child. Of course, these translocations are to be taken seriously. Equally, the truly balanced translocation carrier state (every one of which in the world must have been de novo at some point in the near or distant past) is very familiar, as Chapter 5 attests at length. Very many translocations are indeed balanced, in terms of their functional genetic consequences. Thus, a normal child is very possible, and as the observations have shown, this is considerably the more likely outcome. In Warburton's study, serious malformations were identified in 6% of pregnancies with a de novo simple reciprocal translocation, either at elective termination or at live birth. This is some 3% above the background risk of approximately 3% for malformation and/or serious functional defect that applies to all pregnancies. Thus, we may draw the inference that in approximately 3% of these de novo translocations the chromosomal defect was causative. It seems reasonable to assume that a slightly higher figure, perhaps another percent or so, should apply to the overall risk for not only major malformation but also important functional deficit, which might not become apparent until after babyhood. Normal ultrasonography would be considerably, but not definitively, reassuring.

As mentioned above, microarray studies may well cast light (Lo et al. 2014); although as also mentioned, with microarray as a first-tier study (Wou et al. 2016b), the problem, by virtue of not being recognized, may be avoided.[11] In a study of 14 prenatal diagnoses of de novo simple translocation, the ultrasonography being normal in 12, all proved to be balanced at the level of array-CGH (De Gregori et al. 2007).

DE NOVO BALANCED HETEROLOGOUS ROBERTSONIAN TRANSLOCATION

The great majority of cases will be disomic, non-mosaic, and of biparental inheritance, and a normal phenotype is to be expected. The risk for phenotypic defect over and above the baseline is due to UPD and, theoretically, to occult mosaic trisomy.

Reviewing their own and others' data, accumulating some 102 prenatal cases, Ruggeri et al. (2004) determine a risk for UPD of approximately 3%, based upon the observation of three affected cases (all three due to upd14mat). This figure is slightly higher than earlier estimates, in which results from inherited and de novo cases had been pooled (Silverstein et al. 2002). But because the UPD cases all fell within the de novo group, it may be prudent to regard these separately (and in that case, to see the risk for the inherited form as being very low). Shaffer (2006) combined all studies on heterologous Robertsonian translocations and found that, if all chromosomal combinations are considered, the risk for UPD was 0.8%. If only those imprinted chromosomes are considered (robs that include chromosomes 14 and 15), then the risk of UPD was 0.6%. De novo cases appear to have a twofold increased risk (~2%) compared to maternally inherited Robertsonians (~1%) or paternally inherited (no cases identified in the surveys). Although no cases of paternal UPD were identified in the prenatal surveys, there are single case examples of paternally derived robs and UPD. Given these data, it may be warranted to check for UPD, in the setting of one of the imprintable chromosomes (14 or 15) being a component of the translocation. UPD 15 can be tested at prenatal diagnosis using DNA methylation analysis at the 5′ SNRPN locus (Glenn et al. 2000); amniocytes rather than chorionic villi may be the preferable tissue to test (Silverstein et al. 2002).

DE NOVO BALANCED HOMOLOGOUS ROBERTSONIAN TRANSLOCATION

A chromosome comprising two long arms of the same acrocentric chromosome may be either a homologous Robertsonian translocation or an isochromosome: for example, rob(13q13q),[12] or i(13q).

If the formation of a homologous rob had been through the fusion of the maternal and paternal homologs, which of course must have occurred as a post-fertilization event, then the rearrangement manifestly has to be a true Robertsonian translocation, and the inheritance is *biparental*. In that case, a phenotypically normal child is the expectation, other things being equal (Abrams et al. 2001); infertility would, however, be anticipated (see Chapter 7).

All Robertsonian isochromosomes, and some homologous translocations, will display *uniparental* inheritance. The importance of uniparental disomy depends upon the chromosome involved. In Berend et al.'s (2000) Robertsonian series, there were six identified with an homologous translocation, all de novo, and four of these had UPD, two upd(13)pat, and two upd(14)pat. Barring isozygosity for a single gene mutation, normal outcomes are to be expected following prenatal diagnosis of a Robertsonian translocation (isochromosome) comprising a chromosome not subject to imprinting (chromosomes 13, 21, 22). This is actually recorded for the i(13q) UPD (Berend et al. 1999). No prenatal diagnosis reports exist for i(21q) UPD or i(22q) UPD, but the postnatal state of normality in each of these is known (Engel and Antonarakis 2002). Isodisomy for at least part of the chromosome will exist in the i(13q) UPD, i(21q) UPD, and i(22q) UPD states, and this raises the question of a risk, not readily quantifiable but likely very small, for a Mendelian autosomal recessive disorder due to isozygosity, the parent being heterozygous for the mutation in question. On the other hand, for the imprintable chromosomes 14 and 15, the risk for clinical defect is absolute following prenatal diagnosis of the rea(14) UPD and the rea(15) UPD, and the clinical syndromes of UPD 14 or UPD 15, maternal

---

11 And yet, a new technology may, in its early days, return a question rather than an answer. Rooryck et al. (2010) found an apparently balanced de novo 2;18 translocation in a child with oculo-auriculo-vertebral syndrome and proceeded to a microarray analysis. This showed that each breakpoint was in a gene desert, and no nearby plausible candidate genes that might have been influenced due to a position effect; and furthermore, a microduplication elsewhere on chromosome 18 was identified, not recorded as a known CNV, but which was paternally inherited. What, if any, responsibility these genomic alterations had, severally or separately, for the genesis of the child's phenotype remains, for the moment, speculative. Had this analysis been done at prenatal diagnosis, the interpretation would have been fraught.

12 The formally correct nomenclature is actually der(13;13)(q10;q10).

or paternal, would inevitably ensue (Berend et al. 2000; McGowan et al. 2002).

DE NOVO BALANCED INVERSION

Pathology due to an inversion per se is rare but well recognized. The risk from Warburton (1991) for phenotypic abnormality associated with a de novo inversion, peri- or paracentric, is 9.4%, which is 6%–7% over and above the background risk. The numerator is small, however, and the 95% confidence limits span 2%–25%. Since, in theory, a two-breakpoint inversion should not imply a greater risk than the two-break reciprocal translocation, the figure for this latter category as noted above, namely 3% (or a little above), might reasonably be seen as appropriate also for the inversion. Although if one breakpoint is in an acrocentric short arm, the risk might be that much less (Leach et al. 2005).

DE NOVO BALANCED INSERTION

Only one case is recorded, to our knowledge, of a de novo apparently balanced autosomal interchromosomal insertion detected prenatally (Hashish et al. 1992). The child proved to be phenotypically normal. Van Hemel and Eussen (2000), in their review of nearly 90 families with an interchromosomal insertion, note that of the nine probands with congenital anomalies having a balanced insertion, seven were de novo and only two familial. It might reasonably be suggested that the risk for the interchromosomal insertion (three breakpoints) would be similar or possibly a little greater than the de novo apparently balanced reciprocal translocation (two breakpoints). Recalling the 3% risk figure associated with the latter, perhaps a percent point above this is a fair figure to offer for the risk of "unspecified malformation and/or intellectual deficit."

DE NOVO BALANCED AUTOSOMAL RING CHROMOSOME

The 46,r(A) ring chromosome is discussed in Chapter 11, and the reader is referred to specific instances listed therein. Rings that are truly balanced, reflecting a tip-to-tip telomere fusion, are nevertheless likely to cause growth retardation (or, in the case of r(20), epilepsy). Microarray analysis can reveal a very subtle deletion, which even targeted multiplex ligation-dependent probe analysis (MLPA) and FISH could not detect, as Manolakos et al. (2009) show in a case

of ring 15 chromosome prenatal diagnosis. The prenatally diagnosed r(4) in Akbas et al. (2013) had 4p and 4q deletions of only 130 kb and 2.4 Mb, and this was associated with IUGR. The outlook for the child might be similar to that of the man with a r(4) whose case we mention on p. 213. Equally, array-CGH may demonstrate no apparent loss of material, as Papoulidis et al. (2010) report with a ring 21, the baby subsequently born being assessed as normal.

DE NOVO BALANCED WHOLE-ARM TRANSLOCATION

Very few de novo whole-arm translocations are recorded, "although the existing examples suggest an optimistic prognosis can be given" (Farrell and Fan 1995). A whole-arm X-autosome translocation is mentioned below.

DE NOVO BALANCED COMPLEX REARRANGEMENT

A de novo apparently balanced complex chromosome rearrangement (CCR) has a high risk for intellectual impairment and physical malformation, but equally, normal children have been born. Chen et al. (2006a) and Giardino et al. (2006) reviewed the published cases, in some of which amniocentesis had been triggered by an increased-risk maternal serum screen, or the observation of fetal anomaly on ultrasound. The outcomes were abnormal in about half, the abnormalities ranging from developmental delay to single or multiple malformation. Intuitively, the risk would be greater with a higher number of breakpoints, and Madan et al. (1997) provide support for this view. Microarray analysis may clarify whether a true quantitative imbalance exists; however, a CCR with a breakpoint occurring within a gene might not (as with any such rearrangement) be detected, as exemplified in the t(2;12;18)(q22.3;12q22;q21.33) reported in Engenheiro et al. (2008), in which the 2q22.3 breakpoint disrupted the *ZEB2* gene, causing Mowat-Wilson syndrome. In a report of three CCRs diagnosed prenatally, all proved to be unbalanced upon array-CGH analysis (De Gregori et al. 2007).

DE NOVO BALANCED X-AUTOSOME TRANSLOCATION

In the case of a de novo apparently balanced X-autosome translocation, there are the additional possible complications of (1) gonadal dysfunction if the breakpoint is within one of the critical regions of the X chromosome, and (2) the unpredictability of the patterns of inactivation with the possibility of severe abnormality. On theoretical grounds, the risk may be about twice that for the simple autosomal translocation given earlier (Waters et al. 2001), although Abrams and Cotter (2004), reviewing the literature, arrived at a risk figure as high as 50% (and disregarding a possible risk for reproductive health). Nevertheless, in the case they report, a normal daughter, with follow-up to age 17 months, was born after amniocentesis (for advanced maternal age) had shown a de novo 46,X,t(X;6)(q26;q23) karyotype, with the normal X late replicating. They, and we, hope that further such cases will be reported. Hatchwell et al. (1996) provide the particular example of a severe phenotype associated with a whole-arm X-autosome translocation.

> On the specific issue of an Xp21 breakpoint, the question of Duchenne muscular dystrophy arises. Evans et al. (1993) actually showed normal dystrophin on the invasive procedure of fetal muscle biopsy following detection at amniocentesis of an apparently balanced rcp(X;1) with the X breakpoint at p21, and so predicted the child would not have Duchenne/Becker muscular dystrophy; and their prediction proved to be correct. In a case of de novo 46,X,t(X;9)(p21.3;q22) diagnosed at amniocentesis, Feldman et al. (1999) showed apparent integrity of the dystrophin locus on FISH. Methylation analysis indicated preferential inactivation of the normal X. On these two observations, the couple decided to continue the pregnancy; but fetal demise occurred at 34 weeks, probably due to chorioamnionitis following premature rupture of membranes at 33 weeks. No fetal defects were seen; dystrophin staining of muscle was normal. These days, molecular study would be a simpler approach.

DE NOVO BALANCED Yq-AUTOSOME TRANSLOCATION

The balanced Yq-autosome reciprocal rearrangement, with a 46-chromosome count, has the gonosomal breakpoint in proximal Yq (the breakpoints usually given as q11, q11.2, or q12). Hsu (1994) reviewed 23 reports, in which the usual ascertainment was through infertility (oligospermia/ azoöspermia) in the adult male, with a few being found incidentally, and including one at prenatal diagnosis. Only three, including two from the early 1970s in which the detail of the rearrangement was less certain, were identified through a malformed child. It may be that such translocations should be regarded as conveying no greater risk for an abnormal intellectual phenotype than do reciprocal autosomal translocations, but acknowledging a frequent, perhaps inevitable, compromise of fertility (p. 131). In the particular case of a de novo translocation with Yqh material on the short arm of an acrocentric (which is, to be precise, an *un*balanced rearrangement), this is unlikely to be the basis of any phenotypic defect (p. 133).

MOSAICISM FOR A DE NOVO BALANCED STRUCTURAL REARRANGEMENT

Reciprocal Translocation Mosaicism. True mosaicism for a balanced reciprocal translocation, 46,rcp/46, is very rarely recognized (Fryns and Kleczkowska 1986; Opheim et al. 1995; Leegte et al. 1998). The great majority of this type of mosaicism seen at prenatal diagnosis is level I or II, and this is pseudomosaicism due to in vitro change. Some breakpoints (6p21,13q14) are preferentially involved (Benn and Hsu 1986). In terms of implications for fetal phenotype, it can usually be disregarded. True mosaicism for a reciprocal translocation has been seen at prenatal diagnosis, and Hsu et al. (1996) accumulated 11 examples showing one normal cell line and one with a balanced autosomal translocation. In no instance in which the pregnancy proceeded (nine of the 11) had phenotypic abnormality been observed. Concerning a possible risk for unbalanced progeny in the next generation if the gonad were involved, each such case would need to be individually assessed; the parents would need to know to give their child access to the information in the fullness of time.

Robertsonian Translocation Mosaicism. In four cases in Hsu et al. (1996) of diagnosis at amniocentesis of mosaicism for a balanced heterologous translocation, 45,rob/46, the outcome was normal in all (the mosaicism confirmed postnatally in the two infants studied). The specific translocations were 13q14q, 13q22q, and 14q21q.

Whole-Arm Translocation Mosaicism. The mother reported in Wang et al. (1998) with

46,XX,t(10q;16q)/46,XX mosaicism was normal (although her child was abnormal; see p. 100). We know of one case of level III mosaicism for a balanced whole-arm translocation at amniocentesis, 46,XY,t(1;5)(p10;q10)/46,XY, with 30% of cells in three separate cultures showing the translocation, and confirmed on a cord blood sample at delivery (10 cells out of 50 with the translocation); on follow-up at age 4 years, the child was normal and healthy (D. Grimaldi and B. Richards, personal communication, 2001).

Complex Rearrangement Mosaicism. The only known example to our awareness of de novo mosaicism with an apparently balanced CCR and a normal cell line detected prenatally is that described in Hastings et al. (1999b), 46,XX,t(3;10)(p13;q21.1), inv(6)(p23q12)/46,XX, and this case was associated with fetal abnormality.

Inversion Mosaicism. In four cases in Hsu et al. (1996) of diagnosis at amniocentesis of mosaicism for a balanced inversion (pericentric or paracentric), 46,inv/46, the outcome was normal in all (all four were studied postnatally, with the mosaicism found in only one).

DE NOVO UNBALANCED STRUCTURAL REARRANGEMENT, MODAL NUMBER 46

Autosomal. For any de novo autosomal structural rearrangement in which imbalance is cytogenetically visible, serious phenotypic abnormality is highly likely. Microarray analysis may be used to identify the breakpoints of the rearrangement and aid in the prediction of phenotype. Many cases, indeed most, are unlikely to be exactly the same as those in the literature or on the databases, and the counselor will need to make an informed evaluation. Ultrasonography may clarify the question if abnormalities are seen, but an apparently normal sonogram does not guarantee that the child would be normal (Al-Kouatly et al. 2002). If a "jumping translocation" (p. 226) leads to imbalance, fetal defect is very probable (Annable et al. 2008).

In the *mosaic state*, the risk may be high if pseudomosaicism is judged to be unlikely. Hsu et al. (1992) record 34 cases with at least one cell line having an unbalanced rearrangement (thus, presumed to be a true mosaicism). In follow-up studies, phenotypic abnormality was noted in half and cytogenetic confirmation obtained in 65%. Each rearrangement needs to be considered on its merits. The dilemma of deciding how best to advise couples is illustrated in Cotter et al. (1998). They describe the karyotype 46,XX,der(4)t(4;5)(q34;q12)/46,XX detected at amniocentesis, imparting, in the abnormal cell line, trisomy for most of 5q. This was confirmed on two subsequent amniocenteses, with an average overall of 17% of amniocytes abnormal, but with a 46,XX result on fetal blood sampling, and normal ultrasonography. The parents were advised that "few data were available" to determine risk; they made a decision to continue the pregnancy. In the event, the child appeared normal at birth and at 2-year follow-up; 100 cells at cord blood karyotyping were normal. In contrast, 46,XX,add(15)(p10), t(2;15)(p10;q10)/46,XX mosaicism detected at 30-week prenatal diagnosis (performed due to IUGR), and shown on both amniocentesis and fetal blood sampling, was associated, post termination, with fetal anomalies consistent with a partial trisomy 2p (Pipiras et al. 2004). Cotter et al. rightly call for others' experience in similar cases to be published.

X-Autosomal. Prediction with respect to the unbalanced X-autosome translocation is precarious (and see Chapter 6). Albeit the pattern of inactivation may lessen the effect, and indeed convert an invariably lethal imbalance to a survivable state, the degree to which selective inactivation may occur in fetal tissues is not knowable, and a significant defect remains very probable, the risk as high as 50% (Abrams and Cotter 2004). Had the child with an unbalanced der(X)t(Xp;22q) described on p. 129 (Fig. 6–11) been identified at amniocentesis, and with the DiGeorge critical region intact and no inactivation on the 22q segment, a prediction of typical Turner syndrome might have been reasonable. In the event, this child proved to have a significant mental handicap. Contrary examples in which a prediction of major abnormality would have been mistaken are rare.

Y-Autosomal. Autosomal material attached to the heterochromatin of a Y chromosome is to be seen in essentially the same light, as if it had been a translocation to an autosome (and see Chapter 6). A rare but recurrent unbalanced karyotype seen at prenatal diagnosis is the t(Y;1)(q12;q21) translocation in mosaic state, which endows essentially a 1q trisomy in the tissue with the translocation (Li 2010). The phenotype is lethal. Vice versa, if Y material is attached to an autosome, and if autosomal material is lost at that site, the autosomal monosomy of itself determines phenotypic defect (Klein et al. 2005).

A somewhat different and very rare category is that in which a near-intact Y, missing only part of the pseudoautosomal region, combines with an acrocentric chromosome. Borie et al. (2004) describe the prenatal diagnosis of 45,X,dic(Y;22) (p11.3;p11). Had this dicentric chromosome included all the Yp material, the child might have been normal. But in fact the *SHOX* locus, at Yp11.3 (Fig. 6–1), was deleted, and the otherwise normal male child had short stature.

Yq;15p Variant In the population there is a common variant whereby the heterochromatin of Yq becomes translocated to the short arm of chromosome 15; this occurs in about 1 in 2,000 individuals. Occasionally, translocations with other breakpoints will occur between these two chromosomes, such as the case reported by Chen et al. (2007a), in which the father's karyotype was 46,X,t(Y;15)(q12;p13) and the female fetus inherited the abnormal chromosome 15. Because the derivative chromosome has deleted the repetitive 15 short arm and replaced it with Yq heterochromatin, no phenotypic effect would be expected. The authors suggest that methylation analysis for chromosome 15 should be considered, although in fact no cases of UPD 15 due to this common variant have been reported.

DE NOVO UNBALANCED STRUCTURAL REARRANGEMENT, MODAL NUMBER 47: SUPERNUMERARY CHROMOSOME

A supernumerary chromosome may be of substantial size, and identifiable as to its makeup; or it may be smaller, and its origin uncertain. The latter are referred to as supernumerary marker chromosomes (SMCs), and these have also been described as marker, extra structurally abnormal chromosomes (ESACs), and accessory chromosomes (Hook and Cross 1987). Some as rings and isochromosomes are discussed separately below. The SMCs we mostly consider here are the small SMCs (sSMC); these are defined as structurally abnormal chromosomes that cannot be identified or characterized unambiguously by conventional banding cytogenetics alone,

and which are generally equal in size or smaller than a chromosome 20 in the same metaphase spread. Some are quite harmless, and associated with phenotypic normality, and others are not: They are a very heterogeneous group.

Small SMCs are encountered in about 1 in 1,000 prenatal diagnoses analyzed cytogenetically, frequently in the mosaic state with a normal cell line. Upon the discovery of an sSMC at prenatal diagnosis, an urgent parental chromosome analysis is required. The majority will prove to be de novo,[13] and Liehr et al. (2009a) emphasize the point: De novo sSMCs ascertained at prenatal diagnosis are without phenotypic consequence in about three-fourths of cases. These questions are to be asked: From which chromosome is it derived, and does it comprise euchromatin or heterochromatin? Is it a recognized type of sSMC, for which precedents are recorded? Precise characterization is necessary, and this requires the use of FISH or microarray (Ballif et al. 2006; Pietrzak et al. 2007; Gruchy et al. 2008; Liehr et al. 2009a). On FISH, approximately 80% are shown to derive from one of the acrocentric chromosomes, most commonly chromosome 15 or chromosome 22, and often involving only the pericentromeric region and/or the satellites (Crolla et al. 1998; Lin et al. 2006). Use of microarray as the first-tier prenatal cytogenetic analysis circumvents some of these issues: Small benign SMCs that comprise only heterochromatin will not be detected at all. Larger SMCs will be detected, on microarray, as copy number gains of the relevant chromosomal segment, although cytogenetic analysis may be required to demonstrate that the copy number gain is a result of SMC.

De Novo Identifiable Supernumerary Chromosome of Substantial Size. An additional chromosome which is of sufficient size that it can be characterized on initial routine analysis as a deleted or rearranged form of a specific autosome will imply a very high risk of abnormality, approaching 100%, due to partial trisomy of that chromosome. Once a supernumerary chromosome has been identified, it is no longer referred to as an SMC; it is now described as a ring or derivative—for example, r(7), der(22), or neo(13q31), or whatever may be the precise description.

---

13 Familial SMCs are noted, according to their chromosomal provenance, in Chapter 14; see also Brøndum-Nielsen and Mikkelsen (1995) and Hastings et al. (1999a).

De Novo Small Supernumerary Marker Chromosome. De novo sSMCs have been described for most chromosomes (Hastings et al. 1999a); two-thirds of sSMCs are acrocentric derived (Dalprà et al. 2005). A prenatally diagnosed sSMC, and the child subsequently born being normal, is described in Sung et al. (2009); the sSMC comprised chromosome 10 material (and may actually have been a very small ring). A 21-derived sSMC at amniocentesis, which might otherwise have been interpreted benignly, was seen in a different light due to an accompanying minor 47,XY,+21 cell line, leading to a conclusion that an initially trisomic 21 conception had generated a del(21q) cell line; at post-termination, the fetal karyotype was 47,XY,+21/47,XY,+der(21)/46,XY (Stefanou and Crocker 2004).

De Novo Minute Marker. The *very* small SMC (minSMC) may comprise only centromeric material and be harmless. We discuss a prenatal case on p. 448, a minSMC apparently comprising no more than chromosome 18 centromere; the child turned out to be normal. The tiny bisatellited microchromosome can be thought of as the reciprocal product of the Robertsonian rearrangement; these microchromosomes also are typically harmless (Dalprà et al. 2005; Gruchy et al. 2008).

SMC Outcomes. With precise cytogenetic characterization of an sSMC identified prenatally, using FISH and microarray (Manolakos et al. 2010; Jang et al. 2016), and with concomitant ultrasound examination, it should be possible precisely to categorize the genetic risk. Earlier published reports of liveborn children with various types of SMCs—a notably heterogeneous material—are mostly biased by ascertainment in favor of phenotypic abnormality. Series of prenatally diagnosed fetuses are deficient in that there is usually only a short-term follow-up of liveborn children, while pathological assessments following termination can only show major structural malformations (Warburton 1991). Brøndum-Nielsen and Mikkelsen (1995) report a 10-year experience in Glostrup, Denmark, during which nine de novo SMCs were identified. In seven cases, termination of pregnancy was chosen, with some of these showing defects at pathological examination; and in the two pregnancies continuing, one infant with a minute acrocentric-derived SMC was normal at birth, while one with a ring-like 17 was "slightly retarded" at age 2 years. In the

similar survey of Hastings et al. (1999a), data were presented on 31 prenatally diagnosed SMCs, of which 21 were de novo. In 10 of these 21 proceeding to FISH analysis, six being mosaic, five were shown to be 15-derived and three 14- or 22-derived; the remaining two included a r(8) and a der(16). Of the six in which the pregnancies continued, only the r(8) child was physically and developmentally abnormal. Repeating the point: With FISH and microarray, most sSMCs should admit of precise cytogenomic analysis, and the prenatal advice based upon knowledge of the specific involved segment.

Supernumerary Autosomal Ring Chromosomes. Autosomal ring chromosomes, as a supernumerary 47th chromosome, imply a high risk of phenotypic abnormality. They originate from a variety of chromosomes and contain euchromatin. Certain of these, in which only one arm of the chromosome is represented in the ring, are specifically recorded in association with phenotypic abnormality: r(1p), r(5p), r(7q), r(8q), r(9p), r(10p), r(20p), and r(20q) (Anderlid et al. 2001). The r(8) with an abnormal outcome in Hastings et al. (1999a) is mentioned above. Uniparental disomy may complicate the picture: James et al. (1995) and Anderlid et al. (2001) report supernumerary rings, from chromosomes 6 and 9, associated with UPD 6 and UPD 9, respectively. Very small rings, that might also have been categorized as sSMCs, might not necessarily cause an abnormal phenotype: For example, two infants in Kitsiou-Tzeli et al. (2009) born following prenatal diagnosis of 47,+r(20)/46,N mosaicism were judged normal in early infancy.

Autosomal Isochromosomes. Autosomal isochromosomes are typically seen in the mosaic state as a supernumerary isochromosome (or isodicentric isochromosome), and thus the discovery of 47,+i/46,N (or 47,+idic/46,N) is always a concern, whether at a level II or even level I mosaicism. Such a karyotype raises the prospect of an effective mosaic tetrasomy for the chromosomal arm concerned. A 46-chromosome karyotype in which one homolog is replaced by an isochromosome typically implies a trisomy for one arm of that chromosome, and monosomy for the other. These are certainly rare observations: In an amniocentesis-based survey from Italy, based on slightly less than 90,000 diagnoses, the most frequent were, in order, isochromosomes of 20q, 9p, 18p, and 12p, at approximately 1 in 30,000, 45,000, 45,000, and 90,000, respectively

(Forabosco et al. 2009). Brief commentaries on these, and on certain other isochromosomes, follow.

47,+i(5p) Sijmons et al. (1993) assessed a dysmorphic and neurologically compromised child with a 5p isochromosome in 3/31 lymphocytes and 12/14 skin fibroblasts, and yet upon retrospective checking, only one of 217 cells from a stored short-term CVS culture was 47,XY,+i(5p). We contrast this unfortunate experience with ours of seven cases of i(5p) mosaicism identified at CVS, six of which went on to follow-up amniocentesis (Clement Wilson et al. 2002). Three children were followed up to 2½, 3¼, and 4 years, and their normality was quite apparent. In one of these children, a circumscribed area of the placenta following delivery karyotyped 47,+i(5p), adjacent parts karyotyped 47,+i(5p)/46,N, and most of the placenta (and the child himself) had a normal karyotype. The CVS sampling had presumably needled this small region of confined placental i(5p) mosaicism. One pregnancy tested 100% i(5p) at CVS, and the parents chose termination; no i(5p) cells were detected from fetal skin culture. In another with a 65% load at CVS, a follow-up amniocentesis showed 45% of cells with the isochromosome, and post-termination tissues showed 15%–30%. From the foregoing, we may conclude that a *CVS* diagnosis with a normal follow-up amniocentesis and with normal ultrasonography suggests, but cannot confirm, a normal child. As for the primary detection of i(5p) mosaicism at *amniocentesis*, only four cases are recorded, with all having an abnormal outcome (Reddy and Huang 2003; Grams et al. 2011). Grams et al. reported monozygotic twins who were discordant for i(5p) at CVS and amniocentesis; multiple abnormalities were seen on ultrasound in the affected twin, but the pregnancy ended in spontaneous loss of both twins at 18 weeks gestation.

47,+i(8p) López-Pajares et al. (2003) review the small number of reported cases. Two examples are given of discordance between amniocentesis (normal) and postnatal blood (tetrasomy 8p), an unusual pattern for isochromosomes (but cf. the i(9p) below). A disconcerting story is told in Nucaro et al. (2006): i(8p) mosaicism was seen at long-term cultured (but not short-term) CVS, with a normal result after amniocentesis, but resulting in a child severely retarded and epileptic, and with a 5% level of the i(8p) on blood.

47,+i(9p) The clinical picture and the subtleties of different breakpoints are discussed in Dhandha et al. (2002). Isochromosome mosaicism can be the basis of a false-negative test result at prenatal diagnosis. Thus, Eggermann et al. (1998) reported an abnormal baby born to a 39-year-old mother, in whom amniocentesis at 14 weeks gestation had returned a normal karyotype. On blood analysis, the child had an i(9p) in 32% of cells. From one skin biopsy, 50 cells had a normal karyotype, but on a second biopsy, five out of eight cells showed the i(9p) chromosome. The particular attribute of the i(9p) is for blood, but not skin, to show the abnormality, and this is likely the explanation for its nondetection at amniocentesis. Pertile et al. (1996) support this interpretation, in their follow-up of a (nonmosaic) CVS diagnosis of idic(9)(q13). An extensive search at amniocentesis revealed a single abnormal colony, which might well otherwise have been missed. Finally, fetal blood sampling showed the idic(9) in 8% of cells. A more severe case is recorded in Tang et al. (2004), which showed the isochromosome in all amniocytes at 24 weeks, and in most blood and fibroblast cells from the very malformed infant (who died at 1 month of age).

47,+i(10p) A single case is on record, the diagnosis having been made following the recognition of fetal defects on ultrasonography (Wu et al. 2003).

47,+i(12p), Pallister-Killian Syndrome The 12p isochromosome is the basis of the well-known Pallister-Killian syndrome. The fractions of abnormal cells detected at prenatal diagnosis can vary greatly. Bernert et al. (1992) showed in one example 100% of short-term CVS cells and 10% of amniotic fluid cells having the 47,+i(12p) karyotype, whereas in Kunz et al. (2009), at CVS the isochromosome was seen only in long-term culture; in both cases, the pregnancies were terminated. Horn et al. (1995) reported a pregnancy in which CVS gave a 46,XY result on direct (17 cells) and cultured (eight cells) analysis (and 28 further cells on a retrospective study), and the abnormal newborn baby was 46,XY on a peripheral blood study (100 cells counted); at 18 months, a clinical diagnosis of Pallister-Killian syndrome was made, and the karyotype on skin fibroblast culture was 47,XY,+i(12p)/46,XY, with 85% of cells having the isochromosome. (Had it been an amniocentesis rather than CVS that had been done, abnormal cells would probably have been seen.) Classical karyotyping typically returns a normal result because the i(12p) is lost in stimulated lymphocyte cultures; however, microarray on genomic DNA from whole peripheral blood is able to detect subtle mosaicism (Theisen et al. 2009).

46,i(13q) A de novo "Robertsonian" translocation, leading to trisomy 13, is, in the majority of cases, actually an isochromosome, as discussed above (Bugge et al. 2005).

Isodicentric 15 About half of all SMCs are an idic(15) (also referred to as pseudodicentric 15, or inverted duplication 15; and see p. 323). These are typically dicentric and bisatellited, although one of the centromeres may be suppressed. The smallest ones (smaller than chromosome 21q) appear to be harmless, but larger ones result in the "idic(15) syndrome," characterized by mental defect and autistic features. The boundary between smaller and larger is in 15q12. The use of D15S10 or *SNRPN* FISH probes, which recognize sequences in 15q12q13, enables distinction of harmless and pathogenic chromosomes (Eggermann et al. 2002), a distinction that can also be made using microarray (Wang et al. 2004). Rare idic(15)s have been associated with UPD 15, and it may be warranted to check for this possibility (Hastings et al. 1999a).

47,+i(18p) Schinzel (2001) notes that more than 75 cases of 47,+i(18p) have been recorded. Multiple physical anomalies and a moderate to severe degree of mental retardation characterize the clinical picture. Boyle et al. (2001) emphasize the plausibility of a premeiotic origin, and the caution therefore that gonadal mosaicism may exist in a parent, as they illustrate in their report of affected half-sisters.

46,i(18q) The karyotype produces a combination of monosomy 18p and trisomy 18q. Chen et al. (1998) record that many 18q isochromosomes diagnosed prenatally are associated with very severe malformation, such as holoprosencephaly and cloacal dysgenesis. Levy-Mozziconacci et al. (1996) describe a case presenting at 22 weeks gestation with abnormal ultrasonography, and although the direct CVS was 46,XX in all cells, amniocentesis and fetal blood sampling showed the isochromosome (an isodicentric, in this instance) in all cells: an example of complete CVS-amniocentesis discordance.

46,i(20q) An i(20q) identified at amniocentesis in mosaic form appears most often to be a benign finding; a rather surprising conclusion. It may be an unusual sort of mosaicism in being confined, or largely so, to amniocytes, the abnormal cell line having arisen as a postzygotic event, and its growth perhaps favored in vitro (Robinson et al. 2007). The few reported cases with fetal defect could reflect a tissue distribution which included the fetal anatomy. Goumy et al. (2005) counsel caution, and point to the advisability of careful ultrasonography, targeted in particular to the brain and vertebrae.

46,i(21q) This rearrangement is an isochromosome, not a Robertsonian translocation (Shaffer et al. 1991). The phenotype is that of Down syndrome. Gilardi et al. (2002) report a case in which the isochromosome probably arose postzygotically in an early cell destined to form the lineage of the inner cell mass and the extra-embryonic mesoderm, such that a direct CVS gave a nonmosaic 46,XX result, while long-term CVS and post-termination fetal studies showed nonmosaic 46,XX,i(21q); a similar story comes from Brisset et al. (2003). The i(21q) can also exist in a 47-chromosome karyotype. Nagarsheth and Mootabar (1997) showed a 47,XY,+i(21q)[6]/46,XY[19] karyotype at amniocentesis; the parents elected to continue the pregnancy, and the abnormal child had only one out of 120 peripheral blood lymphocytes with the i(21q), the other 119 being normal. These authors suggest that some previously reported cases of supposed i(12p) mosaicism may have been, in fact, i(21q).

47,+i(22q) A single case of an isochromosome for 22q being detected at amniocentesis is recorded in Guzé et al. (2004). The isochromosome was probably generated postzygotically, with the subsequent production of additional abnormal cell lines. The pregnancy continued to full term: The child had several defects and died on the second day of life.

Isodicentric 22 The bisatellited idic(22) typically, but not invariably, causes cat-eye syndrome (p. 333). If the idic(22) lacks proximal 22q euchromatin, normality is very probable, whereas those containing euchromatin can lead to a phenotype anywhere between full cat-eye syndrome and normality (Crolla et al. 1997).

NORMAL VARIANTS

Chen et al. (2006c) review the question of variants detected at prenatal diagnosis. They identified 16 variants of euchromatin or heterochromatin in 21,832 amniocenteses. Eight of nine euchromatic variants were proven inherited, and seven were C-band positive. The remaining C-band-positive, heterochromatic variants were all inherited from a carrier parent. Concerning the specific case of the nucleolar organizing region translocation, or interstitially inserted satellite, and as noted in

Chapter 17, "genetic counseling should be reassuring" if this is discovered at prenatal diagnosis (Faivre et al. 1999, 2000; Chen et al. 2004b). The Y;15 variant is noted above.

Sex Chromosome Abnormalities

THE CLASSIC FULL ANEUPLOIDIES

A sex chromosome abnormality is not an uncommon discovery at prenatal diagnosis, with an overall incidence of 1 in 250–300 (Linden et al. 2002). The main conditions are XXY, XXX, XYY, and 45,X. As Boyd et al. (2011) write, "The importance of providing parents with accurate information about the frequency of the diagnosis, and the variability of the condition on the basis of outcomes from unbiased population-based follow-up studies on the specific chromosome abnormality, cannot be overemphasized." Two of these aneuploidies (XXY and 45,X) may be firmly predicted in terms of an abnormality of development of the reproductive system: Children with Klinefelter and 45,X Turner syndrome will with near-certainty be infertile.

Some will choose pregnancy termination, although it is of interest that in France, coincident with multidisciplinary centers for prenatal diagnosis being put in place in 1997, the termination rates during the period 1976–2012 fell (from 41% to 12% for XXX, and from 26% to 7% for XYY) (Gruchy et al. 2016), and similar observations are made in some other, but not all, jurisdictions. Liao and Li (2014) wonder if the question can be side-stepped, in the setting of pregnancies tested for some other reason (e.g., thalassemia), by not interrogating the sex chromosomes. For those couples deciding to continue a pregnancy, Robinson et al. (1986) offer a useful commentary. Parents of children predicted to be infertile might feel a sense of loss—a "sadness and regret about their child's anticipated loss and about their own loss of grandchildren" and "concern about their children's wholeness and, by extension, their own." Parents may take some comfort from knowing that infertility is by no means an uncommon problem in the general population, and further comfort from the advice that recent advances in artificial reproductive technology may now enable the infertility to be overcome, in some individuals.

The picture for intellectual and psychological functioning is less predictable. Earlier adult studies defining a strong association with mental deficiency and psychological disturbance were contaminated by ascertainment bias (and counselors' personal experience may have been more with those children whose problems were sufficiently severe that they had come to medical attention). Children identified in newborn populations screened for cytogenetic abnormalities and subsequently followed up constitute a group unbiased in their ascertainment, although perhaps subject to other but less important biases (Puck 1981). Data from the study of such children in several American and European cities, followed from infancy through childhood, adolescence, and young adulthood, have since given a reasonably clear picture of the natural history of the more common sex chromosome aneuploidies (Linden et al. 2002). In general, the IQ averages 10–15 points below that of the siblings. Hook's (1979) early proposition has held up: Some sex chromosome aneuploidies influence brain function in such a way that the development of intellectual capacity, emotional maturity, and speech and language skills are affected to some extent; but none of these effects necessarily occurs, none is specific to sex chromosome aneuploidy, and some may be amenable to corrective intervention. There is considerable overlap with the XX and XY population. Hong and Reiss (2014) reviewed the cognitive and neurological aspects of sex chromosome aneuploidies and noted shared features across the sex chromosome aneuploidies, comprising impairments in executive functioning, motor skills, and higher-order social cognitive ability. Ratcliffe (1999) and Bender et al. (2001) provide long-term follow-up data, well into adulthood. Bender et al. followed eight 45,X, 10 47,XXX, and 11 47,XXY individuals through to an age range of 26–36 years, using siblings as controls, and noted the IQs of the aneuploid groups to be considerably less compared with the sibs. Nevertheless, the variation is wide, and these authors emphasize the point that "sex chromosome aneuploidy does not exert its influence in a vacuum, but rather interacts with the host of other genetic and environmental influences that collectively guide human development." As Le Gall et al. (2017) show, an independent, concomitant CNV can exacerbate the clinical, and especially the neurocognitive phenotype, and may indeed be the more significant factor. Children with sex chromosome aneuploidies seem more susceptible to either the good or the bad effects of a stable or of a dysfunctional family setting, than do their 46,XX and 46,XY siblings (Stewart et al. 1990; Bender et al. 1995). Children identified at prenatal diagnosis, a group biased toward higher socioeconomic status, may do better academically and socially than the cohorts followed from birth, although it was nevertheless true in the study of Linden and Bender (2002) that these children had "a strong risk for developmental problems, particularly for learning disabilities . . . [albeit that] these problems were not often severe." There may, however, be an increased risk for psychosis in childhood and adulthood (Kumra et al. 1998). A pioneering clinic in Colorado, the eXtraordinarY Kids Clinic, providing a multidisciplinary management for children and adolescents with a sex chromosome aneuploidy, was well recieved by parents, and it may offer a model for a similar service in other centers (Tartaglia et al. 2015).

If a couple decides to continue the pregnancy, what should they say to others? Should the family know, should they tell friends, and should school personnel be aware? And when should the child learn about his or her chromosomal condition? Linden et al. (2002) have considered these questions, and in general make a case for openness within the family, but see no need, indeed potential disadvantage, for those outside to be told.

We next outline the predicted outlook for the more commonly encountered sex chromosome aneuploidies. Attention is paid mostly to gonadal function and to intellectual and social development.

XXY (KLINEFELTER SYNDROME)

Almost certainly, the child becomes an infertile adult, although in recent times testicular sperm extraction with in vitro fertilization (IVF) has enabled a small number of men to become fathers (p. 345). Some have used gamete donation from a father or brother. Penile size is usually normal; the testes will be small. Androgen deficiency can be managed by replacement therapy with testosterone.[14] It may be that treatment induces a more masculine body habitus, improved self-esteem, vitality, ability to concentrate, and sexual interest (Nielsen 1990; Winter 1990). Gynecomastia may be present, transiently, in some 50%; if it persists, it can be treated surgically.

As an average statement, verbal IQ is reduced by some 18 points, and performance IQ by 11 points (Leggett et al. 2010). Learning difficulty at school is

to be expected. Of 13 XXY boys studied by Walzer et al. (1990), 11 had persistent reading and spelling problems. Bender et al. (1993) note that a deficit in verbal fluency and reading is "the most homogeneous and consistent cognitive impairment found in any sex chromosome abnormality group," and this may reflect a specific dysfunction of the left cerebral hemisphere. Specific characteristics included a lowered level of motor activity, a pliant disposition, and a cautious approach to new situations; thus, in the classroom setting, they are perceived as "low-key children, well liked by their teachers, and presenting few behavioral management problems." Leggett et al. conclude that these boys "do not usually have major problems with social interaction and adaptation, although they may be timid and unassertive." Speculatively, the neural substrate of this passivity may reside in an underdevelopment of the amygdala, a brain nucleus that underpins aspects of social processing (Patwardhan et al. 2002).

Six Danish XXY boys were followed from birth to age 15–19 years by Nielsen and Wohlert (1991), and all but one needed remedial teaching. Their career plans were carpenter, draughtsman, gardener, unskilled laborer, mechanic, and undecided. Stewart et al. (1990) comment that "XXY boys are unlikely to reach a level of personal and social development that is consistent with their family background." Ratcliffe (1999) commented upon a rate of psychiatric referral being above that of male controls (26% cf. 9%), with the neurotic score (not the antisocial score) being higher. (She also notes anecdotal mention of men from a Klinefelter clinic with professions including physician, engineer, minister, and accountant.) In a summary of psychosocial adaptation from several studies, recurring adjectives to describe the XXY personality were shy, immature, restrained, and reserved. In the Denver study, 11 young adults with XXY "appeared to have met the demands of early adulthood with fair success, although slightly less well than did their siblings"; they appeared to have a diminished insight into their own psychology (Bender et al. 1999). Their mean IQ of 91 compared with 109 in normal male sibling controls. We have noted above the ameliorative effect of growing up in a stable and supportive family.[15] In a cohort of 934 Danish XXY males, the

---

14 A role for testosterone therapy in infancy to mimic the normal "mini-puberty" is controversial, and not routinely recommended (Høst et al. 2014).

15 Besides detection prenatally, the condition may be screened for at different stages of postnatal life. Herlihy et al. (2010) use Klinefelter syndrome as an exemplar of how the pros and cons of diagnosis versus nondiagnosis may be assessed, at different times of life.

incidence of criminal convictions was 1.4 times that of controls, but this difference disappeared after adjusting for socioeconomic indices (Stochholm et al. 2012).

XXX

A full literature review of the XXX syndrome is provided in Otter et al. (2010), and the reader will find this helpful. Physical development of the XXX female is generally unremarkable, although there is a tendency toward tallness. Gross and fine motor skills are likely to be somewhat impaired, and children are awkward and poorly coordinated. Pubertal development and fertility appear, for the most part, uncompromised. In a very few, genitourinary malformations (ovarian, uterine, renal, bladder) are recorded, of which the karyotype may or may not have been causal (Haverty et al. 2004; Linden and Bender 2004).

It is the neural substrate in which the important vulnerability applies (and which may reflect a reduced rate of cell cycles during neurogenesis; Otter et al. 2010). Thus, major concerns in childhood relate to intelligence and language development and poor self-confidence, and, in adulthood, psychosocial maladjustment and, occasionally, frank psychiatric disease. Full scale and verbal IQ is, on average, reduced by some 10–20 points. Language comprehension and use of speech are impaired in over half the cases. Learning difficulty is likely, and many will benefit from additional remedial teaching, but few require education outside the mainstream. In one small study of 11 girls, nine needed special education intervention, and one was placed in a class for retarded children (Bender et al. 1993). While girls who had been diagnosed prenatally do better than those ascertained postnatally (as naturally is to be expected), it remains true that their neurocognitive capacity is somewhat compromised (Wigby et al. 2016).

Harmon et al. (1998) and Bender et al. (1999) reported a longer follow-up in these young women, into adolescence and young adulthood, and documented difficult adaptation to the stresses of life. On a measure of social adjustment (in work, leisure, family, marital, parental), the XXX women scored significantly less well than their sisters. Their mean IQ was 82 (cf. sisters, 103). However, Ratcliffe (1999) described most XXX young women in the Edinburgh survey as "physically attractive, and displaying a common-sense attitude that counterbalanced their low educational achievements" (and relieved to be free of the pressure they had felt while at school). The observations in the similar study of Rovet et al. (1995) were more promising, although, as Harmon et al. point out, this was a group from a higher socioeconomic stratum, and presumably both genetic and environmental factors would have been more favorable. An XXX girl who might otherwise have had an IQ of 130 can yet do well despite a reduction to 110; to the contrary, a drop from 90 to 70 would be a considerable handicap. Many counselors will know from their own experience how variable can be the phenotype.

XYY

The multicenter prospective study documented in Evans et al. (1990) reviewed progress in 39 boys and young men. The particular physical attribute of the XYY male is increased stature. Sexual activity is normal, and fertility is apparently uncompromised. Motor proficiency may be impaired. While the IQ is in the normal range, it is usually lower than those of sibs or controls, and about half of XYY boys have a mild learning difficulty, and may display poor attentiveness and impulsivity in the classroom. There is an overlap in the cognitive profiles between individuals with Klinefelter syndrome and those with XYY syndrome, mainly characterized by deficits in executive function and language-related skills. It may be that the aneuploidy causes a minor and subtle impairment of neurologic maturation, leading to some features of minimal brain dysfunction (Theilgaard 1986). The vignettes from the series of Ratcliffe et al. (1990) of 10 Scottish subjects who had left school give an idea of what XYY young men are capable of: One ran a market stall, two were chefs, and the others were a private in the army, a waiter, a supermarket assistant, a video shop assistant, a technician, a laborer, and one was training as a painter and decorator. In a cohort of children aged 8–16 years selected for the XYY karyotype having been diagnosed prenatally, and of higher socioeconomic status, a considerable range in academic ability was observed, with most coping satisfactorily, and IQs ranging from 100 to 147 (Linden and Bender 2002).

Perhaps the major concern is in psychosocial adaptation. These boys can have a low frustration tolerance, and some are prone to temper tantrums in childhood, progressing to aggressive behavior in teenage, and may need help to learn to cope with this. They may find it difficult to "read" social situations, and antisocial behavior is more common (Ratcliffe 1999). The functioning of the family may be as much an ingredient as the karyotype in psychosocial development. Fryns et al. (1995) identified 50 XYY males among 98,725 patients referred for chromosomal analysis, and they note that this fraction of 50/98,725, approximately 0.05%, is very close to the newborn incidence; they thus drew a conclusion that the XYY phenotype differs little from the norm. They do, however, acknowledge a high (86%) risk for psychosocial pathology in those XYY males with concomitant borderline intelligence or frank mental deficiency. In Ratcliffe's follow-up report into adulthood, some disconcerting data are noted, not incongruent with the conclusions of Fryns et al. Psychiatric referrals were fivefold compared with male controls (47% cf. 9%), and the rate of criminal conviction was fourfold, the mean IQ of those convicted being lower than those who were not (although most offenses were minor and against property rather than persons). More reassuring data come from a cohort of 161 Danish XYY males, in which the incidence of criminal convictions was just 1.42 times that of controls, a difference which disappeared after adjusting for socioeconomic parameters (Stochholm et al. 2012).

45,X (TURNER SYNDROME)

Unlike the foregoing aneuploidies, monosomy X has a very high in utero lethality, peaking at around 12–15 weeks gestation. Spontaneous abortion follows amniocentesis-detected 45,X in three-fourths of cases (Hook 1983). But some survive pregnancy and are born as infants with Turner syndrome. Robinson et al. (1990) note that "variability among 45,X girls is considerable; and precise predictions about any child's prognosis are not possible." They also emphasized that "a supportive environment that provides stimulation and encouragement is of considerable importance." These traits comprise the core phenotype (and a full description is given in Levitsky et al. 2015):

• Gonadal failure with infertility is almost certain (Lippe 1991). In the survey of Sutton et al. (2006), infertility was seen, by the women with Turner syndrome themselves, as the most concerning component of the phenotype. Classically, a spontaneous onset of puberty, with breast development and onset of menses, has been regarded as being very infrequent, although Pasquino et al. (1997) propose that the fraction who enter a spontaneous puberty may be as high as 9%, and they suggest that earlier figures may have been biased downward by a policy, previously, of not karyotyping short girls who had had an onset of menstruation. Childbearing via ovum donation may be successful in some cases. Pavlidis et al. (1995) reviewed sexual functioning in women with Turner syndrome and suggest strategies to avoid possible difficulties.

• Stature will be short. In a study of adult Danish women with Turner syndrome, never having had growth hormone therapy, the average height (with standard deviation) was 147 cm ± 7 cm (4 feet 10 inches ± 2½ inches) (Gravholt and Naeraa 1997), which may be slightly taller than in some other ethnic populations. A useful increment can be achieved with growth hormone treatment.

• Neuropsychological functioning is impaired. The average IQ is reduced compared to siblings. At long-term follow-up in the Denver cohort (Bender et al. 1999), nine young women with 45,X had a mean lower IQ (85) compared with normal female sibling controls (104). Their educational achievements were, however, better than those of the XXX women from the same study: Eight were high school graduates, and five had college degrees. In one notable case, Reiss et al. (1993) report monozygous twins, one nonmosaic 45,X and the other 46,XX, the former's performance IQ being 18 points less than her sister but the verbal IQs practically the same. In fact, girls with Turner syndrome appear possibly to have superior skills in some language domains compared to their 46,XX peers (Temple and Shepherd 2012). Psychological assessment indicates a particular vulnerability in social adaptation (Bender et al. 1999), but women with Turner syndrome do not have diminished empathy or an increase in autistic traits (Lepage et al 2014). Reiss et al. (1993) review aspects of the cognitive-behavioral phenotype and correlate the specific feature of difficulty with visual-spatial appreciation with a lesser volume of the right parietal cerebral cortex. Romans et al. (1998) confirmed and extended this appraisal in a study of 99 subjects with Turner syndrome, in whom they identified diminished abilities on measures of spatial and perceptual skills, visual-motor integration, recognition of facial expressions associated with a particular affect, visual memory, attention, and executive function (the ability to plan, organize, monitor, and execute multistep problem-solving processes); the amygdala (see also "XXY," above) may be a vulnerable neural substrate in this respect (Burnett et al. 2010). These traits are not improved by taking estrogen (Ross et al. 2002).

- Certain physical defects are associated, of which the major are neck webbing and coarctation (narrowing) of the aorta.
- Morbidity in adult life is increased (Gravholt 2001; Swerdlow et al. 2001). Certain common diseases are more frequently seen: obesity, both insulin-dependent and insulin-resistant diabetes, hypothyroidism, heart disease, hypertension, stroke, and liver cirrhosis. Weakness of the bones (osteoporosis) implies a risk for fracture. There may be a place for ongoing hormone replacement therapy.

There is a possibility that Y-chromosome material may be present, even if the karyotype is apparently nonmosaic 45,X. Huang et al. (2002) reviewed 74 cases of 45,X diagnosed prenatally, most having been ascertained via, or discovered with, abnormal fetal ultrasonography. Of six with normal ultrasonography, three showed a male genital phenotype. The explanations, upon more detailed analysis, were as follows: In one, a segment of Yp was translocated to a chromosome 14, shown on FISH with an SRY probe; and in the other two, there was low-level mosaicism for an idic(Y) marker. Apparently normal male children were born. Some women with Turner syndrome who are 45,X on karyotyping may actually show Y sequences on molecular study, and these women do have a greater risk for gonadoblastoma (Mendes et al. 1999).

SEX CHROMOSOME POLYSOMY

Linden et al. (1995) review the phenotypes of 48,XXXX, 48,XXXY, 48,XXYY, 48,XYYY, 49,XXXXX, 49,XXXXY, 49,XXXYY, 49,XXYYY, and 49,XYYYY; and 48,XXYY, 48,XXXX, and 49,XXXXY are also outlined in Visootsak and Graham (2006). The phenotypes may resemble commonly identified traits in the sex chromosome trisomies, such as impairment of language skills, executive function, and social adaption, but with increased severity of these core phenotypic features, and with the addition of delayed developmental milestones and variable intellectual compromise

(Hong and Reiss 2014). While the authors' comment is well taken that the current perception of the seriousness of phenotypic abnormality may have been overstated due to ascertainment bias, and indeed they describe normal (but low) IQs in some of the $2n = 48$ karyotypes, it remains true that most have substantial handicap due to intellectual deficit and abnormal behavior (Cammarata et al. 1999). The very rare 49,XYYYY karyotype is reviewed in Demily et al. (2017); almost as rare is 49,XXXXY, concerning which Peitsidis et al. (2009) review prenatal diagnosis, noting that nuchal thickening is a frequent observation. IQ in both these pentasomies is very low.

X AND Y CHROMOSOME MOSAICISM

True mosaicism involving the sex chromosomes seen at prenatal diagnosis presents a challenge in interpretation, and skilled ultrasonography, with respect to external genital anatomy, is central in determining the fetal gender. The problem is that the tissue analyzed at prenatal diagnosis may or may not reflect the distribution in the gonad. The presence of a Y chromosome in at least some gonadal tissue—or to be precise, the presence of the Y-borne SRY gene—will promote testicular development, which might or might not be complete, and which might or might not secrete male-inducing hormones. Thus, we may observe gender states from normal (although possibly infertile) female, through Turner-like female, genital ambiguity, mixed gonadal dysgenesis, even ovotesticular disorder of sex development (p. 539), to male with incomplete pubertal development, and to normal (although often infertile) male.

XX/XY Mosaicism. At prenatal diagnosis, this is usually pseudomosaicism, resulting from the growth of maternal cells in a 46,XY pregnancy (Worton and Stern 1984). (Obviously, such pseudomosaicism would normally be undetected if the fetus is female.) Level III XX/XY mosaicism, curiously enough, is most likely to indicate a phenotypically normal female fetus in which the XY source is unknown, particularly when the XX cells predominate. A male "vanished twin" is a theoretical possibility (Worton and Stern 1984), and indeed a quite plausible explanation, given the frequency with which a twin pregnancy prior to 7 weeks is followed, some months later, by the birth of a singleton baby (Sampson and de Crespigny 1992). Analysis of placental membranes after delivery in a pregnancy from which one twin has "vanished" can often reveal a fetus papyraceous or a remnant empty sac (Nerlich et al. 1992). One can imagine tissue of the (male) twin remnant having been, by chance, in the path of the amniocentesis needle that sampled cells from the remaining (female) fetus. A girl born following such a prenatal diagnosis (Hunter et al. 1982) was followed through to mid-adolescence, and her development was entirely normal (A. G. W. Hunter, personal communication, 2002). A similar case was studied by I. Hayes and A. George (personal communication, 2009), with an XX:XY ratio of 90:10 on FISH of uncultured amniotic fluid, although nonmosaic 46,XX on cultured cells; ultrasonography indicated female external genital morphology. Following the birth of a normal girl, examination of seven sites from the placenta, and one site each from the cord and sac, all revealed a nonmosaic female sex complement, as did the cord blood sample.

A true fetal XX/XY karyotype is rare indeed, and it is more likely due to the fusion of two conceptuses—that is, XX//XY chimerism (but other mechanisms exist; see Chapter 23). Presumably depending upon the gonadal distribution of XX and XY cells, the genital anatomy will be male, female, or in between. Malan et al. (2007) report XX//XY chimerism at prenatal diagnosis, the child (subjected to pelvic ultrasonography) proving to be an apparently normal girl. Ovotesticular DSD, with imperfect or ambiguous genital anatomy, has been recorded from an XX/XY amniocentesis result, with the same karyotype demonstrated in the child (Amor et al. 1999; Chen et al. 2005b, 2006e; Malan et al. 2007). Yaron et al. (1999) had a case presenting at amniocentesis, with normal male morphology on ultrasound. The XX/XY mosaicism was confirmed on a second amniocentesis, and, in due course, on the normal male newborn infant (including on genital skin). Amor et al. note the point that intellectual compromise is not to be anticipated. Hughes et al. (2006) provide guidelines on management for children with intersex conditions. Infertility is predicted; but remarkably enough, one XX//XY man has fathered a child, following IVF with retrieved sperm (Sugawara et al. 2005).

X/XY Mosaicism. Patients coming to medical attention with 45,X/46,XY mosaicism range in phenotype from females with classical Turner syndrome, through infants with ambiguous genitalia, to normal but infertile males (Telvi et al. 1999; Tho et al. 2007; Lindhardt Johansen et al. 2012). A risk for gonadal tumor applies (Müller and Skakkebæk 1990; Müller et al. 1999). By contrast, a phenotypic male infant is the outcome in the considerable majority (90%–95%) of X/XY gestations detected at prenatal diagnosis—in other words, cases whose ascertainment was unbiased—and going through to birth (Hsu 1994; Huang et al. 2002). Fertility is, however, likely to be compromised, and other manifestations of Turner syndrome, such as short stature and cardiovascular defects, may be present. Van den Berg et al. (2000) report a case in which nonmosaic 45,X was diagnosed at short-term CVS, with a nonmosaic 46,XY karyotype seen on long-term culture. Subsequent amniocentesis revealed a true 45,X/46,XY mosaicism. Post termination, fetal testing showed X/XY mosaicism in all tissues sampled (including gonads). Of 14 pathology studies on fetuses post termination in Chang et al. (1990), two were found to have ovotestes, and one had a "precancerous" lesion. Tosson et al. (2012) offer guidelines for management in childhood and adolescence; growth hormone therapy has been prescribed in some, albeit with uncertain benefit (Bertelloni et al. 2015).

X/XX Mosaicism. In 2002, Huang et al. reported their experience with 17 cases of X/XX mosaicism at amniocentesis. The ratios of X to XX cells ranged from 2:23 to 12:3. One case with IUGR (ratio 6:12) terminated in stillbirth, while the remaining 16 had normal ultrasonography. Of the eight cases continuing to term and for which information was available, two liveborn babies had the features of Turner syndrome (ratios 7:10 and 3:14), with the mosaicism confirmed postnatally in one of these. The remaining six (ratios ranging from 3:15 to 12:8) "reportedly had a normal female phenotype." To quote Huang et al., "The percentage of 45,X cells in amniocytes does not seem to be an indicator of pregnancy outcome, as there was considerable overlap between cases with normal and abnormal outcome." In a unique case of a monozygous twin pregnancy, one fetus showed nuchal swelling and the other appeared normal (Gilbert et al. 2002). Fetal blood sampling showed low-grade 45,X[2]/46,XX[23] mosaicism in the former and a normal 46,XX karyotype in the latter, in contrast to postnatal skin fibroblast karyotyping results of nonmosaic 45,X and 45,X[2]/46,XX[78], respectively.

Tokita and Sybert (2016) followed up 23 females with prenatally diagnosed 45,X/46,XX mosaicism, and noted the importance of accurate counseling in the context of increased detection of this karyotype by noninvasive prenatal testing. Follow-up was until mean age 11 years (range 0.1–27 years), and the mean percent aneuploidy was 42% at prenatal diagnosis and 23% in postnatal blood. Structural heart defects were documented in six females (26%), renal pathology in four (17%), and thyroid dysfunction in three (13%). No 45,X/46,XX female had formal IQ assessment, but persistent learning difficulties were reported in three (13%). Growth was comparable to population norms. Of the six patients older than 16 years, all had completed secondary school, and all had undergone spontaneous puberty. Results were compared with a cohort of 59 females with postnatally ascertained 45,X/46,XX mosaicism. Compared to the prenatally ascertained cohort, postnatally ascertained 45,X/46,XX females had shorter stature and a higher percentage aneuploidy in peripheral blood (40%); they also had a higher frequency of heart defects (39%), renal pathology (43%), and primary amenorrhea (50%). Combined data from both prenatally and postnatally ascertained cohorts suggest that the higher levels of percentage aneuploidy (on blood karyotype) were associated with an increased risk of congenital heart disease and a decreased chance of spontaneous menses, but not with the presence of other complications.

X/XX/XXX, X/XXX, and XXX/XX Mosaicism. One reported case of X/XX/XXX mosaicism illustrates the difficulty in extrapolating the distribution of cell types from one tissue to another (Schwartz and Raffel 1992). Amniocentesis gave the proportions 16:64:20, respectively. Cord blood gave similar findings, although in placental tissue (chorion), the percentages were 2:57:41. The baby appeared normal. Huang et al. (2002) reported a case each of X/XXX and X/XX/XXX mosaicism diagnosed at amniocentesis, the former pregnancy producing a newborn with features of Turner syndrome, and the other a normal female. Sybert (2002) reviewed hers and others' data and concluded that approximately 60% of girls with X/XX/XXX and X/XXX could be predicted to have short stature and that "it is fair to suggest that residual ovarian function is possible, and to caution that premature ovarian failure is common." The IQ in X/XXX, X/XX/XXX, and XXX/XXX mosaicism is not discernibly affected (Netley 1986; Bender et al. 1993). A rare prenatal diagnosis of XX/XXX associated with fetal chylothorax is recorded in Cremonini et al. (2014).

XXY/XY Mosaicism. Verbal IQ may, on average, be slightly lowered in the XXY/XY "partial Klinefelter syndrome" (Netley 1986; Bender et al. 1993).

X/XYY and X/XY/XYY Mosaicism. The X/XYY and X/XY/XYY mosaic states are (necessarily) abnormal in postnatally ascertained cases, but prenatally diagnosed cases have consistently manifested an apparently normal male genital phenotype, albeit that the mosaicism may be confirmed in the child subsequently born (Pettenati et al. 1991; Hsu 1994). Presumably according to the distribution of X and XYY tissues, the gender in X/XYY mosaicism can be of either sex, or there can be ambiguity, these three states documented in one of the earliest reviews (Mulcahy et al. 1977). There is a tumor risk, and gonadoblastoma was identified at gonadectomy in a virilized female with mixed gonadal dysgenesis (Gibbons et al. 1999). Infertility is likely, but it may be treatable (Dale et al. 2002). It is hypothetical whether the XYY line, if involving the brain, would determine an intellect and psyche of the "XYY syndrome."

STRUCTURALLY ABNORMAL SEX CHROMOSOME[16]

X Chromosome Deletion. The possibility of an inherited X-autosome translocation should be checked by doing the mother's karyotype; it may transpire that she has the same karyotype. Cytogenetically visible X chromosome deletions in the female, 46,X,del(Xp) or 46,X,del(Xq), predict the possibility, but not the certainty, of an incomplete form of Turner syndrome and/or premature ovarian failure (Chapter 15). Brown et al. (2001) describe a mother, of tall stature (5 feet 10 inches), having a prenatal diagnosis of del(X)(q22q26); she herself had the same karyotype, and "the parents took comfort in the observation that in the mother the deletion had no apparent phenotypic effect." A normal baby girl was born. Mother and daughter showed completely skewed X-inactivation, the abnormal X being consistently inactive.

---

16 X-autosome and Y-autosome rearrangements are discussed above, under De Novo Rearrangements, Apparently Balanced, and Unbalanced, respectively.

In the male, the 46,Y,del(X) state would be non-viable for all but the very smallest cytogenetically visible deletions, and major abnormality would be probable for those pregnancies that might be viable.

X Chromosome Duplication. De novo X chromosome duplications in the female, 46,X,dup(X), may determine a nil, minor, or major phenotypic impairment, accordingly as the pattern of X-inactivation may or may not be protective, and if a functional disomy is not prevented (Chapter 15). Zhang et al. (1997) provide detail according to the extent and site of the duplication in a review of postnatally diagnosed cases. Normality has been reported with respect to an isodicentric X, idic(X)(q27), comprising practically a double copy of the X, identified prenatally, the abnormal chromosome being late replicating, and indeed one such child was "academically advanced and enrolled in a gifted and talented program"; in contrast, some postnatally diagnosed patients have presented a Turner-like clinical picture (Tsai et al. 2006). In the male, functional disomy for the duplicated segment would likely cause severe defects, often lethal in utero.

X-Y Translocation. The most common form of the t(X;Y) has the X breakpoint at or distal to Xp22, and the Y breakpoint at Yq11.2. The intact sex chromosome may be an X or a Y chromosome, and the two states differ as follows.

46,X,der(X)t(X;Y) A de novo X-Y translocation would be expected to herald a female child, who will likely be short, 150 cm or less in height as an adult (Joseph et al. 1996; Speevak et al. 2001). The site of the breakpoint can be pinpointed using microarray or with probes for two loci (steroid sulfatase, Kallmann syndrome) in Xp22.3; if these loci are present on the der(X)t(X;Y), intelligence and fertility may be intact, and other defects are unlikely. A few de novo cases have been associated with major defects, presumably due to a marginally more proximal Xp breakpoint, with the deletion of crucial genes. Microarray would offer better clarity.

46,Y,der(X)t(X;Y) If the intact sex chromosome is the Y, the child is expected to be male. If the loci noted above are present, the phenotype is likely to be confined to short stature and infertility. A more extensive loss of loci might determine a nullisomy that would cause important malformation and be lethal in utero.

Other rare types include dicentric X;Y translocations, and der(X) and der(Y) chromosomes with a range of p and q arm breakpoints on X and Y (Hsu 1994). The phenotypes are male if *SRY* is present, and otherwise female. Infertility is typical, and, in the male, short stature. In the der(Y) case, in which there may be an effect of functional X disomy, genital anomaly and other malformation is common, as is mental defect. A detailed case is described in Ghosh et al. (2008), in which the recognition of an ultrasound brain anomaly at 21 weeks led to amniocentesis with the discovery of a de novo 46,X,der(Y)t(X;Y) (p22.13;q11.23). The Yqh region was replaced by Xp material, which thus existed in the functionally disomic state.

Other Abnormal X Chromosomes. X chromosome abnormalities are characteristically seen in the mosaic state, the other cell line typically being 45,X (and see Chapter 15). Mosaicism with a large *ring X* or an *Xq isochromosome*, 45,X/46,r(X) and 45,X/46,X,i(Xq), respectively, would lead to variant Turner syndrome. An *Xp isochromosome*, i(Xp), would probably always be lethal because there would be a functional Xp trisomy (Lebo et al. 1999). In an *X inversion*, there may be gonadal insufficiency in the otherwise normal female; and gonadal insufficiency may likewise accompany the de novo intrachromosomal *insertion X*, ins(X) (Grass et al. 1981; Dar et al. 1988; Dahoun et al. 1990). The "tiny ring X" syndrome is discussed on p. 348; a severe phenotype would mostly be the prediction from prenatal diagnosis, but exceptions exist, with a Turner-like picture or, in one extraordinary case, a normal male outcome (Turner et al. 2000; Chen et al. (2006d).

Y Isochromosome. The least rare Y isochromosome (or isodicentric Y) is the 46,X,i(Yq), in which the essential imbalance is a double dose of Yp material, and absence of some or most of Yq.[17] As reviewed in Chapter 15 (p. 349), the condition

---

17 An interesting question, not entirely theoretical in the present context, is what extrapolation, if any, can be made from the XYY syndrome, in which there is a double dose of Yp, but of course also of Yq material. Neas et al. (2005) suggest that trisomy for the pseudoautosomal region PAR1 might lie behind aspects of the cognitive phenotype in the XXX and in some i(Y) karyotypes; and the same might apply to XYY.

may be seen in both nonmosaic and (more usually) mosaic form, the latter with a 45,X cell line. The phenotype in postnatally identified cases has ranged from sterile but otherwise normal male, through female with gonadal dysgenesis, to actual genital ambiguity (Bruyère et al. 2006; DesGroseilliers et al. 2006). In contrast, the outlook from unbiased (i.e., not following an abnormal ultrasound) prenatal diagnosis is markedly in favor of normal male physical development, albeit that infertility will be very probable, and indeed, practically certain. If ultrasonography indicates male genitalia, a normal male phenotype is to be anticipated.

Willis et al. (2006) reviewed 15 cases, with follow-up from 4 months to 9 years: All but one had presented as normal males, and "development has been normal in all cases where follow-up was reported." A similarly optimistic interpretation comes from Bruyère et al. (2006): In a series of 12 cases from these authors, all nine in which diagnosis had been unbiased, and the pregnancies continued, led to births of normal males, and normal development in those who were further followed up. Although a question about cognitive development is not entirely settled (Tuck-Muller et al. 1995; Neas et al. 2005), and few reports give follow-up into adolescence or adulthood, at least anecdotally, many do well.

Y Ring Chromosome. Layman et al. (2009) report their own cases and review the 45,X/46,X,r(Y) karyotype, as identified in males in whom testes were descended. Variable short stature and gonadal failure were typical (and see p. 350). These authors note the confounding factors, in terms of predicting phenotype at prenatal diagnosis, of the bias toward genital abnormality in postnatally identified infants, versus the frequent lack of follow-up in apparently normal males following a prenatal diagnosis, leading to a bias in the other direction.

As for normal Yqh variation identified at prenatal diagnosis, this is reviewed in Cotter and Norton (2005). Microarray will not recognize this. The Y;15 variant is mentioned on p. 133.

22

PREIMPLANTATION GENETIC DIAGNOSIS

CHROMOSOMAL PREIMPLANTATION genetic diagnosis is done in the setting of in vitro fertilization, and in principle it enables an unaffected embryo to be transferred to the uterus, either a few days postconception or following frozen transfer at a subsequent cycle. Thus, for couples facing a high genetic risk, the risk can be bypassed; and the prospect of pregnancy termination for the reason of genetic abnormality can be avoided.

Advances in the late twentieth century in the fields of in vitro fertilization (IVF), human embryo culture, manipulation and cryopreservation, molecular genetics, and fluorescence in situ hybridization (FISH) set the stage for the development of preimplantation genetic diagnosis (PGD). From an essentially research-based exercise in a very few laboratories in the early 1990s, it has progressed to being, in the 2010s, a diagnostic tool available through most larger IVF clinics.

PGD is applied in two main settings: for the diagnosis of chromosome abnormalities and for the detection of a Mendelian condition.[1] Initially, the two categories were distinguished by the methodology applied—FISH in the former, DNA testing in the latter—but DNA-based methodologies are now the mainstay in both categories. Indeed, techniques have converged such that it is possible to accomplish Mendelian and chromosomal PGD with a single test.

There has arisen a praiseworthy tradition of excellent communication between the major centers that do this work, with many contributing their data to an international clearinghouse (under the aegis of ESHRE, the European Society for Human Reproduction and Embryology). Detailed analyses of the accumulated experience of the participating clinics are documented in reports of the ESHRE PGD consortium, which appear in the journal

---

1 PGD can also be used to detect and quantify mutations in the mitochondrial genome.

Human Reproduction (Calhaz-Jorge et al. 2016), and the International Society for Prenatal Diagnosis sponsors a regular conference devoted to PGD. Thus, new knowledge from the leading centers can translate readily into improved services to patients worldwide. Conversely, there is a paucity of large, well-controlled trials of PGD, and meaningful comparison between results published by different IVF clinics is complicated by differences in patient populations, embryology techniques, and molecular testing methods.

PATIENTS AND CIRCUMSTANCES IN WHICH CHROMOSOMAL PREIMPLANTATION GENETIC DIAGNOSIS MAY BE APPROPRIATE

Carriers of Balanced Rearrangements

A parent who is the carrier of a balanced rearrangement typically has a high risk to produce unbalanced embryos, as discussed at length in previous chapters. Particularly in the context of an unfortunate reproductive history, often with several miscarriages, or with one or more terminations following conventional prenatal diagnosis of an unbalanced fetal karyotype, the attraction of PGD is obvious: Only an embryo with a normal or balanced chromosomal constitution is transferred, with the expectation that, for each embryo transferred, there is a good chance of ongoing normal pregnancy. A related benefit for the couple is that they avoid the time, effort, cost, and disappointment of transferring embryos of which many would have been nonviable. Where there exists a risk of a liveborn child with an unbalanced karyotype, this risk is, in principle, eliminated. The two main categories are reciprocal (rcp) and Robertsonian (rob) translocations, although chromosomal PGD can also be applied to pericentric inversions and complex chromosome rearrangements (Scriven et al. 2014).

Preimplantation Genetic Screening

Preimplantation genetic screening is the practice of evaluating embryos for chromosome aneuploidy in chromosomally normal parents. The rationale behind PGS is twofold. First, it is well recognized that the proportion of IVF embryos that result in pregnancy is quite low, in many cases less than 30%. IVF clinics have long sought approaches that will accurately identify, prior to transfer, those embryos with the best chances of resulting in pregnancy.

Second, a substantial number of human embryos are aneuploid, and certain patient populations, including couples of advanced maternal age, or with histories of recurrent miscarriage and repeated implantation failure, may be predisposed to producing aneuploid embryos. Thus, aneuploidy is assumed to be an important reason that many IVF pregnancies fail. Logically, therefore, assessing the chromosome status of embryos, and discarding screened embryos that are aneuploid, should improve the proportion of transferred embryos that result in pregnancy (Weissman et al. 2017).

PGS is also used in the setting of a couple who have had a previously chromosomally abnormal pregnancy, or a previous liveborn child with Down syndrome or other aneuploidy. Here, the risk of recurrence of the specific aneuploidy is usually low, and the benefit of PGS, at least in terms of risk reduction, is small. For couples who are naturally fertile, it is questionable whether such a small risk reduction justifies the use of IVF (with its associated small risks to both mother and baby); but for couples who are already using IVF because of infertility, the addition of PGS may be considered appropriate, and it may give the couple more confidence of a successful outcome.

Gender Selection

Gender diagnosis at PGD, achieved via copy number assessment of the X and Y chromosomes, may be appropriate in the context of a sex-related genetic risk, whether Mendelian or non-Mendelian, an example of the latter being autism (Amor and Cameron 2008). The use of sex-selection PGD in this setting is likely to decline, as direct gene testing becomes feasible for more sex-linked disorders. A notable exception is for males affected by an X-linked disease who wish to avoid transmitting the faulty gene to their (female) offspring, a circumstance in which sex selection can substitute perfectly for a direct gene test.

EMBRYOLOGY PROCEDURES

Those who make the decision to embark upon chromosomal PGD or PGS will need to enroll (if not already) in an IVF program. In IVF, hormone treatment is given to stimulate the ovaries to produce a large number of oöcytes (preferably double figures; but if only a few, this does not per se betoken an increased risk for trisomy; Honorato et al. 2017) in a single menstrual cycle. Ovum "pickup" is conducted by transvaginal endoscopy under ultrasound guidance. The ova are collected, and most commonly fertilization is achieved by the injection of a single sperm into each (intracytoplasmic sperm injection [ICSI]). Although ICSI was originally designed to treat male infertility (which, incidentally, is frequently present in the male heterozygous for a chromosome rearrangement), its use in PGD is for the specific reason of avoiding the risk of DNA contamination from other sperm.

On day 1, approximately 18 hours after exposure to sperm, the oöcytes are checked for the presence of two pronuclei and two polar bodies, as evidence that fertilization[2] has occurred. They are then returned to tissue culture medium; in a few hours syngamy will occur, and during the next 48 hours the first few mitoses will have produced cleavage-stage embryos of six to eight cells.

There are three types of PGD biopsy, done at three sequential stages of gametic and embryonic development: polar body biopsy, blastomere biopsy, and blastocyst (trophectoderm) biopsy. Choosing the ideal stage requires consideration of four main factors: (1) whether the timing of biopsy allows accurate identification of the genetic abnormality (i.e., Is there a risk of false-negative results that could lead to a genetically abnormal embryo being transferred?), (2) whether abnormalities in the biopsy accurately predict abnormalities in the embryo (i.e., Is there a risk of a false-positive result that could lead to a "healthy" embryo being discarded?), (3) whether the timing of biopsy allows sufficient time for genetic testing to be completed prior to embryo transfer (a point that has assumed less importance with the development of improved cryopreservation techniques that permit the freezing of all embryos), and (4) whether the biopsy procedure itself compromises the survival of the embryo (Scott et al. 2013a).

Polar Body Analysis

Polar body (PB) genetic analysis (satisfyingly requiring recall of some elementary facts of biology) has been used for PGD (or "preconception diagnosis") in a few laboratories, and legal or logistic constraints against PGD in some jurisdictions have propelled interest (Landwehr et al. 2008; Vialard et al. 2008; Montag et al. 2009). The process of biopsy is illustrated in Figure 22–1. PB analysis allows a focus on

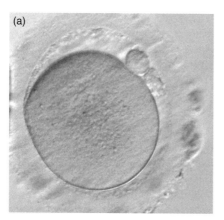 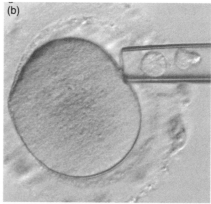

FIGURE 22–1   The process of polar body biopsy. (a) The egg is held in place by a suction pipette, which is applied directly to the zona pellucida (the "shell" that invests the egg itself, seen in dark circular outline). The first and second polar bodies are located in the space between the zona pellucida and the egg's cell membrane. The egg is manipulated so that the polar bodies are at the 1 to 2 o'clock position. (b) The pipette has entered a laser-cut hole in the zona pellucida, and the two polar bodies have been aspirated into its lumen.

Source: From Montag et al., Polar body biopsy: A viable alternative to preimplantation genetic diagnosis and screening, *Reprod Biomed Online* 18 Suppl 1: 6–11, 2009. Courtesy M. Montag, and with the permission of Elsevier.

---

2 Since fertilization in vitro can be observed as it actually happens, the fine detail of the process can be appreciated. The first act is penetration of the ovum by the sperm. To the embryologist, this is only the prelude to conception; the true moment of conception is the point at which the male and female pronuclei fuse, their chromosomes aligning on a common metaphase plate ("syngamy"). Once that event has taken place, the zygote has come into existence. At the first mitosis, it loses that name and becomes, in IVF parlance, a "cleavage-stage embryo," or simply an embryo.

the vulnerable gamete—that is, the ovum—since the great majority of segregation errors occur here, due either to nondisjunction or to premature predivision of sister chromatids. Disomic or nullisomic gametes could be identified and thus excluded from fertilization.

By way of example, imagine that the asterisked gametocyte in Figure 3–3a is the first PB (PB1), and that the two chromosomes shown within it are chromosome 18s—that is, PB1 is disomic 18. The "empty" gamete to the right, therefore, would be a nullisomic 18 oöcyte, and thus of course to be discarded. The reader may also determine, on study of Figure 3–6 with respect to predivision of sister chromatids at meiosis, why analysis of PB2 alone could in some instances mislead. The cell labeled "disomic gamete" in this figure could be the oöcyte, but PB2, represented by the cell next to it, shows a normal monosomy. A nullisomic second PB (PB2) (one of the empty cells in the next row) should provide corroboration. Both PBs together can enable the full picture to be deduced, and the disposition of all four chromatids can be accounted for.

A euploid egg might become, after fertilization, an embryo with some aneuploid cells (i.e., mosaicism, as elsewhere discussed in this chapter). But provided the euploid cell(s) carries on through and gives rise to the inner cell mass, then this transient mosaicism will have been unknown, and unimportant. Thus, a theoretical advantage of PB diagnosis is that the uncertainty relating to aneuploidy screening at PGD, due to biopsy of a possibly unrepresentative aneuploid blastomere, could be avoided (Geraedts et al. 2010).

Potential advantages of PB biopsy are that specimens are obtained earlier and that the biopsy is less disruptive to the embryo. On the other hand, PB is more expensive, given the need to test both polar bodies in every embryo. Abnormalities arising in paternal meiosis, estimated to represent about 10% of aneuploidies (Hassold et al. 2007; Templado et al. 2013), will not be detected.

Cleavage Stage Biopsy (Day-3 Biopsy of a Blastomere)

On day 3, one or at most two cells (blastomeres) are removed from each embryo, under the inverted microscope.[3] This requires a hole to be made in the "shell" (the zona pellucida, which has not yet been cast off), the cells being extracted by very gentle suction. These cells are subject to genetic analysis in order to determine whether or not they have a normal/balanced chromosome constitution or an unbalanced form of the rearrangement. One embryo (sometimes two[4]) shown to be chromosomally normal/balanced is then transferred to the uterus, on day 4 or 5, and with good fortune will develop into a normal infant. The remaining embryos with a normal/balanced chromosomal complement will usually be cryopreserved, in case the first embryo transfer does not result in a pregnancy, and perhaps for a second pregnancy in the future. The process is outlined in Figure 22–2.

Blastocyst Stage Biopsy (Day-5 or -6 Biopsy of Trophectoderm)

If the embryo is incubated for 2 or 3 more days, it advances through the morula (day 4) and early blastocyst (days 5 and 6) stages. There is considerable attrition over the time frame of blastocyst development, with only about half of cleavage-stage embryos surviving to become a blastocyst (Clouston et al. 2002), and this attrition appears preferentially to target aneuploid embryos. Adler et al. (2014), comparing aneuploidy rates from the day-3 cleavage embryo to the day 5 blastocyst, found that the overall proportion of euploid embryos increased from 23% to 32%, indicating loss of at least some aneuploidies by day 5; nevertheless, among the aneuploid embryos that do actually reach day 5 or 6, a wide range of trisomy and monosomy is observed (Rodriguez-Purata et al. 2015) (Fig. 19–3). The foregoing observations suggest that culture to blastocyst, irrespective of any genetic testing, may effectively act as a form of selection in favor of euploid embryos.[5]

---

3 The decision between one versus two blastomere biopsy involves a trade-off: Removal of two blastomeres may increase the likelihood of achieving an accurate PGD result, but it may compromise subsequent embryo development and clinical outcomes (De Vos et al. 2009; Brodie et al. 2012). Analyzing two cells will also be more expensive.

4 If two embryos are transferred, this is not designed to produce twins (for whom there is an increased obstetric risk) but, rather, to improve the odds that one will succeed. PGD may allow a lesser number of embryos to be transferred—ideally just one ("elective single embryo transfer," eSET)—thus reducing the likelihood of multiple pregnancy.

5 This fact should be borne in mind when comparing results of PGD using cleavage-stage cf. blastocyst biopsy.

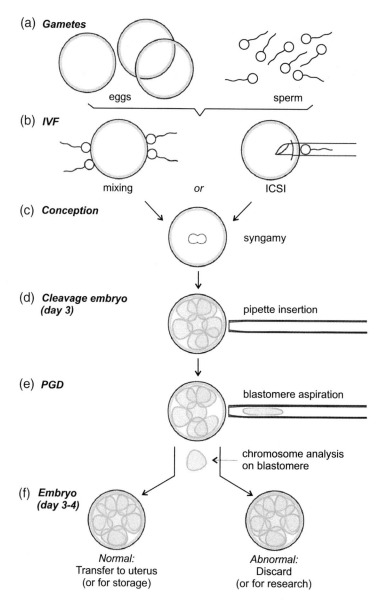

(a) *Gametes*

eggs

sperm

(b) *IVF*

mixing   *or*   ICSI

(c) *Conception*

syngamy

(d) *Cleavage embryo*
    (day 3)

pipette insertion

(e) *PGD*

blastomere aspiration

chromosome analysis
on blastomere

(f) *Embryo*
    (day 3-4)

Normal:
Transfer to uterus
(or for storage)

Abnormal:
Discard
(or for research)

FIGURE 22–2   The process of in vitro fertilization (IVF) (with or without intracytoplasmic sperm injection [ICSI]) and preimplantation genetic diagnosis (PGD) at the day-3 stage. (*a*) Oöcytes are obtained from the woman, and sperm from the man (by testicular aspiration, if necessary). (*b*) Oöcytes and sperm are mixed in vitro; or, single sperm are injected into an oöcyte (ICSI). (*c*) Syngamy, the fusion of male and female pronuclei, occurs. After incubation for 3 days, (*d*) one or two blastomeres are removed from the embryo, and (*e*) these cells are then subject to chromosomal analysis. (*f*) Normal (or balanced) embryos are chosen for transfer to the uterus, or possibly for cryopreservation for a future transfer.[6]

The biopsy procedure involves making a hole in the zona pellucida and allowing a small part of the lining of the blastocele cavity to herniate through ("assisted hatching"); part of this tiny bulge can be excised by laser or teased away by manipulation (Fig. 22–3).

6 The live-birth rate is less when two cells are removed (De Vos et al. 2009).

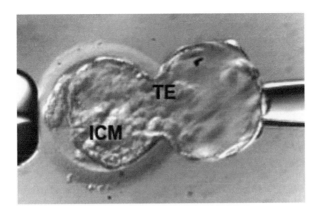

FIGURE 22–3   The process of blastocyst biopsy, at day 5 or 6. The blastocyst is held in place by the suction pipette on the left, which is applied directly to the zona pellucida (the "shell" that invests the blastocyst, "inherited" from the ovum. Trophectoderm (TE) has herniated through a laser-generated hole, visible in this view at 3 o'clock in the zona pellucida; the inner cell mass (ICM) remains comfortably within the zona pellucida. Suction will be applied through the biopsy pipette (right), and approximately five cells from the TE gently teased off.

Source: From McArthur et al., Blastocyst trophectoderm biopsy and preimplantation genetic diagnosis for familial monogenic disorders and chromosomal translocations, *Prenat Diagn* 28: 434-442, 2008. Courtesy R. P. S. Jansen, and with the permission of Wiley-Blackwell.

In theory, implantation should be more successful following blastocyst than cleavage-stage biopsy, and this does indeed appear to be the case (Brezina et al. 2012). One study of particular interest, carried out on couples presenting for IVF, used a novel design whereby two embryos were transferred to the uterus in the same cycle, but with only one of the embryos having been biopsied (Scott et al. 2013c). The embryo biopsy was not for the purpose of selecting embryos for transfer; rather, it was used to DNA-fingerprint embryos so that at birth it could be determined whether the baby had resulted from the biopsied or nonbiopsied embryo. The results showed equivalent implantation for biopsied and nonbiopsied embryos at the blastocyst stage, but reduced implantation for embryos biopsied at cleavage-stage compared to nonbiopsied embryos. From the foregoing, we conclude that clinical pregnancy rates should be higher for biopsied blastocysts than for cleavage-stage embryos. But a note of caution: Replication of data by other groups, to exclude laboratory-specific differences in biopsy technique, is required. Another factor of some controversy is whether "good-looking" blastocysts have a better chance than those of "poor" appearance; while those of better morphology may have an advantage over the "lesser lookers," the latter still have a fair chance of succeeding (Forman 2017; Irani et al. 2017).

Another attraction in delaying PGD until the blastocyst is forming is that cell number has increased, and differentiation between inner cell mass (which develops into the fetus) and trophoblast (which develops into the placenta) has begun, allowing sampling to be focused on the trophectoderm (in a tissue-origin sense, a very early chorionic villus sampling). Trophectoderm biopsy typically involves removal of between two and seven cells, providing more copies of DNA template for use in testing, compared to cleavage-stage biopsy. In an array-based analysis, using embryos from a youngish cohort of couples (average maternal age of 31 years), Johnson et al. (2010) examined blastocysts from which they were able to dissect out the trophectoderm and the inner cell mass. Encouragingly, almost all were concordant as to karyotype between these two tissues—"confined trophectoderm mosaicism" apparently is uncommon—and, perhaps reflecting the younger age profile, the considerable majority (80%) of embryos were euploid.

A counterpoint to the perceived merits of blastocyst biopsy is the fact that some viable embryos may not survive during culture in vitro between the cleavage and blastocyst stages (Glujovsky and Farquar 2016). It is a given that the maternal genital tract offers a better environment than does an IVF container, and a better chance for survival; and so, on this basis, the sooner the embryo could take up residence in its natural home, the better. And a controversial question is whether this longer incubation in vitro might disturb the epigenetic state of the embryo.

GENETIC ANALYSIS OF BIOPSIED CELLS

Various cytogenetic and molecular methods have been used to analyze the biopsied material, with molecular approaches in principle superior, in that copy number analysis of all 24 chromosomes is achievable. In choosing between methods, factors for consideration include the time required to perform the test (and specifically, whether fresh embryo transfer is possible), the ability of the test to detect a range of abnormalities, equipment and reagent cost, and the test complexity (Handyside 2013). Cost of analysis is particularly relevant in PGD (in contrast to prenatal testing or postnatal chromosome analysis) because of the need to test multiple embryos for each IVF cycle, with one or two tests performed per embryo.

Metaphase Chromosome Analysis. The first, and simplest, analysis of chromosomes in human embryos was done by spreading and counting stained metaphase chromosomes on glass slides (Angell et al. 1983). This method provided the earliest evidence of the extent of aneuploidy in human embryos, but the metaphase spreads were too few in number and too poor in quality ever to be of use clinically.

Fluorescence In Situ Hybridization. FISH was the methodology that launched PGD for chromosome abnormalities as a practicable possibility. Chromosome-specific FISH probes applied to the interphase nuclei of human embryos allowed a rapid and targeted assessment of a subset of chromosomes or chromosome regions. Although only about five multicolor FISH probes could be applied at one time, the first set of probes could be washed off and a second round of probes used, allowing analysis of about 10 chromosome loci per cell. Additional testing could be performed if a second cell was biopsied. For the detection of structural rearrangements, the choice of FISH probes for a particular PGD had to consider all possible segregation outcomes. The pattern of FISH signals that each outcome would generate, and the certainty of being able to distinguish a balanced or normal chromosome constitution, needed to be carefully thought through. With most simple reciprocal translocations, three probes would, in general, be required: two that hybridized to a point within the translocated segments, and one to one of the centromeres. Pericentric inversions led only to two unbalanced forms, and these could be accounted for by the use of a subtelomeric probe at either end of the chromosome, and a centromeric probe (Escudero et al. 2001). Observing the number of colored spots in the nucleus of a blastomere removed from the IVF embryo allowed the chromosome complement to be deduced.

For PGS, panels of five to nine FISH probes were the standard methodology for a number of years, targeting the sex chromosomes, and the smaller and acrocentric chromosomes that can result in abnormal but viable pregnancies.

Comparative Genomic Hybridization. The first analysis for the full 24-chromosome copy number was done with comparative genomic hybridization (CGH), a technique using DNA from the embryo and from a karyotypically normal individual, the two samples labeled with different-colored fluorochromes. The two labeled DNAs are then co-hybridized to normal metaphase spreads, and the relative intensity of the two fluorochromes is analyzed. Although this technique could lead to the birth of a healthy child (Wilton et al. 2001), it was too complex and time-consuming for routine application in the clinic.

Array Comparative Genomic Hybridization. Two developments were necessary to allow the more practicable use of CGH: (1) the development of reliable and unbiased methods of whole genome amplification (Handyside et al. 2004) and (2) the hybridization of DNA samples to microarrays rather than to metaphase spreads (hence, array-CGH). Array-CGH analysis is performed by scanning and imaging the array, and measuring the relative intensity of the two hybridization signals (Chapter 2). For PGD use, commercial CGH arrays are available that comprise several thousand fragments of human DNA at approximately 1 Mb intervals, allowing a resolution of approximately 10 Mb. The same CGH arrays can be used for patients with translocations and other chromosome rearrangements, although for translocations with breakpoints near the telomeres, arrays with higher probe density in these regions are needed.[7]

---

7 It is relevant here that translocations for which both translocated segments are very small, which carry the greatest risk of a viable abnormal pregnancy, are also the most difficult to detect, in their unbalanced form, by PGD array-CGH.

Real-Time Quantitative Polymerase Chain Reaction. Real-time quantitative polymerase chain reaction (qPCR) is another methodology enabling 24-chromosome copy number analysis. Treff et al. (2011) developed and used a multiplex PCR reaction to amplify at least two sequences on each arm of each chromosome, an approach that is rapid, inexpensive, and avoids the need for whole genome amplification; however, the technique is low in resolution, and it can only be used on multiple-cell trophectoderm samples.

Single Nucleotide Polymorphism Microarray ("Karyomapping"). Single nucleotide polymorphism (SNP) arrays provide both copy number information and genotyping (Ben-Nagi et al. 2017). To date, the use of SNP-arrays for aneuploidy detection has been confined mainly to multiple-cell trophectoderm biopsies. Compared to array-CGH, more complex bioinformatic analysis can be undertaken, including the incorporation of parental genotypes, which enables the detection of smaller copy number variants, and copy number neutral abnormalities such as uniparental disomy. The experience at Oxford, England, is encouraging: the pregnancy loss rate with SNP-array PGD is only 5%, and this improvement over the background 15–20% almost certainly reflects that chromosomally normal embryos were transferred. At this center, the diagnostic accuracy is very high, above 99% (Wells 2017). Data from SNP-arrays can also be used for linkage analysis for single gene disorders, allowing aneuploidy and single-gene PGD detection to be undertaken in the same test (Natesan et al. 2014). Another potential advantage of SNP-array is that, for translocation carriers, it is possible to distinguish embryos with a normal karyotype from those that have the balanced translocation, via the analysis of family haplotypes, albeit that many translocation patients will not have enough embryos available to allow the luxury of discarding those carrying the translocation.

Next-Generation Sequencing. In next-generation sequencing (massively parallel sequencing, MPS), DNA samples from an embryo biopsy, following whole genome amplification, are fragmented, and the nucleotide sequence is determined (Yin et al. 2013). The number of fragments sequenced from each chromosome (or part of each chromosome) should be proportional to copy number, thus enabling inference of monosomy/disomy/ trisomy of the embryo. Diagnostic accuracy is high (Kung et al. 2015).

Chromosome PGD Results: FISH Versus Molecular Methodology. In principle, discarding embryos with a chromosome complement that could not produce a healthy ongoing pregnancy self-evidently should improve the outcomes of IVF. But this aim would be subverted by a high rate of false-positive or false-negative results, or if the embryo biopsy procedure were to impair the viability of the embryo. We must therefore analyze the outcomes of chromosome PGD testing from these viewpoints, and in particular, we need to address the question of the accuracy of FISH versus microarray. The laboratory requirements differ for aneuploidy screening (PGS) and for specific chromosome rearrangements, and we consider each case separately.

Preimplantation Genetic Screening Outcomes with FISH Although PGS using 5–9 probe FISH was adopted with enthusiasm by many IVF centers, results were disappointing. One large and stringent trial (multicenter, randomized, double-blind controlled), conducted during the period 2003–2007, comparing PGS with standard IVF in 408 women of age range 35–41 years, showed a clear *lessening* in success (a 25% vs. 37% pregnancy rate) in those receiving PGD for aneuploidy screening (PGD-AS) (Mastenbroek et al. 2007). Twisk et al. (2008) reached a similar conclusion against a favorable effect due to PGS. Similarly, FISH PGS from blastocyst biopsy may have *less* success than simple blastocyst transfer (Jansen et al. 2008). In a study of day-3 embryos called as trisomic by FISH, nearly half were actually euploid, when four different sections of the day-5 blastocyst (three from the trophoblast, one from the inner cell mass) were examined by microarray (Northrop et al. 2010); it was also of interest that the normality of the trophoblast in all sections undermined the theory that aneuploid cells might be sequestered to potential placental tissue. A meta-analysis compiling nine published randomized controlled trials concluded that PGS using FISH should not be recommended (Mastenbroek et al. 2011).

With the benefit of hindsight, the major limitation of PGS using FISH could be seen as the FISH technology itself; and the validity of much of the substantial body of literature on FISH PGD is now questioned. First, embryonic aneuploidy occurs for all 23 chromosome pairs, yet only a minority of chromosomes could be tested by FISH. Second, even for the chromosomes that were tested, it was inevitable that a proportion of results would be inaccurate (Wells et al. 2008). Single-cell FISH is a challenging technique, and it cannot achieve 100% of resolvable signal on every chromosomal target. Treff et al. (2010) emphasized the potential for error due to poor spreading and fixation of cells. With 10 or more signals per cell to be interpreted, the error rate compounds. This is not normally a problem for other FISH applications, where many nuclei or metaphases are available for study. In PGD, it is an important, and critical, limitation. The most likely adverse outcomes are wastage of normal embryos (diagnosed as monosomies) and misdiagnosis of embryos with a trisomy as normal.

Preimplantation Genetic Screening Outcomes with Molecular Methodology PGS using either microarray or qPCR are 24-chromosome approaches that avoid the technical limitations of FISH. Scott et al. (2012) undertook a novel prospective blinded study in which 255 embryos were tested by SNP microarray but transferred regardless of genetic status; 41% of embryos predicted to be euploid by SNP-array led to the delivery of healthy children, compared to 28% of embryos overall, indicating a useful benefit of PGS. On the other hand, 4% of embryos predicted to be aneuploid by SNP-array also led to the birth of healthy children, demonstrating that even with SNP-array, the negative predictive value of PGS was less than 100%. This shows that DNA technology will inevitably result in discarding a small proportion of embryos that had the capacity to form healthy children, an awkward point that should be raised in genetic counseling.

A subsequent randomized controlled trial performed by the same group, but using a qPCR-based PGS test, confirmed the benefit of 24-chromosome PGS: 66% of embryos tested to be euploid progressed to delivery, compared to 48% of untested embryos (Scott et al. 2013b). A similar benefit was observed in a retrospective study of qPCR PGS with single embryo transfer, which found an ongoing pregnancy rate of 55% in the PGS group compared to 42% in the control group (Forman et al. 2012). Nevertheless, in a systematic review of 24-chromosome PGS, Lee et al. (2015b) concluded that although most studies demonstrate an improved implantation rate with PGS, there is insufficient published data to evaluate the clinical effectiveness and the cost-effectiveness of PGS.

Preimplantation Genetic Diagnosis Translocation Outcomes with FISH FISH PGD for translocation carriers had considerably better outcomes than did FISH PGS, possibly due to the fact that fewer FISH probes are required for translocation PGD, thereby reducing the likelihood of false-positive and false-negative results. A clear benefit of FISH PGD was observed in terms of a substantially reduced risk of miscarriage and an increased liveborn delivery rate per embryo transferred (Munné 2005; Keymolen et al. 2009). An impressive report comes from Otani et al. (2006), who assessed PGD by FISH in 33 couples having had several miscarriages and no liveborn children, from a total of 117 pregnancies, and one of the couple being a translocation heterozygote. Thus, in their prior reproductive history (typically over several years), there had been a 100% pregnancy loss. Following PGD (an average of 1.24 cycles per patient), a total of 20/88 embryos from rob carriers, and 86/491 from rcp carriers, were diagnosed as normal/balanced (these comprising only 18% of the total, again attesting to the high genetic risk). Of the 19 pregnancies subsequently resulting from transfer of normal/balanced embryos, just one (5%) miscarried; the other 18 pregnancies had either proceeded into the second trimester or culminated in live birth. A 100% loss versus 5% is a notable contrast. This very considerable improvement does imply that many of these couples would otherwise have had no impediment to fertility (although not all couples had been able, at the time of the study, to achieve a pregnancy: as applies, of course, to all IVF).

Preimplantation Genetic Diagnosis Translocation Outcomes with Molecular Methodology The above FISH-based successes notwithstanding, the early results from translocation PGD using microarray indicate that this is, in fact, the superior technique (Treff et al. 2011; Tan et al. 2013). In one of the largest studies to date, Tan et al. retrospectively studied 575 translocation (rcp and rob) couples, comprising 406 couples treated by FISH PGD, and 169 treated with SNP-array PGD. Unlike FISH, SNP-array is able to test simultaneously for unbalanced segregants of the translocation as well as for aneuploidy, and so it was expected that a greater proportion of embryos would be unsuitable for transfer; and yet the opposite has been found. For reciprocal translocations, the proportion of transferrable embryos was 36% in the SNP-array group compared to 20% in the FISH PGD group (it may be that FISH PGD was misclassifying some healthy

	TRANS-LOCATION	BALANCED (%)	ABNORMAL: UNBALANCED TRANSLOCATION (%)	ABNORMAL: ANEUPLOIDY (%)	MEDIAN EMBRYOS TRANSFERRED PER PATIENT	IMPLANTATION RATE (%)	MISCARRIAGE RATE (%)
SNP	rcp	36	52	12	1	59	11
	rob	58	23	19	2	52	12
FISH	rcp	20	80		1	32	16
	rob	36	64		3	28	17

FISH, fluorescence in situ hybridization; rcp, reciprocal; rob, Robertsonian; SNP, single nucleotide polymorphism.
Source: From Tan et al. (2013).

embryos as unbalanced; Table 22–1).[8] And similarly for Robertsonian translocation patients: 58% of embryos in the SNP-array group were transferrable compared to only 36% in the FISH group. Translocation patients treated with SNP-array PGD also had a higher implantation rate and lower miscarriage rate, further supporting the superiority of this methodology. A question does remain: Might there be an aneuploidy unrelated to the translocation chromosomes? This is something that can be detected using a whole genome approach (Ghevaria et al. 2016).

THE PROBLEM OF MOSAICISM AND "CHAOTIC" EMBRYOS

The problem of mosaicism in the early embryo has received considerable attention in the context of PGD. Given that PGD relies on the genetics of the biopsied cell(s) being representative of the embryo as a whole, the presence of mosaicism could lead to incorrect classification of embryos and undermine the PGD strategy.

DAY-3 OR -4 EMBRYO BIOPSY

The six- to eight-cell embryo (the stage at which blastomere sampling is typically done) contains probably only one or two cells whose descendants will go on to form the inner cell mass and

thus, eventually, the embryo proper and the fetus. Chromosome studies on IVF embryos can reveal different chromosome constitutions in different cells, up to the point of "chaotic" embryos in which several cells each have a different aneuploidy, or collection of aneuploidies (Vanneste et al. 2009a, 2009b). It is not necessarily easy to guess (but intelligent guesses can be made), from the observed pattern of the different aneuploidies, what might have been the sequence of events at each individual mitosis that was able to lead to this eventual picture. Munné et al. (2002) list these four main categories: diploid/polyploid mosaicism, chaotic mosaicism, mosaicism due to mitotic nondisjunction, and "split" mosaics with two cell lines that complement each other.

A particular vulnerability may apply to these very early mitoses, before the necessary genes for cell-cycle checkpoint control have fully swung into action, and maternal cytoplasmic factors are still being relied upon (Hardy et al. 2002; Voullaire et al. 2002). Alternatively, or perhaps additionally, there may be a male factor involved, with impairment of the embryo's centrosome function (Rodrigo et al. 2010). This could apply more particularly to cases of a severe spermatogenic defect, with a poor-quality sperm bringing a poor-quality centriole to the embryo, given that the first few mitoses make use of the centriole that came with the sperm (Silber et al. 2003).

---

8 An important caveat here is that embryos tested by SNP-array were tested at blastocyst stage, whereas the embryos tested by FISH were tested at cleavage stage. As noted above, culture to blastocyst selects in favor of euploid embryos (Adler et al. 2014). So the comparison may not be entirely fair.

In a systemic review of chromosome mosaicism in human preimplantation embryos, van Echten-Arends et al. (2011) concluded that 73% of all human embryos were mosaic, of which 80% (59% of all embryos) were diploid-aneuploid mosaic. Such an astonishingly high level of diploid-aneuploid mosaicism, if real, would invalidate the strategy of PGS. But has the problem been overstated? As we discuss above, the power of the microarray has brought a clearer light and has exposed an inherent technical inadequacy in FISH methodology. Mosaicism can certainly happen, but it may be less frequent, and less chaotic, than we had thought in the early 2000s. Treff et al. (2010) proposed that mosaicism at PGD may often be more apparent than real, simply for technical reasons inherent in the methodology. If the same embryos are tested in parallel with FISH and microarray, mosaicism in the latter group falls to much lower levels, in a range of 25%–30% (Northrop et al. 2010; Treff et al. 2010; Fragouli et al. 2011). Moreover, mosaic diploid-aneuploid embryos (those for which there is a high risk of misdiagnosis at PGD) account for only approximately 5% of analyzed embryos (Capalbo et al. 2013).

BLASTOCYST BIOPSY

The biopsy of multiple cells at the blastocyst stage allows a more ready detection of mosaicism. While this may lessen concerns about misdiagnosis, a new question is posed: What to do with embryos in which mosaicism is detected? A conservative approach would be to discard all mosaic embryos, but what if a mosaic embryo is the only embryo available for transfer? A critical observation is that a number of healthy babies have been born following the transfer of mosaic aneuploid blastocysts. Greco et al. (2015) analyzed 3,802 blastocysts by array-CCH and detected chromosomal mosaicism in 181 (4.8%). Eighteen women for whom no euploid embryos were obtained elected to have a mosaic embryo transferred, resulting in the birth of six healthy babies and two additional biochemical pregnancies. Using the more sensitive technique of next generation sequencing, which is able to detect mosaicism down to the level of 20%, Munne et al. (2017) identified mosaicism in 22% of blastocysts tested, comprising mosaic (whole chromosome) aneuploidy in 10%, mosaic segmental aneuploidy in 7%, and complex mosaicism (involving three or more chromosomes) in 5%. When compared to euploid blastocysts, transfer of mosaic blastocysts was associated with a pregnancy rate of 50% (cf. 70% in euploid blastocysts), a miscarriage rate of 25% (cf. 10% in euploid blastocysts), and an ongoing pregnancy rate of 40% (cf. 63% in euploid blastocysts).

In light of these findings, we need to decide upon an appropriate disposition of these mosaic aneuploid blastocysts. Couples could be offered the option of transferring these mosaic embryos, so long as they are aware that, compared to euploid blastocysts, mosaic aneuploid blastocysts have a lower pregnancy rate and may be more likely to miscarry. A more complex question is whether transfer of these embryos carries a risk of the child being born with mosaic (or nonmosaic) aneuploidy. Whether such a risk exists will depend on the nature of the aneuploidy. If the aneuploid cell line is a monosomy (mosaic euploid/monosomy), it can be assumed there is no risk because monosomic cells (other than monosomy X) are not viable. In contrast, trisomic cells may convey a small risk for a mosaic euploid/trisomic child to be born. This risk is presumably highest for mosaic trisomies capable of liveborn viability (13, 18, and 21), but consideration should also be given to trisomies associated with potential for uniparental disomy (e.g., 14 and 15). If couples elect to transfer mosaic aneuploid blastocysts and a pregnancy results, prenatal diagnosis should prudently be offered, preferably by amniocentesis (a confined trophoblast mosaicism might evolve into a confined placental mosaicism at CVS and leave the question unanswered).

GENETIC COUNSELING

PGD is sufficiently complicated, not to mention expensive, that it will not usually be the first option for fertile couples wishing to avoid the birth of a child with a chromosomal disorder. High-risk scenarios, such as one of the couple being a translocation carrier, might, however, warrant consideration sooner rather than later. Women may view access to the procedure as empowering, but equally, may find the process stressful; discarding an embryo with an unbalanced translocation, having had a child with that condition, may raise uncomfortable ambiguities (Karatas et al. 2010). For infertile couples (whether or not there is a chromosomal basis of the infertility) who require an IVF procedure to conceive, advice about a place for PGS will need to be tempered by a continuing understanding of the biology of early human embryo development, and the fact that PGD is, as yet, an imperfect tool for predicting the health and viability of an embryo.

For couples presenting for PGD, on the basis that one of them carries a chromosomal rearrangement, a number of points need to be raised.

THE REASONS FOR CHOOSING PGD

Some couples may have had conventional prenatal diagnosis with successive terminations of pregnancies due to a high-risk translocation and be unwilling to face this prospect again. It may be difficult to distinguish a run of bad luck, with an optimistic outlook for the next pregnancy as a realistic possibility, and therefore allowing the counselor to suggest a further natural attempt. Or, the series of abnormal pregnancies may reflect a strong predisposition of that translocation to generate unbalanced gametes. Avoiding the possibility of termination following conventional prenatal diagnosis is, for those who have had that experience, a strong motivation (Lavery et al. 2002).

THE LIMITED SUCCESS RATE

As discussed above, many IVF/PGD procedures do not produce the desired end result of a "take-home baby," and the figures for PGD pregnancies are fairly similar to those applying to all IVF patients. For couples who require IVF in order to conceive (e.g., when a male translocation carrier also has oligospermia), the benefits of PGD—avoidance of transfer of nonviable embryos and reduced risk of miscarriage—are likely to outweigh the disadvantages, of which financial cost may be prominent. In contrast, couples who would otherwise have no difficulty conceiving may have more difficulty weighing the pros and cons of IVF with PGD, compared to natural conception and conventional prenatal diagnosis (Kanavakis and Traeger-Synodinos 2002). In this comparison, the chances of ultimately having a healthy child may be similar between the two pathways, but the challenges of the two pathways are very different. One study that compared live birth rates in translocation couples who chose PGD, against those choosing natural conception, found no difference in the live birth rate, although the risk of miscarriage was significantly less with PGD (Ikuma et al. 2015). The counselor can help the couple in their decision-making by encouraging them to consider the relative merits and challenges of PGD versus natural conception.

THE OUTLOOK AT PGS

For PGS, a realistic consideration is the likelihood that not one euploid embryo will be obtained from a single IVF stimulation cycle. The risk for this unfortunate circumstance is at its lowest for women in the age range 26–37 years but rises steeply from age 38 years; and, as logically expected, this risk is mirrored by a fall in the positive likelihood of retrieving at least one euploid embryo, according to age (Fig. 22–4) (Franasiak et al. 2014; Demko et al. 2016).

THE QUESTION OF MOSAICISM

With the move toward several-cell (blastocyst) rather than one- or two-cell (cleavage-stage embryo) biopsy, and with the increasing use of molecular methodologies, mosaicism will more often—when it is present—be recognized, or at least suspected. The complexity and inherent imprecision of the interpretation of molecular findings are discussed above and in Scott and Galliano (2016), while Besser and Mounts (2017) rehearse the challenges facing counselors who have the task of conveying these uncertain findings to their patients. These latter authors note that mosaicism for trisomy of one of chromosomes 2, 7, 13, 14, 16, 18, and 21 would raise a particular caution.

THE OUTLOOK FOR TRANSLOCATION CARRIERS

The figures provided elsewhere in this book, with respect to translocation heterozygotes, largely relate to the risk for an unbalanced chromosome complement in either a liveborn child or at conventional prenatal diagnosis. Naturally, the risk that an embryo at PGD will be abnormal is substantially, and often very substantially, higher. Data (FISH analysis) from the embryos of 59 couples, one or the other a rcp heterozygote, are set out in Table 5–2, and the average relative segregant fractions (female;male) were as follows: normal 45%;42%, adjacent-1 28%;35%, adjacent-2 8%;16%, 3:1 19%;7%, and 4:0 0.4%;0.6% (Scriven et al. 2013); thus, slightly more than half were chromosomally imbalanced. These same segregation ratios are shown graphically in Figure 22–5. On microarray PGD, it is helpful to note that an embryo can be shown to be free both of unbalanced segregants due to the translocation, and of coincidental aneuploidy.

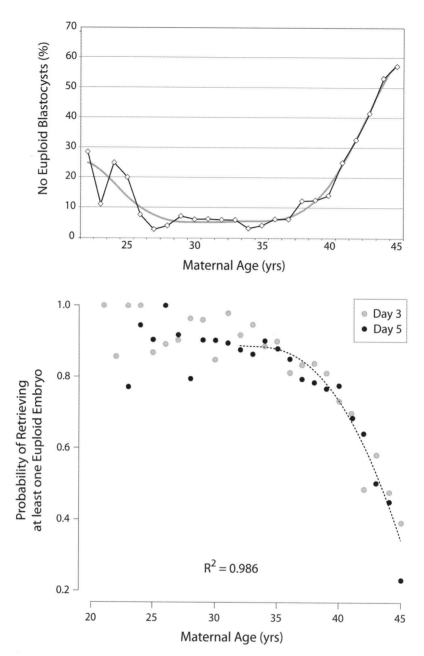

FIGURE 22–4 The relationship between maternal age and the probability (*top*) that *no* euploid blastocysts will be available from a single IVF cycle or (*bottom*) that at least one euploid embryo (day 3 or day 5) will be retrieved. These two studies reflect each other, and they show that the best chances lie between the maternal ages of 26 and 37 years. The odds are slightly less favorable in younger women and much less favorable in older women.

Source: From Franasiak et al., The nature of aneuploidy with increasing age of the female partner: A review of 15,169 consecutive trophectoderm biopsies evaluated with comprehensive chromosomal screening, *Fertil Steril* 101: 656–663.e1, 2014 (also shown as Fig. 19–2), courtesy J. M. Franasiak, and with the permission of Elsevier; and from Demko et al., Effects of maternal age on euploidy rates in a large cohort of embryos analyzed with 24-chromosome single-nucleotide polymorphism-based preimplantation genetic screening, *Fertil Steril* 105: 1307–1313, 2016, courtesy Z. P. Demko, and with the permission of Elsevier, as per the Creative Commons License.

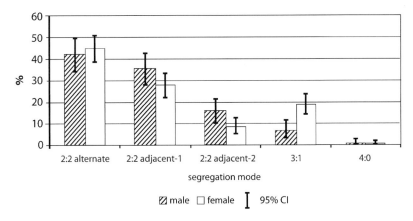

FIGURE 22–5   The range of segregation ratios observed in embryos of "translocation couples," as listed in detail in Table 5–2. CI, confidence interval.

Source: From Scriven et al., Benefits and drawbacks of preimplantation genetic diagnosis (PGD) for reciprocal translocations: Lessons from a prospective cohort study, *Eur J Hum Genet* 21: 1035–1041, 2013. Courtesy P. N. Scriven, and with the permission of Nature Publishing Group.

Table 22–2 summarizes data from three large studies collating results from PGD cycles (microarray analysis), in the setting of reciprocal and Robertsonian translocations. Approximately one-third of embryos successfully biopsied are suitable for transfer. More relevant to the couple is the likelihood of an IVF PGD cycle producing a "take-home baby." Idowu et al. (2015) found that 38% of biopsy cycles, in carriers of balanced translocations, resulted in a live birth, with younger (<35 years) women doing better, at 49%, than older (>35) women, at 23%. Unsurprisingly in the high-risk circumstance of a parental translocation, 30% of biopsied cycles yielded no euploid embryos.

Whereas the proportion of embryos unbalanced for the translocation is fairly constant, independent

Table 22–2. Preimplantation Genetic Diagnosis Observations (Microarray) in Embryos from Translocation Carriers

SOURCE	DAY OF BIOPSY	ARRAY TYPE	EMBRYOS TESTED AND PRODUCING RESULTS	ABNORMAL: UNBALANCED TRANSLOCATION (± OTHER ANEUPLOIDY)	ABNORMAL: OTHER ANEUPLOIDY	EUPLOID EMBRYOS SUITABLE FOR TRANSFER
Reciprocal Translocations						
Tan et al. (2013)	5	SNP	499	261 (52%)	62 (13%)	176 (35%)
Tobler et al. (2014)	3 or 5	SNP or array-CGH	498	154 (31%)	118 (24%)	226 (45%)
Idowu et al. (2015)	3 or 5	SNP	338	186 (55%)	88 (26%)	64 (19%)
Total			1,335	601 (45%)	268 (20%)	466 (35%)
Robertsonian Translocations						
Idowu et al. (2015)			201	16 (8%)	111 (55%)	74 (37%)

array-CGH, array comparative genomic hybridization; SNP, single nucleotide polymorphism.

of parental age, the proportion of aneuploid embryos will naturally increase with advancing maternal age. Hence, for women older than age 35 years, the proportion of tested embryos that are suitable for transfer may be less than 20%, and a probable outcome of a PGD cycle may be that no embryo will be suitable for transfer. When suitable embryos are obtained, the outlook is considerably brighter, regardless of maternal age, with approximately half of transferred euploid embryos leading to the birth of a healthy child (Idowu et al. 2015).

FOLLOW-UP IN THE PREGNANCY

Understandably, some couples will be unenthusiastic about an invasive procedure that could possibly put at risk the pregnancy in which there has been so much investment (Meschede et al. 1998b). Nevertheless, couples need to be aware that chromosomal PGD cannot provide a "guarantee," albeit that the misdiagnosis rate, for whatever reason, is very low, when good-quality embryos are transferred (Wilton et al. 2009). Prenatal testing should be offered. Ultrasonography may be an acceptable, if imperfect, compromise, only proceeding to CVS or amniocentesis if anomalies are detected. Maternal serum screening offers a further possibility, although it is necessary to take account of the fact that pregnancy-associated plasma protein-A (PAPP-A) levels are less in IVF pregnancies, which might otherwise have been interpreted as an increased risk for trisomy 21 (Amor et al. 2009). Noninvasive prenatal testing can target full aneuploidies, but consultation with the laboratory will be required to determine if unbalanced segregants of a translocation are detectable.

NATURE MAY INTERVENE

A natural pregnancy may be achieved while the couple waits for the IVF/PGD preparations to be made. For example, the adjacent-2 karyotype shown in Figure 5–10 came from culture of the products of conception of this couple's third miscarriage, and no normal pregnancies, the woman being a t(13;16) carrier. The outlook did not seem very promising, and plans were being put in place for IVF; but they then reported a naturally conceived pregnancy, in which amniocentesis showed a 46,XY karyotype.

THE CHILDREN RESULTING

Does PGD carry any risks to the embryo and to the child? We may consider three categories of potential risk. First, there is a small risk of an embryo not surviving the biopsy process. With improvements in biopsy technique, this risk is now less than 0.5%; and although it is undoubtedly disappointing for a couple to lose an embryo in this manner, the small risk is unlikely to deter couples from PGD. Second, there is an ongoing question of whether the biopsy procedure itself might lead to reduced viability of biopsied embryos, compared to nonbiopsied embryos. Currently, there is a lack of high-quality studies on this issue; one small randomized clinical trial, as noted also above, found that cleavage-stage (but not blastocyst) biopsy impaired embryonic implantation (Scott et al. 2013c); and there is some evidence that, compared to single blastomere biopsy, biopsy of two blastomeres may have a detrimental effect on subsequent embryo development and clinical outcomes (De Vos et al. 2009).

The third, and most important, question relates to the child born from a PGD pregnancy. It is well recognized that there are differences in health between children conceived by IVF (without PGD) and naturally conceived children. IVF-conceived babies are at increased risk of low birth weight, preterm birth, perinatal mortality, and birth defects (Halliday 2007; Halliday et al. 2010). Nevertheless, it is reassuring that, in the longer term, the health of young adult "IVFlings" appears to be similar to that of their in vivo conceived counterparts (Halliday et al. 2014). For IVF in general, the usual counseling is for an absolute increase of approximately 1% in the risk of congenital abnormalities, compared to background risk.[9] The risk for Beckwith-Wiedemann syndrome in IVF babies generally is noted on p. 412.

It might have been expected that babies conceived using PGD would, at minimum, be exposed to the same risks that have been documented for IVF conception in general, and that additional risks might also be present if there is a detrimental effect of the biopsy process itself. To date, however, outcomes in PGD pregnancies have not been substantially different from those of IVF pregnancies; and thus we may conclude that, in fact, there is likely no detrimental effect of embryo biopsy per

---

9 There is conflicting evidence regarding whether IVF conception increases the risk of chromosome abnormalities in offspring. If such a risk really exists, it is likely to be very low, and therefore IVF conception is not, in itself, an indication for chromosomal PGD.

se. Children born from a PGD pregnancy, a tiny minority group among the large numbers worldwide of "IVFlings," appear to be of essentially normal health (Banerjee et al. 2008; Desmyttere et al. 2009). They may be born slightly earlier, and be a little lighter, than normally conceived babies. These risks, and a risk for perinatal death, may be elevated in the case of a multiple pregnancy (Liebaers et al. 2010). Perhaps unsurprisingly, for a child in whom so much has been invested, PGD infants score well on a scale of "warmth–affection" (measured by observing how infants may be cuddled and kissed, and how positively and kindly spoken to). We can anticipate, in the fullness of time, longer-term studies on the health and development of these "PGD children."

PART SIX

DISORDERS OF SEX DEVELOPMENT

23

CHROMOSOMAL DISORDERS
OF SEX DEVELOPMENT

CHROMOSOMAL SEX is, for the most part, congruently XX female and XY male. The XX and XY embryo are built on a fundamentally similar outline plan, and only as development proceeds do certain modifications evolve. If at any point in this sequential process some genetic instruction is faulty, inappropriate, or cannot be acted on, the direction of anatomical sexual development may proceed imperfectly or completely incongruently. In this chapter, we a focus upon those forms in which classical and molecular cytogenetics comprise key diagnostic investigations. We provide categories for "girls and women" and "boys and men," according to the phenotypes presented, and according to the sex that the individual is regarded as being, by the individual or by the individual's parents. We do not address the question of gender dysphoria, which is more a matter for the psyche.

NOMENCLATURE

These conditions are subsumed under the general heading of disorders of sex development (DSD), a classification that also includes the sex chromosome aneuploidies Turner syndrome and Klinefelter syndrome (Hughes 2008; Kremen et al. 2017). The different chromosomal categories may be indicated by reference to the sex chromosome constitution (XX or XY) and the nature of the gonad (testis, ovary, ovotestis, or dysgenetic/streak). The former expressions XX male, XY female, and hermaphrodite are now referred to as particular types of DSD. Genital ambiguity/intersex is simply denoted XX DSD or XY DSD, according to karyotype; clearly these are rather broad descriptors, and more precise detail might usefully be added in individual cases. With reference to male or female sex, these different levels of definition can apply: gonadal sex (ovary, testis, ovotestis, streak); anatomical/genital sex (structure of the internal and external genital tract); karyotypic sex (46,XX, 46,XY, or other); and behavioral sex (gender identity).

BIOLOGY

Somewhat simplified, the fundamental plan of the reproductive tract is that bilateral gonads, arising from the genital ridge, connect with bilateral paired internal ducts (Müllerian and Wolffian), which enter a midline genital sinus, opening at the perineum. This opening is buttressed on each side by labioscrotal folds and capped above by a phallus. The basic plan of the genital ridge is laid down according to instruction from, in particular, the *WT1* and *SF1* genes. Thereafter, the direction in which gonadal development proceeds is due to the activity of a number of genes on the sexual differentiation pathway (Bashamboo et al. 2017).

The Key Role of the *SRY* Gene

In the *absence* of *SRY*, but with input from *WNT4* and *RSPO1*, the gonad develops into an ovary, and the duct system develops into fallopian tubes and uterus. The genital sinus remains as an opening (the vagina), flanked and surmounted by labia and clitoris. The female state results. If a Y chromosome is *present*—or at least that part of the Y that contains *SRY*, the testis-determining gene—the male direction is taken. Transient expression of the *SRY* gene calls into action *SOX9*, which in turn stimulates the *FGF9* gene; both *FGF9* and *SOX9* suppress *WNT4*, and the gonad becomes a testis. The testis, in turn, secretes hormones, of which androgen influences the genital tract to masculinize, and anti-Müllerian hormone causes regression of the female Müllerian ducts. A vas deferens forms from the duct system. The phallus enlarges. The labioscrotal folds fuse in the midline and accommodate the descending testes. The male state results.

Chromosome Testing in Disorders of Sex Development

Classic cytogenetic testing is necessary to diagnose chromosomal DSDs accurately. A standard microscope karyotype can detect balanced translocations involving the sex chromosomes; and at least 30 cells should be examined in order to check for mosaicism.

The presence of *SRY* is routinely tested with fluorescence in situ hybridization, and chromosome microarray is used for the detection of copy number changes affecting known or postulated DSD genes. Molecular testing for a number of specific DSD genes, per medium of a gene panel or exome sequencing approach, is a suitable adjunctive approach, given the genotypic heterogeneity of the DSDs.

CHROMOSOMAL DISORDERS OF SEX DEVELOPMENT IN GIRLS AND WOMEN

XY Ovarian Disorder of Sexual Development

The 46,XY karyotype in an otherwise normal girl, with (apparently) completely normal female anatomy, is a very rare observation. A single case is reported of a child who was a compound heterozygote for mutations in the *CBX2* gene, discovered only because of a discordant chromosome finding at prenatal diagnosis (Biason-Lauber et al. 2009). The internal genital tract was normal female, the gonads of normal ovarian appearance, and normal upon histology. It may be that *SRY* requires activation by *CBX2* before it can make its male-determining contribution to sexual differentiation.

XY Disorder of Sexual Development, Complete Pure Gonadal Dysgenesis (Swyer Syndrome)

The rare *familial* form provides a unique example of a Mendelian condition that can be inherited in a Y-linked, X-linked recessive, or sex-limited autosomal dominant or recessive mode. In the X-linked forms or autosomal forms, the XY female has a perfectly normal Y chromosome, with a normal *SRY* testis-determining gene; mutation in a gene (whether this be X-linked or autosomal) controls a later event in the testicular developmental pathway.

In the *Y-linked* form, there is a mutation in the *SRY* gene itself. In some Y-hemizygotes, the mutant gene has nevertheless been able to reach a threshold of operation and to induce testis development, while in others with the same mutation, it has not. Thus, for example, an XY male with a mutation in *SRY* may be a normal fertile man, while his XY child may be a daughter. The threshold is apparently all or nothing: Partial expression—that is, an intersex state—does not result (Jäger et al. 1992; Imai et al. 1999). A man may be a gonadal mosaic for an *SRY* deletion, as presumably was the father in Barbosa et al. (1995): Two daughters of his had XY DSD (one with gonadoblastoma) with a deletion of *SRY*, but he himself showed a normal *SRY* result; there were three other normal daughters and six normal sons. Similarly, Schmitt-Ney et al. (1995) describe two XY sisters and their XY half-sister with an *SRY* point mutation, whose father was shown to be mosaic for this mutation. These familial examples notwithstanding, sporadic occurrence is usual, and in approximately 15% of these cases the *SRY* gene has a de novo mutation or rearrangement, that abolishes its function of testis determination. As for the *X chromosome*, duplication of the X-borne gene *NR0B1* (*DAX1*) accounts for some X-linked XY gonadal dysgenesis (Barbaro et al. 2012).

The first *autosomal* gene for an XY DSD to be discovered was *DHH*, at 12q12. Homozygosity for this gene was identified in three of six apparently non-consanguineous Mexican-mestizo women with XY DSD, two of whom, not known to be related, had the same mutation (Canto et al. 2004). (The same gene has been implicated, in heterozygous state, in mixed gonadal dysgenesis; Canto et al. 2005). Other autosomal dominant XY gonadal dysgenesis loci are *NR5A1* (*SF1*) and *MAP3K1* (Pearlman et al. 2010; Philibert et al. 2010).

The gonad in this form of XY DSD is dysgenetic, and it is seen as a "streak." The genital tract feminizes. The lack of female sex hormones causes failure of normal pubertal development. Amenorrhea and failure of pubertal development are the usual complaints that lead these girls to seek medical advice. Gonadectomy is recommended upon diagnosis due to the high risk of gonadoblastoma, a premalignant neoplastic change in the dysgenetic gonad that may progress to dysgerminoma (Huang et al. 2017). Familial ovarian malignancy was a notable observation in a sibship of three XY women (the karyotype presumed in two who had died at ages 19 and 20 years) described in Kempe et al. (2002).

As always, an accurate diagnosis is needed to give useful counseling. It is thus disconcerting that in a review of 48 women carrying a diagnosis of "XY female," undertaken in a specialist clinic, in only half was the description accurate. In about one-third of women, the diagnosis was inaccurate, and in one-eighth, frankly wrong (Minto et al. 2005). Counselors will want to assure themselves that the information they have about a patient is correct, and they should painstakingly review all the test findings, with appropriate expert advice.

XY Disorder of Sexual Development, Complete Androgen Insensitivity Syndrome

This is a Mendelian condition, in which the locus happens to be on the X chromosome. In this disorder, the defect lies further down the developmental path. The gonad becomes a testis and produces testicular secretions, but the genital tract, internal and external, is resistant to the effects of androgen. The inheritance is X-linked recessive, and the locus is the androgen receptor gene at Xq12 (Saranya et al. 2016). The individual appears externally very much as a female, but there is amenorrhea, and pubic and axillary hair is absent. Internally, the vagina is short, and the uterus and tubes are represented only by remnants; the testes may be in the inguinal canal (Boehmer et al. 2001). Malignancy of the gonad, gonadoblastoma or dysgerminoma, is less of a concern than in Swyer syndrome, and is seen in only 1% of patients with complete androgen insensitivity, although a greater risk, 15%, applies in partial insensitivity (Cools et al. 2006).

> One example is on record in which, in a sense, the X-linkage was directly visible to the cytogeneticist; that is, the X chromosome was abnormal, including the region containing the androgen receptor locus. An affected aunt and niece had the karyotype 46,Y,inv(X)(q11.2q27) and the connecting mother was 46,X,inv(X)(q11.2q27) (Xu et al. 2003). A unique case is that of androgen insensitivity due to uniparental disomy X in a woman with the XXY karyotype (Uehara et al. 1999a).

CHROMOSOMAL DISORDERS OF SEX DEVELOPMENT IN BOYS AND MEN

XX Testicular Disorder of Sexual Development

Most males with 46,XX testicular DSD ("XX males," in former parlance) arise from the presence of Yp material (rarely visible cytogenetically) on one of the X chromosomes, from occult XX/XXY mosaicism, or from the inappropriate activity of a gene that is normally switched on only in response to a Y-originating genetic instruction. In approximately three-fourths of cases, the *SRY* gene is present, typically the consequence of an abnormal exchange between the X and Y during meiosis I in gametogenesis in the father, and thus clearly a sporadic event. These are referred to as *SRY*+ XX males, or *SRY*+ XX testicular DSD. Délot and Vilain (2015) provide a full review.

The phenotype in *SRY*+ XX testicular DSD is similar to that of Klinefelter syndrome, presumably reflecting the similar basic genotypes of active X + inactive X + *SRY* in the two conditions; however, the male with XX testicular DSD differs in being of normal height and of unimpaired intelligence (Ferguson-Smith et al. 1990). Margarit et al. (1998) describe six *SRY*+ cases due to translocation of Yp material to Xp22.3, in whom different Y breakpoints could be identified, but whose clinical phenotypes were very similar: normal intelligence, normal stature, and testicular atrophy with azoöspermia. In these *SRY*+ males with XX testicular DSD, a more accurate cytogenetic designation would be 46,X,der(X)t(X;Y)—or more fully 46,X,der(X)t(X;Y)(p22.3;p11.2), albeit the exchange is not usually visible on standard cytogenetics—and so there is reference to this entity also in the section on the X;Y translocation (Chapter 6). Rare cases are known of a male with XX testicular DSD in whom the *SRY* gene had been translocated onto a terminal arm of an autosome (Dauwerse et al. 2006; Queralt et al. 2008).

Males with XX testicular DSD and having no *SRY* gene are denoted *SRY*– (Grinspon and Rey 2016). The fact of male development being able to proceed (to some extent, at least), despite the lack of SRY product, presumably reflects an inappropriate activation of the testis-determining cascade in an otherwise normal 46,XX embryo, either as a sporadic stochastic event or due to some genetic predisposition. Concerning the latter, Jarrah et al. (2000) report an extended inbred kindred with XX individuals of varying degrees of masculinization, and they suggest that in this family, *SRY*– XX maleness and XX ovotesticular DSD represented a continuum of the same disorder. Grigorescu-Sido et al. (2005) describe an *SRY*– XX testicular DSD case with imperfect masculinization, whom they contrasted with the normal maleness of two *SRY*+ XX men. Rare cases may reflect an abnormal dosage of another gene in the sex-determining pathway; *SOX9*, *RSPO1*, and *SOX3* have been implicated in this respect (Parma et al. 2006).

Three cases are reported of males with 47,XXX chromosomes. In one well-studied example, the man was mildly intellectually disabled, with gynecomastia and hypogenitalism, and severe testicular atrophy on biopsy (Ogata et al. 2001). One X of the three was positive for *SRY*. In addition to an Xp-Yp interchange in paternal gametogenesis that produced the *SRY*-positive X chromosome, a coincidental maternal nondisjunction was responsible for a disomic X ovum. Thus, the combination at fertilization was XX(mat) + der(X)t(X;Y)(pat), giving 47,XX,der(X)t(X;Y) and appearing karyotypically as "47,XXX."

XX testicular DSD has been diagnosed prenatally, following the recognition that the chromosomal and ultrasonographic anatomical genders did not match (Trujillo-Tiebas et al. 2006). (This should however be a carefully considered diagnosis, at least for sporadic cases, as mostly the XX "chromosomal sex" will be due to culture of maternal cells; congenital adrenal hyperplasia is another diagnosis to be considered.)

45,X MALE

We refer to this rare disorder on p. 133. Most, quite possibly all, "45,X males" have, in fact, a molecular translocation of the *SRY* gene to an autosome or to the X chromosome (and might therefore be thought of as a type of Y;autosome or X;Y translocation). In some, the underlying constitution might actually be an X/XY mosaicism.

Y ISOCHROMOSOMES

A Y isochromosome, idic(Y)(q11), in mosaic state with a 45,X line, is a rare observation in individuals presenting with a disorder of sex development[1] (Lungeanu et al. 2008). These chromosomes presumably arise in paternal gametogenesis, with loss in an early mitosis of the embryo, to produce the 45,X line.

---

1 The usual presentation with the idic(Yq) is infertility in an otherwise normal male (p. 349).

Ovotesticular Disorders of Sex Development

The term *hermaphroditism*, of classical Greek derivation,[2] has lost favor among those so diagnosed; and the qualifiers "true" and "pseudo" were always somewhat arcane. These days, we speak of ovotesticular DSD. As that descriptor indicates, the defining feature is that the gonads comprise both ovarian and testicular elements: There may be a testis and an ovary, or one or both may be an ovotestis. The most common karyotype is 46,XX (thus, XX ovotesticular DSD), seen in 60%; one-third have mosaicism with one cell line which includes Y chromosomal sequences, mostly 46,XX/46,XY; a few are 46,XY; and other more rare forms are known (Krob et al. 1994; Queipo et al. 2002). Ovotesticular DSD often presents as a problem in determining the sex of a newborn infant (Hadjiathanasiou et al. 1994).

Most of the 46,XX cases test negative on peripheral blood analysis for the *SRY* gene (Grinspon and Rey 2016), and in some of these, the basis of the defect may be sporadic inappropriate activation of the testicular developmental cascade in part of the gonadal tissue during its embryonic formation, as a stochastic event. In some, mutation in *NR5A1* may be the basis (Domenice et al. 2016). An extraordinary case is the family described in Haines et al. (2015), in which a phenotypically normal mother had a child with ovotesticular DSD, initially karyotyping as 46,XX, and mother and child were both subsequently shown to be heterozygous for an insertional translocation, 46,X,ins(X;1)(q27;q25.2q25.3). A 770 kb segment of chromosome 1 at q25.2q25.3 was translocated into the X chromosome, at Xq27, and this site is only 82 kb distant from the *SOX3* gene. *SOX3* may, in certain circumstances, have an *SRY*-like influence; and in this case, the inserted chromatin may have induced, or allowed, inappropriate *SOX3* activity, with its ectopic expression in one gonad (but not the other) producing a testis. Possibly, the mother's normal femaleness may have reflected a favorable X-inactivation. A somewhat similar circumstance is recorded in Ohnesorg et al. (2017), the case of a teenage male presenting with testicular pain, the gonad in fact proving to be an ovotestis. The karyotype was 46,XX, and *SRY*⁻, but upon multiplex ligation-dependent probe analysis (MLPA), he had a de novo ~300 kb duplication which included the upstream regulatory region for *SOX9*, at chr17:71.3-71.6 Mb.

Alternatively, an apparent XX karyotype may harbor Y material, as Margarit et al. (2000) show in a woman reared as a boy with hypospadias, who went on to have gender change surgery after testing "46,XX." Several years later, reanalysis revealed a tiny segment of Yp translocated on to the X long arm, 46,X,der(X),t(X;Y)(q28;p11.31). A more common explanation in the 46,XX case may be cryptic mosaicism within the gonad itself, with an island or islands of tissue containing the *SRY* gene (Ortenberg et al. 2002; Queipo et al. 2002). It is a curious and unexplained fact that ovotesticular DSD (mostly with a 46,XX karyotype) is far more common in the South African Black population than in Europeans (Wiersma 2004; Ganie et al. 2017).

The XX/XY state more usually results due to the fusion of twin XX and XY embryos (XX//XY chimerism). Strain et al. (1998) reported a notable example of iatrogenic ovotesticular DSD, which followed in vitro fertilization, presumably due to an XX and an XY embryo fusing; Malan et al. (2007) reached a similar conclusion in a case diagnosed prenatally, and which could be referred to as "tetragametic chimerism." Another mechanism is that an ovum might divide symmetrically (instead of budding off a polar body), and the two cells are each fertilized by a sperm (Chen et al. 2005c). A further theoretical route is from the postzygotic loss of the X and of the Y in separate cells of an initially 47,XXY conception (Niu et al. 2002). The basis may be molecular, rather than cytogenetic. For example, one nonmosaic 46,XY case had a postzygotic mutation in *SRY* with *SRY*⁺/*SRY*⁻ gonadal mosaicism (Braun et al. 1993). Presumably the *SRY*⁺ line was responsible for the testicular elements in the gonad, and the *SRY*⁻ line for the ovarian elements. A somewhat similar patient is described in Modan-Moses et al. (2003), in whom 46,XX^{SRY+}/45,X^{SRY+}/45,X^{SRY-} mosaicism was associated with a clinical picture of ovotesticular DSD.

Other mosaicisms include XXY/XX, X/XY, and X/X,idic(Yq). Kanaka-Gantenbein et al. (2007) report a boy, regarded as normal except for an undescended left testis, who presented as a 13-year-old with a left scrotal hemorrhage. In fact, the undescended

<hr>

2 In Greek mythology, Hermaphroditus was the son of Aphrodite and Hermes. He was a handsome youth with whom the Naiad nymph Salmacis fell in love, and prayed to be united forever. The gods answered her prayer, and merged their two bodies into one androgynous person.

gonad was an ovary, which had actually ovulated, and presumably this had been the cause of the bleed. There was a left hemi-uterus and fallopian tube; the testis, on the right, was dysgenetic. On both blood and testicular biopsy, the karyotype was 47,XXY/46,XX; as expected, given the presence of a male gonad, albeit an imperfect one, *SRY* and *AZF* loci were present. In another case, a baby girl presenting with clitoral hypertrophy typed 46,XY on blood, but analysis of the removed dysgenetic gonads revealed X/XY mosaicism (Röpke et al. 2007). On histological examination, the gonads contained testicular and ovarian elements: The XY state was observed more in the testicular component of the gonad, while cells with only an X chromosome predominated in the ovarian fraction. Becker and Akhavan (2016) report an infant presenting with genital ambiguity, in whom "the family made an initial gender assignment of female until patient preference could be elicited." The karyotype was 45,X[90]/46,X,idic(Yq)[10]; the isodicentric Y, with two copies of Yp, showed two copies of *SRY*. On laparoscopy, a normal-appearing uterus was seen; on the right, the gonad was an ovotestis, and on the left, the gonad comprised only a "streak" (Fig. 23–1). Prophylactic gonadectomy was done.

A single case is recorded of ovotesticular DSD associated with an autosomal cytogenetic abnormality, and this may reflect the effects of an autosomal gene on the cascade of sexual differentiation (Aleck et al. 1999). This child had ambiguous genitalia, with one ovarian and one testicular-gonad, and karyotyped 46,XX,rec(22)dup(22q) inv(22)(p13q13.1)mat. Testing for *SRY* was negative. Tomaselli et al. (2008) report the first actual autosomal mutation to be recognized, in the *RSPO1* gene, in a woman with ovotesticular DSD, and concomitant palmoplantar hyperkeratosis. This gene is located at 1p34.3; the mutation was in homozygous state, and her parents were first cousins.

Rare *familial* cases of 46,XX ovotesticular DSD may reflect a mutation, whether autosomal or X-linked, such as *RSPO1* or *NR5A1*, that induces the testis developmental cascade to proceed at a post-*SRY* stage (Domenice et al. 2016). Slaney et al. (1998) describe the case of four 46,XX cousins with abnormal sexual differentiation. Three had 46,XX ovotesticular DSD, and one was a 46,XX male. The putative testis-development gene had been transmitted through two mothers. Affected distant relatives due to a familial X;Y translocation are noted on p. 136.

Sterility is almost universal. But of the 11 pregnancies to women with ovotesticular DSD reviewed in Schultz et al. (2009), extraordinarily, all infants were male. The opposite applied to the 46,XY man with ovotesticular DSD reported in Zayed et al. (2008), who had had surgery for removal of an intra-abdominal testicular seminoma, and which included ovarian elements. At the same operation,

(a) (b)

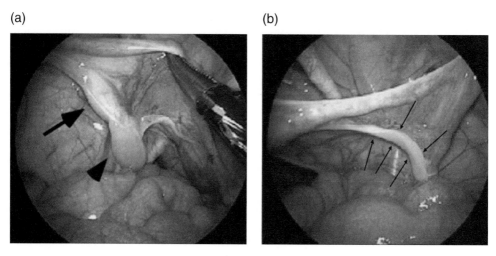

FIGURE 23–1   Gonadal observations at laparoscopy in an infant with an ovotesticular disorder of sex development, having the karyotype 45,X/46,X,idic(Yq). The bilobar-appearing gonad on the child's right (*a*) is in part testicular (arrow) and in part ovarian (arrowhead). The gonad on the left (*b*) is a fibrotic "streak" (the curved structure in mid-field, arrowed).

Source: From Becker and Akhavan, Prophylactic bilateral gonadectomy for ovotesticular disorder of sex development in a patient with mosaic 45,X/46,X,idic(Y)q11.222 karyotype, *Urol Case Rep* 5: 13–16, 2016. Courtesy R.E.N. Becker, and with the permission of Elsevier, per the Creative Commons license.

a uterus and tubes were identified and removed. A few years later, he underwent testicular aspiration of the remaining gonad, which yielded sperm: These were used for intracytoplasmic sperm injection, and eventually a pregnancy resulted—and a normal daughter was born.

MIXED GONADAL DYSGENESIS

Mixed gonadal dysgenesis (MGD) is a phenotype that borders upon that of ovotesticular DSD. One gonad may be a streak (as the case in Figure 23-1, b), and the other of apparently testicular form. The typical karyotype is 45,X/46,XY; the body build and external genital phenotype can range very considerably, from near-normal male, through ambiguity, to Turner-like female. Some with 46,XY on peripheral blood may show X/XY on analysis of the gonad, as Nishina-Uchida et al. (2015) show in an infant presenting as female with clitorimegaly and a gonad in the right labium majus. The removed gonad contained normal-appearing and abnormal testicular elements, undifferentiated gonadal tissue, Wolffian and Müllerian derivatives, and included nests of gonadoblastoma; 46,XY and 45,X cells could be demonstrated. The other gonad was a streak.

RARE DISORDERS OF SEX DEVELOPMENT WITH EXTRAGONADAL DEFECTS

A number of rare conditions exist in which sex reversal coexists with physical, metabolic, and, in some, mental defect. By way of example, one of these is XY female DSD campomelic dysplasia (campomelia refers to long bone bowing) with sex reversal. The usual cause is a mutation within the *SOX9* gene (at 17q24.3q25.1), one of the genes operating on the sexual differentiation pathway and which also influences limb bud mesenchymal development (Wagner et al. 1994). A cytogenetic form of this syndrome is seen in approximately 5% of affected individuals, who have an apparently balanced translocation disrupting the *SOX9* locus at 17q24.3q25.1 (Fig. 14–2).

In the other direction, a chromosomal imbalance may lead to male genital development in the setting of an XX gonosomal complement. Thus, Seeherunvong et al. (2004) describe a child with a chromosome 22 duplication, 46,XX,dup(22) (q11.2q13), who was *SRY*-negative and had male

external genitalia, with intrascrotal gonads, the only genital abnormality being a first-degree hypospadias.

GENETIC COUNSELING

XY Disorder of Sexual Development, Complete Gonadal Dysgenesis (Swyer Syndrome)

FAMILIAL/INHERITED CASES

XY DSD with gonadal dysgenesis, when familial, is mostly inherited as an X-linked recessive, or autosomal dominant or recessive with expression limited to the XY state. Autosomal recessive inheritance would be improbable in a multigenerational family tree, while on the other hand, this mode would be strongly supported in a single affected sibship with more than one affected, and in the setting of parental consanguinity. In the multigenerational scenario, a clear interpretation of autosomal versus X-linkage may not be possible. The risk to the female carrier (as judged by position in the pedigree) to have an affected child would be a simple 25% if the X chromosome is implicated, but not readily calculable if a partially penetrant autosomal gene is the cause. As noted above, more DSD genes are coming to be identified, with gene interrogation "panels" being developed (Eggers et al. 2016), and genetic counseling will be better underpinned as this knowledge evolves. Although the XY female phenotype is close to that of a normal female, but of course associated with infertility, some couples may want to consider prenatal diagnosis. The use of cytogenetics (XY) and ultrasound morphology (female external genitalia) would presumably allow detection of the condition; naturally, diagnosis could be precise if a DSD gene were identified.

The Y-linked form is recognized by the demonstration of an *SRY* mutation carried by the XY girl and her XY father. This circumstance would allow the counselor the rare opportunity to apply principles of Y-linked inheritance with incomplete penetrance to risk estimation. Mutational analysis of the *SRY* gene (including deletion detection) may provide the basis for carrier detection and prenatal or preimplantation diagnosis.

SPORADIC CASES

Advice on the recurrence risk in the sporadic case is less straightforward. If a de novo *SRY* mutation is demonstrated, only paternal testicular mosaicism—which, as noted earlier, has been observed—could imply an increased risk for recurrence. An autosomal recessive form may be identifiable on DSD panel testing. Again, absent the knowledge of a specific gene, prenatal diagnosis by chromosomal/ultrasound gender discordance should be feasible.

For the XY woman herself, assisted conception is possible if a uterus is present, and a handful of successful pregnancy outcomes, using donated gametes, have been reported (Creatsas et al. 2011).

ASPECTS OF MANAGEMENT

Couples electing not to consider prenatal diagnosis (or to continue a pregnancy in which a positive diagnosis has been made) should know of the importance of two particular factors in managing these girls (Jorgensen et al. 2010). First, the psychosexual orientation of these individuals is female. But with secondary sexual characteristics developing incompletely, and infertility being invariable, their self-image is vulnerable. In discussing the condition with parents, the counselor should note the importance of using language that reinforces their view of themselves as girls and women, and the counselor should avoid using such terms as "genetic male." It may be explained to them, beginning in simple terms in childhood, that a genetic factor prevented their ovaries from developing normally (Goodall 1991). As mentioned above, pregnancy may be achievable with in vitro fertilization using a donor ovum. Second, there may be a substantial risk of neoplastic change in the dysgenetic gonad. A gonadoblastoma arises in about half of familial XY gonadal dysgenesis. The gonadoblastoma itself is noninvasive, but it is often associated with malignant elements, most commonly dysgerminoma, which do invade. Thus, and given that the gonad does not usefully contribute in terms of hormone production, early (first decade) gonadectomy is advisable. These and other aspects of management are rehearsed in detail in Jorgensen et al. (2010) and Alhomaidah et al. (2017).

> Considerable publicity in 2009 concerning an athlete who recorded extraordinary times in women's running races at an international meeting put in sharp focus the question of how such people are to be regarded. The unfortunate woman's internal genital state (which apparently included testicular elements) became the subject of public speculation and then of public documentation. The Athletics Federation resolved the issue with some wisdom and imaginativeness, acknowledging her "unfair" but entirely innocent physical advantage as a runner, in allowing her to keep her gold medal, but also awarding a gold medal to the second-placed athlete.

XY Disorder of Sexual Development, Complete Androgen Insensitivity Syndrome

This condition is inherited as an X-linked recessive trait, and the risk of recurrence follows classic Mendelian principles. The carrier may be identified, and preimplantation/prenatal diagnosis accomplished, by molecular analysis of the androgen receptor gene. While complete androgen insensitivity typically has a consistent phenotype within families, allowing for good prediction of the consequences of recurrence, incomplete androgen insensitivity can have variable phenotypes within a family (Boehmer et al. 2001). Issues relating to prenatal diagnosis are discussed in Morel et al. (1994), who also make the interesting but unsurprising point that incomplete forms imply a worse burden than the complete form, with partially virilized males (known as Reifenstein syndrome) having "considerable psychological distress and poor function in their adult life."

Similar considerations with respect to gender orientation in the XY girl, as discussed in the preceding section, apply to complete androgen insensitivity. The risk for neoplastic change in the gonad is less, in the vicinity of 1%, in the case of complete androgen insensitivity syndrome. Thus, gonadectomy may reasonably be delayed to allow spontaneous pubertal feminization (Jorgensen et al. 2010), although regular clinical and imaging checks would be advisable. Lacking a uterus, pregnancy is not possible.

XX Testicular Disorder of Sexual Development

Many XX testicular DSD boys are not diagnosed until after childhood, by which time the parents are likely to have completed their family. Some cases may be recognized at amniocentesis following discordant karyotypic and ultrasonographic sex.

The great majority occur as sporadic events in a family, and in these, the likelihood of recurrence is very small. Concerning the rare case of the SRY⁻ XX male, the application of a DSD panel may allow those cases that would carry a high recurrence risk to be identified. If prenatal diagnosis is requested, and the fetus is 46,XX, testing for *SRY* along with an ultrasound assessment of external genital morphology should enable distinction (Ginsberg et al. 1999).

Ovotesticular Disorder of Sexual Development

The considerable majority of ovotesticular DSD represent sporadic cases, these being characterized by a 46,XX karyotype and absence (at least on peripheral blood analysis) of the *SRY* gene, and presumed to reflect an "accidental" activation of the testis-determining cascade during gonadogenesis, or cryptic intragonadal mosaicism, as discussed above. In some cases, the cytogenetics (46,XY, 46,XX/ 46,XY, or other mosaic karyotype) or molecular genetics (*SRY* mutation that is not present in father) may allow a more secure reassurance of nonrecurrence. Recurrence is very rare; but a positive family history would, of course, imply a high risk. Gene panel testing, and with the *RSPO1* and *NR5A1* genes of particular interest, may aid diagnosis. In the SRY⁻ form, a handful of families are described in which there is also a sib with XX male syndrome, and these cases may speculatively reflect "leaky mutations" in a gene operating at a point downstream in the cascade of sexual differentiation. A familial X;Y translocation is dealt with on its merits.

If the condition is diagnosed prenatally, and the pregnancy continued, counselors should consult Hughes et al. (2006) and Jorgensen et al. (2010) for consensus statements on management of children with DSDs.

PART SEVEN

NOXIOUS AGENTS

24

GONADAL CYTOGENETIC DAMAGE FROM EXPOSURE TO EXTRINSIC AGENTS

IN THIS CHAPTER we review what is known about the effects of some anticancer treatments, and of certain other therapeutic and environmental agents, that could conceivably have an injurious effect upon chromosomal distribution at gametogenesis, or which might cause chromosomal breakage, rearrangement, or copy number variation in the cells of the gonad. In other words, the focus is on factors that might disturb the course of meiosis or that might have clastogenic effects upon the chromosomes of gametocytes. We do not specifically consider other categories of genetic damage, but note that in some human studies, adverse outcomes are lumped within the general category of "congenital abnormalities" without regard to specific genetic (or nongenetic) etiology.

Given the inherent vulnerability of gametogenesis, a logical starting position might have been that any potential damaging agent should be presumed guilty until proven innocent. As discussed in Chapter 19, large fractions of sperm and eggs, in the vicinities of 10%–20%, are chromosomally abnormal due to aneuploidies or structural change acquired, for the most part, during meiosis. If this is what happens naturally, if gametogenesis is so susceptible normally, then surely would not agents known to compromise the integrity of the DNA and of the spindle apparatus (not to mention various artificial dietary and environmental exposures) compound the effect dramatically? Perhaps surprisingly, this seems not to be the case. Gametogenesis—provided the damage is not irreversible—often proceeds normally, or at any rate recovers, even in the setting of some heavy exposures, and no discernible increase in chromosomal abnormality is recorded in the subsequently born children. Nevertheless, if only on the pure grounds of what seems biologically reasonable and plausible, the question is not to be regarded as being closed; and indeed an international workshop was convened in 2013 to address the issue (Yauk et al. 2015). The fact that sperm chromosomes may, with certain agents, show an increased rate of cytogenetic abnormality is a more practical reason for maintaining a cautious view.

Evidence for the existence of human germ cell mutagens is derived from observations in the germ cells (principally sperm, for reasons for accessibility), and in the offspring of individuals who have been exposed to potential germ cell mutagens. We outline the observations and conclusions relating to cancer treatment and radiation exposure, and touch on some environmental and lifestyle factors. The listing is by no means exhaustive.

BIOLOGY AND EPIDEMIOLOGY

Cancer Treatment

A majority of children and young adults who receive modern cancer treatment survive. Some treatments cause sterility, but in quite a number, fertility is unscathed, or at any rate, subsequently recovers (Green et al. 2009, 2010). For those who are potentially capable of having children, the question arises: Could there be an increased risk to have a child with a chromosomal abnormality? For most, in fact, the short answer may be, apparently not. Longer answers follow.

The chemotherapeutic agents and radiation used to rid the body of cancer are essentially cellular toxins, some of which specifically target DNA or the mitotic apparatus. Thus, the starting hypothesis is that the chromosomes in exposed bystander tissues, and thinking specifically of the gonad, could be vulnerable. The fact that these treatments can damage chromosomes is well known, and this is actually the basis of one of the in vitro laboratory tests for ataxia-telangiectasia.[1] Rapidly dividing cells are the most vulnerable to anticancer treatments (this being, of course, the rationale for their use). This would suggest, in theory, a susceptibility for spermatogenesis in the postpubertal male (millions of cell divisions daily); and a relative resistance in the prepubertal male child (male meiosis yet to commence) and in oögenesis from infancy through menopause in the female (cell division in suspension). In the male, the fact of a "blood-testis barrier" may offer a defense (Yauk et al. 2015); a selection against chromosomally imbalanced cells during gametogenesis may be another protective process.

The direct assessment of gametic chromosomes offers insight. Sperm chromosome analysis can be done in men who have survived cancer treatment. Table 24–1 carries a review of 12 such studies and shows that several therapeutic regimens can cause sperm karyotypic defects.[2]

In practice, it is to the experience of the "therapeutic experiments" of oncological medicine that we mostly appeal: the in vivo observations of those who have survived their cancer, recovered from their treatment, and who have gone on to have, or to attempt to have, children. Have the children shown any excess of cytogenetic abnormality? Outcomes from the five largest studies are summarized in Table 24–2. Collectively, these studies report on more than 25,000 children of cancer survivors and show no difference between the prevalence of chromosome abnormalities[3] in the offspring of cancer survivors compared to the offspring of their cancer-free siblings or population controls (Table 24–2). The prevalence of chromosome abnormalities is consistently approximately 1 in 1,000, regardless of the type of cancer, the age of cancer onset, the type and dosage of chemotherapy administered, and the use of radiotherapy. Data about miscarriage rates are in agreement: Green et al. (2009) followed up more than 4,000 pregnancies in which either the mother or the father was a cancer survivor, and they found no increase in the frequency of miscarriage in either group.

SPECIFIC THERAPIES

Chemotherapy. Levy and Stillman (1991) and Arnon et al. (2001) review in detail the effects of various chemotherapeutic regimens upon fertility, in some of which data are also available concerning mutagenicity. The six classes of chemotherapeutic agents are the following: alkylating agents, cisplatin and its analogs, vinca alkaloids, antimetabolites, topoisomerase inhibitors, and "newer agents." In broad terms, the relationship between type of drug

---

1 Radiation and bleomycin, both having potent DNA-breaking properties, cause lymphocyte chromosome rearrangements in normal cells, and considerably more so in ataxia-telangiectasia cells.

2 Male cancer patients may show abnormal sperm genetic studies ahead of having received any treatment, suggesting that there is a harmful effect of the malignant disease per se (Tempest et al. 2008).

3 It is notable that these studies also detected no increase in the prevalence of non-chromosomal birth defects in the offspring of cancer survivors.

Table 24–1. Findings from 12 Sperm Chromosome Studies That Have Been Done in Respect of the Treatment of Certain Cancers, Showing Those Regimens That Are Associated, and Those That Are Not, with Sperm Chromosomal Abnormalities

CANCER	THERAPY	CYTOGENETICS	INCREASED FREQUENCY CHROMOSOME ABNORMALITIES	
			STRUCTURAL	NUMERICAL
Cancer	PEB and D-act and CY-CH-V-MT	Humster	+	+
Testic. ca. (non-sem.)	PVB, PVB and PEB	Humster	+	+
Rhabdomyosarcoma	CYVADIC	Humster	+	−
Ewing sarcoma	VAC	Humster	+	−
Wilms tumor	RT ± D-Act	Humster	+	−
Seminoma	PVB	Humster	−	−
Hodgkin's	MOPP, MOPP and RT	Humster	+	+
Lymphoma	MACOP-B	Humster	−	−
Lymphoma	MACOP-B	FISH	+	−
Embryonal cancer	PEB	FISH	−	+
Embryonal cancer	PEB	Humster	−	−
Hodgkin's	NOVP	FISH	+	+/−
Hodgkin's	Vinb. and RT	FISH	+	++
Testicular cancer (non-sem.)	PEB	FISH	+	++
Testicular cancer (non-sem.)	PEB	FISH	+	+

humster, pseudofertilization human-hamster test. Testic. ca. (non-sem.), testicular cancer, nonseminoma. Treatment regimens: CY-CH-V-MT, cyclophosphamide, chlorambucil, vinblastine, methotrexate; CYVADIC, cyclophosphamide, adriamycin, vincristine, dicarbazine; D-Act, D-actinomycin; FISH, fluorescence in situ hybridization; MACOP-B, methotrexate, doxorubicin, cyclophosphamide, vincristine, prednisone; MOPP, nitrogen mustard, vincristine, procarbazine, prednisone; NOVP, novanthrone (mitoxantrone), vincristine, vinblastine, prednisone; PEB, cisplatin, etoposide, bleomycin; PVB, cisplatin, vinblastine, bleomycin; RT, radiotherapy; VAC, vincristine, adriamycin, cyclophosphamide; vinb., vinblastine.

Source: From the review of De Mas et al. (2001).

and risk for gonadal damage is outlined in Tables 24–3 and 24–4.

Alkylating agents (cyclophosphamide and chlorambucil being major representatives), which have their damaging effect by adding an alkyl group to DNA, can, in the male, cause testicular hypotrophy, with oligospermia or azoöspermia. In follow-up into adulthood, the reproductive potential for males having been treated with an alkylating agent in childhood is considerably reduced, with a relative fertility of 0.4 (Byrne et al. 1987). Levy and Stillman (1991) review a number of papers, which offer a generally optimistic picture for girls in terms of pubertal development, but, as they point out, longer-term studies relating to the specific question of fertility are not so numerous. In one follow-up study, women actually had a relative fertility of 1.0 (Byrne et al. 1987). In adult women who have had chemotherapy with cyclophosphamide for Hodgkin's disease or breast cancer, oöcyte depletion and ovarian failure are documented (Familiari et al. 1993; Goodwin et al. 1999).

Antimetabolites, alkaloids, and antibiotics (including methotrexate, vincristine, actinomycin D) seem not to compromise ovarian function when given alone or as combination therapy, but in conjunction with radiotherapy, some will cause ovarian failure.

Topoisomerase inhibitors affect the integrity of the mechanical apparatus of the meiotic chromosome, including the centromere and the microtubules of the spindle, and they also act directly upon the DNA; mouse studies with etoposide show an actual

Table 24-2. Outcomes from Five Large Studies of the Offspring of Childhood Cancer Survivors

SOURCES	COUNTRY	NO. OF OFFSPRING OF CANCER SURVIVORS	CHROMOSOME ABNORMALITIES		CLASS OF CONTROLS
			CASES (%)	CONTROLS (%)	
Byrne et al. (1998), Meistrich and Byrne (2002)	United States	2,198	0.20	0.10	Siblings
Winther et al. (2004)	Denmark	2,630	0.21	0.21	Siblings
Ståhl et al. (2011)*	Denmark, Sweden	8,670	0.08	0.18	Population
Signorello et al. (2012)	United States	4,699	0.15		None
Seppänen et al. (2016)	Finland	6,862	0.06	0.07	Siblings

*Included only offspring of male cancer survivors.

Table 24-3. Classification of Infertility Risk Induced by Chemotherapy in Females

DEGREE OF RISK	CHEMOTHERAPY TREATMENT
High risk (>80%)	Hemopoietic stem cell transplantation and total body irradiation, radiotherapy to a field including the ovaries
Intermediate risk	CAF, CMF, CEF
Lower risk (<20%)	ABVD, CHOP, CVP, CAF, CMF, CEF, AC
Very low or no risk	Vincristine, methotrexate, fluorouracil
Unknown risk	Taxanes, irinotecan, oxaliplatin, monoclonal antibodies, tyrosine kinase inhibitors

A, adriamycin; B, bleomycin; C, cyclophosphamide; D, dacarbazine; E, epirubicin; F, fluorouracil; H, hydroxydaunorubicin; M, methotrexate; O, vincristine; P, prednisolone; V, vinblastine.

Source: From Zavras et al. (2016).

Table 24-4. Classification of Infertility Risk Induced by Chemotherapy in Males

EFFECT ON SPERM COUNT	CHEMOTHERAPY TREATMENT
Prolonged or permanent azoöspermia	Chlorambucil, cyclophosphamide, procarbazine, melphalan, cisplatin
Azoöspermia likely	Busulphan, ifosfamide, BCNU, CCNU, nitrogen mustard
When used alone, cause only temporary reductions in sperm count; in conjunction with other agents, may be additive in causing azoöspermia	Doxorubicin, thiotepa, cytarabine, vinblastine, vincristine, amsacrine, bleomycin, dacarbazine, duanorubicin, epirubicin, etoposide, fludarabine, fluorouracil, 6-mercaptopurine, methotrexate, mitoxantrone, thioguanine

BCNU, Bis-Chlorethyl-Nitrosourea: CCNU, Cyclonexyl-Chloroethyl-Nitrosourea.

Source: From Zavras et al. (2016)

increase in sperm and zygote aneuploidies (De Mas et al. 2001; Marchetti et al. 2001).

Multiagent chemotherapy is, as would be expected, more damaging, and as illustrated in a group of girls who had succumbed to their cancer, from the observations of ovarian histology postmortem (Nicosia et al. 1985).

Radiotherapy. Fertility is diminished in females who have had radiation therapy to the abdomen, and there is an increased risk of obstetric complication. But their children appear to have no increased incidence of birth defects (Signorello et al. 2012; Seppänen et al. 2016). Martin et al. (1986) studied 13 male cancer patients (mostly seminoma) at intervals up to 36 months after radiotherapy, in whom the doses of testicular radiation were estimated to be in the range 0.4–5.0 Gray. While most were azoöspermic in the first year following treatment, in those in whom spermatogenesis recovered, variable increases in sperm chromosome abnormalities were seen, averaging twofold overall compared with controls, but with wide ranges. The frequencies correlated with the estimated "bystander" testicular radiation (i.e., the extent to which exposure extended beyond the target tissue). Ståhl et al. (2011) studied 2,488 children born one or more years after the diagnosis of testicular cancer in their father. Most fathers would have been treated with radiotherapy, and there was no increased risk of congenital abnormalities in their children compared with children with no paternal history of cancer.

Radioisotopes. Radioiodine is used in thyroid cancer and may cause transient oligospermia and amenorrhea in males and females, respectively, but its use appears to be of no risk for miscarriage, neither for congenital abnormality (Clement et al. 2015).

INFERTILITY ASSOCIATED WITH CANCER THERAPY, AND PRIOR GAMETE BANKING

Preservation of gametes prior to treatment for cancer is a logical management, and sperm banking as "fertility insurance" for boys and men with cancer is now seen as routine (Menon et al. 2009). The American Society of Clinical Oncology recommends that the risk of infertility and options for fertility preservation be discussed with all patients of reproductive age (and with parents or guardians of children and adolescents) prior to commencement of treatment (Loren et al. 2013). All patients who express an interest in fertility preservation should be referred to a reproductive specialist. For adult males, sperm cryopreservation is the only established fertility preservation method, and it should be performed prior to commencement of chemotherapy. Cryopreservation of testicular tissue, which does not require sexual maturity, remains experimental. For adult females, both embryo and oocyte cryopreservation are established methods or fertility preservation, while ovarian tissue cryopreservation remains experimental.

DIAGNOSTIC RADIOLOGY

There is no convincing evidence for an increased risk of chromosome abnormalities in the offspring of parents who have been exposed to diagnostic radiology. A small effect may possibly exist for Down syndrome (DS) with respect to previous X-rays to the abdomen and pelvic area—that is, for X-rays in which the gonads may have been within, or not far off, the field of the film. In a study of 156 mothers and 149 fathers, in whose DS children the "nondisjunctional parent" could be identified (using Q-banding polymorphisms), a history of X-ray exposure was more often recorded in older fathers and in younger mothers (Strigini et al. 1990). The odds ratio for the whole group was 1.85, although the lower limit of the 95% confidence interval was 1.0. If such an effect truly exists in the younger mothers (and the statistics were borderline), it would seem that this slight influence becomes diluted as they get older, and the age effect comes to be predominant.

NONMEDICAL EXPOSURES

Radioactivity. The human germline may be relatively resistant to the damaging effects of radiation, compared with some animal models (Neel et al. 1990; Adriaens et al. 2009).[4] The atomic bomb

---

4 Of historic interest, a very early example of ill health due to radiation exposure is that of Marie Curie, who was awarded the Nobel Prize twice. One daughter of hers was a scientist, and she also won a Nobel Prize, and the other was a skilled pianist and gifted writer. A series of $n = 2$ is very small, but rather evidently there must have been normal chromosomal segregation in the meioses leading to these two daughters.

blasts at Hiroshima and Nagasaki in 1945 were not followed by a statistically significant difference in the rate of chromosome abnormalities in children subsequently conceived, in a study commenced in 1967 (Awa et al. 1987; Neel and Schull 1991; Nakamura 2006). The study population comprised 8,322 individuals born 1946–1972, age range at the time of study 12–38 years, one or both of whose parents were within 2,000 meters of the hypocenter "ATB" (at the time of the bomb), alongside a contemporaneous local control group of 7,976, who were either more than 2,500 meters from the hypocenter or not present in the city. Sex chromosomal abnormalities were seen in 2.28 per 1,000 in the former group and in 3.01 per 1,000 of the latter. The only instance of autosomal trisomy was a 15-year-old with standard trisomy DS, whose father had been exposed at Hiroshima. (Given the structure of this study, deceased younger children and infants with autosomal trisomy were not included, although it is also to be noted that in separate analyses in Neel and Schull, no significant correlation existed between parental exposure ATB and the frequency of stillbirth or congenital malformations.) More children of exposed parents had a small supernumerary abnormal chromosome than in the controls (five cf. two, a difference not specifically commented upon in Awa et al.). Of the balanced structural rearrangements, only two were confirmed as having arisen de novo (one each in the exposed and control groups). An earlier study with specific reference to clinically diagnosed DS in 9-month-old infants, undertaken during 1948–1954 (before the chromosomal basis of DS was known), had shown no increase among offspring of 5,582 exposed cf. 9,452 unexposed mothers, and indeed the figures were in the other direction (0.54 cf. 1.27 per 1,000), and despite the exposed mothers being on average slightly older (Schull and Neel 1962).

The Chernobyl nuclear plant explosion occurred in April 1986, and a cloud of radioactivity was dispersed over Europe. With respect to DS, no subsequent rise in incidence was identified in a number of European countries, apart from small clusters in Berlin and Belarus, the latter of interest in that the peak was confined to January 1997, 9 months after the explosion (Little 1993; Zatsepin et al. 2007). In contrast, Bound et al. (1995) suggest a possible link between events in 1957 (a fire in a nuclear reactor) and the early 1960s (increased levels of fallout from nuclear testing) and peaks of DS prevalence, in 1958 and 1963–1964 in the Fylde district of Lancashire, England. But by no means is a firm case made: *Post hoc* does not necessarily mean *propter hoc*,[5] and some fluctuation is normal. The same 1957 nuclear reactor accident had been proposed as the possible reason for a cluster of six cases of DS among the children of women who had attended the same high school in Dundalk, Ireland, during 1956–1957, when they would have been aged from 12 to 19 years. Of the 387 births to the former pupils from this period, the expectation would have been 0.69 children with DS. However, a stringent review of the evidence, and including molecular analyses that showed one case to have arisen post fertilization, led to the conclusion that, in fact, chance alone was the probable basis for the "cluster" (Dean et al. 2000).

While the germline, at least from the evidence outlined earlier, is apparently resistant, the same cannot be said for the bone marrow. Numerous studies on radiation exposure have shown that stable chromosome rearrangements may be induced, as measured on peripheral blood samples. Indeed, it is proposed that these changes can be used as reliable biomarkers of exposure. Populations in whom this effect has been seen include Russian nuclear plant workers, comparing those exposed to plutonium and those to gamma rays, from 1949 to 1989; New Zealand navy personnel who had served on ships during nuclear bomb testing in the Pacific Ocean in the late 1950s; American radiation technologists who had begun practicing from before 1950 (ages at the time of study 71–90 years); and even astronauts, unprotected by Earth's atmosphere from solar radiation (Durante et al. 2003; Hande et al. 2003; Sigurdson et al. 2008; Wahab et al. 2008). We are unaware of any evidence that individuals exposed in these ways might have acquired any gonadal damage, and that their children could have been at risk for a chromosomal disorder. It would be a massive logistic exercise, but not without interest, if a study could be mounted of descendants of these exposed persons.

Industrial Agents. The male gonad is protected by the blood-testis barrier (Li et al. 2016), but it is prudent to imagine that the protection may not necessarily be absolute. Paternal occupation

---

5 *Post hoc, ergo propter hoc* (Latin) = Something happened after the event, and therefore it must have been due to the event.

provides a surrogate marker for a variety of potential industrial agents. Olshan et al. (1989) assessed the father's occupation for 1,000 DS children born in British Columbia from 1952 through 1973. Seven employment categories out of 59 showed odds ratios in the range 1.4–3.3, the lower confidence limit being not less than 0.9, in certain of which exposure to various industrial agents could plausibly have occurred (including mechanics, janitors, metal workers, sawmillers). But the increases in risk were small, and with 59 items there was of course the possibility of chance fluctuation. One category that might have seemed risky, namely "other chemical workers," in fact had the lowest odds ratio of all (0.2). Exposure to volatile oil (as studied following clean-up after an oil spill at sea) may damage the marrow, with chromosomal breakages observed in peripheral blood, but there is no indication of damage at the level of the gonad (Francés et al. 2016).

Pesticides have biological activity, and it is reasonable to raise a case that distribution across the blood-testis barrier might follow inhalation, or absorption, or ingestion, and that the local effect upon gonadal tissue might be toxic. Perry (2008) has reviewed 30 studies, correlating pesticide exposure with sperm chromosomal abnormality. The methodologies varied, so direct comparisons could not readily be made. Some studies did, and some did not, show an increase in chromosomal defects. Of the numerous agents, the strongest case could be made for carbaryl and fenvalerate, in particular, as potentially causative of autosomal and gonosomal aneuploidy, with sex chromosome disomy the most frequent single abnormality.

The air we breathe, it is suggested, might convey mutagens, in the form of industrial pollutants, and these might reach gonadal tissue (Somers and Cooper 2009). Landfill sites contain toxic matter, which might in theory contaminate the air in nearby residential areas; but in an analysis based upon more than 6,000 such sites throughout the United Kingdom, and comparing populations living within, and beyond 2 kilometers of these sites, in fact no differences in the prevalence of DS were observed (Jarup et al. 2007). However, older mothers living within 1 mile of industrial sites from which solvent and heavy metal emissions are vented may have a slightly increased risk for aneuploidies in their offspring (Brender et al. 2008); in the male, variation in air pollution may affect some aspects of sperm quality, although with no obvious influence

upon disomy or diploidy rates (Rubes et al. 2005). Confirmatory studies are needed.

Bisphenol A (BPA), an estrogenic chemical used widely in plastic manufacture, has been shown to disrupt several different stages of oöcyte development in mice (Susiarjo et al. 2007). The fetal ovaries observed after pregnant mice were treated with low, environmentally relevant doses of BPA during mid-gestation showed synaptic defects and increased levels of recombination. The mature females, exposed as fetuses, went on to have oöcytes and embryos with aneuploidies. There may be further environmental influences on the effect of BPA, in that variations in diet influenced the observation of meiotic abnormalities in exposed mice (Muhlhauser et al. 2009), thus demonstrating the complexities in studying environmental exposures, since even in laboratory animals it is nearly impossible to keep all other variables constant. In a small study in humans, Lathi et al. (2014) found an increased risk of both euploid and aneuploid miscarriage in women with higher serum levels of BPA. Reservations are already held concerning its use in human activity for other health-related reasons, and these data might be seen as one further reason for caution.

Agent Orange (a mixture of phenoxylic herbicides) was used in the Vietnam War as a defoliant spray, and those exposed may have absorbed the chemical via the oral route in particular. A study of New Zealand Vietnam veterans some three or four decades after the war showed an increase in sister chromatid exchanges on blood samples (Rowland et al. 2007). Whether gonadal genetic damage results is controversial (Ngo et al. 2006; Schecter and Constable 2006; Fraser 2009); specifically, we are unaware of any evidence for an increased risk of chromosomal abnormalities in offspring.

Recreational Agents. *Tobacco smoking* in mothers had no influence upon the incidence of DS in the study of Chen et al. (1999a), based upon data of a population case-control analysis in Washington state from 1984 to 1994, and in which they had been at pains to account for a confounding effect of maternal age. The odds ratio was exactly 1.0—that is, no effect either way—for smokers versus nonsmokers. Similar findings are also reported from Sweden, California, and England (Kallen 1997; Torfs and Christianson 2000; Rudnicka et al. 2002). Nevertheless, a tentative role has been proposed for one particular mechanism: trisomy 21 due to nondisjunction in maternal meiosis II (MMII).

In a case-control study in Atlanta, Georgia, cigarette smoking around the time of conception gave an odds ratio of 7.6 in mothers of MMII trisomic offspring, compared with controls, in the <35-year age group (Yang et al. 1999). Very speculatively, smoking might diminish blood flow in the microvasculature of the perifollicular bed, and the resultant hypoxia could compromise some aspect of the oöcyte's functioning as the meiotic process is reactivated.

Alcohol and coffee taken by the mother prior to conceiving might, *prima facie*, actually reduce the DS risk. In the study of Torfs and Christianson (2000), the odds ratios for "high" alcohol and coffee consumption (four or more drinks per week, four or more cups per day) were 0.54 and 0.63, respectively. If these figures really did reflect biological reality, a possible mechanism would be a selective reduction in viability of a trisomic 21, as compared to a normal conceptus.

Concerning spermatogenesis, Shi and Martin (2000b), reviewing the literature, concluded that personal habits with respect to smoking, alcohol, and caffeine ingestion appear not to have any consistent effect upon disomy rates in sperm, although since there were somewhat varying findings in the different studies, it had to be acknowledged that a definitive answer was not at hand. Shi et al. (2001a) proceeded to a study of cigarette smoking and aneuploidy using fluorescence in situ hybridization analysis of sperm, with reference to chromosomes 13, 21, X, and Y. They divided their subjects into nonsmokers, light smokers (<20 cigarettes/day), and heavy smokers (≥20/day). The smokers showed an increase in disomic 13 sperm (0.2% of sperm 24,+13 vs. 0.07% in controls), which was statistically significant. The rates of disomies 21, X, and Y were within the control ranges. Chromosome 13 and, from other studies, chromosome 1 may be more susceptible, as they go through meiotic disjunction, to an untoward influence of toxic substances in cigarette smoke. Since most trisomy 13 is due to a maternal meiotic error, and given that the excess is, in absolute terms, very small, it seems safe to suppose that fathers who smoke contribute disproportionately scarcely, if at all, to the totality of this particular aneuploidy. As for alcohol, the observation of a negative association between sperm disomy frequencies and alcohol consumption in one study[6] (Härkönen et al. 1999), and noting also the figures earlier on maternal consumption, should not at all lead one to advise that couples drink more heavily prior to a planned impregnation.

Second-hand smoke is difficult to assess, outside of controlled animal studies (Hung et al. 2009). A study of four adult male rhesus macaques, exposed to second-hand smoke for 6 months, showed no change in the X:Y ratio in sperm, which may indicate that there is no increase in aneuploidy. In addition, second-hand smoke-exposed pregnancies did not show increased DNA damage in their offspring, as compared to babies born to nonsmoking mothers (de Assis et al. 2009).

GENETIC COUNSELING

As Wyrobek and Adler (1996) commented almost a quarter century ago, "It has been more than half a century [1927] since Muller demonstrated that X-rays can induce germinal mutations in *Drosophila*, yet questions as basic as the existence of even a single human germinal mutagen remain unresolved." McFadden and Friedman, writing in 1997, noted that no environmental agent has been identified in which it could be stated, beyond reasonable doubt, that this agent would cause chromosome abnormalities in the offspring of exposed parents. While some studies, as above, have shown increased rates of aneuploidy in sperm, the practical fact remains that there has been observed no excess in children born with chromosomal syndromes. Only in 2001 could Marchetti et al. claim, with respect to their work on etoposide exposure with a mouse model, that "we know of no other report of an agent for which paternal exposure leads to an increased incidence of aneuploidy in the offspring."

Encouragement can be drawn from this largely negative information, and the counselor will usually be justified in offering substantially reassuring advice from the particular focus of chromosome abnormality. Reference to the commentaries earlier may provide useful supporting information for the individual agent of specific interest. Prenatal diagnosis would be a discretionary option, as would be preimplantation diagnosis for those whose treatment-related infertility required in vitro fertilization.

---

6 But another study showed a positive association with alcohol, as well as with caffeine (Robbins et al. 1997).

But a contrary view is put forward by DeMarini (2012), who argues that the failure to identify any human germ cell mutagens merely reflects methodological challenges of studying germ cell mutagenesis in humans. He points to the fact that in rodents, at least 39 germ cell mutagens have been identified, including ionizing radiation, chemotherapy, tobacco smoke, and air pollution. A further question, in this molecular age, is the susceptibility to de novo generation of copy number variants. Paternal age is one known predisposing factor; but might some environmental agents be causative? Conover and Argueso (2016) draw up a road map of how this matter might be pursued, at this stage simply posing the question, and leaving any answers to come from future research. This chapter is not yet closed.

APPENDIXES

APPENDIX A: IDEOGRAMS OF HUMAN CHROMOSOMES, AND HAPLOID AUTOSOMAL LENGTHS

HAPLOID AUTOSOMAL LENGTH

The concept of the haploid autosomal length (HAL) is discussed in Daniel (1985). To determine the (quantitative) amount of a particular segmental imbalance, as a fraction of the HAL, multiply (*1*) the fraction of the whole chromosome that this segment comprises by (*2*) the HAL of the whole chromosome. The fractions are readily estimated, to a fair approximation, by placing a millimeter rule against the ideogram in Figure A–1. The HAL of the autosome concerned is taken from Table A–1. This table notes also the length in megabases of each chromosome; there is a slight discrepancy between the percentage HAL of each chromosome using this approach, cf. the data in Daniel.

For example, considering the imbalance due to the karyotype of the children pictured in the frontispiece and shown in Figure 4–1, what proportion of the HAL does the segment 4q31.3→qter constitute? First, the segment comprises 18% of the length of chromosome 4: Running a millimeter rule alongside the ideogram of chromosome 4 in Figure A–1, the whole chromosome is 116 mm and the segment is 24 mm, and 24/116 = 21%. Second, from the table, chromosome 4 is 6.30% of the total HAL. Thus, 21% of 6.30% = 1.3% of HAL.

Table A–1. The Nucleotide Content and Percentage of Haploid Autosomal Length (HAL) That Each Chromosome Constitutes

CHROMOSOME	MB (HG38)	HAL % (HG38)	HAL % (DANIEL)
1	248.96	8.66	9.24
2	242.19	8.42	8.02
3	198.30	6.90	6.83
4	190.21	6.62	6.3
5	181.54	6.31	6.08
6	170.81	5.94	5.9
7	159.35	5.54	5.36
8	145.14	5.05	4.93
9	138.39	4.81	4.8
10	133.80	4.65	4.59
11	135.09	4.70	4.61
12	133.28	4.64	4.66
13	114.36	3.98	3.74
14	107.04	3.72	3.56
15	101.99	3.55	3.46
16	90.34	3.14	3.36
17	83.26	2.90	3.46
18	80.37	2.80	2.93
19	58.62	2.04	2.67
20	64.44	2.24	2.56
21	46.71	1.62	1.9
22	50.82	1.77	2.04
Autosomal length	2,875.00	100.00	
X	156.04		
Y	57.23		
Genome	3,088.27		

Source: From Daniel (1985), and UCSC Genome Browser.

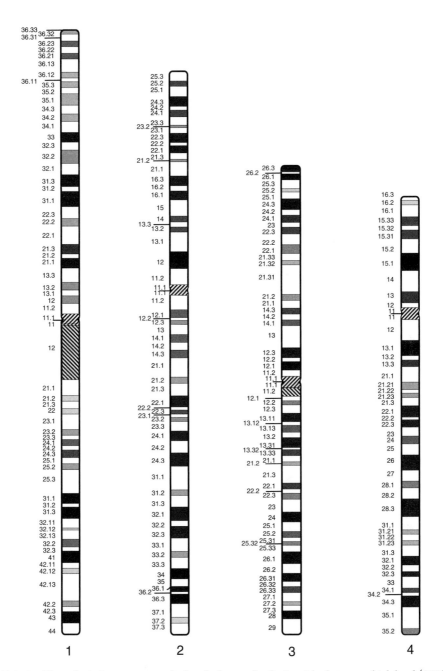

FIGURE A–1 These depictions represent the bands that can be distinguished at a very high level (850 band) of cytogenetic resolution. Different shadings and lengths of bands reflect actual intensities and lengths as observed by the cytogeneticist.

Source: From Chia, in ISCN 2016: An international system for human cytogenomic nomenclature, McGowan-Jordan J, Simons A, Schmid M (eds.), *Cytogenet Genome Res* 149 (1–2), 2016.© Courtesy N. L. Chia.

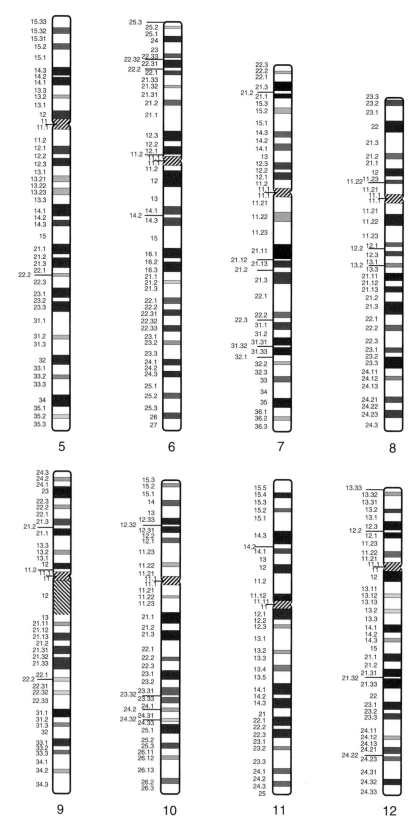

FIGURE A–1 (Continued)

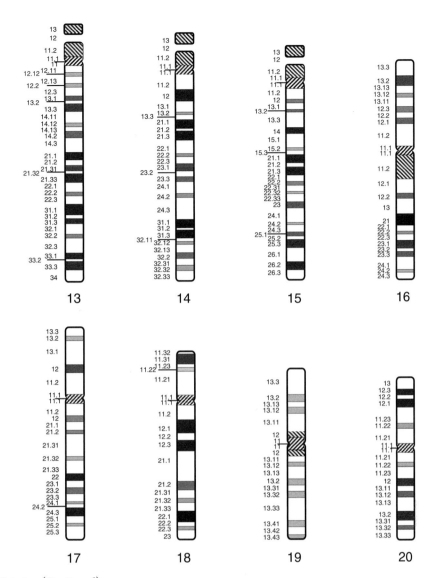

FIGURE A–1 (Continued)

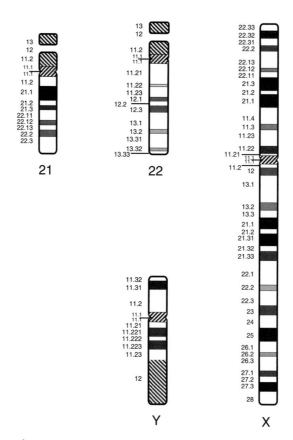

FIGURE A–1 (Continued)

APPENDIX B: CYTOGENETIC ABBREVIATIONS AND NOMENCLATURE

CYTOGENETICS HAS its own jargon and fondness for acronyms, and certain abbreviations are regularly used. The ICSN (itself an abbreviation for International System of Cytogenetic Nomenclature; ISCN, 2016) provides formally approved abbreviations, several of which are set out below (Table B–1); and following this, we list another set of abbreviations (and including a number of clinical expressions), which are used fairly frequently in this book and in many genetics journals, and which should be familiar to the reader (Table B–2):

KARYOTYPE NOMENCLATURE ACCORDING TO THE ISCN

The description of chromosomal constitution in most laboratory reports and in most case reports in the literature is the ISCN (2016) format. First, the diploid number is given. Second, the sex chromosome constitution is given. Thereafter, any abnormality or variant is described. Certain abbreviations are used, as listed above. In structural rearrangements, the position of breakpoints is given by reference to the band involved: short or long arm (p or

Table B–1. SOME ISCN ABBREVIATIONS

add	Additional material of unknown origin
cht	Chromatid
del	Deletion
der	Derivative chromosome
dic	Dicentric chromosome
dn	De novo
dup	Duplication
fis	Fission (at the centromere)
fra	Fragile site
h	Heterochromatin
i	Isochromosome
idem	The same (to avoid repetition of complex description in a mosaic case)
ins	Insertion
dir ins	Direct insertion
inv ins	Inverted insertion
ish	In situ hybridization
inv	Inversion
mar	Marker chromosome
mat	Maternal origin
min	Minute chromosome
minus (−)	Loss of a whole chromosome
mos	Mosaic
neo	Neocentromere
p	Short arm
pat	Paternal origin
plus (+)	Gain of a whole chromosome
q	Long arm
R	Ring
rcp	Reciprocal translocation
rea	Rearrangement
rec	Recombinant chromosome
rob	Robertsonian translocation
solidus (/)	Separates cell lines in describing mosaics. Two, as //, apply to chimersim
t	Translocation
tan	Tandem
tas	Telomeric association
ter	Terminal (end of chromosome arm)
upd	Uniparental disomy

Table B–2. SOME OTHER COMMONLY USED ABBREVIATIONS

abn(X)	An abnormal X chromosome
aCGH	Array comparative genomic hybridization
AFP	Alpha-fetoprotein
arr	Array (microarray)
AS	Angelman syndrome
AT	Ataxia-telangiectasia
BAC	Bacterial artificial chromosome
CGH	Comparative genomic hybridization
CNV	Copy number variant
CpG	Cytosine-guanine DNA sequence
CPM	Confined placental mosaicism
CVS	Chorionic villus sampling
DGS	DiGeorge syndrome
DMR	Differentially methylated region
DS	Down syndrome
ECARUCA	European Cytogeneticists Association Register of Unbalanced Chromosome Aberrations
EEG	Electroencephalogram
ESAC	Extra structurally abnormal chromosome
ESHRE	European Society for Human Reproduction and Embryology
EUCROMIC	European Collaborative Research Group on Mosaicism in CVS
FA	Fanconi anemia
FISH	Fluorescence in situ hybridization
HAL	Haploid autosomal length
ICSI	Intracytoplasmic sperm injection
IUGR	Intrauterine growth retardation
IVF	In vitro fertilization
kb	Kilobases of DNA
LCRs	Low copy repeats

Table B–2. (CONTINUED)

Mb	Megabases of DNA
MCA/MR	Multiple congenital anomalies/mental retardation
MLPA	Multiplex ligation-dependent probe analysis
MRI	Magnetic resonance imaging (an organ imaging modality)
mtDNA	Mitochondrial DNA
NAHR	Nonallelic homologous recombination
NGS	Next-generation sequencing
NHEJ	Nonhomologous end joining
NIPT	Noninvasive prenatal testing
NOR	Nucleolar organizing region
nt	Nucleotide
OMIM	Online Mendelian Inheritance in Man catalog
PAR (1 and 2)	Pseudoautosomal region (primary and secondary)
PB (1 and 2)	Polar body (first and second)
PCD	Premature centromere division
PCR	Polymerase chain reaction
PGD	Preimplantation diagnosis
PGD-AS	Preimplantation diagnosis for aneuploidy screening
PND	Prenatal diagnosis
POF	Premature ovarian failure
PWACR	Prader-Willi/Angelman critical region
PWS	Prader-Willi syndrome
QF-PCR	Quantitative fluorescent polymerase chain reaction
RPL	Recurrent pregnancy loss
SCE	Sister chromatid exchange
SD	Standard deviation
SMC	Supernumerary marker chromosome
snoRNA	Small nucleolar RNA
SNP	Single nucleotide polymorphism
TS	Turner syndrome
UCSC	University of California at Santa Cruz (hosts a Genome Browser)
UPD	Uniparental disomy

q), region, and band or subband(s) within that band. The region is denoted by a digit 1 through 4, the band by a digit 1 through 8, and the subband(s) by digit(s) following a "decimal point." The centromere is p10 or q10. Illustrative examples of commonly described karyotypes follow (Tables B–3 to B–14).

EXAMPLES OF CYTOGENETIC NOMENCLATURE
Normal

Table B–3. Normal

46,XX	Normal female
46,XY	Normal male
46,XX,9qh+	Normal female, additional material in heterochromatic region of chromosome 9 long arm
46,XY,Yqh–	Normal male, deletion of material from heterochromatic region of Y long arm

Abnormal

Table B–4. Sex Chromosome Aneuploidies

45,X	Monosomy X (Turner syndrome)
47,XXY	Klinefelter syndrome
47,XXX	Triple X female
47,XYY	XYY 'syndrome'
48,XXXX, 49,XXXXY	Two of the less rare types of polysomy X
47,XXY/46,XY or mos 47,XXY/46,XY	Mosaic* Klinefelter syndrome
45,X/46,XX	Mosaic Turner syndrome

*In mosaicism, the normal cell line is listed last.

Table B–5. Autosomal Aneuploidies

47,XY,+21	Trisomy 21 (Down syndrome)
47,XX,+21/ 46,XX	Mosaic Down syndrome
47,XX,+18	Trisomy 18 (Edwards syndrome)
47,XY,+13	Trisomy 13 (Patau syndrome)
47,XX,+8/ 46,XX	Mosaic trisomy 8 (Warkany syndrome)
47,XY,+16	Trisomy 16
45,XX,–21	Monosomy 21

Table B–6. Polyploidies

69,XXY	Triploidy
92,XXXX	Tetraploidy

Table B–7. Deletions and Duplications

46,XX,del(4)(p15)	Terminal deletion chromosome 4 short arm (Wolf-Hirschhorn syndrome)
46,XX,del(5)(p13)	Terminal deletion chromosome 5 short arm (cri du chat syndrome)
46,XX,del(18)(q12)	Terminal deletion chromosome 18 long arm
46,XY,dup(17)(p13.3), chr17:0.2-3.0 Mb	Distal duplication of chromosome 17 short arm, band p13.3, which involves the segment encompassed approximately by nucleotides 200,000–3,000,000, 0.2 to 3.0 megabases ("unofficial" nomenclature used in parts of this book)

Reciprocal Translocations

46,XX,t(4;12) (p14;p13)	Reciprocal translocation between chromosome 4 and 12, with breakpoints at p14 in chromosome 4 and p13 in chromosome 12

Table B–7. (CONTINUED)

46,XY,der(12)t(4;12) (p14;p13)mat	Unbalanced complement, having received derivative chromosome 12 in place of normal 12 from translocation carrier mother
47,XX,+der(22) t(11;22)(q23;q11)pat	Unbalanced complement, having received derivative 22 as a supernumerary chromosome from translocation carrier father

Table B–8. FISH Example

46,der(15)t(8;15) (q22.3;q26.2)mat. ish der(15)t(8;15) (qter+;qter-)	Unbalanced complement, having received the derivative 15 in place of a normal 15 from the carrier mother, resulting in partial deletion of 15q and an extra copy of the chromosome 8 segment

Table B–9. Microarray Example

46,der(15)t(8;15) (q22.3;q26.2)mat, arr 8q22.3q24.3 (105,171,556–146,201,91)×3, 15q26.2q26.3 (96,062,102–100,201,136)×1	Unbalanced complement, having received the derivative 15 in place of normal 15 from the carrier mother. On microarray, the extra segment (×3) extends from nucleotides 105,171,556 to 146,201,91 on chromosome 8, and the deleted segment (×1) from 96,062,102 to 100,201,136 on chromosome 15.

Table B–10. Whole-Arm Reciprocal Translocations

46, t(1;9)(p10;p10) — Balanced carrier of translocation having both breakpoints at the centromeres, with exchange of whole short arms. Translocation chromosomes are 9p/1q and 1p/9q.

Table B–11. Robertsonian Translocations

45,XY,der(14;21)(q10;q10) (or replace der with rob) — Balanced carrier of Robertsonian translocation between chromosomes 14 and 21. We sometimes simplify to 45,XY,rob(14;21).

46,XY,der(14;21)(q10;q10)mat,+21 (or replace der with rob) — Unbalanced complement, having received (14;21) Robertsonian chromosome as well as a "free" chromosome 21 from mother (the karyotype of translocation Down syndrome)

Table B–12. Inversions

46,XX,inv(3)(p23q27) — Inversion (pericentric) of chromosome 3, breakpoints at p23 and q27

46,XY,rec(3)dup(3p)inv(3)(p23q27)mat — Recombinant chromosome has been transmitted from mother carrying inversion chromosome 3. There is duplication of the short arm segment distal to p23; and deletion of the long arm segment distal to q27.

46,XY,inv(11)(q13q22) — Inversion (paracentric) of chromosome 11, breakpoints at q13 and q22

Table B–13. Insertions

46,XY,dir ins(10;8)(q21;q21.2q22) — Direct insertion of segment q21.2→q22 of chromosome 8 into q21 of chromosome 10. Segment has original orientation to centromere, namely q21.2 is proximal and q22 distal.

46,XX,inv ins(2)(p13q31q21) — Inverted insertion of segment q31→q21 into band p13. Segment has opposite orientation to centromere, namely q31 is proximal and q21 distal.

Table B–14. Other

46,XY,t(1;18;15)(q32;q21;q24)dn — De novo complex translocation, involving exchanges between three chromosomes, at the breakpoints indicated

46,XX,r(15) — A ring 15 chromosome

46,X,i(Xq) — An isochromosome of the X long arm

46,XX,add(19)(p13) — Additional material of unknown origin attached to band p13 of chromosome 19

46,XY,upd(15)mat — Uniparental disomy for a maternally derived chromosome 15

46,XY,fra(10)(q23.3) — Normal male, fragile site on chromosome 10 long arm at subband 23.3

1(pp)(qqqqqqqqqq) — Multiradial of chromosome 1 comprising two short arms and 10 long arms (informal nomenclature) (see Fig. 16–4)

The nomenclature has evolved to accommodate the growing complexity of cytogenetics, with the earlier nomenclatures issued since the first in 1960, often referred to by the name of the city in which the committee met (Denver, London, Chicago, Paris), and subsequently more anonymously as ISCN (year).

Published papers from the earlier years will, of course, have used the nomenclature of their time. Many old papers remain a valuable resource, particularly case reports. The reader consulting these may therefore need to adjust and learn to handle earlier (generally simpler) versions of cytogenetic nomenclature.

APPENDIX C: DETERMINING 95 PERCENT CONFIDENCE LIMITS, AND THE STANDARD ERROR

CONFIDENCE LIMITS

The "Exact confidence limits for p" tables in Documenta Geigy ("Geigy Scientific Tables," 1982, pp. 89–102) are a useful source of data on confidence limits for the sizes of sample geneticist generally collect. Suppose in a kindred—ascertainment bias having been suitably accounted for—of a total of 54 offspring of translocation carriers were abnormal, and 49 were phenotypically normal. The frequency for abnormality from this particular sample is 9.3% (5/54). Checking in Documenta Geigy under $N = 54$, $x = 5$, we see that the 95% confidence limits are given as 3.08% to 20.30%. In other words, we may take it as close to being sure that the true risk lies in the range 3% to 20%.

STANDARD ERROR

The standard error (SE) is calculated from the simple formula

$$SE = \sqrt{\frac{a(n-a)}{n^3}}$$

where a is the number of abnormals, and n is the total number of offspring after ascertainment correction (Stengel-Rutkowski et al. 1988). Thus, for the preceding example

$$SE = \sqrt{\frac{5(54-5)}{54^3}}$$
$$= 0.039$$

And thus the risk is given as $9.3 \pm 3.9\%$.

REFERENCES

Aalfs CM, Fantes JA, Wenniger-Prick LJ, et al. Tandem duplication of 11p12-p13 in a child with borderline development delay and eye abnormalities: Dose effect of the PAX6 gene product? *Am J Med Genet* 73: 267–271, 1997.

Abaied L, Trabelsi M, Chaabouni M, et al. A novel UBE3A truncating mutation in large Tunisian Angelman syndrome pedigree. *Am J Med Genet* 152A: 141–146, 2010.

Abeliovich D, Dagan J, Lerer I, Silberstein S, Katznelson MB, Frydman M. t(15;21)(q15;q22.1) pat resulting in partial trisomy and partial monosomy of chromosomes 15 and 21 in two offspring. *Am J Med Genet* 66: 45–51, 1996.

Abeliovich D, Dagan J, Levy A, Steinberg A, Zlotogora J. Isochromosome 18p in a mother and her child. *Am J Med Genet* 46: 392–393, 1993.

Abeliovich D, Yagupsky P, Bashan N. 3:1 meiotic disjunction in a mother with a balanced translocation, 46,XX,t(5,14)(p15;q13) resulting in tertiary trisomy and tertiary monosomy offspring. *Am J Med Genet* 12: 83–89, 1982.

Aboura A, Labrune P, Perreaux F, et al. Deletion in the ABL gene resulting from a meiotic recombination of a maternal (3;22;9)(q22;q12;q34.1) translocation. *J Med Genet* 40: e6, 2003.

Abrams DJ, Aronoff AR, Berend SA, Roa BB, Shaffer LG, Geier MR. Prenatal diagnosis of a homologous Robertsonian translocation involving chromosome 15. *Prenat Diagn* 21: 676–679, 2001.

Abrams DJ, Augustyn AM, Geier MR. Prenatally diagnosed mosaic trisomy 17: A case report with two-year follow-up. *Prenat Diagn* 25: 968–969, 2005.

Abrams L, Cotter PD. Prenatal diagnosis of de novo X;autosome translocations. *Clin Genet* 65: 423–428, 2004.

Abramsky L, Chapple J. *Prenatal Diagnosis: The Human Side* (2nd ed.). Cheltenham, UK: Nelson Thornes, 2004.

Abramsky L, Hall S, Levitan J, Marteau TM. What parents are told after prenatal diagnosis of a sex chromosome abnormality: Interview and questionnaire study. *Br Med J* 322: 463–466, 2001.

Abuelo DN, Barsel-Bowers G, Richardson A. Insertional translocations: Report of two new families and review of the literature. *Am J Med Genet* 31: 319–329, 1988.

Acquaviva F, Sana ME, Della Monica M, et al. First evidence of Smith-Magenis syndrome in mother and daughter due to a novel RAI mutation. *Am J Med Genet* 173A: 231–238, 2017.

Adachi M, Tachibana K, Asakura Y, Muroya K, Ogata T. Del(X)(p21.1) in a mother and two daughters: Genotype-phenotype correlation of Turner features. *Hum Genet* 106: 306–310, 2000.

Adeyokunnu AA. The incidence of Down's syndrome in Nigeria. *J Med Genet* 19: 277–279, 1982.

Adhvaryu SG, Peters-Brown T, Livingston E, Qumsiyeh MB. Familial supernumerary marker chromosome evolution through three generations. *Prenat Diagn* 18: 178–181, 1998.

Adler A, Lee HL, McCulloh DH, et al. Blastocyst culture selects for euploid embryos: Comparison of blastomere and trophectoderm biopsies. *Reprod Biomed Online* 28: 485–491, 2014.

Adriaens I, Smitz J, Jacquet P. The current knowledge on radiosensitivity of ovarian follicle development stages. *Hum Reprod Update* 15: 359–377, 2009.

Agathokleous M, Chaveeva P, Poon LC, Kosinski P, Nicolaides KH. Meta-analysis of second-trimester markers for trisomy 21. *Ultrasound Obstet Gynecol* 41: 247–261, 2013.

Aghajanova L, Popwell JM, Chetkowski RJ, Herndon CN. Birth of a healthy child after preimplantation genetic screening of embryos from sperm of a man with non-mosaic Down syndrome. *J Assist Reprod Genet* 32: 1409–1413, 2015.

Aguilera C, Viñas-Jornet M, Baena N, et al. Novel intragenic deletions within the UBE3A gene in two unrelated patients with Angelman syndrome: case report and review of the literature. *BMC Med Genet* 18: 137, 2017.

Aiello V, Astolfi N, Gruppioni R, et al. Paracentric inversion of Yq and review of the literature. *Genet Couns* 18: 379–382, 2007.

Aït Yahya-Graison E, Aubert J, Dauphinot L, et al. Classification of human chromosome 21 gene-expression variations in Down syndrome: Impact on disease phenotypes. *Am J Hum Genet* 81: 475–491, 2007.

Akahoshi K, Fukai K, Kato A, Kimiya S, Kubota T, Spritz RA. Duplication of 15q11.2-q14, including the P gene, in a woman with generalized skin hyperpigmentation. *Am J Med Genet* 104: 299–302, 2001.

Akahoshi K, Spritz RA, Fukai K, Mitsui N, Matsushima K, Ohashi H. Mosaic supernumerary inv dup(15) chromosome with four copies of the P gene in a boy with pigmentary dysplasia. *Am J Med Genet* 126A: 290–292, 2004.

Akbas H, Cine N, Erdemoglu M, et al. Prenatal diagnosis of 4p and 4q subtelomeric microdeletion in de novo ring chromosome 4. *Case Rep Obstet Gynecol* 2013: 248050, 2013.

Akolekar R, Beta J, Picciarelli G, Ogilvie C, D'Antonio F. Procedure-related risk of miscarriage following amniocentesis and chorionic villus sampling: A systematic review and meta-analysis. *Ultrasound Obstet Gynecol* 45: 16–26, 2015.

Akoury E, Gupta N, Bagga R, et al. Live births in women with recurrent hydatidiform mole and two NLRP7 mutations. *Reprod Biomed Online* 31: 120–124, 2015.

Akshoomoff N, Mattson SN, Grossfeld PD. Evidence for autism spectrum disorder in Jacobsen syndrome: Identification of a candidate gene in distal 11q. *Genet Med* 17: 143–148, 2015.

Al Ageeli E, Drunat S, Delanoë C, et al. Duplication of the 15q11-q13 region: Clinical and genetic study of 30 new cases. *Eur J Med Genet* 57: 5–14, 2014.

Alberman E, Mutton D, Morris JK. Cytological and epidemiological findings in trisomies 13, 18, and 21: England and Wales 2004–2009. *Am J Med Genet* 158A: 1145–1150, 2012.

Albers CA, Newbury-Ecob R, Ouwehand WH, Ghevaert C. New insights into the genetic basis of TAR (thrombocytopenia-absent radii) syndrome. *Curr Opin Genet Dev* 23: 316–323, 2013.

Albrecht B, Mergenthaler S, Eggermann K, Zerres K, Passarge E, Eggermann T. Uniparental isodisomy for paternal 2p and maternal 2q in a phenotypically normal female with two isochromosomes, i(2p) and i(2q). *J Med Genet* 38: 214, 2001.

Albrecht U, Sutcliffe JS, Cattanach BM, et al. Imprinted expression of the murine Angelman syndrome gene, *Ube3a*, in hippocampal and Purkinje neurons. *Nat Genet* 17: 75–78, 1997.

Aleck KA, Argueso L, Stone J, Hackel JG, Erickson RP. True hermaphroditism with partial duplication of chromosome 22 and without SRY. *Am J Med Genet* 85: 2–4, 1999.

Aleixandre Blanquer F, Manchón Trives I, Forniés Arnau MJ, Alcaraz Mas LA, Picó Alfonso N, Galán Sánchez F. 3q29 microduplication syndrome. *An Pediatr (Barc)* 75: 409–412, 2011.

Alfarawati S, Fragouli E, Colls P, Wells D. Embryos of Robertsonian translocation carriers exhibit a mitotic interchromosomal effect that enhances genetic instability during early development. *PLoS Genet* 8: e1003025, 2012.

Alfonsi M, Palka C, Morizio E, et al. A new case of pure partial 7q duplication. *Cytogenet Genome Res* 136: 1–5, 2012.

Algar EM, St. Heaps L, Darmanian A, et al. Paternally inherited submicroscopic duplication at 11p15.5 implicates insulin-like growth factor II in overgrowth and Wilms' tumorigenesis. *Cancer Res* 67: 2360–2365, 2007.

Alhomaidah D, McGowan R, Ahmed SF. The current state of diagnostic genetics for conditions affecting sex development. *Clin Genet* 91: 157–162, 2017.

Al-Jasmi F, Abdelhaleem M, Stockley T, Lee KS, Clarke JT. Novel mutation of the perforin gene and maternal uniparental disomy 10 in a patient with familial hemophagocytic lymphohistiocytosis. *J Pediatr Hematol Oncol* 30: 621–624, 2008.

Alkan C, Coe BP, Eichler EE. Genome structural variation discovery and genotyping. *Nat Rev Genet* 12: 363–376, 2011.

Al-Kouatly HB, Chasen ST, Gilbert F, Ahner R, Alonso LM, Chervenak FA. Correlation between rare chromosomal abnormalities and prenatal ultrasound findings. *Am J Med Genet* 107: 197–200, 2002.

Allanson JE, Greenberg F, Smith AC. The face of Smith-Magenis syndrome: A subjective and objective study. *J Med Genet* 36: 394–397, 1999.

Allderdice PW, Ali M, McAlpine PJ. Complementation by two non-homologous recombinant chromosomes 3. *Am J Med Genet* 39: 396–398, 1991.

Allderdice PW, Browne N, Murphy DP. Chromosome 3 duplication q21 leads to qter deletion p25 leads to pter syndrome in children of carriers of a pericentric inversion inv(3) (p25q21). *Am J Hum Genet* 27: 699–718, 1975.

Allderdice PW, Davis JG, Miller OJ, et al. The 13q-deletion syndrome. *Am J Hum Genet* 21: 499–512, 1969.

Allderdice PW, Eales B, Onyett H, et al. Duplication 9q34 syndrome. *Am J Hum Genet* 35: 1005–1019, 1983.

Allen EG, Freeman SB, Druschel C, et al. Maternal age and risk for trisomy 21 assessed by the origin of chromosome nondisjunction: A report from the Atlanta and National Down Syndrome Projects. *Hum Genet* 125: 41–52, 2009.

Allou L, Lambert L, Amsallem D, et al. 14q12 and severe Rett-like phenotypes: New clinical insights and physical mapping of *FOXG1*-regulatory elements. *Eur J Hum Genet* 20: 1216–1223, 2012.

Al-Sarraj Y, Al-Khair HA, Taha RZ, et al. Distal trisomy 10q syndrome, report of a patient with duplicated q24.31-qter, autism spectrum disorder and unusual features. *Clin Case Rep* 2: 201–205, 2014.

Alter BP, Rosenberg PS, Brody LC. Clinical and molecular features associated with biallelic mutations in *FANCD1/BRCA2*. *J Med Genet* 44: 1–9, 2007.

Altiner S, Kutlay NY, Ilhan, O. Constitutional trisomy 8 mosaicism with persistent macrocytosis. *Cytogenet Genome Res* 150: 35–39, 2016.

Alvarez A, del Castillo I, Pera A, et al. Uniparental disomy of chromosome 13q causing homozygosity for the 35delG mutation in the gene encoding connexin26 (*GJB2*) results in prelingual hearing impairment in two unrelated Spanish patients. *J Med Genet* 40: 636–639, 2003.

Alves C, Carvalho F, Cremades N, Sousa M, Barros A. Unique (Y;13) translocation in a male with oligozoospermia: Cytogenetic and molecular studies. *Eur J Hum Genet* 10: 467–474, 2002.

Amarillo IE, O'Connor S, Lee CK, Willing M, Wambach JA. De novo 9q gain in an infant with tetralogy of Fallot with absent pulmonary valve: Patient report and review of congenital heart disease in 9q duplication syndrome. *Am J Med Genet* 167A: 2966–2974, 2015.

American Academy of Pediatrics Committee on Bioethics. Sterilization of women who are mentally handicapped. *Pediatrics* 85: 868–871, 1990.

American College of Obstetricians and Gynecologists Committee on Genetics. Committee Opinion No. 581: The use of chromosomal microarray analysis in prenatal diagnosis. *Obstet Gynecol* 122: 1374–1377, 2013.

American Society of Human Genetics Board of Directors & American College of Medical Genetics Board of Directors. Points to consider: Ethical, legal, and psychosocial implications of genetic testing in children and adolescents. *Am J Hum Genet* 57: 1233–1241, 1995.

American Society for Reproductive Medicine, Practice Committee. Definitions of infertility and recurrent pregnancy loss. *Fertil Steril* 90: S60, 2008.

Amor DJ. Future of whole genome sequencing. *J Paediatr Child Health* 51: 251–254, 2015.

Amor DJ, Bentley K, Ryan J, et al. Human centromere repositioning "in progress." *Proc Natl Acad Sci USA* 101: 6542–6547, 2004.

Amor DJ, Cameron C. PGD gender selection for non-Mendelian disorders with unequal sex incidence. *Hum Reprod* 23: 729–734, 2008.

Amor DJ, Choo KHA. Neocentromeres: Role in human disease, evolution, and centromere study. *Am J Hum Genet* 71: 695–714, 2002.

Amor DJ, De Crespigny L, Gardner RJM. Urinary tract defects and chromosomal disorders. In Flinter F (ed.), *The Genetics of Renal Disease*. Oxford, UK: Oxford University Press, 2003.

Amor D, Delatycki MB, Susman M, et al. 46,XX/46,XY at amniocentesis in a fetus with true hermaphroditism. *J Med Genet* 36: 866–869, 1999.

Amor DJ, Halliday J. A review of known imprinting syndromes and their association with assisted reproduction technologies. *Hum Reprod* 23: 2826–2834, 2008.

Amor DJ, Neo WT, Waters E, Heussler H, Pertile M, Halliday J. Health and developmental outcome of children following prenatal diagnosis of confined placental mosaicism. *Prenat Diagn* 26: 443–448, 2006.

Amor DJ, Woods CG. Pseudotrisomy 13 syndrome in siblings. *Clin Dysmorphol* 9: 115–118, 2000.

Amor DJ, Xu JX, Halliday JL, et al. Pregnancies conceived using assisted reproductive technologies (ART) have low levels of pregnancy-associated plasma protein-A (PAPP-A) leading to a high rate of false-positive results in first trimester screening for Down syndrome. *Hum Reprod* 24: 1330–1338, 2009.

Amyere M, Aerts V, Brouillard P, et al. Somatic uniparental isodisomy explains multifocality of glomuvenous malformations. *Am J Hum Genet* 92: 188–196, 2013.

An Y, Amr SS, Torres A, et al. *SOX12* and *NRSN2* are candidate genes for 20p13 subtelomeric deletions associated with developmental delay. *Am J Med Genet* 162B: 832–840, 2013.

Anahory T, Hamamah S, Andreo B, et al. Sperm segregation analysis of a (13;22) Robertsonian translocation carrier by FISH: A comparison of locus-specific probe and whole chromosome painting. *Hum Reprod* 20: 1850–1854, 2005.

Anderlid BM, Sahlén S, Schoumans J, et al. Detailed characterization of 12 supernumerary ring chromosomes using micro-FISH and search for uniparental disomy. *Am J Med Genet* 99: 223–233, 2001.

Anderson G. Nondirectiveness in prenatal genetics: Patients read between the lines. *Nurs Ethics* 6: 126–136, 1999.

Ang DC, Rodríguez Urrego PA, Prasad V. Placental mesenchymal dysplasia: A potential misdiagnosed entity. *Arch Gynecol Obstet* 279: 937–939, 2009.

Angell R. First-meiotic-division nondisjunction in human oocytes. *Am J Hum Genet* 61: 23–32, 1997.

Angell RR, Aitken RJ, van Look PF, Lumsden MA, Templeton AA. Chromosome abnormalities in human embryos after in vitro fertilization. *Nature* 303: 336–338, 1983.

Anguiano A, Yang X, Felix JK, Hoo JJ. Twin brothers with MIDAS syndrome and XX karyotype. *Am J Med Genet* 119A: 47–49, 2003.

Annable K, Donnenfeld AE, Fischer RL, Knops J. Prenatal diagnosis of a jumping translocation. *Prenat Diagn* 28: 767–769, 2008.

Annunziato AT. DNA packaging: Nucleosomes and cromatin. *Nature Education* 1, 2008.

Antoccia A, Kobayashi J, Tauchi H, Matsuura S, Komatsu K. Nijmegen breakage syndrome and functions of the responsible protein, NBS1. *Genome Dyn* 1: 191–205, 2006.

Anton E, Blanco J, Egozcue J, Vidal F. Risk assessment and segregation analysis in a pericentric inversion inv6p23q25 carrier using FISH on decondensed sperm nuclei. *Cytogenet Genome Res* 97: 149–154, 2002.

Anton E, Blanco J, Egozcue J, Vidal F. Sperm studies in heterozygote inversion carriers: A review. *Cytogenet Genome Res* 111: 297–304, 2005.

Anton E, Blanco J, Vidal F. Meiotic behavior of three D;G Robertsonian translocations: Segregation and interchromosomal effect. *J Hum Genet* 55: 541–545, 2010.

Anton E, Vidal F, Blanco J. Interchromosomal effect analyses by sperm FISH: Incidence and distribution among reorganization carriers. *Syst Biol Reprod Med* 57: 268–278, 2011.

Antonacci F, Dennis MY, Huddleston J, et al. Palindromic GOLGA8 core duplicons promote chromosome 15q13.3 microdeletion and evolutionary instability. *Nat Genet* 46: 1293–1302, 2014.

Antonarakis SE, Avramopoulos D, Blouin JL, Talbot CC, Schinzel AA. Mitotic errors in somatic cells cause trisomy 21 in about 4.5% of cases and are not associated with advanced maternal age. *Nat Genet* 3: 146–150, 1993.

Apacik C, Cohen M, Jakobeit M, et al. Two brothers with multiple congenital anomalies and mental retardation due to disomy (X)(q12→q13.3) inherited from the mother. *Clin Genet* 50: 63–73, 1996.

Aradhya S, Smaoui N, Marble M, Lacassie Y. De novo duplication 11p13 involving the *PAX6* gene in a patient with neonatal seizures, hypotonia, microcephaly, developmental disability and minor ocular manifestations. *Am J Med Genet* 155A: 442–444, 2011.

Archibald AD, Massie J, Smith MJ, Dalton DG, du Sart D, Amor DJ. Population-based genetic carrier screening for cystic fibrosis in Victoria. *Med J Aust* 200: 205–206, 2014.

Ardalan A, Prieur M, Choiset A, Turleau C, Goutieres F, Girard-Orgeolet S. Intrachromosomal insertion mimicking a pericentric inversion: Molecular cytogenetic characterization of a three break rearrangement of chromosome 20. *Am J Med Genet* 138A: 288–293, 2005.

Arens YHJM, Engelen JJM, Govaerts LCP, et al. Familial insertion (3;5)(q25.3;q22.1q31.3) with deletion or duplication of chromosome region 5q22.1-5q31.3 in ten unbalanced carriers. *Am J Med Genet* 130A: 128–133, 2004.

Argiropoulos B, Carter M, Brierley K, et al. Discordant phenotypes in a mother and daughter with mosaic supernumerary ring chromosome 19 explained by a de novo 7q36.2 deletion and 7p22.1 duplication. *Am J Med Genet* 155A: 885–991, 2011.

Arlt MF, Casper AM, Glover TW. Common fragile sites. *Cytogenet Genome Res* 100: 92–100, 2003.

Armstrong L, McGowan-Jordan J, Brierley K, Allanson JE. De novo dup(X)(q22.3q26) in a girl with evidence that functional disomy of X material is the cause of her abnormal phenotype. *Am J Med Genet* 116A: 71–76, 2003.

Arnedo N, Nogués C, Bosch M, Templado C. Mitotic and meiotic behaviour of a naturally transmitted ring Y chromosome: Reproductive risk evaluation. *Hum Reprod* 20: 462–468, 2005.

Arnon J, Meirow D, Lewis-Roness H, Ornoy A. Genetic and teratogenic effects of cancer treatments on gametes and embryos. *Hum Reprod Update* 7: 394–403, 2001.

Asada H, Sueoka K, Hashiba T, Kuroshima M, Kobayashi N, Yoshimura Y. The effects of age and abnormal sperm count on the nondisjunction of spermatozoa. *J Assist Reprod Genet* 17: 51–59, 2000.

Ashley T. Prediction of mammalian meiotic synaptic and recombinational behavior of inversion heterozygotes based on mitotic breakpoint data and the possible evolutionary consequences. *Genetica* 83: 1–7, 1990.

Ashley T, Gaeth AP, Inagaki H, et al. Meiotic recombination and spatial proximity in the etiology of the recurrent t(11;22). *Am J Hum Genet* 79: 524–538, 2006.

Ashton F, O'Connor R, Love JM, et al. Molecular characterisation of a der(Y)t(Xp;Yp) with Xp functional disomy and sex reversal. *Genet Mol Res* 9: 1815–1823, 2010.

Au PY, Argiropoulos B, Parboosingh JS, Innes AM. Refinement of the critical region of 1q41q42 microdeletion syndrome identifies FBXO28 as a candidate causative gene for intellectual disability and seizures. *Am J Med Genet* 164A: 441–448, 2014.

Auerbach AD, Min Z, Ghosh R, et al. Clastogen-induced chromosomal breakage as a marker for first trimester prenatal diagnosis of Fanconi anemia. *Hum Genet* 73: 86–88, 1986.

Austad T. The right not to know—Worthy of preservation any longer? An ethical perspective. *Clin Genet* 50: 85–88, 1996.

Avila M, Kirchhoff M, Marle N, et al. Delineation of a new chromosome 20q11.2 duplication syndrome including the *ASXL1* gene. *Am J Med Genet* 161A: 1594–1598, 2013.

Aviram-Goldring A, Daniely M, Dorf H, Chaki R, Goldman B, Barkai G. Use of interphase fluorescence in situ hybridization in third trimester fetuses with anomalies and growth retardation. *Am J Med Genet* 87: 203–206, 1999.

Awa AA, Honda T, Neriishi S, et al. Cytogenetic study of the offspring of atomic bomb survivors, Hiroshima and Nagasaki. In Obe G, Basler A (eds.), *Cytogenetics: Basic and Applied Aspects*. Berlin: Springer-Verlag, 1987.

Ayukawa H, Tsukahara M, Fukuda M, Kondoh O. Recombinant chromosome 18 resulting from a maternal pericentric inversion. *Am J Med Genet* 50: 323–325, 1994.

Azzi S, Rossignol S, Steunou V, et al. Multilocus methylation analysis in a large cohort of 11p15-related foetal growth disorders (Russell Silver and Beckwith Wiedemann syndromes) reveals simultaneous loss of methylation at paternal and maternal imprinted loci. *Hum Mol Genet* 18: 4724–4733, 2009.

Baarends WM, van der Laan R, Grootegoed JA. DNA repair mechanisms and gametogenesis. *Reproduction* 121: 31–39, 2001.

Baccetti B, Bruni E, Collodel G, et al. 10,15 reciprocal translocation in an infertile man: Ultrastructural and fluorescence in-situ hybridization sperm study: Case report. *Hum Reprod* 18: 2302–2308, 2003.

Baccetti B, Capitani S, Collodel G, Estenoz M, Gambera L, Piomboni P. Infertile spermatozoa in a human carrier of robertsonian translocation 14;22. *Fertil Steril* 78: 1127–1130, 2002.

Bache I, Brondum-Nielsen K, Tommerup N. Genetic counseling in adult carriers of a balanced chromosomal rearrangement ascertained in childhood: Experiences from a nationwide reexamination of translocation carriers. *Genet Med* 9: 185–187, 2007.

Baena N, De Vigan C, Cariati E, et al. Prenatal detection of rare chromosomal autosomal abnormalities in Europe. *Am J Med Genet* 118A: 319–327, 2003.

Baena N, De Vigan C, Cariati E, et al. Turner syndrome: Evaluation of prenatal diagnosis in 19 European registries. *Am J Med Genet* 129A: 16–20, 2004.

Baglietto MG, Caridi G, Gimelli G, et al. *RORB* gene and 9q21.13 microdeletion: Report on a patient with epilepsy and mild intellectual disability. *Eur J Med Genet* 57: 44–46, 2014.

Bagshawe KD, Lawler SD. Unmasking moles. *Br J Obstet Gynaecol* 89: 255–257, 1982.

Bahçe M, Oğur G, Ýmirzalýoõlu N, et al. Repeated fetal loss in two related first cousin marriages with couples all carrying the same translocation t(13q;14q). *Eur J Hum Genet* 4: 35–36, 1996.

Bailey C, Fryer AE, Greenslade M. Warsaw breakage syndrome—A further report, emphasising cutaneous findings. *Eur J Med Genet* 58: 235–237, 2015.

Baillie M. (1799) A series of engravings, accompanied with explanations, which are intended to illustrate the morbid anatomy of some of the most important parts of the human body. Ninth fasciculus. London, UK: W. Bulmer and Co. Facsimile edition prep. H Attwood, Melbourne University Press, 1985.

Baird ML, Heinig JA, Davis D, Sheets K, Kirkpatrick B, Starr DB. Chimeric germline tissue: Alleged father's genetic contribution to child found in semen sample but not in buccal sample. Paper presented at the International Symposium on Human Identification, Grapevine, TX, 2015.

Baker PR, Tsai AC, Springer M, et al. Male with mosaicism for supernumerary ring X chromosome: Analysis of phenotype and characterization of genotype using array comparative genome hybridization. *J Craniofac Surg* 21: 1369–1375, 2010.

Bakhshi S, Joenje H, Schindler D, et al. A case report of a patient with microcephaly, facial dysmorphism, mitomycin-C-sensitive lymphocytes, and susceptibility to lymphoma. *Cancer Genet Cytogenet* 164: 168–171, 2006.

Balakier H, Bouman D, Sojecki A, Librach C, Squire JA. Morphological and cytogenetic analysis of human giant oocytes and giant embryos. *Hum Reprod* 17: 2394–2401, 2002.

Balasubramanian M, Atack E, Smith K, Parker MJ. A novel de novo 20q13.32-q13.33 deletion in a 2-year-old child with poor growth, feeding difficulties and low bone mass. *J Hum Genet* 60: 313–317, 2015.

Balasubramanian M, Barber JCK, Collinson MN, et al. Inverted duplication of 1q32.1 to 1q44 characterized by array CGH and review of distal 1q partial trisomy. *Am J Med Genet* 149A: 793–797, 2009.

Balasubramanian M, Sithambaram S, Smith K. Inherited duplication of the short arm of chromosome 18p11.32-p11.31 associated with developmental delay/intellectual disability. *Clin Dysmorphol* 25: 19–22, 2016.

Balasubramanian M, Smith K, Basel-Vanagaite L, et al. Case series: 2q33.1 microdeletion syndrome—Further delineation of the phenotype. *J Med Genet* 48: 290–298, 2011.

Balcı S, Engiz Ö, Aktaş D, et al. Ring chromosome 4 and Wolf-Hirschhorn syndrome (WHS) in a child with multiple anomalies. *Am J Med Genet* 140: 628–632, 2006.

Balcı S, Unal A, Engiz O, et al. Bilateral periventricular nodular heterotopia, severe learning disability, and epilepsy in a male patient with 46,XY,der(19) t(X;19)(q11.1-11.2;p13.3). *Dev Med Child Neurol* 49: 219–224, 2007.

Balcı S, Zschocke J, Kotzot D. Ergün MA, Spreiz A. Formation of a familial ring chromosome 18 investigated by SNP-array analysis. *Am J Med Genet* 164A: 1854–1856, 2014.

Baldwin EL, May LF, Justice AN, Martin CL, Ledbetter DH. Mechanisms and consequences of small supernumerary marker chromosomes: From Barbara McClintock to modern genetic-counseling issues. *Am J Hum Genet* 82: 398–410, 2008.

Balkan M, Fidanboy M, Isi H, et al. A case of complete tetraploidy in amniocentesis with normal karyotype in subsequent cordocentesis. *J Pediatr Genet* 1: 243–246, 2012.

Ballarati L, Recalcati MP, Bedeschi MF, et al. Cytogenetic, FISH and array-CGH characterization of a complex chromosomal rearrangement carried by a mentally and language impaired patient. *Eur J Med Genet* 52: 218–223, 2009.

Ballarati L, Rossi E, Bonati MT, et al. 13q Deletion and central nervous system anomalies: Further insights from karyotype-phenotype analyses of 14 patients. *J Med Genet* 44: e60, 2007.

Ballesta-Martínez MJ, López-González V, Dulcet LA, et al. Autosomal dominant oculoauriculovertebral spectrum and 14q23.1 microduplication. *Am J Med Genet* 161A: 2030–2035, 2013.

Ballif BC, Kashork CD, Shaffer LG. The promise and pitfalls of telomere region-specific probes. *Am J Hum Genet* 67: 1356–1359, 2000.

Ballif BC, Rorem EA, Sundin K, et al. Detection of low-level mosaicism by array CGH in routine diagnostic specimens. *Am J Med Genet* 140: 2757–2767, 2006.

Ballif BC, Rosenfeld JA, Traylor R, et al. High-resolution array CGH defines critical regions and candidate genes for microcephaly, abnormalities of the corpus callosum, and seizure phenotypes in patients with microdeletions of 1q43q44. *Hum Genet* 131: 145–156, 2012.

Ballif BC, Theisen A, Coppinger J, et al. Expanding the clinical phenotype of the 3q29 microdeletion syndrome and characterization of the reciprocal microduplication. *Mol Cytogenet* 1: 8, 2008.

Ballif BC, Theisen A, Rosenfeld JA, et al. Identification of a recurrent microdeletion at 17q23.1q23.2 flanked by segmental duplications associated with heart defects and limb abnormalities. *Am J Hum Genet* 86: 454–461, 2010.

Ballif BC, Yu W, Shaw CA, Kashork CD, Shaffer LG. Monosomy 1p36 breakpoint junctions suggest pre-meiotic breakage-fusion-bridge cycles are involved in generating terminal deletions. *Hum Mol Genet* 12: 2153–2165, 2003.

Balmer D, Baumer A, Röthlisberger B, Schinzel A. Severe intra-uterine growth retardation in a patient with maternal uniparental disomy 22 and a 22-trisomic placenta. *Prenat Diagn* 19: 1061–1064, 1999.

Baltensperger A, Haischer G, Rohena L. Rare case of live born with confirmed mosaic trisomy 17 and review of the literature. *Clin Case Rep* 4: 420–424, 2016.

Bandyopadhyay R, Berend SA, Page SL, Choo KH, Shaffer LG. Satellite III sequences on 14p and their relevance to Robertsonian translocation formation. *Chromosome Res* 9: 235–242, 2001a.

Bandyopadhyay R, Heller A, Knox-DuBois C, et al. Parental origin and timing of de novo Robertsonian translocation formation. *Am J Hum Genet* 71: 1456–1462, 2002.

Bandyopadhyay R, McCaskill C, Knox-Du Bois C, et al. Mosaicism in a patient with Down syndrome reveals post-fertilization formation of a Robertsonian translocation and isochromosome. *Am J Med Genet* 116A: 159–163, 2003.

Bandyopadhyay R, McQuillan C, Page SL, Choo KHA, Shaffer LG. Identification and characterization of satellite III subfamilies to the acrocentric chromosomes. *Chromosome Res* 9: 223–233, 2001b.

Banerjee I, Shevlin M, Taranissi M, et al. Health of children conceived after preimplantation genetic diagnosis: A preliminary outcome study. *Reprod Biomed Online* 16: 376–381, 2008.

Baptista J, Mercer C, Prigmore E, et al. Breakpoint mapping and array CGH in translocations: Comparison of a phenotypically normal and an abnormal cohort. *Am J Hum Genet* 82: 927–936, 2008.

Baptista MJ, Fairbrother UL, Howard CM, et al. Heterotrisomy, a significant contributing factor to ventricular septal defect associated with Down syndrome? *Hum Genet* 107: 476–482, 2000.

Baralle D, Willatt LR, Shears DJ. Leri-Weill syndrome associated with a pseudodicentric X;Y translocation chromosome and skewed X-inactivation: Implications for genetic counselling. *Am J Med Genet* 95: 391–395, 2000.

Barbaro M, Cook J, Lagerstedt-Robinson K, Wedell A. Multigeneration inheritance through fertile XX carriers of an NR0B1 (DAX1) locus duplication in a kindred of females with isolated XY gonadal dysgenesis. *Int J Endocrinol* 2012: 504904, 2012.

Barbaro M, Oscarson M, Schoumans J, Staaf J, Ivarsson SA, Wedell A. Isolated 46,XY gonadal dysgenesis in two sisters caused by a Xp21.2 interstitial duplication containing the *DAX1* gene. *J Clin Endocrinol Metab* 92: 3305–3313, 2007.

Barber JCK. Directly transmitted unbalanced chromosome abnormalities and euchromatic variants. *J Med Genet* 42: 609–629, 2005.

Barber JCK, Hall V, Maloney VK, et al. 16p11.2-p12.2 duplication syndrome; A genomic condition differentiated from euchromatic variation of 16p11.2. *Eur J Hum Genet* 21: 182–189, 2013.

Barber JCK, Cockwell AE, Grant E, Williams S, Dunn R, Ogilvie CM. Is karyotyping couples experiencing recurrent miscarriage worth the cost? *BJOG* 117: 885–888, 2010.

Barber JCK, Ellis KH, Bowles LV, et al. Adenomatous polyposis coli and a cytogenetic deletion of chromosome 5 resulting from a maternal intrachromosomal insertion. *J Med Genet* 31: 312–316, 1994.

Barber JCK, Rosenfeld JA, Graham JM, et al. Inside the 8p23.1 duplication syndrome; Eight microduplications of likely or uncertain clinical significance. *Am J Med Genet* 167A: 2052–2064, 2015.

Barber JCK, Sharp AJ, Hollox EJ, Tyson C. Copy number variation of the *REXO1L1* gene cluster; Euchromatic deletion variant or susceptibility factor? *Eur J Hum Genet* 25: 8–9, 2016.

Barbosa AS, Ferraz-Costa TE, Semer M, Liberman B, Moreira-Filho CA. XY gonadal dysgenesis and gonadoblastoma: A study in two sisters with a cryptic deletion of the Y chromosome involving the *SRY* gene. *Hum Genet* 95: 63–66, 1995.

Barge-Schaapveld DQCM, Maas SM, Polstra A, Knegt LC, Hennekam RCM. The atypical 16p11.2 deletion: A not so atypical microdeletion syndrome? *Am J Med Genet* 155A: 1066–1072, 2011.

Barišić I, Zergollern L, Mužinić D, Hitrec V. Risk estimates for balanced reciprocal translocation carriers—Prenatal diagnosis experience. *Clin Genet* 49: 145–151, 1996.

Barlow AL, Hultén MA. Combined immunocytogenetic and molecular cytogenetic analysis of meiosis I human spermatocytes. *Chromosome Res* 4: 562–573, 1996.

Barone R, Fichera M, De Grandi M, et al. Familial 18q12.2 deletion supports the role of RNA-binding protein CELF4 in autism spectrum disorders. *Am J Med Genet* 173: 1649–1655, 2017.

Barseghyan K, Sklansky MS, Paquette LB, Randolph LM, Miller DA. Agenesis of the ductus venosus in a fetus with nonmosaic trisomy 22. *Prenat Diagn* 29: 901–902, 2009.

Bartels I, Pütz I, Reintjes N, Netzer C, Shoukier M. Normal intelligence and premature ovarian failure in an adult female with a 7.6 Mb de novo terminal deletion of chromosome 9p. *Eur J Med Genet* 56: 458–462, 2013.

Bartels I, Starke H, Argyriou L, Sauter SM, Zoll B, Liehr T. An exceptional complex chromosomal rearrangement (CCR) with eight breakpoints involving four chromosomes (1;3;9;14) in an azoospermic male with normal phenotype. *Eur J Med Genet* 50: 133–138, 2007.

Bartholdi D, Asadollahi R, Oneda B, et al. Further delineation of genotype-phenotype correlation in homozygous 2p21 deletion syndromes: First description of patients without cystinuria. *Am J Med Genet* 161A: 1853–1859, 2013.

Bartholdi D, Krajewska-Walasek M, Ŏunap K, et al. Epigenetic mutations of the imprinted IGF2-H19 domain in Silver-Russell syndrome (SRS): Results from a large cohort of patients with SRS and SRS-like phenotypes. *J Med Genet* 46: 192–197, 2009.

Bartolini L, Sartori S, Lenzini E, et al. De novo trisomy 20p characterized by array comparative genomic hybridization: Report of a novel case and review of the literature. *Gene* 524: 368–372, 2013.

Bartsch O, König U, Petersen MB, et al. Cytogenetic, FISH and DNA studies in 11 individuals from a family with two siblings with dup(21q) Down syndrome. *Hum Genet* 92: 127–132, 1993.

Basel-Vanagaite L, Davidov B, Friedman J, et al. Amniotic trisomy 11 mosaicism—Is it a benign finding? *Prenat Diagn* 26: 778–781, 2006.

Bashamboo A, Eozenou C, Rojo S, McElreavey K. Anomalies in human sex determination provide unique insights into the complex genetic interactions of early gonad development. *Clin Genet* 91: 143–156, 2017.

Basinko A, Douet-Guilbert N, Parent P, et al. Familial interstitial deletion of the short arm of chromosome 4 (p15.33-p16.3) characterized by molecular cytogenetic analysis. *Am J Med Genet* 146: 899–903, 2008.

Basinko A, Giovannucci Uzielli ML, Scarselli G, Priolo M, Timpani G, De Braekeleer M. Clinical and molecular cytogenetic studies in ring chromosome 5: Report of a child with congenital abnormalities. *Eur J Med Genet* 55: 112–116, 2012.

Basit S, Malibari OI, Al-Balawi AM, Afzal S, Eldardear AE, Ramzan K. Xq21.31-q21.32 duplication underlies intellectual disability in a large family with five affected males. *Am J Med Genet* 170A: 87–93, 2016.

Baskin B, Choufani S, Chen YA, et al. High frequency of copy number variations (CNVs) in the chromosome 11p15 region in patients with Beckwith-Wiedemann syndrome. *Hum Genet* 133: 321–330, 2014.

Bass HN, Sparkes RS, Lessner MM, Fox M, Phoenix B, Bernar J. A family with three independent autosomal translocations associated with 7q32→7qter syndrome. *J Med Genet* 22: 59–63, 1985.

Bassuk AG, Geraghty E, Wu S, et al. Deletions of 16p11.2 and 19p13.2 in a family with intellectual disability and generalized epilepsy. *Am J Med Genet* 161A: 1722–1725, 2013.

Bastepe M, Altug-Teber O, Agarwal C, Oberfield SE, Bonin M, Jüppner H. Paternal uniparental isodisomy of the entire chromosome 20 as a molecular cause of pseudohypoparathyroidism type Ib (PHP-Ib). *Bone* 48: 659–662, 2011.

Bateman MS, Mehta SG, Willatt L, et al. A de novo 4q34 interstitial deletion of at least 9.3 Mb with no discernible phenotypic effect. *Am J Med Genet* 152A: 1764–1769, 2010.

Bates AW. Autopsy on a case of Roberts syndrome reported in 1672: The earliest description? *Am J Med Genet* 117A: 92–96, 2003.

Batstone PJ, Simpson S, Bonthron DT, et al. Effective monosomy or trisomy of chromosome band 2q37.3 due to the unbalanced segregation of a 2;11 translocation. *Am J Med Genet* 118A: 241–246, 2003.

Battaglia A. The inv dup (15) or idic (15) syndrome (tetrasomy 15q). *Orphanet J Rare Dis* 3: 30, 2008.

Battaglia A, Carey JC, South ST. Wolf-Hirschhorn syndrome. In Pagon RA, Adam MP, Ardinger HH, et al. (eds.), *GeneReviews* [Internet]. Seattle, WA: University of Washington, 2015.

Battaglia DE, Goodwin P, Klein NA, Soules MR. Influence of maternal age on meiotic spindle assembly in oocytes from naturally cycling women. *Hum Reprod* 11: 2217–2222, 1996.

Baty BJ, Blackburn BL, Carey JC. Natural history of trisomy 18 and trisomy 13: I. Growth, physical assessment, medical histories, survival, and recurrence risk. *Am J Med Genet* 49: 175–188, 1994.

Baty BJ, Olson SB, Magenis RE, Carey JC. Trisomy 20 mosaicism in two unrelated girls with skin hypopigmentation and normal intellectual development. *Am J Med Genet* 99: 210–216, 2001.

Baumann W, Zabel B, Holl M. Familial pericentric inversion of the X chromosome [inv(X) (p11q28)]. *Ann Génét* 27: 106–108, 1984.

Baumer A, Basaran S, Taralczak M, et al. Initial maternal meiotic I error leading to the formation of a maternal i(2q) and a paternal i(2p) in a healthy male. *Cytogenet Genome Res* 118: 38–41, 2007.

Bayindir B, Dehaspe L, Brison N, et al. Noninvasive prenatal testing using a novel analysis pipeline to screen for all autosomal fetal aneuploidies improves pregnancy management. *Eur J Hum Genet* 23: 1286–1293, 2015.

Beaulieu Bergeron M, Brochu P, Lemyre E, Lemieux N. Correlation of intercentromeric distance, mosaicism, and sexual phenotype: Molecular localization of breakpoints in isodicentric Y chromosomes. *Am J Med Genet* 155A: 2705–2712, 2011.

Becker REN, Akhavan A. Prophylactic bilateral gonadectomy for ovotesticular disorder of sex development in a patient with mosaic 45,X/46,X,idic(Y)q11.222 karyotype. *Urol Case Rep* 5: 13–16, 2016.

Bedoyan JK, Flore LA, Alkatib A, Ebrahim SA, Bawle EV. Transmission of ring chromosome 13 from a mother to daughter with both having a 46,XX, r(13)(p13q34) karyotype. *Am J Med Genet* 129A: 316–320, 2004.

Beekhuis JR, De Wolf BT, Mantingh A, Heringa MP. The influence of serum screening on the amniocentesis rate in women of advanced maternal age. *Prenat Diagn* 14: 199–202, 1994.

Begemann M, Spengler S, Gogiel M, et al. Clinical significance of copy number variations in the 11p15.5 imprinting control regions: New cases and review of the literature. *J Med Genet* 49: 547–553, 2012.

Behnecke A, Hinderhofer K, Jauch A, Janssen JW, Moog U. Silver-Russell syndrome due to maternal uniparental disomy 7 and a familial reciprocal translocation t(7;13). *Clin Genet* 82: 494–498, 2012.

Bekker MN, van den Akker NM, Bartelings MM, et al. Nuchal edema and venous-lymphatic phenotype disturbance in human fetuses and mouse embryos with aneuploidy. *J Soc Gynecol Investig* 13: 209–216, 2006.

Belangero SI, Pacanaro AN, Bellucco FT, et al. Wide clinical variability in cat eye syndrome patients: Four non-related patients and three patients from the same family. *Cytogenet Genome Res* 138: 5–10, 2012.

Belin V, Farhat M, Monset-Couchard M. Intracytoplasmic sperm injection pregnancy with trisomy 20p and monosomy 22q in a newborn resulting from a balanced paternal translocation. *Biol Neonate* 75: 398–401, 1999.

Bell J, Dunlop R, Bryan J. Another paracentric inversion of chromosome 18. *Am J Med Genet* 39: 238, 1991.

Béna F, Gimelli S, Migliavacca E, et al. A recurrent 14q32.2 microdeletion mediated by expanded TGG repeats. *Hum Mol Genet* 19: 1967–1973, 2010.

Ben-Abdallah-Bouhjar I, Hannachi H, Labalme A, et al. Chromosomal microarray analysis of functional Xq27-qter disomy and deletion 3p26.3 in a boy with Prader-Willi like features and hypotonia. *Eur J Med Genet* 55: 461–465, 2012.

Ben-Abdallah-Bouhjar I, Mougou-Zerelli S, Hannachi H, et al. Phenotype and micro-array characterization of duplication 11q22.1-q25 and review of the literature. *Gene* 519: 135–141, 2013.

Ben-Nagi J, Wells D, Doye K, et al. Karyomapping: a single centre's experience from application of methodology to ongoing pregnancy and live-birth rates. *Reprod Biomed Online* 35: 264–271, 2017.

Bender BG, Harmon RJ, Linden MG, Bucher-Bartelson B, Robinson A. Psychosocial competence of unselected young adults with sex chromosome abnormalities. *Am J Med Genet* 88: 200–206, 1999.

Bender BG, Harmon RJ, Linden MG, Robinson A. Psychosocial adaptation of 39 adolescents with sex chromosome abnormalities. *Pediatrics* 96: 302–308, 1995.

Bender BG, Linden MG, Harmon RJ. Neuropsychological and functional cognitive skills of 35 unselected adults with sex chromosome abnormalities. *Am J Med Genet* 102: 309–313, 2001.

Bender BG, Linden MG, Robinson A. Neuropsychological impairment in 42 adolescents with sex chromosome abnormalities. *Am J Med Genet* 48: 169–173, 1993.

Benet J, Oliver-Bonet M, Cifuentes P, Templado C, Navarro J. Segregation of chromosomes in sperm of reciprocal translocation carriers: A review. *Cytogenet Genome Res* 111: 281–290, 2005.

Beneteau C, Baron S, David A, et al. Constitutional telomeric association (Y;7) in a patient with a female phenotype. *Am J Med Genet* 161A: 1436–41, 2013.

Benetti E, Murer L, Bordugo A, Andreetta B, Artifoni L. 10p12.1 deletion: HDR phenotype without DGS2 features. *Exp Mol Pathol* 86: 74–76, 2009.

Benkendorf JL, Prince MB, Rose MA, De Fina A, Hamilton HE. Does indirect speech promote nondirective genetic counseling? Results of a sociolinguistic investigation. *Am J Med Genet* 106: 199–207, 2001.

Benkhalifa M, Janny L, Vye P, Malet P, Boucher D, Menezo Y. Assessment of polyploidy in human morulae and blastocysts using co-culture and fluorescent in-situ hybridization. *Hum Reprod* 8: 895–902, 1993.

Benlian P, Foubert L, Gagne E, et al. Complete paternal isodisomy for chromosome 8 unmasked by lipoprotein lipase deficiency. *Am J Hum Genet* 59: 431–436, 1996.

Benn P. Trisomy 16 and trisomy 16 Mosaicism: A review. *Am J Med Genet* 79: 121–133, 1998.

Benn PA, Hsu LYF. Evidence for preferential involvement of chromosome bands 6p21 and 13q14 in amniotic fluid cell balanced translocation pseudomosaicism. *Clin Genet* 29: 116–121, 1986.

Bens S, Haake A, Tönnies H, et al. A de novo 1.1Mb microdeletion of chromosome 19p13.11 provides indirect evidence for EPS15L1 to be a strong candidate for split hand split foot malformation. *Eur J Med Genet* 54:e501–504, 2011.

Benzacken B, Gavelle FM, Martin-Pont B, et al. Familial sperm polyploidy induced by genetic spermatogenesis failure: Case report. *Hum Reprod* 16: 2646–2651, 2001.

Berend SA, Bejjani BA, McCaskill C, Shaffer LG. Identification of uniparental disomy in phenotypically abnormal carriers of isochromosomes or Robertsonian translocations. *Am J Med Genet* 111: 362–365, 2002a.

Berend SA, Bodamer OAF, Shapira SK, Shaffer LG, Bacino CA. Familial complex chromosomal rearrangement resulting in a recombinant chromosome. *Am J Med Genet* 109: 311–317, 2002b.

Berend SA, Canun S, McCaskill C, Page SL, Shaffer LG. Molecular analysis of mosaicism for two different de novo acrocentric rearrangements demonstrates diversity in Robertsonian translocation formation. *Am J Med Genet* 80: 252–259, 1998.

Berend SA, Feldman GL, McCaskill C, Czarnecki P, Van Dyke DL, Shaffer LG. Investigation of two cases of paternal disomy 13 suggests timing of isochromosome formation and mechanisms leading to uniparental disomy. *Am J Med Genet* 82: 275–281, 1999.

Berend SA, Horwitz J, McCaskill C, Shaffer LG. Identification of uniparental disomy following prenatal detection of Robertsonian translocations and isochromosomes. *Am J Hum Genet* 66: 1787–1793, 2000.

Berg JM, Korossy M. Down syndrome before Down: A retrospect. *Am J Med Genet* 102: 205–211, 2001.

Bergemann E. Manifestation familiale du karyotype triplo-X. Communication préliminaire. *J Génét Hum* 10: 370–371, 1962.

Bergère M, Wainer R, Nataf V, et al. Biopsied testis cells of four 47,XXY patients: Fluorescence in-situ hybridization and ICSI results. *Hum Reprod* 17: 32–37, 2002.

Berghella V, Wapner RJ, Yang-Feng T, Mahoney MJ. Prenatal confirmation of true fetal trisomy 22 mosaicism by fetal skin biopsy following normal fetal blood sampling. *Prenat Diagn* 18: 384–389, 1998.

Berkowitz RS, Bernstein MR, Laborde O, Goldstein DP. Subsequent pregnancy experience in patients with gestational trophoblastic disease. New England Trophoblastic Disease Center, 1965–1992. *J Reprod Med* 39: 228–232, 1994.

Bernard V, Donadille B, Zenaty D, et al. Spontaneous fertility and pregnancy outcomes amongst 480 women with Turner syndrome. *Hum Reprod* 31: 782–788, 2016.

Bernardini L, Capalbo A, D'Avanzo MG, et al. Five cases of supernumerary small ring chromosomes 1: Heterogeneity and genotype-phenotype correlation. *Eur J Med Genet* 50: 94–102, 2007.

Bernasconi F, Karagüzel A, Celep F, et al. Normal phenotype with maternal isodisomy in a female with two isochromosomes: i(2p) and i(2q). *Am J Hum Genet* 59: 1114–1118, 1996.

Berner AL, Bagci S, Wohlleber E, et al. Familial translocation t(6;20)(p21;p13) resulting in partial trisomy 6p and partial monosomy 20p: Report of a new case and review of the literature. *Cytogenet Genome Res* 136: 308–313, 2012.

Bernert J, Bartels I, Gatz G, et al. Prenatal diagnosis of the Pallister-Killian mosaic aneuploidy syndrome by CVS. *Am J Med Genet* 42: 747–750, 1992.

Bernier R, Steinman KJ, Reilly B, et al. Clinical phenotype of the recurrent 1q21.1 copy-number variant. *Genet Med* 18: 341–349, 2016.

Berr C, Borghi E, Rethoré MO, Lejeune J, Alperovitch A. Risk of Down syndrome in relatives of trisomy 21 children: A case-control study. *Ann Génét* 33: 137–140, 1990.

Bersu ET. Anatomical analysis of the developmental effects of aneuploidy in man: The Down syndrome. *Am J Med Genet* 5: 399–420, 1980.

Bertelloni S, Baroncelli GI, Massart F, Toschi B. Growth in boys with 45,X/46,XY mosaicism: Effect of growth hormone treatment on statural growth. *Sex Dev* 9: 183–189, 2015.

Bertelsen B, Nazaryan-Petersen L, Sun W, et al. A germline chromothripsis event stably segregating in 11 individuals through three generations. *Genet Med* 18: 494–500, 2016.

Bertini V, Battini R, Cioni G, Simi P, Valetto A. Molecular cytogenetic characterization of a new case of partial trisomy 13 (13q11q13.2). *Am J Med Genet* 152A: 490–494, 2010.

Bertini V, Orsini A, Mazza R, et al. A 6.5 Mb deletion at 3q24q25.2 narrows Wisconsin syndrome critical region to a 750 kb interval: A potential role for MBNLI. *Am J Med Genet* 173A: 280–284, 2017.

Bertini V, Valetto A, Uccelli A, et al. Molecular cytogenetic characterization of a de novo mosaic supernumerary ring chromosome 7: Report of a new patient. *Am J Med Genet* 146A: 2955–2959, 2008a.

Bertini V, Valetto A, Uccelli A, Tarantino E, Simi P. Ring chromosome 21 and reproductive pattern: A familial case and review of the literature. *Fertil Steril* 90: 2004, e1–5, 2008b.

Bertoli M, Alesi V, Gullotta F, et al. Another patient with 12q13 microduplication. *Am J Med Genet* 161A: 2004–2008, 2013.

Bertossi C, Cassina M, De Palma L, et al. 14q12 duplication including *FOXG1*: Is there a common age-dependent epileptic phenotype? *Brain Dev* 36: 402–407, 2014.

Besser AG, Mounts EL. Counselling considerations for chromosomal mosaicism detected by preimplantation genetic screening. *Reprod Biomed Online* 34: 369–374, 2017.

Bettio D, Baldwin EL, Carrozzo R, et al. Molecular cytogenetic and clinical findings in a patient with a small supernumerary r(8) mosaicism. *Am J Med Genet* 146A: 247–250, 2008.

Bettio D, Levi Setti P, Bianchi P, Grazioli V. Trisomy 18 mosaicism in a woman with normal intelligence. *Am J Med Genet* 120A: 303–304, 2003.

Betts DR, Greiner J, Feldges A, Caflisch U, Niggli FK. Constitutional balanced chromosomal rearrangements and neoplasm in children. *J Pediatr Hematol Oncol* 23: 582–584, 2001.

Beunders G, van de Kamp JM, Veenhoven RH, van Hagen JM, Nieuwint AW, Sistermans EA. A triplication of the Williams-Beuren syndrome region in a patient with mental retardation, a severe expressive language delay, behavioural problems and dysmorphisms. *J Med Genet* 47: 271–275, 2010.

Beverstock GC, Hansson K, Helderman-van den Enden AT, et al. A near false-negative finding of mosaic trisomy 21—A cautionary tale. *Prenat Diagn* 18: 742–746, 1998.

Bevilacqua E, Gil MM, Nicolaides KH, et al. Performance of screening for aneuploidies by cell-free DNA analysis of maternal blood in twin pregnancies. *Ultrasound Obstet Gynecol* 45: 61–66, 2015.

Bianca S, Boemi G, Barrano B, et al. Mosaic trisomy 20: Considerations for genetic counseling. *Am J Med Genet* 146A: 1897–1898, 2008.

Bianchi DW. Fetomaternal cell trafficking: A new cause of disease? *Am J Med Genet* 91: 22–28, 2000.

Bianchi DW, Chudova D, Sehnert AJ, et al. Noninvasive prenatal testing and incidental detection of occult maternal malignancies. *JAMA* 314: 162–169, 2015.

Bianchi DW, Wilkins-Haug LE, Enders AC, Hay ED. Origin of extraembryonic mesoderm in experimental animals: Relevance to chorionic mosaicism in humans. *Am J Med Genet* 46: 542–550, 1993.

Bianco K, Caughey AB, Shaffer BL, Davis R, Norton ME. History of miscarriage and increased incidence of fetal aneuploidy in subsequent pregnancy. *Obstet Gynecol* 107: 1098–1102, 2006.

Biason-Lauber A, Konrad D, Meyer M, DeBeaufort C, Schoenle EJ. Ovaries and female phenotype in a girl with 46,XY karyotype and mutations in the *CBX2* gene. *Am J Hum Genet* 84: 658–663, 2009.

Bielanska M, Tan SL, Ao A. High rate of mixoploidy among human blastocysts cultured in vitro. *Fertil Steril* 78: 1248–1253, 2002a.

Bielanska M, Tan SL, Ao A. Chromosomal mosaicism throughout human preimplantation development in vitro: Incidence, type, and relevance to embryo outcome. *Hum Reprod* 17: 413–419, 2002b.

Biesecker LG, Rosenberg M, Dziadzio L, et al. Detection of a subtle rearrangement of chromosome 22 using molecular techniques. *Am J Med Genet* 58: 389–394, 1995.

Bilimoria KY, Rothenberg JM. Prenatal diagnosis of a trisomy 7/maternal uniparental heterodisomy 7 mosaic fetus. *Am J Med Genet* 118A: 60–63, 2003.

Billuart P, Bienvenu T, Ronce N, et al. Oligophrenin-1 encodes a rhoGAP protein involved in X-linked mental retardation. *Nature* 392: 923–926, 1998.

Binder G, Seidel AK, Martin DD, et al. The endocrine phenotype in Silver-Russell syndrome is defined by the underlying epigenetic alteration. *J Clin Endocrinol Metab* 93: 1402–1407, 2008.

Bint SM, Ogilvie CM, Flinter FA, Khalaf Y, Scriven PN. Meiotic segregation of Robertsonian translocations ascertained in cleavage-stage embryos—Implications for preimplantation genetic diagnosis. *Hum Reprod* 26: 1575–1584, 2011.

Birkebaek NH, Cruger D, Hansen J, Nielsen J, Bruun-Petersen G. Fertility and pregnancy outcome in Danish women with Turner syndrome. *Clin Genet* 61: 35–39, 2002.

Bischoff FZ, Simpson JL. Endocervical fetal trophoblast for prenatal genetic diagnosis. *Curr Opin Obstet Gynecol* 18: 216–220, 2006.

Bisgaard AM, Kirchhoff M, Nielsen JE, et al. Chromosomal deletion unmasking a recessive disease: 22q13 deletion syndrome and metachromatic leukodystrophy. *Clin Genet* 75: 175–179, 2009.

Bispo AV, Burégio-Frota P, Oliveira dos Santos L, et al. Y chromosome in Turner syndrome: Detection of hidden mosaicism and the report of a rare X;Y translocation case. *Reprod Fertil Dev* 26: 1176–1182, 2014.

Bittel DC, Kibiryeva N, Butler MG. Expression of 4 genes between chromosome 15 breakpoints 1 and 2 and behavioral outcomes in Prader-Willi syndrome. *Pediatrics* 118: e1276–1283, 2006.

Bittel DC, Theodoro MF, Kibiryeva N, Fischer W, Talebizadeh Z, Butler MG. Comparison of X-chromosome inactivation patterns in multiple tissues from human females. *J Med Genet* 45: 309–313, 2008.

Bittencourt MC, Morris MA, Chabod J, et al. Fortuitous detection of uniparental isodisomy of chromosome 6. *J Med Genet* 34: 77–78, 1997.

Björck EJ, Anderlid BM, Blennow E. Maternal isodisomy of chromosome 9 with no impact on the phenotype in a woman with two isochromosomes: i(9p) and i(9q). *Am J Med Genet* 87: 49–52, 1999.

Blaicher W, Repa C, Schaller A. Acardiac twin pregnancy: Associated with trisomy 2: Case report. *Hum Reprod* 15: 474–475, 2000.

Blair J, Tolmie J, Hollman AS, Donaldson MD. Phenotype, ovarian function, and growth in patients with 45,X/47,XXX Turner mosaicism: Implications for prenatal counseling and estrogen therapy at puberty. *J Pediatr* 139: 724–728, 2001.

Blanc P, Gouas L, Francannet C, Giollant M, Vago P, Goumy C. Trisomy 20q caused by interstitial duplication 20q13.2: Clinical report and literature review. *Am J Med Genet* 146A: 1307–1311, 2008.

Blanco J, Farreras A, Egozcue J, Vidal F. Meiotic behavior of the sex chromosomes in a 45,X/46,X,r(Y)/46,X,dic r(Y) patient whose semen was assessed by fluorescence in situ hybridization. *Fertil Steril* 79: 913–918, 2003.

Blanco J, Gabau E, Gomez D, et al. Chromosome 21 disomy in the spermatozoa of the fathers of children with trisomy 21, in a population with a high prevalence of Down syndrome: Increased incidence in cases of paternal origin. *Am J Hum Genet* 63: 1067–1072, 1998.

Blassnig-Ezeh A, Bandelier C, Frühmesser A, et al. Severe growth retardation, delayed bone age, and facial dysmorphism in two patients with microduplications in 2p16→p22. *Am J Med Genet* 161A: 3176–3181, 2013.

Blazina Š, Ihan A, Lovrecic L, Hovnik T. 11q terminal deletion and combined immunodeficiency (Jacobsen syndrome): Case report and literature review on immunodeficiency in Jacobsen syndrome. *Am J Med Genet* 170A: 3237–3240, 2016.

Blennow E, Sahlén S, Inzunza J, Hovatta O, Nordenskjöld M, Malmgren H. Single cell CGH analysis of human preimplantation embryos from PGD patients with balanced structural chromosome aberrations. *Ann Génét* 44: s26, 2001.

Bliek J, Snijder S, Maas SM, et al. Phenotypic discordance upon paternal or maternal transmission of duplications of the 11p15 imprinted regions. *Eur J Med Genet* 52: 404–408, 2009.

Bloch EV, DiSalvo M, Hall BD, Epstein CJ. Alternative ways of presenting empiric risks. In Epstein CJ, Curry CJR, Packman S, Sherman S, Hall BD (eds.), Risk, communication, and decision making in genetic counseling. *Birth Defects: Orig Art Series* 15 (5C): 233–244, 1979.

Blouin JL, Binkert F, Antonarakis SE. Biparental inheritance of chromosome 21 polymorphic markers indicates that some Robertsonian translocations t(21;21) occur postzygotically. *Am J Med Genet* 49: 363–368, 1994.

Blumenthal AL, Allanson JE. Turner syndrome in a mother and daughter: r(X) and fertility. *Clin Genet* 52: 187–191, 1997.

Bobabilla-Morales L, Corona-Rivera A, Corona-Rivera JR, et al. Chromosome instability induced in vitro with mitomycin C in five Seckel syndrome patients. *Am J Med Genet* 123A: 148–152, 2003.

Bobrow M, Barby T, Hajianpour A, Maxwell D, Yau SC. Fertility in a male with trisomy 21. *J Med Genet* 29: 141, 1992.

Bocian E, Mazurczak T, Stanczak H. Paracentric inversion inv(18)(q21.1q23) in a woman with recurrent spontaneous abortions. *Am J Med Genet* 35: 592–593, 1990.

Bodri D, Guillén JJ, Schwenn K, Casadesus S, Vidal R, Coll O. Poor outcome in oocyte donation after elective transfer of a single cleavage-stage embryo in Turner syndrome patients. *Fertil Steril* 91: 1489–1492, 2009.

Boehmer ALM, Brinkmann O, Bruggenwirth H, et al. Genotype versus phenotype in families with androgen insensitivity syndrome. *J Clin Endocrinol Metab* 86: 4151–4160, 2001.

Bofinger MK, Needham DF, Saldana LR, Sosnowski JP, Blough RI. 45,X/46,X,r(Y) karyotype transmitted by father to son after intracytoplasmic sperm injection for oligospermia: A case report. *J Reprod Med* 44: 645–648, 1999.

Boghosian-Sell L, Mewar R, Harrison W, et al. Molecular mapping of the Edwards syndrome phenotype to two noncontiguous regions on chromosome 18. *Am J Hum Genet* 55: 476–483, 1994.

Bohers E, Sarafan-Vasseur N, Drouet A, et al. Gradual reduction of BUBR1 protein levels results in premature sister-chromatid separation then in aneuploidy. *Hum Genet* 124: 473–478, 2008.

Boisseau P, Giraud M, Ternisien C, et al. An unexpected transmission of von Willebrand disease type 3: The first case of maternal uniparental disomy 12. *Haematologica* 96: 1567–1568, 2011.

Boivin J, Appleton TC, Baetens P, et al. Guidelines for counselling in infertility: Outline version. *Hum Reprod* 16: 1301–1304, 2001.

Bolor H, Mori T, Nishiyama S, et al. Mutations of the *SYCP3* gene in women with recurrent pregnancy loss. *Am J Hum Genet* 84: 14–20, 2009.

Bonaglia MC, Ciccone R, Gimelli G, et al. Detailed phenotype-genotype study in five patients with chromosome 6q16 deletion: Narrowing the critical region for Prader-Willi-like phenotype. *Eur J Hum Genet* 16: 1443–1449, 2008.

Bonaglia MC, Giorda R, Beri S, et al. Molecular mechanisms generating and stabilizing terminal 22q13 deletions in 44 subjects with Phelan/McDermid syndrome. *PLoS Genet* 7: e1002173, 2011.

Bonaglia MC, Marelli S, Novara F, et al. Genotype-phenotype relationship in three cases with overlapping 19p13.12 microdeletions. *Eur J Hum Genet* 18: 1302–1309, 2010.

Bonaglia MC, Zanotta N, Giorda R, D'Angelo G, Zucca C. Long-term follow-up of a patient with 5q31.3 microdeletion syndrome and the smallest de novo 5q31.2q31.3 deletion involving PURA. *Mol Cytogenet* 8: 89, 2015.

Bonduelle M, Van Assche E, Joris H, et al. Prenatal testing in ICSI pregnancies: Incidence of chromosomal anomalies in 1586 karyotypes and relation to sperm parameters. *Hum Reprod* 17: 2600–2614, 2002.

Bonnet C, Andrieux J, Béri-Dexheimer M, et al. Microdeletion at chromosome 4q21 defines a new emerging syndrome with marked growth restriction, mental retardation and absent or severely delayed speech. *J Med Genet* 47: 377–384, 2010.

Bonnet C, Zix C, Grégoire MJ, et al. Characterization of mosaic supernumerary ring chromosomes by array-CGH: Segmental aneusomy for proximal 4q in a child with tall stature and obesity. *Am J Med Genet* 140: 233–237, 2006.

Bonuccelli A, Valetto A, Orsini A, et al. Maternally derived 15q11.2-q13.1 duplication in a child with Lennox–Gastaut-type epilepsy and dysmorphic

features: Clinical-genetic characterization of the family and review of the literature. *Am J Med Genet* 173A: 556–560, 2017.

Boonen SE, Hoffmann AL, Donnai D, Tümer Z, Ravn K. Diploid/triploid mosaicism: A rare event or an under-diagnosed syndrome? *Eur J Med Genet* 54: 374–375, 2011.

Boonen SE, Mackay DJ, Hahnemann JM, et al. Transient neonatal diabetes, ZFP57, and hypomethylation of multiple imprinted loci: A detailed follow-up. *Diabetes Care* 36: 505–512, 2013.

Boormans EM, Birnie E, Oepkes D, et al. Comparison of multiplex ligation-dependent probe amplification and karyotyping in prenatal diagnosis. *Obstet Gynecol* 115: 297–303, 2010.

Borel C, Cheung F, Stewart H, et al. Evaluation of *PRDM9* variation as a risk factor for recurrent genomic disorders and chromosomal non-disjunction. *Hum Genet* 131: 1519–1524, 2012.

Borgström B, Hreinsson J, Rasmussen C, et al. Fertility preservation in girls with Turner syndrome: Prognostic signs of the presence of ovarian follicles. *J Clin Endocrinol Metab* 94: 74–80, 2009.

Borie C, Léger J, Dupuy O, et al. Translocation (Y;22) resulting in the loss of *SHOX* and isolated short stature. *Am J Med Genet* 125A: 186–190, 2004.

Bos AP, Broers CJ, Hazebroek FW, et al. Avoidance of emergency surgery in newborn infants with trisomy 18. *Lancet* 339: 913–915, 1992.

Bottani A, Robinson WP, DeLozier-Blanchet CD, et al. Angelman syndrome due to paternal uniparental disomy of chromosome 15: A milder phenotype? *Am J Med Genet* 51: 35–40, 1994.

Bouchlariotou S, Tsikouras P, Dimitraki M, et al. Turner's syndrome and pregnancy: Has the 45,X/47,XXX mosaicism a different prognosis? Own clinical experience and literature review. *J Matern Fetal Neonatal Med* 24: 668–672, 2011.

Boudry-Labis E, Demeer B, Le Caignec C, et al. A novel microdeletion syndrome at 9q21.13 characterised by mental retardation, speech delay, epilepsy and characteristic facial features. *Eur J Med Genet* 56: 163–170, 2013.

Boué A, Gallano P. A collaborative study of the segregation of inherited chromosome structural rearrangements in 1356 prenatal diagnoses. *Prenat Diagn* 4 Spec No: 45–67, 1984.

Bouhjar IB, Hannachi H, Zerelli SM, et al. Array-CGH study of partial trisomy 9p without mental retardation. *Am J Med Genet* 155A: 1735–1739, 2011.

Bouman A, Schuitema A, Pfundt R, van de Zande G, Kleefstra T. Clinical delineation of a patient with trisomy 12q23q24. *Eur J Med Genet* 56: 463–469, 2013.

Bound JP, Francis BJ, Harvey PW. Down's syndrome: Prevalence and ionising radiation in an area of north west England 1957–91. *J Epidemiol Community Health* 49: 164–170, 1995.

Bourthoumieu S, Esclaire F, Terro F, et al. "Cri-du-chat" syndrome in a patient born to a mother with a paracentric inversion of chromosome 5q. *Ann Génét* 46: 483–486, 2003.

Bovie C, Holden ST, Schroer A, Smith E, Trump D, Raymond FL. Neurofibromatosis 2 in a patient with a de novo balanced reciprocal translocation 46,X,t(X;22)(p11.2;q11.2). *J Med Genet* 40: 682–684, 2003.

Bowen P, Fitzgerald PH, Gardner RJM, Biederman B, Veale AM. Duplication 8q syndrome due to familial chromosome ins(10;8)(q21;q212q22). *Am J Med Genet* 14: 635–646, 1983.

Bowser-Riley S, Buckton KE, Ratcliffe SG, Syme J. Inheritance of a ring 14 chromosome. *J Med Genet* 18: 209–213, 1981.

Bowser-Riley SM, Griffiths MJ, Creasy MR, et al. Are double translocations double trouble? *J Med Genet* 25: 326–331, 1988.

Boyd LJ, Livingston JS, Brown MG, et al. Meiotic exchange event within the stalk region of an inverted chromosome 22 results in a recombinant chromosome with duplication of the distal long arm. *Am J Med Genet* 138: 355–360, 2005.

Boyd PA, Loane M, Garne E, Khoshnood B, Dolk H; EUROCAT working group. Sex chromosome trisomies in Europe: Prevalence, prenatal detection and outcome of pregnancy. *Eur J Hum Genet* 19: 231–234, 2011.

Boyle J, Sangha K, Dill F, Robinson WP, Yong SL. Grandmaternal origin of an isochromosome 18p present in two maternal half-sisters. *Am J Med Genet* 101: 65–69, 2001.

Boyle MI, Jespersgaard C, Brøndum-Nielsen K, Bisgaard AM, Tümer Z. Cornelia de Lange syndrome. *Clin Genet* 88: 1–12, 2015.

Braddock SR, Henley KM, Potter KL, Nguyen HG, Huang TH. Tertiary trisomy due to a reciprocal translocation of chromosomes 5 and 21 in a four-generation family. *Am J Med Genet* 92: 311–317, 2000.

Braddock SR, South ST, Schiffman JD, et al. Braddock–Carey syndrome: A 21q22 contiguous gene syndrome encompassing *RUNX1*. *Am J Med Genet* 170A: 2580–2586, 2016.

Brady AN, May KM, Fernhoff PM. Mosaic trisomy 4: Long-term outcome on the first reported liveborn. *Am J Med Genet* 132: 411–413, 2005.

Brady P, Brison N, Van Den Bogaert K, et al. Clinical implementation of NIPT—Technical and biological challenges. *Clin Genet* 89: 523–530, 2016.

Brady PD, Delle Chiaie B, Christenhusz G, et al. A prospective study of the clinical utility of prenatal chromosomal microarray analysis in fetuses with ultrasound abnormalities and an exploration of a framework for reporting unclassified variants and risk factors. *Genet Med* 16: 469–476, 2014.

Brahams D. House of Lords upholds decision to sterilise 17-year-old mentally handicapped girl. *Lancet* 1: 1099–1100, 1987.

Brand H, Collins RL, Hanscom C, et al. Paired-duplication signatures mark cryptic inversions and other complex structural variation. *Am J Hum Genet* 97: 170–176, 2015.

Braun A, Kammerer S, Cleve H, Löhrs U, Schwarz HP, Kuhnle U. True hermaphroditism in a 46,XY individual, caused by a postzygotic somatic point mutation in the male gonadal sex-determining locus (*SRY*): Molecular genetics and histological findings in a sporadic case. *Am J Hum Genet* 52: 578–585, 1993.

Braun-Falco M, Schempp W, Nevinny-Stickel-Hinzpeter C, Köhn FM. Azoospermia due to a unique de novo balanced reciprocal translocation (Y;1) (q12;q25). *J Androl* 28: 647–651, 2007.

Breckpot J, Anderlid BM, Alanay Y, et al. Chromosome 22q12.1 microdeletions: Confirmation of the *MN1* gene as a candidate gene for cleft palate. *Eur J Hum Genet* 24: 51–58, 2016.

Breman AM, Chow JC, U'Ren L, et al. Evidence for feasibility of fetal trophoblastic cell-based noninvasive prenatal testing. *Prenat Diagn* 36: 1009–1019, 2016.

Brender JD, Zhan FB, Langlois PH, Suarez L, Scheuerle A. Residential proximity to waste sites and industrial facilities and chromosomal anomalies in offspring. *Int J Hyg Environ Health* 211: 50–58, 2008.

Brewer C, Holloway S, Zawalnyski P, Schinzel A, FitzPatrick D. A chromosomal deletion map of human malformations. *Am J Hum Genet* 63: 1153–1159, 1998.

Brewer C, Holloway S, Zawalnyski P, Schinzel A, FitzPatrick D. A chromosomal duplication map of malformations: Regions of suspected haplo- and triplolethality—and tolerance of segmental aneuploidy—in humans. *Am J Hum Genet* 64: 1702–1708, 1999.

Brewer CM, Grace E, Stark GD, Gregory DW, Howell RT, Fitzpatrick DR. Genomic instability associated with limb defects: Case report and review of the literature. *Clin Dysmorphol* 6: 99–109, 1997.

Brezina PR, Brezina DS, Kearns WG. Preimplantation genetic testing. *BMJ* 345: e5908, 2012.

Brisset S, Aboura A, Audibert F, et al. Discordant prenatal diagnosis of trisomy 21 due to mosaic structural rearrangements of chromosome 21. *Prenat Diagn* 23: 461–469, 2003.

Brisset S, Capri Y, Briand-Suleau A, et al. Inherited 1q21.1q21.2 duplication and 16p11.2 deletion: A two-hit case with more severe clinical manifestations. *Eur J Med Genet* 58: 497–501, 2015.

Brisset S, Izard V, Misrahi M, et al. Cytogenetic, molecular and testicular tissue studies in an infertile 45,X male carrying an unbalanced (Y;22) translocation: Case report. *Hum Reprod* 20: 2168–2172, 2005.

Britt DW, Risinger ST, Miller V, Mans MK, Krivchenia EL, Evans MI. Determinants of parental decisions after the prenatal diagnosis of Down syndrome: Bringing in context. *Am J Med Genet* 93: 410–416, 2000.

Brizot ML, Schultz R, Patroni LT, Lopes LM, Armbruster-Moraes E, Zugaib M. Trisomy 10: Ultrasound features and natural history after first trimester diagnosis. *Prenat Diagn* 21: 672–675, 2001.

Broadbent H, Farran EK, Chin E, et al. Genetic contributions to visuospatial cognition in Williams syndrome: Insights from two contrasting partial deletion patients. *J Neurodev Disord* 6: 18, 2014.

Brock DW. The non-identity problem and genetic harms—The case of wrongful handicaps. *Bioethics* 9: 269–275, 1995.

Brockmann K, Böhm R, Bürger J. Exceptionally mild Angelman syndrome phenotype associated with an incomplete imprinting defect. *J Med Genet* 39: e51, 2002.

Brodie D, Beyer CE, Osborne E, Kralevski V, Rasi S, Osianlis T. Preimplantation genetic diagnosis for chromosome rearrangements—One blastomere biopsy versus two blastomere biopsy. *J Assist Reprod Genet* 29: 821–827, 2012.

Brøndum-Nielsen K, Mikkelsen M. A 10-year survey, 1980–1990, of prenatally diagnosed small supernumerary marker chromosomes, identified by FISH analysis: Outcome and follow-up of 14 cases diagnosed in a series of 12,699 prenatal samples. *Prenat Diagn* 15: 615–619, 1995.

Bronicki LM, Redin C, Drunat S, et al. Ten new cases further delineate the syndromic intellectual disability phenotype caused by mutations in *DYRK1A*. *Eur J Hum Genet* 23: 1482–1487, 2015.

Brown GM, Leversha M, Hultén M, Ferguson-Smith MA, Affara NA, Furlong RA. Genetic analysis of meiotic recombination in humans by use of sperm typing: Reduced recombination within a heterozygous paracentric inversion of chromosome 9q32-q34.3. *Am J Hum Genet* 62: 1484–1492, 1998.

Brown LY, Alonso ML, Yu J, Warburton D, Brown S. Prenatal diagnosis of a familial Xq deletion in a female fetus: A case report. *Prenat Diagn* 21: 27–30, 2001.

Brown N, Burgess T, Forbes R, et al. 5q31.3 Microdeletion syndrome: Clinical and molecular characterization of two further cases. *Am J Med Genet* 161A: 2604–2608, 2013.

Brown S, Gersen S, Anyane-Yeboa K, Warburton D. Preliminary definition of a "critical region" of chromosome 13 in q32: Report of 14 cases with 13q deletions and review of the literature. *Am J Med Genet* 45: 52–59, 1993.

Brown S, Higgins S, Hutchinson R, Bain S, Moore L, Haan E. A case of mosaicism for trisomy of chromosome 5 detected at amniocentesis. *Twin Res Hum Genet* 12: 210, 2009.

Brun JL, Gangbo F, Wen ZQ, et al. Prenatal diagnosis and management of sex chromosome aneuploidy: A report on 98 cases. *Prenat Diagn* 24: 213–218, 2004.

Brun JL, Mangione R, Gangbo F, et al. Feasibility, accuracy and safety of chorionic villus sampling: A report of 10741 cases. *Prenat Diagn* 23: 295–301, 2003.

Brunetti-Pierri N, Paciorkowski AR, Ciccone R, et al. Duplications of *FOXG1* in 14q12 are associated with developmental epilepsy, mental retardation, and severe speech impairment. *Eur J Hum Genet* 19: 102–107, 2011.

Bruno DL, Beddow R, Caramins M, et al. Interpreting clinical microarray genomic data in 2012: What have we learnt and what challenges remain? *Current Topics Genet* 5: 67–79, 2012.

Bruno DL, White SM, Ganesamoorthy D, et al. Pathogenic aberrations revealed exclusively by single nucleotide polymorphism (SNP) genotyping data in 5000 samples tested by molecular karyotyping. *J Med Genet* 48: 831–839, 2011.

Bruns DA. Developmental status of 22 children with trisomy 18 and eight children with trisomy 13: Implications and recommendations. *Am J Med Genet* 167A: 1807–1815, 2015a.

Bruns D, Campbell E. Twenty-five additional cases of trisomy 9 mosaic: Birth information, medical conditions, and developmental status. *Am J Med Genet* 167A: 997–1007, 2015b.

Bruyère H, Robertson G, Wilson RD, Langlois S. Risk of mosaicism and uniparental disomy associated with the prenatal diagnosis of non homologous

Robertsonian translocation carrier. *Am J Hum Genet* 69: 208, 2001.

Bruyère H, Rupps R, Kuchinka BD, Friedman JM, Robinson WP. Recurrent trisomy 21 in a couple with a child presenting trisomy 21 mosaicism and maternal uniparental disomy for chromosome 21 in the euploid cell line. *Am J Med Genet* 94: 35–41, 2000.

Bruyère H, Speevak MD, Winsor EJ, et al. Isodicentric Yp: Prenatal diagnosis and outcome in 12 cases. *Prenat Diagn* 26: 324–329, 2006.

Bryan J, Peters M, Pritchard G, Healey S, Payton D. A second case of intrauterine growth retardation and primary hypospadias associated with a trisomy 22 placenta but with biparental inheritance of chromosome 22 in the fetus. *Prenat Diagn* 22: 137–140, 2002.

Bryant LD, Murray J, Green JM, Hewison J, Sehmi I, Ellis A. Descriptive information about Down syndrome: A content analysis of serum screening leaflets. *Prenat Diagn* 21: 1057–1063, 2001.

Bryman I, Sylvén L, Berntorp K, et al. Pregnancy rate and outcome in Swedish women with Turner syndrome. *Fertil Steril* 95: 2507–2510, 2011.

Brzustowicz LM, Allitto BA, Matseoane D, et al. Paternal isodisomy for chromosome 5 in a child with spinal muscular atrophy. *Am J Hum Genet* 54: 482–488, 1994.

Buckton KE, Newton MS, Collyer S, et al. Phenotypically normal individuals with an inversion (X) (p22q13) and the recombinant (X), dup q. *Ann Hum Genet* 45: 159–168, 1981.

Budowle B, Capt C, Chakraborty R, Ge J. Paternity calculations in a di-spermy case. *Int J Legal Med* 131: 339–343, 2017.

Bugge M, Collins A, Hertz JM, et al. Non-disjunction of chromosome 13. *Hum Mol Genet* 16: 2004–2010, 2007.

Bugge M, Collins A, Petersen MB, et al. Non-disjunction of chromosome 18. *Hum Mol Genet* 7: 661–669, 1998.

Bugge M, deLozier-Blanchet C, Bak M, et al. Trisomy 13 due to rea(13q;13q) is caused by i(13) and not rob(13;13)(q10;q10) in the majority of cases. *Am J Med Genet* 132A: 310–313, 2005.

Buiting K, Clayton-Smith J, Driscoll DJ, et al. Clinical utility gene card for: Angelman syndrome. *Eur J Hum Genet* 23: 2015.

Buiting K, Dittrich B, Gross S, et al. Sporadic imprinting defects in Prader-Willi syndrome and Angelman syndrome: Implications for imprint-switch models, genetic counseling, and prenatal diagnosis. *Am J Hum Genet* 63: 170–180, 1998.

Buiting K, Gross S, Lich C, Gillessen-Kaesbach G, el-Maarri O, Horsthemke B. Epimutations in Prader-Willi and Angelman syndromes: A molecular study of 136 patients with an imprinting defect. *Am J Hum Genet* 72: 571–577, 2003.

Bukovsky A, Caudle MR, Svetlikova M, Upadhyaya NB. Origin of germ cells and formation of new primary follicles in adult human ovaries. *Reprod Biol Endocrinol* 2: 20, 2004.

Bukvic N, Carri VD, Di Cosola ML, et al. Familial X;Y translocation with distinct phenotypic consequences: Characterization using FISH and array CGH. *Am J Med Genet* 152A: 1730–1734, 2010.

Bullman H, Lever M, Robinson DO, Mackay DJ, Holder SE, Wakeling EL. Mosaic maternal uniparental disomy of chromosome 11 in a patient with Silver-Russell syndrome. *J Med Genet* 45: 396–399, 2008.

Burgemeister AL, Daumiller E, Dietze-Armana I, et al. Continuing role for classical cytogenetics: Case report of a boy with ring syndrome caused by complete ring chromosome 4 and review of literature. *Am J Med Genet* 173A: 727–732, 2017.

Burgess T, Brown NJ, Stark Z, et al. Characterization of core clinical phenotypes associated with recurrent proximal 15q25.2 microdeletions. *Am J Med Genet* 164A: 2014, 77–86.

Burke LW, Wiley JE, Glenn CC, et al. Familial cryptic translocation resulting in Angelman syndrome: Implications for imprinting or location of the Angelman gene? *Am J Hum Genet* 58: 777–784, 1996.

Burn J, Baraitser M, Butler LJ. An avoidable recurrence of cri du chat syndrome in the next generation. *Br Med J* 287: 1287–1288, 1983.

Burnett AC, Reutens DC, Wood AG. Social cognition in Turner's syndrome. *J Clin Neurosci* 17: 283–286, 2010.

Burns JP, Koduru PR, Alonso ML, Chaganti RS. Analysis of meiotic segregation in a man heterozygous for two reciprocal translocations using the hamster in vitro penetration system. *Am J Hum Genet* 38: 954–964, 1986.

Burnside RD. 22q11.21 deletion syndromes: A review of proximal, central, and distal deletions and their associated features. *Cytogenet Genome Res* 146: 89–99, 2015.

Burnside RD, Lose EJ, Dominguez MG, et al. Molecular cytogenetic characterization of two cases with constitutional distal 11q duplication/triplication. *Am J Med Genet* 149A: 1516–1522, 2009.

Burnside RD, Pappas JG, Sacharow S, et al. Three cases of isolated terminal deletion of chromosome 8p without heart defects presenting with a mild phenotype. *Am J Med Genet* 161A: 822–828, 2013.

Burnside RD, Spudich L, Rush B, Kubendran S, Schaefer GB. Secondary complex chromosome rearrangement identified by chromosome analysis and FISH subsequent to detection of an unbalanced derivative chromosome 12 by SNP array analysis. *Cytogenet Genome Res* 142: 129–133, 2014.

Burrello N, Calogero AE, De Palma A, et al. Chromosome analysis of epididymal and testicular spermatozoa in patients with azoospermia. *Eur J Hum Genet* 10: 362–366, 2002.

Busche A, Graul-Neumann LM, Zweier C, Rauch A, Klopocki E, Horn D. Microdeletions of chromosome 7p21, including *TWIST1*, associated with significant microcephaly, facial dysmorphism, and short stature. *Eur J Med Genet* 54: 256–261, 2011.

Byers HM, Adam MP, LaCroix A, et al. Description of a new oncogenic mechanism for atypical teratoid rhabdoid tumors in patients with ring chromosome 22. *Am J Med Genet* 173A: 245–249, 2017.

Byrne J, Mulvihill JJ, Myers MH, et al. Effects of treatment on fertility in long-term survivors of childhood or adolescent cancer. *N Engl J Med* 317: 1315–1321, 1987.

Byrne J, Rasmussen SA, Steinhorn SC, et al. Genetic disease in offspring of long-term survivors of childhood and adolescent cancer. *Am J Hum Genet* 62: 45–52, 1998.

Cabrejo L, Guyant-Maréchal L, Laquerrière A, et al. Phenotype associated with APP duplication in five families. *Brain* 129: 2966–2976, 2006.

Cacciagli P, Haddad MR, Mignon-Ravix C, et al. Disruption of the *ATP8A2* gene in a patient with a t(10;13) de novo balanced translocation and a severe neurological phenotype. *Eur J Hum Genet* 18: 1360–1363, 2010.

Caer E, Perrin A, Douet-Guilbert N, Amice V, De Braekeleer M, Morel F. Differing mechanisms of meiotic segregation in spermatozoa from three carriers of a pericentric inversion of chromosome 8. *Fertil Steril* 89: 1637–1640, 2008.

Cafferkey M, Ahn JW, Flinter F, Ogilvie C. Phenotypic features in patients with 15q11.2(BP1-BP2) deletion: Further delineation of an emerging syndrome. *Am J Med Genet* 164A: 1916–1922, 2014.

Cai T, Yu P, Tagle DA, Lu D, Chen Y, Xia J. A de novo complex chromosomal rearrangement with a translocation 7;9 and 8q insertion in a male carrier with no infertility. *Hum Reprod* 16: 59–62, 2001.

Calhaz-Jorge C, de Geyter C, Kupka MS, et al. Assisted reproductive technology in Europe, 2012: Results generated from European registers by ESHRE. *Hum Reprod* 31: 1638–1652, 2016.

Callen DF, Eyre H, Fang YY, et al. Origins of accessory small ring marker chromosomes derived from chromosome 1. *J Med Genet* 36: 847–853, 1999.

Callen DF, Eyre HJ, Ringenbergs ML, Freemantle CJ, Woodroffe P, Haan EA. Chromosomal origin of small ring marker chromosomes in man: Characterization by molecular genetics. *Am J Hum Genet* 48: 769–782, 1991.

Callen DF, Sutherland GR. Normal female carrier and affected male half-sibs with t(X;5)(q13;p15): Location of a gene determining male genital development. *Clin Genet* 30: 59–62, 1986.

Callen DF, Sutherland GR, Carter RF. A fertile man with tdic(Y;22): How a stable neo-X1X2Y sex-determining mechanism could evolve in man. *Am J Med Genet Suppl* 3: 151–155, 1987.

Callen DF, Woollatt E, Sutherland GR. Paracentric inversions in man. *Clin Genet* 28: 87–92, 1985.

Callier P, Faivre L, Pigeonnat S, et al. Contribution of array CGH in prognosis and genetic counselling of prenatally diagnosed supernumerary ring chromosome 20. *Prenat Diagn* 29: 1002–1005, 2009.

Calounova G, Novotna D, Simandlova M, et al. Prader-Willi syndrome due to uniparental disomy in a patient with a balanced chromosomal translocation. *Neuro Endocrinol Lett* 27: 579–585, 2006.

Cammarata M, Di Simone P, Graziano L, Giuffre M, Corsello G, Garofalo G. Rare sex chromosome aneuploidies in humans: Report of six patients with 48,XXYY, 49,XXXXY, and 48,XXXX karyotypes. *Am J Med Genet* 85: 86–87, 1999.

Campbell IM, Yuan B, Robberecht C, et al. Parental somatic mosaicism is underrecognized and influences recurrence risk of genomic disorders. *Am J Hum Genet* 95: 173–182, 2014.

Campbell LE, McCabe KL, Melville JL, Strutt PA, Schall U. Social cognition dysfunction in adolescents with 22q11.2 deletion syndrome (velo-cardio-facial syndrome): Relationship with executive functioning and social competence/functioning. *J Intellect Disabil Res* 59: 845–859, 2015.

Canevini MP, Sgro V, Zuffardi O, et al. Chromosome 20 ring: A chromosomal disorder associated with a particular electroclinical pattern. *Epilepsia* 39: 942–951, 1998.

Cans C, Cohen O, Lavergne C, Mermet MA, Demongeot J, Jalbert P. Logistic regression model to estimate the risk of unbalanced offspring in reciprocal translocations. *Hum Genet* 92: 598–604, 1993.

Canto P, Söderlund D, Reyes E, Méndez JP. Mutations in the desert hedgehog (*DHH*) gene in patients with 46,XY complete pure gonadal dysgenesis. *J Clin Endocrinol Metab* 89: 4480–4483, 2004.

Canto P, Vilchis F, Söderlund D, Reyes E, Méndez JP. A heterozygous mutation in the desert hedgehog gene in patients with mixed gonadal dysgenesis. *Mol Hum Reprod* 11: 833–836, 2005.

Capalbo A, Sinibaldi L, Bernardini L, et al. Interstitial 4q deletion associated with a mosaic complementary supernumerary marker chromosome in prenatal diagnosis. *Prenat Diagn* 33: 782–796, 2013.

Capalbo A, Wright G, Elliott T, Ubaldi FM, Rienzi L, Nagy ZP. FISH reanalysis of inner cell mass and trophectoderm samples of previously array-CGH screened blastocysts shows high accuracy of diagnosis and no major diagnostic impact of mosaicism at the blastocyst stage. *Hum Reprod* 28: 2298–2307, 2013.

Capkova P, Misovicova N, Vrbicka D. Partial trisomy and tetrasomy of chromosome 21 without Down syndrome phenotype and short overview of genotype-phenotype correlation: A case report. *Biomed Pap Med Fac Univ Palacky Olomouc Czech Repub* 158: 321–325, 2014.

Capo-Chichi JM, Bharti SK, Sommers JA, et al. Identification and biochemical characterization of a novel mutation in *DDX11* causing Warsaw breakage syndrome. *Hum Mutat* 34: 103–107, 2013.

Carbone JF, Tuuli MG, Dicke JM, Macones GA, Odibo AO. Revisiting the risk for aneuploidy in fetuses with isolated pyelectasis. *Prenat Diagn* 31: 566–570, 2011.

Cardoso LCA, Moraes L, Camilo MJE, et al. Cytogenetic and molecular studies of an X;21 translocation previously diagnosed as complete monosomy 21. *Eur J Med Genet* 51: 588–597, 2008.

Carella M, Spreafico F, Palumbo O, et al. Constitutional ring chromosome 11 mosaicism in a Wilms tumor patient: Cytogenetic, molecular and clinico-pathological studies. *Am J Med Genet* 152A: 1756–1763, 2010.

Carey JC. Trisomy 18 and 13 syndromes. In Cassidy SB, Allanson JE (eds.), *Management of Genetic Syndromes*. Hoboken, NJ: Wiley-Blackwell, 2010.

Carey JC. Perspectives on the care and management of infants with trisomy 18 and trisomy 13: striving for balance. *Curr Opin Pediatr* 24: 672–678, 2012.

Carey JC, Viskochil DH. Status of the human malformation map: 2007. *Am J Med Genet* 143A: 2868–2885, 2007.

Carey L, Scott F, Murphy K, et al. Prenatal diagnosis of chromosomal mosaicism in over 1600 cases

using array comparative genomic hybridization as a first line test. *Prenat Diagn* 34: 478–486, 2014a.

Carey L, Traversa MV, Wright DC, McArthur SJ, Leigh DA. Identification of a jumping translocation following pre-implantation genetic diagnosis. *Am J Med Genet* 164A: 279–281, 2014b.

Carmany EP, Bawle EV. Microduplication of 4p16.3 due to an unbalanced translocation resulting in a mild phenotype. *Am J Med Genet* 155A: 819–824, 2011.

Carmichael H, Shen Y, Nguyen TT, Hirschhorn JN, Dauber A. Whole exome sequencing in a patient with uniparental disomy of chromosome 2 and a complex phenotype. *Clin Genet* 84: 213–222, 2013.

Carothers AD, Castilla EE, Dutra MG, Hook EB. Search for ethnic, geographic, and other factors in the epidemiology of Down syndrome in South America: Analysis of data from the ECLAMC project, 1967–1997. *Am J Med Genet* 103: 149–156, 2001.

Carothers AD, Hecht CA, Hook EB. International variation in reported livebirth prevalence rates of Down syndrome, adjusted for maternal age. *J Med Genet* 36: 386–393, 1999.

Carp H, Toder V, Aviram A, Daniely M, Mashiach S, Barkai G. Karyotype of the abortus in recurrent miscarriage. *Fertil Steril* 75: 678–682, 2001.

Carrera IA, de Zaldívar MS, Martín R, Begemann M, Soellner L, Eggermann T. Microdeletions of the 7q32.2 imprinted region are associated with Silver-Russell syndrome features. *Am J Med Genet* 170A: 743–749, 2016.

Carter E, Heard P, Hasi M, et al. Ring 18 molecular assessment and clinical consequences. *Am J Med Genet* 167A: 54–63, 2015.

Carter MT, Barrowman NJ, St Pierre SA, Emanuel BS, Boycott KM. Risk of breast cancer not increased in translocation 11;22 carriers: Analysis of 80 pedigrees. *Am J Med Genet* 152A: 212–214, 2010.

Carter MT, St. Pierre SA, Zackai EH, Emanuel BS, Boycott KM. Phenotypic delineation of Emanuel syndrome (supernumerary derivative 22 syndrome): Clinical features of 63 individuals. *Am J Med Genet* 149A: 1712–1721, 2009.

Carvalheira G, Oliveira MM, Takeno S, Lima FT, Meloni VA, Melaragno MI. 19q13.33→qter trisomy in a girl with intellectual impairment and seizures. *Meta Gene* 2: 799–806, 2014.

Carvalho CMB, Lupski JR. Mechanisms underlying structural variant formation in genomic disorders. *Nat Rev Genet* 17: 224–238, 2016.

Carvalho CMB, Vasanth S, Shinawi M, et al. Dosage changes of a segment at 17p13.1 lead to intellectual disability and microcephaly as a result of complex genetic interaction of multiple genes. *Am J Hum Genet* 95: 565–578, 2014.

Carvalho CMB, Zhang F, Lupski JR. Evolution in health and medicine Sackler colloquium: Genomic disorders—A window into human gene and genome evolution. *Proc Natl Acad Sci USA* 107 (Suppl 1): 1765–1771, 2010.

Casper AM, Durkin SG, Arlt MF, Glover TW. Chromosomal instability at common fragile sites in Seckel syndrome. *Am J Hum Genet* 75: 654–660, 2004.

Cassidy SB, Allanson JE (eds.). *Management of Genetic Syndromes.* Hoboken, NJ: Wiley-Blackwell, 2010.

Cassidy SB, Forsythe M, Heeger S, et al. Comparison of phenotype between patients with Prader-Willi syndrome due to deletion 15q and uniparental disomy 15. *Am J Med Genet* 68: 433–440, 1997.

Cassidy SB, Lai LW, Erickson RP, et al. Trisomy 15 with loss of the paternal 15 as a cause of Prader-Willi syndrome due to maternal disomy. *Am J Hum Genet* 51: 701–708, 1992.

Cassidy SB, Whitworth T, Sanders D, Lorber CA, Engel E. Five month extrauterine survival in a female triploid (69,XXX) child. *Ann Génét* 20: 277–279, 1977.

Castanet M, Mallya U, Agostini M, et al. Maternal isodisomy for chromosome 9 causing homozygosity for a novel *FOXE1* mutation in syndromic congenital hypothyroidism. *J Clin Endocrinol Metab* 95: 4031–4036, 2010.

Castella M, Pujol R, Callén E, et al. Chromosome fragility in patients with Fanconi anaemia: Diagnostic implications and clinical impact. *J Med Genet* 48: 242–250, 2011.

Castiglia D, Castori M, Pisaneschi E, et al. Trisomic rescue causing reduction to homozygosity for a novel *ABCA12* mutation in harlequin ichthyosis. *Clin Genet* 76: 392–397, 2009.

Castiglione A, Guaran V, Astolfi L, et al. Karyotype-phenotype correlation in partial trisomies of the short arm of chromosome 6: A family case report and review of the literature. *Cytogenet Genome Res* 141: 243–259, 2013.

Castillo A, Kramer N, Schwartz CE, et al. 19q13.32 microdeletion syndrome: Three new cases. *Eur J Med Genet* 57: 654–658, 2014.

Castorina P, Selicorni A, Bedeschi F, Dalpra L, Larizza L. Genotype-phenotype correlation in two sets of monozygotic twins with Williams syndrome. *Am J Med Genet* 69: 107–111, 1997.

Castronovo C, Rossetti R, Rusconi D, et al. Gene dosage as a relevant mechanism contributing to the determination of ovarian function in Turner syndrome. *Hum Reprod* 29: 368–379, 2014.

Castronovo P, Gervasini C, Cereda A, et al. Premature chromatid separation is not a useful diagnostic marker for Cornelia de Lange syndrome. *Chromosome Res* 17: 763–771, 2009.

Catelani ALPM, Krepischi ACV, Kim CA, et al. Chromosome imbalances in syndromic hearing loss. *Clin Genet* 76: 458–464, 2009.

Caubit X, Gubellini P, Andrieux J, et al. TSHZ3 deletion causes an autism syndrome and defects in cortical projection neurons. *Nat Genet* 48: 1359–1369, 2016.

Causio F, Fischetto R, Leonetti T, Schonauer LM. Ovarian stimulation in a woman with premature ovarian failure and X-autosome translocation: A case report. *J Reprod Med* 45: 235–239, 2000.

Causio F, Fischetto R, Schonauer LM, Leonetti T. Intracytoplasmic sperm injection in infertile patients with structural cytogenetic abnormalities. *J Reprod Med* 44: 859–864, 1999.

Cavadino A, Morris JK. Revised estimates of the risk of fetal loss following a prenatal diagnosis of trisomy 13 or trisomy 18. *Am J Med Genet* 173A: 953–958, 2017.

Ceccarini C, Sinibaldi L, Bernardini L, et al. Duplication 18q21.31-q22.2. *Am J Med Genet* 143A: 343–348, 2007.

Celep F, Karagüzel A, Ozeren M, Bozkaya H. The frequency of chromosomal abnormalities in patients with reproductive failure. *Eur J Obstet Gynecol Reprod Biol* 127: 106–109, 2006.

Cellini E, Disciglio V, Novara F, et al. Periventricular heterotopia with white matter abnormalities associated with 6p25 deletion. *Am J Med Genet* 158A: 1793–1797, 2012.

Cesaretti C, Spaccini L, Righini A, et al. Prenatal detection of 5q14.3 duplication including *MEF2C* and brain phenotype. *Am J Med Genet* 170A: 1352–1357, 2016.

Cetin Z, Mihci E, Yakut S, Keser I, Karauzum SB, Luleci G. Pure and complete 12p trisomy due to a maternal centric fission of chromosome 12. *Am J Med Genet* 155A: 349–352, 2011.

Chan CTJ, Clayton-Smith J, Cheng XJ, et al. Molecular mechanisms in Angelman syndrome: A survey of 93 patients. *J Med Genet* 30: 895–902, 1993.

Chance PF. Inherited focal, episodic neuropathies: hereditary neuropathy with liability to pressure palsies and hereditary neuralgic amyotrophy. *Neuromolecular Med* 8: 159–174, 2006.

Chang HJ, Clark RD, Bachman H. The phenotype of 45,X/46,XY mosaicism: An analysis of 92 prenatally diagnosed cases. *Am J Hum Genet* 46: 156–167, 1990.

Chang LW, Chen PY, Kuo PL, Chang FM. Prenatal diagnosis of a fetus with megacystis and monosomy 21. *Prenat Diagn* 21: 512–513, 2001.

Chang PL, Sauer MV, Brown S. Y chromosome microdeletion in a father and his four infertile sons. *Hum Reprod* 14: 2689–2694, 1999.

Chang YS, Owen JP, Pojman NJ, et al. Reciprocal white matter alterations due to 16p11.2 chromosomal deletions versus duplications. *Hum Brain Mapp* 37: 2833–2848, 2016.

Chantot-Bastaraud S, Ravel C, Berthaut I, et al. Sperm-FISH analysis in a pericentric chromosome 1 inversion, 46,XY,inv(1)(p22q42), associated with infertility. *Mol Hum Reprod* 13: 55–59, 2007.

Chantot-Bastaraud S, Stratmann S, Brioude F, et al. Formation of upd(7)mat by trisomic rescue: SNP array typing provides new insights in chromosomal nondisjunction. *Mol Cytogenet* 10: 28, 2017.

Chatzimichali EA, Brent S, Hutton B, et al. Facilitating collaboration in rare genetic disorders through effective matchmaking in DECIPHER. *Hum Mutat* 36: 941–949, 2015.

Check JH, Katsoff B, Summers-Chase D, Breitbart J. A case report supporting the concept that some women have a predisposition for maternal meiosis errors resulting in digyny. *Clin Exp Obstet Gynecol* 36: 133–134, 2009.

Cheffins T, Chan A, Haan EA, et al. The impact of maternal serum screening on the birth prevalence of Down's syndrome and the use of amniocentesis and chorionic villus sampling in South Australia. *Br J Obstet Gynaecol* 107: 1453–1459, 2000.

Chen CL, Gilbert TJ, Daling JR. Maternal smoking and Down syndrome: The confounding effect of maternal age. *Am J Epidemiol* 149: 442–446, 1999a.

Chen CP, Chang SJ, Chern SR, et al. Rapid diagnosis of pseudomosaicism in a case of level II mosaicism for trisomy 5 in a single colony from an in situ culture of amniocytes and a review of mosaic trisomy 5 at amniocentesis. *Taiwan J Obstet Gynecol* 55: 602–603, 2016a.

Chen CP, Chang TY, Guo WY, et al. Chromosome 17p13.3 deletion syndrome: aCGH characterization, prenatal findings and diagnosis, and literature review. *Gene* 532: 152–159, 2013a.

Chen CP, Chen CY, Chern SR, et al. Molecular cytogenetic characterization of Xp22.32→pter deletion and Xq26.3→qter duplication in a male fetus associated with 46,Y,rec(X)dup(Xq) inv(X) (p22.3q26.3), a hypoplastic left heart, short

stature, and maternal X chromosome pericentric inversion. *Taiwan J Obstet Gynecol* 55: 705–711, 2016b.

Chen CP, Chen M, Su YN, et al. Mosaic small supernumerary marker chromosome 1 at amniocentesis: Prenatal diagnosis, molecular genetic analysis and literature review. *Gene* 529: 169–175, 2013b.

Chen CP, Chen YY, Chern SR, et al. Prenatal diagnosis of mosaic trisomy 2 associated with abnormal maternal serum screening, oligohydramnios, intrauterine growth restriction, ventricular septal defect, preaxial polydactyly, and facial dysmorphism. *Taiwan J Obstet Gynecol* 52: 395–400, 2013c.

Chen CP, Chern SR, Chen LF, Chen WL, Wang W. Prenatal diagnosis of low-level mosaic trisomy 7 by amniocentesis. *Prenat Diagn* 25: 1067–1069, 2005a.

Chen CP, Chern SR, Lee CC, Chang TY, Wang W, Tzen CY. Clinical, cytogenetic, and molecular findings of prenatally diagnosed mosaic trisomy 4. *Prenat Diagn* 24: 38–44, 2004a.

Chen CP, Chern SR, Lee CC, Chen WL, Wang W. Prenatal diagnosis of interstitially satellited 6p. *Prenat Diagn* 24: 430–433, 2004b.

Chen CP, Chern SR, Lee CC, et al. Prenatal diagnosis of de novo t(2;18;14)(q33.1;q12.2;q31.2), dup(5) (q34q34), del(7)(p21.1p21.1), and del(10) (q25.3q25.3) and a review of the prenatally ascertained de novo apparently balanced complex and multiple chromosomal rearrangements. *Prenat Diagn* 26: 138–146, 2006a.

Chen CP, Chern SR, Lee CC, Town DD. Isochromosome 18q in a fetus with congenital megacystis, intra-uterine growth retardation and cloacal dysgenesis sequence. *Prenat Diagn* 18: 1068–1074, 1998.

Chen CP, Chern SR, Lee PY, Town DD, Wang W. Prenatal diagnosis of low-level mosaic trisomy 6 by amniocentesis. *Prenat Diagn* 26: 1093–1096, 2006b.

Chen CP, Chern SR, Sheu JC, et al. Prenatal diagnosis, sonographic findings and molecular genetic analysis of a 46,XX/46,XY true hermaphrodite chimera. *Prenat Diagn* 25: 502–506, 2005b.

Chen CP, Chern SR, Town DD, Wang W, Liao YW. Fetoplacental and fetoamniotic chromosomal discrepancies in prenatally detected mosaic trisomy 9. *Prenat Diagn* 23: 1019–1021, 2003a.

Chen CP, Hwu YM, Yeh LF, Chern SR, Lee CC, Wang W. Successful triplet pregnancy and delivery after oocyte donation in an infertile female with chromosome mosaicism for monosomy X, partial trisomy X, and terminal Xp deletion. *Fertil Steril* 79: 1231–1233, 2003b.

Chen CP, Ko TM, Chern SR, et al. Prenatal diagnosis of low-level mosaicism for trisomy 2 associated with a favorable pregnancy outcome. *Taiwan J Obstet Gynecol* 55: 303–304, 2016c.

Chen CP, Lee CC, Chen WL, Wang W, Tzen CY. Prenatal diagnosis of premature centromere division-related mosaic variegated aneuploidy. *Prenat Diagn* 24: 19–25, 2004c.

Chen CP, Lee CC, Town DD, et al. Detection of euchromatic variants and unusual C band heterochromatin variants at genetic amniocentesis. *Genet Couns* 17: 91–95, 2006c.

Chen CP, Lee CC, Wang W. Prenatal diagnosis of complete trisomy 16q in two consecutive pregnancies. *Prenat Diagn* 24: 928–929, 2004d.

Chen CP, Lin SP, Lin CC, et al. Prenatal diagnosis of low-level mosaicism for a small XIST-negative supernumerary ring X chromosome in a nondysmorphic male fetus. *Prenat Diagn* 26: 387–391, 2006d.

Chen CP, Lin SP, Sheu JC, Wang W, Tzen CY. Neonatal outcome of a prenatally detected 46,XX/46,XY true hermaphrodite. *Prenat Diagn* 26: 185–186, 2006e.

Chen CP, Lin SP, Tsai FJ, Wang TH, Chern SR, Wang W. Characterization of a de novo unbalanced Y;autosome translocation in a 45,X mentally retarded male and literature review. *Fertil Steril* 90: 1198, e11–18, 2008.

Chen CP, Lin YH, Au HK, et al. Chromosome 15q overgrowth syndrome: Prenatal diagnosis, molecular cytogenetic characterization, and perinatal findings in a fetus with dup(15) (q26.2q26.3). *Taiwan J Obstet Gynecol* 50: 359–365, 2011a.

Chen CP, Su YN, Chen YT, Chen WL, Hsu LJ, Wang W. Prenatal diagnosis of directly transmitted benign 4q12-q13.1 quadruplication associated with tandem segmental amplifications of the *LPHN3* gene. *Taiwan J Obstet Gynecol* 50: 401–404, 2011b.

Chen CP, Su YN, Lin CC, et al. Genetic counseling of prenatally detected unbalanced t(Y;15)(q12;p13). *Genet Couns* 18: 455–457, 2007a.

Chen CP, Su YN, Lin SP, et al. Prenatal diagnosis and molecular cytogenetic characterization of a de novo interstitial duplication of 11q (11q22.3→q23.3) associated with abnormal maternal serum biochemistry. *Taiwan J Obstet Gynecol* 52: 120–124, 2013d.

Chen CP, Wang KG, Ko TM, et al. Mosaic trisomy 14 at amniocentesis: Prenatal diagnosis and literature review. *Taiwan J Obstet Gynecol* 52: 446–449, 2013e.

Chen CP, Wang LK, Chern SR, et al. Mosaic trisomy 17 at amniocentesis: Prenatal diagnosis, molecular genetic analysis, and literature review. *Taiwan J Obstet Gynecol* 55: 712–717, 2016d.

Chen CP, Wang YL, Chern SR, et al. Prenatal diagnosis and molecular cytogenetic characterization of low-level true mosaicism for trisomy 21 using uncultured amniocytes. *Taiwan J Obstet Gynecol* 55: 285–287, 2016e.

Chen E, Choe MA, Loughman WD, et al. Recurrent adjacent-2 segregation of a familial t(14;21) (q11.2;q11.2): phenotypic comparison of two brothers and a paternal aunt inheriting the der(14). *Am J Med Genet* 132A: 164–170, 2005c.

Chen H, Young R, Mu X, et al. Uniparental isodisomy resulting from 46,XX,i(1p),i(1q) in a woman with short stature, ptosis, micro/retrognathia, myopathy, deafness, and sterility. *Am J Med Genet* 82: 215–218, 1999b.

Chen K, Chmait RH, Vanderbilt D, Wu S, Randolph L. Chimerism in monochorionic dizygotic twins: Case study and review. *Am J Med Genet* 161A: 1817–1824, 2013f.

Chen M, Yeh GP, Shih JC, Wang BT. Trisomy 13 mosaicism: Study of serial cytogenetic changes in a case from early pregnancy to infancy. *Prenat Diagn* 24: 137–143, 2004e.

Chen SH, Escudero T, Cekleniak NA, Sable DB, Garrisi MG, Munne S. Patterns of ovarian response to gonadotropin stimulation in female carriers of balanced translocation. *Fertil Steril* 83: 1504–1509, 2005d.

Chen Y, Huang J, Liu P, Qiao J. Analysis of meiotic segregation patterns and interchromosomal effects in sperm from six males with Robertsonian translocations. *J Assist Reprod Genet* 24: 406–411, 2007b.

Chen Z, Chen RB, Qiu RZ, Du RF, Lo WHY. Chinese geneticists are far from eugenics movement. *Am J Hum Genet* 65: 1199, 1999.

Chenevix-Trench G, Spurdle AB, Gatei M, et al. Dominant negative ATM mutations in breast cancer families. *J Natl Cancer Inst* 94: 205–215, 2002.

Cheng A, Dinulos MBP, Neufeld-Kaiser W, et al. 6q25.1 (*TAB2*) microdeletion syndrome: Congenital heart defects and cardiomyopathy. *Am J Med Genet* 173A: 1848–1857, 2017.

Cheng DH, Tan YQ, Di YF, Li LY, Lu GX. Crypt Y chromosome fragment resulting from an X;Y translocation in a patient with premature ovarian failure. *Fertil Steril* 92: 828, e3–6, 2009.

Cheng EY, Chen YJ, Disteche CM, Gartler SM. Analysis of a paracentric inversion in human oocytes: Nonhomologous pairing in pachytene. *Hum Genet* 105: 191–196, 1999.

Cheng SF, Rauen KA, Pinkel D, Albertson DG, Cotter PD. Xq chromosome duplication in males: Clinical, cytogenetic and array CGH characterization of a new case and review. *Am J Med Genet* 135A: 308–313, 2005.

Chen-Shtoyerman R, Josefsberg Ben-Yehoshua S, Nissani R, Rosensaft J, Appelman Z. A prevalent Y;15 translocation in the Ethiopian Beta Israel community in Israel. *Cytogenet Genome Res* 136: 171–174, 2012.

Chetaille P, Preuss C, Burkhard S, et al. Mutations in *SGOL1* cause a novel cohesinopathy affecting heart and gut rhythm. *Nat Genet* 46: 1245–1249, 2014.

Chia N, Bousfield L, James S, Nelson J. Report of a severely retarded child with a duplication 18q derived from a paternal paracentric inversion (18q): A note of warning. *Bull Hum Genet Soc Australasia* 6: 48, 1992.

Chia N, Daniel A, Malafiej P, Clarke N, Ades L. A child with a deletion 2q37 found to be a recombinant of a cryptic pericentric inversion: Implications for phenotype and risk of recurrence. *Bull Hum Genet Soc Australasia* 14: 29, 2001.

Chia NL. In ISCN 2016: An international system for human cytogenomic nomenclature, McGowan-Jordan J, Simons A, Schmid M (eds.). *Cytogenet Genome Res* 149 (1–2), 2016.

Chiesa J, Hoffet M, Rousseau O, et al. Pallister-Killian syndrome [i(12p)]: First pre-natal diagnosis using cordocentesis in the second trimester confirmed by in situ hybridization. *Clin Genet* 54: 294–302, 1998.

Chisholm CA, Bray MJ, Karns LB. Successful pregnancy in a woman with Bloom syndrome. *Am J Med Genet* 102: 136–138, 2001.

Cho E, Yang TH, Shin ES, Byeon JH, Kim GH, Eun BL. Saethre-Chotzen syndrome with an atypical phenotype: Identification of *TWIST* microdeletion by array CGH. *Childs Nerv Syst* 29: 2101–2104, 2013a.

Cho SY, Goh DL, Lau KC, Ong HT, Lam CW. Microarray analysis unmasked paternal uniparental disomy of chromosome 12 in a patient with isolated sulfite oxidase deficiency. *Clin Chim Acta* 426: 13–17, 2013b.

Cho SY, Ki CS, Jang JH, et al. Familial Xp22.33-Xp22.12 deletion delineated by chromosomal microarray analysis causes proportionate short stature. *Am J Med Genet* 158A: 1462–1466 2012.

Choi J, Lee H, Lee CG. Partial trisomy of 11q23.3-q25 inherited from a maternal low-level mosaic unbalanced translocation. *Am J Med Genet* 167A: 1859–1864, 2015.

Choufani S, Shapiro JS, Susiarjo M, et al. A novel approach identifies new differentially methylated regions (DMRs) associated with imprinted genes. *Genome Res* 21: 465–476, 2011.

Chowdhury S, Bandholz AM, Parkash S, et al. Phenotypic and molecular characterization of 19q12q13.1 deletions: A report of five patients. *Am J Med Genet* 164A: 62–69, 2014.

Christian SM, Koehn D, Pillay R, MacDougall A, Wilson RD. Parental decisions following prenatal diagnosis of sex chromosome aneuploidy: A trend over time. *Prenat Diagn* 20: 37–40, 2000.

Chu C, Schwartz S, McPherson E. Paternal uniparental isodisomy for chromosome 14 in a patient with a normal 46,XY karyotype. *Am J Med Genet* 127A: 167–171, 2004.

Chuang L, Wakui K, Sue WC, Su MH, Shaffer LG, Kuo PL. Interstitial deletion 11(p11.12p11.2) and analphoid marker formation results in inherited Potocki-Shaffer syndrome. *Am J Med Genet* 133A: 180–183, 2005.

Chudley AE, Bauder F, Ray M, McAlpine PJ, Pena SD, Hamerton JL. Familial mental retardation in a family with an inherited chromosome rearrangement. *J Med Genet* 11: 353–366, 1974.

Chung D, Haynes K, Haynes R. Surviving with trisomy 13: Provider and parent perspectives and the role of the pediatric palliative care program. *Am J Med Genet* 173A: 813–815, 2017.

Ciaccio C, Tucci A, Scuvera G, Estienne M, Esposito S, Milani D. 16p13 microduplication without CREBBP involvement: Moving toward a phenotype delineation. *Eur J Med Genet* 60: 159–162, 2017.

Cifuentes P, Navarro J, Míguez L, Egozcue J, Benet J. Sperm segregation analysis of a complex chromosome rearrangement, 2;22;11, by whole chromosome painting. *Cytogenet Cell Genet* 82: 204–209, 1998.

Cignini P, Dinatale A, D'Emidio L, et al. Prenatal diagnosis of a fetus with de novo supernumerary ring chromosome 16 characterized by array comparative genomic hybridization. *AJP Rep* 1: 29–32, 2011.

Ciocca L, Digilio MC, Lombardo A, et al. Hypoplastic left heart syndrome and 21q22.3 deletion. *Am J Med Genet* 167A: 579–586, 2015.

Cirigliano V, Voglino G, Ordoñez E, et al. Rapid prenatal diagnosis of common chromosome aneuploidies by QF-PCR: Results of 9 years of clinical experience. *Prenat Diagn* 29: 40–49, 2009.

Cirillo E, Giardino G, Gallo V, et al. Intergenerational and intrafamilial phenotypic variability in 22q11.2 deletion syndrome subjects. *BMC Med Genet* 15: 1, 2014.

Cirillo E, Romano R, Romano A, et al. De novo 13q12.3-q14.11 deletion involving *BRCA2* gene in a patient with developmental delay, elevated IgM levels, transient ataxia, and cerebellar hypoplasia, mimicking an A-T like phenotype. *Am J Med Genet* 158A: 2571–2576, 2012.

Città S, Buono S, Greco D, et al. 3q29 microdeletion syndrome: Cognitive and behavioral phenotype in four patients. *Am J Med Genet* 161A: 3018–3022, 2013.

Ciuladaite Z, Preiksaitiene E, Utkus A, Kucinskas V. Relatives with opposite chromosome constitutions, rec(10)dup(10p)inv(10) (p15.1q26.12) and rec(10)dup(10q)inv(10) (p15.1q26.12), due to a familial pericentric inversion. *Cytogenet Genome Res* 144: 109–113, 2014.

Clarke A. The genetic testing of children: Working Party of the Clinical Genetics Society (UK). *J Med Genet* 31: 785–797, 1994.

Clayton EW. Removing the shadow of the law from the debate about genetic testing of children. *Am J Med Genet* 57: 630–634, 1995.

Clayton-Smith J, Giblin C, Smith RA, Dunn C, Willatt L. Familial 3q29 microdeletion syndrome providing further evidence of involvement of the 3q29 region in bipolar disorder. *Clin Dysmorphol* 19: 128–132, 2010

Clayton-Smith J, Laan L. Angelman syndrome: A review of the clinical and genetic aspects. *J Med Genet* 40: 87–95, 2003.

Cleary-Goldman J, D'Alton ME, Berkowitz RL. Prenatal diagnosis and multiple pregnancy. *Semin Perinatol* 29: 312–320, 2005.

Clement SC, Peeters RP, Ronckers CM, et al. Intermediate and long-term adverse effects of radioiodine therapy for differentiated thyroid carcinoma—A systematic review. *Cancer Treat Rev* 41: 925–934, 2015.

Clement Wilson S, Susman M, Bain S, et al. Isochromosome 5p mosaicism at prenatal diagnosis: Observations and outcomes in six cases at chorionic villus sampling and one at amniocentesis. *Prenat Diagn* 22: 681–685, 2002.

Clouston HJ, Herbert M, Fenwick J, Murdoch AP, Wolstenholme J. Cytogenetic analysis of human blastocysts. *Prenat Diagn* 22: 1143–1152, 2002.

Cobben JM, Engelen M, Polstra A. Array CGH on unstimulated blood does not detect all cases of Pallister-Killian syndrome: Buccal smear analysis should remain the diagnostic procedure of first choice. *Am J Med Genet* 161A: 1517–1519, 2013.

Cobben JM, Verheij JBGM, Eisma WH, et al. Bilateral split hand/foot malformation and inv(7) (p22q21.3). *J Med Genet* 32: 375–378, 1995.

Cobben JM, Weiss MM, van Dijk FS, et al. A de novo mutation in *ZMYND11*, a candidate gene for 10p15.3 deletion syndrome, is associated with syndromic intellectual disability. *Eur J Med Genet* 57: 636–638, 2014.

Cockwell AE, Baker SJ, Connarty M, Moore IE, Crolla JA. Mosaic trisomy 6 and maternal uniparental disomy 6 in a 23-week gestation fetus with atrioventricular septal defect. *Am J Med Genet* 140: 624–627, 2006.

Cockwell AE, James RS, Moore IE, Hatchwell E, Crolla JA. Clinical outcomes of adjacent 1 segregation in a familial translocation t(8;18) (p21.3;p11.23). *J Med Genet* 33: 515–517, 1996.

Codina-Pascual M, Oliver-Bonet M, Navarro J, et al. FISH characterization of a dicentric Yq (p11.32) isochromosome in an azoospermic male. *Am J Med Genet* 127A: 302–306, 2004.

Cody JD, Hasi M, Soileau B, et al. Establishing a reference group for distal 18q-: Clinical description and molecular basis. *Hum Genet* 133: 199–209, 2014.

Cody JD, Sebold C, Heard P, et al. Consequences of chromosome 18q deletions. *Am J Med Genet* 169C: 265–280, 2015.

Coe BP, Girirajan S, Eichler EE. A genetic model for neurodevelopmental disease. *Curr Opin Neurobiol* 22: 829–836, 2012.

Coe BP, Witherspoon K, Rosenfeld JA, et al. Refining analyses of copy number variation identifies specific genes associated with developmental delay. *Nat Genet* 46: 1063–1071, 2014.

Cohen MM. *The Child with Multiple Birth Defects* (2nd ed.). New York, NY: Oxford University Press, 1997.

Cohen O, Cans C, Mermet MA, Demongeot J, Jalbert P. Viability thresholds for partial trisomies and monosomies: A study of 1,159 viable unbalanced reciprocal translocations. *Hum Genet* 93: 188–194, 1994.

Cohen O, Simonet M, Cans C, et al. Human reciprocal translocations: A new computer system for genetic counseling. *Ann Génét* 35: 193–201, 1992.

Coles K, Mackenzie M, Crolla J, et al. A complex rearrangement associated with sex reversal and the Wolf-Hirschhorn syndrome: A cytogenetic and molecular study. *J Med Genet* 29: 400–406, 1992.

Collins VR, Muggli EE, Riley M, Palma S, Halliday JL. Is Down syndrome a disappearing birth defect? *J Pediatr* 152: 20–24, 24.e1, 2008.

Collins VR, Webley C, Sheffield LJ, Halliday JL. Fetal outcome and maternal morbidity after early amniocentesis. *Prenat Diagn* 18: 767–772, 1998.

Collinson MN, Fisher AM, Walker J, Currie J, Williams L, Roberts P. Inv(10)(p11.2q21.2), a variant chromosome. *Hum Genet* 101: 175–180, 1997.

Collinson MN, Roberts SE, Crolla JA, Dennis NR. A familial balanced inverted insertion ins(15)(q15q13q11.2) producing Prader-Willi syndrome, Angelman syndrome and duplication of 15q11.2-q13 in a single family: Importance of differentiation from a paracentric inversion. *Am J Med Genet* 126A: 27–32, 2004.

Coman DJ, Gardner RJM. Deletions that reveal recessive genes. *Eur J Hum Genet* 15: 1103–1104, 2007.

Coman D, Gardner RJM, Pertile MD, Kannu P. Trisomy 16 mosaicism at chorionic villus sampling and amniocentesis with a normal physical and intellectual outcome. *Fetal Diagn Ther* 28: 117–118, 2010a.

Coman D, Yaplito-Lee J, La P, et al. Three Mendelian disorders (chronic granulomatous disease, retinitis pigmentosa, ornithine transcarbamylase deficiency) in a young woman with an X chromosome deletion, del(X)(p11.4p21.1). *Mol Genet Metab* 99: 329, 2010b.

Conlin LK, Kramer W, Hutchinson AL, et al. Molecular analysis of ring chromosome 20 syndrome reveals two distinct groups of patients. *J Med Genet* 48: 1–9, 2011.

Conlin LK, Thiel BD, Bonnemann CG, et al. Mechanisms of mosaicism, chimerism and uniparental disomy identified by single nucleotide polymorphism array analysis. *Hum Mol Genet* 19: 1263–1275, 2010.

Conn CM, Cozzi J, Harper JC, Winston RM, Delhanty JD. Preimplantation genetic diagnosis for couples at high risk of Down syndrome pregnancy owing to parental translocation or mosaicism. *J Med Genet* 36: 45–50, 1999.

Conn CM, Harper JC, Winston RM, Delhanty JD. Infertile couples with Robertsonian translocations: Preimplantation genetic analysis of embryos reveals chaotic cleavage divisions. *Hum Genet* 102: 117–123, 1998.

Connerton-Moyer KJ, Nicholls RD, Schwartz S, et al. Unexpected familial recurrence in Angelman syndrome. *Am J Med Genet* 70: 253–260, 1997.

Conover HN, Argueso JL. Contrasting mechanisms of de novo copy number mutagenesis suggest the existence of different classes of environmental copy number mutagens. *Environ Mol Mutagen* 57: 3–9, 2016.

Conrad DF, Pinto D, Redon R, et al. Origins and functional impact of copy number variation in the human genome. *Nature* 464: 704–712, 2010.

Conte RA, Kleyman SM, Kharode C, Verma RS. Delineation of a ring chromosome 16 by the FISH-technique: A case report with review. *Clin Genet* 51: 196–199, 1997.

Conti V, Pantaleo M, Barba C, et al. Focal dysplasia of the cerebral cortex and infantile spasms associated with somatic 1q21.1-q44 duplication including the AKT3 gene. *Clin Genet* 88: 241–247, 2015.

Cools M, Drop SL, Wolffenbuttel KP, Oosterhuis JW, Looijenga LH. Germ cell tumors in the intersex gonad: Old paths, new directions, moving frontiers. *Endocr Rev* 27: 468–484, 2006.

Coonen E, Martini E, Dumoulin JC, et al. Preimplantation genetic diagnosis of a reciprocal translocation t(3;11)(q27.3;q24.3) in siblings. *Mol Hum Reprod* 6: 199–206, 2000.

Cooper GM, Coe BP, Girirajan S, et al. A copy number variation morbidity map of developmental delay. *Nat Genet* 43: 838–846, 2011.

Coppinger J, Alliman S, Lamb AN, Torchia BS, Bejjani BA, Shaffer LG. Whole-genome microarray analysis in prenatal specimens identifies clinically significant chromosome alterations without increase in results of unclear significance compared to targeted microarray. *Prenat Diagn* 29: 1156–1166, 2009.

Coppola A, Ruosi P, Santulli L, et al. Neurological features and long-term follow-up in 15q11.2-13.1 duplication. *Eur J Med Genet* 56: 614–618, 2013a.

Coppola A, Tostevin A, McTague A, Pressler RM, Cross JH, Sisodiya SM. Myoclonic epilepsy in a child with 17q22-q23.1 deletion. *Am J Med Genet* 161A: 2036–2039, 2013b.

Córdova-Fletes C, Rademacher N, Müller I, et al. CDKL5 truncation due to a t(X;2)(p22.1;p25.3) in a girl with X-linked infantile spasm syndrome. *Clin Genet* 77: 92–96, 2010.

Cornelis T, Rayyan M, Devriendt K, Casteels I. Ophthalmological findings in 6p deletion syndrome. *Ophthalmic Genet* 36: 165–167, 2015.

Costa D, Borrell A, Margarit E, et al. Rapid fetal karyotype from cystic hygroma and pleural effusions. *Prenat Diagn* 15: 141–148, 1995.

Cotter DJ, Brotman SM, Wilson Sayres MA. Genetic diversity on the human X chromosome does not support a strict pseudoautosomal boundary. *Genetics* 203: 485–492, 2016.

Cotter PD, Babu A, Willner JP, Desnick RJ. Prenatal diagnosis and outcome of mosaicism for a de novo unbalanced translocation identified in amniocytes. *Prenat Diagn* 18: 857–861, 1998.

Cotter PD, Ko E, Larabell SK, Rademaker AW, Martin RH. Segregation of a supernumerary del(15) marker chromosome in sperm. *Clin Genet* 58: 488–492, 2000.

Cotter PD, Musci TJ. Interphase FISH with chromosome-specific protelomere probes for rapid prenatal diagnosis in a reciprocal translocation carrier. *Prenat Diagn* 21: 171–175, 2001.

Cotter PD, Norton ME. Y chromosome heterochromatin variation detected at prenatal diagnosis. *Prenat Diagn* 25: 1062–1063, 2005.

Cotton AM, Chen CY, Lam LL, Wasserman WW, Kobor MS, Brown CJ. Spread of X-chromosome inactivation into autosomal sequences: role for DNA elements, chromatin features and chromosomal domains. *Hum Mol Genet* 23: 1211–1223, 2014.

Cottrell CE, Mendell J, Hart-Kothari M, et al. Maternal uniparental disomy of chromosome 4 in a patient with limb-girdle muscular dystrophy 2E confirmed by SNP array technology. *Clin Genet* 81: 578–583, 2012.

Court Brown WM, Law P, Smith PG. Sex chromosome aneuploidy and parental age. *Ann Hum Genet* 33: 1–14, 1969.

Courtens W, Grossman D, Van Roy N, et al. Noonan-like phenotype in monozygotic twins with a duplication-deficiency of the long arm of chromosome 18 resulting from a maternal paracentric inversion. *Hum Genet* 103: 497–505, 1998.

Courtens W, Petersen MB, Noël JC, et al. Proximal deletion of chromosome 21 confirmed by in situ hybridization and molecular studies. *Am J Med Genet* 51: 260–265, 1994.

Coussement A, Lochu P, Dupont JM, Choiset A. Inherited interstitial 16q21 deletion of 5.8 Mb without apparent phenotypic effect in three generations of a family: An array-CGH study. *Am J Med Genet* 155A: 2597–2600, 2011.

Coutton C, Bidart M, Rendu J, et al. 190-kb duplication in 1p36.11 including PIGV and ARID1A genes in a girl with intellectual disability and hexadactyly. *Clin Genet* 84: 596–599, 2013.

Coutton C, Devillard F, Vieville G, et al. 17p13.1 microduplication in a boy with Silver-Russell syndrome features and intellectual disability. *Am J Med Genet* 158A: 2564–2570, 2012.

Couzin DA, Watt JL, Stephen GS. Structural rearrangements in the parents of children with primary trisomy 21. *J Med Genet* 24: 280–282, 1987.

Cox DM, Butler MG. The 15q11.2 BP1-BP2 microdeletion syndrome: A review. *Int J Mol Sci* 16: 4068–4082, 2015.

Cozzi J, Conn CM, Harper J, et al. A trisomic germ cell line and precocious chromatid segregation leads to recurrent trisomy 21 conception. *Hum Genet* 104: 23–28, 1999.

Cram DS, Ma K, Bhasin S, et al. Y chromosome analysis of infertile men and their sons conceived through intracytoplasmic sperm injection: Vertical transmission of deletions and rarity of de novo deletions. *Fertil Steril* 74: 909–915, 2000.

Creasy MR. Complex chromosomal rearrangements. *Am J Med Genet* 32: 560, 1989.

Creatsas G, Deligeoroglou E, Tsimaris P, Pantos K, Kreatsa M. Successful pregnancy in a Swyer syndrome patient with preexisting hypertension. *Fertil Steril* 96: e83–85, 2011.

Cremonini G, Poggi A, Capucci R, Vesce F, Patella A, Marci R. Rare case of massive congenital bilateral chylothorax in a hydropic fetus with true mosaicism 47,XXX/46,XX. *J Obstet Gynaecol Res* 40: 259–262, 2014.

Crolla JA. FISH and molecular studies of autosomal supernumerary marker chromosomes excluding those derived from chromosome 15: II. Review of the literature. *Am J Med Genet* 75: 367–381, 1998.

Crolla JA, Howard P, Mitchell C, Long FL, Dennis NR. A molecular and FISH approach to determining karyotype and phenotype correlations in six patients with supernumerary marker(22) chromosomes. *Am J Med Genet* 72: 440–447, 1997.

Crolla JA, van Heyningen V. Frequent chromosome aberrations revealed by molecular cytogenetic studies in patients with aniridia. *Am J Hum Genet* 71: 1138–1149, 2002.

Crone M, Thomas MA. 9p13.1p13.3 interstitial deletion: A case report and further delineation of a rare condition. *Am J Med Genet* 170A: 1095–1098, 2016.

Croonen EA, Nillesen WM, Stuurman KE, et al. Prenatal diagnostic testing of the Noonan syndrome genes in fetuses with abnormal ultrasound findings. *Eur J Hum Genet* 21: 936–942, 2013.

Cross J, Peters G, Wu Z, Brohede J, Hannan GN. Resolution of trisomic mosaicism in prenatal diagnosis: Estimated performance of a 50K SNP microarray. *Prenat Diagn* 27: 1197–1204, 2007.

Crusi A, Engel E. Prenatal diagnosis of 3 cases of ring G chromosomes: One 21 and two 22, one of which was de novo. *Ann Génét* 29: 253–260, 1986.

Csaba A, Bush MC, Saphier C. How painful are amniocentesis and chorionic villus sampling? *Prenat Diagn* 26: 35–38, 2006.

Cubells JF, Deoreo EH, Harvey PD, et al. Pharmacogenetically guided treatment of recurrent rage outbursts in an adult male with 15q13.3 deletion syndrome. *Am J Med Genet* 155A: 805–810,2011.

Cuckle H, Nanchahal K, Wald N. Birth prevalence of Down's syndrome in England and Wales. *Prenat Diagn* 11: 29–34, 1991.

Cui YX, Xia XY, Pan LJ, et al. Gonosomal mosaicism from deleted Y chromosomal nondisjunction. *J Androl* 28: 377–380, 2007.

Cunniff C, Jones KL, Benirschke K. Ovarian dysgenesis in individuals with chromosomal abnormalities. *Hum Genet* 86: 552–556, 1991.

Cupisti S, Conn CM, Fragouli E, et al. Sequential FISH analysis of oocytes and polar bodies reveals aneuploidy mechanisms. *Prenat Diagn* 23: 663–668, 2003.

Curnow KJ, Wilkins-Haug L, Ryan A, et al. Detection of triploid, molar, and vanishing twin pregnancies by a single-nucleotide polymorphism-based noninvasive prenatal test. *Am J Obstet Gynecol* 212: 79.e1–9, 2015.

Curry CJR, Rosenfeld JA, Grant E, et al. The duplication 17p13.3 phenotype: Analysis of 21 families delineates developmental, behavioral and brain abnormalities, and rare variant phenotypes. *Am J Med Genet* 161A: 1833–1852, 2013.

Curtis L, Antonelli E, Vial Y, et al. Prenatal diagnostic indicators of paternal uniparental disomy 14. *Prenat Diagn* 26: 662–666, 2006.

Cutenese C, Mullett M, Hummel M, Wenger SL. Ring chromosome 1 in a newborn. *Clin Dysmorphol* 9: 131–133, 2000.

Cyr AB, Nimmakayalu M, Longmuir SQ, Patil SR, Keppler-Noreuil KM, Shchelochkov OA. A novel 4p16.3 microduplication distal to *WHSC1* and *WHSC2* characterized by oligonucleotide array with new phenotypic features. *Am J Med Genet* 155A: 2224–2228, 2011.

Czakó M, Riegel M, Morava E, Schinzel A, Kosztolányi G. Patient with rheumatoid arthritis and MCA/MR syndrome due to unbalanced der(18) transmission of a paternal translocation t(18;20)(p11.1;p11.1). *Am J Med Genet* 108: 226–228, 2002.

Daber RD, Conlin LK, Leonard LD, et al. Ring chromosome 20. *Eur J Med Genet* 55: 381–387, 2012.

Dahoun S. A second case of (de novo) paracentric inversion of the short arm of the X chromosome. *Ann Génét* 33: 52–55, 1990.

Dai L, Deng Y, Li N, Xie L, Mao M, Zhu J. Discontinuous microduplications at chromosome 10q24.31 identified in a Chinese family with split hand and foot malformation. *BMC Med Genet* 14: 45, 2013.

Daina G, Ramos L, Rius M, et al. Non-meiotic chromosome instability in human immature oocytes. *Eur J Hum Genet* 22: 202–207, 2014.

Dalby S. GIG response to the UK Clinical Genetics Society report "The Genetic Testing of Children." *J Med Genet* 32: 490–491, 1995.

Dale B, Wilding M, De Matteo L, Zullo F. Absence of sperm sex chromosome aneuploidies in an X0/XYY man. *Fertil Steril* 78: 634–636, 2002.

Dale RC, Grattan-Smith P, Nicholson M, Peters GB. Microdeletions detected using chromosome microarray in children with suspected genetic movement disorders: A single-centre study. *Dev Med Child Neurol* 54: 618–623, 2012.

Dallapiccola B, De Filippis V, Notarangelo A, Perla G, Zelante L. Ring chromosome 21 in healthy persons: Different consequences in females and in males. *Hum Genet* 73: 218–220, 1986.

Dallapiccola B, Mastroiacovo P, Gandini E. Centric fission of chromosome no. 4 in the mother of two patients with trisomy 4p. *Hum Genet* 31: 121–125, 1976.

Dalm VASH, Driessen GJA, Barendregt BH, van Hagen PM, van der Burg M. The 11q terminal deletion disorder Jacobsen syndrome is a syndromic primary immunodeficiency. *J Clin Immunol* 35: 761–768, 2015.

Dalprà L, Giardino D, Finelli P, et al. Cytogenetic and molecular evaluation of 241 small supernumerary marker chromosomes: Cooperative study of 19 Italian laboratories. *Genet Med* 7: 620–625, 2005.

Dalzell P, Temple G, Kovacic A, et al. Mosaicism for an unbalanced translocation—Two rare cases (abstract). *Twin Res Hum Genet* 16: 908, 2013.

Danesino C, Pasquali F, Dellavecchia C, Maserati E, Minelli A, Seghezzi L. Constitutional trisomy 8 mosaicism: Mechanism of origin, phenotype variability, and risk of malignancies. *Am J Med Genet* 80: 540, 1998.

Dang V, Surampalli A, Manzardo A, et al. Prader-Willi syndrome due to an unbalanced de novo translocation t(15;19)(q12;p13.3). *Cytogenet Genome Res* 150: 29–34, 2016.

D'Angelo CS, Da Paz JA, Kim CA, et al. Prader-Willi-like phenotype: Investigation of 1p36 deletion in 41 patients with delayed psychomotor development, hypotonia, obesity and/or hyperphagia, learning disabilities and behavioral problems. *Eur J Med Genet* 49: 451–460, 2006.

D'Angelo CS, Moller Dos Santos MF, Alonso LG, Koiffmann CP. Two new cases of 1p21.3 deletions and an unbalanced translocation t(8;12) among individuals with syndromic obesity. *Mol Syndromol* 6: 63–70, 2015.

D'Angelo D, Lebon S, Chen Q, et al. Defining the effect of the 16p11.2 duplication on cognition, behavior, and medical comorbidities. *JAMA Psychiatry* 73: 20–30, 2016.

Daniel A. The size of prometaphase chromosome segments: Tables using percentages of haploid autosome length (750 band stage). *Clin Genet* 28: 216–224, 1985.

Daniel A. Distortion of female meiotic segregation and reduced male fertility in human Robertsonian translocations: Consistent with the centromere model of co-evolving centromere DNA/centromeric histone (CENP-A). *Am J Med Genet* 111: 450–452, 2002.

Daniel A, Athayde N, Ogle R, et al. Prospective ranking of the sonographic markers for aneuploidy: Data of 2143 prenatal cytogenetic diagnoses referred for abnormalities on ultrasound. *Aust NZ J Obstet Gynaecol* 43: 16–26, 2003a.

Daniel A, Hook EB, Wulf G. Collaborative U.S.A. data on prenatal diagnosis for parental carriers of chromosome rearrangements: Risks of unbalanced progeny. In Daniel A (ed.), *The Cytogenetics of Mammalian Autosomal Rearrangements*. New York, NY: Liss, 1988.

Daniel A, Hook EB, Wulf G. Risks of unbalanced progeny at amniocentesis to carriers of chromosome rearrangements: Data from United States and Canadian laboratories. *Am J Med Genet* 33: 14–53, 1989.

Daniel A, Malafiej P. A series of supernumerary small ring marker autosomes identified by FISH with chromosome probe arrays and literature review excluding chromosome 15. *Am J Med Genet* 117A: 212–222, 2003.

Daniel A, Ng A, Kuah KB, Reiha S, Malafiej P. A study of early amniocentesis for prenatal cytogenetic diagnosis. *Prenat Diagn* 18: 21–28, 1998.

Daniel A, St. Heaps L, Sylvester D, Diaz S, Peters G. Two mosaic terminal inverted duplications arising post-zygotically: Evidence for possible formation of neo-telomeres. *Cell Chromosome* 7: 1, 2008.

Daniel A, Wu Z, Bennetts B, et al. Karyotype, phenotype and parental origin in 19 cases of triploidy. *Prenat Diagn* 21: 1034–1048, 2001.

Daniel A, Wu Z, Darmanian A, Collins F, Jackson J. Three different origins for apparent triploid/diploid mosaics. *Prenat Diagn* 23: 529–534, 2003b.

Daniel A, Wu Z, Darmanian A, et al. Issues arising from the prenatal diagnosis of some rare trisomy mosaics—The importance of cryptic fetal mosaicism. *Prenat Diagn* 24: 524–536, 2004.

D'Apice MR, Novelli A, di Masi A, et al. Deletion of *REXO1L1* locus in a patient with malabsorption syndrome, growth retardation, and dysmorphic features: a novel recognizable microdeletion syndrome? *BMC Med Genet* 16: 20, 2015.

Daphnis DD, Fragouli E, Economou K, et al. Analysis of the evolution of chromosome abnormalities in human embryos from day 3 to 5 using CGH and FISH. *Mol Hum Reprod* 14: 117–125, 2008.

Dar H, Tal J, Bar-el H, Halpern I, Sharf M. Paracentric inversion of Xq and ovarian dysfunction. *Am J Med Genet* 29: 167–170, 1988.

Darcy D, Atwal PS, Angell C, Gadi I, Wallerstein R. Mosaic paternal genome-wide uniparental isodisomy with Down syndrome. *Am J Med Genet* 167A: 2463–2469, 2015.

Dastan J, Chijiwa C, Tang F, et al. Exome sequencing identifies pathogenic variants of *VPS13B* in a patient with familial 16p11.2 duplication. *BMC Med Genet* 17: 78, 2016.

Dauwerse JG, Hansson KBM, Brouwers AAM, Peters DJM, Breuning MH. An XX male with the sex-determining region Y gene inserted in the long arm of chromosome 16. *Fertil Steril* 86: 463, e1–5, 2006.

Dave BJ, Olney AH, Zaleski DH, et al. Inherited 14q duplication and 21q deletion: A rare adjacent-2 segregation in multiple family members. *Am J Med Genet* 149A: 2248–2253, 2009.

David D, Marques B, Ferreira C, et al. Co-segregation of trichorhinophalangeal syndrome with a t(8;13)(q23.3;q21.31) familial translocation that appears to increase *TRPS1* gene expression. *Hum Genet* 132: 1287–1299, 2013.

Davidsson J, Collin A, Öreberg M, Gisselsson D. Array-based genotype-phenotype correlation in a case of supernumerary ring chromosome 12. *Clin Genet* 73: 44–49, 2008.

Davidsson J, Jahnke K, Forsgren M, Collin A, Soller M. Dup(19)(q12q13.2): Array-based genotype-phenotype correlation of a new possibly obesity-related syndrome. *Obesity (Silver Spring)* 18: 580–587, 2010.

Davies AF, Kirby TL, Docherty Z, Ogilvie CM. Characterization of terminal chromosome anomalies using multisubtelomere FISH. *Am J Med Genet* 120A: 483–489, 2003.

Davies RW, Lau P, Naing T, et al. A 680 kb duplication at the FTO locus in a kindred with obesity and a distinct body fat distribution. *Eur J Hum Genet* 21: 1417–1422, 2013.

Dawson AJ, Chernos J, McGowan-Jordan J, et al. CCMG guidelines: Prenatal and postnatal diagnostic testing for uniparental disomy. *Clin Genet* 79: 118–124, 2011.

Dayem-Quere M, Giuliano F, Wagner-Mahler K, et al. Delineation of a region responsible for panhypopituitarism in 20p11.2. *Am J Med Genet* 161A: 1547–1554, 2013.

De Assis KR, Ladeira MS, Bueno RC, Dos Santos BF, Dalben I, Salvadori DM. Genotoxicity of cigarette smoking in maternal and newborn lymphocytes. *Mutat Res* 679: 72–78, 2009.

De Braekeleer M, Dao TN. Cytogenetic studies in male infertility: A review. *Hum Reprod* 6: 245–250, 1991.

De Carvalho AFL, da Silva Bellucco FT, Kulikowski LD, Toralles MBP, Melaragno MI. Partial 5p monosomy or trisomy in 11 patients from a family with a t(5;15)(p13.3;p12) translocation. *Hum Genet* 124: 387–392, 2008.

De Crescenzo A, Sparago A, Cerrato F, et al. Paternal deletion of the 11p15.5 centromeric-imprinting control region is associated with alteration of imprinted gene expression and recurrent severe intrauterine growth restriction. *J Med Genet* 50: 99–103, 2013.

De Crespigny L. What's in a name—Is the pregnant woman a mother? Is the fetus a baby? *Aust NZ J Obstet Gynaecol* 36: 435–436, 1996.

De Crespigny L, Chervenak F, McCullough L. Mothers and babies, pregnant women and fetuses. *Br J Obstet Gynaecol* 106: 1235–1237, 1999.

De Crespigny L, Espie M, Holmes S. *Prenatal Testing: Making Choices in Pregnancy*. Ringwood, Victoria, Australia: Penguin Books Australia, 1998.

De Felici M. Origin, migration, and proliferation of human primordial germ cells. In Coticchio G, Albertini DF, De Santis L (eds.), *Oogenesis*, Springer-Verlag, London, 2013.

De Graaf G, Buckley F, Skotko BG. Estimates of the live births, natural losses, and elective terminations with Down syndrome in the United States. *Am J Med Genet* 167A: 756–67, 2015.

De Graaf G, Haveman M, Hochstenbach R, et al. Changes in yearly birth prevalence rates of children with Down syndrome in the period 1986–2007 in The Netherlands. *J Intellect Disabil Res* 55: 462–473, 2011.

De Gregori M, Ciccone R, Magini P, et al. Cryptic deletions are a common finding in "balanced" reciprocal and complex chromosome rearrangements: A study of 59 patients. *J Med Genet* 44: 750–762, 2007.

De Jong A, Dondorp WJ, de Die-Smulders CEM, Frints SGM, de Wert GMWR. Non-invasive prenatal testing: Ethical issues explored. *Eur J Hum Genet* 18: 272–277, 2010.

De Jong A, Dondorp WJ, Macville MVE, de Die-Smulders CEM, van Lith JMM, de Wert GMWR. Microarrays as a diagnostic tool in prenatal screening strategies: Ethical reflection. *Hum Genet* 133: 163–172, 2014.

De la Paz-Gallardo MJ, García FS, de Haro-Muñoz T, et al. Quantitative-fluorescent-PCR versus full karyotyping in prenatal diagnosis of common chromosome aneuploidies in southern Spain. *Clin Chem Lab Med* 53: 1333–1338, 2015.

De Mas P, Daudin M, Vincent MC, et al. Increased aneuploidy in spermatozoa from testicular tumour patients after chemotherapy with cisplatin, etoposide and bleomycin. *Hum Reprod* 16: 1204–1208, 2001.

De Palma A, Burrello N, Barone N, D'Agata R, Vicari E, Calogero AE. Patients with abnormal sperm parameters have an increased sex chromosome aneuploidy rate in peripheral leukocytes. *Hum Reprod* 20: 2153–2156, 2005.

De Pagter MS, van Roosmalen MJ, Baas AF, et al. Chromothripsis in healthy individuals affects multiple protein-coding genes and can result in severe congenital abnormalities in offspring. *Am J Hum Genet* 96: 651–656, 2015.

De Pater JM, Scheres JMJC, Christiaens GCML, Ausems MGEM. Pitfalls in prenatal diagnosis: Cytogenetic analysis in amniocytes fails to detect mosaic r(12). *Prenat Diagn* 23: 65–67, 2003.

De Pater JM, Schuring-Blom GH, van den Bogaard R, et al. Maternal uniparental disomy for chromosome 22 in a child with generalized mosaicism for trisomy 22. *Prenat Diagn* 17: 81–86, 1997.

De Perdigo A, Gabriel-Robez O, Ratomponirina C, Rumpler Y. Synaptonemal complex analysis in a human male carrier of a 4;6 translocation: Heterosynapsis without previous homosynapsis. *Hum Genet* 86: 279–282, 1991.

De Perdigo A, Gabriel-Robez O, Rumpler Y. Correlation between chromosomal breakpoint positions and synaptic behaviour in human males heterozygous for a pericentric inversion. *Hum Genet* 83: 274–276, 1989.

De Ravel TJL, Keymolen K, van Assche E, et al. Post-zygotic origin of isochromosome 12p. *Prenat Diagn* 24: 984–988, 2004.

De Ravel TJL, Legius E, Brems H, Van Hoestenberghe R, Gillis PH, Fryns JP. Hemifacial microsomia in two patients further supporting chromosomal mosaicism as a causative factor. *Clin Dysmorphol* 10: 263–267, 2001.

De Rycke M, Liebaers I, Van Steirteghem A. Epigenetic risks related to assisted reproductive technologies: Risk analysis and epigenetic inheritance. *Hum Reprod* 17: 2487–2494, 2002.

De Silva MG, Elliott K, Dahl HH, et al. Disruption of a novel member of a sodium/hydrogen exchanger family and *DOCK3* is associated with an attention deficit hyperactivity disorder-like phenotype. *J Med Genet* 40: 733–740, 2003.

De Smith AJ, Purmann C, Walters RG, et al. A deletion of the HBII-85 class of small nucleolar RNAs (snoRNAs) is associated with hyperphagia, obesity and hypogonadism. *Hum Mol Genet* 18: 3257–3265, 2009.

De Souza E, Halliday J, Chan A, Bower C, Morris JK. Recurrence risks for trisomies 13, 18, and 21. *Am J Med Genet* 149A: 2716–2722, 2009.

De Villena FPM, Sapienza C. Transmission ratio distortion in offspring of heterozygous female carriers of Robertsonian translocations. *Hum Genet* 108: 31–36, 2001.

De Vos A, Staessen C, De Rycke M, et al. Impact of cleavage-stage embryo biopsy in view of PGD on human blastocyst implantation: A prospective cohort of single embryo transfers. *Hum Reprod* 24: 2988–2996, 2009.

De Vries BBA, Eussen BHJ, van Diggelen OP, et al. Submicroscopic Xpter deletion in a boy with growth and mental retardation caused by a familial t(X;14). *Am J Med Genet* 87: 189–194, 1999.

De Vries FA, Govaerts LC, Knijnenburg J, et al. Another rare prenatal case of post-zygotic mosaic trisomy 17. *Am J Med Genet* 161A: 1196–1199, 2013.

De Vries JWA, Repping S, Oates R, Carson R, Leschot NJ, van der Veen F. Absence of deleted in azoospermia (DAZ) genes in spermatozoa of infertile men with somatic DAZ deletions. *Fertil Steril* 75: 476–479, 2001.

De Wolf V, Brison N, Devriendt K, Peeters H. Genetic counseling for susceptibility loci and neurodevelopmental disorders: The del15q11.2 as an example. *Am J Med Genet* 161A: 2846–2854, 2013.

Dean G, Nevin NC, Mikkelsen M, et al. Investigation of a cluster of children with Down's syndrome born to mothers who had attended a school in Dundalk, Ireland. *Occup Environ Med* 57: 793–804, 2000.

DeBrasi D, Genardi M, D'Agostino A, et al. Double autosomal/gonosomal mosaic aneuploidy: Study of nondisjunction in two cases with trisomy of chromosome 8. *Hum Genet* 95: 519–525, 1995.

Dee SL, Clark AT, Willatt LR, Yates JRW. A case of ring chromosome 2 with growth retardation, mild dysmorphism, and microdeletion of 2p detected using FISH. *J Med Genet* 38: E32, 2001.

Del Gaudio L, Striano S, Coppola A. Severe epilepsy in an adult with partial trisomy 18q. *Am J Med Genet* 164A: 3148–3153, 2014.

Del Porto G, Di Fusco C, Baldi M, Grammatico P, D'Alessandro E. Familial centric fission of chromosome 4. *J Med Genet* 21: 388–391, 1984.

Delahaye A, Khung-Savatovsky S, Aboura A, et al. Pre- and postnatal phenotype of 6p25 deletions involving the *FOXC1* gene. *Am J Med Genet* 158A: 2430–2438, 2012.

Delatycki M, Gardner RJM. Three cases of trisomy 13 mosaicism and a review of the literature. *Clin Genet* 51: 403–407, 1997.

Delatycki MB, Pertile MD, Gardner RJM. Trisomy 13 mosaicism at prenatal diagnosis: Dilemmas in interpretation. *Prenat Diagn* 18: 45–50, 1998.

Delgado S, Velinov M. 7q21.3 Deletion involving enhancer sequences within the gene *DYNC1I1* presents with intellectual disability and split hand-split foot malformation with decreased penetrance. *Mol Cytogenet* 8: 37, 2015.

Delhanty JDA. Inherited aneuploidy: germline mosaicism. *Cytogenet Genome Res* 133: 136–140, 2011.

Delisle MF, Wilson RD. First trimester prenatal diagnosis: Amniocentesis. *Semin Perinatol* 23: 414–423, 1999.

Delobel B, Djlelati R, Gabriel-Robez O, et al. Y-autosome translocation and infertility: Usefulness of molecular, cytogenetic and meiotic studies. *Hum Genet* 102: 98–102, 1998.

Délot EC, Vilain EJ. Nonsyndromic 46,XX testicular disorders of sex development. In Pagon RA, Adam MP, Ardinger HH, et al. (eds.), *GeneReviews*. Seattle, WA: University of Washington, 2015.

DeLozier-Blanchet CD, Roeder E, Denis-Arrue R, et al. Trisomy 12 mosaicism confirmed in multiple organs from a liveborn child. *Am J Med Genet* 95: 444–449, 2000.

Delphin N, Hanein S, Taie LF, et al. Intellectual disability associated with retinal dystrophy in the Xp11.3 deletion syndrome: ZNF674 on trial. Guilty or innocent? *Eur J Hum Genet* 20: 352–356, 2012.

Demaerel W, Hosseinzadeh M, Nouri N, et al. Reciprocal 22q11.2 deletion and duplication in siblings with karyotypically normal parents. *Cytogenet Genome Res* 148: 1–5, 2016.

Demarini DM. Declaring the existence of human germ-cell mutagens. *Environ Mol Mutagen* 53: 166–172, 2012.

Demeer B, Andrieux J, Receveur A, et al. Duplication 16p13.3 and the *CREBBP* gene: Confirmation of the phenotype. *Eur J Med Genet* 56: 26–31, 2013.

Demeestere I, Simon P, Dedeken L, et al. Live birth after autograft of ovarian tissue cryopreserved during childhood. *Hum Reprod* 30: 2107–2109, 2015.

Demily C, Poisson A, Peyroux E, et al. Autism spectrum disorder associated with 49,XYYYY: Case report and review of the literature. *BMC Med Genet* 18: 9, 2017.

Demko ZP, Simon AL, McCoy RC, Petrov DA, Rabinowitz M. Effects of maternal age on euploidy rates in a large cohort of embryos analyzed with 24-chromosome single-nucleotide polymorphism-based preimplantation genetic screening. *Fertil Steril* 105: 1307–1313, 2016.

Denayer E, Brems H, de Cock P, et al. Pathogenesis of vestibular schwannoma in ring chromosome 22. *BMC Med Genet* 10: 97, 2009.

Denes AM, Landin-Wilhelmsen K, Wettergren Y, Bryman I, Hanson C. The proportion of diploid 46,XX cells increases with time in women with Turner syndrome—A 10-year follow-up study. *Genet Test Mol Biomarkers* 19: 82–87, 2015.

Deng C, Yi L, Mu Y, et al. Recent trends in the birth prevalence of Down syndrome in China: Impact of prenatal diagnosis and subsequent terminations. *Prenat Diagn* 35: 311–318, 2015.

Deng HX, Abe K, Kondo I, et al. Parental origin and mechanism of formation of polysomy X: An XXXXX case and four XXXXY cases determined with RFLPs. *Hum Genet* 86: 541–544, 1991.

Denschlag D, Tempfer C, Kunze M, Wolff G, Keck C. Assisted reproductive techniques in patients with Klinefelter syndrome: A critical review. *Fertil Steril* 82: 775–779, 2004.

Depienne C, Nava C, Keren B, et al. Genetic and phenotypic dissection of 1q43q44 microdeletion syndrome and neurodevelopmental phenotypes associated with mutations in *ZBTB18* and *HNRNPU*. *Hum Genet* 136: 463–479, 2017.

DeScipio C, Conlin L, Rosenfeld J, et al. Subtelomeric deletion of chromosome 10p15.3: Clinical findings and molecular cytogenetic characterization. *Am J Med Genet* 158A: 2152–2161, 2012.

DeScipio C, Morrissette JD, Conlin LK, et al. Two siblings with alternate unbalanced recombinants derived from a large cryptic maternal pericentric inversion of chromosome 20. *Am J Med Genet* 152A: 373–382, 2010a.

DeScipio C, Morrissette JD, Conlin LK, et al. Update on "Two Siblings with Alternate Unbalanced Recombinants Derived from a Large Cryptic Maternal Pericentric Inversion of Chromosome 20." *Am J Med Genet* 152A: 1599, 2010b.

DeScipio C, Spinner NB, Kaur M, et al. Fine-mapping subtelomeric deletions and duplications by comparative genomic hybridization in 42 individuals. *Am J Med Genet* 146A: 730–739, 2008.

DesGroseilliers M, Beaulieu Bergeron M, Brochu P, Lemyre E, Lemieux N. Phenotypic variability in isodicentric Y patients: Study of nine cases. *Clin Genet* 70: 145–150, 2006.

Desmyttere S, De Schepper J, Nekkebroeck J, et al. Two-year auxological and medical outcome of singletons born after embryo biopsy applied in preimplantation genetic diagnosis or preimplantation genetic screening. *Hum Reprod* 24: 470–476, 2009.

Destree A, Fourneau C, Dugauquier C, Rombout S, Sartenaer D, Gillerot Y. Prenatal diagnosis of trisomy 6 mosaicism. *Prenat Diagn* 25: 354–357, 2005.

Deveault C, Qian JH, Chebaro W, et al. *NLRP7* mutations in women with diploid androgenetic and triploid moles: a proposed mechanism for mole formation. *Hum Mol Genet* 18: 888–897, 2009.

Devi A, Benn PA. X-chromosome abnormalities in women with premature ovarian failure. *J Reprod Med* 44: 321–324, 1999.

Devillard F, Metzler-Guillemain C, Pelletier R, et al. Polyploidy in large-headed sperm: FISH study of three cases. *Hum Reprod* 17: 1292–1298, 2002.

Devine DH, Whitman-Elia G, Best RG, Edwards JG. Paternal paracentric inversion of chromosome 2: A possible association with recurrent pregnancy loss and infertility. *J Assist Reprod Genet* 17: 293–296, 2000.

Devriendt K, Van Hoestenberghe R, Van Hole C, et al. Submicroscopic deletion in chromosome 22q11 in trizygous triplet siblings and their father: Clinical variability of 22q11 deletion. *Clin Genet* 51: 246–249, 1997.

Devroey P, Wisanto A, Camus M, et al. Oocyte donation in patients without ovarian function. *Hum Reprod* 3: 699–704, 1988.

Dewhurst J. Fertility in 47,XXX and 45,X patients. *J Med Genet* 15: 132–135, 1978.

Dhallan R, Guo X, Emche S, et al. A non-invasive test for prenatal diagnosis based on fetal DNA present in maternal blood: A preliminary study. *Lancet* 369: 474–481, 2007.

Dhakar MB, Ilyas M, Jeong JW, Behen ME, Chugani HT. Frontal aslant tract abnormality on diffusion tensor imaging in an aphasic patient with 49,XXXXY syndrome. *Pediatr Neurol* 55: 64–67, 2016.

Dhandha S, Hogge WA, Surti U, McPherson E. Three cases of tetrasomy 9p. *Am J Med Genet* 113: 375–380, 2002.

Dharmadhikari AV, Gambin T, Szafranski P, et al. Molecular and clinical analyses of 16q24.1 duplications involving *FOXF1* identify an evolutionarily unstable large minisatellite. *BMC Med Genet* 15: 128, 2014.

Di Benedetto D, Musumeci SA, Avola E, et al. Definition of minimal duplicated region encompassing the *XIAP* and *STAG2* genes in the Xq25 microduplication syndrome. *Am J Med Genet* 164A: 1923–1930, 2014.

Di Gregorio E, Riberi E, Belligni, EF, et al. Copy number variants analysis in a cohort of isolated and syndromic developmental delay/intellectual disability reveals novel genomic disorders, position effects and candidate disease genes. *Clin Genet* 92: 415–422, 2017.

Di-Battista A, Meloni VA, da Silva MD, Moysés-Oliveira M, Melaragno MI. Unusual X-chromosome inactivation pattern in patients with Xp11.23-p11.22 duplication: Report and review. *Am J Med Genet* 170A: 3271–3275, 2016.

Diego-Alvarez D, Ramos-Corrales C, Garcia-Hoyos M, et al. Double trisomy in spontaneous miscarriages: Cytogenetic and molecular approach. *Hum Reprod* 21: 958–966, 2006.

Diego-Alvarez D, Rodriguez de Alba M, Cardero-Merlo R, et al. MLPA as a screening method of aneuploidy and unbalanced chromosomal rearrangements in spontaneous miscarriages. *Prenat Diagn* 27: 765–771, 2007.

Digilio MC, Bernardini L, Consoli F, et al. Congenital heart defects in recurrent reciprocal 1q21.1 deletion and duplication syndromes: Rare association with pulmonary valve stenosis. *Eur J Med Genet* 56: 144–149, 2013.

Digilio MC, Bernardini L, Mingarelli R, et al. 3q29 Microdeletion: A mental retardation disorder unassociated with a recognizable phenotype in two mother-daughter pairs. *Am J Med Genet* 149A: 1777–1781, 2009.

Digilio MC, McDonald-McGinn DM, Heike C, et al. Three patients with oculo-auriculo-vertebral spectrum and microdeletion 22q11.2. *Am J Med Genet* 149A: 2860–2864, 2009.

Dilzell K, Darcy D, Sum J, Wallerstein R. Deletion of 7q33-q35 in a patient with intellectual disability and dysmorphic features: Further characterization of 7q interstitial deletion syndrome. *Case Rep Genet* 2015: 131852, 2015.

Dimassi S, Andrieux J, Labalme A, et al. Interstitial 12p13.1 deletion involving *GRIN2B* in three patients with intellectual disability. *Am J Med Genet* 161A: 2564–2569, 2013.

Dimitrov B, Balikova I, de Ravel T, et al. 2q31.1 microdeletion syndrome: Redefining the associated clinical phenotype. *J Med Genet* 48: 98–104, 2011.

Dimitrov BI, de Ravel T, Van Driessche J, et al. Distal limb deficiencies, micrognathia syndrome, and syndromic forms of split hand foot malformation (SHFM) are caused by chromosome 10q genomic rearrangements. *J Med Genet* 47: 103–111, 2010.

Dimitrov BI, Ogilvie C, Wieczorek D, et al. 3p14 deletion is a rare contiguous gene syndrome: Report of 2 new patients and an overview of 14 patients. *Am J Med Genet* 167: 1223–1230, 2015.

Ding Q, Ouyang Q, Xi X, Wang X, Shen Y, Wang H. Maternal chromosome 4 heterodisomy/isodisomy and Bβ chain Trp323X mutation resulting in severe hypodysfibrinogenaemia. *Thromb Haemost* 108: 654–661, 2012.

DiPietro JA, Cristofalo EA, Voegtline KM, Crino J. Isolated prenatal choroid plexus cysts do not affect child development. *Prenat Diagn* 31: 745–749, 2011.

D'Ippolito G, Tirelli A, Giulini S, Volpe A, La Marca A. Hormonal and ultrasound markers of ovarian function in a woman with a balanced 1;11 translocation. *Fertil Steril* 95: 803, e7–8, 2011.

Disciglio V, Lo Rizzo C, Mencarelli MA, et al. Interstitial 22q13 deletions not involving *SHANK3* gene: A new contiguous gene syndrome. *Am J Med Genet* 164A: 1666–1676, 2014.

Disteche CM. Escape from X inactivation in human and mouse. *Trends Genet* 11: 17–22, 1995.

Dixit A, Chandler KE, Lever M, et al. Pseudohypoparathyroidism type 1b due to paternal uniparental disomy of chromosome 20q. *J Clin Endocrinol Metab* 98: E103–E108, 2013a.

Dixit A, McKee S, Mansour S, et al. 7q11.23 microduplication: A recognizable phenotype. *Clin Genet* 83: 155–161, 2013b.

Dixit A, Patel C, Harrison R, et al. 17q12 microdeletion syndrome: Three patients illustrating the phenotypic spectrum. *Am J Med Genet* 158A: 2317–2321, 2012.

Dobek WA, Kim HG, Walls CA, et al. Long-term follow-up of females with unbalanced X;Y translocations—Reproductive and nonreproductive consequences. *Mol Cytogenet* 8: 13, 2015.

Dobyns WB, Mirzaa G, Christian SL, et al. Consistent chromosome abnormalities identify novel polymicrogyria loci in 1p36.3, 2p16.1-p23.1, 4q21.21-q22.1, 6q26-q27, and 21q2. *Am J Med Genet* 146A: 1637–1654, 2008.

Docherty LE, Kabwama S, Lehmann A, et al. Clinical presentation of 6q24 transient neonatal diabetes mellitus (6q24 TNDM) and genotype-phenotype correlation in an international cohort of patients. *Diabetologia* 56: 758–762, 2013.

Doelken SC, Seeger K, Hundsdoerfer P, Weber-Ferro W, Klopocki E, Graul-Neumann L. Proximal and distal 15q25.2 microdeletions-genotype-phenotype delineation of two neurodevelopmental susceptibility loci. *Am J Med Genet* 161A: 218–224, 2013.

Doğer E, Çakiroglu Y, Ceylan Y, Ulak E, Özdamar Ö, Çaliskan E. Reproductive and obstetric outcomes in mosaic Turner's syndrome: A cross-sectional study and review of the literature. *Reprod Biol Endocrinol* 13: 59, 2015.

Doheny KF, Rasmussen SA, Rutberg J, et al. Segregation of a familial balanced (12;10) insertion resulting in Dup(10)(q21.2q22.1) and Del(10)(q21.2q22.1) in first cousins. *Am J Med Genet* 69: 188–193, 1997.

Dohle GR, Halley DJJ, Van Hemel JO, et al. Genetic risk factors in infertile men with severe oligozoospermia and azoospermia. *Hum Reprod* 17: 13–16, 2002.

Dolan M, Berry SA, Rubin KR, Hirsch B. Deletion and duplication of 11p13-11p14: reciprocal aberrations derived from a paternal insertion. *Am J Med Genet* 155A: 2775–2783, 2011.

Dolcetti A, Silversides CK, Marshall CR, et al. 1q21.1 microduplication expression in adults. *Genet Med* 15: 282–289, 2013.

Dolk H, Loane M, Garne E, et al. Trends and geographic inequalities in the prevalence of Down syndrome in Europe, 1980–1999. *Rev Epidemiol Sante Publique* 53: 2S87–2S95, 2005.

Domenice S, Zamboni Machado A, Moraes Ferreira F, et al. Wide spectrum of NR5A1-related phenotypes in 46,XY and 46,XX individuals. *Birth Defects Res C Embryo Today* 108: 309–320, 2016.

Domínguez MG, Rivera H, Aguilar-Lemarroy A, et al. Two familial intrachromosomal insertions with maternal dup(6)(p22.3p25.3) or dup(2) (q24.2q32.1) in recombinant offspring. *Clin Dysmorphol* 26: 209–216, 2017.

Dominguez MG, Rivera H, Vasquez AI, Hernandez-Zaragoza G, Rivas F. Interchange trisomy 21 by t(1;21)(p22;q22)mat. *Genet Couns* 12: 363–367, 2001.

Donaghue C, Mann K, Docherty Z, Mackie Ogilvie C. Detection of mosaicism for primary trisomies in prenatal samples by QF-PCR and karyotype analysis. *Prenat Diagn* 25: 65–72, 2005.

Donate A, Estop AM, Giraldo J, Templado C. Paternal age and numerical chromosome abnormalities in human spermatozoa. *Cytogenet Genome Res* 148: 241–248, 2016.

Dong Z, Jiang L, Yang C, et al. A robust approach for blind detection of balanced chromosomal rearrangements with whole-genome low-coverage sequencing. *Hum Mutat* 35: 625–636, 2014.

Dong Z, Zhang J, Hu P, et al. Low-pass whole-genome sequencing in clinical cytogenetics: A validated approach. *Genet Med* 18: 940–948, 2016.

Donley G. Does the constitution protect abortions based on fetal anomaly? Examining the potential for disability-selective abortion bans in the age of prenatal whole genome sequencing. *Michigan J Gender Law* 20: 291–328, 2013.

Donnai D, Karmiloff-Smith A. Williams syndrome: From genotype through to the cognitive phenotype. *Am J Med Genet* 97: 164–171, 2000.

Donnelly SL, Wolpert CM, Menold MM, et al. Female with autistic disorder and monosomy X (Turner syndrome): Parent-of-origin effect of the X chromosome. *Am J Med Genet* 96: 312–316, 2000.

Doudney K, Bickley V, Robertson M, et al. A diagnosis of Pitt-Hopkins syndrome in a 21 month old child and detection of maternal somatic mosaicism at 18q21.2 (abstract). *Twin Res Hum Genet* 16: 903, 2013.

Draaken M, Reutter H, Schramm C, et al. Microduplications at 22q11.21 are associated with non-syndromic classic bladder exstrophy. *Eur J Med Genet* 53: 55–60, 2010.

Driscoll DJ, Miller JL, Schwartz S, Cassidy SB. Prader-Willi syndrome. In Pagon RA, Adam MP, Ardinger HH, et al. (eds.), *GeneReviews* [Internet]. Seattle, WA: University of Washington, 1993–2016.

Drugan A, Greb A, Johnson MP, et al. Determinants of parental decisions to abort for chromosome abnormalities. *Prenat Diagn* 10: 483–490, 1990.

Du X, An Y, Yu L, et al. A genomic copy number variant analysis implicates the *MBD5* and *HNRNPU* genes in Chinese children with infantile spasms and expands the clinical spectrum of 2q23.1 deletion. *BMC Med Genet* 15: 62, 2014.

Du Sart D, Kalitsis P, Schmidt M. Noninactivation of a portion of Xq28 in a balanced X-autosome translocation. *Am J Med Genet* 42: 156–160, 1992.

Duba HC, Weirich HG, Weirich-Schwaiger H, et al. Chromosomal instability in a woman with infertility and two unaffected brothers: A new familial chromosomal breakage syndrome? *Hum Genet* 100: 431–440, 1997.

Duckett DP, Roberts SH. Adjacent 2 meiotic disjunction. Report of a case resulting from a familial 13q;15q balanced reciprocal translocation and review of the literature. *Hum Genet* 58: 377–386, 1981.

Dufke A, Eggermann K, Balg S, Stengel-Rutkowski S, Enders H, Kaiser P. A second case of inv(4)pat with both recombinants in the offspring: rec dup(4q) in a girl with Wolf-Hirschhorn syndrome and rec dup(4p). *Cytogenet Cell Genet* 91: 85–89, 2000.

Dufke A, Mayrhofer H, Enders H, Kaiser P, Leipoldt M. Unusual chromosomal mosaicism as a cause of mental retardation and congenital malformations in a familial reciprocal translocation carrier, t(17;22)(q24.2;q11.23). *Cytogenet Cell Genet* 93: 168–170, 2001.

Duker NJ. Chromosome breakage syndromes and cancer. *Am J Med Genet* 115: 125–129, 2002.

Duncan FE, Hornick JE, Lampson MA, Schultz RM, Shea LD, Woodruff TK. Chromosome cohesion decreases in human eggs with advanced maternal age. *Aging Cell* 11: 1121–1124, 2012.

Dupont C, Baumann C, Le Du N, et al. *COL2A1* gene disruption by a balanced translocation t(12;15)(q13;q22.2) in familial Stickler syndrome. *Am J Med Genet* 161A: 2663–2665, 2013.

Dupont JM, Cuisset L, Cartigny M, et al. Familial reciprocal translocation t(7;16) associated with maternal uniparental disomy 7 in a Silver-Russell patient. *Am J Med Genet* 111: 405–408, 2002.

Dupont C, Delahaye A, Burglen L, et al. First cryptic balanced reciprocal translocation mosaicism and familial transmission. *Am J Med Genet* 146A: 2971–2974, 2008.

Dupont C, Grati FR, Choy KW, et al. Prenatal diagnosis of 24 cases of microduplication 22q11.2: An investigation of phenotype-genotype correlations. *Prenat Diagn* 35: 35–43, 2015.

Dupont C, Pipiras E, Chantot-Bastaraud S, et al. CGH and direct diagnosis of mosaic structural chromosomal abnormalities: Description of a mosaic ring chromosome 17 and review of the literature. *Eur J Hum Genet* 11: 452–456, 2003.

Dupont JM, Cuisset L, Cartigny M, et al. Familial reciprocal translocation t(7;16) associated with maternal uniparental disomy 7 in a Silver-Russell patient. *Am J Med Genet* 111: 405–408, 2002.

Durante M, Snigiryova G, Akaeva E, et al. Chromosome aberration dosimetry in cosmonauts after single or multiple space flights. *Cytogenet Genome Res* 103: 40–46, 2003.

Durban M, Benet J, Boada M, et al. PGD in female carriers of balanced Robertsonian and reciprocal translocations by first polar body analysis. *Hum Reprod Update* 7: 591–602, 2001.

Duyzend MH, Eichler EE. Genotype-first analysis of the 16p11.2 deletion defines a new type of "autism." *Biol Psychiatry* 77: 769–771, 2015.

Dworschak GC, Crétolle C, Hilger A, et al. Comprehensive review of the duplication 3q syndrome and report of a patient with Currarino syndrome and de novo duplication 3q26.32-q27.2. *Clin Genet* 91: 661–671, 2017.

Dworschak GC, Draaken M, Marcelis C, et al. De novo 13q deletions in two patients with mild anorectal malformations as part of VATER/VACTERL and VATER/VACTERL-like association and analysis of *EFNB2* in patients with anorectal malformations. *Am J Med Genet* 161A: 3035–3041, 2013.

Earhart BA, Williams ME, Zamora I, Randolph LM, Votava-Smith JK, Marcy SN. Phenotype of 7q11.23 duplication: A family clinical series. *Am J Med Genet* 173A: 114–119, 2017.

Eckel H, Wimmer R, Volleth M, Jakubiczka S, Muschke P, Wieacker P. Intrachromosomal triplication 12p11.22-p12.3 and gonadal mosaicism of partial tetrasomy 12p. *Am J Med Genet* 140: 1219–1222, 2006.

Edwards MJ, Park JP, Wurster-Hill DH, Graham JM, Jr. Mixoploidy in humans: Two surviving cases of diploid-tetraploid mixoploidy and comparison with diploid-triploid mixoploidy. *Am J Med Genet* 52: 324–330, 1994.

Egan JF, Smith K, Timms D, Bolnick JM, Campbell WA, Benn PA. Demographic differences in Down syndrome livebirths in the US from 1989 to 2006. *Prenat Diagn* 31: 389–394, 2011.

Egger JIM, Verhoeven WMA, Verbeeck W, de Leeuw N. Neuropsychological phenotype of a patient with a de novo 970 kb interstitial deletion in the distal 16p11.2 region. *Neuropsychiatr Dis Treat* 10: 513–517, 2014.

Eggermann K, Bliek J, Brioude F, et al. EMQN best practice guidelines for the molecular genetic testing and reporting of chromosome 11p15 imprinting disorders: Silver-Russell and Beckwith-Wiedemann syndrome. *Eur J Hum Genet* 24: 1377–1387, 2016.

Eggermann K, Mau UA, Bujdosó G, et al. Supernumerary marker chromosomes derived from chromosome 15: Analysis of 32 new cases. *Clin Genet* 62: 89–93, 2002.

Eggermann T, Begemann M, Binder G, Spengler S. Silver-Russell syndrome: Genetic basis and molecular genetic testing. *Orphanet J Rare Dis* 5: 19, 2010a.

Eggermann T, Curtis M, Zerres K, Hughes HE. Maternal uniparental disomy 16 and genetic counseling: New case and survey of published cases. *Genet Couns* 15: 183–190, 2004.

Eggermann T, Engels H, Heidrich-Kaul C, Moderau I, Schwanitz G. Molecular investigation of the parental origin of a de novo unbalanced translocation 13/18. *Hum Genet* 99: 521–522, 1997.

Eggermann T, Gonzalez D, Spengler S, Arslan-Kirchner M, Binder G, Schonherr N. Broad clinical spectrum in Silver-Russell syndrome and consequences for genetic testing in growth retardation. *Pediatrics* 123: e929–931, 2009.

Eggermann T, Mergenthaler S, Eggermann K, et al. Identification of interstitial maternal uniparental disomy (UPD) (14) and complete maternal UPD(20) in a cohort of growth retarded patients. *J Med Genet* 38: 86–89, 2001.

Eggermann T, Rossier E, Theurer-Mainka U, et al. New case of mosaic tetrasomy 9p with additional neurometabolic findings. *Am J Med Genet* 75: 530–533, 1998.

Eggermann T, Schönherr N, Spengler S, et al. Identification of a 21q22 duplication in a Silver-Russell syndrome patient further narrows down the Down syndrome critical region. *Am J Med Genet* 152A: 356–359, 2010b.

Eggermann T, Spengler S, Bachmann N, et al. Chromosome 11p15 duplication in Silver-Russell syndrome due to a maternally inherited translocation t(11;15). *Am J Med Genet* 152A: 1484–1487, 2010c.

Eggers S, Sadedin S, van den Bergen JA, et al. Disorders of sex development: Insights from targeted gene sequencing of a large international patient cohort. *Genome Biol* 17: 243, 2016.

Eggert M, Müller S, Heinrich U, Mehraein Y. A new familial case of microdeletion syndrome 10p15.3. *Eur J Med Genet* 59: 179–182, 2016.

Egozcue S, Blanco J, Vendrell JM, et al. Human male infertility: Chromosome anomalies, meiotic disorders, abnormal spermatozoa and recurrent abortion. *Hum Reprod Update* 6: 93–105, 2000.

Ehmke N, Karge S, Buchmann J, et al. A de novo nonsense mutation in *ZBTB18* plus a de novo 15q13.3 microdeletion in a 6-year-old female. *Am J Med Genet* 173A: 1251–1256, 2017.

Eichenlaub-Ritter U. Oocyte ageing and its cellular basis. *Int J Dev Biol* 56: 841–852, 2012.

Eid MM, El-Bassyouni HT, Eid OM, et al. Ring chromosome 15: Expanding the phenotype. *Genet Couns* 24: 417–425, 2013.

Ekelund CK, Jørgensen FS, Petersen OB, Sundberg K, Tabor A. Impact of a new national screening policy for Down's syndrome in Denmark: Population based cohort study. *Br Med J* 337: a2547, 2008.

El Chehadeh S, Touraine R, Prieur F, et al. Xq28 duplication including *MECP2* in six unreported affected females: What can we learn for diagnosis and genetic counselling? *Clin Genet* 91: 576–588, 2017.

El Khattabi L, Guimiot F, Pipiras E, et al. Incomplete penetrance and phenotypic variability of 6q16 deletions including *SIM1*. *Eur J Hum Genet* 23: 1010–1018, 2015.

El-Fouly MH, Higgins JV, Kapur S, Sankey BJ, Matisoff DN, Costa-Fox M. DiGeorge anomaly in an infant with deletion of chromosome 22 and dup(9p) due to adjacent type II disjunction. *Am J Med Genet* 38: 569–573, 1991.

Elghezal H, Hidar S, Braham R, Denguezli W, Ajina M, Saad A. Chromosome abnormalities in one thousand infertile males with nonobstructive sperm disorders. *Fertil Steril* 86: 1792–1795, 2006.

Elkins TE, Gafford LS, Wilks CS, Muram D, Golden G. A model clinic approach to the reproductive health concerns of the mentally handicapped. *Obstet Gynecol* 68: 185–188, 1986a.

Elkins TE, Stovall TG, Wilroy S, Dacus JV. Attitudes of mothers of children with Down syndrome concerning amniocentesis, abortion, and prenatal genetic counseling techniques. *Obstet Gynecol* 68: 181–184, 1986b.

Ellaway CJ, Ho G, Bettella E, et al. 14q12 microdeletions excluding *FOXG1* give rise to a congenital variant Rett syndrome-like phenotype. *Eur J Hum Genet* 21: 522–527, 2013.

Elliott M, Bayly R, Cole T, Temple IK, Maher ER. Clinical features and natural history of Beckwith-Wiedemann syndrome: Presentation of 74 new cases. *Clin Genet* 46: 168–174, 1994.

Ellis NA, Ciocci S, German J. Back mutation can produce phenotype reversion in Bloom syndrome somatic cells. *Hum Genet* 108: 167–173, 2001.

Ellison JW, Tekin M, Sikes KS, et al. Molecular characterization of a ring X chromosome in a male with short stature. *Hum Genet* 110: 322–326, 2002.

Emery AEH. *Methodology in Medical Genetics: An Introduction to Statistical Methods.* Edinburgh, UK: Churchill Livingstone, 1986.

Emiliani S, Gonzalez-Merino E, Van den Bergh M, Abramowicz M, Englert Y. Higher degree of chromosome mosaicism in preimplantation embryos from carriers of robertsonian translocation t(13;14) in comparison with embryos from karyotypically normal IVF patients. *J Assist Reprod Genet* 20: 95–100, 2003.

Engel E, Antonarakis SE. *Genomic Imprinting and Uniparental Disomy: Clinical and Molecular Aspects.* New York, NY: Wiley-Liss, 2002.

Engel E, Crippa L, Engel-de Montmollin M, Tran TN, Muhlethaler M. Implications for genetic counselling in regard to sex chromosome aneuploidies diagnosed by amniocentesis. *Ann Génét* 24: 107–109, 1981.

Engelen JJM, Arens YHJM, Gondrie ETCM, Alofs MGP, Loneus WH, Hamers AJH. Intrachromosomal insertion translocation resulting in duplication of chromosome band Yq11.2 in two fertile brothers. *Am J Med Genet* 118A: 287–289, 2003.

Engelen JJM, Marcelis C, Herbergs J, et al. Mosaic telomeric (2;14) association in a child with motor delay. *Am J Med Genet* 92: 318–321, 2000.

Engels H, Eggermann T, Caliebe A, et al. Genetic counseling in Robertsonian translocations der(13;14): Frequencies of reproductive outcomes and infertility in 101 pedigrees. *Am J Med Genet* 146A: 2611–2616, 2008.

Engels H, Schüler HM, Zink AM, et al. A phenotype map for 14q32.3 terminal deletions. *Am J Med Genet* 158A: 695–706, 2012.

Engenheiro E, Moller RS, Pinto M, et al. Mowat-Wilson syndrome: An underdiagnosed syndrome? *Clin Genet* 73: 579–584, 2008.

Englund A, Jonsson B, Zander CS, Gustafsson J, Annerén G. Changes in mortality and causes of death in the Swedish Down syndrome population. *Am J Med Genet* 161A: 642–649, 2013.

Enomoto K, Kishitani Y, Tominaga M, et al. Expression analysis of a 17p terminal deletion, including *YWHAE*, but not *PAFAH1B1*, associated with normal brain structure on MRI in a young girl. *Am J Med Genet* 158A: 2347–2352, 2012.

Eppley S, Hopkin RJ, Mendelsohn B, Slavotinek AM. Clinical Report: Warsaw Breakage Syndrome with small radii and fibulae. *Am J Med Genet* 173A: 3075–3081, 2017.

Epstein CJ. *The Phenotypic Mapping of Down Syndrome and Other Aneuploid Conditions.* New York, NY: Wiley-Liss, 1993.

Epstein CJ. 2001 William Allan Award Address: From Down syndrome to the "human" in "human genetics." *Am J Hum Genet* 70: 300–313, 2002.

Ergin RN, Cigerciogullari E, Alanay Y, Yayla M. A variant case of 6p24 deletion (OMIM #612582). *Genet Couns* 26: 237–241, 2015.

Erickson RP, Hudgins L, Stone JF, Schmidt S, Wilke C, Glover TW. A "balanced" Y;16 translocation associated with Turner-like neonatal lymphedema suggests the location of a potential anti-Turner gene on the Y chromosome. *Cytogenet Cell Genet* 71: 163–167, 1995.

Escribá MJ, Martín J, Rubio C, et al. Heteroparental blastocyst production from microsurgically corrected tripronucleated human embryos. *Fertil Steril* 86: 1601–1607, 2006.

Escudero T, Estop A, Fischer J, Munné S. Preimplantation genetic diagnosis for complex chromosome rearrangements. *Am J Med Genet* 146A: 1662–1669, 2008.

Escudero T, Lee M, Stevens J, Sandalinas M, Munné S. Preimplantation genetic diagnosis of pericentric inversions. *Prenat Diagn* 21: 760–766, 2001.

Esfandiari N, Bunnell ME, Casper RF. Human embryo mosaicism: Did we drop the ball on chromosomal testing? *J Assist Reprod Genet* 33: 1439–1444, 2016.

Eskenazi B, Wyrobek AJ, Kidd SA, et al. Sperm aneuploidy in fathers of children with paternally and maternally inherited Klinefelter syndrome. *Hum Reprod* 17: 576–583, 2002.

Esmer C, Sánchez S, Ramos S, Molina B, Frias S, Carnevale A. DEB test for Fanconi anemia detection in patients with atypical phenotypes. *Am J Med Genet* 124A: 35–39, 2004.

Estop AM, Cieply K, Munne S, Surti U, Wakim A, Feingold E. Is there an interchromosomal effect in reciprocal translocation carriers? Sperm FISH studies. *Hum Genet* 106: 517–524, 2000.

Eto K, Sakai N, Shimada S, et al. Microdeletions of 3p21.31 characterized by developmental delay, distinctive features, elevated serum creatine kinase levels, and white matter involvement. *Am J Med Genet* 161A: 3049–3056, 2013.

European Collaborative Research on Mosaicism in CVS (EUCROMIC). Trisomy 15 CPM: Probable origins, pregnancy outcome and risk of fetal UPD. *Prenat Diagn* 19: 29–35, 1999.

European Polycystic Kidney Disease Consortium. The polycystic kidney disease 1 gene encodes a 14 kb transcript and lies within a duplicated region on chromosome 16. *Cell* 77: 881–894, 1994.

Evans JA, MacDonald K, Hamerton JL. Sex chromosome anomalies: prenatal diagnosis and the need for continued prospective studies. *Birth Defects: Orig Art Series* 26(4): 273–281, 1990.

Evans MI, Farrell SA, Greb A, Ray P, Johnson MP, Hoffman EP. In utero fetal muscle biopsy for the diagnosis of Duchenne muscular dystrophy in a female fetus "suddenly at risk." *Am J Med Genet* 46: 309–312, 1993.

Evans MI, White BJ, Kent SG, Levine MA, Levin SW, Larsen JW. Balanced rearrangement of chromosomes 2, 5, and 13 in a family with duplication 5q and fetal loss. *Am J Med Genet* 19: 783–790, 1984.

Even-Zohar Gross N, Geva-Eldar T, Pollak Y, Hirsch HJ, Gross I, Gross-Tsur V. Attitudes toward prenatal genetic testing and therapeutic termination of pregnancy among parents of offspring with Prader-Willi syndrome. *Eur J Med Genet* 60: 205–211, 2017.

Evers C, Mitter D, Strobl-Wildemann G, et al. Duplication Xp11.22-p14 in females: Does X-inactivation help in assessing their significance? *Am J Med Genet* 167A: 553–562, 2015.

Faivre L, Gosset P, Cormier-Daire V, et al. Overgrowth and trisomy 15q26.1-qter including the IGF1 receptor gene: Report of two families and review of the literature. *Eur J Hum Genet* 10: 699–706, 2002.

Faivre L, Morichon-Delvallez N, Viot G, et al. Prenatal diagnosis of a satellited non-acrocentric chromosome derived from a maternal translocation (10;13)(p13;p12) and review of literature. *Prenat Diagn* 19: 282–286, 1999.

Faivre L, Portnoï MF, Pals G, et al. Should chromosome breakage studies be performed in patients with VACTERL association? *Am J Med Genet* 137: 55–58, 2005.

Faivre L, Radford I, Viot G, et al. Cerebellar ataxia and mental retardation in a child with an inherited satellited chromosome 4q. *Ann Génét* 43: 35–38, 2000.

Falek A, Schmidt R, Jervis GA. Familial de Lange syndrome with chromosome abnormalities. *Pediatrics* 37: 92–101, 1966.

Falik-Borenstein TC, Korenberg JR, Schreck RR. Confined placental chimerism: Prenatal and postnatal cytogenetic and molecular analysis, and pregnancy outcome. *Am J Med Genet* 50: 51–56, 1994.

Falik-Borenstein TC, Pribyl TM, Pulst SM, et al. Stable ring chromosome 21: Molecular and clinical definition of the lesion. *Am J Med Genet* 42: 22–28, 1992.

Familiari G, Caggiati A, Nottola SA, Ermini M, Di Benedetto MR, Motta PM. Ultrastructure of human ovarian primordial follicles after combination chemotherapy for Hodgkin's disease. *Hum Reprod* 8: 2080–2087, 1993.

Fan YS, Siu VM, Jung JH, Farrell SA, Côté GB. Direct duplication of 8p21.3→p23.1: a cytogenetic anomaly associated with developmental delay without consistent clinical features. *Am J Med Genet* 103: 231–234, 2001.

Fannemel M, Barøy T, Holmgren A, et al. Haploinsufficiency of *XPO1* and *USP34* by a de novo 230 kb deletion in 2p15, in a patient with mild intellectual disability and cranio-facial dysmorphisms. *Eur J Med Genet* 57: 513–519, 2014.

Farag TI, Krishna Murthy DS, Al-Awadi SA, et al. Robertsonian translocation t dic (14p;22p) with regular trisomy 21: A possible interchromosomal effect? *Ann Génét* 30: 189–192, 1987.

Farah LMS, Nazareth HRdeS, Dolnikoff M, Delascio D. Balanced homologous translocation t(22q22q) in a phenotypically normal woman with repeated spontaneous abortions. *Humangenetik* 28: 357–360, 1975.

Farah SB, Ramos CF, de Mello MP, et al. Two cases of Y; autosome translocations: A 45,X male and a clinically trisomy 18 patient. *Am J Med Genet* 49: 388–392, 1994.

Faraut T, Mermet MA, Demongeot J, Cohen O. Cooperation of selection and meiotic mechanisms in the production of imbalances in reciprocal translocations. *Cytogenet Cell Genet* 88: 15–21, 2000.

Faravelli F, Murdolo M, Marangi G, Bricarelli FD, Di Rocco M, Zollino M. Mother to son amplification of a small subtelomeric deletion: A new mechanism of familial recurrence in microdeletion syndromes. *Am J Med Genet* 143A: 1169–1173, 2007.

Faria ÁC, Rabbi-Bortolini E, Rebouças MR, et al. Craniosynostosis in 10q26 deletion patients: A consequence of brain underdevelopment or altered suture biology? *Am J Med Genet* 170A: 403–409, 2016.

Farrell SA, Chow G. Intrachromosomal insertion of chromosome 7. *Clin Genet* 41: 299–302, 1992.

Farrell SA, Fan YS. Balanced nonacrocentric whole-arm reciprocal translocations: A de novo case and literature review. *Am J Med Genet* 55: 423–426, 1995.

Farrell SA, Summers AM, Gardner HA, Uchida IA. Balanced complex chromosome rearrangement ascertained through prenatal diagnosis. *Am J Med Genet* 52: 360–361, 1994.

Farwig K, Harmon AG, Fontana KM, Mervis CB, Morris CA. Genetic counseling of adults with Williams syndrome: A first study. *Am J Med Genet* 154C: 307–315, 2010.

Fassihi H, Lu L, Wessagowit V, et al. Complete maternal isodisomy of chromosome 3 in a child with recessive dystrophic epidermolysis bullosa but no other phenotypic abnormalities. *J Invest Dermatol* 126: 2039–2043, 2006.

Favier R, Akshoomoff N, Mattson S, Grossfeld P. Jacobsen syndrome: Advances in our knowledge of phenotype and genotype. *Am J Med Genet* 169C: 239–250, 2015.

Faye-Petersen OM, Kapur RP. Placental mesenchymal dysplasia. *Surg Pathol Clin* 6: 127–151, 2013.

Federman DD. Mapping the X-chromosome: Mapping its p's and q's. *N Engl J Med* 317: 161–162, 1987.

Fedorenko E, Morgan A, Murray E, et al. A highly penetrant form of childhood apraxia of speech due to deletion of 16p11.2. *Eur J Hum Genet* 24: 302–306, 2016.

Feenstra I, Hanemaaijer N, Sikkema-Raddatz B, et al. Balanced into array: Genome-wide array analysis in 54 patients with an apparently balanced de novo chromosome rearrangement and a meta-analysis. *Eur J Hum Genet* 19: 1152–1160, 2011.

Fejgin MD, Arbel-DeRowe Y, Shul N, Amiel A. A false-positive diagnosis of Turner syndrome by amniocentesis. *Prenat Diagn* 17: 88–89, 1997.

Feldman B, Ebrahim SAD, Hazan SL, et al. Routine prenatal diagnosis of aneuploidy by FISH studies in high-risk pregnancies. *Am J Med Genet* 90: 233–238, 2000.

Feldman B, Kramer RL, Ebrahim SAD, Wolff DJ, Evans MI. Prenatal evaluation of a de novo X;9 translocation. *Am J Med Genet* 85: 476–478, 1999.

Feldman GL, Weiss L, Phelan MC, Schroer RJ, Van Dyke DL. Inverted duplication of 8p: Ten new patients and review of the literature. *Am J Med Genet* 47: 482–486, 1993.

Feng R, Yan Z, Li B, et al. Mutations in *TUBB8* cause a multiplicity of phenotypes in human oocytes and early embryos. *J Med Genet* 53: 662–671, 2016.

Fénichel P, Letur H. Procréation et syndrome de Turner: Quelles recommandations avant, pendant et après la grossesse? *Gynécol Obstét Fertil* 36: 891–897, 2008.

Fenu G, Esposito F, Delrio AN, Tedde G. The human gonocytes in the early phases of gonadal differentiation: Observations of one embryo at Carnegie stage 11. *Ital J Anat Embryol* 98: 127–140, 1993.

Ferfouri F, Bernicot I, Schneider A, Haquet E, Hédon B, Anahory T. Is the resulting phenotype of an embryo with balanced X-autosome translocation, obtained by means of preimplantation genetic diagnosis, linked to the X inactivation pattern? *Fertil Steril* 105: 1035–1046, 2016.

Ferfouri F, Clement P, Molina Gomes D, et al. Is classic pericentric inversion of chromosome 2 inv(2)(p11q13) associated with an increased risk of unbalanced chromosomes? *Fertil Steril* 92: 1497, e1–4, 2009.

Ferfouri F, Selva J, Boitrelle F, et al. The chromosomal risk in sperm from heterozygous Robertsonian translocation carriers is related to the sperm count and the translocation type. *Fertil Steril* 96: 1337–1343, 2011.

Ferguson-Smith MA. Prenatal chromosome analysis and its impact on the birth incidence of chromosome disorders. *Br Med Bull* 39: 355–364, 1983.

Ferguson-Smith MA, Cooke A, Affara NA, Boyd E, Tolmie JL. Genotype-phenotype correlations in XX males and their bearing on current theories of sex determination. *Hum Genet* 84: 198–202, 1990.

Fernández RM, Sánchez J, García-Díaz L, et al. Interstitial 10p deletion derived from a maternal ins(16;10)(q22;p13p15.2): Report of the first familial case of 10p monosomy affecting two familial members of different generations. *Am J Med Genet* 170A: 1268–1273, 2016.

Fernández-Rebollo E, Lecumberri B, Garin I, et al. New mechanisms involved in paternal 20q disomy associated with pseudohypoparathyroidism. *Eur J Endocrinol* 163: 953–962, 2010.

Ferraris A, Bernardini L, Sabolic Avramovska V, et al. Dandy-Walker malformation and Wisconsin syndrome: Novel cases add further insight into the genotype-phenotype correlations of 3q23q25 deletions. *Orphanet J Rare Dis* 8: 75, 2013.

Ferrier RA, Lowry RB, Lemire EG, Stoeber GP, Howard J, Parboosingh JS. Father-to-son transmission of an X-linked gene: A case of paternal sex chromosome heterodisomy. *Am J Med Genet* 149A: 2871–2873, 2009.

Field LL, Tobias R, Robinson WP, Paisey R, Bain S. Maternal uniparental disomy of chromosome 1 with no apparent phenotypic effects. *Am J Hum Genet* 63: 1216–1220, 1998.

Fieremans N, Bauters M, Belet S, et al. De novo *MECP2* duplications in two females with intellectual disability and unfavorable complete skewed X-inactivation. *Hum Genet* 133: 1359–1367, 2014.

Figura MG, Coppola A, Bottitta M, et al. Seizures and EEG pattern in the 22q13.3 deletion syndrome: Clinical report of six Italian cases. *Seizure* 23: 774–779, 2014.

Filges I, Kang A, Klug V, et al. aCGH on chorionic villi mirrors the complexity of fetoplacental mosaicism in prenatal diagnosis. *Prenat Diagn* 31: 473–478, 2011.

Filges I, Manokhina I, Peñaherrera MS, et al. Recurrent triploidy due to a failure to complete maternal meiosis II: Whole-exome sequencing reveals candidate variants. *Mol Hum Reprod* 21: 339–346, 2015.

Filges I, Röthlisberger B, Wenzel F, Heinimann K, Huber AR, Miny P. Mosaic ring chromosome 8: Clinical and array-CGH findings in partial trisomy 8. *Am J Med Genet* 146A: 2837–2841, 2008.

Filho AB, Souza J, Faucz FR, et al. Somatic/gonadal mosaicism in a syndromic form of ectrodactyly, including eye abnormalities, documented through array-based comparative genomic hybridization. *Am J Med Genet* 155A: 1152–1156, 2011.

Finucane B. Acculturation in women with mental retardation and its impact on genetic counseling. *J Genet Couns* 7: 31–47, 1998.

Firth H. Chorion villus sampling and limb deficiency—Cause or coincidence? *Prenat Diagn* 17: 1313–1330, 1997.

Fisher RA, Khatoon R, Paradinas FJ, Roberts AP, Newlands ES. Repetitive complete hydatidiform mole can be biparental in origin and either male or female. *Hum Reprod* 15: 594–598, 2000.

Fitzgerald PH, Archer SA, Morris CM. Evidence for the repeated primary non-disjunction of chromosome 21 as a result of premature centromere division (PCD). *Hum Genet* 72: 58–62, 1986.

Flejter WL, Finlinson D, Root S, Nguyen W, Brothman AR, Viskochil D. Familial ring (19) chromosome mosaicism: Case report and review. *Am J Med Genet* 66: 276–280, 1996.

Flipsen-ten Berg K, van Hasselt PM, Eleveld MJ, et al. Unmasking of a hemizygous WFS1 gene mutation by a chromosome 4p deletion of 8.3 Mb in a patient with Wolf-Hirschhorn syndrome. *Eur J Hum Genet* 15: 1132–1138, 2007.

Flori E, Doray B, Rudolf G, et al. Failure of prenatal diagnosis of diploid-triploid mosaicism after amniocentesis. *Clin Genet* 63: 328–331, 2003.

Folsom LJ, Fuqua JS. Reproductive issues in women with Turner syndrome. *Endocrinol Metab Clin North Am* 44: 723–737, 2015.

Fonseca AC, Bonaldi A, Bertola DR, Kim CA, Otto PA, Vianna-Morgante AM. The clinical impact of chromosomal rearrangements with breakpoints upstream of the *SOX9* gene: Two novel de novo balanced translocations associated with acampomelic campomelic dysplasia. *BMC Med Genet* 14: 50, 2013.

Fonseca-Pedrero E, Debbané M, Schneider M, Badoud D, Eliez S. Schizotypal traits in adolescents with 22q11.2 deletion syndrome: Validity, reliability and risk for psychosis. *Psychol Med* 46: 1005–1013, 2016.

Fontana P, Grasso M, Acquaviva F, et al. *SNORD116* deletions cause Prader-Willi syndrome with a mild phenotype and macrocephaly. *Clin Genet* 92: 440–443, 2017.

Forabosco A, Percesepe A, Santucci S. Incidence of non-age-dependent chromosomal abnormalities: A population-based study on 88965 amniocenteses. *Eur J Hum Genet* 17: 897–903, 2009.

Ford CE, Jones KW, Miller OJ, et al. The chromosomes in a patient showing both mongolism and the Klinefelter syndrome. *Lancet* 1: 709–710, 1959.

Ford NM. *When Did I Begin?* Cambridge, UK: Cambridge University Press, 1988.

Foresta C, Ferlin A, Gianaroli L, Dallapiccola B. Guidelines for the appropriate use of genetic tests in infertile couples. *Eur J Hum Genet* 10: 303–312, 2002.

Foresta C, Moro E, Ferlin A. Y chromosome microdeletions and alterations of spermatogenesis. *Endocr Rev* 22: 226–239, 2001.

Forman EJ. Morphology matters: Are all euploid blastocyst created equal? *Fertil Steril* 107: 573–574, 2017.

Forman EJ, Tao X, Ferry KM, Taylor D, Treff NR, Scott RT. Single embryo transfer with comprehensive chromosome screening results in improved ongoing pregnancy rates and decreased miscarriage rates. *Hum Reprod* 27: 1217–1222, 2012.

Forrest LE, Delatycki MB, Skene L, Aitken M. Communicating genetic information in families—A review of guidelines and position papers. *Eur J Hum Genet* 15: 612–618, 2007.

Forrester MB, Merz RD. Epidemiology of triploidy in a population-based birth defects registry, Hawaii, 1986–1999. *Am J Med Genet* 119A: 319–323, 2003a.

Forrester MB, Merz RD. Maternal age-specific Down syndrome rates by maternal race/ethnicity, Hawaii, 1986–2000. *Birth Defects Res* 67: 625–629, 2003b.

Forsberg LA. Loss of chromosome Y (LOY) in blood cells is associated with increased risk for disease and mortality in aging men. *Hum Genet* 136: 657–663, 2017.

Foudila T, Söderström-Anttila V, Hovatta O. Turner's syndrome and pregnancies after oocyte donation. *Hum Reprod* 14: 532–535, 1999.

Fountain MD, Aten E, Cho MT, et al. The phenotypic spectrum of Schaaf-Yang syndrome: 18 new affected individuals from 14 families. *Genet Med* 19: 45–52, 2017.

Fragouli E, Alfarawati S, Daphnis DD, et al. Cytogenetic analysis of human blastocysts with the use of FISH, CGH and aCGH: Scientific data and technical evaluation. *Hum Reprod* 26: 480–490, 2011.

Fragouli E, Alfarawati S, Spath K, et al. The origin and impact of embryonic aneuploidy. *Hum Genet* 132: 1001–1013, 2013.

Fragouli E, Lenzi M, Ross R, Katz-Jaffe M, Schoolcraft WB, Wells D. Comprehensive molecular cytogenetic analysis of the human blastocyst stage. *Hum Reprod* 23: 2596–2608, 2008.

Fragouli E, Wells D, Doshi A, Gotts S, Harper JC, Delhanty JD. Complete cytogenetic investigation of oocytes from a young cancer patient with the use of comparative genomic hybridisation reveals meiotic errors. *Prenat Diagn* 26: 71–76, 2006a.

Fragouli E, Wells D, Thornhill A, et al. Comparative genomic hybridization analysis of human oocytes and polar bodies. *Hum Reprod* 21: 2319–2328, 2006b.

Franasiak JM, Forman EJ, Hong KH, et al. The nature of aneuploidy with increasing age of the female partner: A review of 15,169 consecutive trophectoderm biopsies evaluated with comprehensive chromosomal screening. *Fertil Steril* 101: 656–663.e1, 2014.

Franasiak JM, Olcha M, Shastri S, et al. Embryonic aneuploidy does not differ among genetic ancestry according to continental origin as determined by ancestry informative markers. *Hum Reprod* 31: 2391–2395, 2016.

Francés A, Hildur K, Barberà JA, et al. Persistence of breakage in specific chromosome bands 6 years after acute exposure to oil. *PLoS One* 11: e0159404, 2016.

Fraser FC. Does paternal exposure to Agent Orange cause birth defects? *Am J Med Genet* 149A: 835–836, 2009.

Freitas ÉL, Gribble SM, Simioni M, et al. A familial case with interstitial 2q36 deletion: Variable phenotypic expression in full and mosaic state. *Eur J Med Genet* 55: 660–665, 2012.

Fridman C, Varela MC, Kok F, Diament A, Koiffmann CP. Paternal UPD15: Further genetic and clinical studies in four Angelman syndrome patients. *Am J Med Genet* 92: 322–327, 2000.

Fritz B, Greber-Platzer S, Frischer T, et al. Familial cryptic translocation with del 4q34→qter and dup 12pter→p13 in sibs with tracheal stenosis: Clinical, classical and molecular cytogenetic studies and CGH analyses from archival placental tissues evidencing tertiary trisomy 4 in one abortion specimen. *Am J Med Genet* 94: 271–280, 2000.

Fritz R, Kohan-Ghadr HR, Sacher A, et al. Trophoblast retrieval and isolation from the cervix (TRIC) is unaffected by early gestational age or maternal obesity. *Prenat Diagn* 35: 1218–1222, 2015.

Fryburg JS, Dimaio MS, Yang-Feng TL, Mahoney MJ. Follow-up of pregnancies complicated by placental mosaicism diagnosed by chorionic villus sampling. *Prenat Diagn* 13: 481–494, 1993.

Fryer AE, Ashworth M, Hawe J, Pilling D, Pauling M, Maye U. Isochromosome 20p associated with multiple congenital abnormalities. *Clin Dysmorphol* 14: 49–50, 2005.

Fryns JP, Bulcke J, Hens L, Van den Berghe H. Balanced transmission of centromeric fission products in man. *Hum Genet* 54: 127–128, 1980.

Fryns JP, Kleczkowska A. Reciprocal translocation mosaicism in man. *Am J Med Genet* 25: 175–176, 1986.

Fryns JP, Kleczkowska A. Ring chromosome 21 in the mother and 21/21 translocation in the fetus: Karyotype: 45,XX,-21,-21,+t(21;21)(p11;q11). *Ann Génét* 30: 109–110, 1987.

Fryns JP, Kleczkowska A, Kubień E, Van den Berghe H. On the excess of mental retardation and/or congenital malformations in apparently balanced reciprocal translocations: A critical review of the Leuven data 1966–1991. *Genet Counsel* 2: 185–194, 1992.

Fryns JP, Kleczkowska A, Kubien E, Van den Berghe H. XYY syndrome and other Y chromosome polysomies: Mental status and psychosocial functioning. *Genet Couns* 6: 197–206, 1995.

Fryns JP, Van Buggenhout G. Structural chromosome rearrangements in couples with recurrent fetal wastage. *Eur J Obstet Gynecol Reprod Biol* 81: 171–176, 1998.

Fryns JP, Van den Berghe H, Schrander-Stumpel C. Kabuki (Niikawa-Kuroki) syndrome and paracentric inversion of the short arm of chromosome 4. *Am J Med Genet* 53: 204–205, 1994.

Fryssira H, Makrythanasis P, Kattamis A, et al. Severe developmental delay in a patient with 7p21.1-p14.3 microdeletion spanning the *TWIST* gene and the *HOXA* gene cluster. *Mol Syndromol* 2: 45–49, 2011.

Fukai R, Hiraki Y, Nishimura G, et al. A de novo 1.4-Mb deletion at 21q22.11 in a boy with developmental delay. *Am J Med Genet* 164A: 1021–1028, 2014.

Fukami M, Shima H, Suzuki E, Ogata T, Matsubara K, Kamimaki T. Catastrophic cellular events leading to complex chromosomal rearrangements in the germline. *Clin Genet* 91: 653–660, 2017.

Fukunaga M. Immunohistochemical characterization of p57Kip2 expression in tetraploid hydropic placentas. *Arch Pathol Lab Med* 128: 897–900, 2004.

Fung WL, Butcher NJ, Costain G, et al. Practical guidelines for managing adults with 22q11.2 deletion syndrome. *Genet Med* 17: 599–609, 2015.

Furuya K, Sasaki Y, Takeuchi T, Urita Y. Characteristics of 22q 11.2 deletion syndrome undiagnosed until adulthood: An example suggesting the importance of psychiatric manifestations. *BMJ Case Rep* bcr2014-208903, 2015.

Fusco F, Paciolla M, Chen E, et al. Genetic and molecular analysis of a new unbalanced X;18 rearrangement: Localization of the diminished ovarian reserve disease locus in the distal Xq POF1 region. *Hum Reprod* 26: 3186–3196, 2011.

Fuster C, Miguez L, Miró R, Rigola MA, Perez A, Egozcue J. Familial complex chromosome rearrangement ascertained by in situ hybridisation. *J Med Genet* 34: 164–166, 1997.

Futaki M, Liu JM. Chromosomal breakage syndromes and the *BRCA1* genome surveillance complex. Trends Mol Med 7: 560–565, 2001.

Gabbett MT, Peters GB, Carmichael JM, Darmanian AP, Collins FA. Prader-Willi syndrome phenocopy due to duplication of Xq21.1-q21.31, with array CGH of the critical region. *Clin Genet* 73: 353–359, 2008.

Gabriel AS, Thornhill AR, Ottolini CS, et al. Array comparative genomic hybridisation on first polar bodies suggests that non-disjunction is not the predominant mechanism leading to aneuploidy in humans. *J Med Genet* 48: 433–437, 2011.

Gabriel-Robez O, Rumpler Y. The meiotic pairing behaviour in human spermatocytes carrier of chromosome anomalies and their repercussions on reproductive fitness. I: Inversions and insertions. A European collaborative study. *Ann Génét* 37: 3–10, 1994.

Gabriel-Robez O, Rumpler Y, Ratomponirina C, et al. Deletion of the pseudoautosomal region and lack of sex-chromosome pairing at pachytene in two infertile men carrying an X;Y translocation. *Cytogenet Cell Genet* 54: 38–42, 1990.

Gadancheva VG, Casey JP, Russell JD, McDaid J, Betts DR, Lynch SA. Vocal cord paralysis in association with 9q34 duplication. *Clin Dysmorphol* 23: 105–108, 2014.

Gai D, Haan E, Scholar M, Nicholl J, Yu S. Phenotypes of *AKT3* deletion: A case report and literature review. *Am J Med Genet* 167A: 174–179, 2015.

Gair JL, Arbour L, Rupps R, Jiang R, Bruyère H, Robinson WP. Recurrent trisomy 21: Four cases in three generations. *Clin Genet* 68: 430–435, 2005.

Gajecka M, Gentles AJ, Tsai A, et al. Unexpected complexity at breakpoint junctions in phenotypically normal individuals and mechanisms involved in generating balanced translocations t(1;22)(p36;q13). *Genome Res* 18: 1733–1742, 2008a.

Gajecka M, Mackay KL, Shaffer LG. Monosomy 1p36 deletion syndrome. *Am J Med Genet* 145C: 346–356, 2007.

Gajecka M, Saadeh R, Mackay KL, et al. Clinical and molecular cytogenetic characterization of four patients with unbalanced translocation der(1) t(1;22)(p36;q13). *Am J Med Genet* 146A: 2777–2784, 2008b.

Gajecka M, Saitta SC, Gentles AJ, et al. Recurrent interstitial 1p36 deletions: Evidence for germline mosaicism and complex rearrangement breakpoints. *Am J Med Genet* 152A: 3074–3083, 2010.

Gajecka M, Yu W, Ballif BC, et al. Delineation of mechanisms and regions of dosage imbalance in complex rearrangements of 1p36 leads to a putative gene for regulation of cranial suture closure. *Eur J Hum Genet* 13: 139–149, 2005.

Galvão Gomes A, Paiva Grangeiro CH, Silva LR, et al. Complex mosaic ring chromosome 11 associated with hemizygous loss of 8.6 Mb of 11q24.2qter in atypical Jacobsen syndrome. *Mol Syndromol* 8: 45–49, 2017.

Ganie Y, Aldous C, Balakrishna Y, Wiersma R. Disorders of sex development in children in KwaZulu-Natal Durban South Africa: 20-year experience in a tertiary centre. *J Pediatr Endocrinol Metab* 30: 11–18, 2017.

Garchet-Beaudron A, Dreux S, Leporrier N, Oury JF, Muller F. Second-trimester Down syndrome maternal serum marker screening: A prospective study of 11040 twin pregnancies. *Prenat Diagn* 28: 1105–1109, 2008.

García-Castillo H, Vásquez-Velásquez AI, Rivera H, Barros-Núñez P. Clinical and genetic heterogeneity in patients with mosaic variegated aneuploidy: Delineation of clinical subtypes. *Am J Med Genet* 146A: 1687–1695, 2008.

Garcia-Heras J, Kilani RA, Martin RA, Lamp S. A deletion of proximal 20p inherited from a normal mosaic carrier mother in a newborn with panhypopituitarism and craniofacial dysmorphism. *Clin Dysmorphol* 14: 137–140, 2005.

Garcia-Heras J, Martin JA, Witchel SF, Scacheri P. De novo der(X)t(X;10)(q26;q21) with features of distal trisomy 10q: Case report of paternal origin identified by late replication with BrdU and the human androgen receptor assay (HAR). *J Med Genet* 34: 242–245, 1997.

García-Santiago FA, Martínez-Glez V, Santos F, et al. Analysis of invdupdel(8p) rearrangement: Clinical, cytogenetic and molecular characterization. *Am J Med Genet* 167A: 1018–1025, 2015.

Gardner RJM. Chromosomes and clinical anatomy. *Clin Anat* 29: 540–546, 2016.

Gardner RJM, Chewings WE, Holdaway MD. A ring 15 chromosome in a girl with minor abnormalities. *NZ Med J* 91: 173–174, 1980.

Gardner RJM, Grindley RM, Chewings WE, Clarkson JE. Ring chromosome 1 associated with radial ray defect. *J Med Genet* 21: 400, 1984.

Gardner RJM, Monk NA, Allen GJ, Parslow MI. A three way translocation in mother and daughter. *J Med Genet* 23: 90, 1986a.

Gardner RJM, Monk NA, Clarkson JE, Allen GJ. Ring 21 chromosome: The mild end of the phenotypic spectrum. *Clin Genet* 30: 466–470, 1986b.

Gardner RJM, Rudd NL, Stevens LJ, Worton RG. Autosomal imbalance with a near-normal phenotype: The small effect of trisomy for the short arm of chromosome 18. *Birth Defects Orig Artic Ser* 14: 359–363, 1978.

Gardner RJM, Parslow MI, Veale AMO. The formation of the abnormal chromosome in balanced homologous Robertsonian translocation carriers. *Humangenetik* 21: 270–282, 1974.

Gardner RJM, Veale AMO. De novo translocation Down's syndrome: Risk of recurrence of Down's syndrome. *Clin Genet* 6: 160–164, 1974.

Gardner RJM, Veale AMO, Parslow MI, et al. A survey of 972 cytogenetically examined cases of Down's syndrome. *NZ Med J* 78: 403–409, 1973a.

Gardner RJM, Veale AMO, Sands VE, Holdaway MDH. XXXX syndrome: Case report, and a note on genetic counselling and fertility. *Humangenetik* 17: 323–330, 1973b.

Garin I, Elli FM, Linglart A, et al. Novel microdeletions affecting the GNAS locus in pseudohypoparathyroidism: Characterization of the underlying mechanisms. *J Clin Endocrinol Metab* 100: E681–687, 2015.

Garrett LA, Garner EI, Feltmate CM, Goldstein DP, Berkowitz RS. Subsequent pregnancy outcomes in patients with molar pregnancy and persistent gestational trophoblastic neoplasia. *J Reprod Med* 53: 481–486, 2008.

Gassner R, Metzenbauer M, Hafner E, Vallazza U, Philipp K. Triploidy in a twin pregnancy: Small placenta volume as an early sonographical marker. *Prenat Diagn* 23: 16–20, 2003.

Gat I, AlKudmani B, Wong K, et al. Significant correlation between anti-müllerian hormone and embryo euploidy in a subpopulation of infertile patients. *Reprod Biomed Online* 35: 602–608, 2017.

Gatti R, Perlman S. Ataxia-Telangiectasia. In Pagon RA, Adam MP, Ardinger HH, et al. (eds.), *GeneReviews* [Internet]. Seattle, WA: University of Washington, 2016.

Gau SS, Liao HM, Hong CC, Chien WH, Chen CH. Identification of two inherited copy number variants in a male with autism supports two-hit and compound heterozygosity models of autism. *Am J Med Genet Neuropsychiatr Genet* 159B: 710–717, 2012.

Gautier M, Harper PS. Fiftieth anniversary of trisomy 21: Returning to a discovery. *Hum Genet* 126: 317–324, 2009.

Gazou A, Riess A, Grasshoff U, et al. Xq22.3-q23 deletion including *ACSL4* in a patient with intellectual disability. *Am J Med Genet* 161A: 860–864, 2013.

Geigy Scientific Tables: Introduction to Statistics, Statistical Tables, Mathematical Formulae. Basel, Switzerland: Novartis (formerly Ciba Geigy), 1982.

Gekas J, Thepot F, Turleau C, et al. Chromosomal factors of infertility in candidate couples for ICSI: An equal risk of constitutional aberrations in women and men. *Hum Reprod* 16: 82–90, 2001.

Gendrel AV, Marion-Poll L, Katoh K, Heard E. Random monoallelic expression of genes on autosomes: Parallels with X-chromosome inactivation. *Semin Cell Dev Biol* 56: 100–110, 2016.

Genesio R, Fontana P, Mormile A, et al. Constitutional chromothripsis involving the critical region of 9q21.13 microdeletion syndrome. *Mol Cytogenet* 8: 96, 2015a.

Genesio R, Melis D, Gatto S, et al. Variegated silencing through epigenetic modifications of a large Xq region in a case of balanced X;2 translocation with incontinentia pigmenti-like phenotype. *Epigenetics* 6: 1242–1247, 2011.

Genesio R, Mormile A, Licenziati MR, et al. Short stature and primary ovarian insufficiency possibly due to chromosomal position effect in a balanced X;1 translocation. *Mol Cytogenet* 8: 50, 2015b.

Genesio R, Ronga V, Castelluccio P, et al. Pure 16q21q22.1 deletion in a complex rearrangement possibly caused by a chromothripsis event. *Mol Cytogenet* 6: 29, 2013.

Genest P. Transmission héréditaire depuis 300 ans d'un chromosome Y à satellites dans une lignée familiale. *Ann Génét* 16: 35–38, 1973.

Genest P. Further study on the nature of a multicentury small Y chromosome. *Ann Génét* 24: 165–166, 1981.

Gentile M, Volpe P, Cariola F, et al. Prenatal diagnosis of chromosome 4 mosaicism: Prognostic role of cytogenetic, molecular, and ultrasound/MRI characterization. *Am J Med Genet* 136: 66–70, 2005.

Genuardi M, Tozzi C, Pomponi MG, et al. Mosaic trisomy 17 in amniocytes: Phenotypic outcome, tissue distribution, and uniparental disomy studies. *Eur J Hum Genet* 7: 421–426, 1999.

George AM, Oei P, Winship I. False-positive diagnosis of trisomy 21 using fluorescence in situ hybridisation (FISH) on uncultured amniotic fluid cells. *Prenat Diagn* 23: 302–305, 2003.

Georgiades P, Chierakul C, Ferguson-Smith AC. Parental origin effects in human trisomy for chromosome 14q: Implications for genomic imprinting. *J Med Genet* 35: 821–824, 1998.

Geraedts J, Collins J, Gianaroli L, et al. What next for preimplantation genetic screening? A polar body approach! *Hum Reprod* 25: 575–577, 2010.

Gerkes EH, van der Kevie-Kersemaekers AM, Yakin M, Smeets DFCM, van Ravenswaaij-Arts CMA. The importance of chromosome studies in Roberts syndrome/SC phocomelia and other cohesinopathies. *Eur J Med Genet* 53: 40–44, 2010.

German J. Bloom syndrome: A Mendelian prototype of somatic mutational disease. *Medicine (Baltimore)* 72: 393–406, 1993.

German J, Ellis NA. Bloom syndrome. In Scriver C, Vogelstein B (eds.), *Molecular Metabolic Basis of Inherited Disease.* New York, NY: McGraw Hill, 2000.

German J, Ellis NA. Bloom syndrome. In *The Online Metabolic and Molecular Bases of Inherited Disease*, 2011, Chapter 30. Available at http://www.ommbid.com

German J, Sanz MM, Ciocci S, Ye TZ, Ellis NA. Syndrome-causing mutations of the BLM gene in persons in the Bloom's Syndrome Registry. *Hum Mutat* 28: 743–753, 2007.

Gersen SL, Keagle MB (eds.). *The Principles of Clinical Cytogenetics.* New York, NY: Springer, 2013.

Ghevaria H, SenGupta S, Shmitova N, Serhal P, Delhanty J. The origin and significance of additional aneuploidy events in couples undergoing preimplantation genetic diagnosis for translocations by array comparative genomic hybridization. *Reprod Biomed Online* 32: 178–189, 2016.

Ghosh A, Higgins L, Larkins SA, et al. Prenatal diagnosis and prenatal imaging of a de novo 46,X,der(Y)t(X;Y)(p22.13;q11.23) leading to functional disomy for the distal end of the X chromosome short arm from Xp22.13 in a phenotypically male fetus with posterior fossa abnormalities. *Prenat Diagn* 28: 1068–1071, 2008.

Ghosh S, Feingold E, Dey SK. Etiology of Down syndrome: Evidence for consistent association among altered meiotic recombination, nondisjunction, and maternal age across populations. *Am J Med Genet* 149A: 1415–1420, 2009.

Giacalone JP, Francke U. Common sequence motifs at the rearrangement sites of a constitutional X/autosome translocation and associated deletion. *Am J Hum Genet* 50: 725–741, 1992.

Giambona A, Leto F, Damiani G, et al. Identification of embryo-fetal cells in celomic fluid using morphological and short-tandem repeats analysis. *Prenat Diagn* 36: 973–978, 2016.

Gianaroli L, Magli MC, Cavallini G, et al. Frequency of aneuploidy in sperm from patients with extremely severe male factor infertility. *Hum Reprod* 20: 2140–2152, 2005.

Gianaroli L, Magli MC, Ferraretti AP, et al. Possible interchromosomal effect in embryos generated by gametes from translocation carriers. *Hum Reprod* 17: 3201–3207, 2002.

Giardino D, Corti C, Ballarati L, et al. Prenatal diagnosis of a de novo complex chromosome rearrangement (CCR) mediated by six breakpoints, and a review of 20 prenatally ascertained CCRs. *Prenat Diagn* 26: 565–570, 2006.

Giardino D, Corti C, Ballarati L, et al. De novo balanced chromosome rearrangements in prenatal diagnosis. *Prenat Diagn* 29: 257–265, 2009.

Giardino D, Finelli P, Russo S, et al. Small familial supernumerary ring chromosome 2: FISH characterization and genotype-phenotype correlation. *Am J Med Genet* 111: 319–323, 2002.

Giaroli G, Bass N, Strydom A, Rantell K, McQuillin A. Does rare matter? Copy number variants at 16p11.2 and the risk of psychosis: A systematic review of literature and meta-analysis. *Schizophr Res* 159: 340–346, 2014.

Gibbons B, Tan SY, Yu CC, Cheah E, Tan HL. Risk of gonadoblastoma in female patients with Y chromosome abnormalities and dysgenetic gonads. *J Paediatr Child Health* 35: 210–213, 1999.

Gibbons RJ. α-Thalassemia, mental retardation, and myelodysplastic syndrome. *Cold Spring Harb Perspect Med* 2: a011759, 2012.

Gibbs J, Appleton J, Appleton R. Dyspraxia or developmental coordination disorder? Unravelling the enigma. *Arch Dis Child* 92: 534–539, 2007.

Gidoni YS, Takefman J, Holzer HE, et al. Cryopreservation of a mother's oocytes for possible future use by her daughter with Turner syndrome: Case report. *Fertil Steril* 90: e9–12, 2008.

Gies I, Oates R, De Schepper J, Tournaye H. Testicular biopsy and cryopreservation for fertility preservation of prepubertal boys with Klinefelter syndrome: A pro/con debate. *Fertil Steril* 105: 249–255, 2016.

Giglio S, Broman KW, Matsumoto N, et al. Olfactory receptor-gene clusters, genomic-inversion polymorphisms, and common chromosome rearrangements. *Am J Hum Genet* 68: 874–883, 2001.

Giglio S, Calvari V, Gregato G, et al. Heterozygous submicroscopic inversions involving olfactory receptor-gene clusters mediate the recurrent t(4;8)(p16;p23) translocation. *Am J Hum Genet* 71: 276–285, 2002.

Giglio S, Pirola B, Arrigo G, et al. Opposite deletions/duplications of the X chromosome: two novel reciprocal rearrangements. *Eur J Hum Genet* 8: 63–70, 2000.

Gijsbers AC, Bosch CA, Dauwerse JG, et al. Additional cryptic CNVs in mentally retarded patients with apparently balanced karyotypes. *Eur J Med Genet* 53: 227–233, 2010.

Gil MM, Quezada MS, Revello R, Akolekar R, Nicolaides KH. Analysis of cell-free DNA in maternal blood in screening for fetal aneuploidies: Updated meta-analysis. *Ultrasound Obstet Gynecol* 45: 249–66, 2015.

Gilardi JL, Perrotin F, Paillet C, et al. Prenatal diagnosis of trisomy 21 by i(21q): A rare case of fetoplacental chromosomal discrepancy. *Prenat Diagn* 22: 856–858, 2002.

Gilbert B, Yardin C, Briault S, et al. Prenatal diagnosis of female monozygotic twins discordant for Turner syndrome: Implications for prenatal genetic counselling. *Prenat Diagn* 22: 697–702, 2002.

Gillentine MA, Berry LN, Goin-Kochel RP, et al. The cognitive and behavioral phenotypes of Individuals with *CHRNA7* duplications. *J Autism Dev Disord* 47: 549–562, 2017a.

Gillentine MA, Yin J, Cummock S, Kim JJ, Bajic A, Schaaf CP. *CHRNA7* CNVs: Shared clinical phenotypes mediated by differing molecular mechanisms. Paper presented at the European Human Genetics conference, Copenhagen, 2017b.

Gilling M, Dullinger JS, Gesk S, et al. Breakpoint cloning and haplotype analysis indicate a single origin of the common Inv(10)(p11.2q21.2) mutation among northern Europeans. *Am J Hum Genet* 78: 878–883, 2006.

Gillon R. On sterilising severely mentally handicapped people. *J Med Ethics* 13: 59–61, 1987.

Giltay JC, Kastrop PM, Tiemessen CH, van Inzen WG, Scheres JM, Pearson PL. Sperm analysis in a subfertile male with a Y;16 translocation, using four-color FISH. *Cytogenet Cell Genet* 84: 67–72, 1999.

Gimelbrant A, Hutchinson JN, Thompson BR, Chess A. Widespread monoallelic expression on human autosomes. *Science* 318: 1136–1140, 2007.

Ginsberg NA, Cadkin A, Strom C, Bauer-Marsh E, Verlinsky Y. Prenatal diagnosis of 46,XX male fetuses. *Am J Obstet Gynecol* 180: 1006–1007, 1999.

Ginsburg C, Fokstuen S, Schinzel A. The contribution of uniparental disomy to congenital development defects in children born to mothers at advanced childbearing age. *Am J Med Genet* 95: 454–460, 2000.

Giorda R, Bonaglia MC, Beri S, et al. Complex segmental duplications mediate a recurrent dup(X)(p11.22-p11.23) associated with mental retardation, speech delay, and EEG anomalies in males and females. *Am J Hum Genet* 85: 394–400, 2009.

Giorda R, Bonaglia MC, Milani G, et al. Molecular and cytogenetic analysis of the spreading of X inactivation in a girl with microcephaly, mild dysmorphic features and t(X;5)(q22.1;q31.1). *Eur J Hum Genet* 16: 897–905, 2008.

Girirajan S, Rosenfeld JA, Coe BP, et al. Phenotypic heterogeneity of genomic disorders and rare copy-number variants. *N Engl J Med* 367: 1321–1331, 2012.

Girirajan S, Rosenfeld JA, Cooper GM, et al. A recurrent 16p12.1 microdeletion supports a two-hit model for severe developmental delay. *Nat Genet* 42: 203–209, 2010.

Glass IA, Rauen KA, Chen E, et al. Ring chromosome 15: Characterization by array CGH. *Hum Genet* 118: 611–617, 2006.

Glassford MR, Rosenfeld JA, Freedman AA, Zwick ME, Mulle JG; Unique Rare Chromosome Disorder Support Group. Novel features of 3q29 deletion syndrome: Results from the 3q29 registry. *Am J Med Genet* 170A: 999–1006, 2016.

Glasson EJ, Sullivan SG, Hussain R, Petterson BA, Montgomery PD, Bittles AH. The changing survival profile of people with Down's syndrome: Implications for genetic counselling. *Clin Genet* 62: 390–393, 2002.

Gleeson JG, Allen KM, Fox JW, et al. Doublecortin, a brain-specific gene mutated in human X-linked lissencephaly and double cortex syndrome, encodes a putative signaling protein. *Cell* 92: 63–72, 1998.

Glenn CC, Deng G, Michaelis RC, et al. DNA methylation analysis with respect to prenatal diagnosis of the Angelman and Prader-Willi syndromes and imprinting. *Prenat Diagn* 20: 300–306, 2000.

Glujovsky D, Farquhar C. Cleavage-stage or blastocyst transfer: What are the benefits and harms? *Fertil Steril* 106: 244–250, 2016.

Godo A, Blanco J, Vidal F, Sandalinas M, Garcia-Guixé E, Anton E. Altered segregation pattern and numerical chromosome abnormalities interrelate in spermatozoa from Robertsonian translocation carriers. *Reprod Biomed Online* 31: 79–88, 2015.

Goitia V, Oquendo M, Stratton R. Case of 7p22.1 microduplication detected by whole genome microarray (REVEAL) in workup of child diagnosed with autism. *Case Rep Genet* 2015: 212436, 2015.

Golden WL, Sudduth KW, Burnett SH, Kelly TE. Mosaicism in Prader-Willi syndrome: Detection using fluorescent in situ hybridization. *Am J Med Genet* 85: 424–425, 1999.

Goldman ASH, Hultén MA. Chromosome in situ suppression hybridisation in human male meiosis. *J Med Genet* 29: 98–102, 1992.

Goldman ASH, Martin RH, Johannisson R, et al. Meiotic and sperm chromosome analysis in a male carrier of an inverted insertion (3;10) (q13.2;p14p13). *J Med Genet* 29: 460–464, 1992.

Gole L, Crolla JA, Thomas SN, Jacobs PA, Dennis NR. Characterization of breakpoints in the *GABRG3* and *TSPY* genes in a family with a t(Y;15)(p11.2;q12). *Am J Med Genet* 125A: 177–180, 2004.

Golubovsky MD. Postzygotic diploidization of triploids as a source of unusual cases of mosaicism, chimerism and twinning. *Hum Reprod* 18: 236–242, 2003.

Golzio C, Guirchoun J, Ozilou C, et al. Cytogenetic and histological features of a human embryo with homogeneous chromosome 8 trisomy. *Prenat Diagn* 26: 1201–1205, 2006.

Goodall J. Helping a child to understand her own testicular feminisation. *Lancet* 337: 33–35, 1991.

Goodwin PJ, Ennis M, Pritchard KI, Trudeau M, Hood N. Risk of menopause during the first year after breast cancer diagnosis. *J Clin Oncol* 17: 2365–2370, 1999.

Gordon CT, Attanasio C, Bhatia S, et al. Identification of novel craniofacial regulatory domains located far upstream of *SOX9* and disrupted in Pierre Robin sequence. *Hum Mutat* 35: 1011–1020, 2014.

Gorski JL, Kistenmacher ML, Punnett HH, Zackai EH, Emanuel BS. Reproductive risks for carriers of complex chromosome rearrangements: Analysis of 25 families. *Am J Med Genet* 29: 247–261, 1988.

Goumy C, Beaufrère AM, Francannet C, et al. Prenatal detection of mosaic isochromosome 20q: A fourth report with abnormal phenotype. *Prenat Diagn* 25: 653–655, 2005.

Gradek GA, Kvistad PH, Houge G. Monosomy 8 rescue gave cells with a normal karyotype in a mildly affected man with 46,XY,r(8) mosaicism. *Eur J Med Genet* 49: 292–297, 2006.

Grams SE, Argiropoulos B, Lines M, et al. Genotype-phenotype characterization in 13 individuals with chromosome Xp11.22 duplications. *Am J Med Genet* 170A: 967–977, 2016.

Grams SE, Rand L, Norton ME. Complete isochromosome 5p in one fetus of a monochorionic twin pair. *Prenat Diagn* 31: 605–607, 2011.

Grande M, Sabrià J, Borobio V, et al. Effectiveness of ovarian age as the background risk for aneuploidy screening in an unselected pregnant population. *Reprod Biomed Online* 33: 500–505, 2016.

Grande M, Stergiotou I, Borobio V, Sabrià J, Soler A, Borrell A. Heterotrisomy recurrence risk: a practical maternal age-dependent approach for excess trisomy 21 risk calculation after a previous autosomal trisomy. *J Matern Fetal Neonatal Med* 30: 1613–1615, 2017.

Grange DK, Garcia-Heras J, Kilani RA, Lamp S. Trisomy 20q13→20qter in a girl with multiple congenital malformations and a recombinant chromosome 20 inherited from a paternal inversion (20)(p13q13.1): Clinical report and review of the trisomy 20q phenotype. *Am J Med Genet* 137A: 308–312, 2005.

Grass FS, Schwartz RP, Deal JO, Parke JC, Jr. Gonadal dysgenesis, intra-X chromosome insertion, and possible position effect in an otherwise normal female. *Clin Genet* 20: 28–35, 1981.

Grati FR. Chromosomal mosaicism in human feto-placental development: Implications for prenatal diagnosis. *J Clin Med* 3: 809–837, 2014.

Grati FR. Implications of fetoplacental mosaicism on cell-free DNA testing: a review of a common biological phenomenon. *Ultrasound Obstet Gynecol* 48: 415–423, 2016.

Grati FR, Bajaj K, Malvestiti F, et al. The type of feto-placental aneuploidy detected by cfDNA testing may influence the choice of confirmatory diagnostic procedure. *Prenat Diagn* 35: 994–998, 2015.

Grati FR, Turolla L, D'Ajello P, et al. Chromosome 11 segmental paternal isodisomy in amniocytes from two fetuses with omphalocoele: New highlights on phenotype-genotype correlations in Beckwith-Wiedemann syndrome. *J Med Genet* 44: 257–263, 2007.

Gravholt CH. Medical problems of adult Turner's syndrome. *Horm Res* 56 (Suppl 1): 44–50, 2001.

Gravholt CH, Weis Naeraa R. Reference values for body proportions and body composition in adult women with Ullrich-Turner syndrome. *Am J Med Genet* 72: 403–408, 1997.

Graw SL, Sample T, Bleskan J, Sujansky E, Patterson D. Cloning, sequencing, and analysis of inv8 chromosome breakpoints associated with recombinant 8 syndrome. *Am J Hum Genet* 66: 1138–1144, 2000.

Gray J, Yeo GS, Cox JJ, et al. Hyperphagia, severe obesity, impaired cognitive function, and hyperactivity associated with functional loss of one copy of the brain-derived neurotrophic factor (BDNF) gene. *Diabetes* 55: 3366–3371, 2006.

Grayton HM, Fernandes C, Rujescu D, Collier DA. Copy number variations in neurodevelopmental disorders. *Prog Neurobiol* 99: 81–91, 2012.

Greally JM, Neiswanger K, Cummins JH, et al. A molecular anatomical analysis of mosaic trisomy 16. *Hum Genet* 98: 86–90, 1996.

Greco E, Minasi MG, Fiorentino F. Healthy babies after intrauterine transfer of mosaic aneuploid blastocysts. *N Engl J Med* 373: 2089–2090, 2015.

Green DM, Kawashima T, Stovall M, et al. Fertility of female survivors of childhood cancer: A report from the Childhood Cancer Survivor Study. *J Clin Oncol* 27: 2677–2685, 2009.

Green DM, Kawashima T, Stovall M, et al. Fertility of male survivors of childhood cancer: A report from the Childhood Cancer Survivor Study. *J Clin Oncol* 28: 332–339, 2010.

Green JM, Hewison J, Bekker HL, Bryant LD, Cuckle HS. Psychosocial aspects of genetic screening of pregnant women and newborns: A systematic review. *Health Technol Assess (UK)* 8: No. 33, 2004.

Greger V, Knoll JHM, Wagstaff J, et al. Angelman syndrome associated with an inversion of chromosome 15q11.2q24.3. *Am J Hum Genet* 60: 574–580, 1997.

Gregg AR, Skotko BG, Benkendorf JL, et al. Noninvasive prenatal screening for fetal aneuploidy, 2016 update: A position statement of the American College of Medical Genetics and Genomics. *Genet Med* 18: 1056–1065, 2016.

Gribble SM, Fiegler H, Burford DC, et al. Applications of combined DNA microarray and chromosome sorting technologies. *Chromosome Res* 12: 35–43, 2004.

Griffin DK, Hyland P, Tempest HG, Homa ST. Safety issues in assisted reproduction technology: Should men undergoing ICSI be screened for chromosome abnormalities in their sperm? *Hum Reprod* 18: 229–235, 2003.

Griffiths MJ, Miller PR, Stibbe HM. A false-positive diagnosis of Turner syndrome by amniocentesis. *Prenat Diagn* 16: 463–466, 1996.

Grigorescu-Sido A, Heinrich U, Grigorescu-Sido P, et al. Three new 46,XX male patients: A clinical, cytogenetic and molecular analysis. *J Pediatr Endocrinol Metab* 18: 197–203, 2005.

Grillo L, Reitano S, Belfiore G, et al. Familial 1.1 Mb deletion in chromosome Xq22.1 associated with mental retardation and behavioural disorders in female patients. *Eur J Med Genet* 53: 113–116, 2010.

Grinspon RP, Rey RA. Disorders of sex development with testicular differentiation in *SRY*-negative 46,XX individuals: Clinical and genetic aspects. *Sex Dev* 10: 1–11, 2016.

Groen SE, Drewes JG, de Boer EG, Hoovers JMN, Hennekam RCM. Repeated unbalanced offspring due to a familial translocation involving chromosomes 5 and 6. *Am J Med Genet* 80: 448–453, 1998.

Grønborg S, Kjaergaard S, Hove H, Larsen VA, Kirchhoff M. Monozygotic twins with a de novo 0.32 Mb 16q24.3 deletion, including *TUBB3* presenting with developmental delay and mild facial dysmorphism but without overt brain malformation. *Am J Med Genet* 167A: 2731–2736, 2015.

Gross M, Hanenberg H, Lobitz S, et al. Reverse mosaicism in Fanconi anemia: Natural gene therapy via molecular self-correction. *Cytogenet Genome Res* 98: 126–135, 2002.

Gross SJ, Stosic M, McDonald-McGinn DM, et al. Clinical experience with single-nucleotide polymorphism-based non-invasive prenatal screening for 22q11.2 deletion syndrome. *Ultrasound Obstet Gynecol* 47: 177–183, 2016.

Gross SJ, Tharapel AT, Phillips OP, Shulman LP, Pivnick EK, Park VM. A jumping Robertsonian translocation: A molecular and cytogenetic study. *Hum Genet* 98: 291–296, 1996.

Grossmann V, Höckner M, Karmous-Benailly H, et al. Parental origin of apparently balanced de novo complex chromosomal rearrangements investigated by microdissection, whole genome amplification, and microsatellite-mediated haplotype analysis. *Clin Genet* 78: 548–553, 2010.

Groupe de Cytogénéticiens Français. Pericentric inversions in man: A French collaborative study. *Ann Génét* 29: 129–168, 1986a.

Groupe de Cytogénéticiens Français. Paracentric inversions in man: A French collaborative study *Ann Génét* 29: 169–176, 1986b.

Grover S, Brady S, Chondros P. Sterilisations in girls and young women: Is it still happening? *Aust NZ J Public Health* 26: 273–275, 2002.

Grozeva D, Carss K, Spasic-Boskovic O, et al. De novo loss-of-function mutations in *SETD5*, encoding a methyltransferase in a 3p25 microdeletion syndrome critical region, cause intellectual disability. *Am J Hum Genet* 94: 618–624, 2014.

Gruchy N, Barreau M, Kessler K, Gourdier D, Leporrier N. A paternally transmitted complex chromosomal rearrangement (CCR) involving chromosomes 2, 6, and 18 includes eight breakpoints and five insertional translocations (ITs) through three generations. *Am J Med Genet* 152A: 185–190, 2010.

Gruchy N, Blondeel E, Le Meur N, et al. Pregnancy outcomes in prenatally diagnosed 47,XXX and 47,XYY syndromes: A 30-year French, retrospective, multicentre study. *Prenat Diagn* 36: 523–529, 2016.

Gruchy N, Lebrun M, Herlicoviez M, et al. Supernumerary marker chromosomes management in prenatal diagnosis. *Am J Med Genet* 146A: 2770–2776, 2008.

Grynberg M, Bidet M, Benard J, et al. Fertility preservation in Turner syndrome. *Fertil Steril* 105: 13–19, 2016.

Gu S, Yuan B, Campbell IM, et al. Alu-mediated diverse and complex pathogenic copy-number variants within human chromosome 17 at p13.3. *Hum Mol Genet* 24: 4061–4077, 2015.

Gu W, Zhang F, Lupski JR. Mechanisms for human genomic rearrangements. *Pathogenet* 1: 4, 2008.

Guc-Scekic M, Milasin J, Stevanovic M, Stojanov LJ, Djordjevic M. Tetraploidy in a 26-month-old girl (cytogenetic and molecular studies). *Clin Genet* 61: 62–65, 2002.

Guediche N, Brisset S, Benichou JJ, et al. Chromosomal breakpoints characterization of two supernumerary ring chromosomes 20. *Am J Med Genet* 152A: 464–471, 2010.

Guha S, Rees E, Darvasi A, et al. Implication of a rare deletion at distal 16p11.2 in schizophrenia. *JAMA Psychiatry* 70: 253–260, 2013.

Guichaoua MR, Devictor M, Hartung M, Luciani JM, Stahl A. Random acrocentric bivalent associations in human pachytene spermatocytes: Molecular implications in the occurrence of Robertsonian translocations. *Cytogenet Cell Genet* 42: 191–197, 1986.

Guichaoua MR, Quack B, Speed RM, Noel B, Chandley AC, Luciani JM. Infertility in human males with autosomal translocations: meiotic study of a 14;22 Robertsonian translocation. *Hum Genet* 86: 162–166, 1990.

Guida V, Sinibaldi L, Pagnoni M, et al. A de novo proximal 3q29 chromosome microduplication in a patient with oculo auriculo vertebral spectrum. *Am J Med Genet* 167A: 797–801, 2015.

Guilherme RS, Cernach MC, Sfakianakis TE, et al. A complex chromosome rearrangement involving four chromosomes, nine breakpoints and a cryptic 0.6-Mb deletion in a boy with cerebellar hypoplasia and defects in skull ossification. *Cytogenet Genome Res* 141: 317–323, 2013a.

Guilherme RS, Klein E, Hamid A, et al. Human ring chromosomes—New insights for their clinical significance. *Balkan J Med Genet* 16: 13–20, 2013b.

Guilherme RS, Meloni VF, Kim CA, et al. Mechanisms of ring chromosome formation, ring instability and clinical consequences. *BMC Med Genet* 12: 171, 2011.

Guilherme RS, Meloni VA, Perez AB, et al. Duplication 9p and their implication to phenotype. *BMC Med Genet* 15: 142, 2014.

Guilherme RS, Meloni VA, Takeno SS, et al. Twenty-year cytogenetic and molecular follow-up of a patient with ring chromosome 15: A case report. *J Med Case Rep* 6: 283, 2012.

Guilherme RS, Moysés-Oliveira M, Dantas AG, et al. Position effect modifying gene expression in a patient with ring chromosome 14. *J Appl Genet* 57: 183–187, 2016.

Guimiot F, Dupont C, Fuentes-Duarte A, et al. Maternal transmission of interstitial 8p23.1 deletion detected during prenatal diagnosis. *Am J Med Genet* 161A: 208–213, 2013.

Guioli S, Incerti B, Zanaria E, et al. Kallmann syndrome due to a translocation resulting in an X/Y fusion gene. *Nat Genet* 1: 337–340, 1992.

Gunay-Aygun M, Heeger S, Schwartz S, Cassidy SB. Delayed diagnosis in patients with Prader-Willi syndrome due to maternal uniparental disomy 15. *Am J Med Genet* 71: 106–110, 1997.

Gunn SR, Mohammed M, Reveles XT, et al. Molecular characterization of a patient with central nervous system dysmyelination and cryptic unbalanced translocation between chromosomes 4q and 18q. *Am J Med Genet* 120A: 127–135, 2003.

Gunnarsson C, Graffmann B, Jonasson J. Chromosome r(10)(p15.3q26.12) in a newborn child: Case report. *Mol Cytogenet* 2: 25, 2009.

Guo SW. Cultural difference and the eugenics law. *Am J Hum Genet* 65: 1197–1199, 1999.

Gustashaw KM, Zurcher V, Dickerman LH, Stallard R, Willard HF. Partial X chromosome trisomy with functional disomy of Xp due to failure of X inactivation. *Am J Med Genet* 53: 39–45, 1994.

Guttenbach M, Kohn FM, Engel W, Schmid M. Meiotic nondisjunction of chromosomes 1, 17, 18, X, and Y in men more than 80 years of age. *Biol Reprod* 63: 1727–1729, 2000.

Guvendag Guven ES, Dilbaz S, Ceylaner S, et al. An uncommon complementary isochromosome of 46,XY, i(9)(p10),i(9)(q10) in an infertile oligoasthenoteratozoospermic man. *Fertil Steril* 95: 290, e5–8, 2011.

Guzé C, Qin N, Kelly J, et al. Isochromosome 22 in trisomy 22 mosaic with five cell lines. *Am J Med Genet* 124A: 79–84, 2004.

Gyejye A, Anyane-Yeboa K, Warburton D. Follow-up of 30 children with de novo balanced rearrangements and supernumerary marker chromosomes diagnosed at amniocentesis. *Am J Hum Genet* 69: 208, 2001.

Haas NB, Nathanson KL. Hereditary kidney cancer syndromes. *Adv Chronic Kidney Dis* 21: 81–90, 2014.

Habecker-Green J, Naeem R, Goh W, Pflueger S, Murray M, Cohn G. Reproduction in a patient with trisomy 8 mosaicism: Case report and literature review. *Am J Med Genet* 75: 382–385, 1998.

Hadjiathanasiou CG, Brauner R, Lortat-Jacob S, et al. True hermaphroditism: Genetic variants and clinical management. *J Pediatr* 125: 738–744, 1994.

Hadzsiev K, Dávid D, Szabó G, Czakó M, Melegh B, Kosztolányi G. Partial trisomy of the pericentromeric region of chromosome 5 in a girl with Binder phenotype. *Cytogenet Genome Res* 144: 190–195, 2014.

Hagleitner MM, Lankester A, Maraschio P, et al. Clinical spectrum of immunodeficiency, centromeric instability and facial dysmorphism (ICF syndrome). *J Med Genet* 45: 93–99, 2008.

Hahnemann JM, Nir M, Friberg M, Engel U, Bugge M. Trisomy 10 mosaicism and maternal uniparental disomy 10 in a liveborn infant with severe congenital malformations. *Am J Med Genet* 138A: 150–154, 2005.

Hahnemann JM, Vejerslev LO. European Collaborative Research on Mosaicism in CVS (EUCROMIC)—Fetal and extrafetal cell lineages in 192 gestations with CVS mosaicism involving single autosomal trisomy. *Am J Med Genet* 70: 179–187, 1997.

Haines B, Hughes J, Corbett M, et al. Interchromosomal insertional translocation at Xq26.3 alters *SOX3* expression in an individual with XX male sex reversal. *J Clin Endocrinol Metab* 100: E815–820, 2015.

Hajianpour A, Murer-Orlando M, Docherty Z. Germ line mosaicism for chromosome 5 "cri-du-chat" deletion? *Am J Hum Genet* 49: 217, 1991.

Hale DW. Is X-Y recombination necessary for spermatocyte survival during mammalian spermatogenesis? *Cytogenet Cell Genet* 65: 278–282, 1994.

Hall BD. Recurrence risk in de novo 21q21q translocation Down syndrome. *Am J Med Genet* 22: 417–418, 1985.

Halliday J. Outcomes of IVF conceptions: Are they different? *Best Pract Res Clin Obstet Gynaecol* 21: 67–81, 2007.

Halliday JL, Muller C, Charles T, et al. Offering pregnant women different levels of genetic information from prenatal chromosome microarray: a prospective study. *Eur J Hum Genet*, in press 2018.

Halliday J, Oke K, Breheny S, Algar E, Amor DJ. Beckwith-Wiedemann syndrome and IVF: A case-control study. *Am J Hum Genet* 75: 526–528, 2004.

Halliday JL, Ukoumunne OC, Baker HWG, et al. Increased risk of blastogenesis birth defects, arising in the first 4 weeks of pregnancy, after assisted reproductive technologies. *Hum Reprod* 25: 59–65, 2010.

Halliday JL, Warren R, McDonald G, Rice PL, Bell RJ, Watson LF. Prenatal diagnosis for women aged 37 years and over: To have or not to have. *Prenat Diagn* 21: 842–847, 2001.

Halliday JL, Watson LF, Lumley J, Danks DM, Sheffield LJ. New estimates of Down syndrome risks at chorionic villus sampling, amniocentesis, and livebirth in women of advanced maternal age from a uniquely defined population. *Prenat Diagn* 15: 455–465, 1995.

Halliday J, Wilson C, Hammarberg K, et al. Comparing indicators of health and development of singleton young adults conceived with and without assisted reproductive technology. *Fertil Steril* 101: 1055–1063, 2014.

Hamilton MJ, Newbury-Ecob R, Holder-Espinasse M, et al. Rubinstein-Taybi syndrome type 2: Report of nine new cases that extend the phenotypic and genotypic spectrum. *Clin Dysmorphol* 25: 135–145, 2016.

Hammoud I, Molina Gomes D, Bergere M, Wainer R, Selva J, Vialard F. Sperm chromosome analysis of an infertile patient with a 95% mosaic r(21) karyotype and normal phenotype. *Fertil Steril* 91: 930, e13–15, 2009.

Hamvas A, Nogee LM, Wegner DJ, et al. Inherited surfactant deficiency caused by uniparental disomy of rare mutations in the surfactant protein-B and ATP binding cassette, subfamily a, member 3 genes. *J Pediatr* 155: 854–859.e1, 2009.

Han JC, Thurm A, Golden Williams C, et al. Association of brain-derived neurotrophic factor (BDNF) haploinsufficiency with lower adaptive behaviour and reduced cognitive functioning in WAGR/11p13 deletion syndrome. *Cortex* 49: 2700–2710, 2013.

Han JY, Shin JH, Han MS, Je GH, Shaffer LG. Microarray detection of a de novo der(X)t(X;11) (q28;p13) in a girl with premature ovarian failure and features of Beckwith-Wiedemann syndrome. *J Hum Genet* 51: 641–643, 2006.

Hancarova M, Simandlova M, Drabova J, et al. Chromosome 12q13.13 deletions involving the *HOXC* gene cluster: Phenotype and candidate genes. *Eur J Med Genet* 56: 171–173, 2013.

Hande MP, Azizova TV, Geard CR, et al. Past exposure to densely ionizing radiation leaves a unique permanent signature in the genome. *Am J Hum Genet* 72: 1162–1170, 2003.

Handrigan GR, Chitayat D, Lionel AC, et al. Deletions in 16q24.2 are associated with autism spectrum disorder, intellectual disability and congenital renal malformation. *J Med Genet* 50: 163–173, 2013.

Handyside AH. 24-Chromosome copy number analysis: A comparison of available technologies. *Fertil Steril* 100: 595–602, 2013.

Handyside AH, Robinson MD, Simpson RJ, et al. Isothermal whole genome amplification from single and small numbers of cells: A new era for preimplantation genetic diagnosis of inherited disease. *Mol Hum Reprod* 10: 767–772, 2004.

Hani VH, Park J, Allen EF, Moeschler JB. Paracentric inversion of chromosome 18 with duplication of the inverted material in a child due to maternal paracentric inversion of 18q. *Am J Hum Genet* 57: A115, 1995.

Hannachi H, Mougou S, Benabdallah I, et al. Molecular and phenotypic characterization of ring chromosome 22 in two unrelated patients. *Cytogenet Genome Res* 140: 1–11, 2013.

Hannes FD, Sharp AJ, Mefford HC, et al. Recurrent reciprocal deletions and duplications of 16p13.11: The deletion is a risk factor for MR/MCA while the duplication may be a rare benign variant. *J Med Genet* 46: 223–232, 2009.

Hanson E, Bernier R, Porche K, et al. The cognitive and behavioral phenotype of the 16p11.2 deletion in a clinically ascertained population. *Biol Psychiatry* 77: 785–793, 2015.

Hansson KBM, Gijsbers ACJ, Oostdijk W, et al. Molecular and clinical characterization of patients with a ring chromosome 11. *Eur J Med Genet* 55: 708–714, 2012.

Happle R, König A. Dominant traits may give rise to paired patches of either excessive or absent involvement. *Am J Med Genet* 84: 176–177, 1999.

Hardy K, Wright C, Rice S, et al. Future developments in assisted reproduction in humans. *Reproduction* 123: 171–183, 2002.

Härkönen K, Viitanen T, Larsen SB, Bonde JP, Lähdetie J. Aneuploidy in sperm and exposure to fungicides and lifestyle factors: ASCLEPIOS—A European Concerted Action on Occupational Hazards to Male Reproductive Capability. *Environ Mol Mutagen* 34: 39–46, 1999.

Harmon RJ, Bender BG, Linden MG, Robinson A. Transition from adolescence to early adulthood: Adaptation and psychiatric status of women with 47,XXX. *J Am Acad Child Adolesc Psychiatry* 37: 286–291, 1998.

Harper PS. *First Years of Human Chromosomes: The Beginnings of Human Cytogenetics.* Bloxham, UK: Scion, 2006.

Harper PS. *Practical Genetic Counseling* (7th ed.). London, UK: Hodder Arnold, 2010.

Harris DJ, Hankins L, Begleiter ML. Reproductive risk of t(13q14q) carriers: Case report and review. *Am J Med Genet* 3: 175–181, 1979.

Harris JC. The origin and natural history of autism spectrum disorders. *Nat Neurosci* 19: 1390–1391, 2016.

Harrison KJ, Barrett IJ, Lomax BL, Kuchinka BD, Kalousek DK. Detection of confined placental mosaicism in trisomy 18 conceptions using interphase cytogenetic analysis. *Hum Genet* 92: 353–358, 1993.

Hart SJ, Schoch K, Shashi V, Callanan N. Communication of psychiatric risk in 22q11.2 deletion syndrome: A pilot project. *J Genet Couns* 25: 6–17, 2016.

Hartman RJ, Rasmussen SA, Botto LD, et al. The contribution of chromosomal abnormalities to congenital heart defects: A population-based study. *Pediatr Cardiol* 32: 1147–1157, 2011.

Harton GL, Munné S, Surrey M, et al. Diminished effect of maternal age on implantation after preimplantation genetic diagnosis with array comparative genomic hybridization. *Fertil Steril* 100: 1695–1703, 2013.

Hartwig TS, Sørensen S, Jørgensen FS. The maternal age-related first trimester risks for trisomy 21, 18 and 13 based on Danish first trimester data from 2005 to 2014. *Prenat Diagn* 36: 643–649, 2016.

Hasegawa T, Harada N, Ikeda K, et al. Digynic triploid infant surviving for 46 days. *Am J Med Genet* 87: 306–310, 1999.

Hashemi B, Bassett A, Chitayat D, et al. Deletion of 15q11.2(BP1-BP2) region: Further evidence for lack of phenotypic specificity in a pediatric population. *Am J Med Genet* 167A: 2098–2102, 2015.

Hashish AF, Monk NA, Watt AJ, Gardner RJM. A de novo insertion, detected prenatally, with normal phenotype. *J Med Genet* 29: 351, 1992.

Hasi-Zogaj M, Sebold C, Heard P, et al. A review of 18p deletions. *Am J Med Genet* 169C: 251–264, 2015.

Hassan M, Butler MG. Prader-Willi syndrome and atypical submicroscopic 15q11-q13 deletions with or without imprinting defects. *Eur J Med Genet* 59: 584–589, 2016.

Hassfurther A, Komini E, Fischer J, Leipoldt M. Clinical and genetic heterogeneity of the 15q13.3 microdeletion syndrome. *Mol Syndromol* 6: 222–228, 2016.

Hassold T. Nondisjunction in the human male. *Curr Top Dev Biol* 37: 383–406, 1998.

Hassold T, Arnovitz K, Jacobs PA, May K, Robinson D. The parental origin of the missing or additional chromosome in 45,X and 47,XXX females. *Birth Defects Orig Artic Ser* 26: 297–304, 1990a.

Hassold T, Hall H, Hunt P. The origin of human aneuploidy: Where we have been, where we are going. *Hum Mol Genet* 16: R203–208, 2007.

Hassold T, Hunt P. To err (meiotically) is human: The genesis of human aneuploidy. *Nat Rev Genet* 2: 280–291, 2001.

Hassold T, Hunt PA, Sherman S. Trisomy in humans: Incidence, origin and etiology. *Curr Opin Genet Dev* 3: 398–403, 1993.

Hassold T, Pettay D, May K, Robinson A. Analysis of non-disjunction in sex chromosome tetrasomy and pentasomy. *Hum Genet* 85: 648–650, 1990b.

Hassold T, Sherman S. Down syndrome: Genetic recombination and the origin of the extra chromosome 21. *Clin Genet* 57: 95–100, 2000.

Hastings RJ, Nisbet DL, Waters K, Spencer T, Chitty LS. Prenatal detection of extra structurally abnormal chromosomes (ESACs): New cases and a review of the literature. *Prenat Diagn* 19: 436–445, 1999a.

Hastings RJ, Watson SG, Chitty LS. Prenatal finding of a fetus with mosaicism for two balanced de novo chromosome rearrangements. *Prenat Diagn* 19: 77–80, 1999b.

Hatakeyama C, Gao H, Harmer K, Ma S. Meiotic segregation patterns and ICSI pregnancy outcome of a rare (13;21) Robertsonian translocation carrier: A case report. *Hum Reprod* 21: 976–979, 2006.

Hatchwell E, Robinson D, Crolla JA, Cockwell AE. X inactivation analysis in a female with hypomelanosis of Ito associated with a balanced X;17 translocation: Evidence for functional disomy of Xp. *J Med Genet* 33: 216–220, 1996.

Hattori M, Fujiyama A, Taylor TD, et al. The DNA sequence of human chromosome 21. *Nature* 405: 311–319, 2000.

Hatziioannou AG, Krauss CM, Lewis MB, Halazonetis TD. Familial holoprosencephaly associated with a translocation breakpoint at chromosomal position 7q36. *Am J Med Genet* 40: 201–205, 1991.

Haverty CE, Lin AE, Simpson E, Spence MA, Martin RA. 47,XXX associated with malformations. *Am J Med Genet* 125A: 108–111, 2004.

Havlovicova M, Novotna D, Kocarek E, et al. A girl with neurofibromatosis type 1, atypical autism and mosaic ring chromosome 17. *Am J Med Genet* 143: 76–81, 2007.

He W, Tuck-Muller CM, Martínez JE, Li S, Rowley ER, Wertelecki W. Molecular characterization of a ring chromosome 16 from a patient with bilateral cataracts. *Am J Med Genet* 107: 12–17, 2002.

He WB, Banerjee S, Meng LL, et al. Whole-exome sequencing identifies a homozygous donor splice-site mutation in *STAG3* that causes primary ovarian insufficiency. *Clin Genet*, in press 2018.

Head E, Lott IT, Wilcock DM, Lemere CA. Aging in Down syndrome and the development of Alzheimer's disease neuropathology. *Curr Alzheimer Res* 13: 18–29, 2016.

Heald B, Moran R, Milas M, Burke C, Eng C. Familial adenomatous polyposis in a patient with unexplained mental retardation. *Nat Clin Pract Neurol* 3: 694–700, 2007.

Healy DL, Trounson AO, Andersen AN. Female infertility: Causes and treatment. *Lancet* 343: 1539–1544, 1994.

Hecht F, Hecht BK. Linkage of skeletal dysplasia gene to t(2;8)(q32;p13) chromosome translocation breakpoint. *Am J Med Genet* 18: 779–780, 1984.

Hehir-Kwa JY, Pfundt R, Veltman JA, de Leeuw N. Pathogenic or not? Assessing the clinical relevance of copy number variants. *Clin Genet* 84: 415–421, 2013.

Heide S, Afenjar A, Edery P, et al. Xp21 deletion in female patients with intellectual disability: Two new cases and a review of the literature. *Eur J Med Genet* 58: 341–345, 2015.

Heidemann S, Plendl H, Vater I, et al. Maternal uniparental disomy 15 in a fetus resulting from a balanced familial translocation t(2;15) (p11;q11.2). *Prenat Diagn* 30: 183–185, 2010.

Heilstedt HA, Shapira SK, Gregg AR, Shaffer LG. Molecular and clinical characterization of a patient with duplication of 1p36.3 and metopic synostosis. *Clin Genet* 56: 123–128, 1999.

Heitz E. Das heterochromatin der moose: I. *Jahrb Wiss Botanik* 69: 762–818, 1928.

Helderman-van den Enden ATJM, Madan K, Breuning MH, van der Hout AH, Bakker E, de Die-Smulders CEM, Ginjaar HB. An urgent need for a change in policy revealed by a study on prenatal testing for Duchenne muscular dystrophy. *Eur J Hum Genet* 21: 21–26, 2013.

Hellani A, Lauge A, Ozand P, Jaroudi K, Coskun S. Pregnancy after preimplantation genetic diagnosis for ataxia telangiectasia. *Mol Hum Reprod* 8: 785–788, 2002.

Hellmuth SG, Pedersen LH, Miltoft CB, et al. Increased nuchal translucency thickness and the risk of neurodevelopmental disorders. *Ultrasound Obstet Gynecol* 49: 592–598, 2017.

Hempel M, Rivera Brugués N, Wagenstaller J, et al. Microdeletion syndrome 16p11.2-p12.2: Clinical and molecular characterization. *Am J Med Genet* 149A: 2106–2112, 2009.

Hennebicq S, Pelletier R, Bergues U, Rousseaux S. Risk of trisomy 21 in offspring of patients with Klinefelter's syndrome. *Lancet* 357: 2104–2105, 2001.

Hens K, Dondorp W, Handyside AH, et al. Dynamics and ethics of comprehensive preimplantation genetic testing: A review of the challenges. *Hum Reprod Update* 19: 366–375, 2013a.

Hens K, Dondorp W, de Wert G. Embryos without secrets: An expert panel study on comprehensive embryo testing and the responsibility of the clinician. *Eur J Med Genet* 56: 67–71, 2013b.

Herlihy AS, Halliday J. Is paternal age playing a role in the changing prevalence of Klinefelter syndrome? *Eur J Hum Genet* 16: 1173–1174, 2008.

Herlihy AS, Halliday J, McLachlan R, Cock M, Gillam L. Assessing the risks and benefits of diagnosing genetic conditions with variable phenotypes through population screening: Klinefelter syndrome as an example. *J Comm Genet* 1: 41–46, 2010.

Hernando C, Carrera M, Ribas I, et al. Prenatal and postnatal characterization of Y chromosome structural anomalies by molecular cytogenetic analysis. *Prenat Diagn* 22: 802–805, 2002.

Herrgård E, Mononen T, Mervaala E, et al. More severe epilepsy and cognitive impairment in the offspring of a mother with mosaicism for the ring 20 chromosome. *Epilepsy Res* 73: 122–128, 2007.

Hervé B, Quibel T, Taieb S, Ruiz M, Molina-Gomes D, Vialard F. Are de novo rea(21;21)

chromosomes really de novo? *Clin Case Rep* 3: 786–789, 2015.

Higgins S, Hutchinson R, Gowans L, Friend K, Liebelt J. 46,XY/46,XX chimerism in a healthy male. Poster presented at the Annual Scientific Meeting of the Human Genetics Society of Australasia, 2014.

Hill M, Johnson JA, Langlois S, et al. Preferences for prenatal tests for Down syndrome: An international comparison of the views of pregnant women and health professionals. *Eur J Hum Genet* 24: 968–975, 2016.

Hillman SC, McMullan DJ, Hall G, et al. Use of prenatal chromosomal microarray: Prospective cohort study and systematic review and meta-analysis. *Ultrasound Obstet Gynecol* 41: 610–620, 2013.

Hinds DA, Barnholt KE, Mesa RA, et al. Germ line variants predispose to both *JAK2* V617F clonal hematopoiesis and myeloproliferative neoplasms. *Blood* 128: 1121–1128, 2016.

Hippman C, Oberlander TF, Honer WG, Misri S, Austin JC. Depression during pregnancy: The potential impact of increased risk for fetal aneuploidy on maternal mood. *Clin Genet* 75: 30–36, 2009.

Hiramoto T, Kang G, Suzuki G, et al. Tbx1: Identification of a 22q11.2 gene as a risk factor for autism spectrum disorder in a mouse model. *Hum Mol Genet* 20: 4775–4785, 2011.

Hirsch B, Baldinger S. Pericentric inversion of chromosome 4 giving rise to dup(4p) and dup(4q) recombinants within a single kindred. *Am J Med Genet* 45: 5–8, 1993.

Hirt N, Eggermann K, Hyrenbach S, et al. Genetic dosage compensation via co-occurrence of *PMP22* duplication and *PMP22* deletion. *Neurology* 84: 1605–1606, 2015.

Hitchins MP, Rickard S, Dhalla F, et al. Investigation of *UBE3A* and *MECP2* in Angelman syndrome (AS) and patients with features of AS. *Am J Med Genet* 125A: 167–172, 2004.

Hixon M, Millie E, Judis LA, et al. FISH studies of the sperm of fathers of paternally derived cases of trisomy 21: No evidence for an increase in aneuploidy. *Hum Genet* 103: 654–657, 1998.

Hladilkova E, Barøy T, Fannemel M, et al. A recurrent deletion on chromosome 2q13 is associated with developmental delay and mild facial dysmorphisms. *Mol Cytogenet* 8: 57, 2015.

Hobart HH, Morris CA, Mervis CB, et al. Inversion of the Williams syndrome region is a common polymorphism found more frequently in parents of children with Williams syndrome. *Am J Med Genet* 154C: 220–228, 2010.

Hochstenbach R, Krijtenburg PJ, van der Veken LT, et al. Monosomy 20 mosaicism revealed by extensive karyotyping in blood and skin cells: Case report and review of the literature. *Cytogenet Genome Res* 144: 155–162, 2014.

Hochstenbach R, van Binsbergen E, Engelen J, et al. Array analysis and karyotyping: Workflow consequences based on a retrospective study of 36,325 patients with idiopathic developmental delay in the Netherlands. *Eur J Med Genet* 52: 161–169, 2009.

Hockey KA, Mulcahy MT, Montgomery P, Levitt S. Deletion of chromosome 5q and familial adenomatous polyposis. *J Med Genet* 26: 61–62, 1989.

Höckner M, Spreiz A, Frühmesser A, et al. Parental origin of de novo cytogenetically balanced reciprocal non-Robertsonian translocations. *Cytogenet Genome Res* 136: 242–245, 2012.

Höckner M, Utermann B, Erdel M, Fauth C, Utermann G, Kotzot D. Molecular characterization of a de novo ring chromosome 6 in a growth retarded but otherwise healthy woman. *Am J Med Genet* 146: 925–929, 2008.

Hodge SE. Waiting for the amniocentesis. *N Engl J Med* 320: 63–64, 1989.

Hodgson SV, Fagg NLK, Talbot IC, Wilkinson M. Deletions of the entire *APC* gene are associated with sessile colonic adenomas. *J Med Genet* 31: 426, 1994.

Hoeft F, Barnea-Goraly N, Haas BW, et al. More is not always better: Increased fractional anisotropy of superior longitudinal fasciculus associated with poor visuospatial abilities in Williams syndrome. *J Neurosci* 27: 11960–11965, 2007.

Hoffman TL, Blanco E, Lane A, et al. Glucose metabolism and insulin secretion in a patient with *ABCC8* mutation and Fanconi-Bickel syndrome caused by maternal isodisomy of chromosome 3. *Clin Genet* 71: 551–557, 2007.

Hogart A, Leung KN, Wang NJ, et al. Chromosome 15q11-13 duplication syndrome brain reveals epigenetic alterations in gene expression not predicted from copy number. *J Med Genet* 46: 86–93, 2009.

Hogart A, Wu D, LaSalle JM, Schanen NC. The comorbidity of autism with the genomic disorders of chromosome 15q11.2-q13. *Neurobiol Dis* 38: 181–191, 2010.

Höglund P, Holmberg C, de la Chapelle A, Kere J. Paternal isodisomy for chromosome 7 is compatible with normal growth and development in a patient with congenital chloride diarrhea. *Am J Hum Genet* 55: 747–752, 1994.

Holder JL, Jr., Lotze TE, Bacino C, Cheung SW. A child with an inherited 0.31 Mb microdeletion of chromosome 14q32.33: Further delineation of a critical region for the 14q32 deletion syndrome. *Am J Med Genet* 158A: 1962–1966, 2012.

Hollis ND, Allen EG, Oliver TR, et al. Preconception folic acid supplementation and risk for chromosome 21 nondisjunction: A report from the National Down Syndrome Project. *Am J Med Genet* 161A: 438–444, 2013.

Holmes-Siedle M, Ryynanen M, Lindenbaum RH. Parental decisions regarding termination of pregnancy following prenatal detection of sex chromosome abnormality. *Prenat Diagn* 7: 239–244, 1987.

Homer L, Le Martelot MT, Morel F, et al. 45,X/46,XX mosaicism below 30% of aneuploidy: Clinical implications in adult women from a reproductive medicine unit. *Eur J Endocrinol* 162: 617–623, 2010.

Honeywell C, Argiropoulos B, Douglas S, et al. Apparent transmission distortion of a pericentric chromosome one inversion in a large multi-generation pedigree. *Am J Med Genet* 158A: 1262–1268, 2012.

Hong B, Zunich J, Openshaw A, Toydemir RM. Clinical features of trisomy 12 mosaicism—Report and review. *Am J Med Genet* 173: 1681–1686, 2017.

Hong DS, Reiss AL. Cognitive and neurological aspects of sex chromosome aneuploidies. *Lancet Neurol* 13: 306–318, 2014.

Honorato T, Hoek A, Henningsen AK, et al. Low oocyte yield during IVF treatment and the risk of a trisomic pregnancy. *Reprod Biomed Online* 35: 685–692, 2017.

Hoo JJ, Lorenz R, Fischer A, Fuhrmann W. Tiny interstitial duplication of proximal 7q in association with a maternal paracentric inversion. *Hum Genet* 62: 113–116, 1982.

Hoo JJ, Lowry RB, Lin CC, Haslam RHA. Recurrent de novo interstitial deletion of 16q in two mentally retarded sisters. *Clin Genet* 27: 420–425, 1985.

Hook EB. Exclusion of chromosomal mosaicism: Tables of 90%, 95% and 99% confidence limits and comments on use. *Am J Hum Genet* 29: 94–97, 1977.

Hook EB. Extra sex chromosomes and human behavior: the nature of the evidence regarding XYY, XXY, XXYY and XXX genotypes. In Vallet HL, Porter IH (eds.), *Genetic Mechanisms of Sexual Development*. New York, NY: Academic Press, 1979: 437–463.

Hook EB. Chromosome abnormalities and spontaneous fetal death following amniocentesis:

Further data and associations with maternal age. *Am J Hum Genet* 35: 110–116, 1983.

Hook EB. Chromosome abnormalities: prevalence, risks and recurrence. In Brock DJH, Rodeck CH, Ferguson-Smith MA (eds.), *Prenatal Diagnosis and Screening*. Edinburgh, UK: Churchill Livingstone, 1992.

Hook EB, Cross PK. Interpretation of recent data pertinent to genetic counseling for Down syndrome: Maternal-age-specific-rates, temporal trends, adjustments for paternal age, recurrence risks, risks after other cytogenetic abnormalities, recurrence risk after remarriage. In Willey AM, Carter TP, Kelly S, Porter IH (eds.), *Clinical Genetics: Problems in Diagnosis and Counseling*. New York, NY: Academic Press, 1982.

Hook EB, Cross PK. Rates of mutant and inherited structural cytogenetic abnormalities detected at amniocentesis: Results on about 63,000 fetuses. *Ann Hum Genet* 51: 27–55, 1987.

Hoppman-Chaney N, Wain K, Seger PR, Superneau DW, Hodge JC. Identification of single gene deletions at 15q13.3: Further evidence that *CHRNA7* causes the 15q13.3 microdeletion syndrome phenotype. *Clin Genet* 83: 345–351, 2013.

Horbinski C, Carter EM, Heard PL, et al. Molecular and clinical characterization of a recurrent cryptic unbalanced t(4q;18q) resulting in an 18q deletion and 4q duplication. *Am J Med Genet* 146A: 2898–2904, 2008.

Horigome Y, Kondo I, Kuwajima K, Suzuki T. Familial occurrence of ring chromosome 15. *Clin Genet* 41: 178–180, 1992.

Horike S, Ferreira JCP, Meguro-Horike M, et al. Screening of DNA methylation at the H19 promoter or the distal region of its ICR1 ensures efficient detection of chromosome 11p15 epimutations in Russell-Silver syndrome. *Am J Med Genet* 149A: 2415–2423, 2009.

Horn D, Majewski F, Hildebrandt B, Körner H. Pallister-Killian syndrome: Normal karyotype in prenatal chorionic villi, in postnatal lymphocytes, and in slowly growing epidermal cells, but mosaic tetrasomy 12p in skin fibroblasts. *J Med Genet* 32: 68–71, 1995.

Horsman DE, Dill FJ, McGillivray BC, Kalousek DK. X chromosome aneuploidy in lymphocyte cultures from women with recurrent spontaneous abortions. *Am J Med Genet* 28: 981–987, 1987.

Horsthemke B, Buiting K. Imprinting defects on human chromosome 15. *Cytogenet Genome Res* 113: 292–299, 2006.

Hoshi N, Fujita M, Mikuni M, et al. Seminoma in a postmenopausal woman with a Y;15 translocation in peripheral blood lymphocytes and a t(Y;15)/45,X Turner mosaic pattern in skin fibroblasts. *J Med Genet* 35: 852–856, 1998.

Hosoki K, Takano K, Sudo A, Tanaka S, Saitoh S. Germline mosaicism of a novel *UBE3A* mutation in Angelman syndrome. *Am J Med Genet* 138A: 187–189, 2005.

Høst C, Skakkebæk A, Groth KA, Bojesen A. The role of hypogonadism in Klinefelter syndrome. *Asian J Androl* 16: 185–191, 2014.

Hotz A, Hellenbroich Y, Sperner J, et al. Microdeletion 5q14.3 and anomalies of brain development. *Am J Med Genet* 161A: 2124–2133, 2013.

Houcinat N, Llanas B, Moutton S, et al. Homozygous 16p13.11 duplication associated with mild intellectual disability and urinary tract malformations in two siblings born from consanguineous parents. *Am J Med Genet* 167A: 2714–2719, 2015.

Hovatta O. Ovarian function and in vitro fertilization (IVF) in Turner syndrome. *Pediatr Endocrinol Rev* 9 (Suppl 2): 713–717, 2012.

Howarth ES, Konje JC, Healey KA, Duckett DP, Scudamore IW, Taylor DJ. Invasive testing for the karyotyping of mid-trimester intrauterine fetal death (IUFD): A pilot study. *Prenat Diagn* 22: 453–455, 2002.

Howe K, FitzHarris G. Recent insights into spindle function in mammalian oocytes and early embryos. *Biol Reprod* 89: 71, 2013.

Howell RT, Davies T. Diagnosis of Bloom's syndrome by sister chromatid exchange evaluation in chorionic villus cultures. *Prenat Diagn* 14: 1071–1073, 1994.

Howell RT, McDermott A, Gardner A, Dickinson V. Down's syndrome with a recombinant tandem duplication of chromosome 21 derived from a maternal ring. *J Med Genet* 21: 310–314, 1984.

Hsieh JC, Van Den Berg D, Kang H, Hsieh CL, Lieber MR. Large chromosome deletions, duplications, and gene conversion events accumulate with age in normal human colon crypts. *Aging Cell* 12: 269–279, 2013.

Hsu CC, Lee IW, Su MT, et al. Triple genetic identities for the complete hydatidiform mole, placenta and co-existing fetus after transfer of a single in vitro fertilized oocyte: Case report and possible mechanisms. *Hum Reprod* 23: 2686–2691, 2008.

Hsu LYF. Phenotype/karyotype correlations of Y chromosome aneuploidy with emphasis on structural aberrations in postnatally diagnosed cases. *Am J Med Genet* 53: 108–140, 1994.

Hsu LYF, Benn PA. Revised guidelines for the diagnosis of mosaicism in amniocytes. *Prenat Diagn* 19: 1081–1082, 1999.

Hsu LYF, Kaffe S, Jenkins EC, et al. Proposed guidelines for diagnosis of chromosome mosaicism in amniocytes based on data derived from chromosome mosaicism and pseudomosaicism studies. *Prenat Diagn* 12: 555–573, 1992.

Hsu LYF, Kaffe S, Perlis TE. A revisit of trisomy 20 mosaicism in prenatal diagnosis—An overview of 103 cases. *Prenat Diagn* 11: 7–15, 1991.

Hsu LYF, Perlis TE. United States survey on chromosome mosaicism and pseudomosaicism in prenatal diagnosis. *Prenat Diagn* 4 Spec No: 97–130, 1984.

Hsu LYF, Yu MT, Neu RL, et al. Rare trisomy mosaicism diagnosed in amniocytes, involving an autosome other than chromosomes 13, 18, 20, and 21: Karyotype/phenotype correlations. *Prenat Diagn* 17: 201–242, 1997.

Hsu LYF, Yu MT, Richkind KE, et al. Incidence and significance of chromosome mosaicism involving an autosomal structural abnormality diagnosed prenatally through amniocentesis: A collaborative study. *Prenat Diagn* 16: 1–28, 1996.

Hu H, Yao H, Dong Y, et al. Distinct karyotypes in two offspring of a man with jumping translocation karyotype 45,XY,der(16)t(16;22)(q24;q11.2), -22 [59]/45,XY,der(1)t(1;22)(p36;q11.2), -22 [11]/45,XY,der(22)t(22;22)(p13;q11.2), -22 [10]. *Am J Med Genet* 164A: 2048–2053, 2014.

Hu X, Chen X, Wu B, et al. Further defining the critical genes for the 4q21 microdeletion disorder. *Am J Med Genet* 173A: 120–125, 2017.

Huang B, Thangavelu M, Bhatt S, Sandlin CJ, Wang S. Prenatal diagnosis of 45,X and 45,X mosaicism: The need for thorough cytogenetic and clinical evaluations. *Prenat Diagn* 22: 105–110, 2002.

Huang H, Wang C, Tian Q. Gonadal tumour risk in 292 phenotypic female patients with disorders of sex development containing Y chromosome or Y-derived sequence. *Clin Endocrinol* 86: 621–627, 2017.

Huang L, Tong X, Luo L, et al. Mutation analysis of the *TUBB8* gene in nine infertile women with oocyte maturation arrest. *Reprod Biomed Online* 35: 305–310, 2017.

Huang N, Lee I, Marcotte EM, Hurles ME. Characterising and predicting haploinsufficiency in the human genome. *PLoS Genet* 6: e1001154, 2010.

Huang S, Juneau K, Bogard PE, et al. Identifying Robertsonian translocation carriers by microarray-based DNA analysis. *Fetal Diagn Ther* 40: 59–62, 2016.

Hudson C, Schwanke C, Johnson JP, et al. Confirmation of 6q21-6q22.1 deletion in acro-cardio-facial syndrome and further delineation of this contiguous gene deletion syndrome. *Am J Med Genet* 164A: 2109–2113, 2014.

Hudson DF, Amor DJ, Boys A, et al. Loss of RMI2 increases genome instability and causes a Bloom-like syndrome. *PLoS Genet* 12: e1006483, 2016.

Hughes IA. Disorders of sex development: A new definition and classification. *Best Pract Res Clin Endocrinol Metab* 22: 119–134, 2008.

Hughes IA, Houk C, Ahmed SF, Lee PA. Consensus statement on management of intersex disorders. *Arch Dis Child* 91: 554–563, 2006.

Hui L, Muggli EE, Halliday JL. Population-based trends in prenatal screening and diagnosis for aneuploidy: A retrospective analysis of 38 years of state-wide data. *BJOG* 123: 90–97, 2016a.

Hui L, Tabor A, Walker SP, Kilby MD. How to safeguard competency and training in invasive prenatal diagnosis: "The elephant in the room." *Ultrasound Obstet Gynecol* 47: 8–13, 2016b.

Hultén M, Armstrong S, Challinor P, et al. Genomic imprinting in an Angelman and Prader-Willi translocation family. *Lancet* 338: 638–639, 1991.

Hultén MA, Jonasson J, Iwarsson E, et al. Trisomy 21 mosaicism: We may all have a touch of Down syndrome. *Cytogenet Genome Res* 139: 189–192, 2013.

Hultén MA, Öijerstedt L, Iwarsson E, Jonasson J. Maternal germinal trisomy 21 in Down syndrome. *J Clin Med* 3: 167–175, 2014.

Hung PH, Froenicke L, Lin CY, et al. Effects of environmental tobacco smoke in vivo on rhesus monkey semen quality, sperm function, and sperm metabolism. *Reprod Toxicol* 27: 140–148, 2009.

Hunt PA, Hassold TJ. Sex matters in meiosis. *Science* 296: 2181–2183, 2002.

Hunter A, Brierley K, Tomkins D. 46,XX/46XY chromosome complement in amniotic fluid cell culture followed by the birth of a normal female child. *Prenat Diagn* 2: 127–131, 1982.

Hunter AGW. Down syndrome. In Cassidy SB, Allanson JE (eds.), *Management of Genetic Syndromes*. Hoboken, NJ: Wiley-Blackwell, 2010.

Hunter AGW, Allanson JE. Follow-up study of patients with Wiedemann-Beckwith syndrome with emphasis on the change in facial appearance over time. *Am J Med Genet* 51: 102–107, 1994.

Hunter JE, Allen EG, Shin M, et al. The association of low socioeconomic status and the risk of having a child with Down syndrome: A report from the National Down Syndrome Project. *Genet Med* 15: 698–705, 2013.

Hunter JE, Irving SA, Biesecker LG, et al. A standardized, evidence-based protocol to assess clinical actionability of genetic disorders associated with genomic variation. *Genet Med* 18: 1258–1268, 2016.

Hussain SZ, Evans AL, Ahmed OA, et al. Non-syndromic mental retardation segregating with an apparently balanced t(1;17) reciprocal translocation through three generations. *Am J Med Genet* 95: 99–104, 2000.

Hwang SH, Lee SM, Seo EJ, et al. A case of male infertility with a reciprocal translocation t(X;14)(p11.4;p12). *Korean J Lab Med* 27: 139–142, 2007.

Hysert M, Bruyère H, Côté GB, et al. Prenatal cytogenetic assessment and inv(2)(p11.2q13). *Prenat Diagn* 26: 810–813, 2006.

Ibrahim A, Kirby G, Hardy C, et al. Methylation analysis and diagnostics of Beckwith-Wiedemann syndrome in 1,000 subjects. *Clin Epigenetics* 6: 11, 2014.

Ideraabdullah FY, Vigneau S, Bartolomei MS. Genomic imprinting mechanisms in mammals. *Mutat Res* 647: 77–85, 2008.

Idowu D, Merrion K, Wemmer N, et al. Pregnancy outcomes following 24-chromosome preimplantation genetic diagnosis in couples with balanced reciprocal or Robertsonian translocations. *Fertil Steril* 103: 1037–1042, 2015.

Ikuma S, Sato T, Sugiura-Ogasawara M, Nagayoshi M, Tanaka A, Takeda S. Preimplantation genetic diagnosis and natural conception: A comparison of live birth rates in patients with recurrent pregnancy loss associated with translocation. *PLoS One* 10: e0129958, 2015.

Imai A, Takagi A, Tamaya T. A novel sex-determining region on Y (SRY) missense mutation identified in a 46,XY female and also in the father. *Endocr J* 46: 735–739, 1999.

Imudia AN, Suzuki Y, Kilburn BA, et al. Retrieval of trophoblast cells from the cervical canal for prediction of abnormal pregnancy: A pilot study. *Hum Reprod* 24: 2086–2092, 2009.

Inbar-Feigenberg M, Choufani S, Cytrynbaum C, et al. Mosaicism for genome-wide paternal uniparental disomy with features of multiple imprinting disorders: Diagnostic and management issues. *Am J Med Genet* 161A: 13–20, 2013.

Indrieri A, van Rahden VA, Tiranti V, et al. Mutations in *COX7B* cause microphthalmia with linear skin lesions, an unconventional mitochondrial disease. *Am J Hum Genet* 91: 942–949, 2012.

Ingelfinger FJ. Arrogance. *N Engl J Med* 303: 1507–1511, 1980.

Ioannides Y, Lokulo-Sodipe K, Mackay DJ, Davies JH, Temple IK. Temple syndrome: Improving the recognition of an underdiagnosed chromosome 14 imprinting disorder—An analysis of 51 published cases. *J Med Genet* 51: 495–501, 2014.

Iourov IY, Vorsanova SG, Yurov YB. Single cell genomics of the brain: Focus on neuronal diversity and neuropsychiatric diseases. *Curr Genomics* 13: 477–488, 2012.

Irani M, Reichman D, Robles A, et al. Morphologic grading of euploid blastocysts influences implantation and ongoing pregnancy rates. *Fertil Steril* 107: 664–670, 2017.

Isaacs D. What is the value of a human baby? *J Paediatr Child Health* 38: 608–609, 2002.

ISCN 2016: An international system for human cytogenomic nomenclature. McGowan-Jordan J, Simons A, Schmid M (eds.), *Cytogenet Genome Res* 149 (1–2), 2016.

Iselius L, Lindsten J, Aurias A, et al. The 11q;22q translocation: A collaborative study of 20 new cases and analysis of 110 families. *Hum Genet* 64: 343–355, 1983.

Ishii F, Fujita H, Nagai A, et al. Case report of rec(7)dup(7q)inv(7)(p22q22) and a review of the recombinants resulting from parental pericentric inversions on any chromosomes. *Am J Med Genet* 73: 290–295, 1997.

Ishikawa A, Enomoto K, Tominaga M, et al. Pure duplication of 19p13.3. *Am J Med Genet* 161A: 2300–2304, 2013.

Ishikawa S, Ishikawa M, Tokuda T, et al. Japanese family with an autosomal dominant chromosome instability syndrome: A new neurodegenerative disease? *Am J Med Genet* 94: 265–270, 2000.

Ishikiriyama S, Tonoki H, Shibuya Y, et al. Waardenburg syndrome type I in a child with de novo inversion (2)(q35q37.3). *Am J Med Genet* 33: 505–507, 1989.

Isles AR, Ingason A, Lowther C, et al. Parental origin of interstitial duplications at 15q11.2-q13.3 in schizophrenia and neurodevelopmental disorders. *PLoS Genet* 12: e1005993, 2016.

Isrie M, Froyen G, Devriendt K, et al. Sporadic male patients with intellectual disability: contribution of X-chromosome copy number variants. *Eur J Med Genet* 55: 577–585, 2012.

Itoh N, Becroft DMO, Reeve AE, Morison IM. Proportion of cells with paternal 11p15 uniparental disomy correlates with organ enlargement in Wiedemann-Beckwith syndrome. *Am J Med Genet* 92: 111–116, 2000.

Itsara A, Wu H, Smith JD, et al. De novo rates and selection of large copy number variation. *Genome Res* 20: 1469–1481, 2010.

Iwarsson E, Kvist U, Hultén MA. Disomy 21 in spermatozoa and the paternal origin of trisomy 21 Down syndrome. *Mol Cytogenet* 8: 67, 2015.

Iwarsson E, Sahlén S, Nordgren A. Jumping translocation in a phenotypically normal male: A study of mosaicism in spermatozoa, lymphocytes, and fibroblasts. *Am J Med Genet* 149A: 1706–1711, 2009.

Iype T, Alakbarzade V, Iype M, et al. A large Indian family with rearrangement of chromosome 4p16 and 3p26.3 and divergent clinical presentations. *BMC Med Genet* 16: 104, 2015.

Izumi K, Brooks SS, Feret HA, Zackai EH. 1.9 Mb microdeletion of 21q22.11 within Braddock-Carey contiguous gene deletion syndrome region: Dissecting the phenotype. *Am J Med Genet* 158A: 1535–1541, 2012.

Izumi K, Culler D, Solomon B, Muenke M, Parikh A. Submicroscopic familial chromosomal translocation between 7q and 12p mimicking an autosomal dominant holoprosencephaly syndrome. *Clin Genet* 78: 402–404, 2010.

Jaarola M, Martin RH, Ashley T. Direct evidence for suppression of recombination within two pericentric inversions in humans: A new sperm-FISH technique. *Am J Hum Genet* 63: 218–224, 1998.

Jacobs M, Cooper SA, McGowan R, Nelson SM, Pell JP. Pregnancy outcome following prenatal diagnosis of chromosomal anomaly: A record linkage study of 26,261 pregnancies. *PLoS One* 11: e0166909, 2016.

Jacobs P, Dalton P, James R, et al. Turner syndrome: A cytogenetic and molecular study. *Ann Hum Genet* 61: 471–483, 1997.

Jacobs PA. Recurrence risks for chromosome abnormalities. *Birth Defects Orig Art Series* 15(5C): 71–80, 1979.

Jacobs PA. Mutation rates of structural chromosome rearrangements in man. *Am J Hum Genet* 33: 44–54, 1981.

Jacobs PA, Browne C, Gregson N, Joyce C, White H. Estimates of the frequency of chromosome abnormalities detectable in unselected newborns using moderate levels of banding. *J Med Genet* 29: 103–108, 1992.

Jacobs PA, Strong JA. A case of human intersexuality having a possible XXY sex-determining mechanism. *Nature* 183: 302–303, 1959.

Jacobsen P, Hauge M, Henningsen K, Hobolth N, Mikkelsen M, Philip J. An (11;21) translocation in four generations with chromosome 11 abnormalities in the offspring: A clinical, cytogenetical, and gene marker study. *Hum Hered* 23: 568–585, 1973.

Jacoby RF, Schlack S, Sekhon G, Laxova R. Del(10) (q22.3q24.1) associated with juvenile polyposis. *Am J Med Genet* 70: 361–364, 1997.

Jafari-Ghahfarokhi H, Moradi-Chaleshtori M, Liehr T, Hashemzadeh-Chaleshtori M, Teimori H, Ghasemi-Dehkordi P. Small supernumerary marker chromosomes and their correlation with specific syndromes. *Adv Biomed Res* 4: 140, 2015.

Jäger RJ, Harley VR, Pfeiffer RA, Goodfellow PN, Scherer G. A familial mutation in the testis-determining gene *SRY* shared by both sexes. *Hum Genet* 90: 350–355, 1992.

Jaiswal SK, Sukla KK, Kumari N, Lakhotia AR, Kumar A, Rai AK. Maternal risk for Down syndrome and polymorphisms in the promoter region of the *DNMT3B* gene: A case-control study. *Birth Defects Res A Clin Mol Teratol* 103: 299–305, 2015.

Jalbert P, Jalbert H, Sele B. Types of imbalances in human reciprocal translocations: Risks at birth. In Daniel A (ed.), *The Cytogenetics of Mammalian Autosomal Rearrangements*. New York, NY: Liss, 1988.

Jalbert P, Jalbert H, Sele B, et al. Partial trisomy for the long arms of chromosome no. 5 due to insertion and further "aneusomie de recombinaison." *J Med Genet* 12: 418–423, 1975.

Jalbert P, Sele B, Jalbert H. Reciprocal translocations: A way to predict the mode of imbalanced segregation by pachytene-diagram drawing. *Hum Genet* 55: 209–222, 1980.

Jalil SSA, Mahran MA, Sule M. Placental mesenchymal dysplasia—Can it be predicted prenatally? A case report. *Prenat Diagn* 29: 713–714, 2009.

Jallinoja P, Santalahti P, Toiviainen H, Hemminki E. Acceptance of screening and abortion for Down syndrome among Finnish midwives and public health nurses. *Prenat Diagn* 19: 1015–1022, 1999.

James PA, Gibson K, McGaughran J. Prenatal diagnosis of mosaic trisomy 20 in New Zealand. *Aust NZ J Obstet Gynaecol* 42: 486–489, 2002.

James RS, Ellis K, Pettay D, Jacobs PA. Cytogenetic and molecular study of four couples with multiple trisomy 21 pregnancies. *Eur J Hum Genet* 6: 207–212, 1998.

James RS, Temple IK, Dennis NR, Crolla JA. A search for uniparental disomy in carriers of supernumerary marker chromosomes. *Eur J Hum Genet* 3: 21–26, 1995.

Jamsheer A, Sowinska A, Simon D, Jamsheer-Bratkowska M, Trzeciak T, Latos-Bielenska A. Bilateral radial agenesis with absent thumbs, complex heart defect, short stature, and facial dysmorphism in a patient with pure distal microduplication of 5q35.2-5q35.3. *BMC Med Genet* 14: 13, 2013.

Jang W, Chae H, Kim J, et al. Identification of small marker chromosomes using microarray comparative genomic hybridization and multicolor fluorescent in situ hybridization. *Mol Cytogenet* 9: 61, 2016.

Janke D. Centric fission of chromosome no. 7 in three generations. *Hum Genet* 60: 200–201, 1982.

Jansen RPS, Bowman MC, de Boer KA, Leigh DA, Lieberman DB, McArthur SJ. What next for preimplantation genetic screening (PGS)? Experience with blastocyst biopsy and testing for aneuploidy. *Hum Reprod* 23: 1476–1478, 2008.

Jaques AM, Collins VR, Muggli EE, et al. Uptake of prenatal diagnostic testing and the effectiveness of prenatal screening for Down syndrome. *Prenat Diagn* 30: 522–530, 2010.

Jaques AM, Halliday JL, Bell RJ. Do women know that prenatal testing detects fetuses with Down syndrome? *J Obstet Gynaecol* 24: 647–651, 2004.

Jarrah N, El-Shanti H, Khier A, Obeidat FN, Haddidi A, Ajlouni K. Familial disorder of sex determination in seven individuals from three related sibships. *Eur J Pediatr* 159: 912–918, 2000.

Jarup L, Morris S, Richardson S, et al. Down syndrome in births near landfill sites. *Prenat Diagn* 27: 1191–1196, 2007.

Jaruzelska J, Korcz A, Wojda A, et al. Mosaicism for 45,X cell line may accentuate the severity of spermatogenic defects in men with AZFc deletion. *J Med Genet* 38: 798–802, 2001.

Jay A, Kilby MD, Roberts E, et al. Prenatal diagnosis of mosaicism for partial trisomy 8: A case report including fetal pathology. *Prenat Diagn* 19: 976–979, 1999.

Jean-Marçais N, Decamp M, Gérard M, et al. The first familial case of inherited 2q37.3 interstitial deletion with isolated skeletal abnormalities including brachydactyly type E and short stature. *Am J Med Genet* 167A: 185–189, 2015.

Jedraszak G, Braun K, Receveur A, et al. Growth hormone deficiency and pituitary malformation in a recurrent cat-eye syndrome: A family report. *Ann Endocrinol (Paris)* 76: 629–634, 2015a.

Jedraszak G, Copin H, Demailly M, et al. Azoospermia and trisomy 18p syndrome: A fortuitous association? A patient report and a review of the literature. *Mol Cytogenet* 8: 34, 2015b.

Jedraszak G, Demeer B, Mathieu-Dramard M, et al. Clinical and molecular characterization of the 20q11.2 microdeletion syndrome: Six new patients. *Am J Med Genet* 167A: 504–511, 2015c.

Jeffers MD, O'Dwyer P, Curran B, Leader M, Gillan JE. Partial hydatidiform mole—A common but underdiagnosed condition. A 3-year retrospective clinicopathological and DNA flow cytometric analysis. *Int J Gynec Path* 12: 315–323, 1993.

Jenderny J, Caliebe A, Beyer C, Grote W. Transmission of a ring chromosome 18 from a mother with 46,XX/47,XX, + r(18) mosaicism to her daughter, resulting in a 46,XX,r(18) karyotype. *J Med Genet* 30: 964–965, 1993.

Jenderny J, Schmidt W, Bartsch O. Inheritance of a t(13;14)(q10;q10) Robertsonian translocation with a low level of trisomy 13 mosaicism. *Eur J Pediatr* 169: 789–793, 2010.

Jeon KC, Chen LS, Goodson P. Decision to abort after a prenatal diagnosis of sex chromosome abnormality: A systematic review of the literature. *Genet Med* 14: 27–38, 2012.

Jewell AF, Simpson GF, Pasztor L, Keene CL, Sullivan BA, Schwartz S. Prenatal diagnosis of two cases de novo dup(12p), identified by fluorescence in situ hybridization (FISH). *Am J Hum Genet* 51 (Suppl): 81A, 1992.

Jezela-Stanek A, Kucharczyk M, Pelc M, Chrzanowska KH, Krajewska-Walasek M. Minimal clinical findings in a patient with 15qter microdeletion syndrome: Delineation of the associated phenotype. *Am J Med Genet* 158A: 922–926, 2012.

Ji X, Liang D, Sun R, et al. Molecular characterization of ring chromosome 18 by low-coverage next generation sequencing. *BMC Med Genet* 16: 57, 2015.

Ji Y, Eichler EE, Schwartz S, Nicholls RD. Structure of chromosomal duplicons and their role in mediating human genomic disorders. *Genome Res* 10: 597–610, 2000.

Jiang X, Yu Y, Yang HW, Agar NY, Frado L, Johnson MD. The imprinted gene *PEG3* inhibits Wnt signaling and regulates glioma growth. *J Biol Chem* 285: 8472–8480, 2010.

Jiang YH, Martinez JE, Ou Z, et al. De novo and complex imbalanced chromosomal rearrangements revealed by array CGH in a patient with an abnormal phenotype and apparently "balanced" paracentric inversion of 14(q21q23). *Am J Med Genet* 146A: 1986–1993, 2008.

Jinawath N, Zambrano R, Wohler E, et al. Mosaic trisomy 13: Understanding origin using SNP array. *J Med Genet* 48: 323–326, 2011.

Jobanputra V, Ash E, Anyane-Yeboa K, Warburton D, Levy B. Changes in an inherited ring (22) due to meiotic recombination? Implications for genetic counseling. *Am J Med Genet* 149A: 1310–1314, 2009.

Jobanputra V, Burke A, Kwame AY, et al. Duplication of the *ZIC2* gene is not associated with holoprosencephaly. *Am J Med Genet* 158A: 103–108, 2012.

Jobanputra V, Chung WK, Hacker AM, Emanuel BS, Warburton D. A unique case of der(11)t(11;22), -22 arising from 3:1 segregation of a maternal t(11;22) in a family with co-segregation of the translocation and breast cancer. *Prenat Diagn* 25: 683–686, 2005.

Jobanputra V, Sobrino A, Kinney A, Kline J, Warburton D. Multiplex interphase FISH as a screen for common aneuploidies in spontaneous abortions. *Hum Reprod* 17: 1166–1170, 2002.

Jobling MA, Lo IC, Turner DJ, et al. Structural variation on the short arm of the human Y chromosome: Recurrent multigene deletions encompassing Amelogenin Y. *Hum Mol Genet* 16: 307–316, 2007.

Jobling RK, Kannu P, Licht C, Carter MT. The first report of nephrocalcinosis in a patient with a 16q23.1-16q23.3 deletion, global developmental delay, trigonocephaly, and portocaval shunt. *Clin Dysmorphol* 22: 152–155, 2013.

Joenje H, Arwert F, Kwee ML, Madan K, Hoehn H. Confounding factors in the diagnosis of Fanconi anaemia. *Am J Med Genet* 79: 403–405, 1998.

Joergensen MW, Niemann I, Rasmussen AA, et al. Triploid pregnancies: Genetic and clinical features of 158 cases. *Am J Obstet Gynecol* 211: 370, e1–19, 2014.

Johannisson R, Löhrs U, Wolff HH, Schwinger E. Two different XY-quadrivalent associations and impairment of fertility in men. *Cytogenet Cell Genet* 45: 222–230, 1987.

Johannisson R, Winking H. Synaptonemal complexes of chains and rings in mice heterozygous for multiple Robertsonian translocations. *Chromosome Res* 2: 137–145, 1994.

Johnson DS, Cinnioglu C, Ross R, et al. Comprehensive analysis of karyotypic mosaicism between trophectoderm and inner cell mass. *Mol Hum Reprod* 16: 944–949, 2010.

Johnson JO, Stevanin G, van de Leemput J, et al. A 7.5-Mb duplication at chromosome 11q21-11q22.3 is associated with a novel spastic ataxia syndrome. *Mov Disord* 30: 262–266, 2015.

Johnson L, Barnard JJ, Rodriguez L, et al. Ethnic differences in testicular structure and spermatogenic potential may predispose testes of Asian men to a heightened sensitivity to steroidal contraceptives. *J Androl* 19: 348–357, 1998.

Joly-Helas G, de La Rochebrochard C, Mousset-Siméon N, et al. Complex chromosomal rearrangement and intracytoplasmic sperm injection: A case report. *Hum Reprod* 22: 1292–1297, 2007.

Jones C, Booth C, Rita D, et al. Identification of a case of maternal uniparental disomy of chromosome 10 associated with confined placental mosaicism. *Prenat Diagn* 15: 843–848, 1995.

Jones ML, Murden SL, Brooks C, et al. Disruption of AP3B1 by a chromosome 5 inversion: A new disease mechanism in Hermansky-Pudlak syndrome type 2. *BMC Med Genet* 14: 42, 2013.

Jordan BK, Mohammed M, Ching ST, et al. Up-regulation of WNT-4 signaling and dosage-sensitive sex reversal in humans. *Am J Hum Genet* 68: 1102–1109, 2001.

Jordan VK, Zaveri HP, Scott DA. 1p36 deletion syndrome: An update. *Appl Clin Genet* 8: 189–200, 2015.

Jorgensen PB, Kjartansdóttir KR, Fedder J. Care of women with XY karyotype: A clinical practice guideline. *Fertil Steril* 94: 105–113, 2010.

Jorgez CJ, Rosenfeld JA, Wilken NR, et al. Genitourinary defects associated with genomic deletions in 2p15 encompassing *OTX1*. *PLoS One* 9: e107028, 2014.

Joseph M, Cantú ES, Pai GS, Willi SM, Papenhausen PR, Weiss L. Xp pseudoautosomal gene haploinsufficiency and linear growth deficiency in three girls with chromosome Xp22;Yq11 translocation. *J Med Genet* 33: 906–911, 1996.

Joshi RS, Garg P, Zaitlen N, et al. DNA methylation profiling of uniparental disomy subjects provides a map of parental epigenetic bias in the human genome. *Am J Hum Genet* 99: 555–566, 2016.

Joyce CA, Dennis NR, Cooper S, Browne CE. Subtelomeric rearrangements: Results from a study of selected and unselected probands with idiopathic mental retardation and control individuals by using high-resolution G-banding and FISH. *Hum Genet* 109: 440–451, 2001.

Jurkiewicz D, Kugaudo M, Skórka A, et al. A novel IGF2/H19 domain triplication in the 11p15.5 imprinting region causing either Beckwith-Wiedemann or Silver-Russell syndrome in a single family. *Am J Med Genet* 173A: 72–78, 2017.

Kagami M, Nagai T, Fukami M, Yamazawa K, Ogata T. Silver-Russell syndrome in a girl born after in vitro fertilization: partial hypermethylation at the differentially methylated region of PEG1/MEST. *J Assist Reprod Genet* 24: 131–136, 2007.

Kagami M, Nishimura G, Okuyama T, et al. Segmental and full paternal isodisomy for chromosome 14 in three patients: Narrowing the critical region and implication for the clinical features. *Am J Med Genet* 138A: 127–132, 2005.

Kagan KO, Anderson JM, Anwandter G, Neksasova K, Nicolaides KH. Screening for triploidy by the risk algorithms for trisomies 21, 18 and 13 at 11 weeks to 13 weeks and 6 days of gestation. *Prenat Diagn* 28: 1209–1213, 2008.

Kähkönen M, Kokkonen H-L, Haapala K, Winqvist R, Leisti J. Discrepancy in cytogenetic and DNA analyses of a patient with a deletion of proximal 15q due to familial pericentric inversion and analysis of eight other patients diagnosed to have Prader-Willi syndrome. *Am J Hum Genet* 47: A31, 1990.

Kaiser P. Pericentric inversions: Problems and significance for clinical genetics. *Hum Genet* 68: 1–47, 1984.

Kaiser P. Pericentric inversions: Their problems and clinical significance. In Daniel A (ed.), *The Cytogenetics of Mammalian Autosomal Rearrangements*. New York, NY: Liss, 1988.

Kalantari H, Asia S, Totonchi M, et al. Delineating the association between isodicentric chromosome Y and infertility: A retrospective study. *Fertil Steril* 101: 1091–1096, 2014.

Kallen K. Down's syndrome and maternal smoking in early pregnancy. *Genet Epidemiol* 14: 77–84, 1997.

Kalousek DK. Pathogenesis of chromosomal mosaicism and its effect on early human development. *Am J Med Genet* 91: 39–45, 2000.

Kalousek DK, Langlois S, Robinson WP, et al. Trisomy 7 CVS mosaicism: Pregnancy outcome, placental and DNA analysis in 14 cases. *Am J Med Genet* 65: 348–352, 1996.

Kalscheuer VM, Musante L, Fang C, et al. A balanced chromosomal translocation disrupting *ARHGEF9* is associated with epilepsy, anxiety, aggression, and mental retardation. *Hum Mutat* 30: 61–68, 2009.

Kamiguchi Y, Rosenbusch B, Sterzik K, Mikamo K. Chromosomal analysis of unfertilized human oocytes prepared by a gradual fixation-air drying method. *Hum Genet* 90: 533–541, 1993.

Kanaka-Gantenbein C, Papandreou E, Stefanaki K, et al. Spontaneous ovulation in a true hermaphrodite with normal male phenotype and a rare 46,XX/47,XXY Klinefelter's mosaic karyotype. *Horm Res* 68: 139–144, 2007.

Kanavakis E, Traeger-Synodinos J. Preimplantation genetic diagnosis in clinical practice. *J Med Genet* 39: 6–11, 2002.

Kanduri C, Kantojärvi K, Salo PM, et al. The landscape of copy number variations in Finnish families with autism spectrum disorders. *Autism Res* 9: 9–16, 2016.

Kang SHL, Shaw C, Ou Z, et al. Insertional translocation detected using FISH confirmation of array-comparative genomic hybridization (aCGH) results. *Am J Med Genet* 152A: 1111–1126, 2010.

Kara C, Üstyol A, Yilmaz A, Altundag E, Ogur G. Premature ovarian failure due to tetrasomy X in an adolescent girl. *Eur J Pediatr* 173: 1627–1630, 2014.

Kara N, Okten G, Gunes SO, Saglam Y, Tasdemir HA, Pinarli FA. An epileptic case with mosaic ring chromosome 6 and 6q terminal deletion. *Epilepsy Res* 80: 219–223, 2008.

Karadima G, Bugge M, Nicolaidis P, et al. Origin of nondisjunction in trisomy 8 and trisomy 8 mosaicism. *Eur J Hum Genet* 6: 432–438, 1998.

Kariminejad A, Kariminejad R, Moshtagh A, et al. Pericentric inversion of chromosome 18 in parents leading to a phenotypically normal child with segmental uniparental disomy 18. *Eur J Hum Genet* 19: 555–560, 2011.

Karanjawala ZE, Kääriäinen H, Ghosh S, et al. Complete maternal isodisomy of chromosome 8 in an individual with an early-onset ileal carcinoid tumor. *Am J Med Genet* 93: 207–210, 2000.

Karatas JC, Barlow-Stewart K, Strong KA, Meiser B, McMahon C, Roberts C. Women's experience of pre-implantation genetic diagnosis: A qualitative study. *Prenat Diagn* 30: 771–777, 2010.

Kariminejad A, Kariminejad R, Moshtagh A, et al. Pericentric inversion of chromosome 18 in parents leading to a phenotypically normal child with segmental uniparental disomy 18. *Eur J Hum Genet* 19: 555–560, 2011.

Karp LE. The terrible question. *Am J Med Genet* 14: 1–4, 1983.

Kasher PR, Schertz KE, Thomas M, et al. Small 6q16.1 deletions encompassing *POU3F2* cause susceptibility to obesity and variable developmental delay with intellectual disability. *Am J Hum Genet* 98: 363–372, 2016.

Katari S, Turan N, Bibikova M, et al. DNA methylation and gene expression differences in children conceived in vitro or in vivo. *Hum Mol Genet* 18: 3769–3778, 2009.

Kattera S, Chen C. Normal birth after microsurgical enucleation of tripronuclear human zygotes: Case report. *Hum Reprod* 18: 1319–1322, 2003.

Kaur A, Dhillon S, Garg PD, Singh JR. Ring chromosome 7 in an Indian woman. *J Intellect Dev Disabil* 33: 87–94, 2008.

Kausch K, Haaf T, Köhler J, Schmid M. Complex chromosomal rearrangement in a woman with multiple miscarriages. *Am J Med Genet* 31: 415–420, 1988.

Kawasaki K, Kondoh E, Minamiguchi S, et al. Live-born diploid fetus complicated with partial molar pregnancy presenting with pre-eclampsia, maternal anemia, and seemingly huge placenta: A rare case of confined placental mosaicism and literature review. *J Obstet Gynaecol Res* 42: 911–917, 2016.

Kaya N, Colak D, Albakheet A, et al. A novel X-linked disorder with developmental delay and autistic features. *Ann Neurol* 71: 498–508, 2012.

Kaylor J, Alfaro M, Ishwar A, Sailey C, Sawyer J, Zarate YA. Molecular and cytogenetic evaluation of a patient with ring chromosome 13 and discordant results. *Cytogenet Genome Res* 144: 104–108, 2014.

Kearney HM, Kearney JB, Conlin LK. Diagnostic implications of excessive homozygosity detected by SNP-based microarrays: Consanguinity, uniparental disomy, and recessive single-gene mutations. *Clin Lab Med* 31: 595–613, 2011.

Kee Y, D'Andrea AD. Molecular pathogenesis and clinical management of Fanconi anemia. *J Clin Invest* 122: 3799–3806, 2012.

Keitges EA, Pasion R, Burnside RD, et al. Prenatal diagnosis of two fetuses with deletions of 8p23.1, critical region for congenital diaphragmatic hernia and heart defects. *Am J Med Genet* 161A: 1755–1758, 2013.

Keller MC, McRae AF, McGaughran JM, Visscher PM, Martin NG, Montgomery GW. Non-pathological paternal isodisomy of chromosome 2 detected from a genome-wide SNP scan. *Am J Med Genet* 149A: 1823–1826, 2009.

Kellogg G, Sum J, Wallerstein R. Deletion of 3p25.3 in a patient with intellectual disability and dysmorphic features with further definition of a critical region. *Am J Med Genet* 161A: 1405–1408, 2013.

Kempe A, Engels H, Schubert R, et al. Familial ovarian dysgerminomas (Swyer syndrome) in females associated with 46 XY-karyotype. *Gynecol Endocrinol* 16: 107–111, 2002.

Kennedy RD, D'Andrea AD. The Fanconi Anemia/BRCA pathway: New faces in the crowd. *Genes Dev* 19: 2925–2940, 2005.

Kennedy SJ, Teebi AS, Adatia I, Teshima I. Inherited duplication, dup (8)(p23.1p23.1)pat, in a father and daughter with congenital heart defects. *Am J Med Genet* 104: 79–80, 2001.

Kennerknecht I, Just W, Vogel W. A triploid fetus with a diploid placenta: Proposal of a mechanism. *Prenat Diagn* 13: 885–886, 1993a.

Kennerknecht I, Vogel W, Mehnert K. A modified embryogenic model to explain embryonic/extraembryonic chromosomal inconsistencies. *Prenat Diagn* 13: 1156–1159, 1993b.

Keppler-Noreuil KM, Carroll AJ, Finley SC, et al. Chromosome 18q paracentric inversion in a family with mental retardation and hearing loss. *Am J Med Genet* 76: 372–378, 1998.

Keren B, Chantot-Bastaraud S, Brioude F, et al. SNP arrays in Beckwith-Wiedemann syndrome: An improved diagnostic strategy. *Eur J Med Genet* 56: 546–550, 2013.

Kessler S, Levine EK. Psychological aspects of genetic counseling: IV. The subjective assessment of probability. *Am J Med Genet* 28: 361–370, 1987.

Keymolen K, Staessen C, Verpoest W, et al. A proposal for reproductive counselling in carriers of Robertsonian translocations: 10 years of experience with preimplantation genetic diagnosis. *Hum Reprod* 24: 2365–2371, 2009.

Khalifa M, Stein J, Grau L, et al. Partial deletion of *ANKRD11* results in the KBG phenotype distinct from the 16q24.3 microdeletion syndrome. *Am J Med Genet* 161A: 835–840, 2013.

Kher AS, Chattopadhyay A, Datta S, Kanade S, Sreenivasan VK, Bharucha BA. Familial mosaic Turner syndrome. *Clin Genet* 46: 382–383, 1994.

Kim ED, Bischoff FZ, Lipshultz LI, Lamb DJ. Genetic concerns for the subfertile male in the era of ICSI. *Prenat Diagn* 18: 1349–1365, 1998.

Kim EY, Kim YK, Kim MK, et al. A case of de novo duplication of 15q24-q26.3. *Korean J Pediatr* 54: 267–271, 2011a.

Kim H, Lee KS, Kim AK, et al. A chemical with proven clinical safety rescues Down-syndrome-related phenotypes in through *DYRK1A* inhibition. *Dis Model Mech* 9: 839–848, 2016.

Kim HJ, Cho E, Park JB, Im WY, Kim HJ. A Korean family with KBG syndrome identified by *ANKRD11* mutation, and phenotypic comparison of *ANKRD11* mutation and 16q24.3 microdeletion. *Eur J Med Genet* 58: 86–94, 2015.

Kim JH, Oh PS, Na HY, Kim SH, Cho HC. A case of mosaic ring chromosome 4 with subtelomeric 4p deletion. *Korean J Lab Med* 29: 77–81, 2009.

Kim IW, Khadilkar AC, Ko EY, Sabanegh ES. 47,XYY syndrome and male infertility. *Rev Urol* 15: 188–196, 2013.

Kim JW, Chang EM, Song SH, Park SH, Yoon TK, Shim SH. Complex chromosomal rearrangements in infertile males: Complexity of rearrangement affects spermatogenesis. *Fertil Steril* 95: 352, e1–5, 2011b.

Kim JW, Park SY, Ryu HM, et al. Molecular and clinical characteristics of 26 cases with structural Y chromosome aberrations. *Cytogenet Genome Res* 136: 270–277, 2012.

Kim MY, Seok HH, Kim YS, et al. Molecular genetic and cytogenetic characterization of a partial Xp duplication and Xq deletion in a patient with premature ovarian failure. *Gene* 534: 54–59, 2014.

Kim SR, Shaffer LG. Robertsonian translocations: Mechanisms of formation, aneuploidy, and uniparental disomy and diagnostic considerations. *Genet Test* 6: 163–168, 2002.

King DA, Fitzgerald TW, Miller R, et al. A novel method for detecting uniparental disomy from trio genotypes identifies a significant excess in children with developmental disorders. *Genome Res* 24: 673–687, 2014.

King PH, Waldrop R, Lupski JR, Shaffer LG. Charcot-Marie-Tooth phenotype produced by a duplicated *PMP22* gene as part of a 17p trisomy-translocation to the X chromosome. *Clin Genet* 54: 413–416, 1998.

Kingston HM, Nicolini U, Haslam J, Andrews T. 46,XY/47,XY,+17p+ mosaicism in amniocytes associated with fetal abnormalities despite normal fetal blood karyotype. *Prenat Diagn* 13: 637–642, 1993.

Kircheisen R, Schroeder-Kurth T. Familiäres blasenmolen-syndrom und genetische aspekte dieser gestörten trophoblastentwicklung. *Geburtshilfe Frauenheilkd* 51: 569–571, 1991.

Kirchhoff M, Bisgaard AM, Stoeva R, et al. Phenotype and 244k array-CGH characterization of chromosome 13q deletions: An update of the phenotypic map of 13q21.1-qter. *Am J Med Genet* 149A: 894–905, 2009.

Kirchhoff M, Rose H, Lundsteen C. High resolution comparative genomic hybridisation in clinical cytogenetics. *J Med Genet* 38: 740–744, 2001.

Kirkpatrick G, Chow V, Ma S. Meiotic recombination, synapsis, meiotic inactivation and sperm aneuploidy in a chromosome 1 inversion carrier. *Reprod Biomed Online* 24: 91–100, 2012.

Kirkpatrick G, Ferguson KA, Gao H, et al. A comparison of sperm aneuploidy rates between infertile men with normal and abnormal karyotypes. *Hum Reprod* 23: 1679–1683, 2008.

Kiss A, Rosa RFM, Dibi RP, et al. Chromosomal abnormalities in couples with history of recurrent abortion. *Rev Bras Ginecol Obstet* 31: 68–74, 2009.

Kitsiou-Tzeli S, Manolakos E, Lagou M, et al. Characterization of a prenatally assessed de novo supernumerary minute ring chromosome 20 in a phenotypically normal male. *Mol Cytogenet* 2: 8, 2009.

Kivirikko S, Salonen R, Salo A, von Koskull H. Prenatally detected trisomy 7 mosaicism in a dysmorphic child. *Prenat Diagn* 22: 541–544, 2002.

Klásková E, Tüdös Z, Sobek A, et al. Low-level 45,X/46,XX mosaicism is not associated with congenital heart disease and thoracic aorta dilatation:prospective magnetic resonance imaging and ultrasound study. *Ultrasound Obstet Gynecol* 45: 722–727, 2015.

Kleczkowska A, Fryns JP, Van den Berghe H. Pericentric inversions in man: Personal experience and review of the literature. *Hum Genet* 75: 333–338, 1987.

Kleczkowska A, Fryns JP, Vinken L, van den Berghe H. Effect of balanced X/autosome translocations on sexual and physical development: A personal experience in 4 patients. *Clin Genet* 27: 147–152, 1985.

Kleffmann W, Zink AM, Lee JA, et al. 5q31 microdeletions: Definition of a critical region and analysis of *LRRTM2*, a candidate gene for intellectual disability. *Mol Syndromol* 3: 68–75, 2012.

Klein J, Graham JM, Platt LD, Schreck R. Trisomy 8 mosaicism in chorionic villus sampling: Case report and counselling issues. *Prenat Diagn* 14: 451–454, 1994.

Klein OD, Backstrand K, Cotter PD, Marco E, Sherr E, Slavotinek A. Case report: Y;6 translocation with deletion of 6p. *Clin Dysmorphol* 14: 93–96, 2005.

Knebel S, Pasantes JJ, Thi DA, Schaller F, Schempp W. Heterogeneity of pericentric inversions of the human Y chromosome. *Cytogenet Genome Res* 132: 219–226, 2011.

Knegt AC, Li S, Engelen JJM, Bijlsma EK, Warburton PE. Prenatal diagnosis of a karyotypically normal pregnancy in a mother with a supernumerary neocentric 13q21→13q22 chromosome and balancing reciprocal deletion. *Prenat Diagn* 23: 215–220, 2003.

Knight MA, Hernandez D, Diede SJ, et al. A duplication at chromosome 11q12.2-11q12.3 is associated with spinocerebellar ataxia type 20. *Hum Mol Genet* 17: 3847–3853, 2008.

Knight SJL, Flint J. Perfect endings: A review of subtelomeric probes and their use in clinical diagnosis. *J Med Genet* 37: 401–409, 2000.

Knijnenburg J, van Bever Y, Hulsman LO, et al. A 600 kb triplication in the cat eye syndrome critical region causes anorectal, renal and preauricular anomalies in a three-generation family. *Eur J Hum Genet* 20: 986–989, 2012.

Knoppers BM. "Well-bear and well-rear" in China? *Am J Hum Genet* 63: 686–687, 1998.

Knudson AG, Jr. Mutation and cancer: Statistical study of retinoblastoma. *Proc Natl Acad Sci USA* 68: 820–823, 1971.

Ko DS, Cho JW, Park SY, et al. Clinical outcomes of preimplantation genetic diagnosis (PGD) and analysis of meiotic segregation modes in reciprocal translocation carriers. *Am J Med Genet* 152A: 1428–1433, 2010.

Koç A, Arisoy O, Pala E, et al. Prenatal diagnosis of mosaic ring 22 duplication/deletion with terminal 22q13 deletion due to abnormal first trimester screening and choroid plexus cyst detected on ultrasound. *J Obstet Gynaecol Res* 35: 978–982, 2009.

Koç A, Kan D, Karaer K, et al. An unexpected finding in a child with neurological problems: Mosaic ring chromosome 18. *Eur J Pediatr* 167: 655–659, 2008.

Kohn TP, Kohn JR, Darilek S, Ramasamy R, Lipshultz L. Genetic counseling for men with recurrent pregnancy loss or recurrent implantation failure due to abnormal sperm chromosomal aneuploidy. *J Assist Reprod Genet* 33: 571–576, 2016.

Kojis TL, Gatti RA, Sparkes RS. The cytogenetics of ataxia telangiectasia. *Cancer Genet Cytogenet* 56: 143–156, 1991.

Kokkonen H, Leisti J. An unexpected recurrence of Angelman syndrome suggestive of maternal germ-line mosaicism of del(15)(q11q13) in a Finnish family. *Hum Genet* 107: 83–85, 2000.

Kølvraa S, Singh R, Normand EA, et al. Genome-wide copy number analysis on DNA from fetal cells isolated from the blood of pregnant women. *Prenat Diagn* 36: 1127–1134, 2016.

Komori S, Nakata Y, Sakata K, Kato H, Koyoma K. Analysis for microdeletions of Y chromosome in a single spermatozoon from a man with severe oligozoospermia. *J Hum Genet* 46: 76–79, 2001.

Kompanje EJO. The earliest description of an autopsy on a case of Roberts syndrome reported in 1672: Some additions. *Am J Med Genet* 149A: 1610–1611, 2009.

Kondo Y, Mizuno S, Ohara K, et al. Two cases of partial trisomy 21 (pter-q22.1) without the major features of Down syndrome. *Am J Med Genet* 140: 227–232, 2006.

Kong GW, Cao Y, Huang J, et al. Prenatal detection of 10q22q23 duplications: Dilemmas in phenotype prediction. *Prenat Diagn* 36: 1211–1216, 2016.

Konialis C, Hagnefelt B, Sevastidou S, et al. Uncovering recurrent microdeletion syndromes and subtelomeric deletions/duplications through non-selective application of a MLPA-based extended prenatal panel in routine prenatal diagnosis. *Prenat Diagn* 31: 571–577, 2011.

Koochek M, Harvard C, Hildebrand MJ, et al. 15q duplication associated with autism in a multiplex family with a familial cryptic translocation t(14;15)(q11.2;q13.3) detected using array-CGH. *Clin Genet* 69: 124–134, 2006.

Koolen DA, Dupont J, de Leeuw N, et al. Two families with sibling recurrence of the 17q21.31 microdeletion syndrome due to low-grade mosaicism. *Eur J Hum Genet* 20: 729–733, 2012.

Koolen DA, Pfundt R, Linda K, et al. The Koolen-de Vries syndrome: A phenotypic comparison of patients with a 17q21.31 microdeletion versus a *KANSL1* sequence variant. *Eur J Hum Genet* 24: 652–659, 2016.

Korenberg JR, Chen XN, Schipper R, et al. Down syndrome phenotypes: The consequences of chromosomal imbalance. *Proc Natl Acad Sci USA* 91: 4997–5001, 1994.

Korenromp MJ, Page-Christiaens GCML, van den Bout J, Mulder EJH, Visser GHA. Maternal decision to terminate pregnancy in case of Down syndrome. *Am J Obstet Gynecol* 196: 149.e1–11, 2007.

Korteweg FJ, Bouman K, Erwich JJ, et al. Cytogenetic analysis after evaluation of 750 fetal deaths: Proposal for diagnostic workup. *Obstet Gynecol* 111: 865–874, 2008.

Kosaki R, Migita O, Takahashi T, Kosaki K. Two distinctive classic genetic syndromes, 22q11.2 deletion syndrome and Angelman syndrome, occurring within the same family. *Am J Med Genet* 149A: 702–705, 2009.

Kosho T, Sakazume S, Kawame H, et al. De-novo balanced translocation between 7q31 and 10p14 in a girl with central precocious puberty, moderate mental retardation, and severe speech impairment. *Clin Dysmorphol* 17: 31–34, 2008.

Koskinen S, Onnelainen T, de la Chapelle A, Kere J. A rare reciprocal translocation (12;21) segregating for nine generations. *Hum Genet* 92: 509–512, 1993.

Koster MP, Pennings JL, Imholz S, et al. Proteomics and Down syndrome screening: A validation study. *Prenat Diagn* 30: 1039–1043, 2010.

Kosztolányi G. Does "ring syndrome" exist? An analysis of 207 case reports on patients with a ring autosome. *Hum Genet* 75: 174–179, 1987.

Kosztolányi G, Brecevic L, Bajnòczky K, Schinzel A, Riegel M. Mosaic supernumerary ring chromosome 1 in a three-generational family: 10-year follow-up report. *Eur J Med Genet* 54: 152–156, 2011.

Kosztolányi G, Méhes K, Hook EB. Inherited ring chromosomes: An analysis of published cases. *Hum Genet* 87: 320–324, 1991.

Kotzot D. Abnormal phenotypes in uniparental disomy (UPD): Fundamental aspects and a critical review with bibliography of UPD other than 15. *Am J Med Genet* 82: 265–274, 1999.

Kotzot D. Complex and segmental uniparental disomy (UPD): Review and lessons from rare chromosomal complements. *J Med Genet* 38: 497–507, 2001.

Kotzot D. Review and meta-analysis of systematic searches for uniparental disomy (UPD) other than UPD 15. *Am J Med Genet* 111: 366–375, 2002.

Kotzot D. Complex and segmental uniparental disomy updated. *J Med Genet* 45: 545–556, 2008a.

Kotzot D. Prenatal testing for uniparental disomy: Indications and clinical relevance. *Ultrasound Obstet Gynecol* 31: 100–105, 2008b.

Kotzot D, Hoffmann K, Kujat A, Holland H, Froster UG, Mücke J. Implications of FISH investigations in MIDAS syndrome associated with a 46,XX,t(X;Y) karyotype. *Am J Med Genet* 113: 108–110, 2002.

Kotzot D, Holland H, Keller E, Froster UG. Maternal isochromosome 7q and paternal isochromosome 7p in a boy with growth retardation. *Am J Med Genet* 102: 169–172, 2001.

Kousoulidou L, Tanteles G, Moutafi M, Sismani C, Patsalis PC, Anastasiadou V. 263.4 kb deletion within the *TCF4* gene consistent with Pitt-Hopkins syndrome, inherited from a mosaic parent with normal phenotype. *Eur J Med Genet* 56: 314–318, 2013.

Kowalczyk M, Tomaszewska A, Podbiol-Palenta A, et al. A familial deletion of 16q21 characterized by an SNP array and associated with a normal phenotype. *Am J Med Genet* 161A: 1501–1504, 2013.

Kovaleva NV. Germ-line transmission of trisomy 21: Data from 80 families suggest an implication of grandmaternal age and a high frequency of female-specific trisomy rescue. *Mol Cytogenet* 3: 7, 2010.

Kovaleva NV. Increased risk of tisomy 21 in offspring of carriers of balanced non-contributing autosomal rearrangements is not explained by interchromosomal effect. *Genetika* 49: 259–268, 2013.

Kovaleva NV, Cotter PD. Somatic/gonadal mosaicism for structural autosomal rearrangements: Female predominance among carriers of gonadal mosaicism for unbalanced rearrangements. *Mol Cytogenet* 9: 8, 2016.

Kovaleva NV, Shaffer LG. Under-ascertainment of mosaic carriers of balanced homologous acrocentric translocations and isochromosomes. *Am J Med Genet* 121A: 180–187, 2003.

Kozma C, Slavotinek AM, Meck JM. Segregation of a t(1;3) translocation in multiple affected family

members with both types of adjacent-1 segregants. *Am J Med Genet* 124A: 118–128, 2004.

Kramer RL, Jarve RK, Yaron Y, et al. Determinants of parental decisions after the prenatal diagnosis of Down syndrome. *Am J Med Genet* 79: 172–174, 1998.

Krantz D, Goetzl L, Simpson JL, et al. Association of extreme first-trimester free human chorionic gonadotropin-beta, pregnancy-associated plasma protein A, and nuchal translucency with intrauterine growth restriction and other adverse pregnancy outcomes. *Am J Obstet Gynecol* 191: 1452–1458, 2004.

Krausz C, Casamonti E. Spermatogenic failure and the Y chromosome. *Hum Genet* 136: 637–655, 2017.

Krausz C, McElreavey K. Y chromosome microdeletions in "fertile" males. *Hum Reprod* 16: 1306–1307, 2001.

Kremen J, Chan YM, Swartz JM. Recent findings on the genetics of disorders of sex development. *Curr Opin Urol* 27: 1–6, 2017.

Krieg SA, Lathi RB, Behr B, Westphal LM. Normal pregnancy after tetraploid karyotype on trophectoderm biopsy. *Fertil Steril* 92: 1169, e10, 2009.

Krob G, Braun A, Kuhnle U. True hermaphroditism: geographical distribution, clinical findings, chromosomes and gonadal histology. *Eur J Pediatr* 153: 2–10, 1994.

Kruszka P, Addissie YA, McGinn DE, et al. 22q11.2 deletion syndrome in diverse populations. *Am J Med Genet* 173A: 879–888, 2017.

Krzeminska D, Steinfeld C, Cloez JL, et al. Prenatal diagnosis of Williams syndrome based on ultrasound signs. *Prenat Diagn* 29: 710–712, 2009.

Kubota T, Nonoyama S, Tonoki H, et al. A new assay for the analysis of X-chromosome inactivation based on methylation-specific PCR. *Hum Genet* 104: 49–55, 1999.

Kuchinka BD, Barrett IJ, Moya G, et al. Two cases of confined placental mosaicism for chromosome 4, including one with maternal uniparental disomy. *Prenat Diagn* 21: 36–39, 2001.

Kuechler A, Hauffa BP, Köninger A, et al. An unbalanced translocation unmasks a recessive mutation in the follicle-stimulating hormone receptor (FSHR) gene and causes FSH resistance. *Eur J Hum Genet* 18: 656–661, 2010.

Kuechler A, Zink AM, Wieland T, et al. Loss-of-function variants of *SETD5* cause intellectual disability and the core phenotype of microdeletion 3p25.3 syndrome. *Eur J Hum Genet* 23: 753–760, 2015.

Kühl H, Röttger S, Heilbronner H, Enders H, Schempp W. Loss of the Y chromosomal

PAR2-region in four familial cases of satellited Y chromosomes (Yqs). *Chromosome Res* 9: 215–222, 2001.

Kulharya AS, Mills Lovell C, Flannery DB. Unusual mosaic karyotype resulting from adjacent 1 segregation of t(11;22): Importance of performing skin fibroblast karyotype in patients with unexplained multiple congenital anomalies. *Am J Med Genet* 113: 367–370, 2002.

Kuliev A, Zlatopolsky Z, Kirillova I, Spivakova J, Cieslak Janzen J. Meiosis errors in over 20,000 oocytes studied in the practice of preimplantation aneuploidy testing. *Reprod Biomed Online* 22: 2–8, 2011.

Kuller JA, Meyer WR, Traynor KD, Hartmann KE. Disposition of sperm donors with resultant abnormal pregnancies. *Hum Reprod* 16: 1553–1555, 2001.

Kumar A, Cassidy SB, Romero L, Schwartz S. Molecular cytogenetics of a de novo interstitial deletion of chromosome arm 6q in a developmentally normal girl. *Am J Med Genet* 86: 227–231, 1999.

Kumra S, Wiggs E, Krasnewich D, et al. Brief report: Association of sex chromosome anomalies with childhood-onset psychotic disorders. *J Am Acad Child Adolesc Psychiatry* 37: 292–296, 1998.

Kung A, Munné S, Bankowski B, Coates A, Wells D. Validation of next-generation sequencing for comprehensive chromosome screening of embryos. *Reprod Biomed Online* 31: 760–769, 2015.

Kunz J, Schoner K, Stein W, Rehder H, Fritz B. Tetrasomy 12p (Pallister-Killian syndrome): Difficulties in prenatal diagnosis. *Arch Gynecol Obstet* 280: 1049–1053, 2009.

Kuo PL. Maternal trisomy 21 mosaicism and recurrent spontaneous abortion. *Fertil Steril* 78: 432–433, 2002.

Kupchik GS, Barrett SK, Babu A, Charria-Ortiz G, Velinov M, Macera MJ. Atypical 18p-syndrome associated with partial trisomy 16p in a chromosomally unbalanced child of consanguineous parents with an identical balanced translocation. *Eur J Med Genet* 48: 57–65, 2005.

Kuppermann M, Learman LA, Gates E, et al. Beyond race or ethnicity and socioeconomic status: Predictors of prenatal testing for Down syndrome. *Obstet Gynecol* 107: 1087–1097, 2006.

Kurahashi H, Emanuel BS. Unexpectedly high rate of de novo constitutional t(11;22) translocations in sperm from normal males. *Nat Genet* 29: 139–140, 2001.

Kurahashi H, Inagaki H, Ohye T, et al. The constitutional t(11;22): Implications for a novel mechanism responsible for gross chromosomal rearrangements. *Clin Genet* 78: 299–309, 2010.

Kurahashi H, Sakamoto M, Ono J, Honda A, Okada S, Nakamura Y. Molecular cloning of the chromosomal breakpoint in the *LIS1* gene of a patient with isolated lissencephaly and balanced t(8;17). *Hum Genet* 103: 189–192, 1998.

Kurnit DM, Aldridge JF, Matsuoka R, Matthysse S. Increased adhesiveness of trisomy 21 cells and atrioventricular canal malformations in Down syndrome: A stochastic model. *Am J Med Genet* 20: 385–399, 1985.

Kuroda Y, Ohashi I, Saito T, et al. Deletion of *UBE3A* in brothers with Angelman syndrome at the breakpoint with an inversion at 15q11.2. *Am J Med Genet* 164A: 2873–2878, 2014a.

Kuroda Y, Ohashi I, Tominaga M, et al. De novo duplication of 17p13.1-p13.2 in a patient with intellectual disability and obesity. *Am J Med Genet* 164A: 1550–1554, 2014b.

Kuroda Y, Saito T, Nagai J, et al. Microdeletion of 19p13.3 in a girl with Peutz-Jeghers syndrome, intellectual disability, hypotonia, and distinctive features. *Am J Med Genet* 167A: 389–393, 2015.

Kuroda-Kawaguchi T, Skaletsky H, Brown LG, et al. The AZFc region of the Y chromosome features massive palindromes and uniform recurrent deletions in infertile men. *Nat Genet* 29: 279–286, 2001.

Kurtulgan HK, Özer L, Yildirim ME, et al. Recombinant chromosome with partial 14 q trisomy due to maternal pericentric inversion. *Mol Cytogenet* 8: 92, 2015.

Kvarnung M, Lindstrand A, Malmgren H, et al. Inherited mosaicism for the supernumerary marker chromosome in cat eye syndrome: Inter- and intra-individual variation and correlation to the phenotype. *Am J Med Genet* 158A: 1111–1117, 2012.

La Cour Sibbesen E, Jespersgaard C, Alosi D, Bisgaard AM, Tümer Z. Ring chromosome 9 in a girl with developmental delay and dysmorphic features: Case report and review of the literature. *Am J Med Genet* 161A: 1447–1452, 2013.

Labonne JDJ, Shen Y, Kong IK, Diamond MP, Layman LC, Kim HG. Comparative deletion mapping at 1p31.3-p32.2 implies NFIA responsible for intellectual disability coupled with macrocephaly and the presence of several other genes for syndromic intellectual disability. *Mol Cytogenet* 9: 24, 2016.

Labonne JDJ, Vogt J, Reali L, Kong IK, Layman LC, Kim HG. A microdeletion encompassing PHF21A in an individual with global developmental delay and craniofacial anomalies. *Am J Med Genet* 167A: 3011–3018, 2015.

Lacaria M, Srour M, Michaud JL, et al. Expansion of the clinical phenotype of the distal 10q26.3 deletion syndrome to include ataxia and hyperemia of the hands and feet. *Am J Med Genet* 173: 1611–1619, 2017.

Lacassie Y, Arriaza MI, Vargas A, La Motta I. Ring 2 chromosome: Ten-year follow-up report. *Am J Med Genet* 85: 117–122, 1999.

Lacbawan FL, White BJ, Anguiano A, et al. Rare interstitial deletion (2)(p11.2p13) in a child with pericentric inversion (2)(p11.2q13) of paternal origin. *Am J Med Genet* 87: 139–142, 1999.

Lachlan KL, Youings S, Costa T, Jacobs PA, Thomas NS. A clinical and molecular study of 26 females with Xp deletions with special emphasis on inherited deletions. *Hum Genet* 118: 640–651, 2006.

Lacombe D, Saura R, Taine L, Battin J. Confirmation of assignment of a locus for Rubinstein-Taybi syndrome gene to 16p13.3. *Am J Med Genet* 44: 126–128, 1992.

Lagier-Tourenne C, Ginglinger E, Alembik Y, et al. Two cousins with partial trisomy 12q and monosomy 12p recombinants of a familial pericentric inversion of the chromosome 12. *Am J Med Genet* 125A: 77–85, 2004.

Lahn BT, Ma N, Breg WR, Stratton R, Surti U, Page DC. Xq-Yq interchange resulting in supernormal X-linked gene expression in severely retarded males with 46,XYq- karyotype. *Nat Genet* 8: 243–250, 1994.

Lakovschek IC, Streubel B, Ulm B. Natural outcome of trisomy 13, trisomy 18, and triploidy after prenatal diagnosis. *Am J Med Genet* 155A: 2626–33, 2011.

Lancet editorial. Western eyes on China's eugenics law. *Lancet* 346: 131, 1995.

Landwehr C, Montag M, van der Ven K, Weber RG. Rapid comparative genomic hybridization protocol for prenatal diagnosis and its application to aneuploidy screening of human polar bodies. *Fertil Steril* 90: 488–496, 2008.

Langlois S, Yong PJ, Yong SL, et al. Postnatal follow-up of prenatally diagnosed trisomy 16 mosaicism. *Prenat Diagn* 26: 548–558, 2006.

Lango Allen H, Caswell R, Xie W, et al. Next generation sequencing of chromosomal rearrangements in patients with split-hand/split-foot malformation provides evidence for DYNC1I1 exonic enhancers of DLX5/6

expression in humans. *J Med Genet* 51: 264–267, 2014.

Lathi RB, Liebert CA, Brookfield KF, et al. Conjugated bisphenol A in maternal serum in relation to miscarriage risk. *Fertil Steril* 102: 123–128, 2014.

Lathi RB, Mark SD, Westphal LM, Milki AA. Cytogenetic testing of anembryonic pregnancies compared to embryonic missed abortions. *J Assist Reprod Genet* 24: 521–524, 2007.

Lau NM, Huang JY, MacDonald S, et al. Feasibility of fertility preservation in young females with Turner syndrome. *Reprod Biomed Online* 18: 290–295, 2009.

Lau TK, Fung HYM, Rogers MS, Cheung KL. Racial variation in incidence of trisomy 21: Survey of 57,742 Chinese deliveries. *Am J Med Genet* 75: 386–388, 1998.

Laufer-Cahana A, Krantz ID, Bason LD, Lu FM, Piccoli DA, Spinner NB. Alagille syndrome inherited from a phenotypically normal mother with a mosaic 20p microdeletion. *Am J Med Genet* 112: 190–193, 2002.

Laurell T, Lundin J, Anderlid BM, et al. Molecular and clinical delineation of the 17q22 microdeletion phenotype. *Eur J Hum Genet* 21: 1085–1092, 2013.

Lavery SA, Aurell R, Turner C, et al. Preimplantation genetic diagnosis: Patients' experiences and attitudes. *Hum Reprod* 17: 2464–2467, 2002.

Layman LC. Human gene mutations causing infertility. *J Med Genet* 39: 153–161, 2002.

Layman LC, Tho SPT, Clark AD, Kulharya A, McDonough PG. Phenotypic spectrum of 45,X/46,XY males with a ring Y chromosome and bilaterally descended testes. *Fertil Steril* 91: 791–797, 2009.

Lazier J, Chernos J, Lowry RB. A 2q24.3q31.1 microdeletion found in a patient with Filippi-like syndrome phenotype: A case report. *Am J Med Genet* 164A: 2385–2387, 2014.

Lazzaro SJ, Speevak MD, Farrell SA. Recombinant Down syndrome: A case report and literature review. *Clin Genet* 59: 128–130, 2001.

Le Caignec C, Boceno M, Jacquemont S, Nguyen The Tich S, Rival JM, David A. Inherited ring chromosome 8 without loss of subtelomeric sequences. *Ann Genet* 47: 289–296, 2004.

Le Caignec C, Boceno M, Saugier-Veber P, et al. Detection of genomic imbalances by array based comparative genomic hybridisation in fetuses with multiple malformations. *J Med Genet* 42: 121–128, 2005.

Le Gall J, Nizon M, Pichon O, et al. Sex chromosome aneuploidies and copy-number variants: a further explanation for neurodevelopmental prognosis variability? *Eur J Hum Genet* 25: 930–934, 2017.

Le Guennec K, Quenez O, Nicolas G, et al. 17q21.31 duplication causes prominent tau-related dementia with increased MAPT expression. *Mol Psychiatry* 22: 1119–1125, 2017.

Leach NT, Cole SM, Sandstrom DJ, Weremowicz S. A novel pericentric inversion of chromosome 14 involving the rRNA gene cluster. *Prenat Diagn* 25: 620–621, 2005.

Lebo RV. Prenatal diagnosis of Charcot-Marie-Tooth disease. *Prenat Diagn* 18: 169–172, 1998.

Lebo RV, Milunsky J, Higgins AW, Loose B, Huang XL, Wyandt HE. Symmetric replication of an unstable isodicentric Xq chromosome derived from isolocal maternal sister chromatid recombination. *Am J Med Genet* 85: 429–437, 1999.

Lebre AS, Morinière V, Dunand O, Bensman A, Morichon-Delvallez N, Antignac C. Maternal uniparental heterodisomy of chromosome 17 in a patient with nephropathic cystinosis. *Eur J Hum Genet* 17: 1019–1023, 2009.

Leclercq G, Buvat-Herbaut M, Monnier JC, Vinatier D, Dufour P. Turner's syndrome and pregnancy in donor oocytes and in vitro fertilization: Three case reports. *J Gynecol Obstet Biol Reprod (Paris)* 21: 635–640, 1992.

Leclercq S, Baron X, Jacquemont ML, Cuillier F, Cartault F. Mosaic trisomy 22—Five new cases with variable outcomes: Implications for genetic counselling and clinical management. *Prenat Diagn* 30: 168–172, 2010.

Ledbetter DH, Zachary JM, Simpson JL, et al. Cytogenetic results from the U.S. Collaborative Study on CVS. *Prenat Diagn* 12: 317–345, 1992.

Lee BH, Kasparis C, Chen B, et al. Setleis syndrome due to inheritance of the 1p36.22p36.21 duplication: Evidence for lack of penetrance. *J Hum Genet* 60: 717–722, 2015a.

Lee CG, Cho E, Ahn YM. Maternally inherited autosomal dominant intellectual disability caused by 16p13.3 microduplication. *Eur J Med Genet* 59: 210–214, 2016.

Lee E, Illingworth P, Wilton L, Chambers GM. The clinical effectiveness of preimplantation genetic diagnosis for aneuploidy in all 24 chromosomes (PGD-A): Systematic review. *Hum Reprod* 30: 473–483, 2015b.

Lee CG, Park SJ, Yun JN, Yim SY, Sohn YB. Reciprocal deletion and duplication of 17p11.2-11.2: Korean patients with Smith-Magenis syndrome and Potocki-Lupski syndrome. *J Korean Med Sci* 27: 1586–1590, 2012.

Lee J, Stanley JR, Vaz SA, et al. Down syndrome with pure partial trisomy 21q22 due to a paternal insertion (4;21) uncovered by uncultured amniotic fluid interphase FISH. *Am J Med Genet* 132A: 206–208, 2005.

Lee M, Munné S. Pregnancy after polar body biopsy and freezing and thawing of human embryos. *Fertil Steril* 73: 645–647, 2000.

Lee MH, Park SY, Kim YM, et al. Prenatal diagnosis of a familial complex chromosomal rearrangement involving chromosomes 5, 10, 16 and 18. *Prenat Diagn* 22: 102–104, 2002.

Leegte B, Sikkema-Raddatz B, Hordijk R, et al. Three cases of mosaicism for balanced reciprocal translocations. *Am J Med Genet* 79: 362–365, 1998.

Leffler M, Puusepp S, Žilina O, et al. Two familial microduplications of 15q26.3 causing overgrowth and variable intellectual disability with normal copy number of IGF1R. *Eur J Med Genet* 59: 257–262, 2016.

Lefkowitz RB, Tynan JA, Liu T, et al. Clinical validation of a noninvasive prenatal test for genomewide detection of fetal copy number variants. *Am J Obstet Gynecol* 215: 227.e1–16, 2016.

Lefort G, Blanchet P, Belgrade N, et al. Stable dicentric duplication-deficiency chromosome 14 resulting from crossing-over within a maternal paracentric inversion. *Am J Med Genet* 113: 333–338, 2002.

Lefort G, Blanchet P, Chaze AM, et al. Cytogenetic and molecular study of a jumping translocation in a baby with Dandy-Walker malformation. *J Med Genet* 38: 67–73, 2001.

Légaré F, St-Jacques S, Gagnon S, et al. Prenatal screening for Down syndrome: A survey of willingness in women and family physicians to engage in shared decision-making. *Prenat Diagn* 31: 319–326, 2011.

Leggett V, Jacobs P, Nation K, Scerif G, Bishop DV. Neurocognitive outcomes of individuals with a sex chromosome trisomy: XXX, XYY, or XXY: A systematic review. *Dev Med Child Neurol* 52: 119–129, 2010.

Lehmann KJ, Kovac JR, Xu J, Fischer MA. Isodicentric Yq mosaicism presenting as infertility and maturation arrest without altered SRY and AZF regions. *J Assist Reprod Genet* 29: 939–942, 2012.

Leichtman DA, Schmickel RD, Gelehrter TD, Judd WJ, Woodbury MC, Meilinger KL. Familial Turner syndrome. *Ann Intern Med* 89: 473–476, 1978.

Leisti JT, Kaback MM, Rimoin DL. Human X-autosome translocations: differential inactivation of the X chromosome in a kindred with an X-9 translocation. *Am J Hum Genet* 27: 441–453, 1975.

Lejeune H, Brosse A, Groupe Fertipreserve, Plotton I. Fertilité dans le syndrome de Klinefelter. *Presse Méd* 43: 162–170, 2014.

Lejeune J. Types et contretypes. *J Génét Hum* 15 (Suppl): 20–32, 1966.

Lejeune J. The William Allan Memorial Award Lecture: On the nature of men. *Am J Hum Genet* 22: 121–128, 1970.

Lejeune J, Gautier M, Turpin R. Étude des chromosomes somatiques de neuf enfants mongoliens. *Comp Rend Hebd Séances Acad Sci* 248: 1721–1722, 1959.

Lejeune J, Lafourcade J, Berger R, et al. Trois cas de délétion partielle du bras court d'un chromosome 5. *Comp Rend Hebd Séances Acad Sci* 257: 3098–3102, 1963.

Lemyre E, der Kaloustian VM, Duncan AMV. Stable non-Robertsonian dicentric chromosomes: Four new cases and a review. *J Med Genet* 38: 76–79, 2001.

Lenzi ML, Smith J, Snowden T, et al. Extreme heterogeneity in the molecular events leading to the establishment of chiasmata during meiosis I in human oocytes. *Am J Hum Genet* 76: 112–127, 2005.

Leonard NJ, Tomkins DJ. Diploid/tetraploid/ t(1;6) mosaicism in a 17-year-old female with hypomelanosis of Ito, multiple congenital anomalies, and body asymmetry. *Am J Med Genet* 112: 86–90, 2002.

Leonard S, Bower C, Petterson B, Leonard H. Survival of infants born with Down's syndrome: 1980–96. *Paediatr Perinat Epidemiol* 14: 163–171, 2000.

Lepage JF, Lortie M, Deal CL, Théoret H. Empathy, autistic traits, and motor resonance in adults with Turner syndrome. *Soc Neurosci* 9: 601–609, 2014.

Leroy C, Landais E, Briault S, et al. The 2q37-deletion syndrome: An update of the clinical spectrum including overweight, brachydactyly and behavioural features in 14 new patients. *Eur J Hum Genet* 21: 602–612, 2013.

Lespinasse J, Gicquel C, Robert M, Le Bouc Y. Phenotypic and genotypic variability in monozygotic triplets with Turner syndrome. *Clin Genet* 54: 56–59, 1998.

Lespinasse J, Hoffmann P, Lauge A, et al. Chromosomal instability in two siblings with gonad deficiency: Case report. *Hum Reprod* 20: 158–162, 2005.

Lessel D, Vaz B, Halder S, et al. Mutations in *SPRTN* cause early onset hepatocellular carcinoma, genomic instability and progeroid features. *Nat Genet* 46: 1239–1244, 2014.

Lestner JM, Ellis R, Canham N. Delineating the 17q24.2-q24.3 microdeletion syndrome phenotype. *Eur J Med Genet* 55: 700–704, 2012.

Lestou VS, Desilets V, Lomax BL, et al. Comparative genomic hybridization: A new approach to screening for intrauterine complete or mosaic aneuploidy. *Am J Med Genet* 92: 281–284, 2000.

Letterie GS. Unique unbalanced X;X translocation (Xq22;p11.2) in a woman with primary amenorrhea but without Ullrich-Turner syndrome. *Am J Med Genet* 59: 414–416, 1995.

Levitas AS, Reid CS. An angel with Down syndrome in a sixteenth century Flemish Nativity painting. *Am J Med Genet* 116A: 399–405, 2003.

Levitsky LL, Luria AH, Hayes FJ, Lin AE. Turner syndrome: Update on biology and management across the life span. *Curr Opin Endocrinol Diabetes Obes* 22: 65–72, 2015.

Levy B, Dunn TM, Hirschhorn K, Kardon N. Jumping translocations in spontaneous abortions. *Cytogenet Cell Genet* 88: 25–29, 2000.

Levy B, Sigurjonsson S, Pettersen B, et al. Genomic imbalance in products of conception: Single-nucleotide polymorphism chromosomal microarray analysis. *Obstet Gynecol* 124: 202–209, 2014.

Lévy J, Coussement A, Dupont C, et al. Molecular and clinical delineation of 2p15p16.1 microdeletion syndrome. *Am J Med Genet* 173A: 2081–2087, 2017.

Levy MJ, Stillman RJ. Reproductive potential in survivors of childhood malignancy. *Pediatrician* 18: 61–70, 1991.

Levy-Mozziconacci A, Piquet C, Scheiner C, et al. i(18q) in amniotic and fetal cells with a normal karyotype in direct chorionic villus sampling: Cytogenetics and pathology. *Prenat Diagn* 16: 1156–1159, 1996.

Lewi L, Blickstein I, Van Schoubroeck D, et al. Diagnosis and management of heterokaryotypic monochorionic twins. *Am J Med Genet* 140: 272–275, 2006.

Lewin B. *Genes V*. New York, NY: Oxford University Press, 1994.

Lewis-Jones I, Aziz N, Seshadri S, Douglas A, Howard P. Sperm chromosomal abnormalities are linked to sperm morphologic deformities. *Fertil Steril* 79: 212–215, 2003.

Li C. A prenatally recognizable malformation syndrome associated with a recurrent post-zygotic chromosome rearrangement der(Y)t(Y;1) (q12:q21). *Am J Med Genet* 152A: 2339–2341, 2010.

Li LL, Dong Y, Wang RX, An N, Yun X, Liu RZ. Sperm aneuploidy and implications for genetic counseling in a pedigree of three t(1;3) balanced translocation carriers. *Genet Mol Res* 14: 5003–5009, 2015.

Li M, Squire JA, Weksberg R. Molecular genetics of Wiedemann-Beckwith syndrome. *Am J Med Genet* 79: 253–259, 1998.

Li N, Tang EI, Cheng CY. Regulation of blood-testis barrier by actin binding proteins and protein kinases. *Reproduction* 151: R29–41, 2016.

Li S, Hassed S, Mulvihill JJ, Nair AK, Hopcus DJ. Double trisomy. *Am J Med Genet* 124A: 96–98, 2004.

Li Z, Liu J, Li H, et al. Phenotypic expansion of the interstitial 16p13.3 duplication: A case report and review of the literature. *Gene* 531: 502–505, 2013.

Liang CA, Braddock BA, Heithaus JL, Christensen KM, Braddock SR, Carey JC. Reported communication ability of persons with trisomy 18 and trisomy 13. *Dev Neurorehabil* 18: 322–329, 2015.

Liang D, Wang Y, Ji X, et al. Clinical application of whole-genome low-coverage next-generation sequencing to detect and characterize balanced chromosomal translocations. *Clin Genet* 91: 605–610, 2017.

Liao C, Li DZ. Pregnancy outcome following prenatal diagnosis of sex chromosome abnormalities in Mainland China. *Prenat Diagn* 28: 443–444, 2008.

Liao C, Li DZ. Should sex chromosomes be excluded from use in QF-PCR in prenatal samples with a molecular referral? *Am J Med Genet* 164A: 2404–2406, 2014.

Liao C, Yi CX, Li DZ. Prenatal diagnosis of sex chromosome aneuploidies: Experience at a mainland Chinese hospital. *J Obstet Gynaecol* 33: 827–829, 2013.

Lichtenbelt KD, Hochstenbach R, van Dam WM, Eleveld MJ, Poot M, Beemer FA. Supernumerary ring chromosome 7 mosaicism: Case report, investigation of the gene content, and delineation of the phenotype. *Am J Med Genet* 132A: 93–100, 2005.

Liebaers I, Desmyttere S, Verpoest W, et al. Report on a consecutive series of 581 children born after blastomere biopsy for preimplantation genetic diagnosis. *Hum Reprod* 25: 275–282, 2010.

Lieberman-Aiden E, van Berkum NL, Williams L, et al. Comprehensive mapping of long-range interactions reveals folding principles of the human genome. *Science* 326: 289–293, 2009.

Liehr T. Uniparental disomy—Clinical consequences due to imprinting and activation of recessive genes. *Mol Cytogenet* 7 (Suppl 1): I21, 2014.

Liehr T. Cases with uniparental disomy. http://upd-tl.com/upd.html, 2016a.

Liehr T. Small supernumerary marker chromosomes. http://ssmc-tl.com/sSMC.html, 2016b.

Liehr T, Ewers E, Kosyakova N, et al. Handling small supernumerary marker chromosomes in prenatal diagnostics. *Expert Rev Mol Diagn* 9: 317–324, 2009a.

Liehr T, Stumm M, Wegner RD, et al. 10p11.2 to 10q11.2 is a yet unreported region leading to unbalanced chromosomal abnormalities without phenotypic consequences. *Cytogenet Genome Res* 124: 102–105, 2009b.

Liehr T, Utine GE, Trautmann U, et al. Neocentric small supernumerary marker chromosomes (sSMC)—Three more cases and review of the literature. *Cytogenet Genome Res* 118: 31–37, 2007.

Lim AST, Lim TH, Kee SK, Chieng R, Tay SK. Sperm segregation patterns by fluorescence in situ hybridization studies of a 46,XY,t(2;6) heterozygote giving rise to a rare triploid product of conception with a 69,XXY,t(2;6)(p12;q24) der(6)t(2;6)(p12;q24)pat karyotype. *Am J Med Genet* 117A: 172–176, 2003.

Lim AST, Su LC. Mosaic trisomy 18 male with normal intelligence who fathered a normal baby girl. *Am J Med Genet* 76: 365–366, 1998.

Lim BC, Min BJ, Park WY, et al. A unique phenotype of 2q24.3-2q32.1 duplication: Early infantile epileptic encephalopathy without mesomelic dysplasia. *J Child Neurol* 29: 260–264, 2014.

Lim CK, Cho JW, Kim JY, Kang IS, Shim SH, Jun JH. A healthy live birth after successful preimplantation genetic diagnosis for carriers of complex chromosome rearrangements. *Fertil Steril* 90: 1680–1684, 2008a.

Lim CK, Cho JW, Song IO, Kang IS, Yoon YD, Jun JH. Estimation of chromosomal imbalances in preimplantation embryos from preimplantation genetic diagnosis cycles of reciprocal translocations with or without acrocentric chromosomes. *Fertil Steril* 90: 2144–2151, 2008b.

Lim D, Bowdin SC, Tee L, et al. Clinical and molecular genetic features of Beckwith-Wiedemann syndrome associated with assisted reproductive technologies. *Hum Reprod* 24: 741–747, 2009.

Lim ECP, Ng ISL, Yong MH, Yon HY, Brett MSY, Tan EC. De novo trisomy 12p in twin girls with different levels of mosaicism. *Am J Med Genet* 161A: 1702–1705, 2013.

Lim HH, Kil HR, Koo SH. Incidence, puberty, and fertility in 45,X/47,XXX mosaicism: Report of a patient and a literature review. *Am J Med Genet* 173A: 1961–1964, 2017.

Lim Z, Downs J, Wong K, Ellaway C, Leonard H. Expanding the clinical picture of the *MECP2* duplication syndrome. *Clin Genet* 91: 557–563, 2017.

Lin A, Clasen L, Lee NR, et al. Mapping the stability of human brain asymmetry across five sex-chromosome aneuploidies. *J Neurosci* 35: 140–145, 2015.

Lin CC, Hsieh YY, Wang CH, et al. Prenatal detection and characterization of a small supernumerary marker chromosome (sSMC) derived from chromosome 22 with apparently normal phenotype. *Prenat Diagn* 26: 898–902, 2006.

Lin SP, Huang SY, Tu ME, et al. Netherton syndrome: Mutation analysis of two Taiwanese families. *Arch Dermatol Res* 299: 145–150, 2007.

Lin YH, Chuang L, Lin YM, Teng YN, Kuo PL. Isochromosome of Yp in a man with Sertoli-cell-only syndrome. *Fertil Steril* 83: 764–766, 2005.

Linden MG, Bender BG. Fifty-one prenatally diagnosed children and adolescents with sex chromosome abnormalities. *Am J Med Genet* 110: 11–18, 2002.

Linden MG, Bender BG. Reply to correspondence from Haverty et al.— "47,XXX associated with malformations." *Am J Med Genet* 125A: 112, 2004.

Linden MG, Bender BG, Robinson A. Sex chromosome tetrasomy and pentasomy. *Pediatrics* 96: 672–682, 1995.

Linden MG, Bender BG, Robinson A. Genetic counseling for sex chromosome abnormalities. *Am J Med Genet* 110: 3–10, 2002.

Lindenbaum RH, Clarke G, Patel C, Moncrieff M, Hughes JT. Muscular dystrophy in an X;1 translocation female suggests that Duchenne locus is on X chromosome short arm. *J Med Genet* 16: 389–392, 1979.

Lindenbaum RH, Hultén M, McDermott A, Seabright M. The prevalence of translocations in parents of children with regular trisomy 21: A possible interchromosomal effect? *J Med Genet* 22: 24–28, 1985.

Lindstrand A, Malmgren H, Verri A, et al. Molecular and clinical characterization of patients with overlapping 10p deletions. *Am J Med Genet* 152A: 1233–1243, 2010.

Lindhardt Johansen M, Hagen CP, Rajpert-De Meyts E, et al. 45,X/46,XY mosaicism: Phenotypic characteristics, growth, and reproductive function—A retrospective longitudinal study. *J Clin Endocrinol Metab* 97: E1540–549, 2012.

Linhares ND, Svartman M, Salgado MI, et al. Dental developmental abnormalities in a patient with subtelomeric 7q36 deletion syndrome may confirm a novel role for the SHH gene. *Meta Gene* 2: 16–24, 2014.

Liou JD, Chen CP, Breg WR, Hobbins JC, Mahoney MJ, Yang-Feng TL. Fetal blood sampling and cytogenetic abnormalities. *Prenat Diagn* 13: 1–8, 1993.

Liou JD, Ma YY, Gibson LH, et al. Cytogenetic and molecular studies of a familial paracentric inversion of Y chromosome present in a patient with ambiguous genitalia. *Am J Med Genet* 70: 134–137, 1997.

Lippe B. Turner syndrome. *Endocrinol Metab Clin North Am* 20: 121–152, 1991.

Lisi EC, Hamosh A, Doheny KF, et al. 3q29 interstitial microduplication: A new syndrome in a three-generation family. *Am J Med Genet* 146A(5): 601–609, 2008.

Lissoni S, Baronchelli S, Villa N, et al. Chromosome territories, X;Y translocation and premature ovarian failure: Is there a relationship? *Mol Cytogenet* 2: 19, 2009.

Little J. The Chernobyl accident, congenital anomalies and other reproductive outcomes. *Paediatr Perinat Epidemiol* 7: 121–151, 1993.

Liu JYW, Kasperaviciute D, Martinian L, Thom M, Sisodiya SM. Neuropathology of 16p13.11 deletion in epilepsy. *PLoS One* 7:e34813, 2012.

Liu L, Li XB, Zi XH, et al. A novel hemizygous SACS mutation identified by whole exome sequencing and SNP array analysis in a Chinese ARSACS patient. *J Neurol Sci* 362: 111–114, 2016.

Liu P, Yuan B, Carvalho CMB, et al. An organismal CNV mutator phenotype restricted to early human development. *Cell* 168: 830–842.e7, 2017.

Liu Q, Hesson LB, Nunez AC, et al. A cryptic paracentric inversion of *MSH2* exons 2–6 causes Lynch syndrome. *Carcinogenesis* 37: 10–17, 2016.

Lloveras E, Canellas A, Cirigliano V, Català V, Cerdan C, Plaja A. Supernumerary ring chromosome: An etiology for Pallister-Killian syndrome? *Fetal Diagn Ther* 34: 172–175, 2013.

Lo JO, Shaffer BL, Feist CD, Caughey AB. Chromosomal microarray analysis and prenatal diagnosis. *Obstet Gynecol Surv* 69: 613–621, 2014.

Loeffler J, Soelder E, Erdel M, et al. Muellerian aplasia associated with ring chromosome 8p12q12 mosaicism. *Am J Med Genet* 116A: 290–294, 2003.

Löffler J, Utermann B, Duba HC, Mayr U, Utermann G, Erdel M. Mental and psychomotoric retardation in two brothers with pure partial trisomy 7q32-q34 due to a maternal insertion (14;7). *Am J Med Genet* 91: 291–297, 2000.

Lonardo F, Di Natale P, Lualdi S, et al. Mucopolysaccharidosis type II in a female patient with a reciprocal X;9 translocation and skewed X chromosome inactivation. *Am J Med Genet* 164A: 2627–2632, 2014.

Lonardo F, Perone L, Maioli M, et al. Clinical, cytogenetic and molecular-cytogenetic characterization of a patient with a de novo tandem proximal-intermediate duplication of 16q and review of the literature. *Am J Med Genet* 155A: 769–777, 2011.

López-Expósito I, Bafalliu JA, Santos M, Fuster C, Puche-Mira A, Guillén-Navarro E. Intrachromosomal partial triplication of chromosome 13 secondary to a paternal duplication with mild phenotypic effect. *Am J Med Genet* 146A: 1190–1194, 2008.

López-Pajares I, Delicado A, Lapunzina P, et al. Tetrasomy 8p: Discordance of amniotic fluid and blood karyotypes. *Am J Med Genet* 118A: 353–357, 2003.

López Pajares I, Villa O, Salido M, et al. Euchromatic variant 16p+: Implications in prenatal diagnosis. *Prenat Diagn* 26: 535–538, 2006.

Lorda-Sánchez I, Diego-Alvarez D, Ayuso C, de Alba MR, Trujillo MJ, Ramos C. Trisomy 2 due to a 3:1 segregation in an abortion studied by QF-PCR and CGH. *Prenat Diagn* 25: 934–938, 2005.

Loren AW, Mangu PB, Beck LN, et al. Fertility preservation for patients with cancer: American Society of Clinical Oncology clinical practice guideline update. *J Clin Oncol* 31: 2500–2510, 2013.

Loup V, Bernicot I, Janssens P, et al. Combined FISH and PRINS sperm analysis of complex chromosome rearrangement t(1;19;13): An approach facilitating PGD. *Mol Hum Reprod* 16: 111–116, 2010.

Louvrier C, Egea G, Labalme A, et al. Characterization of a de novo supernumerary neocentric ring chromosome derived from chromosome 7. *Cytogenet Genome Res* 147: 111–117, 2015.

Loviglio MN, Leleu M, Männik K, et al. Chromosomal contacts connect loci associated with autism, BMI and head circumference phenotypes. *Mol Psychiatry* 22: 836–849, 2017.

Lowry RB, Chernos JE, Connelly MS, Wyse JP. Interstitial deletions at 6q14.1q15 associated with developmental delay and a marfanoid phenotype. *Mol Syndromol* 4: 280–284, 2013.

Lowry RB, Sibbald B, Bedard T. *Alberta Congenital Anomalies Surveillance System: Eighth Report 1980–2007.* Edmonton, Alberta, Canada: Alberta Health and Wellness, 2009.

Lowther C, Costain G, Stavropoulos DJ, et al. Delineating the 15q13.3 microdeletion phenotype: A case series and comprehensive review of the literature. *Genet Med* 17: 149–157, 2015.

Lubinsky MS. Kouska's fallacy: The error of the divided denominator. *Lancet* 2: 1449–1450, 1986.

Lubs HA. A marker X chromosome. *Am J Hum Genet* 21: 231–244, 1969.

Lucci-Cordisco E, Zollino M, Baglioni S, et al. A novel microdeletion syndrome with loss of the *MSH2* locus and hereditary non-polyposis colorectal cancer. *Clin Genet* 67: 178–182, 2005.

Luciani JM, Guichaoua MR, Delafontaine D, North MO, Gabriel-Robez O, Rumpler Y. Pachytene analysis in a 17;21 reciprocal translocation carrier: Role of the acrocentric chromosomes in male sterility. *Hum Genet* 77: 246–250, 1987.

Lugli L, Malacarne M, Cavani S, Pierluigi M, Ferrari F, Percesepe A. A 12.4 Mb direct duplication in 19q12-q13 in a boy with cardiac and CNS malformations and developmental delay. *J Appl Genet* 52: 335–339, 2011.

Luijsterburg AJM, van der Zee DC, Gaillard JLJ, et al. Chorionic villus sampling and end-artery disruption of the fetus. *Prenat Diagn* 17: 71–76, 1997.

Luk HM, Ivan Lo FM, Sano S, et al. Silver-Russell syndrome in a patient with somatic mosaicism for upd(11)mat identified by buccal cell analysis. *Am J Med Genet* 170A: 1938–1941, 2016.

Lukusa T, Vermeesch JR, Fryns JP. De novo deletion 7q36 resulting from a distal 7q/8q translocation: Phenotypic expression and comparison to the literature. *Genet Couns* 16: 1–15, 2005.

Lungeanu A, Arghir A, Arps S, et al. Chromosome Y isodicentrics in two cases with ambiguous genitalia and features of Turner syndrome. *Balkan J Med Genet* 11: 8, 2008.

Luo Y, Xu C, Sun Y, Wang L, Chen S, Jin F. Different segregation patterns in five carriers due to a pericentric inversion of chromosome 1. *Syst Biol Reprod Med* 60: 367–372, 2014.

Lupski JR. Genomic disorders ten years on. *Genome Med* 1: 42, 2009.

Lupski JR. Cognitive phenotypes and genomic copy number variations. *JAMA* 313: 2029–2030, 2015.

Lurie IW. Clinical manifestations of partial trisomy 2p. *Cytogenet Genome Res* 144: 28–30, 2014.

Lurie IW. A critical region for ulnar defects in patients with 4q deletions may be narrowed. *Clin Dysmorphol* 25: 133, 2016.

Lustosa-Mendes E, dos Santos AP, Viguetti-Campos NL, Vieira TP, Gil-da-Silva-Lopes VL. A boy with partial dup(18q)/del(18p) due to a maternal pericentric inversion: Genotype-phenotype correlation and risk of recombinant chromosomes based on systematic review of the literature. *Am J Med Genet* 173A: 143–150, 2017.

Luukkonen TM, Pöyhönen M, Palotie A, et al. A balanced translocation truncates Neurotrimin in a family with intracranial and thoracic aortic aneurysm. *J Med Genet* 49: 621–629, 2012.

Lybaek H, Ørstavik KH, Prescott T, et al. An 8.9 Mb 19p13 duplication associated with precocious puberty and a sporadic 3.9 Mb 2q23.3q24.1 deletion containing *NR4A2* in mentally retarded members of a family with an intrachromosomal 19p-into-19q between-arm insertion. *Eur J Hum Genet* 17: 904–910, 2009.

Lybæk H, Øyen N, Fauske L, Houge G. A 2.1 Mb deletion adjacent but distal to a 14q21q23 paracentric inversion in a family with spherocytosis and severe learning difficulties. *Clin Genet* 74: 553–559, 2008.

Ma S, Yuen BH, Penaherrera M, Koehn D, Ness L, Robinson W. ICSI and the transmission of X-autosomal translocation: A three-generation evaluation of X;20 translocation: Case report. *Hum Reprod* 18: 1377–1382, 2003.

Maan AA, Eales J, Akbarov A, et al. The Y chromosome: a blueprint for men's health? *Eur J Hum Genet* 25, 1181–1188, 2017.

Maas NMC, Van Vooren S, Hannes F, et al. The t(4;8) is mediated by homologous recombination between olfactory receptor gene clusters, but other 4p16 translocations occur at random. *Genet Couns* 18: 357–365, 2007.

Maas SM, Shaw AC, Bikker H, et al. Phenotype and genotype in 103 patients with tricho-rhino-phalangeal syndrome. *Eur J Med Genet* 58: 279–92, 2015.

MacArthur JA, Spector TD, Lindsay SJ et al. The rate of nonallelic homologous recombination in males is highly variable, correlated between monozygotic twins and independent of age. *PLoS Genet* 10: e1004195, 2014.

MacDermot KD, Jack E, Cooke A, et al. Investigation of three patients with the "ring syndrome," including familial transmission of ring 5, and estimation of reproductive risks. *Hum Genet* 85: 516–520, 1990.

MacDonald JR, Ziman R, Yuen RK, Feuk L, Scherer SW. The Database of Genomic Variants: A curated collection of structural variation in the human genome. *Nucleic Acids Res* 42: D986–992, 2014.

MacDonald M, Hassold T, Harvey J, Wang LH, Morton NE, Jacobs P. The origin of 47,XXY and 47,XXX aneuploidy: Heterogeneous mechanisms and role of aberrant recombination. *Hum Mol Genet* 3: 1365–1371, 1994.

Machev N, Gosset P, Warter S, Treger M, Schillinger M, Viville S. Fluorescence in situ hybridization sperm analysis of six translocation carriers provides evidence of an interchromosomal effect. *Fertil Steril* 84: 365–373, 2005.

Machiela MJ, Zhou W, Karlins E, et al. Female chromosome X mosaicism is age-related and preferentially affects the inactivated X chromosome. *Nat Commun* 7: 11843, 2016.

Machlitt A, Kuepferling P, Bommer C, Koerner H, Chaoui R. Prenatal diagnosis of trisomy 1q21-qter: Case report and review of literature. *Am J Med Genet* 134A: 207–211, 2005.

Macintosh MCM. Perception of risk. In Grudzinskas JG, Chard T, Chapman M, Cuckle H (eds.), *Screening for Down's syndrome*. Cambridge, UK: Cambridge University Press, 1994.

Mackie FL, Hemming K, Allen S, Morris RK,4, Kilby MD. The accuracy of cell-free fetal DNA-based non-invasive prenatal testing in singleton pregnancies: A systematic review and bivariate meta-analysis. *BJOG* 124: 32–46, 2017.

Mackie Ogilvie C, Watson S, Braude P, Pickering S, Scriven PN. Preimplantation genetic diagnosis for a carrier of a Y;autosome translocation resulting in a healthy male offspring. *Fertil Steril* 94: 1529, e11–14, 2010.

Madan K. Paracentric inversions: A review. *Hum Genet* 96: 503–515, 1995.

Madan K. Balanced complex chromosome rearrangements—Reproductive aspects. A review. *Am J Med Genet* 158A: 947–963, 2012.

Madan K, Hompes PGA, Schoemaker J, Ford CE. X-autosome translocation with a breakpoint in Xq22 in a fertile woman and her 47,XXX infertile daughter. *Hum Genet* 59: 290–296, 1981.

Madan K, Kleinhout J. First trimester abortions associated with a translocation t(1;20)(p36;p11). *Hum Genet* 76: 109, 1987.

Madan K, Lundberg ES. Low grade mosaicism for X aneuploidy in women referred for recurrent abortions. *Eur Cytogeneticists Assoc Newslett* 35: 9–12, 2015.

Madan K, Menko FH. Intrachromosomal insertions: A case report and a review. *Hum Genet* 89: 1–9, 1992.

Madan K, Nieuwint AWM. Reproductive risks for paracentric inversion heterozygotes: Inversion or insertion? That is the question. *Am J Med Genet* 107: 340–343, 2002.

Madan K, Nieuwint AWM, van Bever Y. Recombination in a balanced complex translocation of a mother leading to a balanced reciprocal translocation in the child: Review of 60 cases of balanced complex translocations. *Hum Genet* 99: 806–815, 1997.

Madariaga ML, Rivera H. Familial inv(X) (p22q22): ovarian dysgenesis in two sisters with del Xq and fertility in one male carrier. *Clin Genet* 52: 180–183, 1997.

Maddirevula S, Coskun S, Awartani K, Alsaif H, Abdulwahab FM, Alkuraya FS. The human knockout phenotype of *PADI6* is female sterility caused by cleavage failure of their fertilized eggs. *Clin Genet* 91: 344–345, 2017.

Mademont-Soler I, Morales C, Madrigal I, et al. Prenatal diagnosis of two different unbalanced forms of an inherited (Y;12) translocation. *Am J Med Genet* 149A: 2820–2823, 2009.

Madsen HN, Ball S, Wright D, et al. A reassessment of biochemical marker distributions in trisomy 21-affected and unaffected twin pregnancies in the first trimester. *Ultrasound Obstet Gynecol* 37: 38–47, 2011.

Maeda J, Yamagishi H, Furutani Y, et al. The impact of cardiac surgery in patients with trisomy 18 and trisomy 13 in Japan. *Am J Med Genet* 155A: 2641–2646, 2011.

Magee AC, Humphreys MW, McKee S, Stewart M, Nevin NC. De novo direct duplication 2 (p12→p21) with paternally inherited pericentric inversion 2p11.2 2q12.2. *Clin Genet* 54: 65–69, 1998a.

Magee AC, Nevin NC, Armstrong MJ, McGibbon D, Nevin J. Ullrich-Turner syndrome: Seven pregnancies in an apparent 45,X woman. *Am J Med Genet* 75: 1–3, 1998b.

Magenis E, Webb MJ, Spears B, Opitz JM. Blaschkolinear malformation syndrome in complex trisomy-7 mosaicism. *Am J Med Genet* 87: 375–383, 1999.

Magini P, Poscente M, Ferrari S, et al. Cytogenetic and molecular characterization of a recombinant X chromosome in a family with a severe neurologic phenotype and macular degeneration. *Mol Cytogenet* 8: 58, 2015.

Mahmood R, Brierley CH, Faed MJW, Mills JA, Delhanty JDA. Mechanisms of maternal aneuploidy: FISH analysis of oocytes and polar bodies in patients undergoing assisted conception. *Hum Genet* 106: 620–626, 2000.

Maillard AM, Ruef A, Pizzagalli F, et al. The 16p11.2 locus modulates brain structures common to autism, schizophrenia and obesity. *Mol Psychiatry* 20: 140–147, 2015.

Makrydimas G, Sebire NJ, Thornton SE, Zagorianakou N, Lolis D, Fisher RA. Complete hydatidiform mole and normal live birth: A novel case of confined placental mosaicism: case report. *Hum Reprod* 17: 2459–2463, 2002.

Makrydimas G, Sotiriadis A, Ioannidis JP. Screening performance of first-trimester nuchal translucency for major cardiac defects: A meta-analysis. *Am J Obstet Gynecol* 189: 1330–1335, 2003.

Makrydimas G, Sotiriadis A, Spencer K, Cowans NJ, Nicolaides KH. ADAM12-s in coelomic fluid and maternal serum in early pregnancy. *Prenat Diagn* 26: 1197–1200, 2006.

Malan V, Gesny R, Morichon-Delvallez N, et al. Prenatal diagnosis and normal outcome of a 46,XX/46,XY chimera: A case report. *Hum Reprod* 22: 1037–1041, 2007.

Malinverni ACM, Colovati ME, Perez ABA, et al. Unusual duplication in the pericentromeric region of chromosome 9 in a patient with phenotypic alterations. *Cytogenet Genome Res* 150(2): 100–105, 2017.

Malvestiti F, Agrati C, Grimi B, et al. Interpreting mosaicism in chorionic villi: Results of a monocentric series of 1001 mosaics in chorionic villi with follow-up amniocentesis. *Prenat Diagn* 35: 1117–1127, 2015.

Malvestiti F, De Toffol S, Chinetti S, et al. Prenatal diagnosis of del(4)(q27q31.23), due to a maternal balanced complex chromosome rearrangement, characterized by array-CGH. *Prenat Diagn* 30: 280–283, 2010.

Malzac P, Webber H, Moncla A, et al. Mutation analysis of *UBE3A* in Angelman syndrome patients. *Am J Hum Genet* 62: 1353–1360, 1998.

Mandrile G, Dubois A, Hoffman JD, et al. 3q26.33-3q27.2 microdeletion: A new microdeletion syndrome? *Eur J Med Genet* 56: 216–221, 2013.

Mange A, Desmetz C, Bellet V, Molinari N, Maudelonde T, Solassol J. Proteomic profile determination of autosomal aneuploidies by mass spectrometry on amniotic fluids. *Proteome Sci* 6: 1, 2008.

Mangs AH, Morris BJ. The human pseudoautosomal region (PAR): Origin, function and future. *Curr Genomics* 8: 129–136, 2007.

Manipalviratn S, DeCherney A, Segars J. Imprinting disorders and assisted reproductive technology. *Fertil Steril* 91: 305–315, 2009.

Mann NP, Fitzsimmons J, Fitzsimmons E, Cooke P. Roberts syndrome: Clinical and cytogenetic aspects. *J Med Genet* 19: 116–119, 1982.

Männik K, Mägi R, Macé A, et al. Copy number variations and cognitive phenotypes in unselected populations. *JAMA* 313: 2044–2054, 2015.

Manning M, Hudgins L. Array-based technology and recommendations for utilization in medical genetics practice for detection of chromosomal abnormalities. *Genet Med* 12: 742–745, 2010.

Manolakos E, Kefalas K, Neroutsou R, et al. Characterization of 23 small supernumerary marker chromosomes detected at pre-natal diagnosis: The value of fluorescence in situ hybridization. *Mol Med Rep* 3: 1015–1022, 2010.

Manolakos E, Vetro A, Garas A, et al. Proximal 10q duplication in a child with severe central hypotonia characterized by array-comparative genomic hybridization: A case report and review of the literature. *Exp Ther Med* 7: 953–957, 2014.

Manolakos E, Vetro A, Kitmirides S, et al. Prenatal diagnosis of a fetus with ring chromosome 15 characterized by array-CGH. *Prenat Diagn* 29: 884–888, 2009.

Manolakos E, Vetro A, Papadopoulou E, et al. Partial trisomy 2p and partial monosomy 2q arising from a paternal intrachromosomal 2q-into-2p between-arm insertion and paracentric inversion: Molecular cytogenetic characterization of a four-break rearrangement. *Cytogenet Genome Res* 140: 12–20, 2013.

Mantzouratou A, Mania A, Apergi M, Laver S, Serhal P, Delhanty J. Meiotic and mitotic behaviour of a ring/deleted chromosome 22 in human embryos determined by preimplantation genetic diagnosis for a maternal carrier. *Mol Cytogenet* 2: 3, 2009.

Manvelyan M, Simonyan I, Hovhannisyan G, Aroutiounian R, Hamid AB, Liehr T. A new case of a complex small supernumerary marker chromosome: A der(9)t(7;9)(p22;q22) due to a maternal balanced rearrangement. *J Pediatr Genet* 4: 199–200, 2015.

Mao X. Reply to Guo and to Chen et al. *Am J Hum Genet* 65: 1199–1201, 1999.

Maraia R, Saal HM, Wangsa D. A chromosome 17q de novo paracentric inversion in a patient with campomelic dysplasia: Case report and etiologic hypothesis. *Clin Genet* 39: 401–408, 1991.

Marangi G, Orteschi D, Milano V, Mancano G, Zollino M. Interstitial deletion of 3p22.3p22.2 encompassing *ARPP21* and *CLASP2* is a potential pathogenic factor for a syndromic form of intellectual disability: A co-morbidity model with additional copy number variations in a large family. *Am J Med Genet* 161A: 2890–2893, 2013.

Marangi G, Zollino M. Pitt-Hopkins syndrome and differential diagnosis: A molecular and clinical challenge. *J Pediatr Genet* 4: 168–176, 2015.

Maraschio P, Tupler R, Dainotti E, Cortinovis M, Tiepolo L. Molecular analysis of a human Y;1 translocation in an azoospermic male. *Cytogenet Cell Genet* 65: 256–260, 1994.

Marcelis C, de Blaauw I, Brunner H. Chromosomal anomalies in the etiology of anorectal malformations: A review. *Am J Med Genet* 155A: 2692–2704, 2011.

Marchetti F, Bishop JB, Lowe X, Generoso WM, Hozier J, Wyrobek AJ. Etoposide induces heritable chromosomal aberrations and aneuploidy during male meiosis in the mouse. *Proc Natl Acad Sci USA* 98: 3952–3957, 2001.

Mardy A, Wapner RJ. Confined placental mosaicism and its impact on confirmation of NIPT results.

Am J Med Genet Semin Med Genet 172C: 118–122, 2016.

Margari L, Colonna A, Craig F, et al. Microphthalmia with linear skin defects (MLS) associated with autism spectrum disorder (ASD) in a patient with familial 12.9Mb terminal Xp deletion. *BMC Pediatr* 14: 220, 2014.

Margarit E, Coll MD, Oliva R, Gómez D, Soler A, Ballesta F. SRY gene transferred to the long arm of the X chromosome in a Y-positive XX true hermaphrodite. *Am J Med Genet* 90: 25–28, 2000.

Margarit E, Morales C, Rodríguez-Revenga L, et al. Familial 4.8 MB deletion on 18q23 associated with growth hormone insufficiency and phenotypic variability. *Am J Med Genet* 158A: 611–616, 2012.

Margarit E, Soler A, Carrió A, et al. Molecular, cytogenetic, and clinical characterisation of six XX males including one prenatal diagnosis. *J Med Genet* 35: 727–730, 1998.

Mari F, Novelli A, Romano C, Renieri A. Response to Phelan K. et al.: Letter to the editor regarding Disciglio et al: Interstitial 22q13 deletions not involving *SHANK3* gene: A new contiguous gene syndrome. *Am J Med Genet* 167A: 1681, 2015.

Marignier S, Lesca G, Marguin J, Bussy G, Sanlaville D, des Portes V. Childhood apraxia of speech without intellectual deficit in a patient with cri du chat syndrome. *Eur J Med Genet* 55: 433–436, 2012.

Marinescu RC, Mamunes P, Kline AD, Schmidt J, Rojas K, Overhauser J. Variability in a family with an insertion involving 5p. *Am J Med Genet* 86: 258–263, 1999.

Marion JP, Fernhoff PM, Korotkin J, Priest JH. Pre- and postnatal diagnosis of trisomy 4 mosaicism. *Am J Med Genet* 37: 362–365, 1990.

Mark HFL. *Medical Cytogenetics*. New York, NY: Dekker, 2000.

Mark HFL, Mendoza T, Abuelo D, Beauregard LJ, May JB, LaMarche PH. Reproduction in a woman with low percentage t(21q21q) mosaicism. *J Med Genet* 14: 221–223, 1977.

Maron JL, Bianchi DW. Prenatal diagnosis using cell-free nucleic acids in maternal body fluids: A decade of progress. *Am J Med Genet* 145C: 5–17, 2007.

Marquard K, Westphal LM, Milki AA, Lathi RB. Etiology of recurrent pregnancy loss in women over the age of 35 years. *Fertil Steril* 94: 1473–1477, 2010.

Marshall LS, Simon J, Wood T, et al. Deletion Xq27.3q28 in female patient with global developmental delays and skewed X-inactivation. *BMC Med Genet* 14: 49, 2013.

Marteau T, Drake H, Bobrow M. Counselling following diagnosis of a fetal abnormality: The differing approaches of obstetricians, clinical geneticists, and genetic nurses. *J Med Genet* 31: 864–867, 1994.

Marteau TM, Dormandy E. Facilitating informed choice in prenatal testing: How well are we doing? *Am J Med Genet* 106: 185–190, 2001.

Marteau TM, Nippert I, Hall S, et al. Outcomes of pregnancies diagnosed with Klinefelter syndrome: The possible influence of health professionals. *Prenat Diagn* 22: 562–566, 2002.

Martens M. Developmental and cognitive troubles in Williams syndrome. *Handb Clin Neurol* 111: 291–293, 2013.

Martin CL, Kirkpatrick BE, Ledbetter DH. Copy number variants, aneuploidies, and human disease. *Clin Perinatol* 42: 227–242, vii, 2015.

Martin CL, Warburton D. Detection of chromosomal aberrations in clinical practice: From karyotype to genome sequence. *Annu Rev Genomics Hum Genet* 16: 309–326, 2015.

Martin JR, Wold A, Taylor HS. Ring chromosome 12 and severe oligospermia: A case report. *Fertil Steril* 90: 443, e13–15, 2008.

Martin MM, Vanzo RJ, Sdano MR, Baxter AL, South ST. Mosaic deletion of 20pter due to rescue by somatic recombination. *Am J Med Genet* 170A: 243–248, 2016.

Martin NDT, Smith WR, Cole TJ, Preece MA. New height, weight and head circumference charts for British children with Williams syndrome. *Arch Dis Child* 92: 598–601, 2007.

Martin NJ, Cartwright DW, Harvey PJ. Duplication 5q(5q22→5q33): From an intrachromosomal insertion. *Am J Med Genet* 20: 57–62, 1985.

Martin RH. Sperm chromosome analysis in a man heterozygous for a paracentric inversion of chromosome 7 (q11q22). *Hum Genet* 73: 97–100, 1986.

Martin RH. Sperm chromosome analysis in a man heterozygous for a paracentric inversion of chromosome 14 (q24.1q32.1). *Am J Hum Genet* 64: 1480–1484, 1999.

Martin RH, Greene C, Rademaker A, Barclay L, Ko E, Chernos J. Chromosome analysis of spermatozoa extracted from testes of men with non-obstructive azoospermia. *Hum Reprod* 15: 1121–1124, 2000.

Martin RH, Hildebrand KA, Yamamoto J, et al. The meiotic segregation of human sperm chromosomes in two men with accessory marker chromosomes. *Am J Med Genet* 25: 381–388, 1986.

Martin RH, Ko E, Hildebrand K. Analysis of sperm chromosome complements from a man heterozygous for a robertsonian translocation 45,XY,t(15q;22q). *Am J Med Genet* 43: 855–857, 1992.

Martin RH, Ko E, Rademaker A. Distribution of aneuploidy in human gametes: Comparison between human sperm and oocytes. *Am J Med Genet* 39: 321–331, 1991.

Martin RH, Rademaker A, German J. Chromosomal breakage in human spermatozoa, a heterozygous effect of the Bloom syndrome mutation. *Am J Hum Genet* 55: 1242–1246, 1994.

Martinet D, Vial Y, Thonney F, Beckmann JS, Meagher-Villemure K, Unger S. Fetus with two identical reciprocal translocations: Description of a rare complication of consanguinity. *Am J Med Genet* 140A: 769–774, 2006.

Martínez JE, Tuck-Muller CM, Superneau D, Wertelecki W. Fertility and the cri du chat syndrome. *Clin Genet* 43: 212–214, 1993.

Martinez ME, Cox DF, Youth BP, Hernandez A. Genomic imprinting of *DIO3*, a candidate gene for the syndrome associated with human uniparental disomy of chromosome 14. *Eur J Hum Genet* 24: 1617–1621, 2016.

Martinez-Castro P, Ramos MC, Rey JA, Benitez J, Sanchez Cascos A. Homozygosity for a Robertsonian translocation (13q14q) in three offspring of heterozygous parents. *Cytogenet Cell Genet* 38: 310–312, 1984.

Martínez-Frías ML. The real earliest historical evidence of Down syndrome. *Am J Med Genet* 132A: 231, 2005.

Martínez-Jacobo L, Ortíz-López R, Rizo-Méndez A, et al. Clinical and molecular delineation of duplication 9p24.3q21.11 in a patient with psychotic behavior. *Gene* 560: 124–127, 2015.

Martínez-Juárez A, Uribe-Figueroa L, Quintana-Palma M, Razo-Aguilera G, Sevilla-Montoya R. Pure trisomy 2p syndrome in two siblings with an unbalanced translocation and minimal terminal 12q monosomy characterized by high-density microarray. *Cytogenet Genome Res* 142: 249–254, 2014.

Martínez-Pasarell O, Nogués C, Bosch M, Egozcue J, Templado C. Analysis of sex chromosome aneuploidy in sperm from fathers of Turner syndrome patients. *Hum Genet* 104: 345–349, 1999.

Martinez-Pomar N, Munoz-Saa I, Heine-Suner D, Martin A, Smahi A, Matamoros N. A new mutation in exon 7 of *NEMO* gene: Late skewed X-chromosome inactivation in an incontinentia pigmenti female patient with immunodeficiency. *Hum Genet* 118: 458–465, 2005.

Martorell MR, Martínez-Pasarell O, Lopez O, et al. Chromosome 16 abnormalities in embryos and in sperm from a male with a fragile site at 16q22.1. *Cytogenet Genome Res* 142: 134–139, 2014.

Mascarenhas A, Matoso E, Saraiva J, et al. First prenatally detected small supernumerary neocentromeric derivative chromosome 13 resulting in a non-mosaic partial tetrasomy 13q. *Cytogenet Genome Res* 121: 293–297, 2008.

Mastenbroek S, Twisk M, van der Veen F, Repping S. Preimplantation genetic screening: A systematic review and meta-analysis of RCTs. *Hum Reprod Update* 17: 454–466, 2011.

Mastenbroek S, Twisk M, van Echten-Arends J, et al. In vitro fertilization with preimplantation genetic screening. *N Engl J Med* 357: 9–17, 2007.

Masuno M, Cholsong Y, Kuwahara T, et al. Second meiotic nondisjunction of the rearranged chromosome in a familial reciprocal 5/13 translocation. *Am J Med Genet* 41: 32–34, 1991.

Masuno M, Imaizumi K, Ishii T, Kimura J, Kuroki Y. Supernumerary ring chromosome 5 identified by FISH. *Am J Med Genet* 84: 381, 1999.

Matsui H, Iitsuka Y, Yamazawa K, Tanaka N, Seki K, Sekiya S. Changes in the incidence of molar pregnancies: A population-based study in Chiba Prefecture and Japan between 1974 and 2000. *Hum Reprod* 18: 172–175, 2003.

Matsuo M, Muroya K, Nanao K, et al. Mother and daughter with 45,X/46,X,r(X)(p22.3q28) and mental retardation: Analysis of the X-inactivation patterns. *Am J Med Genet* 91: 267–272, 2000.

Mattina T, Palumbo O, Stallone R, et al. Interstitial 16p13.3 microduplication: Case report and critical review of genotype-phenotype correlation. *Eur J Med Genet* 55: 747–752, 2012.

Mau Kai C, Juul A, McElreavey K, et al. Sons conceived by assisted reproduction techniques inherit deletions in the azoospermia factor (AZF) region of the Y chromosome and the *DAZ* gene copy number. *Hum Reprod* 23: 1669–1678, 2008.

Maurin ML, Labrune P, Brisset S, et al. Molecular cytogenetic characterization of a 4p15.1-pter duplication and a 4q35.1-qter deletion in a recombinant of chromosome 4 pericentric inversion. *Am J Med Genet* 149A: 226–231, 2009.

Maya I, Vinkler C, Konen O, et al. Abnormal brain magnetic resonance imaging in two patients with Smith-Magenis syndrome. *Am J Med Genet* 164A: 1940–1946, 2014.

Mayer A, Fouquet B, Pugeat M, Misrahi M. BMP15 "knockout-like" effect in familial premature ovarian insufficiency with persistent ovarian reserve. *Clin Genet* 92: 208–212, 2017.

McArthur SJ, Leigh D, Marshall JT, Gee AJ, De Boer KA, Jansen RPS. Blastocyst trophectoderm biopsy and preimplantation genetic diagnosis for familial monogenic disorders and chromosomal translocations. *Prenat Diagn* 28: 434–442, 2008.

McCarroll SA. Extending genome-wide association studies to copy-number variation. *Hum Mol Genet* 17: R135–42, 2008.

McClarren J, Donnenfeld AE, Ravnan JB. Prenatal diagnosis of an unexpected interstitial 22q11.2 deletion causing truncus arteriosus and thymic hypoplasia in a ring 22 chromosome derived from a maternally inherited paracentric inversion. *Prenat Diagn* 26: 1212–1215, 2006.

McConkie-Rosell A, Spiridigliozzi GA, Rounds K, et al. Parental attitudes regarding carrier testing in children at risk for fragile X syndrome. *Am J Med Genet* 82: 206–211, 1999.

McCool C, Spinks-Franklin A, Noroski LM, Potocki L. 2017. Potocki-Shaffer syndrome in a child without intellectual disability—The role of *PHF21A* in cognitive function. *Am J Med Genet* 173A: 716–720, 2017.

McCormack A, Claxton K, Ashton F, et al. Microarray testing in clinical diagnosis: An analysis of 5,300 New Zealand patients. *Mol Cytogenet* 9: 29, 2016.

McDermott H, Johnson JL. Is the prevalence of Down syndrome births in Hawai'i increasing? *Hawaii Med J* 70: 72–76, 2011.

McDonald-McGinn DM, Emanuel BS, Zackai EH. 22q11.2 deletion syndrome. In Pagon RA, Adam MP, Ardinger HH, et al. (eds.), *GeneReviews* [Internet]. Seattle, WA: University of Washington, 2013.

McElyea SD, Starbuck JM, Tumbleson-Brink DM, et al. Influence of prenatal EGCG treatment and Dyrk1a dosage reduction on craniofacial features associated with Down syndrome. *Hum Mol Genet* 25: 4856–4869, 2016.

McFadden DE, Friedman JM. Chromosome abnormalities in human beings. *Mutat Res* 396: 129–140, 1997.

McFadden DE, Jiang R, Langlois S, Robinson WP. Dispermy—Origin of diandric triploidy: Brief communication. *Hum Reprod* 17: 3037–3038, 2002.

McFadden DE, Kwong LC, Yam IY, Langlois S. Parental origin of triploidy in human fetuses: Evidence for genomic imprinting. *Hum Genet* 92: 465–469, 1993.

McFadden DE, Langlois S. Parental and meiotic origin of triploidy in the embryonic and fetal periods. *Clin Genet* 58: 192–200, 2000.

McFadden DE, Robinson WP. Phenotype of triploid embryos. *J Med Genet* 43: 609–612, 2006.

McGaughran J, Hadwen T, Clark R. Progressive edema leading to pleural effusions in a female with a ring chromosome 22 leading to a 22q13 deletion. *Clin Dysmorphol* 19: 28–29, 2010.

McGillivray G, Begg L, Billson VR, et al. Trisomy 3: The supported "natural" history. Poster presented at Annual Scientific Meeting of the Human Genetics Society Australasia, 2004.

McGillivray G, Rosenfeld JA, Gardner RJM, Gillam LH. Genetic counselling and ethical issues with chromosome microarray analysis in prenatal testing. *Prenat Diagn* 32: 389–395, 2012.

McGoey RR, Lacassie Y. Paternal balanced reciprocal translocation t(9;22)(q34.3;q11.2) resulting in an infant with features of the 9q subtelomere and the 22q11 deletion syndromes due to 3:1 meiotic segregation and tertiary monosomy. *Am J Med Genet* 149A: 2538–2542, 2009.

McGowan KD, Weiser JJ, Horwitz J, et al. The importance of investigating for uniparental disomy in prenatally identified balanced acrocentric rearrangements. *Prenat Diagn* 22: 141–143, 2002.

McHugh CA, Chen CK, Chow A, et al. The Xist lncRNA interacts directly with SHARP to silence transcription through *HDAC3*. *Nature* 521: 232–236, 2015.

McKenzie LJ, Cisneros PL, Torsky S, et al. Preimplantation genetic diagnosis for a known cryptic translocation: Follow-up clinical report and implication of segregation products. *Am J Med Genet* 121A: 56–59, 2003.

McLysaght A, Makino T, Grayton HM, et al. Ohnologs are overrepresented in pathogenic copy number mutations. *Proc Natl Acad Sci USA* 111: 361–366, 2014.

McWeeney DT, Munné S, Miller RC, et al. Pregnancy complicated by triploidy: A comparison of the three karyotypes. *Am J Perinatol* 26: 641–645, 2009.

Mears AJ, el-Shanti H, Murray JC, McDermid HE, Patil SR. Minute supernumerary ring chromosome 22 associated with cat eye syndrome: Further delineation of the critical region. *Am J Hum Genet* 57: 667–673, 1995.

Mefford HC, Cook J, Gospe SM. Epilepsy due to 20q13.33 subtelomere deletion masquerading as pyridoxine-dependent epilepsy. *Am J Med Genet* 158A: 3190–3195, 2012.

Mefford HC, Rosenfeld JA, Shur N, et al. Further clinical and molecular delineation of the 15q24 microdeletion syndrome. *J Med Genet* 49: 110–118, 2012.

Mefford HC, Sharp AJ, Baker C, et al. Recurrent rearrangements of chromosome 1q21.1 and variable pediatric phenotypes. *N Engl J Med* 359: 1685–1699, 2008.

Mégarbané A, Gosset P, Souraty N, et al. Chromosome 10p11.2-p12.2 duplication: Report of a patient and review of the literature. *Am J Med Genet* 104: 204–208, 2001.

Mehra S, Christ L, Jeng L, Zinn AB, Schwartz S. Characterization of a familial balanced rec(13) in a child with mild MR and his half-sibling with two structurally rearranged chromosomes 13. *Am J Med Genet* 137: 217–221, 2005.

Meiner A, Holland H, Reichenbach H, Horn LC, Faber R, Froster UG. Tetraploidy in a growth-retarded fetus with a thick placenta. *Prenat Diagn* 18: 864–865, 1998.

Meistrich ML, Byrne J. Genetic disease in offspring of long-term survivors of childhood and adolescent cancer treated with potentially mutagenic therapies. *Am J Hum Genet* 70: 1069–1071, 2002.

Mekkawy M, Kamel A, El-Ruby M, et al. Isodicentric Y chromosomes in Egyptian patients with disorders of sex development (DSD). *Am J Med Genet* 158A: 1594–1603, 2012.

Melichar VO, Guth S, Hellebrand H, et al. A male infant with a 9.6 Mb terminal Xp deletion including the OA1 locus: Limit of viability of Xp deletions in males. *Am J Med Genet* 143: 135–141, 2007.

Melis D, Genesio R, Boemio P, et al. Clinical description of a patient carrying the smallest reported deletion involving 10p14 region. *Am J Med Genet* 158A: 832–835, 2012.

Melnyk AR, Ahmed I, Taylor JC. Prenatal diagnosis of familial ring 21 chromosome. *Prenat Diagn* 15: 269–273, 1995.

Melo JB, Estevinho A, Saraiva J, Ramos L, Carreira IM. Cutis aplasia as a clinical hallmark for the syndrome associated with 19q13.11 deletion: The possible role for *UBA2* gene. *Mol Cytogenet* 8: 21, 2015.

Menashe I, Larsen EC, Banerjee-Basu S. Prioritization of copy number variation loci associated with autism from AutDB—An integrative multi-study genetic database. *PLoS One* 8: e66707, 2013.

Mendes JRT, Strufaldi MWL, Delcelo R, et al. Y-chromosome identification by PCR and gonadal histopathology in Turner's syndrome without overt Y-mosaicism. *Clin Endocrinol* 50: 19–26, 1999.

Menon S, Rives N, Mousset-Siméon N, et al. Fertility preservation in adolescent males: Experience over 22 years at Rouen University Hospital. *Hum Reprod* 24: 37–44, 2009.

Mercer CL, Lachlan K, Karcanias A, et al. Detailed clinical and molecular study of 20 females with Xq deletions with special reference to menstruation and fertility. *Eur J Med Genet* 56: 1–6, 2013.

Mercier S, Bresson JL. Analysis of chromosomal equipment in spermatozoa of a 46,XY/47,XY/+8 male by means of multicolour fluorescent in situ hybridization: Confirmation of a mosaicism and evaluation of risk for offspring. *Hum Genet* 99: 42–46, 1997.

Meredith MM, Crabb B, Vargas M, Hirsch BA. Chimerism for 20q11.2 microdeletion of *GDF5* explains discordant phenotypes in monochorionic-diamniotic twins. *Am J Med Genet* 73A: 3182–3188, 2017.

Merrill A, Rosenblum-Vos L, Driscoll DA, Daley K, Treat K. Prenatal diagnosis of Fanconi anemia (Group C) subsequent to abnormal sonographic findings. *Prenat Diagn* 25: 20–22, 2005.

Mertzanidou A, Spits C, Nguyen HT, Van de Velde H, Sermon K. Evolution of aneuploidy up to day 4 of human preimplantation development. *Hum Reprod* 28: 1716–1724, 2013.

Meschede D, Froster UG, Bergmann M, Nieschlag E. Familial pericentric inversion of chromosome 1 (p34q23) and male infertility with stage specific spermatogenic arrest. *J Med Genet* 31: 573–575, 1994.

Meschede D, Lemcke B, Exeler JR, et al. Chromosome abnormalities in 447 couples undergoing intracytoplasmic sperm injection—Prevalence, types, sex distribution and reproductive relevance. *Hum Reprod* 13: 576–582, 1998a.

Meschede D, Lemcke B, Stussel J, Louwen F, Horst J. Strong preference for non-invasive prenatal diagnosis in women pregnant through intracytoplasmic sperm injection (ICSI). *Prenat Diagn* 18: 700–705, 1998b.

Meschede D, Louwen F, Eiben B, Horst J. Intracytoplasmic sperm injection pregnancy with fetal trisomy 9p resulting from a balanced paternal translocation. *Hum Reprod* 12: 1913–1914, 1997.

Meschede D, Louwen F, Nippert I, Holzgreve W, Miny P, Horst J. Low rates of pregnancy termination for prenatally diagnosed Klinefelter syndrome and other sex chromosome polysomies. *Am J Med Genet* 80: 330–334, 1998c.

Meschino WS, Miller K, Bedford HM. Incidental detection of familial APP duplication: An unusual reason for a false positive NIPT result of trisomy 21. *Prenat Diagn* 36: 382–384, 2016.

Meyer E, Lim D, Pasha S, et al. Germline mutation in *NLRP2* (*NALP2*) in a familial imprinting disorder (Beckwith-Wiedemann Syndrome). *PLoS Genet* 5: e1000423, 2009.

Micale M, Insko J, Ebrahim SAD, Adeyinka A, Runke C, Van Dyke DL. Double trisomy revisited—A

multicenter experience. *Prenat Diagn* 30: 173–176, 2010.

Michaelis RC, Velagaleti GVN, Jones C, et al. Most Jacobsen syndrome deletion breakpoints occur distal to *FRA11B*. *Am J Med Genet* 76: 222–228, 1998.

Michelson RJ, Weinert T. Closing the gaps among a web of DNA repair disorders. *Bioessays* 22: 966–969, 2000.

Michie S, Bobrow M, Marteau TM. Predictive genetic testing in children and adults: A study of emotional impact. *J Med Genet* 38: 519–526, 2001.

Middleton FA, Trauzzi MG, Shrimpton AE, et al. Complete maternal uniparental isodisomy of chromosome 4 in a subject with major depressive disorder detected by high density SNP genotyping arrays. *Am J Med Genet* 141B: 28–32, 2006.

Midro AT, Panasiuk B, Stasiewicz-Jarocka B, et al. Risk estimates for carriers of chromosome reciprocal translocation t(4;9)(p15.2;p13). *Clin Genet* 58: 153–155, 2000.

Midro AT, Stengel-Rutkowski S, Stene J. Experiences with risk estimates for carriers of chromosomal reciprocal translocations. *Clin Genet* 41: 113–122, 1992.

Midro AT, Wiland E, Panasiuk B, Lesniewicz R, Kurpisz M. Risk evaluation of carriers with chromosome reciprocal translocation t(7;13)(q34;q13) and concomitant meiotic segregation analyzed by FISH on ejaculated spermatozoa. *Am J Med Genet* 140: 245–256, 2006.

Migeon B. *Females Are Mosaics: X Inactivation and Sex Differences in Disease*. New York, NY: Oxford University Press, 2007.

Migeon BR, Ausems M, Giltay J, et al. Severe phenotypes associated with inactive ring X chromosomes. *Am J Med Genet* 93: 52–57, 2000.

Mihci E, Velagaleti GV, Ensenauer R, Babovic-Vuksanovic D. The phenotypic spectrum of trisomy 2: Report of two new cases. *Clin Dysmorphol* 18: 201–204, 2009.

Mikhaail-Philips MM, Ko E, Chernos J, Greene C, Rademaker A, Martin RH. Analysis of chromosome segregation in sperm from a chromosome 2 inversion heterozygote and assessment of an interchromosomal effect. *Am J Med Genet* 127A: 139–143, 2004.

Mikhaail-Philips MM, McGillivray BC, Hamilton SJ, et al. Unusual segregation products in sperm from a pericentric inversion 17 heterozygote. *Hum Genet* 117: 357–365, 2005.

Mikhaelian M, Veach PM, MacFarlane I, LeRoy BS, Bower M. Prenatal chromosomal microarray analysis: A survey of prenatal genetic counselors' experiences and attitudes. *Prenat Diagn* 33: 371–377, 2013.

Milazzo JP, Rives N, Mousset-Siméon N, Macé B. Chromosome constitution and apoptosis of immature germ cells present in sperm of two 47,XYY infertile males. *Hum Reprod* 21: 1749–1758, 2006.

Milenkovic T, Guc-Scekic M, Zdravkovic D, et al. Molecular analysis of ring Y chromosome in a 10-year-old boy with mixed gonadal dysgenesis and growth hormone deficiency. *Balkan J Med Genet* 14: 71–76, 2011.

Mill P, Lockhart PJ, Fitzpatrick E, et al. Human and mouse mutations in *WDR35* cause short-rib polydactyly syndromes due to abnormal ciliogenesis. *Am J Hum Genet* 88: 508–515, 2011.

Miller DT, Adam MP, Aradhya S, et al. Consensus statement: Chromosomal microarray is a first-tier clinical diagnostic test for individuals with developmental disabilities or congenital anomalies. *Am J Hum Genet* 86: 749–764, 2010.

Miller DT, Shen Y, Weiss LA, et al. Microdeletion/duplication at 15q13.2q13.3 among individuals with features of autism and other neuropsychiatric disorders. *J Med Genet* 46: 242–248, 2009.

Miller JF, Williamson E, Glue J, Gordon YB, Grudzinskas JG, Sykes A. Fetal loss after implantation: A prospective study. *Lancet* 2: 554–556, 1980.

Miller K, Müller W, Winkler L, Hadam MR, Ehrich JHH, Flatz SD. Mitotic disturbance associated with mosaic aneuploidies. *Hum Genet* 84: 361–364, 1990.

Miller K, Pabst B, Ritter H, et al. Chromosome 18 replaced by two ring chromosomes of chromosome 18 origin. *Hum Genet* 112: 343–347, 2003.

Miller K, Reimer A, Schulze B. Tandem duplication chromosome 21 in the offspring of a ring chromosome 21 carrier. *Ann Génét* 30: 180–182, 1987.

Miller KR, Mühlhaus K, Herbst RA, Bohnhorst B, Böhmer S, Arslan-Kirchner M. Patient with trisomy 6 mosaicism. *Am J Med Genet* 100: 103–105, 2001.

Miller OJ, Therman E. *Human Chromosomes* (4th ed.). New York, NY: Springer, 2001.

Miller VL, Ransom SB, Ayoub MA, Krivchenia EL, Evans MI. Fiscal impact of a potential legislative ban on second trimester elective terminations for prenatally diagnosed abnormalities. *Am J Med Genet* 91: 359–362, 2000.

Mills KI, Anderson J, Levy PT, et al. Duplication of 20p12.3 associated with familial

Wolff-Parkinson-White syndrome. *Am J Med Genet* 161A: 137–144, 2013.

Mimouni-Bloch A, Yeshaya J, Kahana S, Maya I, Basel-Vanagaite L. A de-novo interstitial microduplication involving 2p16.1-p15 and mirroring 2p16.1-p15 microdeletion syndrome: Clinical and molecular analysis. *Eur J Paediatr Neurol* 19: 711–715, 2015.

Ming JE, Blagowidow N, Knoll JHM, et al. Submicroscopic deletion in cousins with Prader-Willi syndrome causes a grandmatrilineal inheritance pattern: Effects of imprinting. *Am J Med Genet* 92: 19–24, 2000.

Minto CL, Crouch NS, Conway GS, Creighton SM. XY females: Revisiting the diagnosis. *Br J Obstet Gynaecol* 112: 1407–1410, 2005.

Miryounesi M, Diantpour M, Motevaseli E, Ghafouri-Fard S. Homozygosity for a Robertsonian translocation (13q;14q) in a phenotypically normal 44, XX female with a history of recurrent abortion and a normal pregnancy outcome. *J Reprod Infertil* 17: 184–187, 2016.

Mitchell E, Douglas A, Kjaegaard S, et al. Recurrent duplications of 17q12 associated with variable phenotypes. *Am J Med Genet* 167A: 3038–3045, 2015.

Mitchell JJ, Vekemans M, Luscombe S, et al. U-type exchange in a paracentric inversion as a possible mechanism of origin of an inverted tandem duplication of chromosome 8. *Am J Med Genet* 49: 384–387, 1994.

Mitelman F, Johansson B, Mertens F (Eds.). Mitelman database of chromosome aberrations and gene fusions in cancer. https://cgap.nci.nih.gov/Chromosomes/Mitelman, 2016.

Mitter D, Buiting K, von Eggeling F, et al. Is there a higher incidence of maternal uniparental disomy 14 [upd(14)mat]? Detection of 10 new patients by methylation-specific PCR. *Am J Med Genet* 140: 2039–2049, 2006.

Mitter D, Chiaie BD, Lüdecke HJ, et al. Genotype-phenotype correlation in eight new patients with a deletion encompassing 2q31.1. *Am J Med Genet* 152A: 1213–1224, 2010.

Mitter D, Ullmann R, Muradyan A, et al. Genotype-phenotype correlations in patients with retinoblastoma and interstitial 13q deletions. *Eur J Hum Genet* 19: 947–958, 2011.

Miura K, Obama M, Yun K, et al. Methylation imprinting of *H19* and *SNRPN* genes in human benign ovarian teratomas. *Am J Hum Genet* 65: 1359–1367, 1999.

Miura Y, Hiura M, Torigoe K, et al. Complete paternal uniparental isodisomy for chromosome 1 revealed by mutation analyses of the *TRKA* (*NTRK1*)

gene encoding a receptor tyrosine kinase for nerve growth factor in a patient with congenital insensitivity to pain with anhidrosis. *Hum Genet* 107: 205–209, 2000.

Miyoshi O, Yabe R, Wakui K, et al. Two cases of mosaic RhD blood-group phenotypes and paternal isodisomy for chromosome 1. *Am J Med Genet* 104: 250–256, 2001.

Mizuno S, Fukushi D, Kimura R, et al. Clinical and genomic characterization of siblings with a distal duplication of chromosome 9q (9q34.1-qter). *Am J Med Genet* 155A: 2274–2280, 2011.

Mochizuki J, Saitsu H, Mizuguchi T, et al. Alu-related 5q35 microdeletions in Sotos syndrome. *Clin Genet* 74: 384–391, 2008.

Modan-Moses D, Litmanovitch T, Rienstein S, Meyerovitch J, Goldman B, Aviram-Goldring A. True hermaphroditism with ambiguous genitalia due to a complicated mosaic karyotype: Clinical features, cytogenetic findings, and literature review. *Am J Med Genet* 116A: 300–303, 2003.

Modi DN, Sane S, Bhartiya D. Accelerated germ cell apoptosis in sex chromosome aneuploid fetal human gonads. *Mol Hum Reprod* 9: 219–225, 2003.

Moey C, Hinze SJ, Brueton L, et al. Xp11.2 microduplications including *IQSEC2*, *TSPYL2* and *KDM5C* genes in patients with neurodevelopmental disorders. *Eur J Hum Genet* 24: 373–380, 2016.

Moghadasi S, van Haeringen A, Langendonck L, Gijsbers AC, Ruivenkamp CA. A terminal 3p26.3 deletion is not associated with dysmorphic features and intellectual disability in a four-generation family. *Am J Med Genet* 164A: 2863–2868.

Mokate T, Leask K, Mehta S, et al. Non-mosaic trisomy 22: A report of 2 cases. *Prenat Diagn* 26: 962–965, 2006.

Molina O, Anton E, Vidal F, Blanco J. Sperm rates of 7q11.23, 15q11q13 and 22q11.2 deletions and duplications: A FISH approach. *Hum Genet* 129: 35–44, 2011.

Molina Gomes D, Hammoud I, Bailly M, et al. Preconceptional diagnosis for Robertsonian translocation as an alternative to preimplantation genetic diagnosis in two situations: A pilot study. *J Assist Reprod Genet* 26: 113–117, 2009.

Møller RS, Jensen LR, Maas SM, et multi al. X-linked congenital ptosis and associated intellectual disability, short stature, microcephaly, cleft palate, digital and genital abnormalities define novel Xq25q26 duplication syndrome. *Hum Genet* 133: 625–638, 2014.

Monahan P. Judgements of interest: A doctor's dilemma resolved—Sterilisation of intellectually disabled females. *Australasian J Med Defence Union* 3: 54–55, 1992.

Moncla A, Malzac P, Livet MO, et al. Angelman syndrome resulting from *UBE3A* mutations in 14 patients from eight families: Clinical manifestations and genetic counselling. *J Med Genet* 36: 554–560, 1999.

Monni G, Cau G, Lai R, Demontis G, Usai V. Intracytoplasmic sperm injection and prenatal invasive diagnosis. *Prenat Diagn* 19: 390, 1999.

Monnot S, Giuliano F, Massol C, et al. Partial Xp11.23-p11.4 duplication with random X inactivation: Clinical report and molecular cytogenetic characterization. *Am J Med Genet* 146A: 1325–1329, 2008.

Montag M, van der Ven K, Rösing B, van der Ven H. Polar body biopsy: A viable alternative to preimplantation genetic diagnosis and screening. *Reprod Biomed Online* 18 (Suppl 1): 6–11, 2009.

Mooneyham KA, Holden KR, Cathey S, Dwivedi A, Dupont BR, Lyons MJ. Neurodevelopmental delays and macrocephaly in 17p13.1 microduplication syndrome. *Am J Med Genet* 164A: 2887–2891, 2014.

Moradkhani K, Puechberty J, Bhatt S, et al. Rare Robertsonian translocations and meiotic behaviour: Sperm FISH analysis of t(13;15) and t(14;15) translocations—A case report. *Hum Reprod* 21: 3193–3198, 2006a.

Moradkhani K, Puechberty J, Bhatt S, et al. Meiotic segregation of rare Robertsonian translocations: Sperm analysis of three t(14q;22q) cases. *Hum Reprod* 21: 1166–1171, 2006b.

Morales C, Cuatrecasas E, Mademont-Soler I, et al. Non-mosaic trisomy 20 of paternal origin in chorionic villus and amniotic fluid also detected in fetal blood and other tissues. *Eur J Med Genet* 53: 197–200, 2010.

Morales C, Madrigal I, Esqué T, et al. Duplication/deletion mosaicism of the 7q(21.1→31.3) region. *Am J Med Genet* 143: 179–183, 2007a.

Morales C, Soler A, Bruguera J, et al. Pseudodicentric 22;Y translocation transmitted through four generations of a large family without phenotypic repercussion. *Cytogenet Genome Res* 116: 319–323, 2007b.

Morandi A, Bonnefond A, Lobbens S, et al. A girl with incomplete Prader-Willi syndrome and negative MS-PCR, found to have mosaic maternal UPD-15 at SNP array. *Am J Med Genet* 167A: 2720–2726, 2015.

Morel F, Duguéperoux I, McElreavey K, et al. Transmission of an unbalanced (Y;1) translocation in Brittany, France. *J Med Genet* 39: e52, 2002a.

Morel F, Fellmann F, Roux C, Bresson JL. Meiotic segregation analysis by FISH investigation of spermatozoa of a 46,Y,der(X),t(X;Y) (qter→p22::q11→qter) carrier. *Cytogenet Cell Genet* 92: 63–68, 2001.

Morel F, Laudier B, Guérif F, et al. Meiotic segregation analysis in spermatozoa of pericentric inversion carriers using fluorescence in-situ hybridization. *Hum Reprod* 22: 136–141, 2007.

Morel Y, Mebarki F, Forest MG. What are the indications for prenatal diagnosis in the androgen insensitivity syndrome? Facing clinical heterogeneity of phenotypes for the same genotype. *Eur J Endocrinol* 130: 325–326, 1994.

Mori MA, Huertas H, Pinel I, Giralt P, Martínez-Frías ML. Trisomy 13 in the child of two carriers of a 13/15 translocation. *Am J Med Genet* 20: 17–20, 1985.

Morichon-Delvallez N, Segues B, Pinson MP, et al. Maternal uniparental disomy for chromosome 14 by secondary nondisjunction of an initial trisomy. *Am J Hum Genet* 55 (Suppl): 379A, 1994.

Morisada N, Sekine T, Ishimori S, et al. 16q12 microdeletion syndrome in two Japanese boys. *Pediatr Int* 56:e75–8, 2014.

Morleo M, Franco B. Dosage compensation of the mammalian X chromosome influences the phenotypic variability of X-linked dominant male-lethal disorders. *J Med Genet* 45: 401–8, 2008.

Morris A, Boyd E, Dhanjal S, et al. Two years' prospective experience using fluorescence in situ hybridization on uncultured amniotic fluid cells for rapid prenatal diagnosis of common chromosomal aneuploidies. *Prenat Diagn* 19: 546–551, 1999.

Morris CA, Mervis CB, Paciorkowski AP, et al. 7q11.23 duplication syndrome: Physical characteristics and natural history. *Am J Med Genet* 167A: 2916–2935; 2015.

Morris JK, Alberman E. Trends in Down's syndrome live births and antenatal diagnoses in England and Wales from 1989 to 2008: Analysis of data from the National Down Syndrome Cytogenetic Register. *BMJ* 339: b3794, 2009.

Morris JK, Alberman E, Scott C, Jacobs P. Is the prevalence of Klinefelter syndrome increasing? *Eur J Hum Genet* 16: 163–170, 2008.

Morris JK, De Vigan C, Mutton DE, Alberman E. Risk of a Down syndrome live birth in women 45 years of age and older. *Prenat Diagn* 25: 275–278, 2005a.

Morris JK, Mutton DE, Alberman E. Revised estimates of the maternal age specific live birth prevalence of Down's syndrome. *J Med Screen* 9: 2–6, 2002.

Morris JK, Mutton DE, Alberman E. Recurrences of free trisomy 21: Analysis of data from the National Down Syndrome Cytogenetic Register. *Prenat Diagn* 25: 1120–1128, 2005b.

Morris JK, Wald NJ, Mutton DE, Alberman E. Comparison of models of maternal age-specific risk for Down syndrome live births. *Prenat Diagn* 23: 252–258, 2003.

Mortimer JG, Chewings WE, Gardner RJM. A further report on a kindred with cases of 4p trisomy and monosomy. *Hum Hered* 30: 58–61, 1980.

Mosca SJ, Langevin LM, Dewey D, et al. Copy-number variations are enriched for neurodevelopmental genes in children with developmental coordination disorder. *J Med Genet* 53: 812–819, 2016.

Moysés-Oliveira M, Guilherme R dos S, Dantas AG, et al. Genetic mechanisms leading to primary amenorrhea in balanced X-autosome translocations. *Fertil Steril* 103: 1289–1296.e2, 2015a.

Moysés-Oliveira M, Guilherme RS, Meloni VA, et al. X-linked intellectual disability related genes disrupted by balanced X-autosome translocations. *Am J Med Genet Neuropsychiatr Genet* 168B: 669–677, 2015b.

Mroczkowski HJ, Arnold G, Schneck FX, Rajkovic A, Yatsenko SA. Interstitial 10p11.23-p12.1 microdeletions associated with developmental delay, craniofacial abnormalities, and cryptorchidism. *Am J Med Genet* 164A: 2623–2626, 2014.

Muhlhauser A, Susiarjo M, Rubio C, et al. Bisphenol A effects on the growing mouse oocyte are influenced by diet. *Biol Reprod* 80: 1066–1071, 2009.

Mulcahy MT, Jenkyn J, Mackellar A. 45,X/47,XYY mosaicism. *J Med Genet* 14: 218–221, 1977.

Mulchandani S, Bhoj EJ, Luo M, et al. Maternal uniparental disomy of chromosome 20: A novel imprinting disorder of growth failure. *Genet Med* 18: 309–315, 2016.

Mules EH, Stamberg J. Reproductive outcomes of paracentric inversion carriers: Report of a liveborn dicentric recombinant and literature review. *Hum Genet* 67: 126–131, 1984.

Mulle JG. The 3q29 deletion confers >40-fold increase in risk for schizophrenia. *Mol Psychiatry* 20: 1028–1029, 2015.

Mullegama SV, Elsea SH. Clinical and molecular aspects of MBD5-associated neurodevelopmental disorder (MAND). *Eur J Hum Genet* 24: 1235–1243, 2016.

Mullegama SV, Rosenfeld JA, Orellana C, et multi al. Reciprocal deletion and duplication at 2q23.1 indicates a role for MBD5 in autism spectrum disorder. *Eur J Hum Genet* 22: 57–63, 2014.

Mullen SA, Carvill GL, Bellows S, et al. Copy number variants are frequent in genetic generalized epilepsy with intellectual disability. *Neurology* 81: 1507–1514, 2013.

Muller EA, Aradhya S, Atkin JF, et al. Microdeletion 9q22.3 syndrome includes metopic craniosynostosis, hydrocephalus, macrosomia, and developmental delay. *Am J Med Genet* 158A: 391–399, 2012.

Muller F, Dreux S, Dupoizat H, et al. Second-trimester Down syndrome maternal serum screening in twin pregnancies: impact of chorionicity. *Prenat Diagn* 23: 331–335, 2003.

Muller F, Rebiffé M, Taillandier A, Oury JF, Mornet E. Parental origin of the extra chromosome in prenatally diagnosed fetal trisomy 21. *Hum Genet* 106: 340–344, 2000.

Müller J, Ritzén EM, Ivarsson SA, Rajpert-De Meyts E, Norjavaara E, Skakkebæk NE. Management of males with 45,X/46,XY gonadal dysgenesis. *Horm Res* 52: 11–14, 1999.

Müller J, Skakkebæk NE. Gonadal malignancy in individuals with sex chromosome anomalies. *Birth Defects Orig Artic Ser* 26: 247–255, 1990.

Mundhofir FE, Smeets D, Nillesen W, et al. Monosomy 9pter and trisomy 9q34.11qter in two sisters due to a maternal pericentric inversion. *Gene* 511: 451–454, 2012.

Munné S. Analysis of chromosome segregation during preimplantation genetic diagnosis in both male and female translocation heterozygotes. *Cytogenet Genome Res* 111: 305–309, 2005.

Munné S, Bahçe M, Schimmel T, Sadowy S, Cohen J. Case report: Chromatid exchange and predivision of chromatids as other sources of abnormal oocytes detected by preimplantation genetic diagnosis of translocations. *Prenat Diagn* 18: 1450–1458, 1998a.

Munné S, Blazek J, Large M, et al. Detailed investigation into the cytogenetic constitution and pregnancy outcome of replacing mosaic blastocysts detected with the use of high-resolution next-generation sequencing. *Fertil Steril*, 108: 62–71.e8 2017.

Munné S, Escudero T, Sandalinas M, Sable D, Cohen J. Gamete segregation in female carriers of Robertsonian translocations. *Cytogenet Cell Genet* 90: 303–308, 2000a.

Munné S, Morrison L, Fung J, et al. Spontaneous abortions are reduced after preconception diagnosis of translocations. *J Assit Reprod Genet* 15: 290–296, 1998.

Munné S, Sandalinas M, Escudero T, Fung J, Gianaroli L, Cohen J. Outcome of preimplantation genetic diagnosis of translocations. *Fertil Steril* 73: 1209–1218, 2000b.

Munné S, Sandalinas M, Escudero T, Marquez C, Cohen J. Chromosome mosaicism in cleavage-stage human embryos: Evidence of a maternal age effect. *Reprod Biomed Online* 4: 223–232, 2002.

Muroya K, Yamamoto K, Fukushima Y, Ogata T. Ring chromosome 21 in a boy and a derivative chromosome 21 in the mother: Implication for ring chromosome formation. *Am J Med Genet* 110: 332–337, 2002.

Murphy EA, Chase GA. *Principles of Genetic Counseling.* Chicago, IL: Year Book, 1975.

Murphy SM, Laura M, Fawcett K, et al. Charcot-Marie-Tooth disease: Frequency of genetic subtypes and guidelines for genetic testing. *J Neurol Neurosurg Psychiatry* 83: 706–710, 2012.

Murray J, Cuckle H, Sehmi I, Wilson C, Ellis A. Quality of written information used in Down syndrome screening. *Prenat Diagn* 21: 138–142, 2001.

Mussa A, Russo S, De Crescenzo A, et al. (Epi) genotype-phenotype correlations in Beckwith-Wiedemann syndrome. *Eur J Hum Genet* 24: 183–190, 2016.

Mutter M, Binkert F, Schinzel A. Down syndrome livebirth rate in the eastern part of Switzerland between 1980 and 1996 stays constant in spite of growing numbers of prenatally diagnosed and subsequently terminated cases. *Prenat Diagn* 22: 835–836, 2002.

Myers KA, Wallis MJ, Fitt GJ, Sarnat HB, Newton MR. Blake's pouch cyst in 13q deletion syndrome: Posterior fossa malformations may occur due to disruption of multiple genes. *Am J Med Genet* 173A: 2442–2445, 2017.

Nadal M, Moreno S, Pritchard M, Preciado MA, Estivill X, Ramos-Arroyo MA. Down syndrome: Characterisation of a case with partial trisomy of chromosome 21 owing to a paternal balanced translocation (15;21) (q26;q22.1) by FISH. *J Med Genet* 34: 50–54, 1997.

Nadal M, Valiente A, Domènech A, Pritchard M, Estivill X, Ramos-Arroyo MA. Hereditary neuropathy with liability to pressure palsies: Two cases with a reciprocal translocation t(16;17) (q12;11.2) interrupting the *PMP22* gene. *J Med Genet* 37: 396–398, 2000.

Nagai T, Shimokawa O, Harada N, et al. Postnatal overgrowth by 15q-trisomy and intrauterine growth retardation by 15q-monosomy due to familial translocation t(13;15): Dosage effect of *IGF1R? Am J Med Genet* 113: 173–177, 2002.

Nagarsheth NP, Mootabar H. Prenatal diagnosis of mosaic tetrasomy 21q confirmed by fluorescence in situ hybridization. *Clin Genet* 51: 260–263, 1997.

Nagle C, Hodges R, Wolfe R, Wallace EM. Reporting Down syndrome screening results: Women's understanding of risk. *Prenat Diagn* 29: 234–239, 2009.

Nahata L, Yu RN, Paltiel HJ, et al. Sperm retrieval in adolescents and young adults with Klinefelter syndrome: A prospective, pilot study. *J Pediatr* 170: 260–265.e1–2, 2016.

Nakamura N. Genetic effects of radiation in atomic-bomb survivors and their children: Past, present and future. *J Radiat Res* 47 (Suppl B): B67–73, 2006.

Nap AW, Van Golde RJ, Tuerlings JH, et al. Reproductive decisions of men with microdeletions of the Y chromosome: The role of genetic counselling. *Hum Reprod* 14: 2166–2169, 1999.

Nardmann J, Tranebjærg L, Horsthemke B, Lüdecke HJ. The tricho-rhino-phalangeal syndromes: Frequency and parental origin of 8q deletions. *Hum Genet* 99: 638–643, 1997.

Natacci F, Alfei E, Tararà L, et al. Chromosome 17q21.31 duplication syndrome: Description of a new familiar case and further delineation of the clinical spectrum. *Eur J Paediatr Neurol* 20: 183–187, 2016.

Natera de Benito D, García-Pérez MA, Martínez-Granero MÁ, Izquierdo-López L. A patient with a duplication of chromosome 3p (p24.1p26.2): A comparison with other partial 3p trisomies. *Am J Med Genet* 164A: 548–550, 2014.

Natesan SA, Bladon AJ, Coskun S, et al. Genome-wide karyomapping accurately identifies the inheritance of single-gene defects in human preimplantation embryos in vitro. *Genet Med* 16: 838–845, 2014.

Natsuga K, Nishie W, Arita K, et al. Complete paternal isodisomy of chromosome 17 in junctional epidermolysis bullosa with pyloric atresia. *J Invest Dermatol* 130: 2671–2674, 2010.

Navarro J, Vidal F, Benet J, Templado C, Marina S, Egozcue J. XY-trivalent association and synaptic anomalies in a male carrier of a Robertsonian t(13;14) translocation. *Hum Reprod* 6: 376–381, 1991.

Neal MS, Cowan L, Louis JP, Hughes E, King WA, Basrur PK. Cytogenetic evaluation of human oocytes that failed to complete meiotic maturation in vitro. *Fertil Steril* 77: 844–845, 2002.

Neas KR, Yip MY, James C, Kirk EPE. Patient with a non-mosaic isodicentric Yp and mild developmental delay. *Am J Med Genet* 137: 223–224, 2005.

Neel JV, Schull WJ. *The Children of Atomic Bomb Survivors: A Genetic Study.* Washington, DC: National Academy Press, 1991.

Neel JV, Schull WJ, Awa AA, et al. The children of parents exposed to atomic bombs: Estimates of the genetic doubling dose of radiation for humans. *Am J Hum Genet* 46: 1053–1072, 1990.

Neiswanger K, Hohler PM, Hively-Thomas LB, McPherson EW, Hogge WA, Surti U. Variable outcomes in mosaic trisomy 16: Five case reports and literature analysis. *Prenat Diagn* 26: 454–461, 2006.

Neitzel H, Neumann LM, Schindler D, et al. Premature chromosome condensation in humans associated with microcephaly and mental retardation: A novel autosomal recessive condition. *Am J Hum Genet* 70: 1015–1022, 2002.

Németh AH, Gallen IW, Crocker M, Levy E, Maher E. Klinefelter-like phenotype and primary infertility in a male with a paracentric Xq inversion. *J Med Genet* 39: E28, 2002.

Neri G. A possible explanation for the low incidence of gonosomal aneuploidy among the offspring of triplo-X individuals. *Am J Med Genet* 18: 357–364, 1984.

Neri G, Opitz JM. Down syndrome: Comments and reflections on the 50th anniversary of Lejeune's discovery. *Am J Med Genet* 149A: 2647–2654, 2009.

Neri G, Romana Di Raimo F. Long time no see: The type and contre-type concept. *Eur J Hum Genet* 18: 135–136, 2010.

Nerlich A, Wisser J, Krone S. Placental findings in "vanishing twins." *Geburtshilfe Frauenheilkd* 52: 230–234, 1992.

Ness GO, Lybæk H, Houge G. Usefulness of high-resolution comparative genomic hybridization (CGH) for detecting and characterizing constitutional chromosome abnormalities. *Am J Med Genet* 113: 125–136, 2002.

Netchine I, Rossignol S, Dufourg MN, et al. 11p15 imprinting center region 1 loss of methylation is a common and specific cause of typical Russell-Silver syndrome: Clinical scoring system and epigenetic-phenotypic correlations. *J Clin Endocrinol Metab* 92: 3148–3154, 2007.

Netley CT. Summary overview of behavioural development in individuals with neonatally identified X and Y aneuploidy. *Birth Defects Orig Artic Ser* 22: 293–306, 1986.

Neu RL, Brar HS, Koos BJ. Prenatal diagnosis of inv(X)(q12q28) in a male fetus. *J Med Genet* 25: 52–53, 1988a.

Neu RL, Kousseff BG, Hardy DE, et al. Trisomy 3p23→pter and monosomy 11q23→qter in an infant with two translocation carrier parents. *J Med Genet* 25: 631–633, 1988b.

Neu RL, Valentine FA, Gardner LI. Segregation of a t(14q22q) chromosome in a large kindred. *Clin Genet* 8: 30–36, 1975.

Neumann AA, Robson LG, Smith A. A 15p+ variant shown to be a t(Y;15) with fluorescence in situ hybridisation. *Ann Génét* 35: 227–230, 1992.

Neusser M, Rogenhofer N, Dürl S, et al. Increased chromosome 16 disomy rates in human spermatozoa and recurrent spontaneous abortions. *Fertil Steril* 104: 1130–7, e1–10, 2015.

Nevado J, de Torres ML, Fernández L, et al. Unusual four-generation chromosome-22 rearrangement: When "normality" masks abnormality. *Am J Med Genet* 149A: 1561–1564, 2009.

Newberg MT, Francisco RG, Pang MG, et al. Cytogenetics of somatic cells and sperm from a 46,XY/45,X mosaic male with moderate oligoasthenoteratozoospermia. *Fertil Steril* 69: 146–148, 1998.

Newbury DF, Mari F, Sadighi Akha E, et al. Dual copy number variants involving 16p11 and 6q22 in a case of childhood apraxia of speech and pervasive developmental disorder. *Eur J Hum Genet* 21: 361–365, 2013.

Ngo AD, Taylor R, Roberts CL, Nguyen TV. Association between Agent Orange and birth defects: Systematic review and meta-analysis. *Int J Epidemiol* 35: 1220–1230, 2006.

Nguyen JM, Qualmann KJ, Okashah R, Reilly A, Alexeyev MF, Campbell DJ. 5p deletions: Current knowledge and future directions. *Am J Med Genet Semin Med Genet* 169C: 224–238, 2015.

Nguyen NMP, Khawajkie Y, Mechtouf N, et al. The genetics of recurrent hydatidiform moles: new insights and lessons from a comprehensive analysis of 113 patients. Submitted, 2017.

Nickerson E, Greenberg F, Keating MT, McCaskill C, Shaffer LG. Deletions of the elastin gene at 7q11.23 occur in approximately 90% of patients with Williams syndrome. *Am J Hum Genet* 56: 1156–1161, 1995.

Nicita F, Di Giacomo M, Palumbo O, et al. Neurological features of 14q24-q32 interstitial deletion: Report of a new case. *Mol Cytogenet* 8: 93, 2015.

Nicolaides K, Brizot Mde L, Patel F, Snijders R. Comparison of chorionic villus sampling and amniocentesis for fetal karyotyping at 10–13 weeks' gestation. *Lancet* 344: 435–439, 1994.

Nicosia SV, Matus-Ridley M, Meadows AT. Gonadal effects of cancer therapy in girls. *Cancer* 55: 2364–2372, 1985.

Nielsen J. Follow-up of 25 unselected children with sex chromosome abnormalities to age 12. *Birth Defects Orig Artic Ser* 26: 201–207, 1990.

Nielsen J, Wohlert M. Chromosome abnormalities found among 34,910 newborn children: Results from a 13-year incidence study in Arhus, Denmark. *Hum Genet* 87: 81–83, 1991.

Nielsen J, Wohlert M, Faaborg-Andersen J, et al. (1986). Chromosome examination of 20,222 newborn children: Results from a 7.5-year study in Århus, Denmark. *Birth Defects Orig Art Series* 22(3), 209–219, 1986.

Nielsen KG, Poulsen H, Mikkelsen M, Steuber E. Multiple recurrence of trisomy 21 Down syndrome. *Hum Genet* 78: 103–105, 1988.

Niemczyk M, Ito Y, Huddleston J, et al. Imprinted chromatin around *DIRAS3* regulates alternative splicing of *GNG12-AS1*, a long noncoding RNA. *Am J Hum Genet* 93: 224–235, 2013.

Niessen RC, Jonkman MF, Muis N, Hordijk R, van Essen AJ. Pigmentary mosaicism following the lines of Blaschko in a girl with a double aneuploidy mosaicism: (47,XX,+7/45,X). *Am J Med Genet* 137A: 313–322, 2005.

Nikolaou D, Templeton A. Early ovarian ageing. *Eur J Obstet Gynecol Reprod Biol* 113: 126–133, 2004.

Nimmakayalu M, Horton VK, Darbro B, et al. Apparent germline mosaicism for a novel 19p13.13 deletion disrupting *NFIX* and *CACNA1A*. *Am J Med Genet* 161A: 1105–1109, 2013.

Nishina-Uchida N, Fukuzawa R, Hasegawa Y, Morison IM. Identification of X monosomy cells from a gonad of mixed gonadal dysgenesis with a 46,XY karyotype: case report. *Medicine (Baltimore)* 94: e720, 2015.

Niu DM, Pan CC, Lin CY, Hwang B, Chung MY. Mosaic or chimera? Revisiting an old hypothesis about the cause of the 46,XX/46,XY hermaphrodite. *J Pediatr* 140: 732–735, 2002.

Nizon M, Andrieux J, Rooryck C, et al. Phenotype-genotype correlations in 17 new patients with an Xp11.23p11.22 microduplication and review of the literature. *Am J Med Genet* 167A: 111–122, 2015.

Nogueira C, Marques JS, Nesti C, et al. Identification of maternal uniparental isodisomy of chromosome 10 in a patient with mitochondrial DNA depletion syndrome. *Mol Genet Metab* 110: 493–494, 2013.

Norman AM, Read AP, Clayton-Smith J, Andrews T, Donnai D. Recurrent Wiedemann-Beckwith syndrome with inversion of chromosome (11) (p11.2p15.5). *Am J Med Genet* 42: 638–641, 1992.

Northrop LE, Treff NR, Levy B, Scott RT. SNP microarray-based 24 chromosome aneuploidy screening demonstrates that cleavage-stage FISH poorly predicts aneuploidy in embryos that develop to morphologically normal blastocysts. *Mol Hum Reprod* 16: 590–600, 2010.

Novara F, Alfei E, D'Arrigo S, et al. 5p13 microduplication syndrome: A new case and better clinical definition of the syndrome. *Eur J Med Genet* 56: 54–58, 2013.

Novara F, Rinaldi B, Sisodiya SM, et al. Haploinsufficiency for *ANKRD11*-flanking genes makes the difference between KBG and 16q24.3 microdeletion syndromes: 12 new cases. *Eur J Hum Genet* 25: 694–701, 2017.

Novara F, Stanzial F, Rossi E, et al. Defining the phenotype associated with microduplication reciprocal to Sotos syndrome microdeletion. *Am J Med Genet* 164A: 2084–2090, 2014.

Nowaczyk MJM, Zeesman S, Kam A, Taylor SAM, Carter RF, Whelan DT. Boy with 47,XXY,del(15) (q11.2q13) karyotype and Prader-Willi syndrome: A new case and review of the literature. *Am J Med Genet* 125A: 73–76, 2004.

Nowakowska BA, de Leeuw N, Ruivenkamp CAL, et al. Parental insertional balanced translocations are an important cause of apparently de novo CNVs in patients with developmental anomalies. *Eur J Hum Genet* 20: 166–170, 2012.

Nucaro AL, Meloni M, Pisano T, et al. Familial translocation t(3;10) (p26.3;p12.31) leading to trisomy 10p12.31→pter and monosomy 3p26.3→pter in seven members. *Am J Med Genet* 146A: 3242–3245, 2008.

Nucaro AL, Rossino R, Pruna D, et al. Prenatal diagnosis of a mosaic supernumerary marker iso (8p) (tetrasomy 8p): discordance between chorionic villi culture and amniotic fluid karyotypes. *Prenat Diagn* 26: 418–419, 2006.

Nusbaum C, Zody MC, Borowsky ML, et al. DNA sequence and analysis of human chromosome 18. *Nature* 437: 551–555, 2005.

Oberman LM, Boccuto L, Cascio L, Sarasua S, Kaufmann WE. Autism spectrum disorder in Phelan-McDermid syndrome: Initial characterization and genotype-phenotype correlations. *Orphanet J Rare Dis* 10: 105, 2015.

Odak L, Barisic I, Morozin Pohovski L, Riegel M, Schinzel A. Novel duplication on chromosome 16 (q12.1-q21) associated with behavioral disorder, mild cognitive impairment, speech delay, and dysmorphic features: Case report. *Croat Med J* 52: 415–422, 2011.

O'Donnell L, Soileau BT, Sebold C, Gelfond J, Hale DE, Cody JD. Tetrasomy 18p: Report of cognitive and behavioral characteristics. *Am J Med Genet* 167A: 1474–1482, 2015.

Oegema R, van Zutven LJCM, van Hassel DACM, Huijbregts GCM, Hoogeboom AJM. Unbalanced three-way chromosomal translocation leading to deletion 18q and duplication 20p. *Eur J Med Genet* 55: 265–268, 2012.

Ogasawara M, Aoki K, Okada S, Suzumori K. Embryonic karyotype of abortuses in relation to the number of previous miscarriages. *Fertil Steril* 73: 300–304, 2000.

Ogata T, Kagami M. Kagami-Ogata syndrome: A clinically recognizable upd(14)pat and related disorder affecting the chromosome 14q32.2 imprinted region. *J Hum Genet* 61: 87–94, 2016.

Ogata T, Matsuo M, Muroya K, Koyama Y, Fukutani K. 47,XXX male: A clinical and molecular study. *Am J Med Genet* 98: 353–356, 2001.

Ogur G, Van Assche E, Vegetti W, et al. Chromosomal segregation in spermatozoa of 14 Robertsonian translocation carriers. *Mol Hum Reprod* 12: 209–215, 2006.

Ohira M, Ichikawa H, Suzuki E, et al. A 1.6-Mb P1-based physical map of the Down syndrome region on chromosome 21. *Genomics* 33: 65–74, 1996.

Ohnesorg T, van den Bergen JA, Belluoccio D, et al. A duplication in a patient with 46,XX ovo-testicular disorder of sex development refines the *SOX9* testis-specific regulatory region to 24 kb. *Clin Genet* 92: 347–349, 2017.

Ohnuki Y, Torii C, Kosaki R, et al. Cri-du-chat syndrome cytogenetically cryptic recombination aneusomy of chromosome 5: Implications in recurrence risk estimation. *Mol Syndromol* 1: 95–98, 2010.

Ohtsuka Y, Higashimoto K, Sasaki K, et al. Autosomal recessive cystinuria caused by genome-wide paternal uniparental isodisomy in a patient with Beckwith-Wiedemann syndrome. *Clin Genet* 88: 261–266, 2015.

Ohye T, Inagaki H, Kogo H, et al. Paternal origin of the de novo constitutional t(11;22)(q23;q11). *Eur J Hum Genet* 18: 783–787, 2010.

Õiglane-Shlik E, Puusepp S, Talvik I, et al. Monosomy 1p36—A multifaceted and still enigmatic syndrome: Four clinically diverse cases with shared white matter abnormalities. *Eur J Paediatr Neurol* 18: 338–346, 2014.

Okamoto N, Fujii T, Tanaka J, Saito K, Matsui T, Harada N. A clinical study of patients with pericentromeric deletion and duplication within

16p12.2-p11.2. *Am J Med Genet* 164A: 213–219, 2014.

Okamoto N, Kubota T, Nakamura Y, et al. 22q13 Microduplication in two patients with common clinical manifestations: A recognizable syndrome? *Am J Med Genet* 143A: 2804–2809, 2007.

Oktay K, Bedoschi G, Berkowitz K, et al. Fertility preservation in women with Turner syndrome: A comprehensive review and practical guidelines. *J Pediatr Adolesc Gynecol* 29: 409–416, 2016.

Okumura A, Ishii A, Shimojima K, et al. Phenotypes of children with 20q13.3 microdeletion affecting *KCNQ2* and *CHRNA4*. *Epileptic Disord* 17: 165–171, 2015.

Okun N, Summers AM, Hoffman B, et al. Prospective experience with integrated prenatal screening and first trimester combined screening for trisomy 21 in a large Canadian urban center. *Prenat Diagn* 28: 987–992, 2008.

Olander E, Stamberg J, Steinberg L, Wulfsberg EA. Third Prader-Willi syndrome phenotype due to maternal uniparental disomy 15 with mosaic trisomy 15. *Am J Med Genet* 93: 215–218, 2000.

Oliver-Bonet M, Benet J, Sun F, et al. Meiotic studies in two human reciprocal translocations and their association with spermatogenic failure. *Hum Reprod* 20: 683–688, 2005.

Oliver-Bonet M, Navarro J, Codina-Pascual M, et al. From spermatocytes to sperm: Meiotic behaviour of human male reciprocal translocations. *Hum Reprod* 19: 2515–2522, 2004.

Olshan AF, Baird PA, Teschke K. Paternal occupational exposures and the risk of Down syndrome. *Am J Hum Genet* 44: 646–651, 1989.

Onesimo R, Orteschi D, Scalzone M, et al. Chromosome 9p deletion syndrome and sex reversal: Novel findings and redefinition of the critically deleted regions. *Am J Med Genet* 158A: 2266–2271, 2012.

Ono T, Okuma M, Hamada T, Motohashi N, Moriyama K. A case of ring chromosome 18 syndrome treated with a combined orthodontic-prosthodontic approach. *Cleft Palate Craniofac J* 47: 201–210, 2010.

Opheim KE, Brittingham A, Chapman D, Norwood TH. Balanced reciprocal translocation mosaicism: How frequent? *Am J Med Genet* 57: 601–604, 1995.

Oracova E, Musilova P, Kopecna O, et al. Sperm and embryo analysis in a carrier of supernumerary inv dup(15) marker chromosome. *J Androl* 30: 233–239, 2009.

Ordulu Z, Kammin T, Brand H, et al. Structural chromosomal rearrangements require nucleotide-level resolution: Lessons from next-generation sequencing in prenatal diagnosis. *Am J Hum Genet* 99: 1015–1033, 2016.

Orellana C, Bernabeu J, Monfort S, et al. Duplication of the Williams-Beuren critical region: case report and further delineation of the phenotypic spectrum. *J Med Genet* 45: 187–189, 2008.

Oromendia AB, Amon A. Aneuploidy: Implications for protein homeostasis and disease. *Dis Model Mech* 7: 15–20, 2014.

Ortenberg J, Oddoux C, Craver R, et al. *SRY* gene expression in the ovotestes of XX true hermaphrodites. *J Urol* 167: 1828–1831, 2002.

Osborne CM, Hardisty E, Devers P, et al. Discordant noninvasive prenatal testing results in a patient subsequently diagnosed with metastatic disease. *Prenat Diagn* 33: 609–611, 2013.

Otake K, Uchida K, Inoue M, et al. Congenital diaphragmatic hernia with a pure duplication of chromosome 1q: Report of the first surviving case. *Pediatr Surg Int* 25: 827–831, 2009.

Otani T, Roche M, Mizuike M, Colls P, Escudero T, Munné S. Preimplantation genetic diagnosis significantly improves the pregnancy outcome of translocation carriers with a history of recurrent miscarriage and unsuccessful pregnancies. *Reprod Biomed Online* 13: 869–874, 2006.

Ottaviani V, Bartocci A, Pantaleo M, et al. Myoclonic astatic epilepsy in a patient with a de novo 4q21.22q21.23 microduplication. *Genet Couns* 26: 327–332, 2015.

Otter M, Schrander-Stumpel CTRM, Curfs LMG. Triple X syndrome: A review of the literature. *Eur J Hum Genet* 18: 265–271, 2010.

Ottolini CS, Newnham LJ, Capalbo A, et al. Genome-wide maps of recombination and chromosome segregation in human oocytes and embryos show selection for maternal recombination rates. *Nat Genet* 47: 727–735, 2015.

Ou Z, Martin DM, Bedoyan JK, et al. Branchiootorenal syndrome and oculoauriculovertebral spectrum features associated with duplication of *SIX1*, *SIX6*, and *OTX2* resulting from a complex chromosomal rearrangement. *Am J Med Genet* 146A: 2480–2489, 2008.

Ouldim K, Sbiti A, Natiq A, El-Kerch F, Cherkaoui S, Sefiani A. Unexpected fertility and paternal UPD 22. *Fertil Steril* 90: 2013, e13–15, 2008.

Owen JP, Chang YS, Pojman NJ, et al. Aberrant white matter microstructure in children with 16p11.2 deletions. *J Neurosci* 34: 6214–6223, 2014.

Oyarzabal A, Martínez-Pardo M, Merinero B, et al. A novel regulatory defect in the branched-chain a-keto acid dehydrogenase complex due to a mutation in the *PPM1K* gene causes a mild variant phenotype of maple syrup urine disease. *Hum Mutat* 34: 355–362, 2013.

Ozawa N, Maruyama T, Nagashima T, et al. Pregnancy outcomes of reciprocal translocation carriers who have a history of repeated pregnancy loss. *Fertil Steril* 90: 1301–1304, 2008.

Paciorkowski AR, Keppler-Noreuil K, Robinson L, et al. Deletion 16p13.11 uncovers *NDE1* mutations on the non-deleted homolog and extends the spectrum of severe microcephaly to include fetal brain disruption. *Am J Med Genet* 161A: 1523–1530, 2013.

Pai GS, Shields SM, Houser PM. Segregation of inverted chromosome 13 in families ascertained through liveborn recombinant offspring. *Am J Med Genet* 27: 127–133, 1987.

Pal CV, Eble TN, Burnside RD, Bi W, Patel A, Franco LM. Variable levels of tissue mosaicism can confound the interpretation of chromosomal microarray results from peripheral blood. *Eur J Med Genet* 57: 264–266, 2014.

Palermo GD, Colombero LT, Hariprashad JJ, Schlegel PN, Rosenwaks Z. Chromosome analysis of epididymal and testicular sperm in azoospermic patients undergoing ICSI. *Hum Reprod* 17: 570–575, 2002.

Palka G, Calabrese G, Stuppia L, et al. A woman with an apparent non-mosaic 45,X delivered a 46,X,der(X) liveborn female. *Clin Genet* 45: 93–96, 1994.

Palumbo O, Mattina T, Palumbo P, Carella M, Perrotta CS. A de novo 11p13 microduplication in a patient with some features Invoking Silver-Russell syndrome. *Mol Syndromol* 5: 11–18, 2014.

Palumbo O, Palumbo P, Delvecchio M, et al. Microdeletion of 12q24.31: Report of a girl with intellectual disability, stereotypies, seizures and facial dysmorphisms. *Am J Med Genet* 167A: 438–444, 2015a.

Palumbo O, Palumbo P, Stallone R, Palladino T, Zelante L, Carella M. 8q12.1q12.3 de novo microdeletion involving the *CHD7* gene in a patient without the major features of CHARGE syndrome: Case report and critical review of the literature. *Gene* 513: 209–13, 2013.

Palumbo P, Palumbo O, Leone MP, et al. Maternal uniparental isodisomy (iUPD) of chromosome 4 in a subject with mild intellectual disability and speech delay. *Am J Med Genet* 167A: 2219–2222, 2015b.

Panasiuk B, Danik J, Lurie IW, et al. Reciprocal chromosome translocations involving short arm of chromosome 9 as a risk factor of unfavorable pregnancy outcomes after meiotic malsegregation 2:2. *Adv Med Sci* 54: 203–210, 2009.

Panasiuk B, Leśniewicz R, Spółczyńska A, et al. Translocation form of Wolf-Hirschhorn syndrome—Assessment of recurrence rate probability. *Adv Med Sci* 52 (Suppl 1): 166–170, 2007.

Panasiuk B, Ušinskiené R, Kostyk E, et al. Genetic counselling in carriers of reciprocal chromosomal translocations involving short arm of chromosome X. *Ann Génét* 47: 11–28, 2004.

Pang MG, Hoegerman SF, Cuticchia AJ, et al. Detection of aneuploidy for chromosomes 4, 6, 7, 8, 9, 10, 11, 12, 13, 17, 18, 21, X and Y by fluorescence in-situ hybridization in spermatozoa from nine patients with oligoasthenoteratozoospermia undergoing intracytoplasmic sperm injection. *Hum Reprod* 14: 1266–1273, 1999.

Pangalos C, Théophile D, Sinet PM, et al. No significant effect of monosomy for distal 21q22.3 on the Down syndrome phenotype in "mirror" duplications of chromosome 21. *Am J Hum Genet* 51: 1240–1250, 1992a.

Pangalos CG, Talbot CC, Lewis JG, et al. DNA polymorphism analysis in families with recurrence of free trisomy 21. *Am J Hum Genet* 51: 1015–1027, 1992b.

Paoloni-Giacobino A, Dahoun SP, Sizonenko PC, Stalberg A, Chardonnens D, Campana A. A case of 45,X Turner syndrome with spontaneous ovulation proven by ultrasonography. *Gynecol Endocrinol* 14: 105–110, 2000a.

Paoloni-Giacobino A, Kern I, Rumpler Y, Djlelati R, Morris MA, Dahoun SP. Familial t(6;21) (p21.1;p13) translocation associated with male-only sterility. *Clin Genet* 58: 324–328, 2000b.

Papanikolaou EG, Vernaeve V, Kolibianakis E, et al. Is chromosome analysis mandatory in the initial investigation of normovulatory women seeking infertility treatment? *Hum Reprod* 20: 2899–2903, 2005.

Papavassiliou P, Charalsawadi C, Rafferty K, Jackson-Cook C. Mosaicism for trisomy 21: A review. *Am J Med Genet* 167A: 26–39, 2015.

Papenhausen P, Schwartz S, Risheg H, et al. UPD detection using homozygosity profiling with a SNP genotyping microarray. *Am J Med Genet* 155A: 757–768, 2011.

Papoulidis I, Manolakos E, Siomou E, et al. A fetus with ring chromosome 21 characterized by aCGH shows no clinical findings after birth. *Prenat Diagn* 30: 586–588, 2010.

Papoulidis I, Vetro A, Kefalas K, et al. De novo 15.5-Mb interstitial deletion in 5p in a male ascertained by oligospermia. *Mol Syndromol* 4: 250–254, 2013.

Pardo Vargas RA, Aracena M, Aravena T, et al. Congenital anomalies of poor prognosis: Genetics Consensus Committee. *Rev Chil Pediatr* 87: 422–431, 2016.

Parente DJ, Garriga C, Baskin B, et al. Neuroligin 2 nonsense variant associated with anxiety, autism, intellectual disability, hyperphagia, and obesity. *Am J Med Genet* 173A: 213–216, 2017.

Pareyson D, Testa D, Morbin M, et al. Does CMT1A homozygosity cause more severe disease with root hypertrophy and higher CSF proteins? *Neurology* 60: 1721–1722, 2003.

Park J, Chung KC. New perspectives of Dyrk1A role in neurogenesis and neuropathologic features of Down syndrome. *Exp Neurobiol* 22: 244–248, 2013.

Park JP, Moeschler JB, Hani VH, et al. Maternal disomy and Prader-Willi syndrome consistent with gamete complementation in a case of familial translocation (3;15) (p25;q11.2). *Am J Med Genet* 78: 134–139, 1998.

Park SS, Stankiewicz P, Bi W, et al. Structure and evolution of the Smith-Magenis syndrome repeat gene clusters, SMS-REPs. *Genome Res* 12: 729–738, 2002.

Parker EA, Hovanes K, Germak J, Porter F, Merke DP. Maternal 21-hydroxylase deficiency and uniparental isodisomy of chromosome 6 and X results in a child with 21-hydroxylase deficiency and Klinefelter syndrome. *Am J Med Genet* 140: 2236–2240, 2006.

Parma P, Radi O, Vidal V, et al. R-spondin1 is essential in sex determination, skin differentiation and malignancy. *Nat Genet* 38: 1304–1309, 2006.

Parmar RC, Muranjan MN, Kotvaliwale S, Sharma S, Bharucha BA. Ring chromosome 12 with variable phenotypic features: Clinical report and review of the literature. *Am J Med Genet* 117A: 275–277, 2003.

Parrott A, James J, Goldenberg P, et al. Aortopathy in the 7q11.23 microduplication syndrome. *Am J Med Genet* 167A: 363–370; 2015.

Paskulin GA, Riegel M, Machado Rosa RF, Graziadio C, Gazzola Zen PR. Interstitial deletion of 7q31.32→q33 secondary to a paracentric inversion of a maternal chromosome 7. *Eur J Med Genet* 54: 181–185, 2011.

Pasquier L, Fradin M, Chérot E, et al. Karyotype is not dead (yet)! *Eur J Med Genet* 59: 11–15, 2016.

Pasquini L, Tondi F, Pontello V, Filippeschi M. First trimester diagnosis of hypotriploidy (68,XX) with elevated fetal head to trunk volume ratio and small placental volume. *Prenat Diagn* 30: 589–590, 2010.

Pasquino AM, Passeri F, Pucarelli I, Segni M, Municchi G. Spontaneous pubertal development in Turner's syndrome: Italian Study Group for Turner's Syndrome. *J Clin Endocrinol Metab* 82: 1810–1813, 1997.

Passarge E. Emil Heitz and the concept of heterochromatin: Longitudinal chromosome differentiation was recognized fifty years ago. *Am J Hum Genet* 31: 106–115, 1979.

Patel ZM, Madon P. Interchange trisomy 22 in a live born resulting from 3:1 segregation in a t(15;22) (p12;q13) carrier mother. *Indian J Pediatr* 71: 1042, 2004.

Patwardhan AJ, Brown WE, Bender BG, Linden MG, Eliez S, Reiss AL. Reduced size of the amygdala in individuals with 47,XXY and 47,XXX karyotypes. *Am J Med Genet* 114: 93–98, 2002.

Pauli RM, Pagon RA, Hall JG. Trisomy 18 in sibs and maternal chromosome 9 variant. *Birth Defects Orig Artic Ser* 14: 297–301, 1978.

Pavlidis K, McCauley E, Sybert VP. Psychosocial and sexual functioning in women with Turner syndrome. *Clin Genet* 47: 85–89, 1995.

Pavone P, Praticò AD, Falsaperla R, et al. A girl with a 14.7 Mb 3q26.32-q28 duplication: A new report of 3q duplication syndrome and a literature review. *Clin Dysmorphol* 25: 121–127, 2016.

Pazooki M, Lebbar A, Roubergues A, Baverel F, Letessier D, Dupont JM. Pure familial 6q21q22.1 duplication in two generations. *Eur J Med Genet* 50: 60–65, 2007.

Pearlman A, Loke J, Le Caignec C, et al. Mutations in *MAP3K1* cause 46,XY disorders of sex development and implicate a common signal transduction pathway in human testis determination. *Am J Hum Genet* 87: 898–904, 2010.

Pebrel-Richard C, Debost-Legrand A, Eymard-Pierre E, et al. An unusual clinical severity of 16p11.2 deletion syndrome caused by unmasked recessive mutation of *CLN3*. *Eur J Hum Genet* 22: 369–373, 2014.

Peddibhotla S, Khalifa M, Probst FJ, et al. Expanding the genotype-phenotype correlation in subtelomeric 19p13.3 microdeletions using high resolution clinical chromosomal microarray analysis. *Am J Med Genet* 161A: 2953–2963, 2013.

Peitsidis P, Manolakos E, Peitsidou A, et al. Pentasomy 49,XXXXY diagnosed in utero: Case report and systematic review of antenatal findings. *Fetal Diagn Ther* 26: 1–5, 2009.

Pelias MZ, Shaw MW. Torts of wrongful birth and wrongful life: A review. *Am J Medi Genet* 25: 71–80, 1986.

Pellestor F, Andréo B, Anahory T, Hamamah S. The occurrence of aneuploidy in human: Lessons from the cytogenetic studies of human oocytes. *Eur J Med Genet* 49: 103–116, 2006.

Pellestor F, Imbert I, Andréo B, Lefort G. Study of the occurrence of interchromosomal effect in spermatozoa of chromosomal rearrangement carriers by fluorescence in-situ hybridization and primed in-situ labelling techniques. *Hum Reprod* 16: 1155–1164, 2001.

Pellestor F, Puechberty J, Weise A, et al. Meiotic segregation of complex reciprocal translocations: Direct analysis of the spermatozoa of a t(5;13;14) carrier. *Fertil Steril* 95: 2433, e17–22, 2011.

Pellicer A, Rubio C, Vidal F, et al. In vitro fertilization plus preimplantation genetic diagnosis in patients with recurrent miscarriage: An analysis of chromosome abnormalities in human preimplantation embryos. *Fertil Steril* 71: 1033–1039, 1999.

Penacho V, Galán F, Martín-Bayón TA, et al. Prenatal diagnosis of a female fetus with ring chromosome 9, 46,XX,r(9)(p24q34), and a de novo interstitial 9p deletion. *Cytogenet Genome* 144: 275–279, 2014.

Penrose LS. The relative effects of paternal and maternal age in mongolism. *J Genet* 27: 219–224, 1933.

Penrose LS. The relative aetiological importance of birth order and maternal age in mongolism. *Proc Roy Soc B* 115: 431–450, 1934.

Penrose LS. Some notes on heredity counseling. *Acta Genet Stat Med* 6: 35–40, 1956.

Perche O, Haddad G, Menuet A, et al. Dysregulation of *FOXG1* pathway in a 14q12 microdeletion case. *Am J Med Genet* 161A: 3072–3077, 2013.

Pergament E. By 2020 … *Prenat Diagn* 30: 710–711, 2010.

Pergament E, Confino E, Zhang JX, Roscetti L, Xien Chen P, Wellman D. Recurrent triploidy of maternal origin. *Prenat Diagn* 20: 561–563, 2000.

Periquito I, Carrusca C, Morgado J, Robalo B, Pereira C, de Lurdes Sampaio M. Familial Turner syndrome: The importance of information. *J Pediatr Endocrinol Metab* 29: 617–620, 2016.

Perrin A, Douet-Guilbert N, Le Bris MJ, et al. Segregation of chromosomes in sperm of a t(X;18)(q11;p11.1) carrier inherited from his mother: Case report. *Hum Reprod* 23: 227–230, 2008.

Perrin A, Douet-Guilbert N, Le Bris MJ, et al. Increased aneuploidy rates in spermatozoa of a male carrier of a trisomy 18 mosaicism. *Int J Androl* 32: 231–234, 2009a.

Perrin A, Vialard F, Douet-Guilbert N, et al. Meiotic segregation of X-autosome translocation in two carriers and implications for assisted reproduction. *Reprod Biomed Online* 18: 850–855, 2009b.

Perry J, Slater HR, Choo KHA. Centric fission—Simple and complex mechanisms. *Chromosome Res* 12: 627–640, 2004.

Perry J, White SM, Nouri S, et al. Unstable Robertsonian translocations der(13;15)(q10;q10): Heritable chromosome fission without phenotypic effect in two kindreds. *Am J Med Genet* 136: 25–30, 2005.

Perry MJ. Effects of environmental and occupational pesticide exposure on human sperm: A systematic review. *Hum Reprod Update* 14: 233–242, 2008.

Persutte WH, Lenke RR. Failure of amniotic-fluid-cell growth: Is it related to fetal aneuploidy? *Lancet* 345: 96–97, 1995.

Pertile MD, Halks-Miller M, Flowers N, et al. Rare autosomal trisomies, revealed by maternal plasma DNA sequencing, suggest increased risk of feto-placental disease. *Sci Transl Med* 9:1240, 2017.

Pertile MD, Ryan JT, Kelley JL, Webber LM. Prenatal diagnosis of tetrasomy 9p. *Bull Hum Genet Soc Australasia* 9: 43, 1996.

Pescucci C, Caselli R, Grosso S, et al. 2q24-q31 deletion: Report of a case and review of the literature. *Eur J Med Genet* 50: 21–32, 2007.

Peter B, Lancaster H, Vose C, Fares A, Schrauwen I, Huentelman M. Two unrelated children with overlapping 6q25.3 deletions, motor speech disorders, and language delays. *Am J Med Genet* 173A: 2659–2669, 2017.

Petersen MB, Adelsberger PA, Schinzel AA, Binkert F, Hinkel GK, Antonarakis SE. Down syndrome due to de novo Robertsonian translocation t(14q;21q): DNA polymorphism analysis suggests that the origin of the extra 21q is maternal. *Am J Hum Genet* 49: 529–536, 1991.

Petersen OB, Vogel I, Ekelund C, et al. Potential diagnostic consequences of applying non-invasive prenatal testing: Population-based study from a country with existing first-trimester screening. *Ultrasound Obstet Gynecol* 43: 265–271. 2014.

Petignat P, Billieux MH, Blouin JL, Dahoun S, Vassilakos P. Is genetic analysis useful in the routine management of hydatidiform mole? *Hum Reprod* 18: 243–249, 2003.

Petit F, Holder-Espinasse M, Duban-Bedu B, et al. Trisomy 7 mosaicism prenatally misdiagnosed and maternal uniparental disomy in a child with pigmentary mosaicism and Russell-Silver syndrome. *Clin Genet* 81: 265–271, 2012.

Petković I, de Capoa A, Giancotti P, Barišić I. Unusual segregation of t(11;22) resulting from crossing-over followed by 3:1 disjunction at meiosis I. *Clin Genet* 50: 515–519, 1996.

Petrova E, Neuner C, Haaf T, et al. A boy with an LCR3/4-flanked 10q22.3q23.2 microdeletion and uncommon phenotypic features. *Mol Syndromol* 5: 19–24, 2014.

Pettenati MJ, Rao PN, Phelan MC, et al. Paracentric inversions in humans: A review of 446 paracentric inversions with presentation of 120 new cases. *Am J Med Genet* 55: 171–187, 1995.

Pettenati MJ, Rao PN, Weaver RG, Thomas IT, McMahan MR. Inversion (X)(p11.4q22) associated with Norrie disease in a four generation family. *Am J Med Genet* 45: 577–580, 1993.

Pettenati MJ, Von Kap-Herr C, Jackle B, et al. Rapid interphase analysis for prenatal diagnosis of translocation carriers using subtelomeric probes. *Prenat Diagn* 22: 193–197, 2002.

Pettenati MJ, Wheeler M, Bartlett DJ, et al. 45,X/47,XYY mosaicism: Clinical discrepancy between prenatally and postnatally diagnosed cases. *Am J Med Genet* 39: 42–47, 1991.

Pfeiffer RA, Loidl J. Mirror image duplications of chromosome 21: Three new cases and discussion of the mechanisms of origin. *Hum Genet* 62: 361–363, 1982.

Pflueger S, Golden J, Troiano R, Gasparini R, Marini T. Fission of familial (13;22) Robertsonian translocation resulting in fetal mosaicism. *Am J Hum Genet* 49: 283, 1991.

Phelan K, Boccuto L, Rogers RC, Sarasua SM, McDermid HE. Letter to the editor regarding Disciglio et al.: Interstitial 22q13 deletions not involving *SHANK3* gene: A new contiguous gene syndrome. *Am J Med Genet* 167A: 1679–1680, 2015.

Phelan MC. Additional studies warranted to confirm monosomy 21. *Prenat Diagn* 22: 160–161, 2002.

Phelan MC, Crawford EC, Bealer DM. Mental retardation in South Carolina III: Chromosome aberrations. *Proc Greenwood Genet Center* 15: 45–60, 1996.

Phelan MC, Rogers RC, Stevenson RE. Multiple, compound, and complex chromosome rearrangements. *Proc Greenwood Genet Center* 9: 19–37, 1990.

Phelan MC, Stevenson RE, Anderson EV, Jr. Recombinant chromosome 9 possibly derived from breakage and reunion of sister chromatids within a paracentric inversion loop. *Am J Med Genet* 46: 304–308, 1993.

Philibert P, Leprieur E, Zenaty D, et al. Steroidogenic factor-1 (SF-1) gene mutation as a frequent cause of primary amenorrhea in 46,XY female adolescents with low testosterone concentration. *Reprod Biol Endocrinol* 8: 28, 2010.

Philipp T, Philipp K, Reiner A, Beer F, Kalousek DK. Embryoscopic and cytogenetic analysis of 233 missed abortions: Factors involved in the pathogenesis of developmental defects of early failed pregnancies. *Hum Reprod* 18: 1724–1732, 2003.

Piard J, Mignot B, Arbez-Gindre F, et al. Severe sex differentiation disorder in a boy with a 3.8 Mb 10q25.3-q26.12 microdeletion encompassing *EMX2*. *Am J Med Genet* 164A: 2618–2622, 2014.

Piccione M, Antona V, Antona R, et al. Array-CGH defined chromosome 1p duplication in a patient with autism spectrum disorder, mild mental deficiency, and minor dysmorphic features. *Am J Med Genet* 152A: 486–489, 2010.

Piccione M, Serra G, Consiglio V, et al. 14q13.1-21.1 deletion encompassing the *HPE8* locus in an adolescent with intellectual disability and bilateral microphthalmia, but without holoprosencephaly. *Am J Med Genet* 158A: 1427–1433, 2012.

Pietrzak J, Mrasek K, Oberszytn E, et al. Molecular cytogenetic characterization of eight small supernumerary marker chromosomes originating from chromosomes 2, 4, 8, 18, and 21 in three patients. *J Appl Genet* 48: 167–175, 2007.

Pilling S, Baron-Cohen S, Megnin-Viggars O, Lee R, Taylor C; Guideline Development Group. Recognition, referral, diagnosis, and management of adults with autism: summary of NICE guidance. *BMJ* 344:e4082, 2012.

Pinho MJ, Neves R, Costa P, et al. Unique t(Y;1) (q12;q12) reciprocal translocation with loss of the heterochromatic region of chromosome 1 in a male with azoospermia due to meiotic arrest: A case report. *Hum Reprod* 20: 689–696, 2005.

Pinto MR, Fonseca e Silva ML, Aguiar J, Quelhas I, Lima MR. Supernumerary ring chromosome 20 in a mother and her child. *Am J Med Genet* 133A: 193–196, 2005.

Pinto Leite R, Pinto M. Prenatal detection of an inverted X chromosome in a male fetus. *Prenat Diagn* 21: 233, 2001.

Pipiras E, Dupont C, Chantot-Bastaraud S, et al. Structural chromosomal mosaicism and prenatal diagnosis. *Prenat Diagn* 24: 101–103, 2004.

Pirollo LM, Salehi LB, Sarta S, et al. A new case of prenatally diagnosed pentasomy X: Review of the literature. *Case Rep Obstet Gynecol* 2015: 935202, 2015.

Pivnick EK, Wilroy RS, Summitt JB, Tucker B, Herrod HG, Tharapel AT. Adjacent-2 disjunction of a maternal t(9;22) leading to duplication 9pter→q22 and deficiency of 22pter→q11.2. *Am J Med Genet* 37: 92–96, 1990.

Pizzo L, Andrieux J, Amor DJ, Girirajan S. Clinical utility gene card for: 16p12.2 microdeletion. *Eur J Hum Genet* 25: 2017.

Plaisancié J, Bouneau L, Cances C, et al. Distal 10q monosomy: New evidence for a neurobehavioral condition? *Eur J Med Genet* 57: 47–53, 2014.

Plaja A, Lloveras E, Martinez-Bouzas C, et al. Trisomy 18p caused by a supernumerary marker with a chromosome 13/21 centromere: A possible recurrent chromosome aberration. *Am J Med Genet* 161A: 2363–2368, 2013.

Plaja A, Mediano C, Cano L, et al. Prenatal diagnosis of a rare chromosomal instability syndrome: Variegated aneuploidy related to premature centromere division (PCD). *Am J Med Genet* 117A: 85–86, 2003.

Plotton I, Giscard d'Estaing S, Cuzin B, et al. Preliminary results of a prospective study of testicular sperm extraction in young versus adult patients with nonmosaic 47,XXY Klinefelter syndrome. *J Clin Endocrinol Metab* 100: 961–967, 2015.

Pober BR. Williams-Beuren syndrome. *N Engl J Med* 362: 239–252, 2010.

Podolska A, Kobelt A, Fuchs S, et al. Functional monosomy of 6q27-qter and functional disomy of Xpter-p22.11 due to X;6 translocation with an atypical X-inactivation pattern. *Am J Med Genet* 173A: 1334–1341, 2017.

Poirsier C, Landais E, Bednarek N, et al. Report on 3 patients with 12p duplication including *GRIN2B*. *Eur J Med Genet* 57: 185–194, 2014.

Pollin TI, Dobyns WB, Crowe CA, Ledbetter DH, Bailey-Wilson JE, Smith AC. Risk of abnormal pregnancy outcome in carriers of balanced reciprocal translocations involving the Miller-Dieker syndrome (MDS) critical region in chromosome 17p13.3. *Am J Med Genet* 85: 369–375, 1999.

Poot M. Beware of hemizygous deletions that may unmask deleterious variants. *Mol Syndromol* 3: 45–46, 2012.

Poot M, Haaf T. Mechanisms of origin, phenotypic effects and diagnostic Implications of complex chromosome rearrangements. *Mol Syndromol* 6: 110–134, 2015.

Popovici C, Busa T, Boute O, et al. Whole *ARX* gene duplication is compatible with normal intellectual development. *Am J Med Genet* 164A: 2324–2327, 2014.

Portnoï MF. Microduplication 22q11.2: A new chromosomal syndrome. *Eur J Med Genet* 52: 88–93, 2009.

Portnoï MF, Chantot-Bastaraud S, Christin-Maitre S, et al. Familial Turner syndrome with an X;Y translocation mosaicism: Implications for genetic counseling. *Eur J Med Genet* 55: 635–640, 2012.

Posmyk R, Lesniewicz R, Gogiel M, et al. The smallest de novo deletion of 20q11.21-q11.23 in a girl with feeding problems, retinal dysplasia, and skeletal abnormalities. *Am J Med Genet* 164A: 1056–1061, 2014.

Potocki L, Bi W, Treadwell-Deering D, et al. Characterization of Potocki-Lupski syndrome (dup(17)(p11.2p11.2)) and delineation of a dosage-sensitive critical interval that can convey an autism phenotype. *Am J Hum Genet* 80: 633–649, 2007.

Potocki L, Chen KS, Park SS, et al. Molecular mechanism for duplication 17p11.2—The homologous recombination reciprocal of the Smith-Magenis microdeletion. *Nat Genet* 24: 84–87, 2000.

Potok O, Schlade-Bartusiak K, Perrier R, et al. Paternal uniparental isodisomy for chromosome 14 in a child with normal karyotype, resulting from malsegregation of maternal Robertsonian translocation. *Eur J Hum Genet* 17 (Supp 2): P03.147, 2009.

Póvoa A, Ramalho C, Torgal A, et al. Positive biochemical screening for trisomy 18: On the path of trisomy 9. *Prenat Diagn* 28: 162–164, 2008.

Pradhan M, Dalal A, Khan F, Agrawal S. Fertility in men with Down syndrome: A case report. *Fertil Steril* 86: 1765, e1–3, 2006.

Prasad C, Wagstaff J. Genotype and phenotype in Angelman syndrome caused by paternal UPD 15. *Am J Med Genet* 70: 328–329, 1997.

Preis S, Majewski F. Monozygotic twins concordant for Rubinstein-Taybi syndrome: Changing phenotype during infancy. *Clin Genet* 48: 72–75, 1995.

Price HA, Roberts SH, Laurence KM. Homozygous paracentric inversion 12 in a mentally retarded boy: A case report and review of the literature. *Hum Genet* 75: 101–108, 1987.

Price N, Bahra M, Griffin D, Hanna G, Stock A. Cornelia de Lange Syndrome in association with a balanced reciprocal translocation involving chromosomes 3 and 5. *Prenat Diagn* 25: 602–603, 2005.

Priola V, De Vivo A, Imbesi G, Azzerboni A, Triolo O. Trisomy 9 associated with maternal serum screening results positive for trisomy 18: Case report and review of the literature. *Prenat Diagn* 27: 1167–1169, 2007.

Pritchard MA, Kola I. The "gene dosage effect" hypothesis versus the "amplified developmental instability" hypothesis in Down syndrome. *J Neural Transm Suppl* 57: 293–303, 1999.

Probst FJ, James RA, Burrage LC, et al. De novo deletions and duplications of 17q25.3 cause susceptibility to cardiovascular malformations. *Orphanet J Rare Dis* 10: 75, 2015.

Prontera P, Buldrini B, Aiello V, et al. Trisomy 15 mosaicism owing to familial reciprocal translocation t(1;15): Implication for prenatal diagnosis. *Prenat Diagn* 26: 571–576, 2006.

Prontera P, Ottaviani V, Isidori I, Stangoni G, Donti E. Xq12-q13.3 duplication: Evidence of a recurrent syndrome. *Ann Neurol* 72: 821–822, 2012.

Prontera P, Stangoni G, Ardisia C, Rogaia D, Mencarelli A, Donti E. Trisomy 2 mosaicism with caudal dysgenesis, Hirschsprung disease, and micro-anophthalmia. *Am J Med Genet* 155A: 928–930, 2011.

Puck MH. Some considerations bearing on the doctrine of self-fulfilling prophecy in sex chromosome aneuploidy. *Am J Med Genet* 9: 129–137, 1981.

Punnett A, Teshima I, Heon E, et al. Unique insertional translocation in a childhood Wilms' tumor survivor detected when his daughter developed bilateral retinoblastoma. *Am J Med Genet* 120A: 105–109, 2003.

Purandare SM, Lee J, Hassed S, et al. Ring chromosome 9 [r(9)(p24q34)]: A report of two cases. *Am J Med Genet* 138A: 229–235, 2005.

Purvis-Smith SG, Saville T, Manass S, et al. Uniparental disomy 15 resulting from "correction" of an initial trisomy 15. *Am J Hum Genet* 50: 1348–1350, 1992.

Putoux A, Labalme A, André JM, et al. Jacobsen and Beckwith-Wiedemann syndromes in a child with mosaicism for partial 11pter trisomy and partial 11qter monosomy. *Am J Med Genet* 161A: 331–337, 2013.

Puvabanditsin S, Garrow E, Razi S, et al. A Y/15 translocation in a 45,X male with Prader-Willi syndrome. *Genet Couns* 18: 417–421, 2007.

Qi Z, Jeng LJ, Slavotinek A, Yu J. Haploinsufficiency and triploinsensitivity of the same 6p25.1p24.3 region in a family. *BMC Med Genomics* 8: 38, 2015.

Qian J, Cheng Q, Murdoch S, et al. The genetics of recurrent hydatidiform moles in China: Correlations between *NLRP7* mutations, molar genotypes and reproductive outcomes. *Mol Hum Reprod* 17: 612–619, 2011.

Qiao Y, Badduke C, Tang F, et al. Whole exome sequencing of families with 1q21.1 microdeletion or microduplication. *Am J Med Genet* 173A: 1782–1791, 2017.

Qin Y, Jiao X, Simpson JL, Chen ZJ. Genetics of primary ovarian insufficiency: New developments and opportunities. *Hum Reprod Update* 21: 787–808, 2015.

Quack B, Speed RM, Luciani JM, Noel B, Guichaoua M, Chandley AC. Meiotic analysis of two human reciprocal X-autosome translocations. *Cytogenet Cell Genet* 48: 43–47, 1988.

Quan F, Janas J, Toth-Fejel S, Johnson DB, Wolford JK, Popovich BW. Uniparental disomy of the entire X chromosome in a female with Duchenne muscular dystrophy. *Am J Hum Genet* 60: 160–165, 1997.

Queipo G, Zenteno JC, Peña R, et al. Molecular analysis in true hermaphroditism: Demonstration of low-level hidden mosaicism for Y-derived sequences in 46,XX cases. *Hum Genet* 111: 278–283, 2002.

Quéméner-Redon S, Bénech C, Audebert-Bellanger S, et al. A small de novo 16q24.1 duplication in a woman with severe clinical features. *Eur J Med Genet* 56: 211–215, 2013.

Queralt R, Madrigal I, Vallecillos MA, et al. Atypical XX male with the *SRY* gene located at the long arm of chromosome 1 and a 1qter microdeletion. *Am J Med Genet* 146A: 1335–1340, 2008.

Quigley DI, McDonald MT, Krishnamuthy V, et al. Triploid mosaicism in a 45,X/69,XXY infant. *Am J Med Genet* 138A: 171–174, 2005.

Quilter CR, Svennevik EC, Serhal P, et al. Cytogenetic and Y chromosome microdeletion screening of a random group of infertile males. *Fertil Steril* 79: 301–307, 2003.

Quinonez SC, Gelehrter TD, Uhlmann WR. A Marfan syndrome-like phenotype caused by a neocentromeric supernumerary ring chromosome 15. *Am J Med Genet* 173A: 268–273, 2017a.

Quinonez SC, Hedera P, Barr M, et al. Maternal intrachromosomal insertional translocation leads to recurrent 1q21.3q23.3 deletion in two siblings. *Am J Med Genet* 158A: 2591–2601, 2012.

Quinonez SC, Park JM, Rabah R, et al. 9p partial monosomy and disorders of sex development: Review and postulation of a pathogenetic mechanism. *Am J Med Genet* 161A: 1882–1896, 2013.

Quinonez SC, Seeley AH, Lam C, Glover TW, Barshop BA, Keegan CE. Paracentric inversion of chromosome 21 leading to disruption of the *HLCS* gene in a family with holocarboxylase synthetase deficiency. *JIMD Rep* 34: 55–61, 2017b.

Quintela I, Fernandez-Prieto M, Gomez-Guerrero L, et al. A 6q14.1-q15 microdeletion in a male patient with severe autistic disorder, lack of oral language, and dysmorphic features with concomitant presence of a maternally inherited Xp22.31 copy number gain. *Clin Case Rep* 3: 415–423, 2015.

Qumsiyeh MB, Kim KR, Ahmed MN, Bradford W. Cytogenetics and mechanisms of spontaneous abortions: Increased apoptosis and decreased cell proliferation in chromosomally abnormal villi. *Cytogenet Cell Genet* 88: 230–235, 2000.

Rabinowitz M, Ryan A, Gemelos G, et al. Origins and rates of aneuploidy in human blastomeres. *Fertil Steril* 97: 395–401, 2012.

Raca G, Artzer A, Thorson L, et al. Array-based comparative genomic hybridization (aCGH) in the genetic evaluation of stillbirth. *Am J Med Genet* 149A: 2437–2443, 2009.

Rajangam S, Michaelis RC, Velagaleti GVN, et al. Down syndrome with biparental inheritance of der(14q21q) and maternally derived trisomy 21: Confirmation by fluorescent in situ hybridization and microsatellite polymorphism analysis. *Am J Med Genet* 70: 43–47, 1997.

Rajcan-Separovic E, Qiao Y, Tyson C, et al. Genomic changes detected by array CGH in human embryos with developmental defects. *Mol Hum Reprod* 16: 125–134, 2010.

Rajcan-Separovic E, Robinson WP, Stephenson M, et al. Recurrent trisomy 15 in a female carrier of der(15)t(Y;15)(q12;p13). *Am J Med Genet* 99: 320–324, 2001.

Ralph A, Scott F, Tiernan C, et al. Maternal uniparental isodisomy for chromosome 14 detected prenatally. *Prenat Diagn* 19: 681–684, 1999.

Ramachandram S, Keng WT, Ariffin R, Ganesan V. A mother with variant Turner syndrome and two daughters with trisomy X: A case report. *J Genet* 92: 313–316, 2013.

Ramalingam A, Zhou XG, Fiedler SD, et al. 16p13.11 duplication is a risk factor for a wide spectrum of neuropsychiatric disorders. *J Hum Genet* 56: 541–544, 2011.

Ramírez-Velasco A, Rivera H. A further rec(X) dup p and compilation of 23 cases. Comment on "Molecular Genetic and Cytogenetic Characterization of a Partial Xp Duplication and Xq Deletion in a Patient with Premature Ovarian Failure" by Kim et al. *Gene* 548: 155–157, 2014.

Ramocki MB, Bartnik M, Szafranski P, et al. Recurrent distal 7q11.23 deletion including *HIP1* and *YWHAG* identified in patients with intellectual disabilities, epilepsy, and neurobehavioral problems. *Am J Hum Genet* 87: 857–865, 2010.

Ramsay L, Howe DT, Wellesley D. Parental attitude to participating in long-term follow-up studies of their children's health after in utero diagnosis of abnormalities. *Prenat Diagn* 29: 207–212, 2009.

Rao R, Platt LD. Ultrasound screening: Status of markers and efficacy of screening for structural abnormalities. *Semin Perinatol* 40: 67–78, 2016.

Rapp R. *Testing Women, Testing the Fetus: The Social Impact of Amniocentesis in America*. New York, NY: Routledge, 1999.

Ratcliffe S. Long-term outcome in children of sex chromosome abnormalities. *Arch Dis Child* 80: 192–195, 1999.

Ratcliffe SG, Butler GE, Jones M. Edinburgh study of growth and development of children with sex chromosome abnormalities: IV. *Birth Defects Orig Artic Ser* 26: 1–44, 1990.

Rauch A, Dörr HG. Chromosome 5q subtelomeric deletion syndrome. *Am J Med Genet* 145C: 372–376, 2007.

Rauen KA, Bitts SM, Li L, Golabi M, Cotter PD. Tandem duplication mosaicism: Characterization of a mosaic dup(5q) and review. *Clin Genet* 60: 366–370, 2001.

Rauen KA, Golabi M, Cotter PD. Fertility in a female with mosaic trisomy 8. *Fertil Steril* 79: 206–208, 2003.

Raun N, Mailo J, Spinelli E, et al. Quantitative phenotypic and network analysis of 1q44 microdeletion for microcephaly. *Am J Med Genet* 173A: 972–977, 2017.

Ravel C, Berthaut I, Bresson JL, Siffroi JP. Prevalence of chromosomal abnormalities in phenotypically normal and fertile adult males: large-scale survey of over 10,000 sperm donor karyotypes. *Hum Reprod* 21: 1484–1489, 2006a.

Ravel C, Chantot-Bastaraud S, Siffroi JP, Escalier D, Antoine JM, Mandelbaum J. Tail stump syndrome associated with chromosomal translocation in two brothers attempting intracytoplasmic sperm injection. *Fertil Steril* 86: 719, e1–7, 2006b.

Raziel A, Friedler S, Schachter M, Kasterstein E, Strassburger D, Ron-El R. Increased frequency of female partner chromosomal abnormalities in patients with high-order implantation failure after in vitro fertilization. *Fertil Steril* 78: 515–519, 2002.

Redaelli S, Sala E, Roncaglia N, et al. Severe intrauterine growth restriction and trisomy 15 confined placental mosaicism: A case report and review of literature. *Prenat Diagn* 25: 140–147, 2005.

Reddy KS. Double trisomy in spontaneous abortions. *Hum Genet* 101: 339–345, 1997.

Reddy KS. Triple aneuploidy in spontaneous abortions. *Clin Genet* 56: 103–104, 1999.

Reddy KS, Huang B. Prenatal management of mosaic tetrasomy 5p. *Prenat Diagn* 23: 82–85, 2003.

Reddy KS, Mak L. Mosaic unbalanced structural abnormalities confirmed using FISH on buccal mucosal cells. *Ann Génét* 44: 37–40, 2001.

Reddy KS, Sulcova V. Pathogenetics of 45,X/46,XY gonadal mosaicism. *Cytogenet Cell Genet* 82: 52–57, 1998.

Reddy KS, Sulcova V, Siassi B. Two sibs with Wolf-Hirschhorn and DiGeorge deletions resulting from an unbalanced chromosome rearrangement, 45,XX/XY, der(4)t(4;22) (p16.3;q11.2) mat,-22. *J Med Genet* 33: 852–855, 1996.

Reddy KS, Sulcova V, Young H, Blancato JK, Haddad BR. De novo mosaic add(3) characterized to be trisomy 14q31-qter using spectral karyotyping and subtelomeric probes. *Am J Med Genet* 82: 318–321, 1999.

Reddy UM, Page GP, Saade GR, et al. Karyotype versus microarray testing for genetic abnormalities after stillbirth. *N Engl J Med* 367: 2185–2193, 2012.

Redin C, Brand H, Collins RL, et al. The genomic landscape of balanced cytogenetic abnormalities associated with human congenital anomalies. *Nat Genet*, 49: 36–45, 2017.

Rees E, Kirov G, Sanders A, et al. Evidence that duplications of 22q11.2 protect against schizophrenia. *Mol Psychiatry* 19: 37–40, 2014a.

Rees E, Walters JT, Chambert KD, et al. CNV analysis in a large schizophrenia sample implicates deletions at 16p12.1 and SLC1A1 and duplications at 1p36.33 and *CGNL1*. *Hum Mol Genet* 23: 1669–1676, 2014b.

Reid R, Sepulveda W, Kyle PM, Davies G. Amniotic fluid culture failure: Clinical significance and association with aneuploidy. *Obstet Gynecol* 87: 588–592, 1996.

Reinehr T, Jauch A, Zoll B, Engel U, Bartels I, Andler W. Short stature in a mother and daughter caused by familial der(X)t(X;X)(p22.1-3;q26). *Am J Med Genet* 102: 81–85, 2001.

Reish O, Wolach B, Amiel A, Kedar I, Dolfin T, Fejgin M. Dilemma of trisomy 20 mosaicism detected prenatally: Is it an innocent finding? *Am J Med Genet* 77: 72–75, 1998.

Reiss AL, Freund L, Plotnick L, et al. The effects of X monosomy on brain development: Monozygotic twins discordant for Turner's syndrome. *Ann Neurol* 34: 95–107, 1993.

Reittinger AM, Helm BM, Boles DJ, Gadi IK, Schrier Vergano SA. A prenatal diagnosis of mosaic trisomy 5 reveals a postnatal complete uniparental disomy of chromosome 5 with multiple congenital anomalies. *Am J Med Genet* 173A: 2528–2533, 2017.

Ren H, Chow V, Ma S. Meiotic behaviour and sperm aneuploidy in an infertile man with a mosaic 45,X/46,XY karyotype. *Reprod Biomed Online* 31: 783–789, 2015.

Renault NK, Pritchett SM, Howell RE, et al. Human X-chromosome inactivation pattern distributions fit a model of genetically influenced choice better than models of completely random choice. *Eur J Hum Genet* 21: 1396–1402, 2013.

Rendeiro P, Gonçalves R, Freixo JP, et al. A case of parental transmission of Koolen-de Vries syndrome. Poster presented at the American College of Medical Genetics meeting, Tampa, 2016.

Renshaw R, Ellis K, Jacobs P, Morris J. Antenatal screening for Down syndrome: A quantitative demonstration of the improvements over the past 20 years. *J Health Serv Res Policy* 18: 195–201, 2013.

Rentmeester CA. Value neutrality in genetic counseling: An unattained ideal. *Med Health Care Philos* 4: 47–51, 2001.

Repnikova EA, Astbury C, Reshmi SC, et al. Microarray comparative genomic hybridization and cytogenetic characterization of tissue-specific mosaicism in three patients. *Am J Med Genet* 158A: 1924–1933, 2012.

Rethoré MO, Blois MC, Peeters M, Popowski P, Pangalos C, Lejeune J. Pure partial trisomy of the short arm of chromosome 5. *Hum Genet* 82: 296–298, 1989.

Revah-Politi A, Ganapathi M, Bier L, et al. Loss-of-function variants in *NFIA* provide further support that *NFIA* is a critical gene in 1p32-p31 deletion syndrome: A four patient series. *Am J Med Genet* 173A: 3158–3164, 2017.

Ricard-Mousnier B, N'Guyen S, Dubas F, Pouplard F, Guichet A. Ring chromosome 17 epilepsy may resemble that of ring chromosome 20 syndrome. *Epileptic Disord* 9: 327–331, 2007.

Riccaboni A, Lalatta F, Caliari I, Bonetti S, Somigliana E, Ragni G. Genetic screening in 2,710 infertile candidate couples for assisted reproductive techniques: Results of application of Italian guidelines for the appropriate use of genetic tests. *Fertil Steril* 89: 800–808, 2008.

Rice AM, McLysaght A. Dosage sensitivity is a major determinant of human copy number variant pathogenicity. *Nat Commun* 8: 14366, 2017.

Richards EG, Zaveri HP, Wolf VL, Kang SH, Scott DA. Delineation of a less than 200 kb minimal deleted region for cardiac malformations on chromosome 7p22. *Am J Med Genet* 155A: 1729–1734, 2011.

Richards S, Aziz N, Bale S, et al. Standards and guidelines for the interpretation of sequence variants: A joint consensus recommendation of the American College of Medical Genetics and Genomics and the Association for Molecular Pathology. *Genet Med* 17: 405–424, 2015.

Rickman L, Fiegler H, Shaw-Smith C, et al. Prenatal detection of unbalanced chromosomal rearrangements by array CGH. *J Med Genet* 43: 353–361, 2006.

Riegel M, Wisser J, Baumer A, Schinzel A. Postzygotic isochromosome formation as a cause for false-negative results from chorionic villus chromosome examinations. *Prenat Diagn* 26: 221–225, 2006.

Riehmer V, Erger F, Herkenrath P, et al. A heritable microduplication encompassing *TBL1XR1* causes a genomic sister-disorder for the 3q26.32 microdeletion syndrome. *Am J Med Genet* 173A: 2132–2138, 2017.

Rieubland C, Francis D, Houben L, Corrie S, Bankier A, White SM. Two cases of trisomy 16 mosaicism ascertained postnatally. *Am J Med Genet* 149A: 1523–1528, 2009.

Rigola MA, Baena N, Català V, et al. A 11.7-Mb paracentric Inversion in chromosome 1q detected in prenatal diagnosis associated with familial intellectual disability. *Cytogenet Genome Res* 146: 109–114, 2015.

Riley KN, Catalano LM, Bernat JA, et al. Recurrent deletions and duplications of chromosome 2q11.2 and 2q13 are associated with variable outcomes. *Am J Med Genet* 167A: 2664–2673, 2015.

Rink BD, Norton ME. Screening for fetal aneuploidy. *Semin Perinatol* 40: 35–43, 2016.

Ritter DI, Haines K, Cheung H, et al. Identifying gene disruptions in novel balanced de novo constitutional translocations in childhood cancer patients by whole-genome sequencing. *Genet Med* 17: 831–835, 2015.

Rittinger O, Krabichler B, Kronberger G, Kotzot D. Clinical, cytogenetic, and molecular findings in a patient with a 46,XX,del(18)(q22)/ 46,XX,idic(18)(q22) karyotype. *Eur J Med Genet* 58: 603–607, 2015.

Rivas F, García-Esquivel L, Rivera H, Jimenez ME, Gonzalez RM, Cantú JM. Inv(4)(p16q21): A five-generation pedigree with 24 carriers and no recombinants. *Clin Genet* 31: 97–101, 1987.

Rivera H, Cantú JM. Centric fission consequences in man. *Ann Génét* 29: 223–225, 1986.

Rivera H, Domínguez MG, Vásquez-Velásquez AI, Lurie IW. De novo dup p/del q or dup q/del p rearranged chromosomes: Review of 104 cases of a distinct chromosomal mutation. *Cytogenet Genome Res* 141: 58–63, 2013.

Rives N, Siméon N, Milazzo JP, Barthélémy C, Macé B. Meiotic segregation of sex chromosomes in mosaic and non-mosaic XYY males: Case reports and review of the literature. *Int J Androl* 26: 242–249, 2003.

Rizzolio F, Bione S, Sala C, et al. Chromosomal rearrangements in Xq and premature ovarian failure: Mapping of 25 new cases and review of the literature. *Hum Reprod* 21: 1477–1483, 2006.

Rizzolio F, Pramparo T, Sala C, et al. Epigenetic analysis of the critical region I for premature ovarian failure: Demonstration of a highly heterochromatic domain on the long arm of the mammalian X chromosome. *J Med Genet* 46: 585–592, 2009.

Robberecht C, Voet T, Zamani Esteki M, Nowakowska BA, Vermeesch JR. Nonallelic homologous recombination between retrotransposable elements is a driver of de novo unbalanced translocations. *Genome Res* 23: 411–418, 2013.

Robbins WA, Vine MF, Truong KY, Everson RB. Use of fluorescence in situ hybridization (FISH) to assess effects of smoking, caffeine, and alcohol on aneuploidy load in sperm of healthy men. *Environ Mol Mutagen* 30: 175–183, 1997.

Roberts E, Dunlop J, Davis GS, Churchill D, Davison EV. A further case of confined placental mosaicism for trisomy 2 associated with adverse pregnancy outcome. *Prenat Diagn* 23: 564–565, 2003.

Roberts JL, Buckley RH, Luo B, et al. CD45-deficient severe combined immunodeficiency caused by uniparental disomy. *Proc Natl Acad Sci USA* 109: 10456–10461, 2012.

Roberts P, Williams J, Sills MA. A case of two inversion (10) recombinants in a family. *J Med Genet* 26: 461–464, 1989.

Robertson S, Savulescu J. Is there a case in favour of predictive genetic testing in young children? *Bioethics* 15: 26–49, 2001.

Robinson A, Bender BG, Borelli JB, Puck MH, Salbenblatt JA, Winter JSD. Sex chromosomal aneuploidy: Prospective and longitudinal studies. *Birth Defects Orig Artic Ser* 22: 23–71, 1986.

Robinson A, Bender BG, Linden MG, Salbenblatt JA. Sex chromosome aneuploidy: The Denver Prospective Study. *Birth Defects Orig Artic Ser* 26: 59–115, 1990.

Robinson WP. Mechanisms leading to uniparental disomy and their clinical consequences. *Bioessays* 22: 452–459, 2000.

Robinson WP, Barrett IJ, Bernard L, et al. Meiotic origin of trisomy in confined placental mosaicism is correlated with presence of fetal uniparental disomy, high levels of trisomy in trophoblast, and increased risk of fetal intrauterine growth restriction. *Am J Hum Genet* 60: 917–927, 1997.

Robinson WP, Bernasconi F, Basaran S, et al. A somatic origin of homologous Robertsonian translocations and isochromosomes. *Am J Hum Genet* 54: 290–302, 1994.

Robinson WP, Bernasconi F, Lau A, McFadden DE. Frequency of meiotic trisomy depends on involved chromosome and mode of ascertainment. *Am J Med Genet* 84: 34–42, 1999.

Robinson WP, Binkert F, Bernasconi F, Lorda-Sánchez I, Werder EA, Schinzel AA. Molecular studies of chromosomal mosaicism: Relative frequency of chromosome gain or loss and possible role of cell selection. *Am J Hum Genet* 56: 444–451, 1995.

Robinson WP, Binkert F, Gine R, et al. Clinical and molecular analysis of five inv dup(15) patients. *Eur J Hum Genet* 1: 37–50, 1993.

Robinson WP, Christian SL, Kuchinka BD, et al. Somatic segregation errors predominantly contribute to the gain or loss of a paternal chromosome leading to uniparental disomy for chromosome 15. *Clin Genet* 57: 349–358, 2000.

Robinson WP, Kuchinka BD, Bernasconi F, et al. Maternal meiosis I non-disjunction of chromosome 15: Dependence of the maternal age effect on level of recombination. *Hum Mol Genet* 7: 1011–1019, 1998.

Robinson WP, McFadden DE, Barrett IJ, et al. Origin of amnion and implications for evaluation of the fetal genotype in cases of mosaicism. *Prenat Diagn* 22: 1076–1085, 2002.

Robinson WP, McFadden DE, Stephenson MD. The origin of abnormalities in recurrent aneuploidy/polyploidy. *Am J Hum Genet* 69: 1245–1254, 2001.

Robinson WP, McGillivray B, Friedman JM. Pregnancy and postnatal outcome of mosaic isochromosome 20q. *Prenat Diagn* 27: 143–145, 2007.

Robinson WP, McGillivray B, Lewis ME, Arbour L, Barrett I, Kalousek DK. Prenatally detected trisomy 20 mosaicism. *Prenat Diagn* 25: 239–244, 2005.

Rodrigo L, Peinado V, Mateu E, et al. Impact of different patterns of sperm chromosomal abnormalities on the chromosomal constitution of preimplantation embryos. *Fertil Steril* 94: 1380–1386, 2010.

Rodriguez JD, Bhat SS, Meloni I, et al. Intellectual disability, midface hypoplasia, facial hypotonia, and Alport syndrome are associated with a deletion in Xq22.3. *Am J Med Genet* 152A: 713–717, 2010.

Rodríguez L, Diego-Alvarez D, Lorda-Sánchez I, et al. A small and active ring X chromosome in a female with features of Kabuki syndrome. *Am J Med Genet* 146A: 2816–2821, 2008.

Rodriguez-Purata J, Lee J, Whitehouse M, et al. Embryo selection versus natural selection: How do outcomes of comprehensive chromosome screening of blastocysts compare with the analysis of products of conception from early pregnancy loss (dilation and curettage) among an assisted reproductive technology population? *Fertil Steril* 104: 1460–1466.e1–12, 2015.

Rodriguez-Revenga L, Badenas C, Madrigal I, et al. 46,XY,18q+/46,XY,18q- mosaicism in a fragile X prenatal diagnosis. *Prenat Diagn* 25: 448–450, 2005.

Rogers JC, Harris DJ, Pasztor LM. Reciprocal translocation 4;11 with both adjacent-1 segregants viable within a family. *Clin Genet* 51: 250–256, 1997.

Rogers JF. Clinical delineation of proximal and distal partial 13q trisomy. *Clin Genet* 25: 221–229, 1984.

Rogers JG, Voullaire L, Gold H. Monozygotic twins discordant for trisomy 21. *Am J Med Genet* 11: 143–146, 1982.

Rohayem J, Fricke R, Czeloth K, et al. Age and markers of Leydig cell function, but not of Sertoli cell function predict the success of sperm retrieval in adolescents and adults with Klinefelter's syndrome. *Andrology* 3: 868–875, 2015.

Romain DR, Columbano-Green LM, Whyte S, et al. Familial paracentric inversion of 1p. *Am J Med Genet* 14: 629–634, 1983.

Romans SM, Stefanatos G, Roeltgen DP, Kushner H, Ross JL. Transition to young adulthood in Ullrich-Turner syndrome: Neurodevelopmental changes. *Am J Med Genet* 79: 140–147, 1998.

Ronzoni L, Grassi FS, Pezzani L, et al. 7p22.1 microduplication syndrome: Refinement of the critical region. *Eur J Med Genet* 60: 114–117, 2017.

Ronzoni L, Tagliaferri F, Tucci A, Baccarin M, Esposito S, Milani D. Interstitial 6q25 microdeletion syndrome: *ARID1B* is the key gene. *Am J Med Genet* 170A: 1257–1261, 2016.

Rooryck C, VuPhi Y, Souakri N, et al. Characterization of a de novo balanced translocation t(9;18)(p23;q12.2) in a patient with oculoauriculovertebral spectrum. *Eur J Med Genet* 53: 104–107, 2010.

Röpke A, Kalinski T, Mohnike K, et al. Distribution of sex chromosomes in dysgenetic gonads of mixed type. *Cytogenet Genome Res* 116: 146–151, 2007.

Rose CSP, Patel P, Reardon W, Malcolm S, Winter RM. The *TWIST* gene, although not disrupted in Saethre-Chotzen patients with apparently balanced translocations of 7p21, is mutated in familial and sporadic cases. *Hum Mol Genet* 6: 1369–1373, 1997.

Rosenbusch B. Co-existence of a diploid hydatidiform mole and a normal fetus: Mysterious events at the pronuclear stage. *Hum Reprod* 23: 2876–2877, 2008.

Rosenbusch B, Schneider M, Gläser B, Brucker C. Cytogenetic analysis of giant oocytes and zygotes to assess their relevance for the development of digynic triploidy. *Hum Reprod* 17: 2388–2393, 2002.

Rosenfeld JA, Ballif BC, Lucas A, et al. Small deletions of *SATB2* cause some of the clinical features of the 2q33.1 microdeletion syndrome. *PLoS One* 4: e6568, 2009.

Rosenfeld JA, Coe BP, Eichler EE, Cuckle H, Shaffer LG. Estimates of penetrance for recurrent pathogenic copy-number variations, *Genet Med* 15: 478–481, 2013.

Rosenfeld JA, Fox JE, Descartes M, et al. Clinical features associated with copy number variations of the 14q32 imprinted gene cluster. *Am J Med Genet* 167A: 345–353, 2015.

Rosenfeld JA, Kim KH, Angle B, et al. Further evidence of contrasting phenotypes caused by reciprocal deletions and duplications: Duplication of *NSD1* causes growth retardation and microcephaly. *Mol Syndromol* 3: 247–254, 2012a.

Rosenfeld JA, Traylor RN, Schaefer GB, et al. Proximal microdeletions and microduplications of 1q21.1 contribute to variable abnormal phenotypes. *Eur J Hum Genet* 20: 754–761, 2012b.

Rosenkrantz JL, Carbone L. Investigating somatic aneuploidy in the brain: Why we need a new model. *Chromosoma* 126:337–350, 2017.

Rosenmann A, Wahrman J, Richler C, Voss R, Persitz A, Goldman B. Meiotic association between the XY chromosomes and unpaired autosomal elements as a cause of human male sterility. *Cytogenet Cell Genet* 39: 19–29, 1985.

Ross JL, Stefanatos GA, Kushner H, Zinn A, Bondy C, Roeltgen D. Persistent cognitive deficits in adult women with Turner syndrome. *Neurology* 58: 218–225, 2002.

Rossi E, Messa J, Zuffardi O. Ring syndrome: Still true? *J Med Genet* 45: 766–768, 2008a.

Rossi E, Riegel M, Messa J, et al. Duplications in addition to terminal deletions are present in a proportion of ring chromosomes: Clues to the mechanisms of formation. *J Med Genet* 45: 147–154, 2008b.

Rothenmund H, Chudley AE, Dawson AJ. Familial transmission of a small supernumerary marker

chromosome 8 identified by FISH: An update. *Am J Med Genet* 72: 339–342, 1997.

Röthlisberger B, Kotzot D. Recurrence risk in de novo structural chromosomal rearrangements. *Am J Med Genet* 143A: 1708–1714, 2007.

Röthlisberger B, Kotzot D, Brecevic L, et al. Recombinant balanced and unbalanced translocations as a consequence of a balanced complex chromosomal rearrangement involving eight breakpoints in four chromosomes. *Eur J Hum Genet* 7: 873–883, 1999.

Rothman BK. *The Tentative Pregnancy: Prenatal Diagnosis and the Future of Motherhood.* London, UK: Pandora Press, 1988.

Rougeulle C, Lalande M. Angelman syndrome: How many genes to remain silent? *Neurogenet* 1: 229–237, 1998.

Rovet J, Netley C, Bailey J, Keenan M, Stewart D. Intelligence and achievement in children with extra X aneuploidy: A longitudinal perspective. *Am J Med Genet* 60: 356–363, 1995.

Rowe LR, Lee JY, Rector L, et al. U-type exchange is the most frequent mechanism for inverted duplication with terminal deletion rearrangements. *J Med Genet* 46: 694–702, 2009.

Rowland RE, Edwards LA, Podd JV. Elevated sister chromatid exchange frequencies in New Zealand Vietnam War veterans. *Cytogenet Genome Res* 116: 248–251, 2007.

Rowsey R, Kashevarova A, Murdoch B, et al. Germline mosaicism does not explain the maternal age effect on trisomy. *Am J Med Genet* 161A: 2495–2503, 2013.

Rubes J, Selevan SG, Evenson DP, et al. Episodic air pollution is associated with increased DNA fragmentation in human sperm without other changes in semen quality. *Hum Reprod* 20: 2776–2783, 2005.

Rubio C, Simón C, Vidal F, et al. Chromosomal abnormalities and embryo development in recurrent miscarriage couples. *Hum Reprod* 18: 182–188, 2003.

Rudnicka AR, Wald NJ, Huttly W, Hackshaw AK. Influence of maternal smoking on the birth prevalence of Down syndrome and on second trimester screening performance. *Prenat Diagn* 22: 893–897, 2002.

Ruggeri A, Dulcetti F, Miozzo M, et al. Prenatal search for UPD 14 and UPD 15 in 83 cases of familial and de novo heterologous Robertsonian translocations. *Prenat Diagn* 24: 997–1000, 2004.

Rumpler Y. Meiotic studies in animal models. *Ann Génét* 44: s18, 2001.

Rusconi D, Negri G, Colapietro P, et al. Characterization of 14 novel deletions underlying

Rubinstein-Taybi syndrome: An update of the *CREBBP* deletion repertoire. *Hum Genet* 134: 613–626, 2015.

Rushton DI. Examination of products of conception from previable human pregnancies. *J Clin Pathol* 34: 819–835, 1981.

Russell LM, Strike P, Browne CE, Jacobs PA. X chromosome loss and ageing. *Cytogenet Genome Res* 116: 181–185, 2007.

Russell MW, Raeker MO, Geisler SB, et al. Functional analysis of candidate genes in 2q13 deletion syndrome implicates *FBLN7* and *TMEM87B* deficiency in congenital heart defects and *FBLN7* in craniofacial malformations. *Hum Mol Genet* 23: 4272–4284, 2914.

Russo S, Finelli P, Recalcati MP, et al. Molecular and genomic characterisation of cryptic chromosomal alterations leading to paternal duplication of the 11p15.5 Beckwith-Wiedemann region. *J Med Genet* 43: e39, 2006.

Saadallah N, Hultén M. A complex three breakpoint translocation involving chromosomes 2, 4, and 9 identified by meiotic investigations of a human male ascertained for subfertility. *Hum Genet* 71: 312–320, 1985.

Sabbaghian M, Meybodi AM, Rahimian M, Sadighi Gilani MA. Occurrence of 47,X,i(X)(q10),Y Klinefelter variant with hypogonadotropic hypogonadism. *Fertil Steril* 96: e115–117, 2011.

Sacharow S, Li D, Fan YS, Tekin M. Familial 16q24.3 microdeletion involving *ANKRD11* causes a KBG-like syndrome. *Am J Med Genet* 158A: 547–552, 2012.

Sachs ES, Jahoda MGJ, Los FJ, Pijpers L, Wladimiroff JW. Trisomy 21 mosaicism in gonads with unexpectedly high recurrence risks. *Am J Med Genet Suppl* 7: 186–188, 1990.

Sago H, Chen E, Conte WJ, et al. True trisomy 2 mosaicism in amniocytes and newborn liver associated with multiple system abnormalities. *Am J Med Genet* 72: 343–346, 1997.

Sahinturk S, Ozemri Sag S, Ture M, et al. A fertile patient with 45X/47XXX mosaicism. *Genet Couns* 26: 29–34, 2015.

Sahnane N, Bernasconi B, Carnevali I, et al. Disruption of the *APC* gene by t(5;7) translocation in a Turcot family. *Cancer Genet* 209: 107–111, 2016.

Sahoo T, Bacino CA, German JR, et al. Identification of novel deletions of 15q11q13 in Angelman syndrome by array-CGH: Molecular characterization and genotype-phenotype correlations. *Eur J Hum Genet* 15: 943–949, 2007.

Sahoo T, del Gaudio D, German JR, et al. Prader-Willi phenotype caused by paternal deficiency for the HBII-85 C/D box small nucleolar RNA cluster. *Nat Genet* 40: 719–721, 2008.

Sahoo T, Dzidic N, Strecker MN, et al. Comprehensive genetic analysis of pregnancy loss by chromosomal microarrays: Outcomes, benefits, and challenges. *Genet Med* 19: 83–89, 2017.

Sahoo T, Theisen A, Sanchez-Lara PA, et al. Microdeletion 20p12.3 involving *BMP2* contributes to syndromic forms of cleft palate. *Am J Med Genet* 155A: 1646–1653, 2011.

Saitoh S, Buiting K, Cassidy SB, et al. Clinical spectrum and molecular diagnosis of Angelman and Prader-Willi syndrome patients with an imprinting mutation. *Am J Med Genet* 68: 195–206, 1997.

Saito-Ohara F, Fukuda Y, Ito M, et al. The Xq22 inversion breakpoint interrupted a novel Ras-like GTPase gene in a patient with Duchenne muscular dystrophy and profound mental retardation. *Am J Hum Genet* 71: 637–645, 2002.

Saitta SC, Harris SE, McDonald-McGinn DM, et al. Independent de novo 22q11.2 deletions in first cousins with DiGeorge/velocardiofacial syndrome. *Am J Med Genet* 124A: 313–317, 2004.

Sajan SA, Fernandez L, Nieh SE, et al. Both rare and de novo copy number variants are prevalent in agenesis of the corpus callosum but not in cerebellar hypoplasia or polymicrogyria. *PLoS Genet* 9: e1003823, 2013.

Sakazume S, Kido Y, Murakami N, Matsubara T, Numabe H. Additional patients with 4q deletion: Severe growth delay and polycystic kidney disease associated with 4q21q22 loss. *Pediatr Int* 57: 880–883, 2015.

Sakazume S, Ohashi H, Sasaki Y, et al. Spread of X-chromosome inactivation into chromosome 15 is associated with Prader-Willi syndrome phenotype in a boy with a t(X;15)(p21.1;q11.2) translocation. *Hum Genet* 131: 121–130, 2012.

Salas-Labadía C, Cervantes-Barragán DE, Cruz-Alcívar R, et al. Cytogenomic and phenotypic analysis in low-level monosomy 7 mosaicism with non-supernumerary ring chromosome 7. *Am J Med Genet* 164A: 1765–1769, 2014.

Salo P, Ignatius J, Simola KOJ, Tahvanainen E, Kaariainen H. Clinical features of nine males with molecularly defined deletions of the Y chromosome long arm. *J Med Genet* 32: 711–715, 1995.

Salomon LJ, Bernard JP, Nizard J, Ville Y. First-trimester screening for fetal triploidy at 11 to 14 weeks: a role for fetal biometry. *Prenat Diagn* 25: 479–483, 2005.

Salpietro V, Ruggieri M, Mankad K, et al. A de novo 0.63 Mb 6q25.1 deletion associated with growth failure, congenital heart defect, underdeveloped cerebellar vermis, abnormal cutaneous elasticity and joint laxity. *Am J Med Genet* 167A: 2042–2051, 2015.

Samango-Sprouse C, Kirkizlar E, Hall MP, et al. Incidence of X and Y chromosomal aneuploidy in a large child bearing population. *PLoS One* 11:e0161045, 2016.

Samplaski MK, Lo KC, Grober ED, Millar A, Dimitromanolakis A, Jarvi KA. Phenotypic differences in mosaic Klinefelter patients as compared with non-mosaic Klinefelter patients. *Fertil Steril* 101: 950–955, 2014.

Sampson A, de Crespigny LC. Vanishing twins: The frequency of spontaneous fetal reduction of a twin pregnancy. *Ultrasound Obstet Gynecol* 2: 107–109, 1992.

Sánchez J, Fernández R, Madruga M, Bernabeu-Wittel J, Antiñolo G, Borrego S. Somatic and germ-line mosaicism of deletion 15q11.2-q13 in a mother of dyzigotic twins with Angelman syndrome. *Am J Med Genet* 164A: 370–376, 2014.

Sánchez JM, Franzi L, Collia F, De Díaz SL, Panal M, Dubner M. Cytogenetic study of spontaneous abortions by transabdominal villus sampling and direct analysis of villi. *Prenat Diagn* 19: 601–603, 1999.

Sanlaville D, Prieur M, de Blois MC, et al. Functional disomy of the Xq28 chromosome region. *Eur J Hum Genet* 13: 579–585, 2005.

Sanlaville D, Schluth-Bolard C, Turleau C. Distal Xq duplication and functional Xq disomy. *Orphanet J Rare Dis* 4: 4, 2009.

Saranya B, Bhavani G, Arumugam B, Jayashankar M, Santhiya ST. Three novel and two known androgen receptor gene mutations associated with androgen insensitivity syndrome in sex-reversed XY female patients. *J Genet* 95: 911–921, 2016.

Sarno AP, Moorman AJ, Kalousek DK. Partial molar pregnancy with fetal survival: An unusual example of confined placental mosaicism. *Obstet Gynecol* 82: 716–719, 1993.

Sarri C, Gyftodimou J, Avramopoulos D, et al. Partial trisomy 17q22-qter and partial monosomy Xq27-qter in a girl with a de novo unbalanced translocation due to a postzygotic error: Case report and review of the literature on partial trisomy 17qter. *Am J Med Genet* 70: 87–94, 1997.

Sasaki K, Okamoto N, Kosaki K, et al. Maternal uniparental isodisomy and heterodisomy on chromosome 6 encompassing a *CUL7* gene mutation causing 3M syndrome. *Clin Genet* 80: 478–483, 2011.

Sasaki T, Tonoki H, Soejima H, Niikawa N. A 4 Mb cryptic deletion associated with inv(8)(q13.1q24.11) in a patient with trichorhinophalangeal syndrome type I. *J Med Genet* 34: 335–339, 1997.

Sato K, Iwakoshi M, Shimokawa O, et al. Angelman syndrome caused by an identical familial 1,487-kb deletion. *Am J Med Genet* 143: 98–101, 2007.

Saugier-Veber P, Doummar D, Barthez MA, et al. Myoclonus dystonia plus syndrome due to a novel 7q21 microdeletion. *Am J Med Genet* 152A: 1244–1249, 2010.

Saura R, Traore W, Taine L, et al. Prenatal diagnosis of trisomy 9: Six cases and a review of the literature. *Prenat Diagn* 15: 609–614, 1995.

Savage AR, Petersen MB, Pettay D, et al. Elucidating the mechanisms of paternal non-disjunction of chromosome 21 in humans. *Hum Mol Genet* 7: 1221–1227, 1998.

Savarese M, Grandone A, Perone L, et al. Familial trisomy 6p in mother and daughter. *Am J Med Genet* 161A: 1675–1681, 2013.

Savarirayan R, Bankier A. Acampomelic campomelic dysplasia with de novo 5q;17q reciprocal translocation and severe phenotype. *J Med Genet* 35: 597–599, 1998.

Savulescu J, Kahane G. The moral obligation to create children with the best chance of the best life. *Bioethics* 23: 274–290, 2009.

Savva GM, Morris JK, Mutton DE, Alberman E. Maternal age-specific fetal loss rates in Down syndrome pregnancies. *Prenat Diagn* 26: 499–504, 2006.

Savva GM, Walker K, Morris JK. The maternal age-specific live birth prevalence of trisomies 13 and 18 compared to trisomy 21 (Down syndrome). *Prenat Diagn* 30: 57–64, 2010.

Sawyer JR, Binz RL, Swanson CM, Lim C. De novo proximal duplication of 1(q12q22) in a female infant with multiple congenital anomalies. *Am J Med Genet* 143A: 338–342, 2007.

Sawyer JR, Swanson CM, Wheeler G, Cunniff C. Chromosome instability in ICF syndrome: Formation of micronuclei from multibranched chromosomes 1 demonstrated by fluorescence in situ hybridization. *Am J Med Genet* 56: 203–209, 1995.

Schaaf CP, Wiszniewska J, Beaudet AL. Copy number and SNP arrays in clinical diagnostics. *Annu Rev Genomics Hum Genet* 12: 25–51, 2011.

Schaap AHP, van der Pol HG, Boer K, Leschot NJ, Wolf H. Long-term follow-up of infants after transcervical chorionic villus sampling and after amniocentesis to compare congenital abnormalities and health status. *Prenat Diagn* 22: 598–604, 2002.

Schecter A, Constable JD. Commentary: Agent Orange and birth defects in Vietnam. *Int J Epidemiol* 35: 1230–1232, 2006.

Scheffer I, Brett EM, Wilson J, Baraitser M. Angelman's syndrome. *J Med Genet* 27: 275–277, 1990.

Scherer SW, Gripp KW, Lucena J, et al. Observation of a parental inversion variant in a rare Williams-Beuren syndrome family with two affected children. *Hum Genet* 117: 383–388, 2005.

Scheuerle A, Heller K, Elder F. Complete trisomy 1q with mosaic Y;1 translocation: A recurrent aneuploidy presenting diagnostic dilemmas. *Am J Med Genet* 138A: 166–170, 2005.

Scheuvens R, Begemann M, Soellner L, et al. Maternal uniparental disomy of chromosome 16 (upd(16) mat): Clinical features are rather caused by (hidden) trisomy 16 mosaicism than by upd(16) mat itself. *Clin Genet* 92: 45–51, 2017.

Schiff JD, Palermo GD, Veeck LL, Goldstein M, Rosenwaks Z, Schlegel PN. Success of testicular sperm extraction and intracytoplasmic sperm injection in men with Klinefelter syndrome. *J Clin Endocrinol Metab* 90: 6263–6267, 2005.

Schinzel A. *Catalogue of Unbalanced Chromosome Aberrations in Man.* New York, NY: de Gruyter, 2001.

Schinzel AA, Adelsberger PA, Binkert F, Basaran S, Antonarakis SE. No evidence for a paternal interchromosomal effect from analysis of the origin of nondisjunction in Down syndrome patients with concomitant familial chromosome rearrangements. *Am J Hum Genet* 50: 288–293, 1992.

Schinzel AA, Riegel M, Baumer A, et al. Long-term follow-up of four patients with Langer-Giedion syndrome: Clinical course and complications. *Am J Med Genet* 161A: 2216–2225, 2013.

Schinzel AA, Robinson WP, Binkert F, Torresani T, Werder EA. Exclusively paternal X chromosomes in a girl with short stature. *Hum Genet* 92: 175–178, 1993.

Schlade-Bartusiak K, Brown L, Lomax B, et al. BPES with atypical premature ovarian insufficiency, and evidence of mitotic recombination, in a woman with trisomy X and a translocation t(3;11)(q22.3;q14.1). *Am J Med Genet* 158A: 2322–2327, 2012.

Schlessel JS, Brown WT, Lysikiewicz A, Schiff R, Zaslav AL. Monozygotic twins with trisomy 18: A report of discordant phenotype. *J Med Genet* 27: 640–642, 1990.

Schlessinger D, Mandel JL, Monaco AP, Nelson DL, Willard HF. Report and abstracts of the fourth international workshop on human X chromosome mapping 1993. *Cytogenet Cell Genet* 64: 147–194, 1993.

Schluth-Bolard C, Delobel B, Sanlaville D, et al. Cryptic genomic imbalances in de novo and inherited apparently balanced chromosomal rearrangements: Array CGH study of 47 unrelated cases. *Eur J Med Genet* 52: 291–296, 2009.

Schluth-Bolard C, Sanlaville D, Labalme A, et al. 17p13.1 microdeletion involving the *TP53* gene in a boy presenting with mental retardation but no tumor. *Am J Med Genet* 152A: 1278–1282, 2010.

Schluth-Bolard C, Till M, Rafat A, et al. Monosomy 19pter and trisomy 19q13-qter in two siblings arising from a maternal pericentric inversion: Clinical data and molecular characterization. *Eur J Med Genet* 51: 622–630, 2008.

Schmiady H, Neitzel H. Arrest of human oocytes during meiosis I in two sisters of consanguineous parents: First evidence for an autosomal recessive trait in human infertility: Case report. *Hum Reprod* 17: 2556–2559, 2002.

Schmickel RD. Contiguous gene syndromes: A component of recognizable syndromes. *J Pediatr* 109: 231–241, 1986.

Schmidt M, Du Sart D. Functional disomies of the X chromosome influence the cell selection and hence the X inactivation pattern in females with balanced X-autosome translocations: A review of 122 cases. *Am J Med Genet* 42: 161–169, 1992.

Schmidt T, Bartels I, Liehr T, Burfeind P, Zoll B, Shoukier M. A family with an inverted tandem duplication 5q22.1q23.2. *Cytogenet Genome Res* 139: 65–70, 2013

Schmidt T, Bierhals T, Kortüm F, et al. Branchio-otic syndrome caused by a genomic rearrangement: Clinical findings and molecular cytogenetic studies in a patient with a pericentric inversion of chromosome 8. *Cytogenet Genome Res* 142: 1–6, 2014.

Schmitt-Ney M, Thiele H, Kaltwasser P, Bardoni B, Cisternino M, Scherer G. Two novel *SRY* missense mutations reducing DNA binding identified in XY females and their mosaic fathers. *Am J Hum Genet* 56: 862–869, 1995.

Schmitz D, Henn W, Netzer C. Commentary: No risk, no objections? Ethical pitfalls of cell-free fetal DNA and RNA testing. *Br Med J* 339: b2690, 2009.

Schmutz SM, Pinno E. Morphology alone does not make an isochromosome. *Hum Genet* 72: 253–255, 1986.

Schneider M, Forrester S, Crain V, Kimonis V. A further case of coincidental Prader-Willi and Klinefelter syndromes. *Am J Med Genet* 126A: 213–214, 2004.

Scholz NB, Bolund L, Nyegaard M, et al. Triploidy—Observations in 154 diandric cases. *PLoS One* 10: e0142545, 2015.

Schönewolf-Greulich B, Ravn K, Hamborg-Petersen B, Brøndum-Nielsen K, Tümer Z. Segregation of a 4p16.3 duplication with a characteristic appearance, macrocephaly, speech delay and mild intellectual disability in a 3-generation family. *Am J Med Genet* 161A: 2358–2362, 2013.

Schönherr N, Meyer E, Roos A, Schmidt A, Wollmann HA, Eggermann T. The centromeric 11p15 imprinting centre is also involved in Silver-Russell syndrome. *J Med Genet* 44: 59–63, 2007.

Schoolcraft WB, Keller JL, Schlenker T. Excellent embryo quality obtained from vitrified oocytes. *Reprod Biomed Online* 19: 820–823, 2009.

Schorderet DF, Friedman C, Disteche CM. Pericentric inversion of the X chromosome: Presentation of a case and review of the literature. *Ann Génét* 34: 98–103, 1991.

Schouten JP, McElgunn CJ, Waaijer R, Zwijnenburg D, Diepvens F, Pals G. Relative quantification of 40 nucleic acid sequences by multiplex ligation-dependent probe amplification. *Nucleic Acids Res* 30: e57, 2002.

Schramm C, Draaken M, Bartels E, et al. De novo duplication of 18p11.21-18q12.1 in a female with anorectal malformation. *Am J Med Genet* 155A: 445–449, 2011.

Schull WJ, Neel JV. Maternal radiation and mongolism. *Lancet* 279: 537–538, 1962.

Schultz BAH, Roberts S, Rodgers A, Ataya K. Pregnancy in true hermaphrodites and all male offspring to date. *Obstet Gynecol* 113: 534–536, 2009.

Schulz S, Gerloff C, Ledig S, et al. Prenatal diagnosis of Roberts syndrome and detection of an *ESCO2* frameshift mutation in a Pakistani family. *Prenat Diagn* 28: 42–45, 2008.

Schwaibold EM, Zoll B, Burfeind P, et al. A 3p interstitial deletion in two monozygotic twin brothers and an 18-year-old man: Further characterization and review. *Am J Med Genet* 161A: 2634–2640, 2013.

Schwartz S, Raffel LJ. Prenatal detection of 45,X/46,XX/47,XXX mosaicism through amniocentesis: Mosaicism confirmed in cord blood, amnion, and chorion. *Prenat Diagn* 12: 1043–1046, 1992.

Schwarzbraun T, Obenauf AC, Langmann A, et al. Predictive diagnosis of the cancer prone Li-Fraumeni syndrome by accident: New challenges through whole genome array testing. *J Med Genet* 46: 341–344, 2009.

Schwendemann WD, Contag SA, Wax JR, et al. Sonographic findings in trisomy 9. *J Ultrasound Med* 28: 39–42, 2009.

Schwinger E, Mikkelsen M, Niesen M. Familial balanced (7;11;21) translocation and Down's syndrome in two siblings. *Clin Genet* 7: 304–307, 1975.

Scott JA, Wenger SL, Steele MW, Chakravarti A. Down syndrome consequent to a cryptic maternal 12p;21q chromosome translocation. *Am J Med Genet* 56: 67–71, 1995.

Scott KL, Hong KH, Scott RT. Selecting the optimal time to perform biopsy for preimplantation genetic testing. *Fertil Steril* 100: 608–614, 2013a.

Scott RH, Douglas J, Baskcomb L, et al. Constitutional 11p15 abnormalities, including heritable imprinting center mutations, cause nonsyndromic Wilms tumor. *Nat Genet* 40: 1329–1334, 2008a.

Scott RH, Douglas J, Baskcomb L, et al. Methylation-specific MLPA (MS-MLPA) robustly detects and distinguishes 11p15 abnormalities associated with overgrowth and growth retardation. *J Med Genet* 45: 106–113, 2008b.

Scott RT, Ferry K, Su J, Tao X, Scott K, Treff NR. Comprehensive chromosome screening is highly predictive of the reproductive potential of human embryos: A prospective, blinded, nonselection study. *Fertil Steril* 97: 870–875, 2012.

Scott RT, Galliano D. The challenge of embryonic mosaicism in preimplantation genetic screening. *Fertil Steril* 105: 1150–1152, 2016.

Scott RT, Upham KM, Forman EJ, et al. Blastocyst biopsy with comprehensive chromosome screening and fresh embryo transfer significantly increases in vitro fertilization implantation and delivery rates: A randomized controlled trial. *Fertil Steril* 100: 697–703, 2013b.

Scott RT, Upham KM, Forman EJ, Zhao T, Treff NR. Cleavage-stage biopsy significantly impairs human embryonic implantation potential while blastocyst biopsy does not: A randomized and paired clinical trial. *Fertil Steril* 100: 624–630, 2013c.

Scott Schwoerer J, Laffin J, Haun J, Raca G, Friez MJ, Giampietro PF. *MECP2* duplication: Possible cause of severe phenotype in females. *Am J Med Genet* 164A: 1029–1034, 2014.

Scriven PN. X;autosome translocations do not follow the normal rules and more caution is advised for PGD. *Hum Reprod Online* November 2013, in response to Van Echten-Arends et al., Preimplantation genetic diagnosis for X; autosome translocations: Lessons from a case of misdiagnosis. *Hum Reprod* 28: 3141–3145, 2013.

Scriven PN, Bint SM, Davies AF, Ogilvie CM. Meiotic outcomes of three-way translocations ascertained in cleavage-stage embryos: Refinement of reproductive risks and implications for PGD. *Eur J Hum Genet* 22: 748–753, 2014.

Scriven PN, Flinter FA, Khalaf Y, Lashwood A, Mackie Ogilvie C. Benefits and drawbacks of preimplantation genetic diagnosis (PGD) for reciprocal translocations: Lessons from a prospective cohort study. *Eur J Hum Genet* 21: 1035–1041, 2013.

Scriven PN, Handyside AH, Mackie Ogilvie C. Chromosome translocations: Segregation modes and strategies for preimplantation genetic diagnosis. *Prenat Diagn* 18: 1437–1449, 1998.

Searle CJ, Smith K, Daniels G, Maher EJ, Quarrell O. Cell-free fetal DNA sex determination identified a maternal *SRY* gene with a known X chromosome deletion. *Prenat Diagn* 33: 612–613, 2013.

Sebire NJ, Lindsay I. p57^KIP2 immunostaining in the diagnosis of complete versus partial hydatidiform moles. *Histopathology* 48: 873–874, 2006.

Sebire NJ, May PC, Kaur B, Seckl MJ, Fisher RA. Abnormal villous morphology mimicking a hydatidiform mole associated with paternal trisomy of chromosomes 3,7,8 and unipaternal disomy of chromosome 11. *Diagn Pathol* 11: 20, 2016.

Sebire NJ, Snijders RJ, Santiago C, Papapanagiotou G, Nicolaides KH. Management of twin pregnancies with fetal trisomies. *Br J Obstet Gynaecol* 104: 220–222, 1997.

Sebold C, Roeder E, Zimmerman M, et al. Tetrasomy 18p: Report of the molecular and clinical findings of 43 individuals. *Am J Med Genet* 152A: 2164–2172, 2010.

Sebold C, Soileau B, Heard P, et al. Whole arm deletions of 18p: Medical and developmental effects. *Am J Med Genet* 167A: 313–323, 2015.

Seckl MJ, Fisher RA, Salerno G, et al. Choriocarcinoma and partial hydatidiform moles. *Lancet* 356: 36–39, 2000.

Seeherunvong T, Perera EM, Bao Y, et al. 46,XX sex reversal with partial duplication of chromosome arm 22q. *Am J Med Genet* 127A: 149–151, 2004.

Seemanová E, Sperling K, Neitzel H, et al. Nijmegen breakage syndrome (NBS) with neurological abnormalities and without chromosomal instability. *J Med Genet* 43: 218–224, 2006.

Seghezzi L, Maserati E, Minelli A, et al. Constitutional trisomy 8 as first mutation in multistep carcinogenesis: Clinical, cytogenetic, and molecular data on three cases. *Genes Chromosomes Cancer* 17: 94–101, 1996.

Seidel J, Schiller S, Kelbova C, et al. Brachytelephalangic dwarfism due to the loss of *ARSE* and *SHOX* genes resulting from an X;Y translocation. *Clin Genet* 59: 115–121, 2001.

Seller MJ, Mazzaschi R, Ogilvie CM, Mohammed S. A trisomy 2 fetus with severe neural tube defects and other abnormalities. *Clin Dysmorphol* 13: 25–27, 2004.

Seppänen VI, Artama MS, Malila NK, et al. Risk for congenital anomalies in offspring of childhood, adolescent and young adult cancer survivors. *Int J Cancer* 139: 1721–1730, 2016.

Sepulveda W, Be C, Youlton R, Carstens E, Reyes M. Nuchal translucency thickness and outcome in chromosome translocation diagnosed in the first trimester. *Prenat Diagn* 21: 726–728, 2001.

Severino M, Accogli A, Gimelli G, et al. Clinico-radiological and molecular characterization of a child with ring chromosome 2 presenting growth failure, microcephaly, kidney and brain malformations. *Mol Cytogenet* 8: 17, 2015.

Sgardioli IC, Simioni M, Viguetti-Campos NL, Prota JR, Gil-da-Silva-Lopes VL. A new case of partial 14q31.3-qter trisomy due to maternal pericentric inversion. *Gene* 523: 192–194, 2013.

Shaaya EA, Pollack SF, Boronat S, Davis-Cooper S, Zella GC, Thibert RL. Gastrointestinal problems in 15q duplication syndrome. *Eur J Med Genet* 58: 191–193, 2015.

Shaffer BL, Caughey AB, Norton ME. Variation in the decision to terminate pregnancy in the setting of fetal aneuploidy. *Prenat Diagn* 26: 667–671, 2006.

Shaffer LG. Risk estimates for uniparental disomy following prenatal detection of a nonhomologous Robertsonian translocation. *Prenat Diagn* 26: 303–307, 2006.

Shaffer LG, Bui TH. Molecular cytogenetic and rapid aneuploidy detection methods in prenatal diagnosis. *Am J Med Genet* 145C: 87–98, 2007.

Shaffer LG, Coppinger J, Alliman S, et al. Comparison of microarray-based detection rates for cytogenetic abnormalities in prenatal and neonatal specimens. *Prenat Diagn* 28: 789–795, 2008.

Shaffer LG, Dabell MP, Fisher AJ, et al. Experience with microarray-based comparative genomic hybridization for prenatal diagnosis in over 5000 pregnancies. *Prenat Diagn* 32: 976–985, 2012.

Shaffer LG, Hecht JT, Ledbetter DH, Greenberg F. Familial interstitial deletion 11(p11.12p12) associated with parietal foramina, brachymicrocephaly, and mental retardation. *Am J Med Genet* 45: 581–583, 1993.

Shaffer LG, Jackson-Cook CK, Meyer JM, Brown JA, Spence JE. A molecular genetic approach to the identification of isochromosomes of chromosome 21. *Hum Genet* 86: 375–382, 1991.

Shaffer LG, McCaskill C, Adkins K, Hassold TJ. Systematic search for uniparental disomy in early fetal losses: The results and a review of the literature. *Am J Med Genet* 79: 366–372, 1998.

Shaffer LG, McCaskill C, Egli CA, Baker JC, Johnston KM. Is there an abnormal phenotype associated with maternal isodisomy for chromosome 2 in the presence of two isochromosomes? *Am J Hum Genet* 61: 461–462, 1997.

Shahwan A, Green AJ, Carey A, Stallings RL, O'Flaherty OC, King MD. Malignant refractory epilepsy in identical twins mosaic for a supernumerary ring chromosome 19. *Epilepsia* 45: 997–1000, 2004.

Shalev E, Zalel Y, Weiner E, Cohen H, Shneur Y. The role of cordocentesis in assessment of mosaicism found in amniotic fluid cell culture. *Acta Obstet Gynecol Scand* 73: 119–122, 1994.

Shamonki MI, Jin H, Haimowitz Z, Liu L. Proof of concept: Preimplantation genetic screening without embryo biopsy through analysis of cell-free DNA in spent embryo culture media. *Fertil Steril* 106: 1312–1318, 2016.

Shanske A, Ellison J, Vuguin P, et al. Deletion of the pseudoautosomal region in a male with a unique Y;13 translocation and short stature. *Am J Med Genet* 82: 34–39, 1999.

Shanske AL, Leonard J, Nahum O, Coppock DL, Levy B. Delineation of the breakpoints of pure duplication 3q due to a de novo duplication event using SOMA. *Am J Med Genet* 152A: 3185–3188, 2010.

Shapira SK, McCaskill C, Northrup H, et al. Chromosome 1p36 deletions: The clinical phenotype and molecular characterization of a common newly delineated syndrome. *Am J Hum Genet* 61: 642–650, 1997.

Shapiro BL. Whither Down syndrome critical regions? *Hum Genet* 99: 421–423, 1997.

Sharp A, Kusz K, Jaruzelska J, Szarras-Czapnik M, Wolski J, Jacobs P. Familial X/Y translocations associated with variable sexual phenotype. *J Med Genet* 41: 440–444, 2004.

Sharp A, Robinson D, Jacobs P. Age- and tissue-specific variation of X chromosome inactivation ratios in normal women. *Hum Genet* 107: 343–349, 2000.

Shashi V, Golden WL, Allinson PS, Blanton SH, von Kap-Herr C, Kelly TE. Molecular analysis of recombination in a family with Duchenne muscular dystrophy and a large pericentric X chromosome inversion. *Am J Hum Genet* 58: 1231–1238, 1996.

Sheath KL, Asquith PM, Zhang L, Aftimos S. Prenatal diagnosis of trisomy 3 mosaicism in a fetus with severe IUGR. *Prenat Diagn* 30: 803–805, 2010.

Sherard J, Bean C, Bove B, et al. Long survival in a 69,XXY triploid male. *Am J Med Genet* 25: 307–312, 1986.

Sheridan MB, Kato T, Haldeman-Englert C, et al. A palindrome-mediated recurrent translocation with 3:1 meiotic nondisjunction: The t(8;22)(q24.13;q11.21). *Am J Hum Genet* 87: 209–218, 2010.

Sherman SL, Iselius L, Gallano P, et al. Segregation analysis of balanced pericentric inversions in pedigree data. *Clin Genet* 30: 87–94, 1986.

Sherman SL, Petersen MB, Freeman SB, et al. Non-disjunction of chromosome 21 in maternal meiosis I: Evidence for a maternal age-dependent mechanism involving reduced recombination. *Hum Mol Genet* 3: 1529–1535, 1994.

Sheth J, Joshi R, Sheth F. Ring chromosome 9 in a dysmorphic child. *Indian J Pediatr* 74: 507–508, 2007.

Shi Q, Ko E, Barclay L, Hoang T, Rademaker A, Martin R. Cigarette smoking and aneuploidy in human sperm. *Mol Reprod Dev* 59: 417–421, 2001.

Shi Q, Martin RH. Spontaneous frequencies of aneuploid and diploid sperm in 10 normal Chinese men: Assessed by multicolor fluorescence in situ hybridization. *Cytogenet Cell Genet* 90: 79–83, 2000a.

Shi Q, Martin RH. Aneuploidy in human sperm: A review of the frequency and distribution of aneuploidy, effects of donor age and lifestyle factors. *Cytogenet Cell Genet* 90: 219–226, 2000b.

Shi Q, Martin RH. Aneuploidy in human spermatozoa: FISH analysis in men with constitutional chromosomal abnormalities, and in infertile men. *Reproduction* 121: 655–666, 2001.

Shi Q, Spriggs E, Field LL, et al. Absence of age effect on meiotic recombination between human X and Y chromosomes. *Am J Hum Genet* 71: 254–261, 2002.

Shim SH, Lee CH, Lee JY, et al. A de novo centric fission of chromosome 11 in a patient with recurrent miscarriages. *J Korean Med Sci* 22: 146–148, 2007.

Shimada S, Maegaki Y, Osawa M, Yamamoto T. Mild developmental delay and obesity in two patients with mosaic 1p36 deletion syndrome. *Am J Med Genet* 164A: 415–420, 2014.

Shimada S, Okamoto N, Hirasawa K, et al. Clinical manifestations of Xq28 functional disomy involving *MECP2* in one female and two male patients. *Am J Med Genet* 161A: 1779–1785, 2013.

Shimojima K, Okamoto N, Tamasaki A, Sangu N, Shimada S, Yamamoto T. An association of 19p13.2 microdeletions with Malan syndrome and Chiari malformation. *Am J Med Genet* 167A: 724–30, 2015.

Shimokawa O, Kurosawa K, Ida T, et al. Molecular characterization of inv dup del(8p): Analysis of five cases. *Am J Med Genet* 128A: 133–137, 2004.

Shinawi M, Liu P, Kang SH, et al. Recurrent reciprocal 16p11.2 rearrangements associated with global developmental delay, behavioural problems, dysmorphism, epilepsy, and abnormal head size. *J Med Genet* 47: 332–341, 2010.

Shiohama T, Fujii K, Hino M, et al. Coexistence of neuroblastoma and ganglioneuroma in a girl with a hemizygous deletion of chromosome 11q14.1-23.3. *Am J Med Genet* 170A: 492–497, 2016.

Shirai K, Higashi Y, Shimojima K, Yamamoto T. An Xq22.1q22.2 nullisomy in a male patient with severe neurological impairment. *Am J Med Genet* 173A: 1124–1127, 2017.

Shobha Rani A, Jyothi A, Reddy PP, Reddy OS. Reproduction in Down's syndrome. *Int J Gynaecol Obstet* 31: 81–86, 1990.

Shohat M, Legum C, Romem Y, Borochowitz Z, Bach G, Goldman B. Down syndrome prevention program in a population with an older maternal age. *Obstet Gynecol* 85: 368–373, 1995.

Shoukier M, Wickert J, Schröder J, et al. A 16q12 microdeletion in a boy with severe psychomotor delay, craniofacial dysmorphism, brain and limb malformations, and a heart defect. *Am J Med Genet* 158A: 229–235, 2012.

Shuib S, McMullan D, Rattenberry E, et al. Microarray based analysis of 3p25-p26 deletions (3p-syndrome). *Am J Med Genet* 149A: 2099–2105, 2009.

Shuster E. Microarray genetic screening: A prenatal roadblock for life? *Lancet* 369: 526–529, 2007.

Shuttleworth GE. Mongolian imbecility. *Br Med J* 2: 661–665, 1909.

Sifakis S, Eleftheriades M, Kappou D, et al. Prenatal diagnosis of proximal partial trisomy 1q confirmed by comparative genomic hybridization array: Molecular cytogenetic analysis, fetal pathology and review of the literature. *Birth Defects Res A Clin Mol Teratol* 100: 284–293, 2014.

Sifakis S, Karkaletsi M, Christopoulou S, et al. Distinctive pattern of first trimester maternal serum biochemical markers in trisomy 22 pregnancies. *Prenat Diagn* 28: 1174–1176, 2008.

Siggberg L, Ala-Mello S, Jaakkola E, et al. Array CGH in molecular diagnosis of mental retardation—A study of 150 Finnish patients. *Am J Med Genet* 152A: 1398–1410, 2010.

Signorello LB, Mulvihill JJ, Green DM, et al. Congenital anomalies in the children of cancer survivors: A report from the childhood cancer survivor study. *J Clin Oncol* 30: 239–245, 2012.

Sigurdardottir S, Goodman BK, Rutberg J, Thomas GH, Jabs EW, Geraghty MT. Clinical, cytogenetic, and fluorescence in situ hybridization findings in two cases of "complete ring" syndrome. *Am J Med Genet* 87: 384–390, 1999.

Sigurdson AJ, Bhatti P, Preston DL, et al. Routine diagnostic X-ray examinations and increased frequency of chromosome translocations among U.S. radiologic technologists. *Cancer Res* 68: 8825–8831, 2008.

Sijmons RH, Leegte B, van Lingen RA, et al. Tetrasomy 5p mosaicism in a boy with delayed growth, hypotonia, minor anomalies, and an additional isochromosome 5p [46,XY/47,XY, + i(5p)]. *Am J Med Genet* 47: 559–562, 1993.

Sikkema-Raddatz B, Bouman K, Verschuuren-Bemelmans CC, de Jong B. Trisomy 12 mosaicism in CVS culture confirmed in the fetus. *Prenat Diagn* 19: 1176–1177, 1999.

Sikkema-Raddatz B, Castedo S, Te Meerman GJ. Probability tables for exclusion of mosaicism in prenatal diagnosis. *Prenat Diagn* 17: 115–118, 1997a.

Sikkema-Raddatz B, Verschuuren-Bemelmans CC, Kloosterman M, de Jong B. A 46,XX,der(13;14) (q10;q10),+21 child born after a 45,XX,der(13;14)(q10;q10) chromosomal finding in CVS. *Prenat Diagn* 17: 1086–1088, 1997b.

Silber S, Escudero T, Lenahan K, Abdelhadi I, Kilani Z, Munné S. Chromosomal abnormalities in embryos derived from testicular sperm extraction. *Fertil Steril* 79: 30–38, 2003.

Silverstein S, Lerer I, Sagi M, Frumkin A, Ben-Neriah Z, Abeliovich D. Uniparental disomy in fetuses diagnosed with balanced Robertsonian translocations: Risk estimate. *Prenat Diagn* 22: 649–651, 2002.

Sim JC, White SM, Lockhart PJ. *ARID1B*-mediated disorders: Mutations and possible mechanisms. *Intractable Rare Dis Res* 4: 17–23, 2015.

Singh PP, Arora J, Isambert H. Identification of ohnolog genes originating from whole genome duplication in early vertebrates, based on synteny comparison across multiple genomes. *PLoS Comput Biol* 11: e1004394, 2015.

Singh R, Gardner RJM, Crossland KM, Scheffer IE, Berkovic SF. Chromosomal abnormalities and epilepsy: A review for clinicians and gene hunters. *Epilepsia* 43: 127–140, 2002a.

Singh S, Aftimos S, George A, Love DR. Interstitial deletion of 10q23.1 and confirmation of three 10qdel syndromes. *Singapore Med* J 52:e143–46, 2011.

Singh SM, Murphy B, O'Reilly R. Monozygotic twins with chromosome 22q11 deletion and discordant phenotypes: Updates with an epigenetic hypothesis. *J Med Genet* 39:e71, 2002b.

Sinnerbrink IB, Sherwen A, Meiser B, et al. Long-term health and development of children diagnosed prenatally with a de novo apparently balanced chromosomal rearrangement. *Prenat Diagn* 33: 831–838, 2013.

Šípek A, Panczak A, Mihalová R, et al. Pericentric inversion of human chromosome 9 epidemiology study in Czech males and females. *Folia Biol (Praha)* 61: 140–146, 2015.

Sirchia SM, Garagiola I, Colucci G, et al. Trisomic zygote rescue revealed by DNA polymorphism analysis in confined placental mosaicism. *Prenat Diagn* 18: 201–206, 1998.

Sismani C, Anastasiadou V, Kousoulidou L, et al. 9 Mb familial duplication in chromosome band Xp22.2-22.13 associated with mental retardation, hypotonia and developmental delay, scoliosis, cardiovascular problems and mild dysmorphic facial features. *Eur J Med Genet* 54: e510–515, 2011.

Sivak LE, Esbenshade J, Brothman AR, Issa B, Lemons RS, Carey JC. Multiple congenital anomalies in a man with (X;6) translocation. *Am J Med Genet* 51: 9–12, 1994.

Skakkebæk NE, Giwercman A, de Kretser D. Pathogenesis and management of male infertility. *Lancet* 343: 1473–1479, 1994.

Sklower Brooks SS, Genovese M, Gu H, Duncan CJ, Shanske A, Jenkins EC. Normal adaptive function with learning disability in duplication 8p including band p22. *Am J Med Genet* 78: 114–117, 1998.

Skotko BG, Kishnani PS, Capone GT. Prenatal diagnosis of Down syndrome: How best to deliver the news. *Am J Med Genet* 149A: 2361–2367, 2009.

Skraban CM, Wells CF, Markose P, et al. *WDR26* haploinsufficiency causes a recognizable syndrome of intellectual disability, seizures, abnormal gait, and distinctive facial features. *Am J Hum Genet* 101: 139–148, 2017.

Skuse DH, James RS, Bishop DVM, et al. Evidence from Turner's syndrome of an imprinted X-linked locus affecting cognitive function. *Nature* 387: 705–708, 1997.

Slaney SF, Chalmers IJ, Affara NA, Chitty LS. An autosomal or X linked mutation results in true hermaphrodites and 46,XX males in the same family. *J Med Genet* 35: 17–22, 1998.

Slater H, Shaw JH, Bankier A, Forrest SM, Dawson G. UPD 13: No indication of maternal or paternal imprinting of genes on chromosome 13. *J Med Genet* 32: 493, 1995.

Slater H, Shaw JH, Dawson G, Bankier A, Forrest SM. Maternal uniparental disomy of chromosome 13 in a phenotypically normal child. *J Med Genet* 31: 644–646, 1994.

Slater HR, Nouri S, Earle E, Lo AW, Hale LG, Choo KHA. Neocentromere formation in a stable ring 1p32-p36.1 chromosome. *J Med Genet* 36: 914–918, 1999.

Slater HR, Ralph A, Daniel A, Worthington S, Roberts C. A case of maternal uniparental disomy of chromosome 9 diagnosed prenatally and the related problem of residual trisomy. *Prenat Diagn* 20: 930–932, 2000.

Slavotinek A, Gaunt L, Donnai D. Paternally inherited duplications of 11p15.5 and Beckwith-Wiedemann syndrome. *J Med Genet* 34: 819–826, 1997.

Slim R, Ao A, Surti U, et al. Recurrent triploid and dispermic conceptions in patients with *NLRP7* mutations. *Placenta* 32: 409–412, 2011.

Slim R, Mehio A. The genetics of hydatidiform moles: New lights on an ancient disease. *Clin Genet* 71: 25–34, 2007.

Sloter E, Nath J, Eskenazi B, Wyrobek AJ. Effects of male age on the frequencies of germinal and heritable chromosomal abnormalities in humans and rodents. *Fertil Steril* 81: 925–943, 2004.

Smeets DFCM, Hamel BCJ, Nelen MR, et al. Prader-Willi syndrome and Angelman syndrome in cousins from a family with a translocation between chromosomes 6 and 15. *N Engl J Med* 326: 807–811, 1992.

Smigiel R, Marcelis C, Patkowski D, et al. Oesophageal atresia with tracheoesophageal fistula and anal atresia in a patient with a de novo microduplication in 17q12. *Eur J Med Genet* 57: 40–43, 2014.

Smith A, Deng ZM, Beran R, Woodage T, Trent RJ. Familial unbalanced translocation t(8;15) (p23.3;q11) with uniparental disomy in Angelman syndrome. *Hum Genet* 93: 471–473, 1994.

Smith A, Robson L. Low frequency of inherited deletions of 22q11. *Am J Med Genet* 85: 513–514, 1999.

Smith A, Watt AJ, Cummins M, Gardner RJM, Wilson M. A small one-band paracentric inversion inv (4) (p15.3p16.3). *Ann Génét* 35: 161–163, 1992.

Smith ACM, Spuhler K, Williams TM, McConnell T, Sujansky E, Robinson A. Genetic risk for recombinant 8 syndrome and the transmission rate of balanced inversion 8 in the Hispanic population of the southwestern United States. *Am J Hum Genet* 41: 1083–1103, 1987.

Smith AW, Holden KR, Dwivedi A, Dupont BR, Lyons MJ. Deletion of 16q24.1 supports a role for the *ATP2C2* gene in specific language impairment. *J Child Neurol* 30: 517–521, 2015.

Smith K, Lowther G, Maher E, Hourihan T, Wilkinson T, Wolstenholme J. The predictive value of findings of the common aneuploidies, trisomies 13, 18 and 21, and numerical sex chromosome abnormalities at CVS: Experience from the ACC U.K. collaborative study. *Prenat Diagn* 19: 817–826, 1999.

Smith MJ, Creasy MR, Clarke A, Upadhyaya M. Sex ratio and absence of uniparental disomy in spontaneous abortions with a normal karyotype. *Clin Genet* 53: 258–261, 1998.

Smrcek JM, Germer U, Krokowski M, et al. Prenatal ultrasound diagnosis and management of body stalk anomaly: Analysis of nine singleton and two multiple pregnancies. *Ultrasound Obstet Gynecol* 21: 322–328, 2003.

Snape K, Hanks S, Ruark E, et multi al. Mutations in *CEP57* cause mosaic variegated aneuploidy syndrome. *Nat Genet* 43: 527–529, 2011.

Snijders AM, Nowak N, Segraves R, et al. Assembly of microarrays for genome-wide measurement of DNA copy number. *Nat Genet* 29: 263–264, 2001.

Snijders RJM, Sebire NJ, Nicolaides KH. Maternal age and gestational age-specific risk for chromosomal defects. *Fetal Diagn Ther* 10: 356–367, 1995.

Snijders RJM, Sundberg K, Holzgreve W, Henry G, Nicolaides KH. Maternal age- and gestation-specific risk for trisomy 21. *Ultrasound Obstet Gynecol* 13: 167–170, 1999.

Soares SR, Templado C, Blanco J, Egozcue J, Vidal F. Numerical chromosome abnormalities in the spermatozoa of the fathers of children with trisomy 21 of paternal origin: Generalised tendency to meiotic non-disjunction. *Hum Genet* 108: 134–139, 2001a.

Soares SR, Vidal F, Bosch M, et al. Acrocentric chromosome disomy is increased in spermatozoa from fathers of Turner syndrome patients. *Hum Genet* 108: 499–503, 2001b.

Soblet J, Dimov I, Graf von Kalckreuth C, et al. *BCL11A* frameshift mutation associated with dyspraxia and hypotonia affecting the fine, gross, oral, and speech motor systems. *Am J Med Genet* 176A: 201–208, 2018.

Sobotka V, Vozdova M, Heracek J, Rubes J. A rare Robertsonian translocation rob(14;22) carrier with azoospermia, meiotic defects, and testicular sperm aneuploidy. *Syst Biol Reprod Med* 61: 245–250, 2015.

Sodré CP, Guilherme RS, Meloni VF, et al. Ring chromosome instability evaluation in six patients with autosomal rings. *Genet Mol Res* 9: 134–143, 2010.

Soemedi R, Topf A, Wilson IJ, et al. Phenotype-specific effect of chromosome 1q21.1 rearrangements and GJA5 duplications in 2436 congenital heart disease patients and 6760 controls. *Hum Mol Genet* 21: 1513–1520, 2012.

Sohn YB, Lee CG, Ko JM, et al. Clinical and genetic spectrum of 18 unrelated Korean patients with Sotos syndrome: Frequent 5q35 microdeletion and identification of four novel *NSD1* mutations. *J Hum Genet* 58: 73–77, 2013.

Solé M, Blanco J, Valero O, Vergés L, Vidal F, Sarrate Z. Altered bivalent positioning in metaphase I human spermatocytes from Robertsonian translocation carriers. *J Assist Reprod Genet* 34: 131–138, 2017.

Soler A, Badenas C, Margarit E, et al. A 92,XXXY miscarriage consecutive to a digynic triploid pregnancy. *Cytogenet Genome Res* 149: 258–261, 2016.

Soler A, Margarit E, Queralt R, et al. Paternal isodisomy 13 in a normal newborn infant after trisomy rescue evidenced by prenatal diagnosis. *Am J Med Genet* 90: 291–293, 2000.

Soler A, Salami C, Balmes I, et al. Pericentric X chromosome in a family. *Clin Genet* 20: 234–235, 1981.

Soler A, Sánchez A, Carrió A, et al. Recombination in a male carrier of two reciprocal translocations involving chromosomes 14, 14′, 15, and 21 leading to balanced and unbalanced rearrangements in offspring. *Am J Med Genet* 134A: 309–314, 2005.

Somers CM, Cooper DN. Air pollution and mutations in the germline: Are humans at risk? *Hum Genet* 125: 119–130, 2009.

Somprasit C, Aguinaga M, Cisneros PL, et al. Paternal gonadal mosaicism detected in a couple with recurrent abortions undergoing PGD: FISH analysis of sperm nuclei proves valuable. *Reprod Biomed Online* 9: 225–230, 2004.

Song J, Li X, Sun L, et al. A family with Robertsonian translocation: A potential mechanism of speciation in humans. *Mol Cytogenet* 9: 48, 2016.

Sosoi S, Streata I, Tudorache S, et al. Prenatal and postnatal findings in a 10.6 Mb interstitial deletion at 10p11.22-p12.31. *J Hum Genet* 60: 183–185, 2015.

Souka AP, Von Kaisenberg CS, Hyett JA, Sonek JD, Nicolaides KH. Increased nuchal translucency with normal karyotype. *Am J Obstet Gynecol* 192: 1005–1021, 2005.

South ST, Lamb AN. Detecting genomic imbalances in prenatal diagnosis: Main hurdles and recent advances. *Expert Opin Med Diagn* 3: 227–235, 2009.

South ST, Rope AF, Lamb AN, et al. Expansion in size of a terminal deletion: A paradigm shift for parental follow-up studies. *J Med Genet* 45: 391–395, 2008a.

South ST, Swensen JJ, Maxwell T, Rope A, Brothman AR, Chen Z. A new genomic mechanism leading to cri-du-chat syndrome. *Am J Med Genet* 140: 2714–2720, 2006.

South ST, Whitby H, Maxwell T, Aston E, Brothman AR, Carey JC. Co-occurrence of 4p16.3 deletions with both paternal and maternal duplications of 11p15: Modification of the Wolf-Hirschhorn syndrome phenotype by genetic alterations predicted to result in either a Beckwith-Wiedemann or Russell-Silver phenotype. *Am J Med Genet* 146A: 2691–2697, 2008b.

Sowińska-Seidler A, Socha M, Jamsheer A. Split-hand/foot malformation—Molecular cause and implications in genetic counseling. *J Appl Genet* 55: 105–115, 2014.

Sparago A, Cerrato F, Vernucci M, Ferrero GB, Silengo MC, Riccio A. Microdeletions in the human *H19* DMR result in loss of *IGF2* imprinting and Beckwith-Wiedemann syndrome. *Nat Genet* 36: 958–960, 2004.

Sparkes RL, Shetty S, Chernos JE, Mefford HC, Micheil Innes A. Interstitial deletion of 11q in a mother and fetus: Implications of directly transmitted chromosomal imbalances for prenatal genetic counseling. *Prenat Diagn* 29: 283–286, 2009.

Spazzapan P, Arnaud E, Baujat G, et al. Clinical and neuroradiological features of the 9p deletion syndrome. *Childs Nerv Syst* 32: 327–335, 2016.

Speed RM. Meiotic configurations in female trisomy 21 foetuses. *Hum Genet* 66: 176–180, 1984.

Speevak MD, Farrell SA. Charcot-Marie-Tooth 1B caused by expansion of a familial myelin protein zero (MPZ) gene duplication. *Eur J Med Genet* 56: 566–569, 2013.

Speevak MD, Farrell SA, Chadwick D. Molecular and cytogenetic characterization of a prenatally ascertained de novo (X;Y) translocation. *Am J Med Genet* 98: 107–108, 2001.

Speevak MD, Smart C, Unwin L, Bell M, Farrell SA. Molecular characterization of an inherited ring (19) demonstrating ring opening. *Am J Med Genet* 121A: 141–145, 2003.

Spena S, Duga S, Asselta R, et al. Congenital afibrinogenaemia caused by uniparental isodisomy of chromosome 4 containing a novel 15-kb deletion involving fibrinogen Aalpha-chain gene. *Eur J Hum Genet* 12: 891–898, 2004.

Spencer K. What is the true fetal loss rate in pregnancies affected by trisomy 21 and how does this influence whether first trimester detection rates are superior to those in the second trimester? *Prenat Diagn* 21: 788–789, 2001.

Spencer K. Aneuploidy screening in the first trimester. *Am J Med Genet* 145C: 18–32, 2007.

Spencer K, Kagan KO, Nicolaides KH. Screening for trisomy 21 in twin pregnancies in the first trimester: An update of the impact of chorionicity on maternal serum markers. *Prenat Diagn* 28: 49–52, 2008.

Spencer K, Pertile MD, Bonacquisto L, et al. First trimester detection of trisomy 16 using combined biochemical and ultrasound screening. *Prenat Diagn* 34: 291–295, 2014.

Spencer K, Staboulidou I, Nicolaides KH. First trimester aneuploidy screening in the presence of a vanishing twin: Implications for maternal serum markers. *Prenat Diagn* 30: 235–240, 2010.

Spinner NB, Saitta SC, Delaney DP, et al. Intracytoplasmic sperm injection (ICSI) with transmission of a ring(Y) chromosome and ovotesticular disorder of sex development in offspring. *Am J Med Genet* 146A: 1828–1831, 2008.

Spittel H, Kubek F, Kreskowski K, et al. Mitotic stability of small supernumerary marker chromosomes: A study based on 93 immortalized cell lines. *Cytogenet Genome Res* 142: 151–160, 2014.

Srebniak MI, Diderich KE, Noomen P, Dijkman A, de Vries FA, van Opstal D. Abnormal non-invasive prenatal test results concordant with karyotype of cytotrophoblast but not reflecting abnormal fetal karyotype. *Ultrasound Obstet Gynecol* 44: 109–111, 2014.

Srinivasan A, Bianchi DW, Huang H, Sehnert AJ, Rava RP. Noninvasive detection of fetal subchromosome abnormalities via deep sequencing of maternal plasma. *Am J Hum Genet* 92: 167–176, 2013.

Staals JE, Schrander-Stumpel CT, Hamers G, Fryns JP. Prenatal diagnosis of trisomy 12 mosaicism:

Normal development of a 3 years old female child. *Genet Couns* 14: 233–237, 2003.

Stabile M, Angelino T, Caiazzo F, et al. Fertility in a i(Xq) Klinefelter patient: Importance of XIST expression level determined by qRT-PCR in ruling out Klinefelter cryptic mosaicism as cause of oligozoospermia. *Mol Hum Reprod* 14: 635–640, 2008.

Staebler M, Donner C, Van Regemorter N, et al. Should determination of the karyotype be systematic for all malformations detected by obstetrical ultrasound? *Prenat Diagn* 25: 567–573, 2005.

Staessen C, Tournaye H, Van Assche E, et al. PGD in 47,XXY Klinefelter's syndrome patients. *Hum Reprod Update* 9: 319–330, 2003.

Stagi S, Lapi E, Pantaleo M, et al. A *SOX3* (Xq26.3-27.3) duplication in a boy with growth hormone deficiency, ocular dyspraxia, and intellectual disability: A long-term follow-up and literature review. *Hormones (Athens)* 13: 552–560, 2014.

Stagi S, Lapi E, Pantaleo M, et al. A new case of de novo 6q24.2-q25.2 deletion on paternal chromosome 6 with growth hormone deficiency: A twelve-year follow-up and literature review. *BMC Med Genet* 16: 69, 2015.

Stahl BC, Patil SR, Syrop CH, Sparks AE, Wald M. Supernumerary minute ring chromosome 14 in a man with primary infertility and left varicocele. *Fertil Steril* 87: 1213, e1–3, 2007.

Ståhl O, Boyd HA, Giwercman A, et al. Risk of birth abnormalities in the offspring of men with a history of cancer: A cohort study using Danish and Swedish national registries. *J Natl Cancer Inst* 103: 398–406, 2011.

Stalker HJ, Gray BA, Zori RT. Dominant transmission of a previously unidentified 13/17 translocation in a five-generation family with Robin cleft and other skeletal defects. *Am J Med Genet* 103: 339–341, 2001.

Stalker HJ, Williams CA. Genetic counseling in Angelman syndrome: The challenges of multiple causes. *Am J Med Genet* 77: 54–59, 1998.

Stallard R, Krueger S, James RS, Schwartz S. Uniparental isodisomy 13 in a normal female due to transmission of a maternal t(13q13q). *Am J Med Genet* 57: 14–18, 1995.

Stamberg J, Thomas GH. Unusual supernumerary chromosomes: Types encountered in a referred population, and high incidence of associated maternal chromosome abnormalities. *Hum Genet* 72: 140–144, 1986.

Stankiewicz P, Brozek I, Hélias-Rodzewicz Z, et al. Clinical and molecular-cytogenetic studies in seven patients with ring chromosome 18. *Am J Med Genet* 101: 226–239, 2001a.

Stankiewicz P, Kuechler A, Eller CD, et al. Minimal phenotype in a girl with trisomy 15q due to t(X;15)(q22.3;q11.2) translocation. *Am J Med Genet* 140: 442–452, 2006.

Stankiewicz P, Rujner J, Löffler C, et al. Alagille syndrome associated with a paracentric inversion 20p12.2p13 disrupting the *JAG1* gene. *Am J Med Genet* 103: 166–171, 2001b.

Stankiewicz P, Sen P, Bhatt SS, et al. Genomic and genic deletions of the *FOX* gene cluster on 16q24.1 and inactivating mutations of *FOXF1* cause alveolar capillary dysplasia and other malformations. *Am J Hum Genet* 84: 780–791, 2009.

Stankiewicz P, Thiele H, Baldermann C, et al. Phenotypic findings due to trisomy 7p15.3-pter including the *TWIST* locus. *Am J Med Genet* 103: 56–62, 2001c.

Stankiewicz P, Thiele H, Schlicker M, et al. Duplication of Xq26.2-q27.1, including *SOX3*, in a mother and daughter with short stature and dyslalia. *Am J Med Genet* 138: 11–17, 2005.

Staples AJ, Sutherland GR, Haan EA, Clisby S. Epidemiology of Down syndrome in South Australia, 1960–89. *Am J Hum Genet* 49: 1014–1024, 1991.

Starbuck JM, Cole TM, Reeves RH, Richtsmeier JT. The Influence of trisomy 21 on facial form and variability. *Am J Med Genet* 173A: 2861–2872, 2017.

Stark Z, Gillam L, Walker SP, McGillivray G. Ethical controversies in prenatal microarray. *Curr Opin Obstet Gynecol* 25: 133–137, 2013.

Starr LJ, Truemper EJ, Pickering DL, Sanger WG, Olney AH. Duplication of 20qter and deletion of 20pter due to paternal pericentric inversion: Patient report and review of 20qter duplications. *Am J Med Genet* 164A: 2020–2024, 2014.

Stasiewicz-Jarocka B, Haus O, Van Assche E, et al. Genetic counseling in carriers of reciprocal chromosomal translocations involving long arm of chromosome 16. *Clin Genet* 66: 189–207, 2004.

Stasiewicz-Jarocka B, Raczkiewicz B, Kowalczyk D, Zawada M, Midro AT. Genetic risk of families with t(1;2)(q42;q33) GTG, RHG, QFQ, FISH. *Ginekol Pol* 71: 1262–1272, 2000.

Stefanou EG, Crocker M. A chromosome 21-derived minute marker in a mosaic trisomy 21 background: Implications for risk assessments in marker chromosome cases. *Am J Med Genet* 127A: 191–193, 2004.

Stefanou EG, Crocker M, Boon A, Stewart H. Cryptic mosaicism for monosomy 20 identified in renal tract cells. *Clin Genet* 70: 228–232, 2006.

Stefanova I, Jenderny J, Kaminsky E, et al. Mosaic and complete tetraploidy in live-born infants: two new patients and review of the literature. *Clin Dysmorphol* 19: 123–127, 2010.

Stefansson H, Meyer-Lindenberg A, Steinberg S, et al. CNVs conferring risk of autism or schizophrenia affect cognition in controls. *Nature* 505: 361–366, 2014.

Stein QP, Boyle JG, Crotwell PL, et al. Prenatally diagnosed trisomy 20 mosaicism associated with arachnoid cyst of basal cistern. *Prenat Diagn* 28: 1169–1170, 2008.

Steinbach P. Excess of mental retardation and/or congenital malformation in reciprocal translocations in man. *Hum Genet* 73: 379, 1986.

Steinberg C, Zackai EH, Eunpu DL, Mennuti MT, Emanuel BS. Recurrence rate for de novo 21q21q translocation Down syndrome: A study of 112 families. *Am J Med Genet* 17: 523–530, 1984.

Steinberg Warren N, Soukup S, King JL, St JDP. Prenatal diagnosis of trisomy 20 by chorionic villus sampling (CVS): A case report with long-term outcome. *Prenat Diagn* 21: 1111–1113, 2001.

Steinbusch CVM, van Roozendaal KEP, Tserpelis D, et al. Somatic mosaicism in a mother of two children with Pitt-Hopkins syndrome. *Clin Genet* 83: 73–77, 2013.

Steiner B, Masood R, Rufibach K, et al. An unexpected finding: younger fathers have a higher risk for offspring with chromosomal aneuploidies. *Eur J Hum Genet* 23: 466–472, 2015.

Steinman KJ, Spence SJ, Ramocki MB, et al. 16p11.2 deletion and duplication: Characterizing neurologic phenotypes in a large clinically ascertained cohort. *Am J Med Genet* 170A: 2943–2955, 2016.

Stelzer Y, Sagi I, Yanuka O, Eiges R, Benvenisty N. The noncoding RNA IPW regulates the imprinted *DLK1-DIO3* locus in an induced pluripotent stem cell model of Prader-Willi syndrome. *Nat Genet* 46: 551–557, 2014.

Stemkens D, Broekmans FJ, Kastrop PM, Hochstenbach R, Smith BG, Giltay JC. Variant Klinefelter syndrome 47,X,i(X)(q10),Y and normal 46,XY karyotype in monozygotic adult twins. *Am J Med Genet* 143A: 1906–1911, 2007.

Stene J. Detection of higher recurrence risk for age-dependent chromosome abnormalities with an application to trisomy G1 (Down's syndrome). *Hum Hered* 20: 112–122, 1970.

Stene J. Comments on methods and results in: Sherman et al., "Segregation Analysis of Balanced Pericentric Inversions in Pedigree Data." *Clin Genet* 30: 95–107, 1986.

Stene J, Stene E, Mikkelsen M. Risk for chromosome abnormality at amniocentesis following a child with a non-inherited chromosome aberration: A European collaborative study on prenatal diagnoses 1981. *Prenat Diagn* 4: Spec No. 81–95, 1984.

Stene J, Stengel-Rutkowski S. Genetic risks of familial reciprocal and Robertsonian translocation carriers. In Daniel A (ed.), *The Cytogenetics of Mammalian Autosomal Rearrangements*. New York, NY: Liss, 1988.

Stengel-Rutkowski S, Stene J, Gallano P. Risk estimates in balanced parental reciprocal translocations. *Monogr Ann Génétique* 1–147, 1988.

Stephenson MD, Awartani KA, Robinson WP. Cytogenetic analysis of miscarriages from couples with recurrent miscarriage: A case-control study. *Hum Reprod* 17: 446–451, 2002.

Stern C, Pertile M, Norris H, Hale L, Baker HGW. Chromosome translocations in couples with in-vitro fertilization implantation failure. *Hum Reprod* 14: 2097–2101, 1999.

Stern S, Biron D, Moses E. Transmission of trisomy decreases with maternal age in mouse models of Down syndrome, mirroring a phenomenon in human Down syndrome mothers. *BMC Genet* 17: 105, 2016.

Stetten G, Escallon CS, South ST, McMichael JL, Saul DO, Blakemore KJ. Reevaluating confined placental mosaicism. *Am J Med Genet* 131: 232–239, 2004.

Stevens SJC, Smeets EEJGL, Blom E, et al. Identical cryptic partial monosomy 20pter and trisomy 20qter in three adult siblings due to a large maternal pericentric inversion: Detection by MLPA and breakpoint mapping by SNP array analysis. *Am J Med Genet* 149A: 2226–2230, 2009.

Stevenson DA, Brothman AR, Chen Z, Bayrak-Toydemir P, Longo N. Paternal uniparental disomy of chromosome 14: Confirmation of a clinically-recognizable phenotype. *Am J Med Genet* 130A: 88–91, 2004.

Stewart DA, Bailey JD, Netley CT, Park E. Growth, development, and behavioral outcome from mid-adolescence to adulthood in subjects with chromosome aneuploidy: The Toronto Study. *Birth Defects Orig Artic Ser* 26: 131–188, 1990.

Stipoljev F, Stanojevic M, Kurjak A. Familial pericentric inversion of chromosome 4: inv(4)(p16.1q12). *Clin Genet* 61: 386–388, 2002.

Stochholm K, Bojesen A, Jensen AS, Juul S, Gravholt CH. Criminality in men with Klinefelter's syndrome and XYY syndrome: A cohort study. *BMJ Open* 2: e000650, 2012.

Stoklasova J, Kaprova J, Trkova M, et al. A rare variant of Turner syndrome in four sequential generations: Effect of the interplay of growth hormone treatment and estrogens on body proportion. *Horm Res Paediatr* 86: 349–356, 2016

Stokman MF, Oud MM, van Binsbergen E, et al. De novo 14q24.2q24.3 microdeletion including *IFT43* is associated with intellectual disability, skeletal anomalies, cardiac anomalies, and myopia. *Am J Med Genet* 170: 1566–1569, 2016.

Stokowski R, Wang E, White K, et al. Clinical performance of non-invasive prenatal testing (NIPT) using targeted cell-free DNA analysis in maternal plasma with microarrays or next generation sequencing (NGS) is consistent across multiple controlled clinical studies. *Prenat Diagn* 35: 1243–1246, 2015.

Strain L, Dean JCS, Hamilton MPR, Bonthron DT. A true hermaphrodite chimera resulting from embryo amalgamation after in vitro fertilization. *N Engl J Med* 338: 166–169, 1998.

Strain L, Warner JP, Johnston T, Bonthron DT. A human parthenogenetic chimaera. *Nat Genet* 11: 164–169, 1995.

Strazisar M, Cammaerts S, van der Ven K, et al. *MIR137* variants identified in psychiatric patients affect synaptogenesis and neuronal transmission gene sets. *Mol Psychiatry* 20: 472–481, 2015.

Strehle EM, Yu L, Rosenfeld JA, et al. Genotype-phenotype analysis of 4q deletion syndrome: Proposal of a critical region. *Am J Med Genet* 158A: 2139–2151, 2012.

Streuli I, Fraisse T, Ibecheole V, Moix I, Morris MA, de Ziegler D. Intermediate and premutation *FMR1* alleles in women with occult primary ovarian insufficiency. *Fertil Steril* 92: 464–470, 2009.

Strigini P, Pierluigi M, Forni GL, et al. Effect of X-rays on chromosome 21 nondisjunction. *Am J Med Genet Suppl* 7: 155–159, 1990.

Stumm M, Müsebeck J, Tönnies H, et al. Partial trisomy 9p12p21.3 with a normal phenotype. *J Med Genet* 39: 141–144, 2002.

Stuppia L, Calabrese G, Borrelli P, et al. Loss of the *SHOX* gene associated with Leri-Weill dyschondrosteosis in a 45,X male. *J Med Genet* 36: 711–713, 1999.

Stuppia L, Gatta V, Calabrese G, et al. A quarter of men with idiopathic oligo-azoospermia display chromosomal abnormalities and microdeletions of different types in interval 6 of Yq11. *Hum Genet* 102: 566–570, 1998.

Su MT, Liang YL, Chen JC, Sun HS, Chang FM, Kuo PL. Non-mosaic uniparental trisomy 16 presenting with asplenia syndrome and placental abruption: A case report and literature review. *Eur J Med Genet* 56: 197–201, 2013.

Su PH, Lee IC, Yang SF, Ng YY, Liu CS, Chen JY. Nine genes that may contribute to partial trisomy (6)(p22→pter) and unique presentation of persistent hyperplastic primary vitreous with retinal detachment. *Am J Med Genet* 158A: 707–712, 2012.

Sudha T, Gopinath PM. Homologous Robertsonian translocation (21q21q) and abortions. *Hum Genet* 85: 253–255, 1990.

Sudhir N, Kaur T, Beri A, Kaur A. Cytogenetic analysis in couples with recurrent miscarriages: A retrospective study from Punjab, north India. *J Genet* 95: 887–894, 2016.

Sudik R, Jakubiczka S, Nawroth F, Gilberg E, Wieacker PF. Chimerism in a fertile woman with 46,XY karyotype and female phenotype. *Hum Reprod* 16: 56–58, 2001.

Sugawara N, Kimura Y, Araki Y. Case report: A successful pregnancy outcome in a patient with non-mosaic Turner syndrome (45, X) via in vitro fertilization. *Hum Cell* 26: 41–43, 2013.

Sugawara N, Tokunaga Y, Maeda M, Komaba R, Araki Y. A successful pregnancy outcome using frozen testicular sperm from a chimeric infertile male with a 46,XX/46,XY karyotype: Case report. *Hum Reprod* 20: 147–148, 2005.

Sukenik-Halevy R, Sukenik S, Koifman A, et al. Clinical aspects of prenatally detected congenital heart malformations and the yield of chromosomal microarray analysis. *Prenat Diagn* 36: 1185–1191, 2016.

Šumanovic-Glamuzina D, Lozic B, Iwanowski PS, et al. Limited survivability of unbalanced progeny of carriers of a unique t(4;19)(p15.32;p13.3): a study in multiple generations. *Mol Cytogenet* 10: 29, 2017.

Sun F, Oliver-Bonet M, Turek PJ, Ko E, Martin RH. Meiotic studies in an azoospermic human translocation (Y;1) carrier. *Mol Hum Reprod* 11: 361–364, 2005.

Sun K, Jiang P, Chan KC, et al. Plasma DNA tissue mapping by genome-wide methylation sequencing for noninvasive prenatal, cancer, and transplantation assessments. *Proc Natl Acad Sci USA* 112: E5503–5512, 2015.

Sundvall L, Lund H, Niemann I, Jensen UB, Bolund L, Sunde L. Tetraploidy in hydatidiform moles. *Hum Reprod* 28: 2010–2020, 2013.

Sung PL, Chang SP, Wen KC, et al. Small supernumerary marker chromosome originating from chromosome 10 associated with an apparently normal phenotype. *Am J Med Genet* 149A: 2768–2774, 2009.

Surace C, Berardinelli F, Masotti A, et al. Telomere shortening and telomere position effect in mild ring 17 syndrome. *Epigenetics Chromatin* 7: 1, 2014.

Susanne GO, Sissel S, Ulla W, Charlotta G, Sonja OL. Pregnant women's responses to information about an increased risk of carrying a baby with Down syndrome. *Birth* 33: 64–73, 2006.

Susiarjo M, Hassold TJ, Freeman E, Hunt PA. Bisphenol A exposure in utero disrupts early oogenesis in the mouse. *PLoS Genet* 3: e5, 2007.

Sutherland GR. Rare fragile sites. *Cytogenet Genome Res* 100: 77–84, 2003.

Sutherland GR, Baker E. The clinical significance of fragile sites on human chromosomes. *Clin Genet* 58: 157–161, 2000.

Sutherland GR, Callen DF, Gardner RJM. Paracentric inversions do not normally generate monocentric recombinant chromosomes. *Am J Med Genet* 59: 390–392, 1995.

Sutherland GR, Gardiner AJ, Carter RF. Familial pericentric inversion of chromosome 19, inv(19) (p13q13) with a note on genetic counseling of pericentric inversion carriers. *Clin Genet* 10: 54–59, 1976.

Sutherland GR, Hecht F. *Fragile Sites on Human Chromosomes* (Oxford Monographs on Medical Genetics). New York, NY: Oxford University Press, 1985.

Sutton EJ, Young J, McInerney-Leo A, Bondy CA, Gollust SE, Biesecker BB. Truth-telling and Turner Syndrome: The importance of diagnostic disclosure. *J Pediatr* 148: 102–107, 2006.

Sutton VR, McAlister WH, Bertin TK, et al. Skeletal defects in paternal uniparental disomy for chromosome 14 are re-capitulated in the mouse model (paternal uniparental disomy 12). *Hum Genet* 113: 447–451, 2003.

Sutton VR, Shaffer LG. Search for imprinted regions on chromosome 14: Comparison of maternal and paternal UPD cases with cases of chromosome 14 deletion. *Am J Med Genet* 93: 381–387, 2000.

Swerdlow AJ, Hermon C, Jacobs PA, et al. Mortality and cancer incidence in persons with numerical sex chromosome abnormalities: A cohort study. *Ann Hum Genet* 65: 177–188, 2001.

Swillen A, Devriendt K, Vantrappen G, et al. Familial deletions of chromosome 22q11: The Leuven experience. *Am J Med Genet* 80: 531–532, 1998.

Swinkels MEM, Simons A, Smeets DF, et al. Clinical and cytogenetic characterization of 13 Dutch patients with deletion 9p syndrome: Delineation of the critical region for a consensus phenotype. *Am J Med Genet* 146A: 1430–1438, 2008.

Sybert VP. Phenotypic effects of mosaicism for a 47,XXX cell line in Turner syndrome. *J Med Genet* 39: 217–220, 2002.

Sybert VP. Turner Syndrome. In Cassidy SB, Allanson JE (eds.), *Management of Genetic Syndromes* (2nd edn.). Hoboken, NJ: John Wiley & Sons, 2005.

Szafranski P, Dharmadhikari AV, Wambach JA, et al. Two deletions overlapping a distant *FOXF1* enhancer unravel the role of lncRNA LINC01081 in etiology of alveolar capillary dysplasia with misalignment of pulmonary veins. *Am J Med Genet* 164A: 2013–2019, 2014.

Szafranski P, Gambin T, Dharmadhikari AV, et al. Pathogenetics of alveolar capillary dysplasia with misalignment of pulmonary veins. *Hum Genet* 135: 569–586, 2016.

Szafranski P, Von Allmen GK, Graham BH, et al. 6q22.1 microdeletion and susceptibility to pediatric epilepsy. *Eur J Hum Genet* 23: 173–179, 2015.

Sztainberg Y, Zoghbi HY. Lessons learned from studying syndromic autism spectrum disorders. *Nature Neurosci* 19, 1408–1417, 2016.

Tabet AC, Aboura A, Gérard M, et al. Molecular characterization of a de novo 6q24.2q25.3 duplication interrupting *UTRN* in a patient with arthrogryposis. *Am J Med Genet* 152A: 1781–1788, 2010.

Tabet AC, Pilorge M, Delorme R, et al. Autism multiplex family with 16p11.2p12.2 microduplication syndrome in monozygotic twins and distal 16p11.2 deletion in their brother. *Eur J Hum Genet* 20: 540–546, 2012.

Tabet AC, Verloes A, Pilorge M, et al. Complex nature of apparently balanced chromosomal rearrangements in patients with autism spectrum disorder. *Mol Autism* 6: 19, 2015.

Tabolacci E, Zollino M, Lecce R, et al. Two brothers with 22q13 deletion syndrome and features suggestive of the Clark-Baraitser syndrome. *Clin Dysmorphol* 14: 127–132, 2005.

Tachdjian G, Aboura A, Benkhalifa M, et al. De novo interstitial direct duplication of Xq21.1q25 associated with skewed X-inactivation pattern. *Am J Med Genet* 131: 273–280, 2004.

Tagaya M, Mizuno S, Hayakawa M, Yokotsuka T, Shimizu S, Fujimaki H. Recombination of a maternal pericentric inversion results in 22q13 deletion syndrome. *Clin Dysmorphol* 17: 19–21, 2008.

Takahashi K, Sasaki A, Wada S, et al. The outcomes of 31 cases of trisomy 13 diagnosed in utero with various management options. *Am J Med Genet* 173A: 966–971, 2017.

Takenouchi T, Miura K, Uehara T, Mizuno S, Kosaki K. Establishing SON in 21q22.11 as a cause a new syndromic form of intellectual disability: Possible contribution to Braddock-Carey syndrome phenotype. *Am J Med Genet* 170: 2587–2590, 2016.

Takenouchi T, Yagihashi T, Tsuchiya H, et al. Tissue-limited ring chromosome 18 mosaicism as a cause of Pitt-Hopkins syndrome. *Am J Med Genet* 158A: 2621–2623, 2012.

Takeuchi A, Ehara H, Ohtani K, et al. Live birth prevalence of Down syndrome in Tottori, Japan, 1980–1999. *Am J Med Genet* 146A: 1381–1386, 2008.

Talkowski ME, Mullegama SV, Rosenfeld JA, et al. Assessment of 2q23.1 microdeletion syndrome implicates *MBD5* as a single causal locus of intellectual disability, epilepsy, and autism spectrum disorder. *Am J Hum Genet* 89: 551–563, 2011.

Tamagaki A, Shima M, Tomita R, et al. Segregation of a pure form of spastic paraplegia and NOR insertion into Xq11.2. *Am J Med Genet* 94: 5–8, 2000.

Tamura M, Isojima T, Kawashima M, et al. Detection of hereditary 1,25-hydroxyvitamin D-resistant rickets caused by uniparental disomy of chromosome 12 using genome-wide single nucleotide polymorphism array. *PLoS One* 10: e0131157, 2015.

Tan TY, Aftimos S, Worgan L, et al. Phenotypic expansion and further characterisation of the 17q21.31 microdeletion syndrome. *J Med Genet* 46: 480–489, 2009.

Tan TY, Gordon CT, Amor DJ, Farlie PG. Developmental perspectives on copy number abnormalities of the 22q11.2 region. *Clin Genet* 78: 201–218, 2010.

Tan WH, Bird LM, Thibert RL, Williams CA. If not Angelman, what is it? A review of Angelman-like syndromes. *Am J Med Genet* 164A: 975–992, 2014.

Tan YQ, Tan K, Zhang SP, et al. Single-nucleotide polymorphism microarray-based preimplantation genetic diagnosis is likely to improve the clinical outcome for translocation carriers. *Hum Reprod* 28: 2581–2592, 2013.

Tan-Sindhunata G, Castedo S, Leegte B, et al. Molecular cytogenetic characterization of a small, familial supernumerary ring chromosome 7 associated with mental retardation and an abnormal phenotype. *Am J Med Genet* 92: 147–152, 2000.

Tang W, Boyd BK, Hummel M, Wenger SL. Prenatal diagnosis of tetrasomy 9p. *Am J Med Genet* 126A: 328, 2004.

Tartaglia NR, Howell S, Sutherland A, Wilson R, Wilson L. A review of trisomy X (47,XXX). *Orphanet J Rare Dis* 5: 8, 2010.

Tartaglia NR, Howell S, Wilson R, et al. The eXtraordinarY Kids Clinic: An interdisciplinary model of care for children and adolescents with sex chromosome aneuploidy. *J Multidiscip Healthc* 8: 323–334, 2015.

Tassano E, Biancheri R, Denegri L, et al. Heterozygous deletion of *CHL1* gene: Detailed array-CGH and clinical characterization of a new case and review of the literature. *Eur J Med Genet* 57: 626–629, 2014.

Tatton-Brown K, Douglas J, Coleman K, et al. Multiple mechanisms are implicated in the generation of 5q35 microdeletions in Sotos syndrome. *J Med Genet* 42: 307–313, 2005.

Tatton-Brown K, Pilz DT, Örstavik KH, et al. 15q overgrowth syndrome: a newly recognized phenotype associated with overgrowth, learning difficulties, characteristic facial appearance, renal anomalies and increased dosage of distal chromosome 15q. *Am J Med Genet* 149A: 147–154, 2009.

Taylor AMR. Chromosome instability syndromes. *Best Pract Res Clin Haematol* 14: 631–644, 2001.

Tekin M, Jackson-Cook C, Buller A, et al. Fluorescence in situ hybridization detectable mosaicism for Angelman syndrome with biparental methylation. *Am J Med Genet* 95: 145–149, 2000.

Tello C, Darling A, Lupo V, Ortez CI, Pérez-Dueñas B, Espinós C. Twin-sisters with *PLA2G6*-associated neurodegeneration due to paternal isodisomy of the chromosome 22 following in vitro fertilization. *Clin Genet* 92: 117–118, 2017.

Telvi L, Lebbar A, Del Pino O, Barbet JP, Chaussain JL. 45,X/46,XY mosaicism: Report of 27 cases. *Pediatrics* 104: 304–308, 1999.

Tempest HG, Ko E, Chan P, Robaire B, Rademaker A, Martin RH. Sperm aneuploidy frequencies analysed before and after chemotherapy in testicular cancer and Hodgkin's lymphoma patients. *Hum Reprod* 23: 251–258, 2008.

Tempest HG, Simpson JL. Why are we still talking about chromosomal heteromorphisms? *Reprod Biomed Online* 35: 1–2, 2017.

Templado C, Donate A, Giraldo J, Bosch M, Estop A. Advanced age increases chromosome structural abnormalities in human spermatozoa. *Eur J Hum Genet* 19: 145–151, 2011.

Templado C, Uroz L, Estop A. New insights on the origin and relevance of aneuploidy in human spermatozoa. *Mol Hum Reprod* 19: 634–643, 2013.

Temple CM, Shephard EE. Exceptional lexical skills but executive language deficits in school starters and young adults with Turners syndrome: Implications for X chromosome effects on brain function. *Brain Lang* 120: 345–359, 2012.

Temple IK, Gardner RJ, Robinson DO, et al. Further evidence for an imprinted gene for neonatal diabetes localised to chromosome 6q22-q23. *Hum Mol Genet* 5: 1117–21, 1996.

Ten SK, Chin YM, Noor PJ, Hassan K. Cytogenetic studies in women with primary amenorrhea. *Singapore Med J* 31: 355–359, 1990.

Tennakoon J, Kandasamy Y, Alcock G, Koh TH. Edwards syndrome with double trisomy. *Singapore Med J* 49: e190–191, 2008.

Termsarasab P, Yang AC, Reiner J, Mei H, Scott SA, Frucht SJ. Paroxysmal kinesigenic dyskinesia caused by 16p11.2 microdeletion. *Tremor Other Hyperkinet Mov* 4: 274, 2014.

Terribas E, Bonache S, García-Arévalo M, et al. Changes in the expression profile of the meiosis-involved mismatch repair (MMR) genes in impaired human spermatogenesis. *J Androl* 31: 346–357, 2010.

Terzoli G, Lalatta F, Lobbiani A, Simoni G, Colucci G. Fertility in a 47,XXY patient: Assessment of biological paternity by deoxyribonucleic acid fingerprinting. *Fertil Steril* 58: 821–822, 1992.

Terzoli G, Rossella F, Biscaglia M, Simoni G. True fetal mosaicism revealed by a single abnormal colony in amniocyte culture. *Prenat Diagn* 10: 273–274, 1990.

Teshima IE, Winsor EJT, Van Allen MI. Trisomy 18 and a constitutional maternal translocation (2;18). *Am J Med Genet* 43: 759–761, 1992.

Teyssier M, Gaucherand P, Buenerd A. Prenatal diagnosis of a tetraploid fetus. *Prenat Diagn* 17: 474–478, 1997.

Teyssier M, Moreau N. Familial transmission of deleted chromosome 22 [r(22)p0?] in two normal women. *Ann Génét* 28: 116–118, 1985.

Teyssier M, Rafat A, Pugeat M. Case of (Y;1) familial translocation. *Am J Med Genet* 46: 339–340, 1993.

Thapa M, Asamoah A, Gowans GC, et al. Molecular characterization of distal 4q duplication in two patients using oligonucleotide array-based comparative genomic hybridization (oaCGH) analysis. *Am J Med Genet* 164A: 1069–1074, 2014.

Tharapel AT, Elias S, Shulman LP, Seely L, Emerson DS, Simpson JL. Resorbed co-twin as an explanation for discrepant chorionic villus results: Non-mosaic 47,XX,+16 in villi (direct and culture) with normal (46,XX) amniotic fluid and neonatal blood. *Prenat Diagn* 9: 467–472, 1989.

Tharapel AT, Michaelis RC, Velagaleti GVN, et al. Chromosome duplications and deletions and their mechanisms of origin. *Cytogenet Cell Genet* 85: 285–290, 1999.

Tharapel AT, Tharapel SA, Bannerman RM. Recurrent pregnancy losses and parental chromosome abnormalities: A review. *Br J Obstet Gynaecol* 92: 899–914, 1985.

Tharapel SA, Lewandowski RC, Tharapel AT, Wilroy RS, Jr. Phenotype-karyotype correlation in patients trisomic for various segments of chromosome 13. *J Med Genet* 23: 310–315, 1986.

Theilgaard A. Psychologic study of XYY and XXY men. *Birth Defects Orig Artic Ser* 22: 277–292, 1986.

Theisen A, Rosenfeld JA, Farrell SA, et al. aCGH detects partial tetrasomy of 12p in blood from Pallister-Killian syndrome cases without invasive skin biopsy. *Am J Med Genet* 149A: 914–918, 2009.

Therman E, Laxova R, Susman B. The critical region on the human Xq. *Hum Genet* 85: 455–461, 1990.

Therman E, Susman B, Denniston C. The nonrandom participation of human acrocentric chromosomes in Robertsonian translocations. *Ann Hum Genet* 53: 49–65, 1989.

Thevenon J, Callier P, Andrieux J, et al. 12p13.33 microdeletion including *ELKS/ERC1*, a new locus associated with childhood apraxia of speech. *Eur J Hum Genet* 21: 82–88, 2013.

Thevenon J, Callier P, Poquet H, et al. 3q27.3 microdeletional syndrome: A recognisable clinical entity associating dysmorphic features, marfanoid habitus, intellectual disability and psychosis with mood disorder. *J Med Genet* 51: 21–27, 2014.

Thiede C, Prange-Krex G, Freiberg-Richter J, Bornhäuser M, Ehninger G. Buccal swabs but not mouthwash samples can be used to obtain pretransplant DNA fingerprints from recipients of allogeneic bone marrow transplants. *Bone Marrow Transplant* 25: 575–577, 2000.

Thienpont B, Béna F, Breckpot J, et al. Duplications of the critical Rubinstein-Taybi deletion region on chromosome 16p13.3 cause a novel recognisable syndrome. *J Med Genet* 47: 155–161, 2010.

Thierry G, Bénéteau C, Pichon O, et al. Molecular characterization of 1q44 microdeletion in 11 patients reveals three candidate genes for intellectual disability and seizures. *Am J Med Genet* 158A: 1633–1640, 2012.

Tho SP, Jackson R, Kulharya AS, Reindollar RH, Layman LC, McDonough PG. Long-term follow-up and analysis of monozygotic twins concordant for 45,X/46,XY peripheral blood karyotype but discordant for phenotypic sex. *Am J Med Genet* 143A: 2616–2622, 2007.

Thomas NS, Maloney V, Bryant V, et al. Breakpoint mapping and haplotype analysis of three reciprocal translocations identify a novel recurrent translocation in two unrelated families: t(4;11)(p16.2;p15.4). *Hum Genet* 125: 181–188, 2009.

Thomas NS, Morris JK, Baptista J, Ng BL, Crolla JA, Jacobs PA. De novo apparently balanced translocations in man are predominantly paternal in origin and associated with a significant increase in paternal age. *J Med Genet* 47: 112–115, 2010.

Tiepolo L, Zuffardi O. Localization of factors controlling spermatogenesis in the nonfluorescent portion of the human Y chromosome long arm. *Hum Genet* 34: 119–124, 1976.

Tihy F, Lemieux N, Lemyre E. Complex chromosome rearrangement and recombinant balanced translocation in a mother and a daughter with the same phenotypic abnormalities. *Am J Med Genet* 135: 317–319, 2005.

Tillisch DL. Chromosome deletions. Looking beyond disability. *Lancet* 358 (Suppl): S10, 2001.

Tinkle BT, Walker ME, Blough-Pfau RI, Saal HM, Hopkin RJ. Unexpected survival in a case of prenatally diagnosed non-mosaic trisomy 22: Clinical report and review of the natural history. *Am J Med Genet* 118A: 90–95, 2003.

Tiranti V, Lamantea E, Uziel G, et al. Leigh syndrome transmitted by uniparental disomy of chromosome 9. *J Med Genet* 36: 927–928, 1999.

Tischkowitz MD, Hodgson SV. Fanconi anaemia. *J Med Genet* 40: 1–10, 2003.

Tobler KJ, Brezina PR, Benner AT, Du L, Xu X, Kearns WG. Two different microarray technologies for preimplantation genetic diagnosis and screening, due to reciprocal translocation imbalances, demonstrate equivalent euploidy and clinical pregnancy rates. *J Assist Reprod Genet* 31: 843–850, 2014.

Tobler KJ, Zhao Y, Ross R, et al. Blastocoel fluid from differentiated blastocysts harbors embryonic genomic material capable of a whole-genome deoxyribonucleic acid amplification and comprehensive chromosome microarray analysis. *Fertil Steril* 104: 418–425, 2015.

Tokita MJ, Chow PM, Mirzaa G, et al. Five children with deletions of 1p34.3 encompassing *AGO1* and *AGO3*. *Eur J Hum Genet* 23: 761–765, 2015.

Tokita MJ, Sybert VP. Postnatal outcomes of prenatally diagnosed 45,X/46,XX. *Am J Med Genet* 170A: 1196–1201, 2016.

Tomaselli S, Megiorni F, De Bernardo C, et al. Syndromic true hermaphroditism due to an R-spondin1 (*RSPO1*) homozygous mutation. *Hum Mutat* 29: 220–226, 2008.

Tomaszewska A, Podbiol-Palenta A, Boter M, et al. Deletion of 14.7 Mb 2q32.3q33.3 with a marfanoid phenotype and hypothyroidism. *Am J Med Genet* 161A: 2347–2351, 2013.

Tomkins DJ. Unstable familial translocations: A t(11;22)mat inherited as a t(11;15). *Am J Hum Genet* 33: 745–751, 1981.

Tommerup N. Mendelian cytogenetics: Chromosome rearrangements associated with Mendelian disorders. *J Med Genet* 30: 713–727, 1993.

Tommerup N, Fonseca AC, Mehrjouy MM, et al. Interpretation of NGS-mapped chromosomal breakpoints: The importance of healthy controls. Poster presented at the European Human Genetics conference, Copenhagen, 2017.

Tonk V, Schultz RA, Christian SL, Kubota T, Ledbetter DH, Wilson GN. Robertsonian (15q;15q) translocation in a child with Angelman syndrome: Evidence of uniparental disomy. *Am J Med Genet* 66: 426–428, 1996.

Tonk VS, Jesurun CA, Morgan DL, Lockhart LH, Velagaleti GV. Molecular cytogenetic characterization of a recombinant chromosome rec(22)dup(22q)inv(22)(p13q12.2). *Am J Med Genet* 124A: 92–95, 2004.

Torfs CP, Christianson RE. Anomalies in Down syndrome individuals in a large population-based registry. *Am J Med Genet* 77: 431–438, 1998.

Torfs CP, Christianson RE. Effect of maternal smoking and coffee consumption on the risk of having a recognized Down syndrome pregnancy. *Am J Epidemiol* 152: 1185–1191, 2000.

Torisu H, Yamamoto T, Fujiwaki T, et al. Girl with monosomy 1p36 and Angelman syndrome due to unbalanced der(1) transmission of a maternal translocation t(1;15)(p36.3;q13.1). *Am J Med Genet* 131: 94–98, 2004.

Torniero C, Dalla Bernardina B, Novara F, et al. Dysmorphic features, simplified gyral pattern and 7q11.23 duplication reciprocal to the Williams-Beuren deletion. *Eur J Hum Genet* 16: 880–887, 2008.

Torres F, Barbosa M, Maciel P. Recurrent copy number variations as risk factors for neurodevelopmental disorders: Critical overview and analysis of clinical implications. *J Med Genet* 53: 73–90, 2016.

Tosca L, Brisset S, Petit FM, et al. Recurrent 70.8 Mb 4q22.2q32.3 duplication due to ovarian germinal mosaicism. *Eur J Hum Genet* 18: 882–888, 2010.

Tosson H, Rose SR, Gartner LA. Description of children with 45,X/46,XY karyotype. *Eur J Pediatr* 171: 521–529, 2012.

Tosur M, Geary CA, Matalon R, et al. Persistence of müllerian duct structures in a genetic male with distal monosomy 10q. *Am J Med Genet* 167A: 791–796, 2015.

Tóth A, Gaál M, László J. Familial pericentric inversion of the Y chromosome. *Ann Génét* 27: 60–61, 1984.

Toth A, Jessberger R. Oogenesis: Ageing oocyte chromosomes rely on amazing protein stability. *Curr Biol* 26:R329–331, 2016.

Towner DR, Shaffer LG, Yang SP, Walgenbach DD. Confined placental mosaicism for trisomy 14 and maternal uniparental disomy in association with elevated second trimester maternal serum human chorionic gonadotrophin and third trimester fetal growth restriction. *Prenat Diagn* 21: 395–398, 2001.

Tran THT, Zhang Z, Yagi M, et al. Molecular characterization of an X(p21.2;q28) chromosomal inversion in a Duchenne muscular dystrophy patient with mental retardation reveals a novel long non-coding gene on Xq28. *J Hum Genet* 58: 33–39, 2013.

Tranebjaerg L, Petersen A, Hove K, Rehder H, Mikkelsen M. Clinical and cytogenetic studies in a large (4;8) translocation family with pre- and postnatal Wolf syndrome. *Ann Génét* 27: 224–229, 1984.

Trask BJ. Human cytogenetics: 46 chromosomes, 46 years and counting. *Nat Rev Genet* 3: 769–778, 2002.

Travan L, Naviglio S, De Cunto A, et al. Phenotypic expression of 19q13.32 microdeletions: Report of a new patient and review of the literature. *Am J Med Genet* 173: 1970–1974, 2017.

Treff NR, Levy B, Su J, Northrop LE, Tao X, Scott RT. SNP microarray-based 24 chromosome aneuploidy screening is significantly more consistent than FISH. *Mol Hum Reprod* 16: 583–589, 2010.

Treff NR, Northrop LE, Kasabwala K, Su J, Levy B, Scott RT. Single nucleotide polymorphism microarray-based concurrent screening of 24-chromosome aneuploidy and unbalanced translocations in preimplantation human embryos. *Fertil Steril* 95: 1606–1612.e1–2, 2011.

Trimborn M, Grueters A, Neitzel H, Tönnies H. First small supernumerary ring chromosome carrying 10q euchromatin in a patient with mild phenotype characterized by molecular cytogenetic techniques and review of the literature. *Cytogenet Genome Res* 108: 278–282, 2005.

Tropeano M, Ahn JW, Dobson RJ, et al. Male-biased autosomal effect of 16p13.11 copy number variation in neurodevelopmental disorders. *PLoS One* 8: e61365, 2013.

Tropeano M, Howley D, Gazzellone MJ, et al. Microduplications at the pseudoautosomal *SHOX* locus in autism spectrum disorders and related neurodevelopmental conditions. *J Med Genet* 53: 536–47, 2016.

Trujillo-Tiebas MJ, González-González C, Lorda-Sánchez I, Querejeta ME, Ayuso C, Ramos C. Prenatal diagnosis of 46, XX male fetus. *J Assist Reprod Genet* 23: 253–254, 2006.

Tsai AC, Fine CA, Yang M, Walton CS, Beischel L, Johnson JP. De novo isodicentric X chromosome: 46,X,idic(X)(q24), and summary of literature. *Am J Med Genet* 140: 923–930, 2006.

Tsai AC, Gibby T, Beischel L, McGavran L, Johnson JP. A child with Angelman syndrome and trisomy 13 findings due to associated paternal UPD 15 and segmental UPD 13. *Am J Med Genet* 126A: 208–212, 2004.

Tsai LP, Liao HM, Chen YJ, Fang JS, Chen CH. A novel microdeletion at chromosome 2q31.1-31.2 in a three-generation family presenting duplication of great toes with clinodactyly. *Clin Genet* 75: 449–456, 2009.

Tseng LH, Chuang SM, Lee TY, Ko TM. Recurrent Down's syndrome due to maternal ovarian trisomy 21 mosaicism. *Arch Gynecol Obstet* 255: 213–216, 1994.

Tsezou A, Hadjiathanasiou C, Gourgiotis D, et al. Molecular genetics of Turner syndrome: Correlation with clinical phenotype and response to growth hormone therapy. *Clin Genet* 56: 441–446, 1999.

Tsilchorozidou T, Menko FH, Lalloo F, et al. Constitutional rearrangements of chromosome 22 as a cause of neurofibromatosis 2. *J Med Genet* 41: 529–534, 2004.

Tucker ME, Garringer HJ, Weaver DD. Phenotypic spectrum of mosaic trisomy 18: Two new patients, a literature review, and counseling issues. *Am J Med Genet* 143: 505–517, 2007.

Tuck-Muller CM, Chen H, Martínez JE, et al. Isodicentric Y chromosome: Cytogenetic, molecular and clinical studies and review of the literature. *Hum Genet* 96: 119–129, 1995.

Tuğ E, Karacaaltincaba D, Yirmibeş Karaoğuz M, Saat H, Özek A. Confirmation of the prenatal mosaic trisomy 2 via fetal USG and cytogenetic analyses. *J Matern Fetal Neonatal Med* 18: 1–12, 2016.

Tupler R, Barbierato L, Larizza D, Sampaolo P, Piovella F, Maraschio P. Balanced autosomal translocations and ovarian dysgenesis. *Hum Genet* 94: 171–176, 1994.

Turleau C. Monosomy 18p. *Orphanet J Rare Dis* 3: 4, 2008.

Turner C, Dennis NR, Skuse DH, Jacobs PA. Seven ring (X) chromosomes lacking the *XIST* locus, six with an unexpectedly mild phenotype. *Hum Genet* 106: 93–100, 2000.

Turner G. Finding genes on the X chromosome by which homo may have become sapiens. *Am J Hum Genet* 58: 1109–1110, 1996.

Turner JMA. Meiotic sex chromosome inactivation. *Development* 134: 1823–1831, 2007.

Turner TN, Yi Q, Krumm N, et al. denovo-db: A compendium of human de novo variants. *Nucleic Acids Res* 45: D804–811, 2017.

Turnpenny PD, Pigott RW. Deletion 22q11 syndrome: Acknowledging a lost eponym as we say farewell to an acronym. *J Med Genet* 38: 271–273, 2001.

Tüysüz B, Collin A, Arapoglu M, Suyugül N. Clinical variability of Waardenburg-Shah syndrome in patients with proximal 13q deletion syndrome including the endothelin-B receptor locus. *Am J Med Genet* 149A: 2290–2295, 2009.

Twisk M, Mastenbroek S, Hoek A, et al. No beneficial effect of preimplantation genetic screening in women of advanced maternal age with a high risk for embryonic aneuploidy. *Hum Reprod* 23: 2813–2817, 2008.

Tyler CT, Rice GM, Grady M, Raca G. Mild clinical presentation in a child with prenatally diagnosed 45,X/47,XX,+18 mosaicism. *Am J Med Genet* 149A: 2588–2592, 2009.

Tyshchenko N, Lurie I, Schinzel A. Chromosomal map of human brain malformations. *Hum Genet* 124: 73–80, 2009.

Tyson C, Dawson AJ, Bal S, et al. Molecular cytogenetic investigation of two patients with Y chromosome rearrangements and intellectual disability. *Am J Med Genet* 149A: 490–495, 2009.

Tyson C, Sharp AJ, Hrynchak M, et al. Expansion of a 12-kb VNTR containing the *REXO1L1* gene cluster underlies the microscopically visible euchromatic variant of 8q21.2. *Eur J Hum Genet* 22: 458–463, 2014.

Tzancheva M, Kaneva R, Kumanov P, Williams G, Tyler-Smith C. Two male patients with ring Y: Definition of an interval in Yq contributing to Turner syndrome. *J Med Genet* 36: 549–553, 1999.

Uchida IA, Freeman VCP. Trisomy 21 Down syndrome: II. Structural chromosome

rearrangements in the parents. *Hum Genet* 72: 118–122, 1986.

Uehara S, Nata M, Obara Y, Niinuma T, Funato T, Yajima A. A Turner syndrome woman with a ring X chromosome [45,X/46,X,r(X)(p22.3q27)] whose child also had a ring X chromosome. *Fertil Steril* 67: 576–579, 1997.

Uehara S, Tamura M, Nata M, et al. Complete androgen insensitivity in a 47,XXY patient with uniparental disomy for the X chromosome. *Am J Med Genet* 86: 107–111, 1999a.

Uehara S, Yaegashi N, Maeda T, et al. Risk of recurrence of fetal chromosomal aberrations: Analysis of trisomy 21, trisomy 18, trisomy 13, and 45,X in 1,076 Japanese mothers. *J Obstet Gynaecol Res* 25: 373–379, 1999b.

Uematsu A, Yorifuji T, Muroi J, et al. Parental origin of normal X chromosomes in Turner syndrome patients with various karyotypes: Implications for the mechanism leading to generation of a 45,X karyotype. *Am J Med Genet* 111: 134–139, 2002.

Uhlmann F. SMC complexes: From DNA to chromosomes. *Nat Rev Mol Cell Biol* 17: 399–412, 2016.

Ulker V, Gurkan H, Tozkir H, et al. Novel *NLRP7* mutations in familial recurrent hydatidiform mole: Are *NLRP7* mutations a risk for recurrent reproductive wastage? *Eur J Obstet Gynecol Reprod Biol* 170: 188–192, 2013.

Ulm JE. Recurrent trisomies: Chance or inherited predisposition? *J Genet Counsel* 8: 109–117, 1999.

Urban M, Bommer C, Tennstedt C, et al. Ring chromosome 6 in three fetuses: Case reports, literature review, and implications for prenatal diagnosis. *Am J Med Genet* 108: 97–104, 2002.

Urioste M, Martínez-Frías ML, Bermejo E, et al. Short rib-polydactyly syndrome and pericentric inversion of chromosome 4. *Am J Med Genet* 49: 94–97, 1994.

Uroz L, Templado C. Meiotic non-disjunction mechanisms in human fertile males. *Hum Reprod* 27: 1518–1524, 2012.

Urquhart E. Clairvoyance. *Am J Med Genet* 170A: 1242–1244, 2016.

Urquhart JE, Williams SG, Bhaskar SS, Bowers N, Clayton-Smith J, Newman WG. Deletion of 19q13 reveals clinical overlap with Dubowitz syndrome. *J Hum Genet* 60: 781–785, 2015.

Usui D, Shimada S, Shimojima K, et al. Interstitial duplication of 2q32.1-q33.3 in a patient with epilepsy, developmental delay, and autistic behavior. *Am J Med Genet* 161A: 1078–1084, 2013.

Utami KH, Hillmer AM, Aksoy I, et al. Detection of chromosomal breakpoints in patients with developmental delay and speech disorders. *PLoS One* 9: e90852, 2014.

Uyar A, Seli E. The impact of assisted reproductive technologies on genomic imprinting and imprinting disorders. *Curr Opin Obstet Gynecol* 26: 210–221, 2014.

Valerio G, Franzese A, Salerno M, et al. Beta-cell dysfunction in classic transient neonatal diabetes is characterized by impaired insulin response to glucose but normal response to glucagon. *Diabetes Care* 27: 2405–2458, 2004.

Valetto A, Bertini V, Toschi B, Simi P. A 47,XX,+der(21)t(8;21)(q24.2;q21.1) karyotype in a patient with mild intellectual disability, cleft lip, Hashimoto thyroiditis and hirsutism. *Am J Med Genet* 161A: 2389–2392, 2013.

Valetto A, Orsini A, Bertini V, et al. Molecular cytogenetic characterization of an interstitial deletion of chromosome 21 (21q22.13q22.3) in a patient with dysmorphic features, intellectual disability and severe generalized epilepsy. *Eur J Med Genet* 55: 362–366, 2012.

Vals MA, Kahre T, Mee P, et al. Familial 1.3-Mb 11p15.5p15.4 duplication in three generations causing Silver-Russell and Beckwith-Wiedemann syndromes. *Mol Syndromol* 6: 147–151, 2015.

Van Bon BWM, Coe BP, Bernier R, et al. Disruptive de novo mutations of *DYRK1A* lead to a syndromic form of autism and ID. *Mol Psychiatry* 21: 126–132, 2016.

Van Bon BWM, Mefford HC, Menten B, et al. Further delineation of the 15q13 microdeletion and duplication syndromes: A clinical spectrum varying from non-pathogenic to a severe outcome. *J Med Genet* 46: 511–523, 2009.

Van Buggenhout G, Fryns JP. Angelman syndrome (AS, MIM 105830). *Eur J Hum Genet* 17: 1367–1373, 2009.

Van Buggenhout G, Van Ravenswaaij-Arts C, Mc Maas N, et al. The del(2)(q32.2q33) deletion syndrome defined by clinical and molecular characterization of four patients. *Eur J Med Genet* 48: 276–289, 2005.

Van de Laar I, Rabelink G, Hochstenbach R, Tuerlings J, Hoogeboom J, Giltay J. Diploid/triploid mosaicism in dysmorphic patients. *Clin Genet* 62: 376–382, 2002.

Van den Berg C, Van Opstal D, Brandenburg H, Los FJ. Case of 45,X/46,XY mosaicism with non-mosaic discordance between short-term villi

(45,X) and cultured villi (46,XY). *Am J Med Genet* 93: 230–233, 2000.

Van den Berg C, Van Opstal D, Polak-Knook J, Galjaard RJ. (Potential) false-negative diagnoses in chorionic villi and a review of the literature. *Prenat Diagn* 26: 401–408, 2006.

Van den Berg DJ, Francke U. Roberts syndrome: A review of 100 cases and a new rating system for severity. *Am J Med Genet* 47: 1104–1123, 1993.

Van den Berg IM, Laven JSE, Stevens M, et al. X chromosome inactivation is initiated in human preimplantation embryos. *Am J Hum Genet* 84: 771–779, 2009.

Van den Berg L, de Waal HD, Han JC, et al. Investigation of a patient with a partial trisomy 16q including the fat mass and obesity associated gene (*FTO*): Fine mapping and *FTO* gene expression study. *Am J Med Genet* 152A: 630–637, 2010.

Van den Boogaard ML, Thijssen PE, Aytekin C, et al. Expanding the mutation spectrum in ICF syndrome: Evidence for a gender bias in *ICF2*. *Clin Genet* 92: 380–387, 2017.

Van den Veyver IB, Patel A, Shaw CA, et al. Clinical use of array comparative genomic hybridization (aCGH) for prenatal diagnosis in 300 cases. *Prenat Diagn* 29: 29–39, 2009.

Van der Aa N, Vandeweyer G, Reyniers E, et al. Haploinsufficiency of CMIP in a girl with autism spectrum disorder and developmental delay due to a de novo deletion on chromosome 16q23.2. *Autism Res* 5: 277–281, 2012.

Van der Burgt CJAM, Merkx GFM, Janssen AH, Mulder JC, Suijkerbuijk RF, Smeets DFCM: Partial trisomy for 5q and monosomy for 12p in a liveborn child as a result of a complex five breakpoint chromosome rearrangement in a parent. *J Med Genet* 29: 739–741, 1992.

Van der Crabben SN, Hennus MP, McGregor GA, et al. Destabilized *SMC5/6* complex leads to chromosome breakage syndrome with severe lung disease. *J Clin Invest* 126: 2881–2892, 2016.

Van der Lelij P, Chrzanowska KH, Godthelp BC, et al. Warsaw breakage syndrome, a cohesinopathy associated with mutations in the XPD helicase family member *DDX11/ChlR1*. *Am J Hum Genet* 86: 262–266, 2010.

Van der Veken LT, Dieleman MMJ, Douben H, et al. Low grade mosaic for a complex supernumerary ring chromosome 18 in an adult patient with multiple congenital anomalies. *Mol Cytogenet* 3: 13, 2010.

Van der Ven K, Peschka B, Montag M, Lange R, Schwanitz G, van der Ven HH. Increased frequency of congenital chromosomal aberrations in female partners of couples undergoing intracytoplasmic sperm injection. *Hum Reprod* 13: 48–54, 1998.

Van der Werf IM, Buiting K, Czeschik C, et al. Novel microdeletions on chromosome 14q32.2 suggest a potential role for non-coding RNAs in Kagami-Ogata syndrome. *Eur J Hum Genet* 24: 1724–1729, 2016.

Van Dijck A, van der Werf IM, Reyniers E, et al. Five patients with a chromosome 1q21.1 triplication show macrocephaly, increased weight and facial similarities. *Eur J Med Genet* 58: 503–508, 2015.

Van Dyke DL, Weiss L, Roberson JR, Babu VR. The frequency and mutation rate of balanced autosomal rearrangements in man estimated from prenatal genetic studies for advanced maternal age. *Am J Hum Genet* 35: 301–308, 1983.

Van Echten-Arends J, Mastenbroek S, Sikkema-Raddatz B, et al. Chromosomal mosaicism in human preimplantation embryos: A systematic review. *Hum Reprod Update* 17: 620–627, 2011.

Van Haelst MM, Van Opstal D, Lindhout D, Los FJ. Management of prenatally detected trisomy 8 mosaicism. *Prenat Diagn* 21: 1075–1078, 2001.

Van Hemel JO, Eussen HJ. Interchromosomal insertions: Identification of five cases and a review. *Hum Genet* 107: 415–432, 2000.

Van Hummelen P, Manchester D, Lowe X, Wyrobek AJ. Meiotic segregation, recombination, and gamete aneuploidy assessed in a t(1;10) (p22.1;q22.3) reciprocal translocation carrier by three- and four-probe multicolor FISH in sperm. *Am J Hum Genet* 61: 651–659, 1997.

Van Karnebeek CDM, Hennekam RCM. Associations between chromosomal anomalies and congenital heart defects: A database search. *Am J Med Genet* 84: 158–166, 1999.

Van Kogelenberg M, Ghedia S, McGillivray G, et al. Periventricular heterotopia in common microdeletion syndromes. *Mol Syndromol* 1: 35–41, 2010.

Van Opstal D, van den Berg C, Galjaard RJH, Los FJ. Follow-up investigations in uncultured amniotic fluid cells after uncertain cytogenetic results. *Prenat Diagn* 21: 75–80, 2001.

Van Rahden VA, Fernandez-Vizarra E, Alawi M, et al. Mutations in *NDUFB11*, encoding a complex I component of the mitochondrial respiratory chain, cause microphthalmia with linear skin defects syndrome. *Am J Hum Genet* 96: 640–650, 2015.

Van Saen D, Gies I, De Schepper J, Tournaye H, Goossens E. Can pubertal boys with Klinefelter syndrome benefit from spermatogonial stem cell banking? *Hum Reprod* 27: 323–330, 2012a.

Van Saen D, Tournaye H, Goossens E. Presence of spermatogonia in 47,XXY men with no spermatozoa recovered after testicular sperm extraction. *Fertil Steril* 97: 319–323, 2012b.

Van Silfhout AT, van den Akker PC, Dijkhuizen T, et al. Split hand/foot malformation due to chromosome 7q aberrations (*SHFM1*): Additional support for functional haploinsufficiency as the causative mechanism. *Eur J Hum Genet* 17: 1432–1438, 2009.

Vanlerberghe C, Petit F, Malan V, et al. 15q11.2 microdeletion (BP1-BP2) and developmental delay, behaviour issues, epilepsy and congenital heart disease: A series of 52 patients. *Eur J Med Genet* 58: 140–147, 2015.

Vanneste E, Voet T, Le Caignec C, et al. Chromosome instability is common in human cleavage-stage embryos. *Nat Med* 15: 577–583, 2009a.

Vanneste E, Voet T, Melotte C, et al. What next for preimplantation genetic screening? High mitotic chromosome instability rate provides the biological basis for the low success rate. *Hum Reprod* 24: 2679–2682, 2009b.

Varela M, Shapira E, Hyman DB. Ullrich-Turner syndrome in mother and daughter: Prenatal diagnosis of a 46,X,del(X)(p21) offspring from a 45,X mother with low-level mosaicism for the del(X)(p21) in one ovary. *Am J Med Genet* 39: 411–412, 1991.

Varela MC, Simões-Sato AY, Kim CA, Bertola DR, De Castro CI, Koiffmann CP. A new case of interstitial 6q16.2 deletion in a patient with Prader-Willi-like phenotype and investigation of *SIM1* gene deletion in 87 patients with syndromic obesity. *Eur J Med Genet* 49: 298–305, 2006.

Vargiami E, Ververi A, Kyriazi M, et al. Severe clinical presentation in monozygotic twins with 10p15.3 microdeletion syndrome. *Am J Med Genet* 164A: 764–768, 2014.

Varley JM. Patterns of silver staining of human chromosomes. *Chromosoma* 61: 207–214, 1977.

Varvagiannis K, Stefanidou A, Gyftodimou Y, et al. Pure de novo partial trisomy 6p in a girl with craniosynostosis. *Am J Med Genet* 161A: 343–351, 2013.

Vassos E, Collier DA, Holden S, et al. Penetrance for copy number variants associated with schizophrenia. *Hum Mol Genet* 19: 3477–3481, 2010.

Vauhkonen AE, Sankila EM, Simola KOJ, de la Chapelle A. Segregation and fertility analysis in an autosomal reciprocal translocation, t(1;8) (q41;q23.1). *Am J Hum Genet* 37: 533–542, 1985.

Vaz I, Larkins SA, Norman A, Green SH. Mild developmental delay due to ring chromosome 19 mosaicism. *Dev Med Child Neurol* 41: 48–50, 1999.

Vázquez-Cárdenas A, Vásquez-Velásquez AI, Barros-Núñez P, Mantilla-Capacho J, Rocchi M, Rivera H. Familial whole-arm translocations (1;19), (9;13), and (12;21): A review of 101 constitutional exchanges. *J Appl Genet* 48: 261–268, 2007.

Vears DF, Delany C, Massie J, Gillam L. Parents' experiences with requesting carrier testing for their unaffected children. *Genet Med* 18: 1199–1205, 2016.

Vega H, Trainer AH, Gordillo M, et al. Phenotypic variability in 49 cases of *ESCO2* mutations, including novel missense and codon deletion in the acetyltransferase domain, correlates with *ESCO2* expression and establishes the clinical criteria for Roberts syndrome. *J Med Genet* 47: 30–37, 2010.

Vegetti W, Van Assche E, Frias A, et al. Correlation between semen parameters and sperm aneuploidy rates investigated by fluorescence in-situ hybridization in infertile men. *Hum Reprod* 15: 351–365, 2000.

Velagaleti GVN, Lockhart LH, Schmalstieg FC, Goldman AS. Trisomy 4 pter-q12 and monosomy of chromosome 13 pter-q12 in a male with deficiency of all blood lymphocyte populations. *Am J Med Genet* 102: 139–145, 2001.

Veld PA, Weber RF, Los FJ, et al. Two cases of Robertsonian translocations in oligozoospermic males and their consequences for pregnancies induced by intracytoplasmic sperm injection. *Hum Reprod* 12: 1642–1644, 1997.

Vendola C, Canfield M, Daiger SP, et al. Survival of Texas infants born with trisomies 21, 18, and 13. *Am J Med Genet* 152A: 360–366, 2010.

Venter PA, Dawson B, Du Toit JL, et al. A familial paracentric inversion: A short review of the current status. *Hum Genet* 67: 121–125, 1984.

Vera-Carbonell A, López-González V, Bafalliu JA, et al. Pre- and postnatal findings in a patient with a novel rec(8)dup(8q)inv(8)(p23.2q22.3) associated with San Luis Valley syndrome. *Am J Med Genet* 161A: 2369–2375, 2013.

Vera-Carbonell A, López-González V, Bafalliu JA, et al. Clinical comparison of 10q26 overlapping deletions: Delineating the critical region for urogenital anomalies. *Am J Med Genet* 167A: 786–790, 2015.

Vergés L, Molina O, Geán E, Vidal F, Blanco J. Deletions and duplications of the 22q11.2 region in spermatozoa from DiGeorge/velocardiofacial fathers. *Mol Cytogenet* 7: 86, 2014.

Vergult S, Hoogeboom AJM, Bijlsma EK, et al. Complex genetics of radial ray deficiencies: Screening of a cohort of 54 patients. *Genet Med* 15: 195–202, 2013a.

Vergult S, Leroy B, Claerhout I, Menten B. Familial cases of a submicroscopic Xp22.2 deletion: Genotype-phenotype correlation in microphthalmia with linear skin defects syndrome. *Mol Vis* 19: 311–318, 2013b.

Verhoeven WMA, Egger JIM, van den Bergh JPW, van Beek R, Kleefstra T, de Leeuw N. A 12q24.31 interstitial deletion in an adult male with *MODY3*: Neuropsychiatric and neuropsychological characteristics. *Am J Med Genet* 167A: 169–173, 2015.

Verhoeven WMA, Tuinier S, Curfs LMG. Prader-Willi syndrome: The psychopathological phenotype in uniparental disomy. *J Med Genet* 40: e112, 2003.

Verlinsky Y, Cieslak J, Kuliev A. Similar frequencies of meiosis I & II aneuploidies in IVF patients of advanced maternal age. *Ann Génét* 44: s124, 2001a.

Verlinsky Y, Rechitsky S, Schoolcraft W, Strom C, Kuliev A. Preimplantation diagnosis for Fanconi anemia combined with HLA matching. *J Am Med Assoc* 285: 3130–3133, 2001b.

Verloes A, Gillerot Y, Van Maldergem L, et al. Major decrease in the incidence of trisomy 21 at birth in south Belgium: Mass impact of triple test? *Eur J Hum Genet* 9: 1–4, 2001.

Verma RS, Rodriguez J, Dosik H. The clinical significance of pericentric inversion of the human Y chromosome: A rare "third" type of heteromorphism. *J Hered* 73: 236–238, 1982.

Vermeesch JR, Petit P, Speleman F, Devriendt K, Fryns JP, Marynen P. Interstitial telomeric sequences at the junction site of a jumping translocation. *Hum Genet* 99: 735–737, 1997.

Vermeiden JP, Bernardus RE. Are imprinting disorders more prevalent after human in vitro fertilization or intracytoplasmic sperm injection? *Fertil Steril* 99: 642–651, 2013.

Vernon HJ, Bytyci Telegrafi A, Batista D, Owegi M, Leigh R. 6p25 microdeletion: White matter abnormalities in an adult patient. *Am J Med Genet* 161A: 1686–1689, 2013.

Verp MS, Bombard AT, Simpson JL, Elias S. Parental decision following prenatal diagnosis of fetal chromosome abnormality. *Am J Med Genet* 29: 613–622, 1988.

Vetro A, Dehghani MR, Kraoua L, et al. Testis development in the absence of *SRY*: Chromosomal rearrangements at *SOX9* and *SOX3*. *Eur J Hum Genet* 23: 1025–1032, 2015.

Vialard F, Hammoud I, Molina-Gomes D, et al. Gamete cytogenetic study in couples with implantation failure: Aneuploidy rate is increased in both couple members. *J Assist Reprod Genet* 25: 539–545, 2008.

Vialard F, Nouchy M, Malan V, Taillemite JL, Selva J, Portnoï MF. Whole-arm translocations between chromosome 1 and acrocentric G chromosomes are associated with a poor prognosis for spermatogenesis: Two new cases and review of the literature. *Fertil Steril* 86: 1001, e1–5, 2006.

Vichinsartvichai P. Primary ovarian insufficiency associated with autosomal abnormalities: From chromosome to genome-wide and beyond. *Menopause* 23: 806–815, 2016.

Vičić A, Roje D, Strinić T, Stipoljev F. Trisomy 1 in an early pregnancy failure. *Am J Med Genet* 146A: 2439–2441, 2008.

Vicidomini C, Ponzoni L, Lim D, et al. Pharmacological enhancement of mGlu5 receptors rescues behavioral deficits in *SHANK3* knock-out mice. *Mol Psychiatr* 22: 689–702, 2017.

Vickers S, Dahlitz M, Hardy C, Kilpatrick M, Webb T. A male with a de novo translocation involving loss of 15q11q13 material and Prader-Willi syndrome. *J Med Genet* 31: 478–481, 1994.

Vieira GH, Rodriguez JD, Carmona-Mora P, et al. Detection of classical 17p11.2 deletions, an atypical deletion and *RAI1* alterations in patients with features suggestive of Smith-Magenis syndrome. *Eur J Hum Genet* 20: 148–154, 2012.

Vieira JP, Lopes F, Silva-Fernandes A, et al. Variant Rett syndrome in a girl with a pericentric X-chromosome inversion leading to epigenetic changes and overexpression of the *MECP2* gene. *Int J Dev Neurosci* 46: 82–87, 2015.

Vignoli A, Bisulli F, Darra F, et al. Epilepsy in ring chromosome 20 syndrome. *Epilepsy Res* 128: 83–93, 2016.

Villa N, Bentivegna A, Ertel A, et al. A de novo supernumerary genomic discontinuous ring chromosome 21 in a child with mild intellectual disability. *Am J Med Genet* 155A: 1425–1431, 2011.

Villavicencio-Lorini P, Klopocki E, Trimborn M, Koll R, Mundlos S, Horn D. Phenotypic variant of brachydactyly-mental retardation syndrome in a family with an inherited interstitial 2q37.3 microdeletion including *HDAC4*. *Eur J Hum Genet* 21: 743–748, 2013.

Visootsak J, Graham JM. Klinefelter syndrome and other sex chromosomal aneuploidies. *Orphanet J Rare Dis* 1: 42, 2006.

Vissers LELM, van Ravenswaaij CMA, Admiraal R, et al. Mutations in a new member of the chromodomain gene family cause CHARGE syndrome. *Nat Genet* 36: 955–957, 2004.

Vockley J, Inserra JA, Breg WR, Yang-Feng TL. "Pseudomosaicism" for 4p- in amniotic fluid cell culture proven to be true mosaicism after birth. *Am J Med Genet* 39: 81–83, 1991.

Voiculescu I, Barbi G, Wolff G, Steinbach P, Back E, Schempp W. Familial pericentric inversion of chromosome 12. *Hum Genet* 72: 320–322, 1986.

Vona B, Nanda I, Neuner C, et al. Terminal chromosome 4q deletion syndrome in an infant with hearing impairment and moderate syndromic features: Review of literature. *BMC Med Genet* 15: 72, 2014.

Vorstman JA, Breetvelt EJ, Duijff SN, et al. Cognitive decline preceding the onset of psychosis in patients with 22q11.2 deletion syndrome. *JAMA Psychiatry* 72: 377–385, 2015.

Voullaire L, Collins V, Callaghan T, McBain J, Williamson R, Wilton L. High incidence of complex chromosome abnormality in cleavage embryos from patients with repeated implantation failure. *Fertil Steril* 87: 1053–1058, 2007.

Voullaire L, Gardner RJM, Vaux C, Robertson A, Oertel R, Slater H. Chromosomal duplication of band 10p14 segregating through four generations. *J Med Genet* 37: 233–237, 2000a.

Voullaire LE, Slater HR, Petrovic V, Choo KHA. A functional marker centromere with no detectable alpha-satellite, satellite III, or CENP-B protein: Activation of a latent centromere? *Am J Hum Genet* 52: 1153–1163, 1993.

Voullaire L, Slater H, Williamson R, Wilton L. Chromosome analysis of blastomeres from human embryos by using comparative genomic hybridization. *Hum Genet* 106: 210–217, 2000b.

Voullaire L, Wilton L, McBain J, Callaghan T, Williamson R. Chromosome abnormalities identified by comparative genomic hybridization in embryos from women with repeated implantation failure. *Mol Hum Reprod* 8: 1035–1041, 2002.

Vozdova M, Heracek J, Sobotka V, Rubes J. Testicular sperm aneuploidy in non-obstructive azoospermic patients. *Hum Reprod* 27: 2233–2239, 2012.

Vozdova M, Horinova V, Wernerova V, et al. der(4) t(Y;4): Three-generation transmission and sperm meiotic segregation analysis. *Am J Med Genet* 155A: 1157–1161, 2011.

Vranekovic J, Božovic IB, Grubic Z, et al. Down syndrome: Parental origin, recombination, and maternal age. *Genet Test Mol Biomarkers* 16: 70–73, 2012.

Vreeburg M, van Steensel MA. Genodermatoses caused by genetic mosaicism. *Eur J Pediatr* 171: 1725–1735, 2012.

Wagner T, Wirth J, Meyer J, et al. Autosomal sex reversal and campomelic dysplasia are caused by mutations in and around the *SRY*-related gene *SOX9*. *Cell* 79: 1111–1120, 1994.

Wagstaff J, Hemann M. A familial "balanced" 3;9 translocation with cryptic 8q insertion leading to deletion and duplication of 9p23 loci in siblings. *Am J Hum Genet* 56: 302–309, 1995.

Wahab MA, Nickless EM, Najar-M'Kacher R, Parmentier C, Podd JV, Rowland RE. Elevated chromosome translocation frequencies in New Zealand nuclear test veterans. *Cytogenet Genome Res* 121: 79–87, 2008.

Wakeling EL, Abu-Amero S, Alders M, et al. Epigenotype-phenotype correlations in Silver-Russell syndrome. *J Med Genet* 47: 760–768, 2010.

Wakui K, Gregato G, Ballif BC, et al. Construction of a natural panel of 11p11.2 deletions and further delineation of the critical region involved in Potocki-Shaffer syndrome. *Eur J Hum Genet* 13: 528–540, 2005.

Walczak C, Enders H, Grissinger K, Dufke A. Retrospective diagnosis of trisomy 15 in formalin-fixed, paraffin-embedded placental tissue in a newborn girl with Prader-Willi syndrome. *Prenat Diagn* 20: 914–916, 2000.

Walczak-Sztulpa J, Wisniewska M, Latos-Bielenska A, et al. Chromosome deletions in 13q33-34: Report of four patients and review of the literature. *Am J Med Genet* 146: 337–342, 2008.

Walker AP, Bocian M. Partial duplication 8q12→q21.2 in two sibs with maternally derived insertional and reciprocal translocations: Case reports and review of partial duplications of chromosome 8. *Am J Med Genet* 27: 3–22, 1987.

Walkinshaw SA. Fetal choroid plexus cysts: Are we there yet? *Prenat Diagn* 20: 657–662, 2000.

Walknowska J, Conte FA, Grumbach MM. Practical and theoretical implications of fetal-maternal lymphocyte transfer. *Lancet* 1: 1119–1122, 1969.

Wallace BMN, Hultén MA. Triple chromosome synapsis in oocytes from a human foetus with trisomy 21. *Ann Hum Genet* 47: 271–276, 1983.

Wallace WHB, Kelsey TW. Human ovarian reserve from conception to the menopause. *PLoS One* 5: e8772, 2010.

Wallerstein R, Oh T, Durcan J, Abdelhak Y, Clachko M, Aviv H. Outcome of prenatally diagnosed trisomy 6 mosaicism. *Prenat Diagn* 22: 722–724, 2002.

Wallerstein R, Twersky S, Layman P, et al. Long term follow-up of developmental delay in a child with prenatally-diagnosed trisomy 20 mosaicism. *Am J Med Genet* 137: 94–97, 2005.

Wallerstein R, Yu MT, Neu RL, et al. Common trisomy mosaicism diagnosed in amniocytes involving chromosomes 13, 18, 20 and 21: Karyotype-phenotype correlations. *Prenat Diagn* 20: 103–122, 2000.

Walters, S. (1995). Down's tests are a right. *Sunday Age* (Melbourne), July 23, 1995.

Walters-Sen LC, Windemuth K, Angione K, Nandhlal J, Milunsky JM. Familial transmission of 5p13.2 duplication due to maternal der(X)ins(X;5). *Eur J Med Genet* 58: 305–309, 2015.

Walzer S, Bashir AS, Silbert AR. Cognitive and behavioral factors in the learning disabilities of 47,XXY and 47,XYY boys. *Birth Defects Orig Artic Ser* 26: 45–58, 1990.

Wang BT, Chong TP, Boyar FZ, et al. Abnormalities in spontaneous abortions detected by G-banding and chromosomal microarray analysis (CMA) at a national reference laboratory. *Mol Cytogenet* 7: 33, 2014a.

Wang D, Zeesman S, Tarnopolsky MA, Nowaczyk MJ. Duplication of *AKT3* as a cause of macrocephaly in duplication 1q43q44. *Am J Med Genet* 161A: 2016–2019, 2013a.

Wang JC, Dang L, Fisker T. Chromosome 6 between-arm intrachromosomal insertion with intrasegmental double inversion: A four-break model. *Am J Med Genet* 152A: 209–211, 2010a.

Wang JC, Fisker T, Dang L, Teshima I, Nowaczyk MJM. 4.3-Mb triplication of 4q32.1-q32.2: Report of a family through two generations. *Am J Med Genet* 149A: 2274–2279, 2009a.

Wang JCC, Mamunes P, Kou SY, Schmidt J, Mao R, Hsu WT. Centromeric DNA break in a 10;16 reciprocal translocation associated with trisomy 16 confined placental mosaicism and maternal uniparental disomy for chromosome 16. *Am J Med Genet* 80: 418–422, 1998.

Wang L, Iqbal F, Li G, et al. Abnormal meiotic recombination with complex chromosomal rearrangement in an azoospermic man. *Reprod Biomed Online* 30: 651–658, 2015.

Wang M, Lu S, Zhu Y, Li H. *ADAM12* is an effective marker in the second trimester of pregnancy for prenatal screening of Down syndrome. *Prenat Diagn* 30: 561–564, 2010b.

Wang NJ, Liu D, Parokonny AS, Schanen NC. High-resolution molecular characterization of 15q11-q13 rearrangements by array comparative genomic hybridization (array CGH) with detection of gene dosage. *Am J Hum Genet* 75: 267–281, 2004.

Wang P, Carrion P, Qiao Y, et al. Genotype-phenotype analysis of 18q12.1-q12.2 copy number variation in autism. *Eur J Med Genet* 56: 420–425, 2013b.

Wang W, Hu Y, Zhu H, Li J, Zhu R, Wang YP. A case of an infertile male with a small supernumerary marker chromosome negative for M-FISH and containing only heterochromatin. *J Assist Reprod Genet* 26: 291–295, 2009b.

Wang Y, Chen Y, Tian F, et al. Maternal mosaicism is a significant contributor to discordant sex chromosomal aneuploidies associated with noninvasive prenatal testing. *Clin Chem* 60: 251–259, 2014b.

Wang Y, Zhang B, Zhang L, et al. The 3D Genome Browser: a web-based browser for visualizing 3D genome organization and long-range chromatin interactions. *BioRχiv*, in press 2018.

Wang Z, Cody JD, Leach RJ, O'Connell P. Gene expression patterns in cell lines from patients with 18q- syndrome. *Hum Genet* 104: 467–475, 1999.

Wapner RJ, Martin CL, Levy B, et al. Chromosomal microarray versus karyotyping for prenatal diagnosis. *N Engl J Med* 367: 2175–2184, 2012.

Warburton D. Genetic factors influencing aneuploidy frequency. In Dellarco VL, Voytek PE, Hollaender A (eds.), *Aneuploidy: Etiology and Mechanisms.* New York, NY: Plenum, 1985.

Warburton D. De novo balanced chromosome rearrangements and extra marker chromosomes identified at prenatal diagnosis: Clinical significance and distribution of breakpoints. *Am J Hum Genet* 49: 995–1013, 1991.

Warburton D. Trisomy 7 mosaicism: Prognosis after prenatal diagnosis. *Prenat Diagn* 22: 1239–1240, 2002.

Warburton D, Byrne J, Canki N. *Chromosome Anomalies and Prenatal Development: An Atlas* (Oxford Monographs on Medical Genetics No. 20). New York, NY: Oxford University Press, 1991.

Warburton D, Dallaire L, Thangavelu M, Ross L, Levin B, Kline J. Trisomy recurrence: A reconsideration based on North American data. *Am J Hum Genet* 75: 376–385, 2004.

Warburton D, Kline J, Kinney A, Yu CY, Levin B, Brown S. Skewed X chromosome inactivation and trisomic spontaneous abortion: No association. *Am J Hum Genet* 85: 179–193, 2009.

Warsof SL, Larion S, Abuhamad AZ. Overview of the impact of noninvasive prenatal testing on diagnostic procedures. *Prenat Diagn* 35: 972–979, 2015.

Waters JJ, Campbell PL, Crocker AJM, Campbell CM. Phenotypic effects of balanced X-autosome translocations in females: A retrospective survey of 104 cases reported from UK laboratories. *Hum Genet* 108: 318–327, 2001.

Watkins C, Lazzarini A, McCormack M, Reid CS. Genetic counseling for the mildly mentally retarded client: Three case reports. In Zellers N (ed.), *Strategies for Genetic Counseling: Tools for Professional Advancement.* New York, NY: Human Services Press, 1989: 219–234.

Watson CM, Crinnion LA, Harrison SM, et al. A chromosome 7 pericentric inversion defined at single-nucleotide resolution using diagnostic whole genome sequencing in a patient with hand-foot-genital syndrome. *PLoS One* 11: e0157075, 2016.

Watson P. Legal and ethical issues in wrongful life actions. *Melbourne Univ Law Rev* 26: 14, 2002.

Watt AJ, Devereux FJ, Monk NA, Myers CJ, Gardner RJM. The phenotype in placental trisomy 7. *Aust NZ J Obstet Gynaecol* 31: 246–248, 1991.

Watt JL, Ward K, Couzin DA, Stephen GS, Hill A. A paracentric inversion of 7q illustrating a possible interchromosomal effect. *J Med Genet* 23: 341–344, 1986.

Wattanasirichaigoon D, Promsonthi P, Chuansumrit A, et al. Maternal uniparental disomy of chromosome 16 resulting in hemoglobin Bart's hydrops fetalis. *Clin Genet* 74: 284–287, 2008.

Wawrocka A, Sikora A, Kuszel L, Krawczynski MR. 11p13 deletions can be more frequent than the *PAX6* gene point mutations in Polish patients with aniridia. *J Appl Genet* 54: 345–351, 2013.

Webb GC, Voullaire LE, Rogers JG. Duplication of a small segment of 5p due to maternal recombination within a paracentric shift. *Am J Med Genet* 30: 875–881, 1988.

Webb T. Inv dup(15) supernumerary marker chromosomes. *J Med Genet* 31: 585–594, 1994.

Webb T, Clayton-Smith J, Cheng XJ, et al. Angelman syndrome with a chromosomal inversion 15 inv(p11q13) accompanied by a deletion in 15q11q13. *J Med Genet* 29: 921–924, 1992.

Weber W. France's highest court recognises "the right not to be born." *Lancet* 358: 1972, 2001.

Webster A, Schuh M. Mechanisms of aneuploidy in human eggs. *Trends Cell Biol* 27: 55–68, 2017.

Wegner RD, Entezami M, Knoll U, Horn D, Sohl S, Becker R. Prenatal diagnosis of fetal trisomy 6 mosaicism and phenotype of the affected newborn. *Am J Med Genet* 124A: 85–88, 2004.

Wegner RD, Kistner G, Becker R, et al. Fetal 46,XX/69,XXY mixoploidy: Origin and confirmation by analysis of fetal urine cells. *Prenat Diagn* 29: 287–289, 2009.

Wei HJ, Chiang HS, Lin WM, Wen JY. Pregnancy after preimplantation genetic diagnosis by fluorescence in situ hybridization using 18-, X-, and Y-chromosome probes in an infertile male with mosaic trisomy 18. *J Assist Reprod Genet* 17: 229–231, 2000.

Weil D, Wang I, Dietrich A, Poustka A, Weissenbach J, Petit C. Highly homologous loci on the X and Y chromosomes are hot-spots for ectopic recombinations leading to XX maleness. *Nat Genet* 7: 414–419, 1994.

Weiner DJ, Wigdor EM, Ripke S, et al. Polygenic transmission disequilibrium confirms that common and rare variation act additively to create risk for autism spectrum disorders. *Nat Genet* 49: 978–985, 2017.

Weissman A, Shoham G, Shoham Z, Fishel S, Leong M, Yaron Y. Preimplantation genetic screening: results of a worldwide web-based survey. *Reprod Biomed Online* 35: 693–700, 2017.

Weisz B, Rodeck CH. An update on antenatal screening for Down's syndrome and specific implications for assisted reproduction pregnancies. *Hum Reprod Update* 12: 513–518, 2006.

Weksberg R, Shuman C, Beckwith JB. Beckwith-Wiedemann syndrome. *Eur J Hum Genet* 18: 8–14, 2010.

Welham A, Barth B, Moss J, et al. Behavioral characteristics associated with 19p13.2 microdeletions. *Am J Med Genet* 167A: 2334–2343, 2015.

Wells D. Karyo- and meio-mapping for human embryo selection. Paper presented at the European Human Genetics conference, Copenhagen, 2017.

Wells D, Alfarawati S, Fragouli E. Use of comprehensive chromosomal screening for embryo assessment: microarrays and CGH. *Mol Hum Reprod* 14: 703–710, 2008.

Wells D, Kaur K, Grifo J, et al. Clinical utilisation of a rapid low-pass whole genome sequencing technique for the diagnosis of aneuploidy in human embryos prior to implantation. *J Med Genet* 51: 553–562, 2014.

Wenger SL, Boone LY, Cummins JH, et al. Newborn infant with inherited ring and de novo interstitial deletion on homologous chromosome 22s. *Am J Med Genet* 91: 351–354, 2000.

Wenger SL, Sell SL, Painter MJ, Steele MW. Inherited unbalanced subtelomeric translocation in a child with 8p- and Angelman syndromes. *Am J Med Genet* 70: 150–154, 1997.

Wenger SL, Steele MW, Boone LY, Lenkey SG, Cummins JH, Chen XQ. "Balanced" karyotypes in six abnormal offspring of balanced reciprocal translocation normal carrier parents. *Am J Med Genet* 55: 47–52, 1995.

Wentzel C, Annerén G, Thuresson AC. A maternal de novo non-reciprocal translocation results in a 6q13-q16 deletion in one offspring and a 6q13-q16 duplication in another. *Eur J Med Genet* 57: 259–263, 2014.

Wentzel C, Rajcan-Separovic E, Ruivenkamp CA, et al. Genomic and clinical characteristics of six patients with partially overlapping interstitial deletions at 10p12p11. *Eur J Hum Genet* 19: 959–964, 2011.

Weremowicz S, Sandstrom DJ, Morton CC, Niedzwiecki CA, Sandstrom MM, Bieber FR. Fluorescence in situ hybridization (FISH) for rapid detection of aneuploidy: Experience in 911 prenatal cases. *Prenat Diagn* 21: 262–269, 2001.

Werner-Lin A, Barg FK, Kellom KS, et al. Couple's narratives of communion and isolation following abnormal prenatal microarray testing results. *Qual Health Res* 26: 1975–1987, 2016a.

Werner-Lin A, McCoyd JL, Bernhardt BA. Balancing genetics (science) and counseling (art) in prenatal chromosomal microarray testing. *J Genet Couns* 25: 855–867, 2016b.

Werner-Lin A, Walser S, Barg FK, Bernhardt BA. "They can't find anything wrong with him, yet": Mothers' experiences of parenting an infant with a prenatally diagnosed copy number variant (CNV). *Am J Med Genet* 173A: 444–451, 2017.

Wessels MW, Los FJ, Frohn-Mulder IME, Niermeijer MF, Willems PJ, Wladimiroff JW. Poor outcome in Down syndrome fetuses with cardiac anomalies or growth retardation. *Am J Med Genet* 116A: 147–151, 2003.

Wheeler M, Peakman D, Robinson A, Henry G. 45,X/46,XY mosaicism: Contrast of prenatal and postnatal diagnosis. *Am J Med Genet* 29: 565–571, 1988.

White LM, Treat K, Leff A, Styers D, Mitchell M, Knoll JHM. Exclusion of uniparental inheritance of chromosome 15 in a fetus with a familial dicentric (Y;15) translocation. *Prenat Diagn* 18: 111–116, 1998.

Whiteford ML, Baird C, Kinmond S, Donaldson B, Davidson HR. A child with bisatellited, dicentric chromosome 15 arising from a maternal paracentric inversion of chromosome 15q. *J Med Genet* 37: E11, 2000.

Wieczorek D, Prott EC, Robinson WP, Passarge E, Gillessen-Kaesbach G. Prenatally detected trisomy 4 and 6 mosaicism—Cytogenetic results and clinical phenotype. *Prenat Diagn* 23: 128–133, 2003.

Wieland I, Schanze D, Schanze I, Volleth M, Muschke P, Zenker M. A cryptic unbalanced translocation der(4)t(4;17)(p16.1;q25.3) identifies Wittwer syndrome as a variant of Wolf-Hirschhorn syndrome. *Am J Med Genet* 164A: 3213–3214.

Wierenga KJ, Jiang Z, Yang AC, Mulvihill JJ, Tsinoremas NF. A clinical evaluation tool for SNP arrays, especially for autosomal recessive conditions in offspring of consanguineous parents. *Genet Med* 15: 354–60, 2013.

Wiersma R. True hermaphroditism in southern Africa: The clinical picture. *Pediatr Surg Int* 20: 363–368, 2004.

Wigby K, D'Epagnier C, Howell S, et al. Expanding the phenotype of triple X syndrome: A comparison of prenatal versus postnatal diagnosis. *Am J Med Genet* 170A: 2870–2881, 2016.

Wiktor AE, Van Dyke DL. Detection of low level sex chromosome mosaicism in Ullrich-Turner syndrome patients. *Am J Med Genet* 138A: 259–261, 2005.

Wiland E, Hobel CJ, Hill D, Kurpisz M. Successful pregnancy after preimplantation genetic diagnosis for carrier of t(2;7)(p11.2;q22) with high rates of unbalanced sperm and embryos: A case report. *Prenat Diagn* 28: 36–41, 2008.

Wiland E, Midro AT, Panasiuk B, Kurpisz M. The analysis of meiotic segregation patterns and aneuploidy in the spermatozoa of father and son with translocation t(4;5)(p15.1;p12) and the prediction of the individual probability rate for unbalanced progeny at birth. *J Androl* 28: 262–272, 2007.

Wilbur AK. Possible case of Rubinstein-Taybi syndrome in a prehistoric skeleton from west-central Illinois. *Am J Med Genet* 91: 56–61, 2000.

Wiley JE, Madigan M, Christie JD, Smith AW. Dispermic chimerism with two abnormal cell lines, 47,XY, +21 and 47,XX, +12. *Am J Med Genet* 107: 64–66, 2002.

Wilkins EJ, Archibald AD, Sahhar MA, White SM. "It wasn't a disaster or anything": Parents' experiences of their child's uncertain chromosomal microarray result. *Am J Med Genet* 170A: 2895–2904, 2016.

Willemsen MH, Vallès A, Kirkels LAMH, et al. Chromosome 1p21.3 microdeletions comprising *DPYD* and *MIR137* are associated with intellectual disability. *J Med Genet* 48: 810–818, 2011.

Willemsen MH, Vulto-van Silfhout AT, Nillesen WM, et al. Update on Kleefstra syndrome. *Mol Syndromol* 2: 202–212, 2012.

Williams C, Sandall J, Lewando-Hundt G, Heyman B, Spencer K, Grellier R. Women as moral pioneers? Experiences of first trimester antenatal screening. *Soc Sci Med* 61: 1983–1992, 2005.

Williams J, Dear PRF. An unbalanced t(X;10) mat translocation in a child with congenital abnormalities. *J Med Genet* 24: 633, 1987.

Williamson EM, Miller JF, Seabright M. Pericentric inversion (13) with two different recombinants in the same family. *J Med Genet* 17: 309–312, 1980.

Willis MJH, Bird LM, Dell'Aquilla M, Jones MC. Natural history of prenatally diagnosed 46,X,isodicentric Y. *Prenat Diagn* 26: 134–137, 2006.

Willis MJH, Bird LM, Dell'Aquilla M, Jones MC. Expanding the phenotype of mosaic trisomy 20. *Am J Med Genet* 146: 330–336, 2008.

Wilson GR, Sim JC, McLean C, et al. Mutations in RAB39B cause X-linked intellectual disability and early-onset Parkinson disease with α-synuclein pathology. *Am J Hum Genet* 95: 729–735, 2014.

Wilson M, Peters G, Bennetts B, et al. The clinical phenotype of mosaicism for genome-wide paternal uniparental disomy: Two new reports. *Am J Med Genet* 146A: 137–148, 2008.

Wilson MG, Lin MS, Fujimoto A, Herbert W, Kaplan FM. Chromosome mosaicism in 6,000 amniocenteses. *Am J Med Genet* 32: 506–513, 1989.

Wilson ND, Ross LJN, Close J, Mott R, Crow TJ, Volpi EV. Replication profile of *PCDH11X* and *PCDH11Y*, a gene pair located in the non-pseudoautosomal homologous region Xq21.3/Yp11.2. *Chromosome Res* 15: 485–498, 2007.

Wilton L. Preimplantation genetic diagnosis for aneuploidy screening in early human embryos: A review. *Prenat Diagn* 22: 512–518, 2002.

Wilton L, Thornhill A, Traeger-Synodinos J, Sermon KD, Harper JC. The causes of misdiagnosis and adverse outcomes in PGD. *Hum Reprod* 24: 1221–1228, 2009.

Wilton L, Williamson R, McBain J, Edgar D, Voullaire L. Birth of a healthy infant after preimplantation confirmation of euploidy by comparative genomic hybridization. *N Engl J Med* 345: 1537–1541, 2001.

Wimalasundera RC, Gardiner HM. Congenital heart disease and aneuploidy. *Prenat Diagn* 24: 1116–1122, 2004.

Wimplinger I, Rauch A, Orth U, Schwarzer U, Trautmann U, Kutsche K. Mother and daughter with a terminal Xp deletion: Implication of chromosomal mosaicism and X-inactivation in the high clinical variability of the microphthalmia with linear skin defects (MLS) syndrome. *Eur J Med Genet* 50: 421–431, 2007.

Winter JSD. Androgen therapy in Klinefelter syndrome during adolescence. *Birth Defects Orig Artic Ser* 26: 235–245, 1990.

Winther JF, Boice JD, Jr., Mulvihill JJ, et al. Chromosomal abnormalities among offspring of childhood-cancer survivors in Denmark: A population-based study. *Am J Hum Genet* 74: 1282–1285, 2004.

Witters I, Chabchoub E, Vermeesch JR, Fryns JP. Submicroscopic distal deletion of the long arm of chromosome 13(13q34) with corpus callosum agenesis. *Am J Med Genet* 149A: 1834–1836, 2009.

Witters I, Devriendt K, Legius E, et al. Rapid prenatal diagnosis of trisomy 21 in 5049 consecutive uncultured amniotic fluid samples by fluorescence in situ hybridisation (FISH). *Prenat Diagn* 22: 29–33, 2002.

Witters I, Fryns JP. Follow-up of a child with trisomy 17 mosaicism. *Prenat Diagn* 28: 1080, 2008.

Witteveen JS, Willemsen MH, Dombroski TC, et al. Haploinsufficiency of *MeCP2*-interacting transcriptional co-repressor *SIN3A* causes mild intellectual disability by affecting the development of cortical integrity. *Nat Genet* 48: 877–887, 2016.

Wójcik C, Volz K, Ranola M, Kitch K, Karim T, O'Neil J, Smith J, Torres-Martinez W. Rubinstein-Taybi syndrome associated with Chiari type I malformation caused by a large 16p13.3 microdeletion: A contiguous gene syndrome? *Am J Med Genet* 152A: 479–483, 2010.

Wolff DJ, Miller AP, Van Dyke DL, Schwartz S, Willard HF. Molecular definition of breakpoints associated with human Xq isochromosomes: Implications for mechanisms of formation. *Am J Hum Genet* 58: 154–160, 1996.

Wolstenholme J. Confined placental mosaicism for trisomies 2, 3, 7, 8, 9, 16, and 22: Their incidence, likely origins, and mechanisms for cell lineage compartmentalization. *Prenat Diagn* 16: 511–524, 1996.

Wolstenholme J, Angell RR. Maternal age and trisomy—A unifying mechanism of formation. *Chromosoma* 109: 435–438, 2000.

Wolstenholme J, Brummitt JA, English CJ, Goodship JA. Prenatal detection of multiple copies of a familial supernumerary marker chromosome. *Prenat Diagn* 12: 1067–1071, 1992.

Wolstenholme J, Webb AL, English CJ, Evans J. Prenatal diagnosis of chromosome 22 mosaicism with extensive investigation of placental and fetal tissues. *Ann Génét* 44 (Suppl 1): 14s, 2001a.

Wolstenholme J, White I, Sturgiss S, Carter J, Plant N, Goodship JA. Maternal uniparental heterodisomy for chromosome 2: Detection through "atypical" maternal AFP/hCG levels, with an update on a previous case. *Prenat Diagn* 21: 813–817, 2001b.

Won RH, Currier RJ, Lorey F, Towner DR. The timing of demise in fetuses with trisomy 21 and trisomy 18. *Prenat Diagn* 25: 608–611, 2005.

Woodage T, Prasad M, Dixon JW, et al. Bloom syndrome and maternal uniparental disomy for chromosome 15. *Am J Hum Genet* 55: 74–80, 1994.

Woods CG, Bankier A, Curry J, et al. Asymmetry and skin pigmentary anomalies in chromosome mosaicism. *J Med Genet* 31: 694–701, 1994.

Woods CG, Noble J, Falconer AR. A study of brothers with Klinefelter syndrome. *J Med Genet* 34: 702, 1997.

Worsham MJ, Miller DA, Devries JM, et al. A dicentric recombinant 9 derived from a paracentric inversion: Phenotype, cytogenetics, and molecular analysis of centromeres. *Am J Hum Genet* 44: 115–123, 1989.

Worton RG, Stern R. A Canadian collaborative study of mosaicism in amniotic fluid cell cultures. *Prenat Diagn* 4: Spec No. 131–144, 1984.

Wou K, Hyun Y, Chitayat D, et al. Analysis of tissue from products of conception and perinatal losses using QF-PCR and microarray: A three-year retrospective study resulting in an efficient protocol. *Eur J Med Genet* 59: 417–424, 2016a.

Wou K, Levy B, Wapner RJ. Chromosomal microarrays for the prenatal detection of microdeletions and microduplications. *Clin Lab Med* 36: 261–276, 2016b.

Wright DJ, Day FR, Kerrison ND, et al. Genetic variants associated with mosaic Y chromosome loss highlight cell cycle genes and overlap with cancer susceptibility. *Nat Genet* 49: 674–679, 2017.

Writzl K, Knegt AC. 6p21.3 microdeletion involving the *SYNGAP1* gene in a patient with intellectual disability, seizures, and severe speech impairment. *Am J Med Genet* 161A: 1682–1685, 2013.

Wu C, Wang L, Iqbal F, et al. Preferential Y-Y pairing and synapsis and abnormal meiotic recombination in a 47,XYY man with non obstructive azoospermia. *Mol Cytogenet* 9: 9, 2016a.

Wu DJ, Wang NJ, Driscoll J, et al. Autistic disorder associated with a paternally derived unbalanced translocation leading to duplication of chromosome 15pter-q13.2: A case report. *Mol Cytogenet* 2: 27, 2009.

Wu L, Liu J, Lv W, Wen J, Xia Y, Liang D. An Xp21.3p11.4 duplication observed in a boy with intellectual deficiency and speech delay and his asymptomatic mother. *Birth Defects Res A* 97: 467–470, 2013.

Wu T, Yin B, Zhu Y, et al. Molecular cytogenetic analysis of early spontaneous abortions conceived from varying assisted reproductive technology procedures. *Mol Cytogenet* 9: 79, 2016b.

Wu YC, Yu MT, Chen LC, Chen CL, Yang ML. Prenatal diagnosis of mosaic tetrasomy 10p associated with megacisterna magna, echogenic focus of left ventricle, umbilical cord cysts and distal arthrogryposis. *Am J Med Genet* 117A: 278–281, 2003.

Wyrobek AJ, Adler ID. Detection of aneuploidy in human and rodent sperm using FISH and applications of sperm assays of genetic damage in heritable risk evaluation. *Mutat Res* 352: 173–179, 1996.

Xanthopoulou L, Mantzouratou A, Mania A, et al. Male and female meiotic behaviour of an intrachromosomal insertion determined by preimplantation genetic diagnosis. *Mol Cytogenet* 8: 2, 2010.

Xiao P, Liu P, Weber JL, Papasian CJ, Recker RR, Deng HW. Paternal uniparental isodisomy of the entire chromosome 3 revealed in a person with no apparent phenotypic disorders. *Hum Mutat* 27: 133–137, 2006.

Xu F, Zhang YN, Cheng DH, et al. The first patient with a pure 1p36 microtriplication associated with severe clinical phenotypes. *Mol Cytogenet* 7: 64, 2014.

Xu J, Chernos J, Roland B. Trisomy 16pter to 16q12.1 and monosomy 22pter to 22q11.2 resulting from adjacent-2 segregation of a maternal complex chromosome rearrangement. *Am J Med Genet* 73: 327–329, 1997.

Xu J, Fang R, Chen L, et al. Noninvasive chromosome screening of human embryos by genome sequencing of embryo culture medium for in vitro fertilization. *Proc Natl Acad Sci USA* 113: 11907–11912, 2016.

Xu W, Robert C, Thornton PS, Spinner NB. Complete androgen insensitivity syndrome due to X chromosome inversion: A clinical report. *Am J Med Genet* 120A: 434–436, 2003.

Yaegashi N, Senoo M, Uehara S, et al. Age-specific incidences of chromosome abnormalities at the second trimester amniocentesis for Japanese mothers aged 35 and older: Collaborative study of 5484 cases. *J Hum Genet* 43: 85–90, 1998.

Yakut S, Cetin Z, Sanhal C, Karaman B, Mendilcioglu I, Karauzum SB. Prenatal diagnosis of de novo pericentric inversion inv(2)(p11.2q13). *Genet Couns* 26: 243–247, 2015a.

Yakut S, Clarck OA, Sanhal C, et al. A familial interstitial 4q35 deletion with no discernible clinical effects. *Am J Med Genet* 167A: 1836–1841, 2015b.

Yamamoto T, Dowa Y, Ueda H, et al. Tetralogy of Fallot associated with pulmonary atresia and major aortopulmonary collateral arteries in a patient with interstitial deletion of 16q21-q22.1. *Am J Med Genet* 146A: 1575–1580, 2008.

Yamamoto T, Wilsdon A, Joss S, et al. An emerging phenotype of Xq22 microdeletions in females with severe intellectual disability, hypotonia and behavioral abnormalities. *J Hum Genet* 59: 300–306, 2014.

Yamanaka M, Setoyama T, Igarashi Y, et al. Pregnancy outcome of fetuses with trisomy 18 identified by prenatal sonography and chromosomal analysis in a perinatal center. *Am J Med Genet* 140: 1177–1182, 2006.

Yamazawa K, Ogata T, Ferguson-Smith AC. Uniparental disomy and human disease: An overview. *Am J Med Genet Semin Med Genet* 154C: 329–334, 2010.

Yan D, Ouyang XM, Angeli SI, Du LL, Liu XZ. Paternal uniparental disomy of chromosome 13 causing homozygous 35delG mutation of the *GJB2* gene and hearing loss. *Am J Med Genet* 143A: 385–386, 2007.

Yang C, Chapman AG, Kelsey AD, Minks J, Cotton AM, Brown CJ. X-chromosome inactivation: Molecular mechanisms from the human perspective. *Hum Genet* 130: 175–185, 2011.

Yang Q, Sherman SL, Hassold TJ, et al. Risk factors for trisomy 21: Maternal cigarette smoking and oral contraceptive use in a population-based case-control study. *Genet Med* 1: 80–88, 1999.

Yang SP, Bidichandani SI, Figuera LE, et al. Molecular analysis of deletion (17)(p11.2p11.2) in a family segregating a 17p paracentric inversion: Implications for carriers of paracentric inversions. *Am J Hum Genet* 60: 1184–1193, 1997.

Yang Y, Yang C, Zhu Y, et al. Intragenic and extragenic disruptions of *FOXL2* mapped by whole genome low-coverage sequencing in two BPES families with chromosome reciprocal translocation. *Genomics* 104: 170–176, 2014.

Yang YF, Ai Q, Huang C, et al. A 1.1Mb deletion in distal 13q deletion syndrome region with congenital heart defect and postaxial polydactyly: Additional support for a CHD locus at distal 13q34 region. *Gene* 528: 51–54, 2013.

Yang YJ, Yao X, Guo J, et al. Trisomy 3 mosaicism in a 5-year-old boy with multiple anomalies: A very rare case. *Am J Med Genet* 170A: 1590–1594, 2016.

Yapan C, Beyazyurek C, Ekmekci C, Kahraman S. The largest paracentric inversion, the highest rate of recombinant spermatozoa—Case report: 46,XY, inv(2)(q21.2q37.3) and literature review. *Balkan J Med Genet* 17: 55–62, 2014.

Yardin C, Esclaire F, Gilbert B, Brosset P, Hugon J, Barthe D. Identical chromosome imbalance in two siblings born to a mother with a double reciprocal translocation. *Ann Genet* 40: 232–234, 1997.

Yardin C, Esclaire F, Terro F, Baclet MC, Barthe D, Laroche C. First familial case of ring chromosome

18 and monosomy 18 mosaicism. *Am J Med Genet* 104: 257–259, 2001.

Yaron Y, Feldman B, Kramer RL, et al. Prenatal diagnosis of 46,XY/46,XX mosaicism: A case report. *Am J Med Genet* 84: 12–14, 1999.

Yaron Y, Hyett J, Langlois S. Current controversies in prenatal diagnosis 2: For those women screened by NIPT using cell free DNA, maternal serum markers are obsolete. *Prenat Diagn* 36: 1167–1171, 2016.

Yauk CL, Aardema MJ, Benthem JV, et al. Approaches for identifying germ cell mutagens: Report of the 2013 IWGT workshop on germ cell assays. *Mutat Res Genet Toxicol Environ Mutagen* 783: 36–54, 2015.

Ye Y, Qian Y, Xu C, Jin F. Meiotic segregation analysis of embryos from reciprocal translocation carriers in PGD cycles. *Reprod Biomed Online* 24: 83–90, 2012.

Yenamandra A, Deangelo P, Aviv H, Suslak L, Desposito F. Interstitial insertion of Y-specific DNA sequences including *SRY* into chromosome 4 in a 45,X male child. *Am J Med Genet* 72: 125–128, 1997.

Yeung A, Francis D, Giouzeppos O, Amor DJ. Pallister-Killian syndrome caused by mosaicism for a supernumerary ring chromosome 12p. *Am J Med Genet* 149A: 505–509, 2009.

Yeung KS, Chee YY, Luk HM, et al. Spread of X inactivation on chromosome 15 is associated with a more severe phenotype in a girl with an unbalanced t(X; 15) translocation. *Am J Med Genet* 164A: 2521–2528, 2014.

Yin X, Tan K, Vajta G, et al. Massively parallel sequencing for chromosomal abnormality testing in trophectoderm cells of human blastocysts. *Biol Reprod* 88: 69, 2013.

Yokoyama Y, Narahara K, Teraoka M, et al. Cryptic pericentric inversion of chromosome 17 detected by fluorescence in situ hybridization study in familial Miller-Dieker syndrome. *Am J Med Genet* 71: 236–237, 1997.

Yong PJ, Barrett IJ, Kalousek DK, Robinson WP. Clinical aspects, prenatal diagnosis, and pathogenesis of trisomy 16 mosaicism. *J Med Genet* 40: 175–182, 2003.

Yong PJ, Langlois S, von Dadelszen P, Robinson W. The association between preeclampsia and placental trisomy 16 mosaicism. *Prenat Diagn* 26: 956–961, 2006.

Yong PJ, Marion SA, Barrett IJ, Kalousek DK, Robinson WP. Evidence for imprinting on chromosome 16: The effect of uniparental disomy on the outcome of mosaic trisomy 16 pregnancies. *Am J Med Genet* 112: 123–132, 2002.

Yoon PW, Freeman SB, Sherman SL, et al. Advanced maternal age and the risk of Down syndrome characterized by the meiotic stage of chromosomal error: A population-based study. *Am J Hum Genet* 58: 628–633, 1996.

Youings S, Ellis K, Ennis S, Barber J, Jacobs P. A study of reciprocal translocations and inversions detected by light microscopy with special reference to origin, segregation, and recurrent abnormalities. *Am J Med Genet* 126A: 46–60, 2004.

Yu N, Kruskall MS, Yunis JJ, et al. Disputed maternity leading to identification of tetragametic chimerism. *N Engl J Med* 346: 1545–1552, 2002.

Yu S, Cox K, Friend K, et al. Familial 22q11.2 duplication: A three-generation family with a 3-Mb duplication and a familial 1.5-Mb duplication. *Clin Genet* 73: 160–164, 2008.

Yu S, Yi H, Wang Z, Dong J. Screening key genes associated with congenital heart defects in Down syndrome based on differential expression network. *Int J Clin Exp Pathol* 8: 8385–8393, 2015.

Yu YR, You LR, Yan YT, Chen CM. Role of *OVCA1/DPH1* in craniofacial abnormalities of Miller-Dieker syndrome. *Hum Mol Genet* 23: 5579–5596, 2014.

Yuan B, Harel T, Gu S, et al. Nonrecurrent 17p11.2p12 rearrangement events that result in two concomitant genomic disorders: The *PMP22-RAI1* contiguous gene duplication syndrome. *Am J Hum Genet* 97: 691–707, 2015.

Yuan B, Neira J, Gu S, et al. Nonrecurrent *PMP22-RAI1* contiguous gene deletions arise from replication-based mechanisms and result in Smith-Magenis syndrome with evident peripheral neuropathy. *Hum Genet* 135: 1161–1174, 2016.

Yue Y, Farcas R, Thiel G, et al. De novo t(12;17)(p13.3;q21.3) translocation with a breakpoint near the 5′ end of the *HOXB* gene cluster in a patient with developmental delay and skeletal malformations. *Eur J Hum Genet* 15: 570–577, 2007.

Yurov YB, Vorsanova SG, Liehr T, Kolotii AD, Iourov IY. X chromosome aneuploidy in the Alzheimer's disease brain. *Mol Cytogenet* 7: 20, 2014.

Zackai EH, Emanuel BS. Site-specific reciprocal translocation, t(11;22) (q23;q11), in several unrelated families with 3:1 meiotic disjunction. *Am J Med Genet* 7: 507–521, 1980.

Zahed L, Der Kaloustian V, Batanian JR. Familial complex chromosome rearrangement giving rise to balanced and unbalanced recombination products. *Am J Med Genet* 79: 30–34, 1998.

Zalel Y, Shapiro I, Weissmann-Brenner A, Berkenstadt M, Leibovitz Z, Bronshtein M. Prenatal sonographic features of triploidy at 12–16 weeks. *Prenat Diagn* 36: 650–655, 2016.

Zaragoza MV, Keep D, Genest DR, Hassold T, Redline RW. Early complete hydatidiform moles contain inner cell mass derivatives. *Am J Med Genet* 70: 273–277, 1997.

Zaragoza MV, Surti U, Redline RW, Millie E, Chakravarti A, Hassold TJ. Parental origin and phenotype of triploidy in spontaneous abortions: Predominance of diandry and association with the partial hydatidiform mole. *Am J Hum Genet* 66: 1807–1820, 2000.

Zarrei M, MacDonald JR, Merico D, Scherer SW. A copy number variation map of the human genome. *Nat Rev Genet* 16: 172–183, 2015.

Zarrei M, Merico D, Kellam B, et al. A de novo deletion in a boy with cerebral palsy suggests a refined critical region for the 4q21.22 microdeletion syndrome. *Am J Med Genet* 173A: 1287–1293, 2017.

Zaslav AL, Blumenthal D, Willner JP, Pierno G, Jacob J, Fox JE. Prenatal diagnosis of trisomy 4 mosaicism. *Am J Med Genet* 95: 381–384, 2000.

Zaslav AL, Fallet S, Blumenthal D, Jacob J, Fox J. Mosaicism with a normal cell line and an unbalanced structural rearrangement. *Am J Med Genet* 82: 15–19, 1999.

Zaslav AL, Fallet S, Brown S, et al. Prenatal diagnosis of low level trisomy 15 mosaicism: Review of the literature. *Clin Genet* 53: 286–292, 1998.

Zaslav AL, Fox JE, Jacob J, et al. Significance of a prenatally diagnosed del(10)(q23). *Am J Med Genet* 107: 174–176, 2002.

Zaslav AL, Pierno G, Davis J, et al. Prenatal diagnosis of trisomy 3 mosaicism. *Prenat Diagn* 24: 693–696, 2004.

Zatsepin I, Verger P, Robert-Gnansia E, et al. Down syndrome time-clustering in January 1987 in Belarus: Link with the Chernobyl accident? *Reprod Toxicol* 24: 289–295, 2007.

Zavras N, Siristatidis C, Siatelis A, Koumarianou A. Fertility risk assessment and preservation in male and female prepubertal and adolescent cancer patients. *Clin Med Insights Oncol* 10: 49–57, 2016.

Zayed F, Ghalayini I, Matalka I. A male phenotype (XY) hermaphrodite treated for seminoma, fathered a healthy child by IVF-ICSI technique. *J Assist Reprod Genet* 25: 345–348, 2008.

Zech NH, Wisser J, Natalucci G, Riegel M, Baumer A, Schinzel A. Monochorionic-diamniotic twins discordant in gender from a naturally conceived pregnancy through postzygotic sex chromosome loss in a 47,XXY zygote. *Prenat Diagn* 28: 759–763, 2008.

Zeesman S, McCready E, Sadikovic B, Nowaczyk MJ. Prader-Willi syndrome and Tay-Sachs disease in association with mixed maternal uniparental isodisomy and heterodisomy 15 in a girl who also had isochromosome Xq. *Am J Med Genet* 167A: 180–184, 2015.

Zenker M, Wermuth B, Trautmann U, et al. Severe, neonatal-onset OTC deficiency in twin sisters with a de novo balanced reciprocal translocation t(X;5)(p21.1;q11). *Am J Med Genet* 132A: 185–188, 2005.

Zeschnigk M, Albrecht B, Buiting K, et al. IGF2/H19 hypomethylation in Silver-Russell syndrome and isolated hemihypoplasia. *Eur J Hum Genet* 16: 328–334, 2008.

Zhang A, Weaver DD, Palmer CG. Molecular cytogenetic identification of four X chromosome duplications. *Am J Med Genet* 68: 29–38, 1997.

Zhang B, Willing M, Grange DK, et al. Multigenerational autosomal dominant inheritance of 5p chromosomal deletions. *Am J Med Genet* 170: 583–593, 2016a.

Zhang F, Khajavi M, Connolly AM, Towne CF, Batish SD, Lupski JR. The DNA replication FoSTeS/MMBIR mechanism can generate genomic, genic and exonic complex rearrangements in humans. *Nat Genet* 41: 849–853, 2009.

Zhang F, Seeman P, Liu P, et al. Mechanisms for nonrecurrent genomic rearrangements associated with *CMT1A* or *HNPP*: Rare CNVs as a cause for missing heritability. *Am J Hum Genet* 86: 892–903, 2010.

Zhang K, Song F, Zhang D, et al. Chromosome r(3)(p25.3q29) in a patient with developmental delay and congenital heart defects: A case report and a brief literature review. *Cytogenet Genome Res* 148: 6–13, 2016b.

Zhang M, Fan HT, Zhang QS, et al. Genetic screening and evaluation for chromosomal abnormalities of infertile males in Jilin Province, China. *Genet Mol Res* 14: 16178–16184, 2015.

Zhang R, Chen X, Li P, et al. Molecular characterization of a novel ring 6 chromosome using next generation sequencing. *Mol Cytogenet* 9: 33, 2016c.

Zhang Y, Zhu S, Wu J, Liu S, Sun X. Quadrivalent asymmetry in reciprocal translocation carriers predicts meiotic segregation patterns in cleavage stage embryos. *Reprod Biomed Online* 29: 490–498, 2014.

Zhang Z, Gao H, Li S, Hong M, Liu R. Chromosomal abnormalities in patients with recurrent spontaneous abortions in northeast China. *J Reprod Med* 56: 321–324, 2011.

Zhou W, Machiela MJ, Freedman ND, et al. Mosaic loss of chromosome Y is associated with common variation near *TCL1A*. *Nat Genet* 48: 563–568, 2016.

Ziats MN, Goin-Kochel RP, Berry LN, et al. The complex behavioral phenotype of 15q13.3 microdeletion syndrome. *Genet Med* 18: 1111–1118, 2016.

Zietkiewicz E, Wojda A, Witt M. Cytogenetic perspective of ageing and longevity in men and women. *J Appl Genet* 50: 261–273, 2009.

Žilina O, Reimand T, Tammur P, Tillmann V, Kurg A, Õunap K. Patient with dup(5)(q35.2-q35.3) reciprocal to the common Sotos syndrome deletion and review of the literature. *Eur J Med Genet* 56: 202–206, 2013.

Zinn AR, Ouyang B, Ross JL, Varma S, Bourgeois M, Tonk V. Del (X)(p21.2) in a mother and two daughters with variable ovarian function. *Clin Genet* 52: 235–239, 1997.

Zirn B, Arning L, Bartels I, et al. Ring chromosome 22 and neurofibromatosis type II: Proof of two-hit model for the loss of the *NF2* gene in the development of meningioma. *Clin Genet* 81: 82–87, 2012.

Zollino M, Marangi G, Ponzi E, et al. Intragenic *KANSL1* mutations and chromosome 17q21.31 deletions: broadening the clinical spectrum and genotype-phenotype correlations in a large cohort of patients. *J Med Genet* 52: 804–814, 2015.

Zollino M, Orteschi D, Marangi G, et al. A case of Beckwith-Wiedemann syndrome caused by a cryptic 11p15 deletion encompassing the centromeric imprinted domain of the *BWS* locus. *J Med Genet* 47: 429–432, 2010a.

Zollino M, Orteschi D, Neri G. Phenotypic map in ring 14 syndrome. *Am J Med Genet* 152A: 237, 2010b.

Zollino M, Ponzi E, Gobbi G, Neri G. The ring 14 syndrome. *Eur J Med Genet* 55: 374–380, 2012.

Zollino M, Tiziano F, Di Stefano C, Neri G. Partial duplication of the long arm of chromosome 15: Confirmation of a causative role in craniosynostosis and definition of a 15q25-qter trisomy syndrome. *Am J Med Genet* 87: 391–394, 1999.

Zou YS, Newton S, Milunsky JM. A complex maternal rearrangement results in a pure 10.8 Mb duplication of the 5q13.1-q14.1 region in an affected son. *Am J Med Genet* 152A: 498–503, 2010.

Zuffardi O, Bonaglia M, Ciccone R, Giorda R. Inverted duplications deletions: underdiagnosed rearrangements? *Clin Genet* 75: 505–513, 2009.

Zufferey F, Sherr EH, Beckmann ND, et al. A 600 kb deletion syndrome at 16p11.2 leads to energy imbalance and neuropsychiatric disorders. *J Med Genet* 49: 660–668, 2012.

Zühlke C, Thies U, Braulke I, Reis A, Schirren C. Down syndrome and male fertility: PCR-derived fingerprinting, serological and andrological investigations. *Clin Genet* 46: 324–326, 1994.

Zung A, Petek E, Ben-Zeev B, Schwarzbraun T, Ben-Yehoshua SJ. MODY type 2 in Greig cephalopolysyndactyly syndrome (GCPS) as part of a contiguous gene deletion syndrome. *Am J Med Genet* 155A: 2469–2472, 2011.

Zwanenburg RJ, Bocca G, Ruiter SAJ, et al. Is there an effect of intranasal insulin on development and behaviour in Phelan-McDermid syndrome? A randomized, double-blind, placebo-controlled trial. *Eur J Hum Genet* 24: 1696–1701, 2016.

INDEX